Handbook of Experimental Pharmacology

Continuation of Handbuch der experimentellen Pharmakologie

Vol. 52

Snake Venoms

Contributors

E. X. Albuquerque · C. A. Alper · A. Bdolah · A. L. Bieber
G. M. Böhm · I. L. Bonta · V. Boonpucknavig · P. Boquet
R. A. Bradshaw · C. H. Campbell · C. C. Chang · P. A. Christensen
E. Condrea · P. Efrati · A. T. Eldefrawi · M. E. Eldefrawi
R. A. Hogue-Angeletti · S. Iwanaga · E. Karlsson · C.Y. Lee
S. Y. Lee · B. W. Low · S. A. Minton · A. Ohsaka · C. Ouyang
H. A. Reid · P. Rosenberg · A. M. Rothschild · Z. Rothschild
F. E. Russell · Y. Sawai · W. H. Seegers · V. Sitprija · D. J. Strydom
T. Suzuki · G. L. Underwood · B. B. Vargaftig

Editor

Chen-Yuan Lee

With 208 Figures

Springer-Verlag Berlin Heidelberg New York 1979

CHEN-YUAN LEE, MD, Professor
National Taiwan University, College of Medicine,
No. 1. Jen Ai Road, 1st Section, Taipei, Taiwan, Republic of China

ISBN-13: 978-3-642-66915-6 e-ISBN-13: 978-3-642-66913-2
DOI: 10.1007/978-3-642-66913-2

Library of Congress Cataloging in Publication Data. Main entry under title: Snake venoms. (Handbook of experimental pharmacology: New Series; v. 52). Includes bibliographies and index. 1. Snake venom. 2. Snake venom – Physiological effect. 3. Snake venom – Toxicology. I. Albuquerque, E. X. II. Lee, Chen Yuan, 1915–. III. Series: Handbuch der experimentellen Pharmakologie: New series; v. 52. QP905.H3 vol. 52 615'.1'08s [615'.36] 78-14789.

Softcover reprint of the hardcover 1st edition 1979

2122/3130-543210

Preface

The past decade has been a period of explosion of knowledge on the chemistry and pharmacology of snake toxins. Thanks to the development of protein chemistry, nearly a hundred snake toxins have been purified and sequenced, representing one of the largest families of sequenced proteins. Moreover, the mode of action of these toxins has been largely elucidated by the concerted efforts of pharmacologists, electrophysiologists, and biochemists. As a result of these studies, some of the snake toxins, e.g., α-bungarotoxin and cobra neurotoxins, have been extensively used as specific markers in the study of the acetylcholine receptors. Indeed, without the discovery of these snake toxins, our knowledge of the structure and function of nicotinic acetylcholine receptors would not have advanced so rapidly.

The contribution of snake venom research to the biomedical sciences is not limited to the study of cholinergic receptors. Being one of the most concentrated enzyme sources in nature, snake venoms are also valuable tools in biochemical research. Venom phosphodiesterase, for example, has been widely used for structural studies of nucleic acids; proteinase, for the sequence studies of proteins and peptides; phospholipase A_2, for lipid research; and L-amino acid oxidase for identifying optical isomers of amino acids. Furthermore, snake venoms have proven to be useful agents for clarifying some basic concepts on blood coagulation and some venom enzymes, e.g., thrombin-like enzymes and procoagulants have been used as therapeutic agents. The discovery of bradykinin as a hypotensive peptide released by the venom of *Bothrops jararaca* is another important contribution derived from venom research. Other components of certain snake venoms, e.g., presynaptic neurotoxins, crotamine, cardiotoxins, etc., are of current interest as potential tools for studies of transmitter release, ion channel, and biomembrane structure.

The present treatise is an attempt to offer a comprehensive review of the entire field of snake venom research. The volume is devided into four parts. Part I starts with the history of venom research, followed by a chapter on the distribution of venomous snakes and another on their venom glands. Part II deals with chemistry and biochemistry of snake venoms, including enzymes, snake toxins, nerve growth factors, and metal and nonprotein constituents in snake venoms. One special chapter is devoted to the three-dimensional structure of postsynaptic toxins and another to the evolution of snake toxins. Part III describes the pharmacologic effects of snake toxins and enzymes, especially phospholipase A_2, on nerve, muscle, circulatory system, blood vessels, blood cells, blood coagulation, etc. One chapter specially deals with the use of snake toxins for the study of the acetylcholine receptor, and another for the study of microvessel damage. Part IV describes the immunologic and clinical aspects, including antigenic properties of snake venoms, production of antivenin, common antigens, vaccination, snake venoms and compliment system, and the symptomatology, pathology, and treatment of snake bites. One chapter is devoted to nephrotoxicity of snake venoms.

A variety of descriptive terms, such as neurotoxins (α-neurotoxins, postsynaptic or curaremimetic neurotoxins, and presynaptic neurotoxins), cardiotoxins (cytotoxins, direct lytic factors, membrane active toxins, etc.), myotoxins, myonecrotic toxins, vasculotoxins, etc., are used by different authors in this volume. The editor is aware of the increasing criticism among toxinologists concerning use of such phenomenological nomenclature. At the fifth International Symposium on Animal, Plant and Microbial Toxins, Costa Rica, 1976, a round table discussion on "Nomenclature of Naturally Occurring Peptides" was held and consequently an International Committee on this problem was formed. Since, so far, no agreement on the nomenclature system has been reached, the editor believes that there is no alternative but to use such phenomenological nomenclature, provided that the name used is well-defined and not confused with another.

The contributors of this volume are highly qualified specialists in their specific areas of research. The editor wishes to thank his collaborators who have not only contributed important chapters but have also cooperated fully in the final preparation of this volume. It is hoped that this volume will be a most comprehensive reference book on snake venoms and serve as a stimulating guide for future research not only to toxinologists but also to investigators of other disciplines.

The editor cannot conclude this preface without expressing his deepest gratitude to Dr. BERNHARD WITKOP, Chief of the Laboratory of Chemistry, NIADD, and Dr. M. D. LEAVITT, Jr., Director of Fogarty International Center, National Institutes of Health, Bethesda, Maryland, U.S.A., who invited him to participate in the Scholors-in-Residence Program from July 1976 to February 1977, during which period the manuscripts of most chapters of this volume were edited. Had the editor not been given this opportunity of sabbatical leave, it would not have been possible to accomplish such a heavy task for a busy administrator as a dean of a medical school. The editor is grateful also to Mrs. M. SWENSON for her secretarial help during his stay at the Stone House, Fogarty International Center.

September 1978, Taipei CHEN-YUAN LEE

Table of Contents

Part I: History, Ecological and Zoological Aspects

CHAPTER 1

CHAPTER 2

CHAPTER 3

Part II: Chemistry and Biochemistry of Snake Venoms

CHAPTER 4

Enzymes in Snake Venom. S. IWANAGA and T. SUZUKI. With 25 Figures

CHAPTER 5

Chemistry of Protein Toxins in Snake Venoms. E. KARLSSON. With 11 Figures

CHAPTER 6

The Three-Dimensional Structure of Postsynaptic Snake Neurotoxins: Consideration of Structure and Function. BARBARA W. LOW. With 11 Figures

CHAPTER 7

The Evolution of Toxins Found in Snake Venoms. D. J. STRYDOM. With 6 Figures

CHAPTER 8

Nerve Growth Factors in Snake Venoms. R. A. HOGUE-ANGELETTI and R. A. BRADSHAW. With 5 Figures

CHAPTER 9

Metal and Nonprotein Constituents in Snake Venoms. A. L. BIEBER. With 1 Figure

Part III: Pharmacology of Snake Venoms

CHAPTER 10

The Action of Snake Venoms on Nerve and Muscle. C. CHIUNG CHANG. With 3 Figures

CHAPTER 11

The Use of Snake Toxins for the Study of the Acetylcholine Receptor and its Ion-Conductance Modulator. E. X. ALBUQUERQUE, A. T. ELDEFRAWI, and M. E. ELDEFRAWI. With 3 Figures

CHAPTER 12

Pharmacology of Phospholipase A_2 from Snake Venoms. P. ROSENBERG

CHAPTER 13

Hemolytic Effects of Snake Venoms. E. CONDREA. With 6 Figures

CHAPTER 14

Hemorrhagic, Necrotizing and Edema-Forming Effects of Snake Venoms.
A. OHSAKA. With 34 Figures

CHAPTER 15

Cardiovascular Effects of Snake Venoms. C. Y. LEE and S. Y. LEE

CHAPTER 16

Liberation of Pharmacologically Active Substances by Snake Venoms.
A. M. ROTHSCHILD and Z. ROTHSCHILD. With 4 Figures

CHAPTER 17

Snake Venoms as an Experimental Tool to Induce and Study Models of Microvessel Damage. I. L. BONTA, B. B. VARGAFTIG, and G. M. BÖHM. With 21 Figures

CHAPTER 18

Snake Venoms and Blood Coagulation. W. H. SEEGERS and C. OUYANG. With 9 Figures

Part IV: Immunological and Clinical Aspects

CHAPTER 19

Immunological Properties of Snake Venoms. P. BOQUET. With 7 Figures.

CHAPTER 20

Production and Standardization of Antivenin. P.A. CHRISTENSEN. With 2 Figures

CHAPTER 24

Symptomatology, Pathology, and Treatment of the Bites of Elapid Snakes.
C.H. CAMPBELL. With 2 Figures

CHAPTER 26

Symptomatology, Pathology, and Treatment of the Bites of Viperid Snakes.
P. EFRATI. With 8 Figures

CHAPTER 27

The Clinical Problem of Crotalid Snake Venom Poisoning. F. E. RUSSELL

CHAPTER 28

Snake Venoms and Nephrotoxicity. V. SITPRIJA and V. BOONPUCKNAVIG. With 17 Figures.

List of Contributors

E. X. ALBUQUERQUE, Professor, Dept. of Pharmacology and Exp. Therapeutics, School of Medicine, University of Maryland, 660W Redwood St., Baltimore, Md. 21201, USA

C. A. ALPER, MD., Center of Blood Research, 800 Huntington Avenue, Boston, Mass. 02115, USA

A. BDOLAH, Professor, Dept. of Zoology, Faculty of Life Sciences, Tel Aviv University, Ramat-Aviv, Tel Aviv, Israel

A. L. BIEBER, Professor, Dept. of Chemistry, Arizona State University, Tempe, Ariz. 85281, USA

G. M. BÖHM, Professor, Departamento de Morfologia, Faculdade de Medicina, Caixa Postal 301, Ribeirão Preto, Estado São Paulo, Brazil

I. L. BONTA, Professor, Dept. of Pharmacology, Medical Faculty, Erasmus University, P.O. Box 1738, Rotterdam, The Netherlands

V. BOONPUCKNAVIG, Professor, Dept. of Pathology, Ramathibodi Hospital, Mahidol University, Bangkok, Thailand

P. BOQUET, Professor, Institut Pasteur, Annex de Garches, F-92380 (Hauts-de-Seine) Garches

R. A. BRADSHAW, PhD., Dept. of Biological Chemistry, Washington University, School of Medicine, 660 S. Euclid Avenue. St. Louis MO 63110, USA

C. H. CAMPBELL, MD., F.R.A.C.P., School of Public Health and Tropical Medicine, The University of Sydney, Sydney N.S.W., 2006, Australia

C. C. CHANG, Professor, Pharmacological Institute, College of Medicine, National Taiwan University, Taipei, Taiwan, ROC

P. A. CHRISTENSEN, Dr., The South African Institute for Medical Research, Hospital Street, Johannesburg, South Africa

ELEONORA CONDREA, Professor, Rogoff-Wellcome Medical Research Institute, Beilinson, Medical Center, Petah-Tikva, Israel

P. EFRATI, Professor, Dept. of Medicine B, Kaplan Hospital, P.O.B. 1, Rehovot, Israel

AMIRA T. ELDEFRAWI, PhD., Dept. of Pharmacology and Exp. Therapeutics, School of Medicine, University of Maryland, 660 W Redwood St., Baltimore, Md. 21201, USA

M. E. Eldefrawi, Professor, Dept. of Pharmacology and Exp. Therapeutics, University of Maryland, School of Medicine, Baltimore, Md. 21201, USA

Ruth A. Hogue-Angeletti, PhD., Division of Neuropathology, University of Pennsylvania, School of Medicine, Philadelphia, PA 19185, USA

S. Iwanaga, PhD., Division of Plasma Proteins, Institute for Protein Research, Osaka University, Suita, Osaka-565, Japan

E. Karlsson, PhD., Biokemiska Institutionen, Box 531, 751 23 Uppsala 1, Sweden

C. Y. Lee, Professor, Pharmacological Institute, College of Medicine, National Taiwan University, No. 1, Jen Ai Road, 1st Section, Taipei, Taiwan, ROC

Shu-Yue Lee, MD., Dept. of Clinical Pathology, College of Medicine, National Taiwan University, No. 1, Jen Ai Road, 1st Section, Taipei, Taiwan, ROC

Barbara W. Low, Professor, Dept. of Biochemistry, College of Physicians and Surgeons, Columbia University, New York, NY 10032, USA

S. A. Minton, Professor, Dept. of Microbiology, Indiana University, School of Medicine, 1100 West Mich. Street, Indianapolis, Indiana 46202, USA

A. Ohsaka, PhD., National Institute of Health, The 2nd Dept. of Bacteriology, 10–35, Kamiosaki, 2-chome Shinagawaku, Tokyo, Japan

C. Ouyang, Professor, Pharmacological Institute, College of Medicine, National Taiwan University, Taipei, Taiwan, ROC

H. A. Reid, Dr., Liverpool School of Tropical Medicine, Pembroke Place, Liverpool L3 & QA, England

P. Rosenberg, Professor, Section of Pharmacology and Toxicology, School of Pharmacy, The University of Connecticut, Storrs, Conn. 06268, USA

A. M. Rothschild, Professor, Dept. of Pharmacology, Universidade de São Paulo, Faculdade de Medicina de Ribeirão Preto 14.100 S.P., Brazil

Zuleika Rothschild, Professor, Dept. of Biochemistry, School of Pharmacy Universidade de São Paulo, Ribeirão Preto, 14.100, S.P., Brazil

F. E. Russell, Professor, Laboratory of Neurological Research, University of Southern California, Los Angeles, Calif. 90033, USA

Y. Sawai, MD., The Japan Snake Institute, Yabuzuka Honmachi, Nitta-gun, Gunma Prefecture 379-23, Japan

W. H. Seegers, Professor, Department of Physiology, Thrombosis Specialized Center of Research, Wayne State University, School of Medicine, Detroit, Mich. 48201, USA

V. Sitprija, Professor, Dept. of Medicine, Chulalongkorn Hospital, Chulalongkorn University, Bangkok, Thailand

D. J. Strydom, PhD., National Chemical Research Laboratory of the South African Council for Scientific and Industrial Research, P.O. Box 395, Pretoria, Republic of South Africa

T. Suzuki, Professor, Division of Plasma Proteins, Institute for Protein Research, Osaka University, Suita, Osaka-565, Japan

G. L. Underwood, D.Sc., City of London Polytechnic, Old Castle Street, London, E 1 7NT, England

B. B. Vargaftig, MD., Centre de Recherche Merrell Int., 16, Rue d'Ankara, F-6700 Strasbourg

Part I

History, Ecological and Zoological Aspects

CHAPTER 1

History of Snake Venom Research

P. BOQUET

In ancient civilizations, the snake embodied the spirit of the earth. It was god and at the fount of all cosmogonies. According to the beliefs of the Egyptians, *Atoum*, the snake, after leaving the primordial waters, gave the day to the gods, who, in their turn, created Geb and Nout, the air and the earth. *Atoum* was "the one who remains," i.e., the one who was "on this side" and the one who will be "beyond."

The barque of the sun, whose story is told in the book of the dead, traveled across sandy areas infested with snakes. After a long voyage, it sailed in the body of a snake, emerging through the mouth. Then the scarab appeared, in all its glory: the image of a radiant sun.

Uraeus, the gold cobra, symbol of sovereignty, knowledge, and life, shone on the forehead of the goddess *Isis*. It was to become the emblem of sacred power of the royal line which was tragically extinguished with Cleopatra Ptolemy.

In the language of the Chaldeans, one single word meant both "life and snake."

In ancient Greek civilization, *Archeloos*, the river god, metamorphosed from a snake to a bull and from a bull to a man.

At this time, the snake was the attribute of *Athena*. It represented the spirit of air and earth and was the symbol of fecundity, health, continuity, and eternity.

Sick people, hoping for a cure, flocked to the temples of *Asklepios* at Epidaurus, Rhodes, Cnides, and Cos, where snakes were carefully tended. A single touch of their tongues was supposed to give sight to the blind. The snake is, then, at the very foundation of medicine.

Snakes moult several times a year. In the eyes of man, obsessed by images of ageing and death, this periodic rejuvenation seemed to suggest immortality, and it was this theme of immortality which was developed in the moving epic of Gilgamesh. Gilgamesh, a shepherd from Ourouk, discovered a shrub whose sap made man immortal. He cut a twig from it, which he took at the price of memorable labours, but on his way home, a snake stole the marvellous plant from him.

In biblical tales, the serpent encouraged the woman to pick the fruit from the tree of knowledge of good and evil (FRASER, 1924).

Aaron, the brother of Moses, turned rods into snakes, and Yahve ordained Moses to place a bronze snake on a staff. Anyone who was the victim of snake poisoning was saved when he saw this symbol.

Curiously, the rainbow has often been compared with a serpent quenching its thirst in the sea.

The snake, as a divinity ruling the water and the rain, so necessary for fertility, is represented as a dragon in China and in America as a feathered serpent, rather like a snake of clouds with a beard of rain. It incarnates the "Quetzalcoatl" of the toltecs whose sacrifice brings good fortune to men. In the same image, it appears as a rapacious bird and a snake, the bird tearing the serpent to pieces with its claws; the blood of the snake gives birth to man (Chevalier, 1973).

The "*Ouroboros*" of Africa is a snake which bites its own tail off; since it fertilizes itself it is considered a "source of Life." Being venomous, it is also a "source of death," but the cycle is not interrupted by death, and the "*Ouroboros*" is an expression of the idea of life and death followed by resurrection. Similarly, the ancient Egyptians associated the likeness of the snake with the concept of ceaselessness and for the African people, it evoked concepts of time and space (Chevalier, 1973).

In the religion inspired by the Tantras of India, it symbolized power and also the aggressive forces of the gods of darkness.

The Upanishads tell the story of Kaleyeni, the king of the serpents. Kaleyeni met Krishna and demanded that he should worship the most horrible of all snakes, the one which devoured men. Krishna became violently angry and cut off the snake's head, then went to the banks of the river Ganges to purify himself (Chevalier, 1973). The cult of snake worship persists even today in some regions of India.

From the Far East, comes a familiar image: that of Buddha protected by the shadow of a cobra with seven heads.

In Europe, Christianity has expurgated ancient beliefs and blames the snake for all sins as it is the original seducer and the incarnation of the devil. Its image is associated with the damnable science. However, Bruno (1971) reports that in a village, east of Rome, which is still very primitive, Catholicism and the cult of snake worship are incorporated with no apparent difficulty.

Jung (1964) tells the curious story of the chemist Kekule who, in the 19th century, came to define the molecular structure of benzene. Influenced by the memory of ancient symbols, he was dreaming one night of a snake holding its tail in its mouth and, on awakening from this dream, related the circular shape of the snake to the cyclic structure of benzene.

Banished from Eden, loathed by man, and condemned to crawl eternally in the dust, the snake sadly carries its sense of shame and produces its venom. However, a few great minds felt interested in it.

Four centuries before the birth of Christ, Aristotle described it in his "history of animals," a tentative classification of the then known animals. The elder Pliny, writing 100 years before the birth of Christ, made a note of it, and Avicenne carefully described the symptoms of snake venom poisoning. However, 200 years earlier, Hannibal of Carthage had put it to an unusual use. He turned it to good account as an offensive weapon and had earthenware pots containing living venomous snakes thrown at the Roman ships. Terrified by this unexpected bombardment, the sailors fled. Wishing to avoid a similar mishap in the future, General Caius Claudius Neron, who was responsible for military operations, asked his doctor, Andromachus to find a substance which would serve to protect his men. Certain that the snake itself must contain an antidote, Andromachus mixed the flesh of Roman snakes with other substances and developed an antidote to the venom called "Theriaque." Some historians, however, give credit of discovery of this drug to Galen.

During the Middle Ages, there is little mention of the snake, but in the 13th century, Marco Polo reported that in the kingdom of Mutfile, there were many diamonds to be found, "but there are so many enormous snakes and other kinds of vermin, because of the heat, that they are a real wonder. And these are the most poisonous snakes in the world, so the men who go there run great risks, and are very frightened" (AT'SERSTEVENS, 1955). At that time, the Chinese pharmacopoeia had several remedies based on parts of snakes, particularly bile.

In the 16th century, VAN HELMONT proposed his phlogistic theory. In "Orthus Medicinae," which was published after his death (1648), he considered snake venoms "irritated spirits" which the beast threw out when biting and which were "so cold" that they coagulated the blood in the veins and arrested the circulation.

Moïse CHARAS (1685), charged by the College of Apothecaries of Paris to ensure preparation of "Theriaque" in his dispensary at the sign of the "Golden Serpent," agreed with the opinion of VAN HELMONT. He produced not only "Theriaque," but also "Orvietan," which had a more simple composition, and the "Bezoard" containing snake liver powder and snake fat.

I cannot resist quoting a few lines from the book by Marie PHISALIX (1940), "The Vipers in France." The picturesque turn of phrase and detail in documentation employed by the author merit the attention of the reader.

> All these preparations were until the time of Louis XIV, sold with a great deal of stagy eloquence, by charlatans, on market days and fair days at the Place Dauphine, and the Pont Neuf ... In his dispensary, CHARAS received live vipers and there ... he applied all the dreadful treatments that the imagination of an artist apothecary could conceive, ... pounded alive and put into poultices, dried and reduced to a powder, burnt and reduced to cinders, distilled to collect the stable salt, and more important, the volatile salt, plunged alive into olive oil and macerated in wine, in aromatic vinegars, dissolved over boiling water to obtain the fat, eaten raw or cooked, drunk down in soup, in wine, in elixir, in pills, in electuaries, applied as pomades, as unguents, as poultices and plasters, and even more preparations ... vipers have been used continuously for more than twenty centuries to treat, even if they did not cure, venom poisonings, infections, illnesses, epidemics, oedemas and many different chronic states. What a glorious career! Could any other medicament match it?

Following this impressive list, Marie PHISALIX adds that VALLOT, the first doctor of the King (Louis XIV) administered viper powder added to olive oil to the Duchess of Orleans, "Madame" (Henrietta of England) who said she was poisoned. Unfortunately, the remedy was too late since "Madame" died a few hours later.

A controversy arose between CHARAS and REDI (REDI, 1664). CHARAS, a supporter of the phlogistic theory, considered that the bite of a viper was only dangerous if the animal was irritated. The Florentine, REDI, who was not concerned with current theories but followed observations and facts, stated positively that the juice emitted from the poison fangs of a snake, dead or alive, caused lethal injury. A century had to pass before, in FONTANA'S beautiful book published in 1781, the results of an experiment confirming the observation of REDI were reported putting an end to the myth of "irritated spirits."

Several years earlier, however, BUFFON (1749), impressed by the observations made by LEEUWENHOEK, proposed that the activity of the vipers' venom was due to its containing microscopic "animalcules."

It was at this stage that LINNAEUS (1758) defined the order of snakes. From LINNAEUS' time until the beginning of the 19th century, the term was applied to a heterogeneous assemblage of various species including the lizards. WAGLER (1830) eliminated improper members from the order of "snakes." DUMERIL and BIBRON (1854) divided this order according to the dental structure. Lastly, LACEPEDE (1855) wrote a natural history of snakes.

At the end of the 18th century, LAVOISIER developed chemistry into an experimental science. In the 19th century, under the influence of Claude BERNARD, the science of physiology progressed, and the understanding of structures, functions, and "milieu" were correlated in a system of defining the essential conditions for maintaining life.

Some time after mineral chemistry was developed, the chemistry of substances transformed by living matter, incorrectly called organic chemistry, began to progress. CHEVREUL, DUMAS, LIEBIG, and WÖHLER developed the ground on which, little by little, the young science of biological chemistry advanced. DARWIN drew attention to the problem of the origin of species. PASTEUR, who was followed by EHRLICH and BORDET, was the genius who opened up the fields of bacteriological and immunological sciences. Progressively, the edifice of knowledge appeared from the fogs of metaphysics.

The theory of "irritated spirits" which communicated their "fire" to the saliva of the snake was followed by descriptions of objective observations and reports of experiments whose precision became greater as the methods of exploration developed.

Chemists were among the first to consider the venoms with interest, and they endeavored to define their composition. They submitted venoms to the actions of the common reagents and attempted to extract the toxic constituents. They observed that certain of the reagents destroyed the venoms while others caused precipitation of the toxic components.

In 1843, Lucien BONAPARTE, brother of Napoleon, precipitated the venom of *Vipera berus* with alcohol and then with ether and obtained a toxic powder which he called "Viperine." Lucien BONAPARTE, who had a remarkable knack for observation, compared "Viperine" to digestive ferments.

Several years later, in the USA, MITCHELL (1860, 1868) treated a *Crotalus* venom with boiling water and then with alcohol. He dried the precipitate which formed, measured its toxicity on animals, and named it "Crotaline."

In 1878, new progress was made in the research when PELDER proposed that venoms were protein-like substances. In collaboration with REICHERT, MITCHELL (1883, 1886) established shortly afterwards that "Crotaline" was not a homogeneous substance. He then separated the venom of *Crotalus adamanteus* into "peptone venom" and "globulin venom," by submitting it to dialysis across a semipermeable membrane. By boiling venom, he managed to extract a precipitate which he considered to be like an albumin. During the same period, WOLFENDEN (1886b) who supported the hypothesis of the protein-like constitution of the venoms, invalidated the conclusions of GAUTHIER (1881), on their alkaloid nature and those of BLYTH (1877) on the existence of a "cobric acid."

A conflict then arose among the chemists. WOLFENDEN (1886a) and KANTHACK (1892) claimed that the peptone venom of MITCHELL and REICHERT was an albumose. MARTIN and SMITH (1892) finally established that the toxic constituents of cobra venom from India, and of *Pseudechis porphyriacus* from Australia, also belonged to the group of albumoses. The observations of FAUST (1907) caused a temporary suspension of the battle, but added the term "Ophiotoxin" to the already long list of names given to substances extracted from venoms. After heating a solution of Indian cobra venom, FAUST treated the precipitate obtained with acidulated water and in this way obtained "Ophiotoxin." He submitted it to analysis and defined its composition as $C_{17}H_{26}O_{10}$. FAUST likened "Ophiotoxin" to the substances of the "Sapotoxins" group.

During the following 25 years, knowledge of the chemical nature of snake venom toxins did not progress greatly. However, in 1893, MARTIN reported an important finding. Using a filter under 50 atm of pressure, he separated *Pseudechis porphyriacus* venom into two fractions. One of these produced hemorrhages when it was injected into animals, while the other arrested respiration.

It is at this point that the physiologists, whose experimental techniques had made great progress since the beginning of the 19th century, intervened. In 1860, MITCHELL, observing the effects of *Crotalus* bites on frogs and rabbits, reported that intoxication by the venom of these reptiles was characterized by paralysis. In the work published with REICHERT (1886) following a long series of experiments, he concluded that the venoms of *Crotalus adamanteus*, *Agkistrodon piscivorus*, and *Naja tripudians* irritated nerve terminals and depressed the nerve centers. However, FAYRER (1868–1869) expressed a different opinion when he described the paralysis and asphyxia following a cobra bite. Working in collaboration with BRUNTON (BRUNTON and FAYRER, 1874), he attributed these phenomena to motor nerve paralysis consequent to a lesion of the motor end plate. He compared this lesion to that produced by curare whose mechanism of action had been described by CLAUDE BERNARD. WALL (1883), then RAGOTZI (1890) confirmed the observations of BRUNTON and FAYRER (1874). RAGOTZI specified that it was the phrenic nerve terminals which were very rapidly affected by cobra venom.

ELLIOT et al. (1905) likewise established that the paralysis produced by *Bungarus coeruleus* venom was comparable to that seen in animals poisoned with curare. They did, however, admit that the venom also affected the respiratory center. At the same time, FRASER and ELLIOT (1905) reported that the venom of *Hydrophiidae* paralyzed the neuromuscular junctions and confirmed the earlier finding of RAGOTZI that this paralysis selectively attacked the muscles dependent on the phrenic nerve.

Thus, the existence of a curarizing toxin in the venom of *Elapidae* and *Hydrophiidae* was recognized at the end of the 19th century. Attention was then drawn to other symptoms of venom poisoning. However, the question was still debated by some experimenters whether the respiratory paralysis produced by these venoms is, at least in part, due to a central effect (ROGERS, 1904a, b; ELLIOT, 1905; FRASER and GUNN, 1909; ACTON and KNOWLES, 1921; EPSTEIN, 1930; CHOPRA and ISWARIAH, 1931; VENKATACHALAM and RATNAGIRISWARAN, 1934) or entirely to a peripheral action (ARTHUS, 1910; CUSHNY and YAGI, 1918; KELLAWAY et al., 1932; KELLAWAY, 1937).

Examination of victims of snake bites encouraged the physiologists to reproduce experimentally, in animals, the phenomena which they observed in man, with a view to study them more closely. Since these phenomena were the results of an alteration of one or several functions, they then tried to dissociate each symptom of poisoning and relate it to the function which was disturbed. Then they improved their understanding of the situation by in vitro experiments on selected biological systems.

The various observations on animals bitten by venomous snakes, which had been amassed over the years, led to the general conclusion that venoms had an effect on the circulating blood. The often arbitrary interpretations of these observations led to opposing views.

As early as 1737, GEOFFROY and HUNAULT observed that the blood from cats and dogs bitten by vipers did not coagulate. However, FONTANA in 1787, trying to inject a rabbit in the jugular vein with a small quantity of the same venom, caused its immediate death and, on opening the vessels of the animal, found that the blood was coagulated.

It was at the end of the 19th century that the two activities of viper venom, anticoagulant at low doses and coagulant at high doses, were described by PHISALIX (1899).

Similarly, BRAINARD (1854), in the United States, drew attention to the incoagulability of the blood from animals which died after protacted suffering from intoxication by *Crotalidae* venom. Later, MITCHELL (1860) remarked that the toxic secretion of *Crotalus adamanteus* prevented normal blood from clotting in vitro. However, very diverse observations were published on the subject. According to MARTIN (1893) from Sydney, the venom of certain *Elapidae*, such as *Pseudechis porphyriacus* and *Notechis scutatus*, coagulated the blood in the vessels when injected at high doses, but at low doses, it rendered the blood incoagulable. In contrast, the venom of Indian cobra tested at any dose inhibited blood coagulation in vivo and in vitro (CUNNINGHAM, 1895; STEPHENS and MYERS, 1898; ROGERS, 1904a).

The first attempts at classification of venoms according to their actions on plasma were made by LAMB (1901–1903) and subsequently by NOC (1904). LAMB considered that venoms which were coagulant included, among the *Viperidae* venoms, those of *Vipera russellii* and *Echis carinatus*, among the *Crotalidae* those of *Lachesis gramineus* and *Crotalus adamanteus* and finally, among the *Elapidae*, those of *Pseudechis porphyriacus* and *Acanthophis antarcticus* of Australia.

One important point noted by LAMB (1901) was that RUSSELL's viper venom coagulated citrated plasma which is not itself spontaneously coagulable. NOC confirmed these findings and discovered that the venom of Asian and African Elapidae prevented the coagulation of citrated plasma to which calcium chloride had been added in a proportion such that the control plasma readily coagulated. MORAWITZ (1904, 1905) then defined, in his basic studies, the essential mechanism of the phenomenon of blood coagulation. His theory was later confirmed. It was the essential element of the development of our knowledge on the transformation of fibrinogen to fibrin and the formation of a clot. The "serozyme" of serum acting with the "cytozyme" from the platelets caused thrombin formation, thrombin being the factor reacting on fibrinogen. NOC (1904) presumed that venoms inducing coagulation contributed to the formation of an activated thrombin in the blood but he did not exclude the possibility that these venoms could actually contain a preformed thrombin. According to MELLAMBY (1909), the coagulant action of some venoms was considerably increased by calcium. The problem was clarified by ARTHUS (1912b) and his co-worker STAWSKA (1910). According to these workers, the venoms of *Crotalidae* acted as if they contained a thrombin and RUSSELL's viper venom accelerated the transformation of prothrombin to thrombin.

Soon after this, MARTIN (1905), followed by HOUSSAY working with SORDELLI and NEGRETE (1918, 1919), demonstrated that the coagulating factors in venoms did not pass dialyzing membranes.

The anticoagulant action of venomous secretions of snakes was attributed to the dissolution of fibrin by "ferments" (MITCHELL and STEWARD, 1898; NOC, 1904), to the precipitation of fibrinogen on the red blood cells and vascular endothelia (HOUSSAY and SORDELLI, 1918), or to the action of an "antikinase" (MORAWITZ, 1904).

These observations on the initiation of the blood clotting phenomenon by venoms led to the postulate that these substances contained "ferments," i.e., principles comparable to digestive juices or to those diastases which had been discussed greatly since their discovery in 1833 by PAYEN and PERSOZ. Already in 1843, as previously mentioned, Lucien Bonaparte had established a relationship between "Viperine" and "ferments." Seventeen years later, MITCHELL, in the United States, considered that "Crotaline," the substance which he had extracted from *Crotalidae* venom, was related to pepsin and ptyalin. VIAUD GRAND-MARAIS (1867–1869) attributed the properties of a ferment to "Nagine," which he had extracted from cobra venom. In 1884, DE LACERDA managed to coagulate milk and dissolve fibrin and egg white with *Bothrops* venom. PHISALIX (1897) established that a component of viper venom, "Echidnase," digested the tissues in a manner similar to that of a diastase. FLEXNER and NOGUCHI (1902) observed that *Crotalus* venom was able to modify proteins. NOC (1904) attributed these phenomena to proteolysis. He came to the conclusion that the most strongly proteolytic venoms were those of the *Crotalus*, while those of the *Elapidae* were generally only weakly proteolytic. Finally, DELEZENNE (DELEZENNE and LEDEBT, 1912) claimed that the venom of *Lachesis* contained a kinase which activated the pancreatic juice and in experiments with MOREL (1919), he observed that the toxic secretion of snakes was able to cause the catalytic breakdown of nucleic acids.

MITCHELL (1860–1868), then MITCHELL and REICHERT (1883–1886) attributed the hemorrhages produced by *Crotalus* venoms to their content of substances destroyed by heat and alcohol. They noted that these hemorrhage-producing substances did not cross dialysis membranes. Their observations were later confirmed by FLEXNER and NOGUCHI (1902).

An early experiment of FONTANA (1781) had demonstrated that the mammalian red blood cells were not altered when collected and mixed with *Vipera aspis* venom. In 1884, however, DE LACERDA found that the cells were deformed and even fragmented when the venom from *Lachesis* was added to them. MITCHELL alone (1868) and subsequently in collaboration with REICHERT (1883–1886) and STEWART (1898), studying the properties of *Crotalus adamanteus* venom, confirmed the observation made by DE LACERDA. FEOKTISTOW (1888) described the lysis of red blood cells in a solution of viper or crotal venom. According to RAGOTZI (1890), the hemoglobin diffused out of frog red blood cells treated with venom, and MARTIN (1893) made a similar observation.

It was about 1898 that MYERS caused the lysis of red blood cells in vitro by adding a small amount of horse serum to a nonlytic dose of cobra venom. He made, at this time, a distinction between cobralysin and cobranervine, cobralysin being responsible for hemolysis.

In a similar line of work, FLEXNER and NOGUCHI (1902) made an important observation: red blood cells devoid of all traces of serum were not lysed by snake venom but on the addition of a small quantity of fresh serum to the envenomated cells, lysis occurred. A substance called "seric alexine" or complement, responsible for the phenomenon of hemolysis by immune sera, had been discovered a few years before by BORDET (1899a, b; 1901) and by EHRLICH and MORGENROTH (1900). Was it responsible for this effect? CALMETTE (1902, 1907) subsequently demonstrated that "alexine" was not the active substance, since guinea-pig serum retained its properties after being heated, a treatment which resulted in the destruction of "alexine." KYES (1902, 1903) suggested that the factor responsible for the lytic phenomenon was lecithin of serum transformed into "lecithid venom." Study of this phenomenon was developed by DUNGERN and COCA (1907, 1908). These workers found that antivenom sera were without action on the "lecithid venom." They expressed the opinion that the "lecithid venom" was not a combination of venom and lecithin and proposed that the venom contained a lipase which cleaved the oleic acid of lecithin, giving rise to hemolytic substances. DELEZENNE and LEDEBT (1911, 1912) later showed that a "diastase" of the venom transformed the lecithin of egg yolk or serum to hemolytic lysolecithin under certain conditions.

Thus, at the beginning of the 20th century, it appeared that snake venoms could be distinguished from each other by their properties. They contained diverses protein-like substances: some were toxic, others comparable to "ferments" or "diastases." These results encouraged ARTHUS (1912a) to propose a physiological classification of these substances considering the dominant characteristics produced by venom poisoning. He stated that the venoms of *Naja tripudians*, *Crotalus adamanteus*, and *Vipera russellii* represented respectively curarizing, depressor, and coagulating types of venoms and according to this observation considered that the different snake venoms could be divided into three principal groups.

Following the experiments at Pouilly-le-Fort, where Pasteur elegantly demonstrated the usefulness of vaccination with mild bacteria, SEWALL (1887) in the United States observed that the pigeons he had injected with doses of *Crotalidae* venom which were too low to cause death resisted the injection several weeks later of a quantity of the same venom which was capable of killing untreated pigeons.

Soon after the discovery of antitoxins by BEHRING and KITASATO (1890), PHISALIX and BERTRAND (1894), and independently, CALMETTE (1894), on immunizing guinea pigs and rabbits by the injections of sublethal doses of viper and cobra venoms found that the serum of these animals acquired the property of neutralizing these same venoms. CALMETTE (1896) established then the fundamental principles of antivenom serotherapy. Later, RAMON (1924), by treating viper venom with formalin, supressed its toxicity without destroying its immunogenic power. A new stage has been reached in the field of research on toxic secretions of snake venoms.

Biochemistry, physiology, pharmacology, and immunology, which have progressed so far in the 20th century, have enriched our knowledge of the composition of venoms, the structure of their constituents, the disturbances which they produce in organic functions and the reactions by which they bring into play, under certain conditions, mechanisms for safeguarding life.

Each of the following chapters will consider these subjects separately.

In conclusion, we think that it is useful to quote these few lines from the beautiful work of J. B. DE LACERDA on snake venoms, which was published in 1884 in Rio de Janeiro:

> Les théories s'écroulent avec le progrès de la science et les doctrines s'évanouissent; seul les faits restent et il est toujours facile d'en verifier la réalité en les reproduisant, en quelque temps que ce soit, dans des conditions identiques. Le lecteur doit accepter cet écrit comme un recueil de faits provoqués par l'expérience...

References

Acton, H. W., Knowles, R.: The Practice of Medicine in the Tropics. In: Byam, W., Archibald, R. G. (Eds.). London: Frowde, Hodder, and Stoughton 1921

Arthus, M.: Venin de Cobra et curare. C.R. Acad. Sci. (Paris) **151**, 91—94 (1910)

Arthus, M.: Physiologie comparée des intoxications par les venins de serpents. Arch. int. Physiol. **11**, 285—316 (1912a)

Arthus, M.: Etude sur les venins de serpents. IV. Venins coagulants et anaphylaxie. Arch. int. Physiol. **12**, 369—394 (1912b)

At'Serstevens, A.: Le Livre de Marco Polo ou le Divisement du Monde. Paris: Albin Michel 1955

Behring, E. von, Kitasato, S.: Über das Zustandekommen der Diphtheriae Immunität und der Tetanus-Immunität bei Thieren. Dtsch. med. Wschr. **16**, 1113—1114 (1890)

Blyth, A. W.: Poison of the cobra de Capello. Analyst (Lond.) **1**, 204—207 (1877)

Bonaparte, L. L.: Richerche chimiche sul veleno della vipera. Estratto della Gazzetta Toscana del Scienze Medico-fisiche, pp. 1—11 (1843)

Bordet, J.: Mecanisme de l'agglutination. Ann. Inst. Pasteur **13**, 225—250 (1899a)

Bordet, J.: Agglutination et dissolution des globules rouges par le serum. Ann. Inst. Pasteur **13**, 273—297 (1899b)

Bordet, J.: Sur le mode d'action des sérums cytolytiques et sur l'unité de l'alexine dans un même sérum. Ann. Inst. Pasteur **15**, 303—318 (1901)

Brainard, D.: On the nature and cure of the bite of serpents and the wounds of poisoned arrows. Smithsonian Reports 1854

Brazil, V.: La Défense Contre l'Ophidisme, 2nd Ed. Sao Paulo: Weiss 1914

Bruno, S.: Il serpente nel folklore e nelle usanze magiche e religiose della Marsica. Universo **51**, 443—460 (1971)

Brunton, T. L., Fayrer, J.: On the nature and physiological action of the poison of *Naja tripudians* and other indian venomous snakes. Proc. R. Soc. (Lond.) [Biol.] **22**, 68—133 (1874)

Buffon, G. L. de: Histoire naturelle générale et particulière. Paris: Imprimerie royale 1769—1770

Calmette, A.: Contribution à l'étude du venin des serpents. Immunisation des animaux et traitement de l'envenimation. Ann. Inst. Pasteur **8**, 275—291 (1894)

Calmette, A.: The treatment of animals poisoned with snake venom by the injection of antivenomous serum. Lancet **1896 II**, 449—450

Calmette, A.: Sur l'action hémolytique du venin de Cobra. C.R. Acad. Sci. (Paris) **134**, 1446—1447 (1902)

Calmette, A.: Les Venins, les Animaux Venimeux et la Sérothérapie Antivenimeuse. Paris: Masson 1907

Charas, M.: Nouvelles Expériences sur la Vipère. Paris: Laurent d'Houry 1669

Charas, M.: La Thériaque d'Andromachus. Paris: Laurent d'Houry 1685

Chevalier, J., Cheerbrant, A., Berleni, M.: Dictionnaire des Symboles. Paris: Seghers 1973

Chopra, R. N., Iswariah, Y.: An experimental investigation into the action of the venom of the indian cobra *(Naja naja tripudians)*. Indian J. Med. Res. **18**, 1113—1125 (1931)

Cunningham, D. D.: The physiological action of snake venom. Sci. Mem. Med. Officers (Army of India) **9**, 1 (1895)

Cushny, A. R., Yagi, S.: On the action of cobra venom. Phil. Trans. R. Soc. Lond. [Biol.] **208**, 1—18 (1918)

Delezenne, C.: Sur l'action kinasique des venins. C.R. Acad. Sci. (Paris) **135**, 329—331 (1902)

Delezenne, C., Ledebt, S.: Formation de substances hemolytiques et toxiques aux dépens du vitellus de l'oeuf soumis à l'action du venin de cobra. C.R. Acad. Sci. (Paris) **153**, 81—84 (1911a)

Delezenne, C., Ledebt, S.: Action du venin de cobra sur le sérum de cheval. Ses rapports avec l'hémolyse. C.R. Acad. Sci. (Paris) **152**, 790—792 (1911b)

Delezenne, C., Ledebt, S.: Nouvelle contribution à l'étude des substances hémolytiques dérivées du sérum et du vitellus de l'oeuf soumis à l'action du venin de cobra. C.R. Acad. Sci. (Paris) **155**, 1101—1103 (1912)

Delezenne, C., Morel, H.: Action catalytique des venins de serpents sur les acides nucléiques. C.R. Acad. Sci. (Paris) **168**, 244—246 (1919)

Deoras, P. J.: Snakes of India. New Delhi: National Book Trust 1963

Dumeril, A. M. C., Bibron, G.: Erpétologie Générale ou Histoire Naturelle Complète des Reptiles. Paris: Librairie Encyclopédique Roret 1854
Dungern, E. von, Coca, A. F.: Über Hämolyse durch Schlangengift. Münch. med. Wschr. **54**, 2317—2321 (1907)
Dungern, E. von, Coca, A. F.: Über Hämolyse durch Kombination von Oelsäure oder Oelsäure Natrium und Kobra-gift. Biochem. Z. **12**, 407—421 (1908)
Ehrlich, P., Morgenroth, J.: Über Hämolysin. Klin. Wschr. **21**, 453—458, 681—687 (1900)
Elliot, R. H.: A contribution to the study of the action of Indian cobra poison. Phil. Trans. R. Soc. Lond. [Biol.] **197**, 361—406 (1905)
Elliot, R. H., Sillar, W. C., Carmichael, G. S.: On the action of the venom of *Bungarus coeruleus* (the common Krait). Phil. Trans. R. Soc. Lond. [Biol.] **197**, 327—345 (1905)
Encyclopedie de la Pleiade: Histoire de la Science. Paris: Gallimard 1957
Epstein, D.: The pharmacology of the venom of cape cobra *(Naja flava)*. Quart. J. exp. Physiol. **20**, 7—19 (1930)
Faust, E. S.: Über das Ophiotoxin aus dem Gift der Ostindischen Brillen-Schlange cobra di Capello. Arch. Pharmakol. exp. Pathol. **56**, 236—260 (1907)
Fayrer, J.: On the action of cobra poison. Edinb. Med. J. **14**, 522—529, 915—923, 926—1011 (1868—1869)
Fayrer, J.: Deaths from snakebites; a trial condensed from the session's report. Ind. Med. Gaz. **4**, 156 (1869)
Feoktistow, A. E.: Eine vorläufige Mitteilung über die Wirkung des Schlangengiftes auf den Thierischen Organismus. Mem. Acad. Imper. Sci. (Saint-Petersbourg) **36**, 1—22 (1888)
Flexner, S., Noguchi, H.: Snake venom in relation to haemolysis, bacteriolysis, and toxicity. J. exp. Med. **6**, 277—301 (1902)
Flexner, S., Noguchi, H.: Plurality of cytolysins in snake venom. J. Path. **10**, 111—124 (1905)
Fontana, F.: Traité sur le Venin de la Vipère, Florence, 1781, quoted by M. Phisalix in "les Vipères de France." Paris: Stock 1940
Fraser, J. C.: Le Rameau d'Or. Paris: L. Geuthner 1924
Fraser, T. R., Elliot, R. H.: Contributions to the study of the action of sea-snake venoms. Part. I. Venoms of *Enhydrina valakadien* and *Enhydris curtus*. Phil. Trans. R. Soc. Lond. [Biol.] **197**, 249—279 (1905)
Fraser, T. R., Gunn, J. A.: The action of the venom of *Sepedon haemachatus* of South Africa. Proc. R. Soc. Lond. [Biol.] **81**, 80—81 (1909)
Gauthier, A.: Sur le venin de *Naja tripudians* de l'Inde. Bull. Acad. Med. (Paris) **10**, 947—958 (1881)
Geoffroy, E. F., Hunauld, I.: Mémoire dans lequel on examine si l'huile d'olive est un spécifique contre la morsure de vipères. Paris 1737, quoted by M. Phisalix in "Les Animaux Venimeux et les venins." Paris: Masson 1922
Helmont, F. M. Van: Discussion on the opinion that the virulence of viper venom is due to the animal being angry. Orthus Medicinae Amsterdam (1648), quoted in "Histoire de la Science," Encyclopédie de la Pléiade. Paris: Gallimard 1957
Houssay, B. A., Sordelli, A.: Action in vitro des venins de serpents sur la coagulation du sang. C.R. Soc. Biol. (Paris) **81**, 12—14 (1918)
Houssay, B. A., Sordelli, A.: Action des venins sur la coagulation sanguine. J. Physiol. Path. Gen. **18**, 781—811 (1919 a)
Houssay, B. A., Sordelli, A.: Estudios sobre los venenos de serpientes. V. Influenza de los venenos de serpientes sobre la coagulation de la sangre. Action in vivo. Rev. Inst. Bact. (Buenos Aires) **2**, 151—188 (1919 b)
Jung, L. G.: L'Homme et Ses Symboles. Paris: R. Laffont 1964
Kanthack, A. A.: On the nature of cobra poison. J. Physiol. (Lond.) **13**, 272 (1892)
Kaufmann, M.: Du Venin de la Vipère. Paris: Masson 1889
Kellaway, C. H.: Snake venoms: their peripheral action. Johns Hopkins Med. J. **40**, 18—39 (1937)
Kellaway, C. H., Cherry, R. O., Williams, F. E.: The peripheral action of australian snake venoms. Aust. J. exp. Biol. med. Sci. **10**, 181—194 (1932)
Kyes, P.: Über die Wirkungsweise des Cobragiftes. Klin. Wschr. **39**, 886—918 (1902)
Kyes, P.: Über die Isolierung von Schlangengift-Lecithidien. Klin. Wschr. **42—43**, 1—16 (1903)
Lacepede, B.: Histoire Naturelle des Serpents. Paris: A. G. Demarest 1855

Lacerda, J. B. de: Leçons sur le Venin des Serpents du Brésil. Rio de Janeiro: Lombaerts 1884
Lacerda, J. B. de: Adisamento as investigaçoes experimentais sobre a açao do veneno da *Bothrops jararaca*. Exame clinico e microscopico do veneno. Arq. Mus. Nacional (Rio de Janeiro) **2**, 15—17 (1877)
Lamb, G.: On the action of snake venom on the coagulability of the blood. Ind. Med. Gaz. **36**, 443—455 (1901)
Lamb, G.: On the action of the venom of the cobra *(Naja tripudians)* and the Daboia *(Vipera Russellii)* on the red corpuscules and on the blood plasma. Sci. Mem. Med. Sanit. Dep. Gov. (India) **4**, 1—45 (1903)
Lamb, G., Hanna, W.: Some observations on the poison of Russel's viper *(Daboia Russellii)*. J. Path. **8**, 1—33 (1902)
Linnaeus, C. von: Systema naturae per regna tria naturae, secudum classes, ordines, genera, species, cum characteribus differentiis, synonymus, locis. 10th ed. Holmia: Laurentius Salvius 1758
Martin, C. J.: On some effects upon the blood produced by the injection of the Australian black snake *(Pseudechis porphyriacus)*. J. Physiol. (Lond.) **15**, 380 (1893)
Martin, C. J.: An explanation of the marked difference in the effects produced by subcutaneous and intraveinous injections of the venom of australian snakes. Proc. R. Soc. N.S. Wales, 1896, quoted by M. Phisalix in "Les Animaux Venimeux et les Venins." Paris: Masson 1922
Martin, C. J.: Note on a method of separating colloïds from cristalloïds by filtration. Proc. R. Soc. N.S. Wales, 1896, quoted by M. Phisalix in "Les Animaux Venimeux et les Venins." Paris: Masson 1922
Martin, C. J., Smith, J. M. C. G.: The venom of the Australian black snake. Proc. Soc. N.Y. Wales **26**, 240—264 (1892)
Mellamby, J.: The coagulation of blood. The action of snake venom, peptone and leech extract. J. Physiol. **38**, 442—503 (1909)
Minton, S. A., Jr., Minton, M. R.: Venomous Reptiles. New York: Charles Scriber's 1969
Mitchell, S. W.: Research upon the venom of the rattlesnake, with an investigation of the anatomy and physiology of the organs concerned. Smithsonian Contrib. Knowl. **12**, 1 (1860)
Mitchell, S. W.: Experimental contribution to the toxicity of rattlesnake venom. N.Y. Med. J. **6**, 289—322 (1868)
Mitchell, S. W., Reichert, E. T.: Preliminary report on the venoms of serpents. Med. News (Philad.) **42**, 469 (1883)
Mitchell, S. W., Reichert, E. T.: Researchs upon the venoms of poisonous serpents. Smithonian Contrib. Knowl. **26**, 1—186 (1886)
Mitchell, S. W., Stewart, A. H.: A contribution to the study of action of the venom of the *Crotalus adamanteus* upon the blood. Trans. College of Physicians, Philadelphia, 1898, 3rd Ser., No. 19, p. 105, quoted by M. Phisalix in "Les Animaux Venimeux et les Venins." Paris: Masson 1922
Morawitz, P.: Über die gerinnungshemmende Wirkung des Kobragiftes. Dtsch. Arch. med. Klin. (Leipzig) **80**, 340 (1904)
Morawitz, P.: Die Chemie der Blutgerinnung. Ergeb. Physiol. **4**, 307 (1905)
Myers, W.: Cobra poison in relation to Wasserman's new theory of immunity. Lancet **1898 II**, 23—24
Noc, F.: Sur quelques propriétés physiologiques des différents venins de serpents. Ann. Inst. Pasteur **18**, 387—406 (1904)
Noguchi, H.: Snake Venoms. Washington, D.C.: Carnegie Institution 1909
Payen, A., Persoz, J.: Mémoire sur la diastase. Les principaux produits de ses réactions et leurs applications aux arts industriels. Ann. Chim. Phys. **53**, 73 (1833), quoted by Y. Schaeffer in "Les Ferments." Paris: Masson 1929
Pelder, A.: On cobra venom. Proc. roy. Soc. Lond. [Biol.] **27**, 17 (1878)
Phisalix, C.: Nouveaux procédés de séparation de l'echidnase et de l'echnidnovaccin du venin de vipères. C.R. Congr. Med. (Moscva) (1897)
Phisalix, C.: Venin et coagulabilité du sang chez la vipère. C.R. Soc. Biol. (Paris) **51**, 834—837 (1899)
Phisalix, C., Bertrand, G.: Sur la propriété antitoxique du sang des animaux vaccinés contre le venin de vipère. C.R. Acad. Sci. (Paris) **118**, 356—358 (1894)

Phisalix, M.: Les Animaux Venimeux et les Venins. Paris: Masson 1922
Phisalix, M.: Vipères de France. Paris: Stock 1940
Ragotzi, V.: Über die Wirkung des Giftes der *Naja tripudians*. Arch. Pathol. Anat. Physiol. **122**, 201—234 (1890)
Ramon, G.: Des anatoxines. C.R. Acad. Sci. (Paris) **178**, 1436—1439 (1924)
Redi, F.: Observatione Intorno Alle Vipera. Florence 1664
Redi, F.: Epistolas ad aliquas oppositionas factas in suas observationes circa viperas. Scriptae ad D. Alex. Mous et D. Abb. Bondelot. Amsterdam 1675
Rogers, L.: The physiological action and antidotes of colubrine and viperine snake venom. Phil. Trans. roy. Soc. Lond. [Biol.] **197**, 123—191 (1904a)
Rogers, L.: L'action des venins de serpents sur l'organisme. Rev. Sci. **1**, 377—378 (1904b)
Rosenfeld, G., Kelen, E. M. A.: Bibliography of Animals-Venoms, Envenomations and Treatment. Sao Paulo: Instituto Pinheiros 1969
Sewall, H.: Experiments on the preventive inoculations of rattle-snake venoms. J. Physiol. (Lond.) **8**, 203—210 (1887)
Stawska, B.: Etude que le venin de cobra. Thèse: Lausanne 1910
Stephens, J. W. W., Myers, W.: The action of cobra poison on the blood; a contribution to the study of passive immunity. J. Path. **5**, 279—301 (1898)
Venkatachalam, K., Ratnagiriswaran, A. N.: Some experimental observations on the venom of the Indian cobra. Ind. J. Med. Res. **22**, 289—294 (1934)
Viaud Grand-Marais, A.: Etude Médicale sur les Serpents de la Vendée et de la Loire Inférieure. Imp. Vve Mellinet Edit., Nantes (1860—1868)
Wagler, J.: Natürliches System der Amphibien, mit vorangehender Classification der Säugethiere und Vögel. München 1830
Wall, A. J.: Indian Snake Poisons. Their Nature and Effects. London: W. H. Allen 1883
Wolfenden, R. N.: On the nature and action of the venom of poisonous snakes. I. The venom of indian cobra *(Naja tripudians)*. J. Physiol. (Lond.) **7**, 326—364 (1886a)
Wolfenden, R. N.: On "cobric acid" a so-called constituent of cobra venom. J. Physiol. (Lond.) **7**, 365 (1886b)

CHAPTER 2

Classification and Distribution of Venomous Snakes in the World

G. UNDERWOOD

The systematics of snakes in general and of poisonous snakes in particular can be extremely confusing, especially to those not experienced in the complexities of taxonomy. There are three main sources of this confusion.

1. Different names have been applied to the same form and the same name to different forms; the former has particularly affected poisonous snakes because they attracted the attention of early workers.

2. There are no agreed criteria for the recognition of subspecies. This has led to the naming of trivial local variant populations on the one hand and to the lumping of significantly different populations on the other hand. This is of some importance in the present connection because intraspecific geographic variation in snake venom is known. Subspecies are often recognized on the basis of a few external features, sometimes on color pattern alone. Several studies have shown that, within a species, different characteristics may show discordant patterns of geographic variation. This means that one or a few characteristics can be misleading as a guide to the overall affinities of populations.

3. There is even less agreement about the classification of snakes in general and poisonous snakes in particular than there is about subspecies. Indeed, arranging the genera in alphabetic order has the merit that it does not mislead by appearing to be natural.

Poisonous snakes have bedeviled the classification of higher snakes in general. Because people sometimes die when bitten by snakes, the venom apparatus and in particular the dentition have attracted much interest. The classification and evolution of higher snakes came to be seen in terms of a progression from harmless forms with simple teeth and no venom glands, through various intermediate stages, to the vipers with their elaborate venom injection apparatus. Much snake taxonomy to this day rests upon dentition and external features, to the neglect of other aspects.

With the uncertainties of their systematics in mind, I would urge investigators of snake venom to give full information about the origin of their material. Indeed, it is a good practice to put examples of specimens used into a museum collection and to cite the registration numbers.

Within the higher snakes, or *Caenophidia*, there are four types defined by maxillary dentition, which have sometimes been accorded formal taxonomic status. The *Aglypha* have solid maxillary teeth which may be of equal size, may be evenly graded with the largest posterior or may have the posterior ones abruptly enlarged and fang-like, and may also have anterior fangs (ANTHONY, 1955; Fig. 1 I, II, and V). Only a few of these are known to be venomous. The *Opisthoglypha* have the posterior teeth grooved for the conduction of venom, they are nearly always enlarged, sometimes

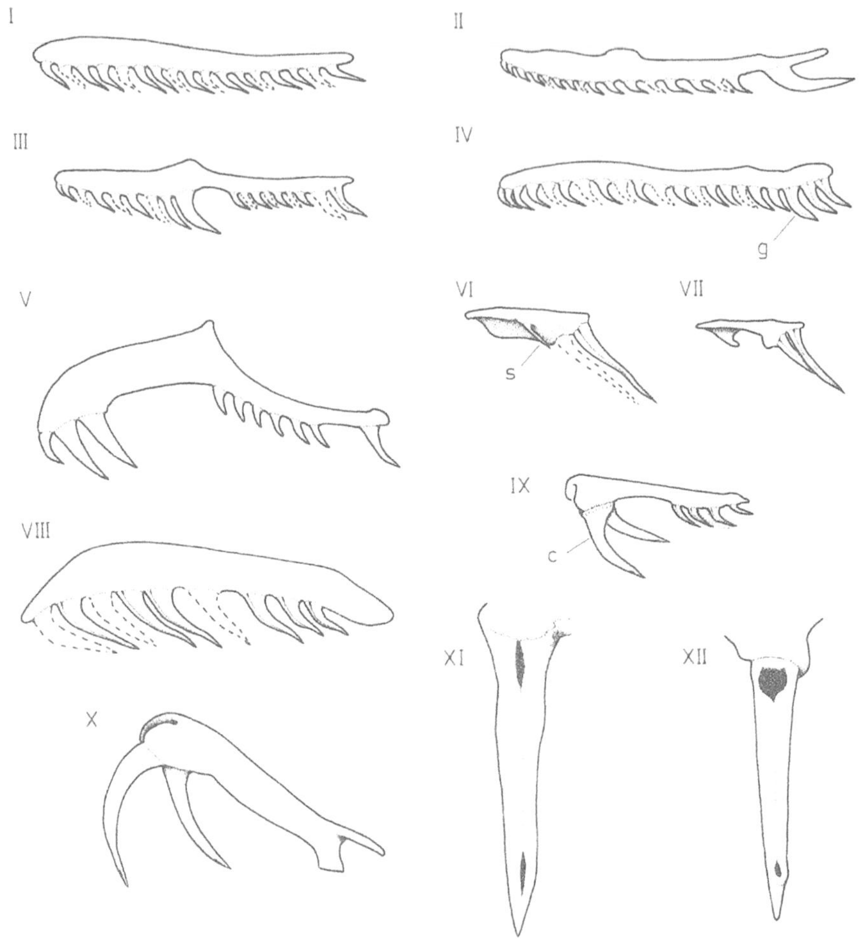

Fig. 1 I—X. Left maxillae of snakes. I. *Elaphe longissima, Colubrinae*, Mediterranean; teeth all similar, aglyphous. II. *Rhabdophis tigrina, Natricinae*, E. Asia: posterior tooth separated by a diastema and greatly enlarged, aglyphous. III. *Ahetulla nasuta, Colubrinae*, S. Asia; posterior teeth enlarged and grooved, small teeth behind diastema grooved, enlarged median tooth faintly grooved. IV. *Oxybelis fulgida, Colubrinae*, Trop. America; three enlarged, grooved posterior teeth, no diastema. V. *Lycodon aulicus, Lycodontinae*, S. Asia; strongly differentiated teeth but aglyphous. VI. *Tomodon dorsatus, Xenodontinae*, S. America; two very large grooved posterior fangs preceded by two solid teeth. VII. *Opisthoplus degener, Xenodontinae*, S. America; like *Tomodon* but no solid teeth precede fangs. After HOGE. VIII. *Ogmodon vitianus, Elapinae*, Fiji; teeth all similar and grooved. IX. *Austrelaps (Denisonia) superba, Elapinae*, Australia; two canaliculate fangs (c) followed by diastema and small grooved teeth. X. *Dendroaspis jamesoni, Elapinae*, Africa; anterior end raised, long curved canaliculate fangs, no other teeth. XI and XII. Anterior views of right fangs. XI. *Naja haje, Elapinae*, N. Africa; elongate opening at tip. XII. *Hemachatus haemachatus, Elapinae*, Africa; rounded opening at tip of fang of spitting cobra

greatly. Most commonly there are two grooved teeth, but sometimes three or four, in series. Often the anterior of two grooved teeth is offset towards the midline, sometimes they form a transverse pair. Occasionally, more anterior teeth are also grooved, and even teeth on the lower jaw. These, however, are not known to be associated with differentiated glands (Fig. 1 III and IV). In some, the anterior teeth are reduced in number, in *Opisthoplus* missing altogether (HOGE, 1957; Fig. 1 VI and VII). All opisthoglyphous snakes are presumably venomous, only the African *Dispholidus* and *Thelotornis* are known to be dangerous to man, however. The *Proteroglypha* have anterior maxillary teeth which are deeply grooved, usually with the edges fused to enclose a canal. There are usually smaller teeth behind the fangs up to about eight in number, sometimes these are grooved (Fig. 1 IX and X). All of these are venomous and many are dangerous. A few species of cobras are of interest for their ability to "spit" their venom; it is in fact ejected in the form of fine droplets, rather like a scent spray. The aperture at the tip of the fang is usually elongated, in "spitting" forms it is rounded (BOGERT, 1943; Fig. 1 XI and XII). The *Solenoglypha* have fangs which are tubular, usually with complete fusion of the groove; there are no solid teeth on the maxilla. The maxilla is hinged so that the teeth can be erected when biting (KARDONG, 1974). All of these forms are venomous, many of them dangerously so.

To avoid involvement in some of the uncertainties surrounding higher snakes, I continue to use the artificial "family *Colubridae*" here; to indicate some of the directions in which its analysis may go, I divide it into subfamilies. It is only fair to point out that the views implied or expressed are personal and, in their totality, unlikely to be shared by any other student of the group. Students of snake venom should be prepared occasionally to find that their observations do not conform with this, or indeed with any systematic arrangement. Because there are several clear cases of affinity between aglyphous and opisthoglyphous forms, the condition of the teeth can be an uncertain guide to snakes of toxicologic interest.

The upper jaw of higher snakes consists of four paired bones (Fig. 2 I), the toothless premaxilla is functionally part of the skeleton of the snout. The maxilla is moveably attached to the prefrontal which is itself attached to the braincase. The palatine tooth row is continuous with the pterygoid tooth row. A lateral process of the palatine attaches to the prefrontal and approaches a mesial process of the maxilla. A mesial process of the palatine arches over the choanal passage and attaches by a ligament to the vomer. The junction between palatine and pterygoid usually permits some flexion. The pterygoid extends back, resting against the floor of the braincase, and the posterior end attaches by a ligament to the quadrate, from which the lower jaw is suspended. The ectopterygoid runs forward from a firm attachment to the pterygoid to a flexible attachment to the posterior end of the maxilla (Fig. 3 I).

Several muscles attach to the upper jaw. From the dorsal side of the braincase in the temporal region originates the *M. levator pterygoidei*, which descends backward to insert on the dorsal face of the pterygoid, and the *M. retractor pterygoidei*, which descends forward to insert on the pterygoid and palatine bones. A *M. protractor pterygoidei* originates on the floor of the braincase and passes back to insert on the mesial face of the pterygoid, some fibers may also reach the quadrate. The *M. pterygoideus* has its origin on the ectopterygoid and passes back to insert on the ventral side of the retroarticular process of the lower jaw; this muscle evidently contributes to the force of the bite when the mouth is closed. In vipers, some of the fibers may originate on the maxilla (HAAS, 1973).

Forward thrust of the pterygoid pushes forward the upper jaw bones as a whole, thus advancing the grip of the recurved teeth. At the same time, the thrust of the ectopterygoid against the posterior end of the maxilla tends to rotate the latter on

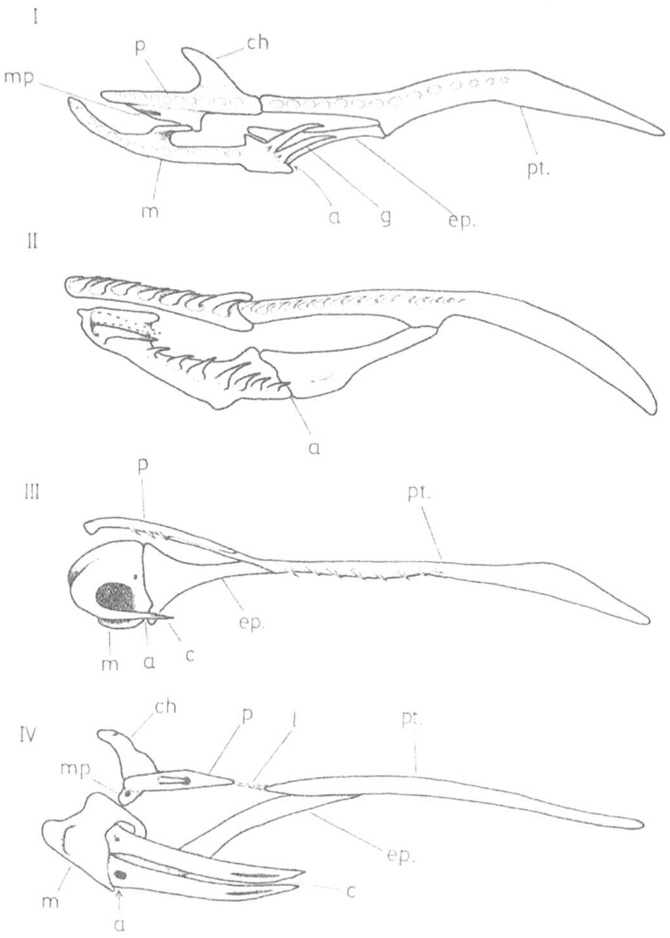

Fig. 2I—IV. Right upper jaws of snakes in ventral view. *a:* articulation between ectopterygoid and maxilla, *c:* canaliculate fang, *ch:* choanal process of palatine, *ep:* ectopterygoid bone, *g:* grooved fang, *m:* maxilla, *mp:* maxillary process of palatine, *p:* palatine bone, *pt:* pterygoid bone. I. *Pseudoboa neuwiedii*, *Pseudoboinae*, S. America; an opisthoglyphous colubrid showing usual relationships of bones; teeth other than fangs omitted for clarity. II. *Hydrophis cyanocinctus*, *Hydrophiinae*, W. Pacific; fangs followed by small grooved teeth, processes of palatine reduced. III. *Vipera russellii*, *Viperinae*, S. Asia; hinged maxilla, palatine reduced. IV. *Atractaspis bibroni*, *Atractaspidinae*, C. Africa; hinged maxilla, gap between palatine and pterygoid bridged by ligament (*l*); palatine retains processes

the prefrontal, increasing the gape and thus the capacity of posterior fangs to gain a purchase on the prey. A measure of rotation of the maxilla is thus important to opisthoglyphous snakes to facilitate penetration of the venom. The freedom of the pterygoid to thrust forward is limited in most snakes by the attachments of the palatine, laterally to the prefrontal and mesially, via the choanal process, to the vomer. The choanal process of the palatine is reduced or absent in several stocks of aglyphous and opisthoglyphous snakes; this may allow greater freedom of move-

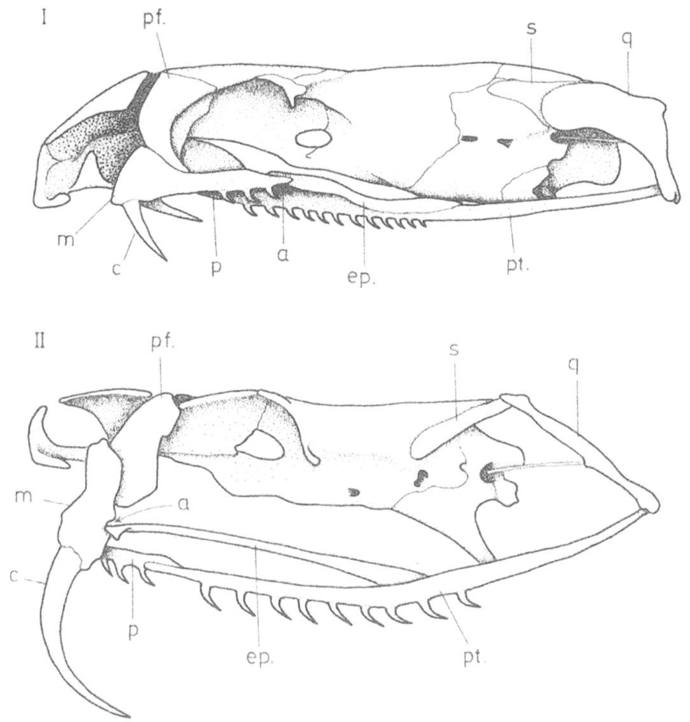

Fig. 3 I and II. Left side of skull with lower jaw removed. I. *Bungarus caeruleus*, *Elapinae*, S. Asia; faintly grooved teeth behind fangs, little movement of maxilla. II. *Vipera russellii*, *Viperinae*, S. Asia; fang partly erected on hinged maxilla, prefrontal also movable

ment of the palatine and pterygoid and thus of rotation of the maxilla. In *Dendroaspis*, the Australian *Elapinae*, and the *Hydrophiinae*, the maxillary process of the palatine is absent as well as the choanal process (Fig. 2 II). In the *Viperidae*, the palatine is effectively no more than a forward continuation of the pterygoid, without bony processes (Fig. 2 III; 3). An alternative way of increasing the mobility of the pterygoid, with rotation of the maxilla, is to loosen its link with the palatine, as in the *Aparallactinae*. Movement of the pterygoid does not now entail movement of the palatine, which is thus free to retain its processes. This trend culminates in the *Atractaspidinae* in which there is a gap between palatine and pterygoid (Fig. 2 IV). In the *Atractaspidinae*, the *Viperidae*, and the *Elapidae* portions of the adductor mandibulae muscles are variously involved in forming compressor glandulae muscles. Outside these groups, apart from *Dispholidus*, no muscle fiber insertions on the venom glands have been reported (HAAS, 1973; KOCHVA and GANS, 1970).

The groups of snakes discussed here are arranged informally in three grades, based mainly on features of the braincase and retina (UNDERWOOD, 1967a, b, 1970). Again, it is only fair to add that this view may be shared by no other student of the group. In the first grade, the orbits are usually small and separated by the full width of the braincase. The retina resembles that of the primitive boid snakes with a high proportion of closely packed rods and a minority of simple cones. The outer (visual cell) nuclei outnumber the inner nuclei (bipolar, horizontal, and amacrine cells) by about 2:1. The impression is given of a visual system with a low threshold of sensitivity but transmission of little detailed information. The pupil usually closes to a vertical ellipse. Included in this grade are the opisthoglyphous *Pseudoboinae* and *Aparallactinae*, the solenoglyphous *Atractaspidinae* as well as aglyphous groups *(Pareinae, Xenodermatinae)*. As survivors of an early *Caenophidian* radiation, these are divergent groups which have few features in common. What is rather strongly indicated is that differentiated venom glands, in association with grooved maxillary teeth, evolved early in the history of the *Caenophidia*. This in turn gives rise to a suspicion that some aglyphous groups may have lost grooved teeth and venom in association with feeding on innocuous prey. The initial function of venom was, fairly surely, to aid in subduing prey, thus reducing the hazards of tackling relatively large prey able to defend themselves.

In the second grade, the orbits are usually larger and may approach one another in the midline. The retina retains densely packed rods but there are up to three types of cones, including double cones, often in a second tier distal (scleral) to the rods. The outer nuclei usually outnumber the inner nuclei but may be somewhat fewer. The pupil usually closes to a vertical slit. The impression given is that the visual system has been elaborated over the preceding grade with an increase in resolution but a continuing adaptation to low levels of illumination. In this grade are included the opisthoglyphous *Boiginae* and *Homalopsinae* as well as some aglyphous groups *(Lycodontinae, Dipsadinae, Dasypeltinae)*.

In the third grade, the orbits are usually large, sometimes there is an interorbital septum of peculiarly ophidian type. The retina has a minority of rods, or none at all, in combination with up to three cone types. The visual cells are never arranged in two tiers. The outer nuclei are outnumbered by the inner nuclei by from 5:1 to 9:1. The impression given is of a high resolution retina operating at relatively high levels of illumination. The pupil is usually circular. In at least one stock, there has been reversion to nocturnal habits with conversion of cones into rodlike cells but retention of the high proportion of inner nuclei and presumably, therefore, of high resolution. This grade includes the proteroglyphous *Elapidae*, the mixed aglyphous and opisthoglyphous *Xenodontinae*, *Natricinae*, and *Colubrinae* as well as some purely aglyphous forms.

It is probable that the transition from second grade to third grade has taken place more than once. Indeed, the family *Viperidae* appears to be transitional. The *Crotalinae* have numerous densely packed rods together with large single and double cones; the outer nuclei somewhat outnumber the inner nuclei. In the *Viperinae* we see a reduced proportion of rods, down to about half, and a gradation from two tiers to a single tier—with the inner nuclei outnumbering the outer. The retention of the more primitive retinal pattern by the *Crotalinae* is presumably related to the development of the infrared-sensitive pit organ which facilitates the location of warm blooded prey in total darkness (BARRETT, 1970).

Three major divisions of the "*Colubridae*" are recognized by a number of workers on the basis of characters of the hemipenis. In the *Xenodontinae*, the hemipenis is typically divided, the *sulcus spermaticus* runs distally and forks on the shaft, each branch sulcus passes up the *outer* face of each lobe ("centrifugal" pattern of McDOWELL, 1961). These lobes may be lost with either the sulcus remaining forked or the

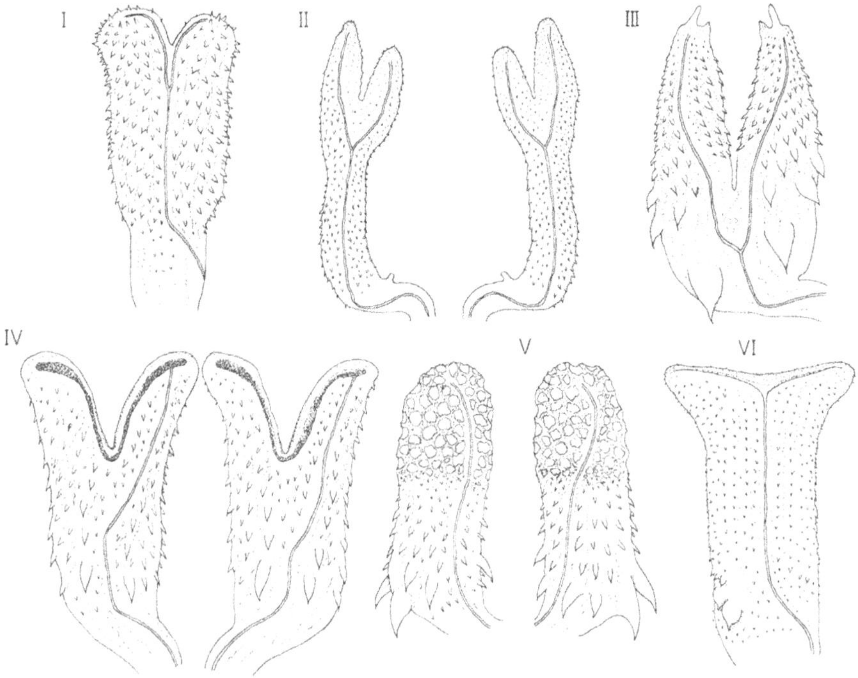

Fig. 4 I—VI. Hemipenes, erected and viewed from behind. I. *Micrurus spixii*, *Elapinae*, S. America; right side organ, bilobed, sulcus forks on shaft and runs onto lobes. After DOWLING. II. *Enhydrina schistosa*, *Hydrophiinae*, Indian Ocean and W. Pacific; both organs, lobes unequal but pair of organs symmetric. III. *Vipera berus*, *Viperinae*, Palearctic; deeply bilobed, each lobe terminates in an awn. IV. *Coronella austriaca*, *Colubrinae*, Europe; bilobed, unbranched sulcus to *left* lobe of *both* organs, pair of organs asymmetric. Specimen prepared by Dr. R. Duguy. V. *Thelotornis kirtlandi*, *Colubrinae*, Africa; simple organ, unbranched sulci asymmetric. Partly after DOMERGUE (1955) and DOUCET (1963). VI. *Natrix natrix*, *Natricinae*, Palearctic; bilobed, sulcus runs to cleft between lobes. After DOWLING

undivided sulcus terminating on the tip of the hemipenis. This type of hemipenis is also shown by *Pseudoboinae*, *Aparallactinae*, *Atractaspidinae*, *Boiginae*, *Homalopsinae*, *Viperidae*, and *Elapidae* (Fig. 4 I–III).

In the *Natricinae*, the hemipenis is typically divided, the sulcus runs into the cleft between the lobes and there it divides; the branch sulci run up the *inner* faces of the lobes ("centripetal" pattern of MCDOWELL, 1961). The branch sulci may be lost so that the sulcus terminates in the cleft and further the lobes may be reduced so that only a small cleft remains (Fig. 4 VI), in some the sulcus extends onto the right hand lobe of both organs (ROSSMANN and EBERLE, 1977).

In the *Colubrinae* the hemipenis may be bilobed, but the sulcus spermaticus is always undivided. The sulcus runs to the outside of the *left* hand lobe of *both* hemipenes so that they do not show mirror image symmetry (DOWLING and SAVAGE, 1960). The lobes may be reduced or absent; in the latter case, the *sulcus spermaticus* still passes to the left side of the simple organ (Fig. 4 IV and V).

Several other features should be mentioned for their use in snake systematics. The anterior trunk vertebrae bear ventral processes known as hypapophyses (HOFF-

STETTER and GASC, 1969). In many snakes at about the level of the heart these processes disappear. In some stocks, the hypapophyses continue onto the posterior trunk vertebrae. Attempts to interpret the presence of posterior hypapoplyses as primitive and their absence as derived have been inconclusive. Posterior hypapophyses are absent in *Pseudoboinae*, *Aparallactinae*, and *Atractaspidinae*. They are present in only a few of the *Boiginae* but in all of the *Homalopsinae*. These processes are well-developed in the *Viperidae* and *Elapidae*. They are present in some *Xenodontinae*, nearly all *Natricinae* and some *Colubrinae*.

The head scales of most *Caenophidia* include nine large symmetric shields. This pattern is so widely distributed, including groups outside the *Caenophidia*, that it appears to be primitive (MARX and RABB, 1965). Also seemingly primitive for the *Caenophidia* are presence of a loreal scale between the nostril and the eye and contact of the labial scales with the eye. On the trunk and tail, the scales are arranged in rows. Usually the number of scale rows is at a maximum on the neck, falls slowly to the cloaca, and then more rapidly to the tip of the tail. In burrowing snakes including the *Aparallactinae* and *Atractaspidinae*, the symmetric head shields may be reduced in number, the loreal scale lost, and the number of scale rows uniform from neck to cloaca. In some of the *Homalopsinae* and *Hydrophiinae*, the head shields are somewhat broken up; in most of the *Viperidae* they are nearly completely broken up and the head is covered with small irregular scales. In most of the *Viperinae*, the number of scale rows increases to a maximum at midbody and then declines toward the cloaca. Higher snakes generally have transversely enlarged scales beneath the belly and similar, but paired, scales beneath the tail. In the burrowing *Aparallactinae* and *Atractaspidinae* and the aquatic *Homalopsinae*, the belly scales are somewhat reduced. In most of the *Hydrophiinae*, the belly scales are greatly reduced or undifferentiated from the dorsal scales.

The scales of many snakes are macroscopically smooth, including secretive and burrowing forms like the *Aparallactinae* and *Atractaspidinae* and the elapines *Calliophis* and *Micrurus*. On the other hand, many have median longitudinal keels on the scales. Smooth scales may have microscopic striations. Scanning electron microscopy is beginning to reveal a wealth of surface fine structure which promises to be systematically significant.

The scales of snakes show the presence of two types of underlying sense organs: pits and tubercles (UNDERWOOD, 1967a). Circumstantial evidence suggests that the pits may be thermoreceptors and the tubercles tactile (NOBLE, 1937). Pits are shallow depressions, from about 50–300 μ in diameter; they are found, either singly or in pairs, near the apex of the trunk and tail scales, are rarely found on subcaudal scales, and have never been seen on belly scales. On the head, pits are often found on the loreal and temporal regions and around the eye, more rarely they are found on the underside of the head or on the frontal scale. Tubercles are smaller than pits, about 10–25 μ in diameter, and more sharply defined by an annular depression around a raised center. Tubercles are usually found on the snout, chin, and top of the head. Less commonly tubercles extend onto the trunk, belly, and tail scales. On these scales, they are found nearer to the centers of the scales than to the edges.

The lungs of snakes are primitively paired but the left is always the smaller. In the *Caenophidia*, the left lung is very rarely more than 1 or 2% of the length of the right; in many stocks, including *Viperinae* and many *Crotalinae*, *Homalopsinae*, and *Hydro-*

phiinae it is absent. In *Boiginae, Elapinae, Xenodontinae, Natricinae,* and *Colubrinae,* some are with and some without. The sharp boundary between trachea and lung is often lost with simple expansion of the former into the latter at the level of the heart. This is sometimes accompanied by extension of the vascularization of the lung proper into the roof of the trachea, forming a tracheal lung. The trachea may extend, as an intrapulmonary bronchus, past the heart into the right lung.

Where the tracheal lung is well-developed, the gap between heart and liver is usually closed. There is a well-developed tracheal lung in *Homalopsinae,* most *Viperinae, Crotalinae,* and *Hydrophiinae;* in the latter there is also an intrapulmonary bronchus. The *Xenodontinae, Natricinae* and *Colubrinae* are variable in this respect. A curious feature of *Ophiophagus* is the presence of nonvascular air sacs in the roof of the trachea.

Most snakes lay eggs. In *Vipera palaestinae,* the embryos are at a fairly advanced stage of development when the eggs are laid (KOCHVA, 1963). Some are ovoviviparous, i.e., the eggs are retained until development is complete and the young emerge from the egg membranes immediately after they are laid. In a number of different snake stocks, a simple allantoic placenta is formed, so that they are truly viviparous.

In reviewing the venomous snakes, I mention the genera of opisthoglyphous forms and the species of members of dangerously venomous groups. For many which may be dangerous to man we lack precise information; some may indeed have caused deaths but be unrecorded because there was no precise identification. There is a small but distinct possibility that anyone who handles snakes may accidentally furnish the first firm evidence that a particular species can be dangerous. For forms known to be dangerous, I give the length of a large specimen.

The *Pseudoboinae* include three closely related neotropical genera, *Pseudoboa, Oxyrhopus,* and *Clelia,* other genera may belong. They are opisthoglyphous with no obvious adaptations for rotation of the maxilla. On present rather limited evidence, these appear to be the most conservative of the lower *Caenophidia.* Some of the species are coral snake mimics. *Clelia cloelia,* the mussurana, grows to a large size and eats other snakes, including vipers.

The *Aparallactinae* are African forms, nearly all of them opisthoglyphous. Some of them are fairly highly modified burrowers. Each maxilla is short with a transverse pair of fangs. Some species of *Aparallactus* lack grooves, presumably secondarily. The food includes small, secretive vertebrates, including amphisbenians, and arthropods, including centipedes. The included genera are *Chilorhinophis, Cynodontophis, Elapocalamus, Melanocalamus, Miodon, Polemon, Amblyodipas, Calamelaps, Choristocalamus, Elapotinus, Macrelaps, Micrelaps, Xenocalamus, Aparallactus, Brachyophis,* and *Hypoptophis* (DE WITTE and LAURENT, 1947).

The *Atractaspidinae,* or mole vipers, have only one included genus, *Atractaspis.* Although long included in the Viperidae, there is now little doubt that they are related to the Aparallactinae, which they resemble in many external features and mode of life. They are, however, sufficiently different in the venom apparatus to be put in a separate group (BOURGEOIS, 1965; KOCHVA and WOLLBERG, 1970). They have a transverse pair of canaliculate fangs on an otherwise toothless maxilla. They do not appear to erect the fangs or to strike with open mouth (VISSER, 1975). The fangs can be bared on either side separately without opening the mouth. There are several records of persons who have held the snake "safely" behind the head but

Table 1. Systematics of poisonous snakes

Family	SubfamilJTribe	Genera
Colubridae		
	Pseudoboinae	3 genera (see p. 23)
	Aparallactinae	16 genera (see p. 23)
	Atractaspidinae	*Atractaspis*
	Boiginae	27 genera (see p. 25)
	Homalopsinae	10 genera (see p. 25)
	Xenodontinae	11 opisthoglyphous genera (see p. 29)
	Natricinae	1 opisthoglyphous species (see p. 34)
	Colubrinae	*Dispholidus*, *Thelotornis* plus 9 other opisthoglyphous genera (see p. 34)
Viperidae		
	Azemiopinae	*Azemiops*
	Viperinae	*Adenorphinus, Atheris, Bitis, Causus, Cerastes, Echis, Eristicophis, Pseudocerastes, Vipera*
	Crotalinae	*Agkistrodon, Bothrops, Crotalus, Lachesis, Sistrurus, Trimeresurus*
Elapidae		
	Elapinae	*Acanthophis, Aspidelaps, Aspidomorphus, Austrelaps, Boulengerina, Bungarus, Cacophis, Calliophis, Cryptophis, Demansia, Dendroaspis, Denisonia, Drysdalia, Echiopsis, Elapognathus, Elapsoidea, Furina, Glyphodon, Hemachatus, Hemiaspis, Homoroselaps, Hoplocephalus, Leptomicrurus, Loveridgelaps, Maticora, Micropechis, Micruroides, Micrurus, Naja, Notechis, Ogmodon, Ophiophagus, Oxyuranus, Parademansia, Paranaja, Parapistocalamus, Pseudechis, Pseudonaja, Rhinhoplocephalus, Simoselaps, Solomonelaps, Suta, Toxicocalamus, Tropidechis, Vermicella, Walterinnesia*
	Laticaudinae	*Laticauda*
	Hydrophiinae	
	Ephalophiini	*Aipysurus, Emydocephalus, Ephalophis, Hydrelaps, Parahydrophis*
	Hydrophiini	*Acalyptophis, Enhydrina, Hydrophis, Kerilia, Kolpophis, Pelamis, Thalassophis*

nevertheless had a finger stabbed by a fang with a sideway and backward turn of the snake's head. Some are seriously, although not dangerously, poisonous to man. *A. microlepidota* and *A. engaddensis* have greatly elongated venom glands (KOCHVA et al., 1967). The genus has been reviewed by LAURENT (1950). *A. microlepidota* is widely distributed from Mauritania to southern Arabia, *leucomelas*, *engdahli*, and *scorteccii* occur in Somalia, *engaddensis* in Israel and Sinai. *A. irregularis* and *aterrima* extend from tropical west Africa to Tanzania, *dahomeyensis* is in west Africa only. Centered on the Zaire-Cameroon area are *A. congica*, *boulengeri*, *reticulata*, *battersbyi*, and *coalescens*, and *corpulenta* which extends westward to the Ivory Coast. *A. bibroni* is widely distributed in southern and east Africa, *duerdeni* is confined to Botswana.

The *Boiginae* are a heterogeneous opithoglyphous group with an obliquely transverse pair of fangs on the maxilla. Most have the head clearly distinct from the neck. They are of terrestrial or arboreal and usually of nocturnal habits; the pupil usually closes to a vertical slit. The following genera are provisionally included: the Mediterranean and Middle-eastern *Macropisthodon* and *Telescopus*, the African *Chamaetortus*, *Crotaphopeltis*, and *Dipsadoboa*, the Sokotran *Ditypophis*, the Madagascan *Alluaudina*, *Ithycyphus*, *Langaha*, *Lycodryas*, and *Madagascarophis*, the Oriental *Psammodynastes*, the African, Oriental, and Australasian *Boiga*, and the neotropical *Barbourina*, *Imantodes*, *Leptodeira*, *Manolepis*, *Opisthoplus*, *Phimophis*, *Rhachidelus*, *Rhinobothryum*, *Siphlophis*, *Tachymenis*, *Thamnodynastes*, and *Tripanurgos*. *Tomodon* has a short maxilla with long fangs, *Opisthoplus* is similar but has no solid teeth before the fangs (HOGE, 1957; Fig. 1 VI and VII).

The *Homalopsinae* appear to be aquatic relatives of the *Boiginae*. They are more stoutly built and have the eyes and nostrils more dorsally placed. They are found in lowland freshwaters and brackish waters from peninsular India to Australasia. They eat mainly fish and frogs. There are ten included genera: *Bitia*, *Cantoria*, *Cerberus*, *Enhydris*, *Erpeton*, *Fordonia*, *Gerardia*, *Heurnia*, *Homalopsis*, and *Myron* (GYI, 1970).

It now seems likely that the *Viperidae* are derivatives of fairly early *Caenophidian* stock (HAAS, 1973; UNDERWOOD, 1970). As yet, however, we lack any clear indication of their affinities. They are one of the major groups of venomous snakes, many are dangerous to man. They have a transverse pair of canaliculate fangs on the maxilla which are replaced alternately. Throughout the family, the triangular head is set off from the neck. The eyes have a vertical elliptic or vertical slit pupil. Some of them, particularly at temperate latitudes, are more or less diurnal and bask in the sun.

The *Azemiopinae* (LIEM et al., 1971) have only one species, the little known *Azemiops feae* of the mountains of northern Indochina. In several respects, it is more primitive than other vipers.

The *Viperinae*, or Old World vipers, occur in Africa and Eurasia. They show a wide adaptive radiation in Africa. In most forms, the head is covered by small keeled scales like those on the body. In *Pseudocerastes*, *Eristicophis*, and all species of *Bitis* there are supranasal sacs. They lie just beneath the skin on the dorsal side of the nostril. They have an innervation which suggests a sensory function, but there does not appear to be any direct evidence (PARKER, 1932). These sacs are weakly indicated in *Causus*, *Vipera lebetina*, and *V. russellii*.

The genus *Vipera* ranges through much of Eurasia. All the species are terrestrial and nearly all are viviparous. *Vipera berus* and *ursini* retain symmetric head shields and appear to be primitive. *V. berus* (ca. 600 mm) extends from Great Britain to Sakhalin and reaches the Artic circle. *V. ursini* (ca. 450 mm) has a more southerly fragmented distribution from France to Mongolia. *V. seoanei* of the Iberian peninsula is now separated as a full species (SAINT-GIRONS and DUGUY, 1976). *V. latastei* (ca. 550 mm) occurs around the western Mediterranean and *V. aspis* is found in France, Switzerland, and Italy. Bites of the foregoing can be painful but are rarely dangerous. *V. ammodytes* (ca. 750 mm) ranges from the Balkans through Turkey to the Caucasus, and *V. kaznakovi* (ca. 600 mm) is confined to the Caucasus; the bites of these two species are reported to be dangerous.

The second group of *Vipera* species consists of larger forms ranging from the Mediterranean to the Oriental region. *V. xanthina* (ca. 900 mm) occurs around the eastern Mediterranean, the status of some subspecies is uncertain; *palaestinae* is often recognized as a distinct species. *V. latifii*, recently described from the Elburz mountains, is near to *xanthina*. *V. lebetina* (ca. 900 mm) ranges from Morocco through Anatolia to Kazakhstan; again there are subspecies of uncertain status. *V. russellii* (ca. 1300 mm) is a large and systematically somewhat isolated species. It extends from Iran to Taiwan, is absent from the Malay peninsula and Greater Sunda islands, save for an isolated population in Java, but is present in the Lesser Sunda islands. The bites of these three species are dangerous.

Apparently related to the above are two desert vipers: *Pseudocerastes persicus* (ca. 850 mm) and *Eristicophis macmahoni* (ca. 600 mm) found in Iran and Baluchistan. Bites are rare but may be dangerous.

There are a further two genera of the Sahara-Arabian desert belt, *Cerastes* and *Echis*; they appear to be related to one another and probably closer to the African than to the Eurasian stocks. They have strongly keeled scales which are serrated on the flanks. When provoked they gather the body into figure of eight coils and rub the sides together producing a hissing noise. *Cerastes vipera* (ca. 450 mm) is confined to the Sahara, *C. cerastes* (ca. 600 mm) extends into Arabia. *Echis coloratus* occurs in northeast Africa and Arabia; *E. carinatus* (ca. 600 mm) extends right across northern Africa to peninsular India and Sri Lanka; it shows geographic variation; the specific status of some populations has still to be resolved. *Echis* are known to be viviparous. They are irritable snakes which bite readily, the bite of *Echis* is dangerous, *Cerastes* less so.

The African forms appear to comprise a separate group of viperine snakes. The species of the genus *Causus* are primitive in several respects. They range across equatorial Africa. Although of nocturnal habits, they have round pupils. They eat mainly toads. Unlike most vipers, they are oviparous. *C. lichtensteini* and *C. defilippi* are more primitive species; *C. resimus* and *C. rhombeatus* are remarkable for the great extent of the venom glands beneath the skin back toward the heart.

The most primitive *Bitis* appears to be the poorly known *B. worthingtoni* of east Africa.

Bitis arietans (ca. 1200 mm), the puff adder, is found throughout Africa and the Arabian peninsula in all types of dry country between forest and sandy desert. *B. gabonica* (ca. 1500 mm), the gaboon viper, occurs in rain forests from equatorial Africa south to Natal. *B. nasicornis* (ca. 1150 mm), the rhinoceros viper, has a similar distribution but is restricted to damper situations. Bites by *arietans* are fairly common, by the other two less common. All three are dangerous; *gabonica* has particularly long fangs. *B. atropos* (ca. 400 mm) is found in rocky and grassy situations in mountainous areas in southern Africa; the bite can be dangerous. From veldt to desert in southern Africa are found the small species *caudalis*, *cornuta*, *heraldica*, *peringueyi*, *schneideri*, and *xeropaga;* only the bite of *caudalis* ca. 400 mm) is known sometimes to be dangerous. HAACKE (1975) gives information on the ecology of some species.

In equatorial Africa are found the small nocturnal tree vipers of the genus *Atheris* (ca. 600 mm). They have a slender body, very distinct head, very strongly keeled scales, and are generally green in color. Bites are rare and none of the seven species (*ceratophora*, *chloroechis*, *desaixi*, *hispidus*, *katangensis*, *nitschei*, and *squamiger*) is known to be dangerous. The little known *Adenorhinus barbouri* of Tanganyika is believed to be terrestrial and to feed on soft-bodied invertebrates.

Two terrestrial species are currently placed in the genus *Atheris* but do not appear to be close to the other species or to one another. *A. hindii* is found in Kenya, *A. superciliaris* in swampy terrain in Tanganyika and Mozambique.

The *Crotalinae*, or pit vipers, are readily distinguished from the *Viperinae* by the pit organ between the eye and the nostril.

Amongst the more primitive crotalines are the species of *Agkistrodon*. BRATTSTROM (1964) divides *Agkistrodon* into two groups. *A. acutus* (ca. 1100 mm) of Indochina and southern China is ovoviviparous and a dangerous species. Related to it are the semiaquatic *A. piscivorous* (ca. 1100 mm) of the southern USA and *A. bilineatus* (ca. 900 mm) from Mexico to Nicaragua; their bites are often reported to be dangerous. The remaining *Agkistrodon* form the second group. *A. (Calloselasma) rhodostoma* (ca. 800 mm) extends from Indochina to Sumatra and Java. Bites are fairly common and often dangerous. *A. hypnale* and *himalayana* of India and Sri Lanka are not reported to be dangerous. *A. halys* (ca. 700 mm) extends from the Caucasus to China and *A. blomhoffi* occurs in eastern China and Japan; bites of these are common but few are dangerous. The Chinese *monticola* and *strauchi*, Manchurian *saxatilis*, and Korean *caliginosus* are not well-known (GLOYD, 1972). *A. contortrix* (ca. 900 mm), the copperhead, of eastern North America is responsible for fairly numerous bites which are, however, rarely dangerous.

Lachesis muta (ca. 2000 mm), the bushmaster, ranges in forested country from Nicaragua to northwestern South America and the Amazon basin. The modified tail tip with a number of rows of small scales and a terminal spine is thought to be related to the rattle of *Crotalus*. Bites of this large nocturnal viper are rare but dangerous when they occur.

The rattlesnakes are believed by BRATTSTROM (1964) to be related to *Agkistrodon* and *Lachesis*. They are readily distinguished by the rattle. They are usually placed into two genera: *Sistrurus* with nine symmetric head shields and *Crotalus* with small irregular scales on the head. They are extensively discussed by KLAUBER (1972). BRATTSTROM (1964) makes a phyletic analysis. *Sistrurus catenatus* (ca. 700 mm) of central USA is sometimes dangerous. *S. miliarius* occurs in southern USA and *S. ravus* in southern Mexico. The poorly known *C. stejnegeri* of central Mexico is believed to be the most primitive *Crotalus*; BRATTSTROM (1964) puts *polystictus* near to it. The *triseriatus* group consists entirely of Mexican species arranged in three subgroups: *lannomi*, *polystictus*, *willardi*, and *lepidus*; *pricei*, *pusillus*, and *triseriatus*; *transversus* and *intermedius*. The *atrox* group has a more northerly distribution. *C. adamanteus* (ca. 1700 mm), the eastern diamondback, found in dry lowland country in the eastern USA is a very dangerous species. *C. atrox* (ca. 1700 mm), the western diamondback, found in similar terrain from southern USA through Mexico is also dangerous. In Baja California and adjacent islands *ruber*, *exsul*, and *tortugensis* are to be found. The *viridis* group also has a northerly distribution. *C. viridis* (ca. 1200 mm) of western North America and *C. cerastes* (ca. 600 mm), the sidewinder, of the deserts of the southwestern USA sometimes inflict a dangerous bite. In Baja California and adjacent islands *mitchelli*, *enyo*, and *catalinensis* and in northern Mexico *tigris* and *scutulatus* are to be found. The *durissus* group has a very wide distribution. In wooded country in central and eastern USA is the timber rattler, *C. horridus* (ca. 1200 mm), a moderately dangerous species. *Molossus* inhabits northern Mexico. More widely distributed, mainly in dry country, in Mexico is *C. basiliscus* (ca. 1500 mm) which is probably dangerous. The most dangerous species of rattlesnake, *C. durissus* (ca. 1500 mm), is distributed over dry country from southern Mexico, through Central America, northern and eastern South America to south of the Amazon basin. It is readily provoked and has a highly toxic venom. Several subspecies are recognized, including *C. d. terrificus*, found south of the isthmus of Panama. *C. vegrandis* is confined to Venezuela and *C. unicolor* to the island of Aruba.

The genus *Trimeresurus* has about 30 species in the oriental region, most are arboreal, many are green. Some are very poorly known and some are of uncertain systematic status. *Trimeresurus* appears to be close to the New World *Bothrops*. Indeed, MASLIN (1942) includes *T. wagleri* and *T. philippinensis* in *Bothrops;* BRATTSTROM (1964) regards *wagleri* as overall the most primitive crotaline and puts the two species in the subgenus *Tropidolaemus. T. wagleri* is a widespread, common, green, arboreal species in Indochina, Malaya, Sumatra, Borneo, Celebes, and the Lesser Sunda islands whose bite is often dangerous; *philippinensis*, widespread in the Philippines, is closely related. Where information is available, the bites of most of the remaining species are not known to be dangerous. BRATTSTROM makes two major divisions. The first division, with spines on the hemipenis, includes five of MASLIN's groups. Grouped with *puniceus* of southeast Asia are the Indochinese *cornutus* and *kanburiensis*, *gracilis* of Taiwan, and *malabaricus* and *trigonocephalus* of the Indian *peninsula* and Sri Lanka, respectively. *T. gramineus* of the Indian peninsula is classified with *stejnegeri* of southern China and southeast Asia. The *jerdoni* group consists of *strigatus* of southern India, *jerdoni* of China and Indochina, *kaulbacki* of upper Burma and *flavoviridis* (ca. 1500 mm) of the Ryukyu islands; bites of the latter are sometimes dangerous. *T. elegans* of the Ryukyu islands is grouped with *mucrosquamatus* (ca. 1000 mm) of southeastern China, this latter is also sometimes dangerous. The *monticola* group consists of stout-bodied terrestrial forms in southeast Asia and the Ryukyu islands: *monticola*, *tonkinensis*, *chaseni*, and *okinavensis*.

BRATTSTROM's second major division, without spines on the hemipenis, includes three of MASLIN's groups. The *albolabris* group ranges through southern India *(macrolepis)*, the Nicobar Islands *(labialis)* and southeastern China to Timor *(albolabris, popeorum, fasciatus)*. The species of the *purpureomaculatus* group spread over the Indian peninsula, the Nicobar Islands, and the eastern Himalayas to Sumatra *(cantori, erythrurus, huttoni, purpureomaculatus)*. *T. sumatranus* of Sumatra and Borneo is grouped with *flavomaculatus* of the Philippines. Much of this differs from the views of SMITH (1943) concerning affinities.

The genus *Bothrops* is also poorly analyzed. HOGE (1966) recognizes more species than previous workers; BRATTSTROM (1942) makes a tentative phyletic analysis. BRATTSTROM has a separate subgenus, *Bothriechis*, for the mostly arboreal *schlegeli*, *bicolor*, *brachystoma*, *dunni*, *lateralis*, *nigroviridis*, and the terrestrial *nummifer* in the area from Mexico to northwestern South America. A tentative group of small "hog-nosed pit vipers" includes *lansbergi*, *nasuta*, and *ophryomegas* in the area from Central America to northwestern South America and *cotiara* and *itapetiningae* south of the Amazon basin. The remaining forms are mainly large and terrestrial. The most widely distributed is the barba amarilla, *Bothrops atrox* (ca. 2000 mm). There are two forms: *asper* in Mexico and Central America and *atrox* in northern South America and the Amazon basin. Formerly regarded as subspecies, HOGE (1966) raises them to the rank of full species. They are primarily forest inhabitants. Bites are numerous and dangerous. The remaining forms are less widespread, some of them have very limited known ranges; an asterisk indicates those grouped here by BRATTSTROM (1964). In Mexico there are *barbouri*, *melanurus*, *sphenophrys*, and *yucatanicus*. In Central America, **godmani*, **picadoi*, and *supraciliaris*. In northwestern South America, *albocarinatus*, *alticola*, *andianus*, *barnetii*, *lojanus*, *oligolepis*, *peruvianus*, *pictus*, *punctatus*, *roedingeri*, *sanctaecrucis*, and *xanthogrammus*. In South America north of the Amazon basin, *colombiensis*, *lichenatus*, *medusa*, *pifanoi*, and *venezuelae*. In and around the Amazon basin, **bilineatus*, *brazili*, **castelnaudi*, *hyoprorus*, *iglesiasi*, *marajoensis*, *microphthalmus*, *neglectus*, and *pulcher*. South of the Amazon basin, beyond the range of *atrox*, the list includes several dangerous species. **B. alternatus* (ca. 1200 mm) is found near water; bites are common and effects are severe but not usually lethal. **B. jajaraca* (ca. 1200 mm) occurs in open country; bites are common and sometimes dangerous. **B. jararacussu* (ca. 1200 mm) is found in or near water; bites are not very common but very dangerous. **B. neuwiedi* (ca. 900 mm) occurs in open country; bites are fairly common and may be dangerous. Also in this area are *ammodytoides*, *erythromelas*, *fonsecai*, **insularis*, *marajo*, *megaera*, *moojeni*, and *pirajoi*. In the Antilles, two species with dangerous bites are to be found: on St. Lucia the terrestrial *B. caribbaeus* (ca. 1200 mm) and on Martinique **B. lanceolatus* (ca. 1500 mm) of arboreal propensities.

The *Xenodontinae*, as here understood, are heterogeneous. The genera closely related to *Xenodon* are few in number and divergent from the main lines of snake descent; there are, however, several larger groups of genera which appear to be broadly related. The subfamily also forms a convenient holding group for a number of forms at about the same evolutionary grade but of presently indeterminate affinities. Few generalizations can be made about so heterogeneous an assemblage. There are several genera of opisthoglyphous forms. In the neotropical region are *Erythrolamprus*, *Conophis*, *Philodryas*, *Coniophanes*, *Ialtris*, *Conopsis*, and *Tantilla*.

The aglyphous *Alsophis portoricensis* has been reported to be venomous (HEATWOLE and BANUCHI, 1966). In Africa, *Amplorhinus* and *Geodipsas* are to be found. There do not appear to be any oriental opisthoglyphs.

The family *Elapidae* is the second major group of venomous snakes. The sea snakes are often put into a separate family, sometimes with two subfamilies. As the affinity of the laticaudine sea snakes with the *Hydrophiinae* is in doubt, I suggest that three subfamilies of the *Elapidae* are preferable at present.

In the organization of the retina, the *Elapidae* clearly belong to the third grade, suggesting primary adaptation to good visual discrimination in daylight. Although there are numerous secretive and nocturnal forms, there are no obvious modifications of the retina known which implies that the primary sensory cues are not visual. Some features suggest that the *Elapidae* originated from secretive stock, assignable to the *Xenodontinae*. The absence of a loreal scale is a feature often found in secretive and fossorial forms; the absence of scale pits is a stronger indication of such habits. MINTON and COSTA (1975) cite immunologic evidence of natricine affinity. This recalls DOWLING'S (1975) observation that the branch sulci of the elapid hemipenis are "subcentrifugal." In the warm, mainly tropical parts of the world, the *Elapidae* show a wide distribution; the need exists for further systematic analysis.

The *Elapinae* range from fossorial, through secretive, surface living, arboreal, aquatic, and nocturnal, to diurnal habits and from forest to desert habitats; all types are found in Africa. *Homorelaps lacteus* and *H. dorsalis* of southern Africa are small and secretive. This genus was, for some time known as *Elaps*, the type genus of the family; it is hoped that a ruling of the International Commission for Zoological Nomenclature will restrict the name *Elaps* to the New World coral snakes. McDOWELL (1968) questions the elapid affinities of these snakes and would classify them near to the *Aparallactinae* (see, however, KOCHVA and WOLLBERG, 1970).

Elapsoidea, with six species now recognized (BROADLEY, 1971), occurs in tropical and warm southern Africa, most reach about 600 mm, *sundevalli* about 1000 mm. The widely distributed species are *semiannulata*, *sundevalli*, and *loveridgei*, more limited are *guentheri*, *laticincta*, and *nigra* of secretive and nocturnal habits; bites are rare but may be dangerous. There are two species of *Aspidelaps*, *scutatus*, and *lubricus* (ca. 750 mm), in southern Africa; they are shallow burrowers in loose soil, neither is known to be dangerous. In central Africa is the small secretive *Paranaja multifasciata* (ca. 600 mm); it is not known to be dangerous. *Boulengerina annulata* (ca. 2500 mm) occurs in lakes and rivers from Lake Tanganyika to Nigeria. Despite the large size, there appear to be no definite records of dangerous bites; the smaller *B. christyi* is little known. Six species of cobras of the genus *Naja* are known. *N. nivea* (ca. 1500 mm) of southern Africa has highly toxic venom and bites are very dangerous. *N. melanoleuca* (ca. 2000 mm) occurs in forest through tropical Africa, bites are uncommon but dangerous when they do occur. There are two African spitting cobras in savanna country, *N. mossambica* (ca. 1500 mm) in Mali, northeast Africa, and southern Africa and *N. nigricollis* (ca. 1800 mm) from Senegal to east Africa at tropical latitudes and in southwestern Africa (BROADLEY, 1968; BROADLEY and COCK, 1974). Defense by spitting, aimed at the eyes up to about 2 m, is commoner than by biting, both are dangerous. *Naja haje* (ca. 1800 mm) ranges from around the Sahara into Arabia and south to Botswana. Bites are fairly common and dangerous. The oriental common cobra, *Naja naja* (ca. 1500 mm) ranges from Iran to Taiwan. It seems likely that some of the subspecies will be recognized as species. *Oxiana* is found in the west, *naja* in the Indian peninsula, *kaouthia* throughout Indochina, and *atra* in southern China. *Sputatrix* in southeast Asia and the forms in the Philippines show spitting modification of the fangs. Bites are fairly common and often dangerous. The ringkals, *Hemachatus haemachatus* (ca. 1200 mm) is the most specialized spitting cobra. It is found in open country in southern Africa and the bite can also be dangerous. There are four species of mambas of the genus *Dendroaspis*. They are slender, fast moving snakes. The most dangerous and most terrestrial in habits is *D. polylepis* (ca. 3000 mm), the black mamba; it occurs in open country in eastern and southern Africa. The other three mambas are more definitely arboreal: *D. angusticeps* (ca. 2400 mm) in dry forests in east Africa, *D. jamesoni* (ca. 2000 mm) in rain forests of equatorial Africa, and *D. viridis* (ca. 2000 mm) in similar terrain in west Africa.

In dry country from Egypt to the Persian gulf, *Walterinnesia aegyptia* (ca. 1000 mm) is to be found. Bites are rare but the venom is dangerously toxic.

The oriental elapids, apart from *Naja* appear to form a natural group in which there is no reduction in the number of scale rows in the posterior half of the body. *Ophiophagus hannah* (ca. 4000 mm), the king cobra, inhabits forested country from peninsular India to the Philippines. Bites are uncommon but dangerous when they occur. The kraits of the genus *Bungarus* are all, as far as known, of secretive habits and placid disposition. They do not bite readily but the venom is highly toxic and bites are dangerous when they occur. In Sri Lanka and peninsular India are found *B. ceylonicus, walli, lividus* and the widespread *caeruleus* (ca. 1200 mm) which is found also in the Andaman Islands. In the area from the eastern Himalayas through Indo-China to southern China are found *B. bungaroides, niger, magnimaculatus*, and the widespread *multicinctus* (ca. 1000 mm) and *fasciatus* (ca. 1800 mm), the last of which is found also in eastern India and southeast Asia. In south east Asia are found *B. flaviceps, candidus* and *javanicus*. The oriental coral snakes of the genus *Calliophis* are very secretive and bites are so rare that the danger has not been assessed. Most are small but a few reach a length of about 1100 mm. They extend from Sri Lanka and peninsular India to south east Asia, the Philippines and Taiwan. Twelve species are recognized: *C. beddomei, bibroni, boettgeri, calligaster, gracilis, iwasaki, kelloggii, macclellandii, maculiceps, melanurus, nigrescens*, and *sauteri*. *Maticora*, with two species *bivirgata* and *intestinalis*, are slender snakes reaching a length of about 1500 mm with very long venom glands lying inside the body cavity. Because of their secretive habits, bites are rare but are known to be dangerous. They occur in south east Asia, Celebes, and the Philippines.

The New World elapids, the coral snakes, form a homogeneous group of three genera. They are of interest because they form part of an elaborate ring of coral-snake mimics. Some of the members of the ring are rearfanged (*Pseudoboa, Erythrolamprus*) and presumably have some protection in their own right; others are aglyphous and completely inoffensive. They are of secretive habits and, in general, of placid disposition, so bites are rare. However, the venoms are highly toxic and some of the bites which do occur result in deaths. They range from the southern United States to Northern Argentina. There has been little systematic analysis of the coral snakes above the species level and the three genera may prove to be artificial. *Micruroides* with one species, *euryxanthus*, is found in southwestern USA and adjacent Mexico. The genus *Micrurus* has about 40 recognized species, *Leptomicrurus* has three. Found in Mexico are *M. bernadi, bogerti, browni, diastema, distans, elegans, ephippifer, fitzingeri, laticollaris, latifasciatus, limbatus, nuchalis*, and *proximans*; from Mexico to northwestern South America is *M. nigrocinctus*. Within the area of Central America *M. alleni, clarki, hippocrepis, mipartitus, ruatanus, stewarti*, and *stuarti* are to be found. Northwestern South America is inhabited by *M. ancoralis, annellatus, bocourti, carinicauda, dissoleucus, dumerili, hollandi, isozonus, margaritiferus, mertensi, mipartitus, nigrocinctus, peruvianus, putumayensis*, and *spurelli*. In northern South America are found *L. collaris, M. averyi, hemprichi, psyches, langsdorffi, lemniscatus, spixii*, and *surinamensis*, the latter four also extend into the Amazon basin. In and around the Amazon basin are *M. balzani, corallinus, decoratus, filiformis, steindachneri, tschudii*, and *L. narduccii*. South of the Amazon basin are *M. frontalis, ibiboca*, and *pyrrhocryptus*.

The Australasian elapids are in an untidy state. There has been general agreement recently that a number of the older generic groupings, such as *Aspidomorphus*,

Demansia, and *Denisonia*, were artificial. WORRELL (1961 a, 1961 b, 1963 b) extensively rearranged the genera on the basis of limited evidence. MCDOWELL (1967, 1969 b, 1970) brought additional evidence to bear and partly rearranged WORRELL'S treatment. MCDOWELL was primarily concerned with analysis of the New Guinea and Solomon Island elapids and thoroughly considered only those Australian forms which were directly related. He thus left a number of Australian forms in a state of uncertainty. COGGER (1975), in a popular work, partly accepted and partly changed MCDOWELL'S treatment and revived a number of old generic names. As MCDOWELL'S treatment is based on a wide range of characteristics other than external features and dentition, I follow his classification as far as possible, utilizing COGGER'S revived generic names where appropriate; old generic names are in parenthesis. MCDOWELL (1976) thinks that *Parapistocalamus hedigeri* of Bougainville may be related to *Laticauda*. The *Vermicella* group, considered primitive by MCDOWELL includes *V. annulata* of Australia, *Solomonelaps (Denisonia) par*, and *Loveridgelaps (Micropechis) elapoides* of the Solomon Islands and *Ogmodon vitianus* of Fiji. Left over after the formation of MCDOWELL'S generic groups are the members of the *Glyphodon* series, all Australian: *Cacophis (Aspidomorphus) harriettae*, *kreffti*, and *squamulosus*, *Cryptophis (Denisonia) nigrescens* and *pallidiceps* (eastern), *Drysdalia (Denisonia) coronoides* (southern), *Elapognathus minor* (southwestern), *Furina (Aspidomorphus) christieanus* and *diadema*, *Glyphodon barnardi*, *dunmalli*, and *tristis* (eastern), *Pseudonaja (Demansia) guttata*, *modesta*, *nuchalis*, and *textilis* (ca. 1800 mm). The latter, in Australia and New Guinea, is readily provoked and has a dangerous venom. The *Simoselaps (Rhynchoelaps)* group consists of *Simoselaps*, with Australian species *(Vermicella) bimaculata (V.) calonota*, *(Brachyurophis) australis*, *(B.) fasciolatus*, *(B.) semifasciatus*, *(B.) warro*, and *bertholdi*, and *Toxicocalamus* with New Guinea species *(Apistocalamus) grandis*, *(A.) holopelturus*, *(A.) loriae*, *(A.) spilolepidotus*, *(Ultrocalamus) buergersi*, *(U.) preussi*, *longissimus*, *misimae*, and *stanleyanus*. Not explicitly grouped but agreeing with one another in some features are: *Acanthophis antarcticus* (ca. 600 mm) and *A. pyrrhus*, the former is known to be very dangerous; *Denisonia maculata* and *fasciata* and the arboreal *Hoplocephalus bitorquata*, *stephensi*, and *bungaroides* (ca. 1200 mm), the latter bites readily and may sometimes be dangerous. Somewhat more clearly grouped by jaw muscle peculiarities are the Australian *Echiopsis (Brachyaspis) curta*, *Notechis scutatus* (ca. 1500 mm) which has a very serious bite, *N. (Denisonia) coronatus*, *Tropidechis stanleyanus*, and *T. carinatus* (ca. 1200 mm), which has inflicted fatal bites, the little known *Parademansia microlepidota*, and the taipan *Oxyuranus scutellatus* (ca. 2100 mm). If provoked, this latter is an extremely dangerous snake with highly toxic venom.

The *Pseudechis* group is clearly defined. *Austrelaps (Denisonia) superba* (ca. 1500 mm) occurs in southeast Australia; bites are few but dangerous. *Micropechis ikaheka* (ca. 1200 mm) of New Guinea is so secretive that bites are rare, but they can be dangerous. *Pseudechis australis* (ca. 1800 mm) occurs in northern Australia and New Guinea. If provoked, it bites hard but rarely with dangerous effects. *P. papuanus* (ca. 1200 mm) is confined to New Guinea, although not well-known its venom is known to be dangerous. *P. porphyriacus* (ca. 1800 mm) occurs in wet and forested country in the south and east of Australia. It is rarely provoked to bite and the bites are only occasionally dangerous. Five species of *Suta (Denisonia)* occur in Australia;

carpentariae, flagellum, punctata, suta, gouldi, and *nigrostriata;* one species, *S. boschmai* occurs in New Guinea.

The *Demansia* group is also well-defined. *D. olivacea* (ca. 1500 mm) occurs in open country in northern Australia and New Guinea. Bites are uncommon but may be dangerous. Other Australian species are *D. atra, ornaticeps, psammophis,* and *torquata.* In Australia are found the swamp dwelling *Hemiaspis (Denisonia) daemeli* and *signata* and the little known *Rhinhoplocephalus bicolor.* Three species of *Aspidomorphus, lineaticollis, muelleri,* and *schlegeli,* are found in New Guinea.

The marine snakes are in some ways better classified than the Australian terrestrial elapids; they are also the object of better defined disagreements. SMITH (1926) recognized a family *Hydrophiidae* with a subfamily *Laticaudinae* for *Laticauda, Aipysurus,* and *Emydocephalus.* This is followed by some at present, but in 1967 McDOWELL brought forward evidence to support inclusion of the latter two genera in the Hydrophiinae whilst linking *Laticauda* with the oriental *Calliophis* and other terrestrial elapids. BURGER and NATSUNO (1974) reviewed the evidence, redefined some genera, and proposed a new classification with *Laticauda* alone in a separate family and the Hydrophiidae in two subfamilies. As McDOWELL's investigations have tended to reduce the gaps between *Laticauda,* terrestrial elapids, and other sea snakes, I prefer to lower the family groups by one rank; I follow nearly all the genera of BURGER and NATSUNO.

The *Laticaudinae* has only the genus *Laticauda.* The most obvious aquatic modification is the flattened tail, they spend time ashore where they lay their eggs. Three species occur in warm seas from the Bay of Bengal to the western Pacific: *L. colubrina, L. laticaudata,* and *L. semifasciata. L. crockeri* occurs in a freshwater lake on Rennel Island (Solomon Islands).

The *Hydrophiinae* are completely aquatic and, being viviparous, breed in the water. The nostrils are dorsal and valvular; the body and the tail are laterally compressed. McDOWELL suggests that the *Hydrophiinae* may have originated from *Hemiaspis*-like members of the Australian *Demansia* stock. If further work supports this view, then it should be possible to reconstruct hydrophine phylogeny in some detail from the surviving forms. The *Ephalophiini* are primitive hydrophines, small in size, and retaining enlarged scales on the belly and underside of the tail. *Hydrelaps darwiniensis* and *Ephalophis greyi* are found in shallow waters in northern Australia. *Aipysurus,* with the species *apraefrontalis, duboisi, eydouxi, foliosquama, fuscus, laevis,* and *tenuis, Emydocephalus,* with *annulatus* and *ijimae,* and *Parahydrophis mertoni* are found between southeast Asia and northern Australia. The *Hydrophiini* are more highly modified with greatly reduced belly scales. Some are large and have highly toxic venom. They are, in general, disinclined to bite but accidents occur, especially to fishermen. Most species occur between southeast Asia and northern Australia. *Acalyptophis peroni* (ca. 900 mm) is rare but may be dangerous. *Lapemis* includes *L. curtus* (ca. 800 mm) and *viperinus;* the former extends westward to the Arabian Gulf and can be dangerous. *Kerilia jerdoni Kolpophis annandalei* and *Thalassophis anomalus* are not known to be dangerous. *Enhydrina schistosa* (ca. 1200 mm), widespread and common from the Arabian Gulf to northern Australia, is the most frequent cause of serious sea snakebites; the venom is extremely toxic. It has recently been included in *Hydrophis,* but COGGER argues reasonably for its retention. *Hydrophis* now includes about 25 species following McDOWELL's supression of several other genera. Some *Hydrophis* have very small heads and slender necks and feed on eels in crevices (VORIS, 1974). Some of the larger headed species sometimes inflict dangerous bites. *H. cyanocinctus* (ca. 1600 mm), from the Persian Gulf to the lesser Sunda Islands, appears to be the most dangerous; *H. spiralis* (ca. 1800 mm), with a similar distribution and *H. ornatus* (ca. 900 mm), which reaches the Central Pacific, occasionally cause serious accidents. Other species are: *melanocephalus, elegans, klossi, melanosoma, torquatus, stricticollis, mamillaris, caerulescens, lapemoides, belcheri, bituberculatus, inornatus, kingi, nigrocincta, major, stokesi* and the small headed forms *cantoris, gracilis, parviceps, obscurus, fasciatus*, and *brooki*. *Pelamis platurus* is the most truly oceanic of the sea snakes, it extends from the Arabian Gulf to the western seaboard of the Americas. There is no certain record of dangerous bites. In a work edited by DUNSON (1975), many aspects of sea snake biology are reviewed.

The *Natricinae*, as here understood, occur in Eurasia, Africa, Australasia, and North America. Only one natricine, *Rhabdophis (Balanophis) ceylonensis* is opisthoglyphous.

The *Colubrinae*, in the restricted sense used here, are widespread, occurring in the warm parts of all continents and extending into temperate latitudes in the northern hemisphere. Most are diurnal, with a round pupil, but there are some secondarily nocturnal forms. Most are terrestrial or arboreal, few secretive, none fossorial or aquatic. The opisthoglyphous genera are mostly African. There is a group of terrestrial African genera related to *Psammophis* (which also reaches the oriental region): *Dromophis, Hemiragerrhis, Malpolon* (also around the Mediterranean), *Psammophylax*, and *Rhamphiophis*.

Also in Africa are the only two opisthoglyphous snakes known to be dangerous to man, both are arboreal. *Dispholidus typus* has three long, grooved fangs. It shows clear affinity with the more primitive aglyphous genus *Thrasops*, also arboreal. *Thelotornis kirtlandi* shows no clear affinity with African forms; it appears to be related to the opisthoglyphous arboreal genus *Ahaetulla (=Dryophis)* which is widely distributed in the oriental region. Also in the oriental region is the opisthoglyphous arboreal *Chrysopelea*. The only opisthoglyphous New World genus is the arboreal *Oxybelis*.

There is little doubt that the primary function of snake venom is to subdue prey. Most snakes eat small vertebrates and some eat prey, such as rodents, which are capable of inflicting serious injury. Rapid dispatch of the prey through the injection of venom, therefore, greatly reduces the hazard to the snake. The viperid stab and withdrawal is more effective in this respect than the elapid bite and chew. Natural selection, therefore, probably favors rapid action of the venom on the preferred prey. On the other hand, the function of the venom in relation to large animals such as man is secondary and defensive. If the venom rapidly produces painful effects, it is unlikely to be important whether or not it results in death. Indeed, many poisonous snakes have warning signals, the effectiveness of which would seem to depend upon the surviving large animals learning to avoid the snakes concerned. The details of the effects of the venom on a person are, therefore, unlikely to have much significance in nature.

It is a safe rule that venomous snakes do not attack people; they bite defensively when threatened and sometimes only after a warning signal has failed to deter. Nearly all cases of snake bite are the result of accidental encounters.

The hazards of snake bite depend upon a combination of factors involving the habits of snakes and of people. Clearly a snake such as *Echis carinatus*, which is widespread and common, active in the open, occurs in areas where much peasant agriculture is pursued, is readily provoked to bite, and produces a highly toxic venom in some quantity, represents an important hazard. On the other hand, although a bite of *Bothrops insularis* is extremely serious for someone landing on the small uninhabited island of Queimada Grande, its contribution to the snakebite danger in Brazil is almost zero.

Poisonous snakes of secretive or burrowing habits represent the least overall danger. Active in the litter of the forest floor or in burrows, these snakes rarely expose themselves and usually shun light so that the chances of accidental encounters by day are very small. Some may move on the surface by night, especially in wet weather, and occasionally they may find their way into houses and hide, for example, under bedding. Amongst the dangerously poisonous snakes, the African *Atractaspis* and *Elapsoidea*, the oriental *Bungarus*, *Calliophis*, and *Maticora*, and the New World *Micrurus* fall into this category. Some of these snakes are brilliantly colored but do not emit active or audible signals. If abroad at night, they are easily stepped upon without any warning.

Snakes active on the surface present a greater hazard, and diurnal ones more so than nocturnal. Man-made situations such as farms, which attract prey, are also liable to attract predators. Diurnal species are more likely to be encountered in the open than are nocturnal. By day, the nocturnal forms may be accidentally encountered in hiding, sometimes in houses or farm buildings. Both diurnal and nocturnal forms are a hazard to forestry workers. Some forms which move around mainly at night may be encountered basking in the sun by day. Some tend to diurnal habits in cool weather and nocturnal in hot; this applies particularly to species of *Crotalus*, *Agkistrodon*, and *Vipera* in temperate latitudes. Amongst the diurnal forms are the African *Hemachatus* and some of the *Naja*, the oriental *Ophiophagus*, and Australian *Pseudonaja textilis*, *Oxyuranus*, and *Pseudechis*. The nocturnal forms include the African *Bitis*, the oriental *Vipera russelli* and *Trimeresurus*, the New World *Bothrops*, and the Australian *Acanthophis* and *Notechis*. In deserts, snakes, like most animals, are not active by day but liable to be found half buried in sand in the shade of bushes. This holds true for some of the African *Bitis*, *Cerastes*, and a few rattlesnakes. Some poisonous snakes are found in swampy ground and are, therefore, not much of a hazard to most people. In Africa, there are the fully aquatic *Boulengerina*, not known to be dangerous.

Venomous tree snakes are rather narrowly confined to the tropics. Again some are diurnal and some nocturnal. They present the danger of bites to the upper parts of the body not normally covered by protective clothing. The arboreal vipers, *Atheris*, *Trimeresurus*, and *Bothrops* are nocturnal and do not move very actively through trees, at any rate by day. The Australian *Hoplocephalus* are also nocturnal, but the African mambas are diurnal and disconcertingly agile in their movements through trees. *Dispholidus* and *Thelotornis* are also diurnal. The marine *Laticauda* comes ashore mainly at night. The other sea snakes are more or less helpless out of water. They are obviously a serious danger to fishermen who catch them in their nets. Some, however, come close inshore in shallow water and represent a hazard to bathers who may blunder into them.

By far the most useful single work is the U.S. Department of Navy (1968) publication on the poisonous snakes of the world. KLEMMER (1963) gives a world list of poisonous species and lists many of the nomenclatorial synonyms. DOWLING and MINTON (1975) have recently reviewed the subject of snake bites.

There are many works on particular regions. The following is a list of the more recent ones: Africa, Central—LAURENT (1956a and b, 1964); Africa, East—LOVERIDGE (1957); Africa, Southern—FITZSIMONS (1962, 1975), VISSER (1966); Africa, West—ANGEL (1933); Afghanistan—LEVITON (1970); Antilles—LAZELL (1964); Arabia—CORKILL and COCHRANE (1965); Argentina—FREIBERG (1968); Australia—WORRELL (1963a), COGGER (1975); Belize—SCHMIDT (1941); Borneo—HAILE (1958); Brazil—SANTOS (1955); Cambodia—SAINT-GIRONS (1972); Chiapas—ALVAREZ DEL TORO (1960); China—POPE (1935); Colombia—DUNN (1944); Costa Rica—PICADO (1931); TAYLOR (1951); Ecuador—PETERS (1960); Egypt—MARX (1956); El Salvador—MERTENS (1952a); Europe—HELLMICH (1956), STEWARD (1971); Ghana—CANSDALE (1961); Guatemala—STUART (1963); Hong Kong—ROMER (1961); Indo-Australian Archipelago—DE ROOIJ (1917), DE HAAS (1950); Indochina—BOURRET (1936); Israel—MENDELSOHN (1965); Ivory Coast—DOUCET (1963); Japan—STEJNEGER (1907); Libya—KRAMER and SCHNURRENBERGER (1963); Malawi—SWEENEY (1961); Malaya—TWEEDIE (1954); Mauritania—VILLIERS (1950); Mexico—SMITH and TAYLOR (1945); Morocco—SAINT-GIRONS (1956); Neotropical Region—PETERS and OREJAS-MIRANDA (1970); Nepal—SWAN and LEVITON (1962); North America—WRIGHT and WRIGHT (1957); Oriental Region—SMITH (1943); Pacific Islands—LOVERIDGE (1945), WERLER and KEEGAN (1963); Pakistan—MINTON (1966); Rhodesia—BROADLEY and COCK (1974); Somalia—PARKER (1949); Surinam—BRONGERSMA (1966); Taiwan—KUNTZ (1963); Thailand—TAYLOR (1965); Trinidad—MOLE (1924); Turkey—MERTENS (1952b); Uganda—PITMAN (1974); U.S.S.R.—TERENTJEV and CHERNOV (1949); Venezuela—ROZE (1966); Viet Nam, South—CAMPDEN-MAIN (1970).

References

Alvarez del Toro, M.: Los Reptiles de Chiapas. Inst. Zool. Estado, Tuxtla Gutierrez, Chiapas, Mexico, 1960

Amaral, A. do: Lista remissiva dos ophidios da regiao neotropical. Mem. Inst. Butantan **4**, 127—271 (1930)

Anderson, S. C.: Amphibians and reptiles from Iran. Proc. Calif. Acad. Sci. **31**, 417—498 (1963)

Angel, F.: Les Serpents de l'Afrique Occidentale Française. Paris: Larose 1933

Anthony, J.: Essai sur l'évolution anatomique de l'appareil vénimeux des Ophidiens. Ann. Sci. Nat. [Zoologie] **17**, 7—53 (1955)

Barrett, R.: The pit organs of snakes. In: Gans, C., Parsons, T. (Eds.): Biology of the Reptilia. London-New York: Academic Press 1970

Bogert, C. M.: Dentitional phenomena in cobras and other elapids with notes on adaptive modifications of fangs. Bull. Amer. Mus. Hist. **81**, 285—360 (1943)

Bons, J., Girot, B.: Clé illustrée des reptiles du Maroc. Trav. Inst. Sci. Cherifien Ser. Zool. **26**, 1—62 (1962)

Bourgeois, M.: Contribution à la morphologie comparée du crane des ophidiens de l'Afrique Centrale. Publ. Univ. Off. Congo. **18**, 1—293 (1965)

Bourret, R.: Les Serpents de l'Indochine. Toulouse: H. Basuyau 1936

Brattstrom, B. H.: Evolution of the pit vipers. Trans. San Diego Soc. nat. Hist. **13**, 185—268 (1964)

Broadley, D. G.: A Review of the African Cobras of the Genus *Naja* (Serpentes, Elapinae) Misc. Publ. nat. Mus. S. Rhodesia **3**, 1—14 (1968)

Broadley, D. G.: A revision of the African snake genus *Elapsoidea* Bocage (Elapidae). Occ. Pap. nat. Mus. Rhod. B. **4**, 577—626 (1971)

Broadley, D. G., Cock, E. V.: Snakes of Rhodesia. Salisbury: Longman 1974

Brongersma, L. D.: Poisonous snakes of Surinam. Mem. Inst. Butantan **33**, 73—79 (1966)

Burger, W. L., Natsuno, T.: A new genus for the Arafura smooth sea-snake and redefinitions of other sea-snake genera. Snake **6**, 61—75 (1974)

Campden-Main, S. M.: A Field Guide to the Snakes of South Vietnam. Washington: U.S. Natl. Mus. 1970

Cansdale, G. S.: West Africa Snakes. London: Longmans Green 1961

Cogger, H. G.: Reptiles and Amphibians of Australia. Sydney-Wellington-London: Reed 1975

Corkill, N. L., Cochrane, J. A.: The snakes of the Arabian peninsula and Socotra. J. Bombay Nat. Hist. Soc. **62**, 475—506 (1965)

Doucet, J.: Les serpents de la republique de Côte d'Ivoire. Acta Tropica **20**, 201—340 (1963)

Dowling, H. G.: Snake venoms and venomous snakes. In: Dowling, H. G. (Ed.): 1974 HISS Yearbook of Herpetology. New York: Amer. Mus. Nat. Hist. 1975

Dowling, H. G., Minton, S. A.: Snakebite. In: Dowling, H. G. (Ed.): 1974 HISS Yearbook of Herpetology. New York: Amer. Mus. Nat. Hist. 1975

Dowling, H. G., Savage, J. M.: A guide to the snake hemipenis: a survey of basic structure and systematic characteristics. Zoologica **45**, 17—28 (1960)

Dunn, E. R.: Los generos de anfibios y reptiles de Colombia, III. Reptiles; orden de las serpientes. Caldasia **3**, 155—224 (1944)

Dunson, W. A. (Ed.): The Biology of Sea Snakes. Baltimore-London-Tokyo: University Park Press 1975

Fitzsimons, V. F. M.: Snakes of Southern Africa. London: Macdonald 1962

Fitzsimons, V. F. M.: A Field Guide to the Snakes of Southern Africa. London: Collins 1975

Freiberg, M. A.: Ofidios ponzoñosos de la Argentina. Ciencia Investigación **24**, 338—353 (1968)

Gloyd, H. K.: The Korean snakes of the genus *Agkistrodon* (Crotalinae). Proc. Biol. Soc. (Wash.) **85**, 557—578 (1972)

Gyi, K. K.: A revision of the Colubrid snakes of the sub-family *Homalopsinae*. Univ. Kansas Publ. Mus. nat. Hist. **20**, 47—223 (1970)

Haacke, W. B.: Description of a new adder *(Viperidae reptilia)* from southern Africa with a discussion of related forms. Cimbebasia [A] **4**, 116—127 (1975)

Haas, C. P. J. de: Checklist of the snakes of the Indo-Australian archipelago. Treubia **20**, 511—625 (1950)

Haas, G.: Muscles of the jaws and associated structures in the *Rhynchocephalia* and *Squamata*. In: Gans, C., Parsons, T. (Eds.): Biology of the Reptilia. London-New York: Academic Press 1973

Haile, N. S.: The snakes of Borneo with a key to the species. Sarawak Mus. J. **8**, 743—771 (1958)

Heatwole, H., Banuchi, I. B.: Envenomation by the colubrid snake, *Alsophis portoricensis*. Herpetologica **22**, 132—134 (1966)

Hellmich, W.: Die Lurche und Kriechtiere Europas. Heidelberg: Carl Winter 1956

Hoffstetter, R., Gasc, J. P.: Vertebrae and ribs of modern reptiles. In: Gans, C., Parsons, T. (Eds.): Biology of the Reptilia. London-New York: Academic Press 1969

Hoge, A. R.: Notes sur la position systematique de *Opisthoplus degener* Peters 1882 et *Leimadophis regina macrosoma* Amaral 1935 (Serpentes). Mem. Inst. Butantan **28**, 67—72 (1957)

Hoge, A. R.: Preliminary account of neotropical Crotalinae (Serpentes, Viperidae). Mem. Inst. Butantan **32**, 109—184 (1966)

Kardong, K. V.: Kinesis of the jaw apparatus during the strike in the cottonmouth snake, *Agkistrodon piscivorous*. Forma Functio **7**, 327—354 (1974)
Khalaf, K. T.: Reptiles of Iraq With Some Notes on the Amphibians. Baghdad: Ministry of Education 1959
Kinghorn, J. R.: The Snakes of Australia, 2nd Ed. Sydney: Angus & Robertson 1956
Klauber, L.: Rattlesnakes. Berkeley-Los Angeles: Univ. California 1972
Klemmer, K.: Liste der rezenten Giftschlangen. In: Die Giftschlangen der Erde. Marburg: Behringwerk-Mitteilungen N. G. Elwert 1963
Kochva, E.: Development of the venom gland and trigeminal muscles in *Vipera palaestinae*. Acta Anat. **52**, 49—89 (1963)
Kochva, E., Gans, C.: Salivary glands of snakes. Clin. Toxicol. **3**, 363—387 (1970)
Kochva, E., Shayer-Wollberg, M., Sobol, R.: The special pattern of the venom gland in *Atractaspis* and its bearing on the taxonomic status of the genus. Copeia **1967**, 763—772
Kochva, E., Wollberg, S. H.: The salivary glands of *Aparallactinae (Colubridae)* and the venom glands of *Elaps (Elapidae)* in relation to the taxonomic status of this genus. Zool. J. Linn. Soc. **49**, 217—224 (1970)
Kramer, E., Schnurrenberger, H.: Systematik, Verbreitung und Ökologie der Libyschen Schlangen. Rev. Suisse Zool. **70**, 453—568 (1963)
Kuntz, R. E.: The Snakes of Taiwan. Taipei: U.S. Naval. Med. Res. Unit 1963, No. 2
Laurent, R.: Revision du genre *Atractaspis*. Mem. Inst. Roy. nat. Belg. [2] **38** (1950)
Laurent, R. F.: Contribution a l'herpetologie de la region des Grands Lacs de l'Afrique central. Pts. 1—3. Ann. Mus. R. Congo Belg. **48**, 1—390 (1956a)
Laurent, R. F.: Esquisse d'une faune herpetologique du Ruanda-Urundi. Bull. nat. Belges **1956**, 280—287 (1956b)
Laurent, R. F.: Reptiles et amphibiens de l'Angola. Pub. Culturais Mus. Dundo **67**, 1—165 (1964)
Lazell, Jr., J. D.: The Lesser Antillean representatives of *Bothrops* and *Constrictor*. Bull. Mus. Comp. Zool. **132**, 245—273 (1964)
Lecuru-Renous, S., Platel, R.: La Vipère Aspic Doin-Deren. Paris: 1970
Leviton, A. E.: Keys to the dangerous venomous terrestrial snakes of the Philippine Islands. Silliman J. **8**, 98—106 (1961)
Leviton, A. E.: The amphibians and reptiles of Afghanistan. A check list and key to the Herpetofauna. Proc. Calif. Acad. Sci. **37**, 163—206 (1970)
Liem, K. F., Marx, H., Rabb, G.: The viperid snake *Azemiops*, its comparative cephalic anatomy and phylogenetic position in relation to *Viperinae* and *Crotalinae*. Fieldana [Zool.] **59**, 65—126 (1971)
Loveridge, A.: Reptiles of the Pacific World. New York: Macmillan 1945
Loveridge, A.: Check list of the reptiles and amphibians of East Africa (Uganda, Kenya, Tanganyika, Zanzibar). Bull. Mus. Comp. Zool. **117**, 153—362 (1957)
Manaças, S.: Ofidios de Moçambique. Mem. Junta. Invest. Ultram. **8**, 135—160 (1956)
Marx, H.: Keys to the Lizards and Snakes of Egypt. Cairo: Research Dept. NM 005 050.39.45, NAMRU-3, 1956
Marx, H., Rabb, G.: Relationships and zoogeography of the viperine snakes (Family *Viperidae*). Fieldiana [Zool.] **44**, 161—206 (1965)
Marx, H., Rabb, G.: Character analysis: an empirical approach applied to advanced snakes. J. Zool. (Lond.) **161**, 525—548 (1970)
Maslin, T. P.: Evidence for the separation of the crotalid genera *Trimeresurus* and *Bothrops*. Key to the genus *Trimeresurus*. Copeia **1942**, 18—24
McDowell, S. B.: Review of Malnate: "Systematic division and evolution of the colubrid snake genus *Natrix*, with comments on the sub-family Natricinae." Copeia **1961**, 502—506
McDowell, S. B.: *Aspidomorphus*, a genus of New Guinea snakes of the family *Elapidae*, with notes on related genera. J. Zool. (Lond.) **151**, 497—543 (1967)
McDowell, S. B.: Affinities of the snakes usually called *Elaps lacteus* and *E. dorsalis*. J. Linn. Soc. (Zool.) **47**, 561—578 (1968)
McDowell, S. B.: Notes on the Australian sea-snake *Ephalophis greyi* M. Smith (Serpentes; *Elapidae, Hydrophiinae*) and the origin and classification of sea-snakes. Zool. J. Linn. Soc. **48**, 333—349 (1969a)

McDowell, S. B.: *Toxicocalamus*, a New Guinea genus of snakes of the family *Elapidae*. J. Zool. (Lond.) **159**, 443—511 (1969 b)
McDowell, S. B.: On the status and relationships of the Solomon island elapid snakes. J. Zool. (Lond.) **161**, 145—190 (1970)
McDowell, S. B.: The genera of sea-snakes of the *Hydrophis* group (Serpentes: *Elapidae*). Trans. Zool. Soc. (Lond.) **32**, 189—247 (1972)
Mendelssohn, H.: On the biology of the venomous snakes of Israel. Israel J. Zool. **14**, 185—212 (1965)
Mertens, R.: Die Amphibien and Reptilien von El Salvador, aufgrund der Reisen von R. Mertens und A. Zilch. Abh. Senckenbergischen Ges. **487**, 1—120 (1952 a)
Mertens, R.: Amphibien und Reptilien aus der Türkei. Rev. Fac. Sci. Univ. (Istanbul) [B] **1**, 41—75 (1952 b)
Minton, Jr., S. A.: A contribution to the herpetology of West Pakistan. Bull. Amer. Mus. nat. Hist. **134**, 27—184 (1966)
Minton, S. A., Costa, M. S. da: Serological relationships of sea-snakes and their evolutionary implication. In: Dunson, W. A. (Ed.): Biology of Sea-Snakes, pp. 33—35. Baltimore-London-Tokyo: University Park Press 1975
Mole, R. R.: The Trinidad Snakes. Proc. Zool. Soc. (Lond.) **1924**, 235—278 (1924)
Noble, G. K.: The sense organs involved in the courtship of *Storeria*, *Thamnophis* and other Snakes. Bull. Amer. Mus. Nat. Hist. **73**, 673—725 (1937)
Parker, H. W.: Scientific results of the Cambridge expedition to the East African lakes. J. Linn. Soc. Zool. **38**, 213—229 (1932)
Parker, H. W.: The snakes of Somaliland and the Sokotra Islands. Zool. Verh. Rijksmus. Nat. Hist. (Leiden) **6**, 1—115 (1949)
Peters, J. A.: The snakes of Ecuador: a checklist and key. Bull. Mus. Comp. Zool. **122**, 491—541 (1960)
Peters, J. A., Orejas-Miranda, B.: Catalogue of the neotropical Squamata. I. Snakes. Bull. U.S. Nat. Mus. **297**, i—viii, 1—347 (1970)
Picado, C.: Serpientes Venenosas de Costa Rica. San Jose (Costa Rica): Imprenta Alsina 1931
Pitman, C. R. S.: A Guide to the Snakes of Uganda. Rev. Ed. Codicote: Wheldon and Wesley 1974
Pope, C. H.: The Reptiles of China. In: Natl. Hist. Centr. Asia. New York, 1935, Vol. X
Romer, J. D.: Annotated checklist with keys to the snakes of Hong Kong. Mem. Hong Kong Nat. Hist. Soc. **5**, 1—14 (1961)
Rooij, N. de: The Reptiles of the Indo-Austrian Archipelago. II. Ophidia. Leiden: E. J. Brill 1917
Rossman, D. A., Eberle, W. G.: Partition of the genus *Natrix*, with preliminary observations on evolutionary trends in natricine snakes. Herpetologica **33**, 34—43 (1977)
Roze, J. A.: La Taxonomia y Zoogeographia de los Ofidios de Venezuela. Caracas: Universidad Central de Venezuela 1966
Roze, J. A.: A check list of the New World venomous coral snakes *(Elapidae)* with description of new forms. Am. Mus. Novitates **2287**, 1—60 (1967)
Saint-Girons, H.: Les serpents du Maroc. Var. Sci. Sci. nat. Psyc. (Maroc.) **8**, 1—29 (1956)
Saint-Girons, H.: Les serpents du Cambodge. Mem. Mus. nat. d'Hist. Nat. [A] **74**, 1—170 (1972)
Saint-Girons, H., Duguy, R.: Ecologie et position systématique de *Vipera seoanei* Lataste, 1879. Bull. Soc. Zool. France **101**, 325—339 (1976)
Santos, E.: Anfibios e Repteis do Brasil (Vida e Costumes). 2nd Ed. Rio de Janeiro: F. Briguiet 1955
Schmidt, K. P.: The amphibians and reptiles of British Honduras. Zool. Ser. Field Mus. nat. Hist. **22**, 475—510 (1941)
Smith, H. M., Taylor, E. H.: An annotated checklist and key to the snakes of Mexico. Bull. U.S. Nat. Mus. **187**, 1—239 (1945)
Smith, M. A.: A Monograph of the Sea-Snakes. London: Taylor & Francis 1926
Smith, M. A.: The fauna of British India including Ceylon and Burma. Reptilia and Amphibia. III. Serpentes. London: Taylor & Francis 1943
Stejneger, L.: Herpetology of Japan and adjacent territory. Bull. U.S. Nat. Mus. **58**, 1—577 (1907)
Steward, J. W.: The Snakes of Europe. Newton Abbot: David & Charles 1971
Stuart, L. C.: A checklist of the herpetofauna of Guatemala. Misc. Pub. Mus. Zool. Univ. Michigan **122**, 1—150 (1963)

Swan, L. W., Leviton, A. E.: The herpetology of Nepal: a history, checklist and zoogeographical analysis of the herpetofauna. Proc. Calif. Acad. Sci. **32**, 103—147 (1962)
Sweeney, R. C. H.: Snakes of Nyasaland. Zomba (Nyasaland): Nyasaland Soc. and Nyasaland Govt. 1961
Taylor, E. H.: A brief review of the snakes of Costa Rica. Univ. Kansas Sci. Bull. **34**, 3—88 (1951)
Taylor, E. H.: The serpents of Thailand and adjacent waters. Univ. Kansas Sci. Bull. **45**, 609—1096 (1965)
Terentjev, P. V., Chernov, S. A.: Apredelitelji Presmykajuschcichsja i Semnowodnych. 3rd Ed. Moscow: Government Printing Office 1949
Tweedie, M. W. F.: The Snakes of Malaya. Singapore: Government Printing Office 1954
Underwood, G.: A Contribution to the Classification of Snakes. London: British Museum (Natural History) 1967a
Underwood, G.: A comprehensive approach to the classification of higher snakes. Herpetologica **23**, 161—168 (1967b)
Underwood, G.: The eye. In: Gans, C., Parsons, T. (Eds.): Biology of the Reptilia. London-New York: Academic Press 1970
U.S.A. Department of the Navy: Poisonous Snakes of the World. Washington, D.C.: U.S. Govt. Printing Office 1968
Villiers, A.: Contribution a l'étude du peuplement de la Mauritanie. Ophidiens. Bull. Inst. Fr. d'Afrique Noir **12**, 984—998 (1950)
Visser, J.: Poisonous Snakes of Southern Africa and the Treatment of Snakebite. Capetown: Howard Timmins 1966
Visser, J.: *Atractaspis*, how does it bite? J. Herp. Ass. Africa **14**, 18—22 (1975)
Voris, H. K.: The role of sea-snakes (Hydrophiidae) in the trophic structure of coastal ocean communities. J. Marine Biol. Ass. India **14**, 429—442 (1974)
Werler, J. E., Keegan, H. L.: Venomous snakes of the Pacific area. In: Keegan, H. L., McFarlane, W. V. (Eds.): Venomous and Poisonous Animals and Noxious Plants of the Pacific Region. Oxford: Pergamon Press 1963
Witte, G. F. de, Laurent, R.: Revision d'un groupe de Colubridae Africains. Mem. Mus. Roy. Hist. Nat. Belgique **29**, 1—134 (1947)
Worrell, E.: A new generic name for a nominal species of *Denisonia*. Proc. roy Zool. Soc. N.S.W. 1958—1959, 54—55 (1961a)
Worrell, E.: Herpetological name changes. W. Aust. Nat. **8**, 18—27 (1961b)
Worrell, E.: Dangerous Snakes of Australia and New Guinea, 5th Ed. Sydney: Angus & Robertson 1963a
Worrell, E.: A new elapine generic name. Aust. Reptile Park Rec. No. **1**, 2—7 (1963b)
Worrell, E.: Reptiles of Australia. Sydney: Angus & Robertson 1963b
Wright, A. H., Wright, A. A.: Handbook of Snakes of the United States and Canada. New York: Comstock 1957

CHAPTER 3

The Venom Glands of Snakes and Venom Secretion

A. BDOLAH

A. Introduction

The origin of snake venom has been variously ascribed to different body organs. The idea that the venom virulence depends on the snake's anger led to a famous controversy in the late 17th century. REDI, an Italien biologist, ascribed the dangerous nature of the venom to the yellow liquid issuing from the fangs, while the French chemist, CHARAS, maintained that the virulence lies in the anger of the snake. Needless to say, Redi's ideas eventually prevailed; they were supported by his own experiments and later by the studies of FONTANA (1787), who first described the histology of a viper's venom gland (for references, see KLAUBER, 1956; MINTON and MINTON, 1969).

It has been repeatedly reported in the ancient and newer literature that the blood of snakes is toxic to animals. MINTON (1973) found, indeed, precipitin-cross reactions between antivenins and snake sera. However, the serum components reacting with antivenins were not identic to major venom components, and most of the reactions were attributed to blood contamination in the venom used for immunization.

Although the existence of common antigens in blood and venom cannot be ruled out, it does not necessarily mean that the source of venom antigens is in the blood or vice versa.

Today, we know that the yellow liquid which is produced by the venom glands contains an impressive variety of toxic, enzymic, and other components. The venom is accumulated in the lumina of the glands and is expelled during the bite. Earlier work on the structure and function of the venom glands has been extensively reviewed by GANS and ELLIOTT (1968), KOCHVA and GANS (1970), and KOCHVA (1977).

B. General Morphology and Histology

In the present review, three types of venom glands will be discussed. The glands of *Elapidae* (including cobras and sea snakes), the glands of the genus *Atractaspis* (mole viper), and the glands of *Viperidae* (true vipers and pit vipers).

The general structural pattern of the venom gland is characteristic for each of these groups, although in each of these groups there are species that have long glands that surpass the head region considerably.

I. Venom Glands of Elapidae

BOBEAU (1936) furnished an early description of the elapid venom glands. More recently, a detailed report on the structure of several venom glands of elapid species

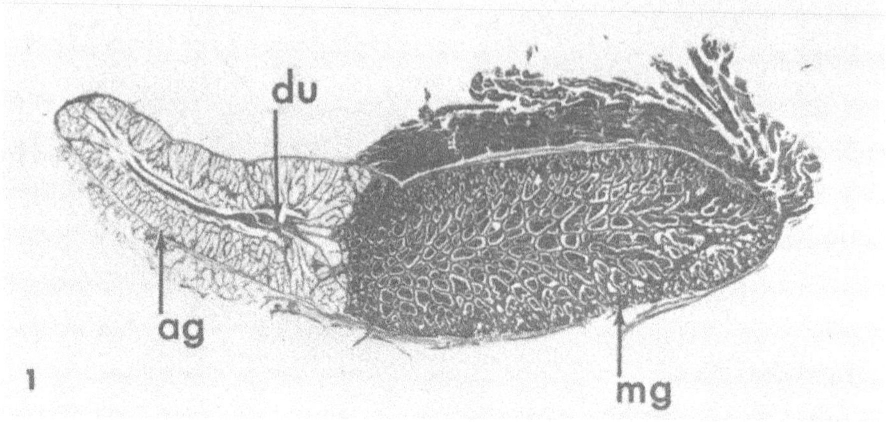

Fig. 1. Venom gland of *Walterinnesia aegyptia*. Sagittal section. *mg* main gland; *ag* accessory gland; *du* duct (courtesy of Prof. E. KOCHVA) (× 12)

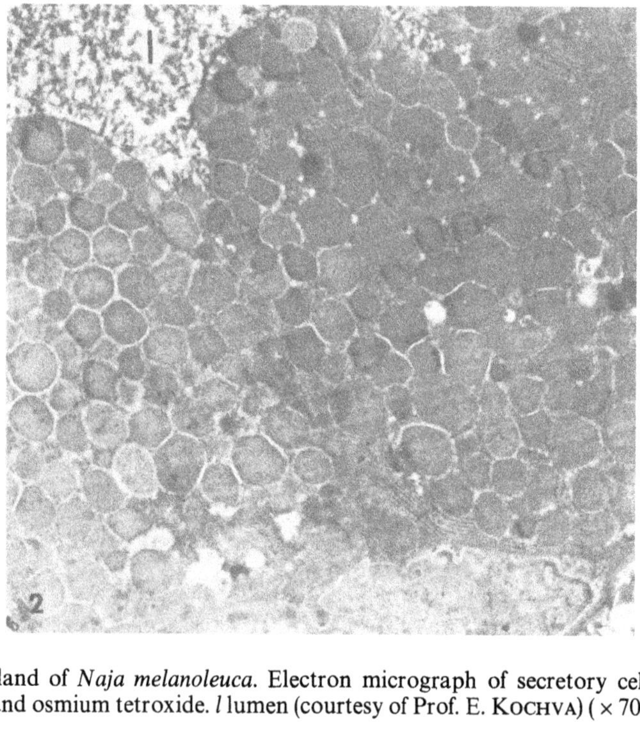

Fig. 2. Venom gland of *Naja melanoleuca*. Electron micrograph of secretory cells. Fixed with glutaraldehyde and osmium tetroxide. *l* lumen (courtesy of Prof. E. KOCHVA) (× 7000)

(including sea snakes) and their emptying mechanism has been published by ROSENBERG (1967). A few other reports were published later (BAWA et al., 1971; MAYS, 1971; BURNS and PICKWELL, 1972).

The venom gland of *Elapidae* is enclosed in a tough capsule of connective tissue, more compactly built than that of viperid snakes. It may be divided into a posterior main gland and an anterior secretory duct with an accessory mucous gland (Fig. 1).

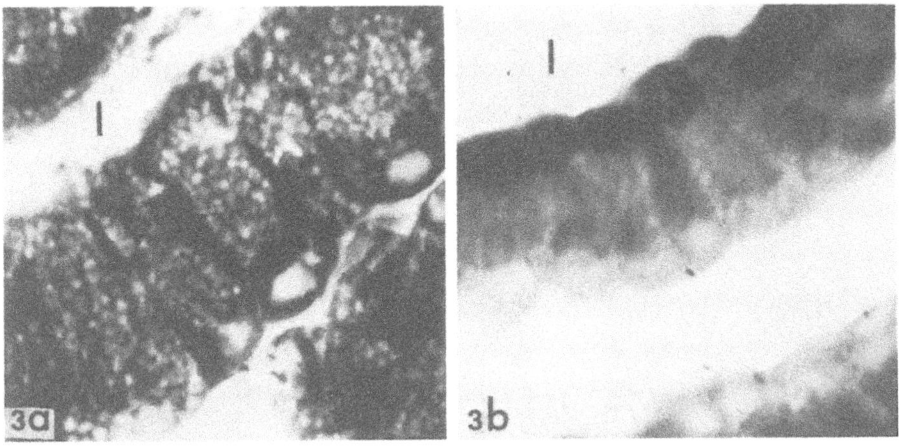

Fig. 3a and b. Venom gland of *Walterinnesia aegyptia*. Stained for (a) L-amino acid oxidase (AVRAMEAS and URIEL, 1965) and (b) for phosphodiesterase (SIERAKOWSKA and SHUGAR, 1963). *l* lumen (courtesy of Prof. E. KOCHVA) (×1500)

The framework of the main gland is organized into many contiguous tubules which may be simple or compound. The tubules usually run in a posteroanterior direction, converge toward the center of the gland, and open into a rather small lumen.

The secretory epithelium is of a serous nature. The height of the cells most probably changes with the stage of secretion. However, no systematic studies on the correlation between the morphology of the cells of elapid venom glands and their secretory stage have yet been published. Secretory cells of *Naja melanoleuca* at the resting stage appear to be loaded with granules that differ in structure and number from those found in viperid venom glands (Fig. 2).

In the venom gland of *Walterinnesia*, enzymes found in the venom (phosphodiesterase and L-amino acid oxidase) can be demonstrated histochemically (Fig. 3). In a gland homogenate of *N. melanoleuca*, up to 40% of the phosphodiesterase is associated with cell particles (BDOLAH, unpublished).

The cells of the accessory glands of *Elapidae* are usually PAS-positive and their secretion contains sialomucins (ROSENBERG, 1967).

II. Venom Glands of Viperidae

The venom glands of the two viperid subfamilies (*Viperinae* and *Crotalinae*) are generally similar in shape and structure. In more than 20 species studied so far, a remarkable uniformity in glandular structure has been shown (KOCHVA and GANS, 1970). Only the mole vipers of the genus *Atractaspis* have different venom glands (KOCHVA et al., 1967).

The most conspicuous feature of the venom glands of the mole vipers is the absence of differentiated accessory glands found in the "genuine" vipers. The structure of both short and long glands of various species consists of large numbers of radial tubules surrounding a central lumen. The tubules are essentially unbranched, and their luminal ends consist of a mucous epithelium (KOCHVA et al., 1967).

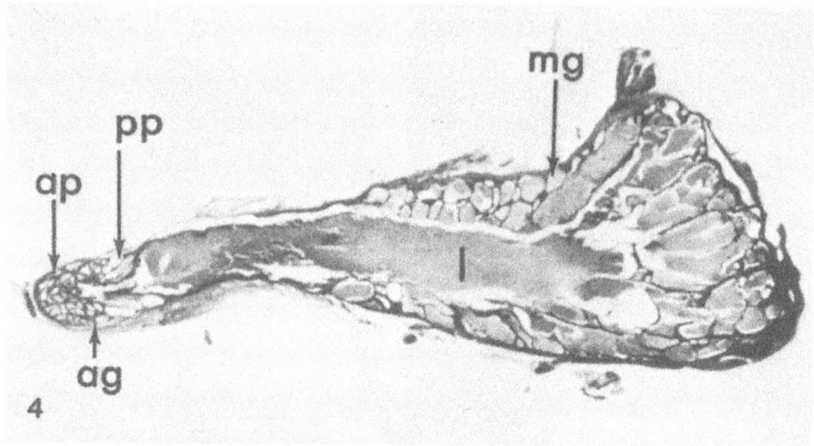

Fig. 4. Venom gland of *Vipera palaestinae*. Sagittal section. Note the two distinct parts of the accessory gland. *ag* accessory gland, *ap* anterior part of ag, *pp* posterior part of ag, *l* lumen, *mg* main gland (courtesy of Prof. E. KOCHVA) (× 20)

Preliminary results also indicate that the pattern of enzymic activities in the venom of *Atractaspis* differs from that of other viperid venom. Thus, the venom of *A. engaddensis* has a relatively high alkaline monophosphatase activity, while arginine ester hydrolase activity, which is very high in venoms of other vipers, cannot be detected in the venom of *Atractaspis* (BDOLAH, unpublished).

The first detailed account of the venom glands of a true viper was published by WOLTER (1924) for *Vipera berus*. This was followed more recently by publications on the histochemistry and electron microscopy of venom glands in *Agkistrodon* (GENNARO et al., 1960, 1963, 1968; ODOR and GENNARO, 1960; ODOR, 1965) and by histologic and histochemical surveys on glands of viperine and crotaline snakes (GANS and KOCHVA, 1965; KOCHVA and GANS, 1965, 1966, 1967).

The venom glands of vipers have four distinct regions: the main gland, which occupies the posterior two-thirds of the gland, the primary duct, the accessory glands, and the secondary duct that leads to the fang sheath (Fig. 4).

The accessory glands show two distinct parts. The anterior part is lined by a typical mucous epithelium that contains goblet cells (GENNARO et al., 1963; KOCHVA and GANS, 1965, 1966; ODOR, 1965). The posterior part is lined with a flat to cuboid epithelium, the shape of which seems to be correlated with the secretory stage.

The function of the accessory glands remains to be clarified. According to GENNARO et al. (1963), an extract of this gland slightly enhanced the toxicity of the main gland homogenate (see also GANS and ELLIOT, 1968). However, mixing experiments failed to show any inhibition or activation of enzymes in the venom of *V. palaestinae* by homogenate of washed accessory glands (SHKOLNIK, GEFEN, and BDOLAH, unpublished).

The main part of the viperid venom gland is made of repeatedly branched tubules arranged around a large central lumen, in which considerable amounts of venom may be stored (see below). The tubules consist mainly of the typical secretory cells.

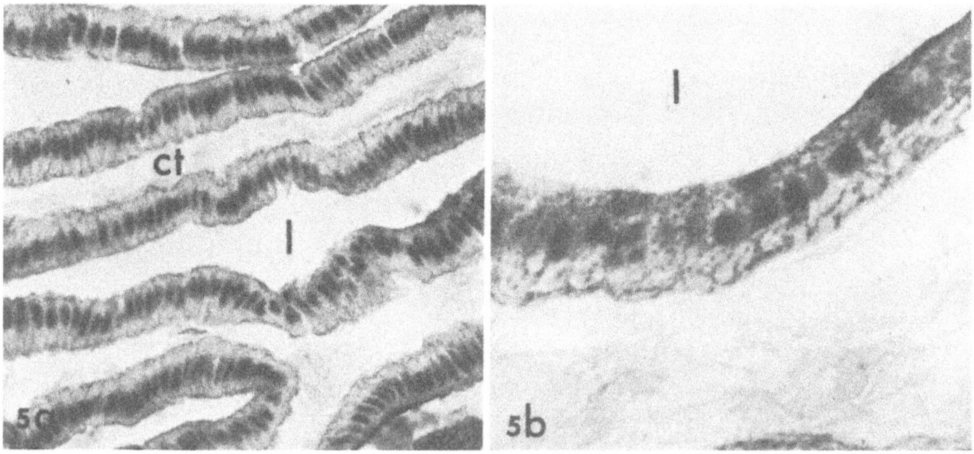

Fig. 5a and b. Venom gland of *Vipera palaestinae*. 2 days after milking. Stained for (a) L-amino acid oxidase (× 300) and for (b) phosphodiesterase (× 700). *ct* connective tissue, *l* lumen

Several other cell types have been described (WOLTER, 1924; ODOR and GENNARO, 1960; ODOR, 1965; BEN-SHAUL et al., 1971; WARSHAWSKY et al., 1972, 1973).

In the venom gland of *V. palaestinae*, a uniform coloration of the secretory epithelium is found when histochemical techniques for certain enzymes of the venom are used (Fig. 5). Similar histochemical evidence, which shows that secretory proteins originate from the secretory cell proper, has been found in venom glands of other species (SOBOL-BROWN, 1974). Venom enzymes and other venom proteins have also been traced in the secretory epithelium by immunohistochemical techniques (SHAHAM and KOCHVA, 1969; SHAHAM et al., 1974) (Fig. 6).

C. The Fine Structure of the Secretory Cell During the Venom Regeneration Cycle

Morphologic changes in the secretory epithelium of the venom gland after expulsion of venom were already noticed by VELIKII (1890) in *Vipera ammodytes*. More recently, the correlation between the size of the cells and the secretory stage of the gland has been studied in several venom glands of vipers (BEN SHAUL et al., 1971; ROTENBERG et al., 1971; SCHAEFFER et al., 1972a, b; ORON and BDOLAH, 1973; DE LUCCA et al., 1974). Synchronization of the secretory cells by the complete removal of venom from the gland lumina (by manual milking; KLAUBER, 1956) is essential for studying the venom regeneration cycle. In snakes that remain unmilked for a long period of time (1–3 months) the glands are filled with venom, and the cells are cuboid to flat. The apex of the cells is usually not much higher than the level of the nucleus, the rough endoplasmic reticulum (RER) is made of closely packed membranes and several electron-opaque vesicles are seen (Fig. 7).

After milking, the secretory cells increase in size and assume a columnar shape (Fig. 8). In *Vipera palaestinae* (ROTENBERG et al., 1971) and in *Crotalus durissus terrifi-*

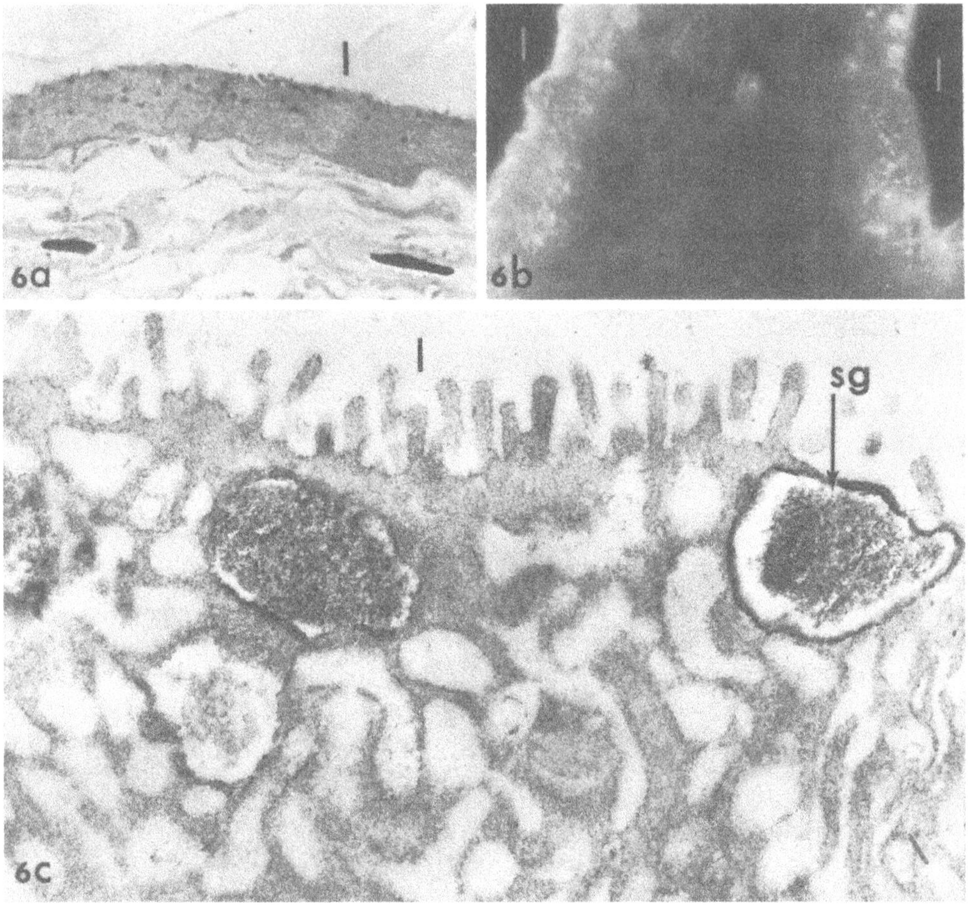

Fig. 6a–c. Localization of venom antigens in the venom gland of *Vipera palaestinae* (2 days after milking) with labeled antibodies. (a) and (b) light microscopy. (a) Peroxidase labeled gamma-globulins, antiserum against arginine ester hydrolase, epon sections (1 μm) (×630). (b) Fluorescein labeled gamma-globulins, antiserum against L-amino acid oxidase, cryostat sections (6 μm) (×700) *l* lumen. (c) Electron micrograph. Venom gland treated with peroxidase labeled gamma-globulins, antiserum against phosphodiesterase, *sg* secretory granules (×18000)

cus (DE LUCCA et al., 1974), the cells reach a maximum height in about 4 days post milking. In *V. palaestinae*, the greatest amount of ribonucleic acid (RNA) per gland is found at this stage (ROTENBERG et al., 1971); indeed, most of the cell volume is occupied by the RER with its distended intracisternal space. WARSHAWSKY et al. (1972, 1973) reported the existence of dense intracisternal granules, which had no limiting membrane, in the venom gland of *Crotalus*. Such granules have not been observed in *V. palaestinae* or *V. ammodytes*.

A well-developed Golgi apparatus becomes most conspicuous at the active stage of secretion, but relatively few large vesicles are found in the secretory cell. This is in contradistinction to the well-known mammalian digestive glands which are loaded

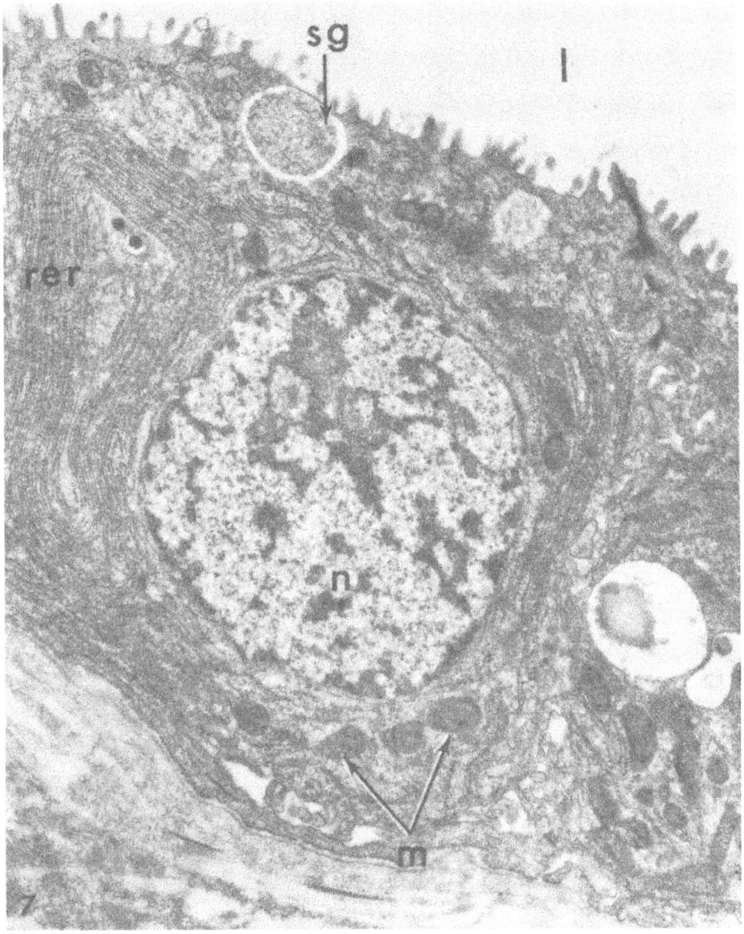

Figs. 7–9. Venom gland of *Vipera palaestinae*. Electron micrographs. Fixed with glutaraldehyde and osmium tetroxide. *n* nucleus, *m* mitochondria, *rer* rough endoplasmic reticulum, *ci* intracisternal space of rer, *g* Golgi complex, *gs* Golgi saccules, *gv* Golgi vesicles, *ly* lysosomes, *cv* condensing vacuole, *sg* secretory granules, *l* lumen, *BC* blood cells

Fig. 7. Secretory cells of a gland unmilked for 2 months. Note the packed pattern of the endoplasmic reticulum. (×9500)

with secretory vesicles when not stimulated to secrete (AMSTERDAM et al., 1969; MELDOLESI, 1976). Some large vesicles in the venom gland cell, usually of low electron density, are closely associated with the Golgi saccules (Fig. 9) and are highly reminiscent of the condensing vacuoles of the pancreas (PALADE, 1975). Vesicles of variable density are also found close to the apical membrane.

Secretory cells in glands at longer intervals after milking decrease in height; the RER is again more closely packed and they gradually assume the organization of the quiescent stage (BEN-SHAUL et al., 1971; ORON and BDOLAH, 1973).

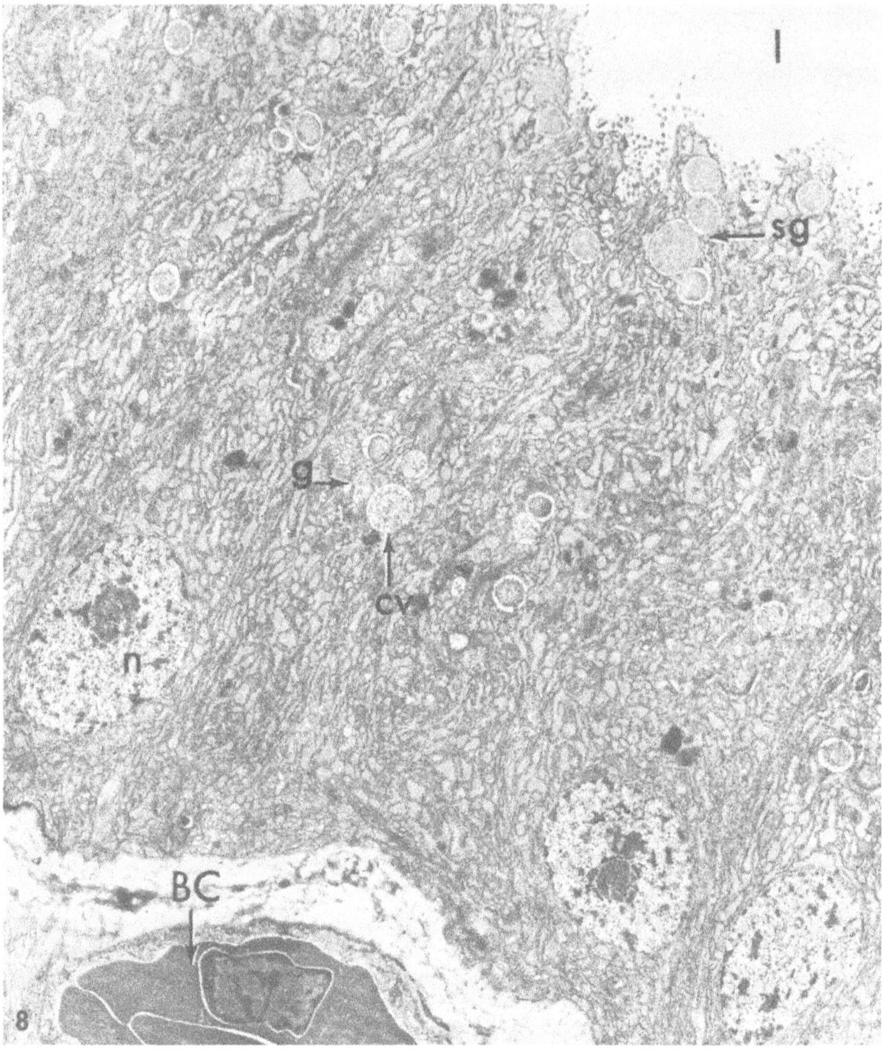

Fig. 8. Secretory cells with a typical columnar shape. 5 days after milking (× 3300)

The fact that the total population of vesicles in the viperid venom gland cell accounts for only 4% of the cell volume, while most of its volume is occupied by the RER (including the cisternae) (ORON and BDOLAH, 1976), raised the question of whether secretory products are stored intracellularly within the vesicles. Recent immunocytochemical studies (SHAHAM et al., 1974) clearly showed that the vesicles found in the venom gland are, indeed, genuine membrane-bound secretory granules (Fig. 6c). Several venom antigens have been traced to the same granules. It is, therefore, suggested that the different venom components are packed in the same granules and also use the same intracellular pathways.

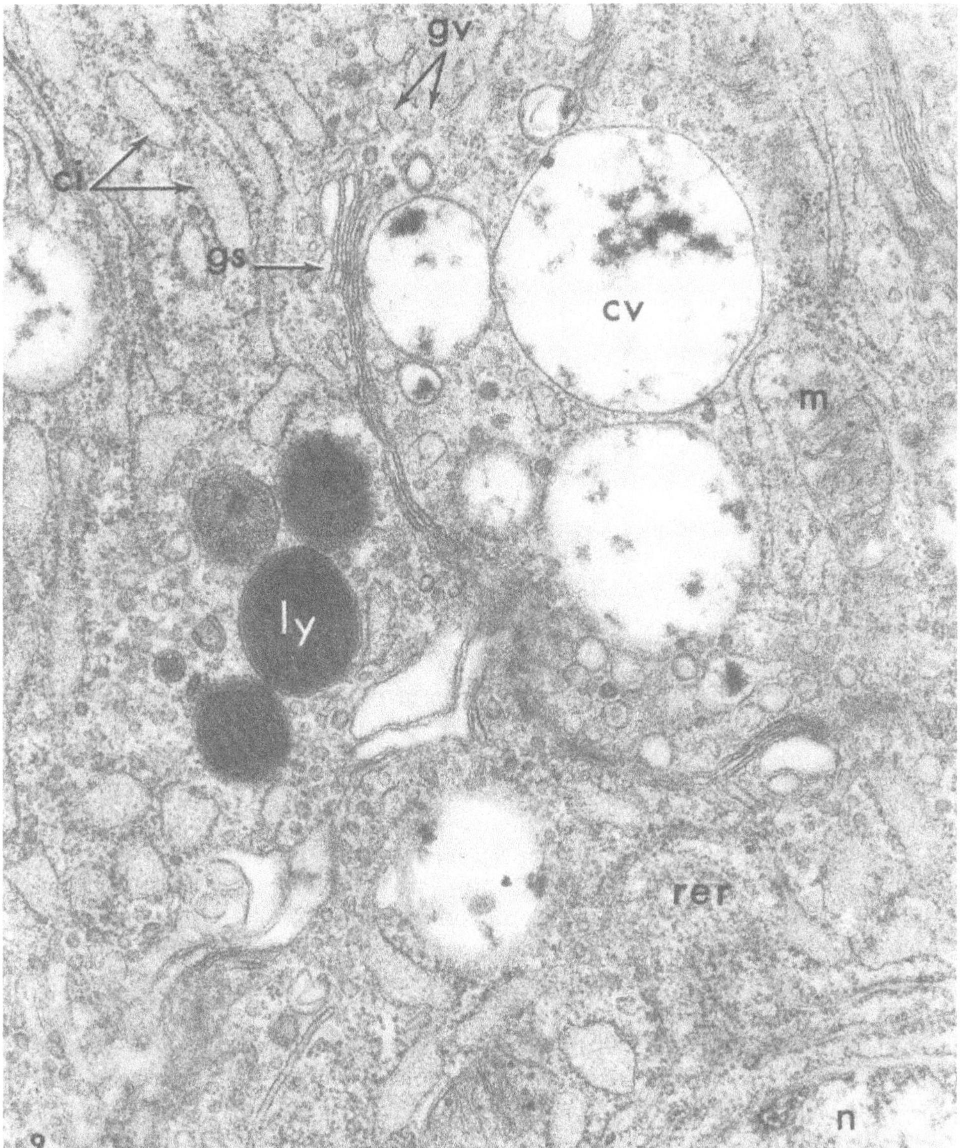

Fig. 9. Golgi zone in a secretory cell 5 days after milking. (× 28000)

D. Intracellular Transport of Venom Proteins

The sequence of events in protein synthesis and secretion in the venom gland of *C. durissus terrificus* was studied by WARSHAWSKY et al. (1973). It was concluded that the intracellular transport of venom proteins is similar to that described in mammalian glands (PALADE, 1975) except that it occurs more slowly. More than 8 h (at

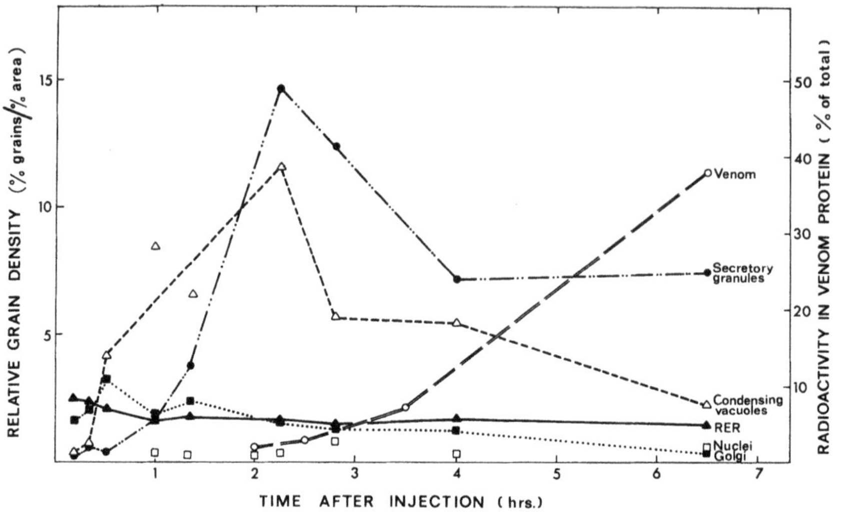

Fig. 10. Kinetics of intracellular transport of labeled proteins in the venom gland of *Vipera palaestinae*. Relative grain density of silver grains at various time intervals after injection of (^{3}H)-L-leucine into the blood system of the snake. Radioactivity in venom was estimated by scintillation counting

about 24° C) are required for the label to appear in the venom after an intraperitoneal injection of the precursor.

Recent autoradiographic study with the venom gland of *V. palaestinae* has shown that the slow intracellular transport found in *Crotalus* is not necessarily typical for other viperid snakes. The kinetics of the intracellular transport were studied in *V. palaestinae* with the venom gland at the active stage (4 days post milking at 30° C) (ORON and BDOLAH, 1976). As expected, the label first appears in the RER (Fig. 10) and then in the Golgi complex with a concomitant increase of grain density over the so-called condensing vacuoles. At 2–3 h after administration of the labeled precursor, the highest grain density is found in the secretory granules. Later, a decline in the labeling of these granules is evident, and at the same time (about 3 h after the injection) radioactive proteins appear in the venom. It is thus concluded that in the secretory cell of the viper's venom gland, exportable proteins are transported from the RER via the Golgi complex into the condensing vacuoles. These vacuoles are probably transformed into the more dense secretory granules which are the immediate source of the secreted venom. The relatively small number of granules found in these cells is a result of a continuous secretion from this pool into the lumen.

According to WARSHAWSKY et al. (1973), in the venom gland of *Crotalus* the intracisternal granules become more frequently labeled when a substantial fraction of the labeled venom has already been secreted. This should involve an additional pathway that would lead to the accumulation of proteins in the cisternae. However, it seems unlikely that such a pathway exists in the venom gland of *V. palaestinae*. Analysis of autoradiograms of this gland shows that not more than 10% of the grains over the RER could be attributed to cisternal contents at any of the time intervals studied.

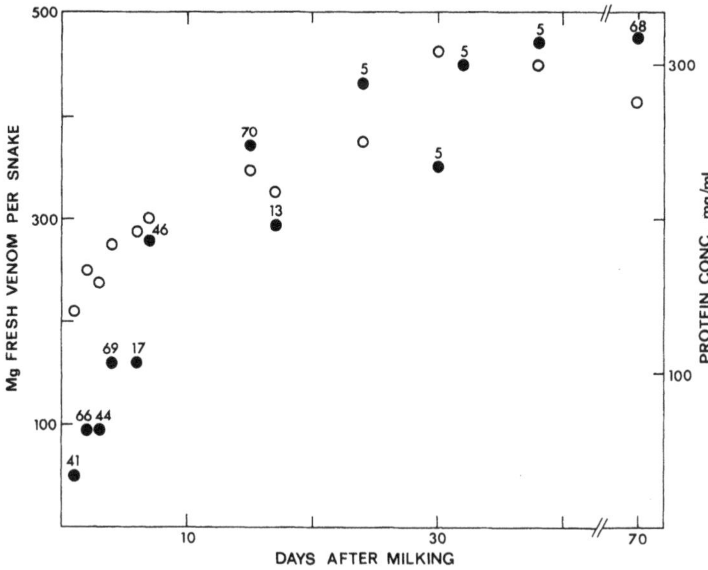

Fig. 11. Accumulation of venom (●) and protein concentration of venom (○) in *Vipera palaestinae*. Composite graph based on the work done in the author's laboratory during the last 17 years. Each dot shows the average of number of samples, as indicated

E. Venom Synthesis and Secretion

I. The Venom Regeneration Cycle

In the venom glands of vipers, most of the venom is stored extracellularly, a considerable amount of venom being accumulated in the extended gland lumina (SOBOL-BROWN et al., 1975). The removal of the venom from the gland lumina causes a renewal of venom production. The kinetics of venom accumulation have been followed in several viperid snakes (KOCHVA, 1960; ROTENBERG et al., 1971; ORON and BDOLAH, 1973; DE LUCCA et al., 1974).

In *V. palaestinae*, the rate of venom accumulation is rapid during the 1st week after milking. It slows down later, and from about 1 month onward the accumulation of venom practically stops (Fig. 11). The concentration of the venom increases with the time after milking and achieves a maximum of close to 300 mg protein per ml.

From this data it could be assumed that there is a cycle of activity in the venom gland whereby the synthetic apparatus of the secretory cell is first activated and later suppressed. Indeed, the incorporation of ^{32}P into RNA in the venom gland of *V. palaestinae* corroborates this assumption; a cyclic pattern of RNA synthesis was observed with the highest incorporation rate in 1–4 days after milking (ROTENBERG et al., 1971). A similar pattern was evident in protein synthesis in the glands of *V. palastinae*, *V. ammodytes* (ORON and BDOLAH, 1973), and *C. durissus terrificus* (DE LUCCA et al., 1974). In *V. ammodytes*, the highest rate of protein synthesis is evident at about 1 week after milking (Fig. 12). At this stage, most of the labeled proteins are precipitable by venom antiserum and can therefore be considered venom proteins. During the 1st day after milking, only 25% of the incorporated label is found in

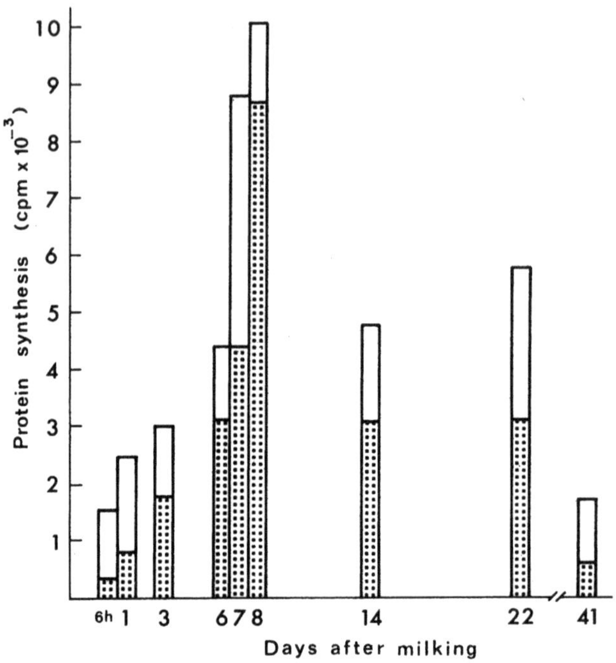

Fig. 12. Incorporation of (^{14}C)-amino acids into total and venom proteins as a function of time after milking in the venom gland of *Vipera ammodytes*. Snakes were not milked or fed for 2 months. One gland of each snake was milked while the contralateral one remained unmilked. The values of total protein synthesis (columns) or venom synthesis (shaded area) were normalized according to the deviation of the control unmilked gland

venom proteins; most of the proteins synthesized at this stage are probably structural proteins, which are needed for the building of the synthetic apparatus.

The control mechanisms operating in synthesis and secretion in the venom glands are not well-understood. Sectioning of the main nerve supply to the venom gland does not affect venom production, protein concentration, or enzyme activities of the venom (ALLON, 1973). It may thus be assumed that the control of venom production and secretion occurs in the glands themselves. It is evident that the amount of venom present in the lumina of the gland regulates the synthetic activity of the secretory epithelium and also its morphologic structure (see above). It might be speculated that the release of pressure after milking activates the synthetic apparatus in the secretory cells (see also WOLTER, 1924), although the influence of chemical stimuli cannot be ruled out at present. Applying external hydrostatic pressure to the venom gland by implanting inflated balloons underneath the skin showed, indeed, reduction of venom synthesis and secretion (ALLON, 1973).

Under natural conditions vipers usually have glands filled with venom, and during the bite only about 10% of the available venom is injected (KOCHVA, 1960; ALLON and KOCHVA, 1974). The venom spent in the bite seems to be derived from only a few tubules. Preliminary autoradiographic studies with glands after a bite indicate that only the epithelial cells of the tubules from which venom had been

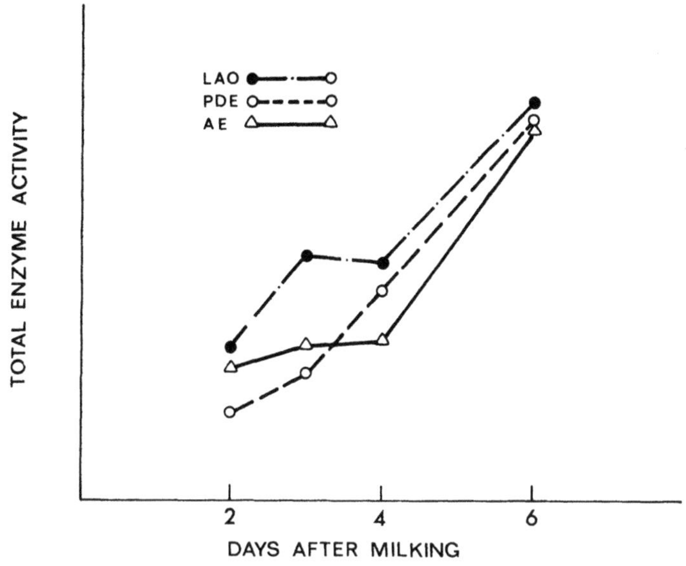

Fig. 13. Accumulation patterns of L-amino acid oxidase (LAO), phosphodiesterase (PDE), and arginine ester hydrolase (AE) in the venom of *Vipera palaestinae*

withdrawn are activated (KOCHVA et al., 1975). This provides the snake with a rather simple method for control of venom replenishment, which operates at the level of the tubule.

II. Synthesis and Secretion of Different Venom Components

Enzymes found in the venom have been used as markers in the study of the secretory process. In *Bothrops jararaca* repeated milking at 3–4-day intervals caused a decrease in venom yield and an unparalleled regeneration of several enzymes in the venom (SCHENBERG et al., 1970). SOBOL-BROWN et al. (1975) have shown in *V. palaestinae* that following milking, protein concentration and enzyme activities increase in the venom and reach a plateau at the longer intervals. The detailed kinetics of accumulation of total protein, L-amino acid oxidase (LAO), phosphodiesterase (PDE), and arginine ester hydrolase (AE) during the first 2 weeks after milking show a linear trend. However, fluctuations from linearity are evident during the shorter intervals; thus, a significant increase in secretion of LAO is evident during the 3rd day after milking, while the fluctuations of PDE shows an opposite direction (Fig. 13). No significant changes are found in the total activities of these enzymes in gland homogenates from snakes 2–15 days after milking. These results, and the fact that only a very small amount of venom is stored in this gland intracellularly, lead to the conclusion that the nonparallel accumulation of the enzymes results from nonparallel changes in their rate of synthesis during the pertinent intervals (SOBOL-BROWN et al., 1975). Direct evidence for asynchronous synthesis of venom components has been obtained recently, when the incorporation of a labeled amino acid into venom proteins was measured in glands at the 2nd day, versus glands at the 4th day, post milking (ORON and BDOLAH, in preparation).

III. Total Venom Yield and the Amount of Venom Expelled During the Bite

The highest records of venom yield (1.5 g dry weight) have been reported for some very large viperid species (BÜCHERL, 1963; MINTON and MINTON, 1969; KAISER and MICHL, 1971). There is some difficulty in comparing the average venom yield of different species. The technique used for milking the snake, manual or electric (see GANS and ELLIOTT, 1968), might influence the yield of venom, and data do not always include concentration of the venom or its dry weight. General information on venom yield, lethality, and the size of the snake has recently been collected by MINTON and MINTON (1969). Positive correlation between the size of the snake (probably reflects the age of the snake) and its venom yield was found by KLAUBER (1956) in *Crotalus*. Similar results have recently been obtained for *V. palaestinae* (LIFSHITZ, 1977).

KLAUBER (1956) found a decline in venom production by rattlesnakes in captivity and attributed it to the adverse conditions. However, in the Serpentarium of Tel-Aviv University, specimens of *V. palaestinae* have been kept in individual cages for many years; some of them have gone through 30 monthly milkings without a decrease in venom yield (KOCHVA, 1960).

The determination of the quantity of venom injected is most important for the evaluation of the danger of a snakebite. Snakes do not inject all the venom found in their glands in a single bite. According to ACTON and KNOWLES (1914), cobras use about 60% of their venom. FAIRLEY and SPLATT (1929) reported that in Australian poisonous snakes up to 80% of the venom might be spent in a bite. It is generally believed that in elapid snakes, which tend to bite and hold on, a larger amount of venom is injected (MINTON and MINTON, 1969). KLAUBER(1956) reports that rattlesnakes use considerably less than half of their venom in a single bite. The quantities of venom injected into prey by *V. palaestinae* have been measured by weighing mice before and after a bite (KOCHVA, 1960) or by estimating radioactivity in mice and rats after a bite by ^{14}C-labeled snakes (ALLON and KOCHVA, 1974). The amounts of venom injected were variable, and in most cases about 10% of the available venom was spent. Similar results were obtained for two species of *Trimeresurus* (KONDO et al., 1972).

GENNARO et al. (1961) stated that in *Agkistrodon piscivorus* the amount of venom injected into a rat is higher than that injected into a mouse. According to ALLON and KOCHVA (1974), the amounts of venom injected into prey of different size (mice or rats) by *V. palaestinae* are extremely variable; it is, therefore, concluded that the size of the prey does not necessarily influence the amount of venom injected by the snake.

F. Concluding Remarks

The occurrence of oral glands in snakes is probably connected with their adaptation to the swallowing of a large prey (GANS, 1961). The highly differentiated venom glands, which give the snake the ability to immobilize its prey, have been developed in several groups of snakes. The patterns of gland growth during later embryonic development in *Viperidae* and *Elapidae* (KOCHVA and GANS, 1970) and the general architecture of the venom apparatus in adult snakes point to major differences between these two groups.

The fine structure of the secretory cells and the venom regeneration cycle have been extensively studied only in viperid venom glands. It becomes apparent that activation of the secretory epithelium in these glands induces an accelerated rate of protein synthesis, which is followed by secretion of venom into the gland lumen. Very little secretion is stored intracellularly and it seems that the secretion rate is correlated to the rate of venom production.

From the few ultrastructural studies of elapid venom glands, it appears that the secretory cells of these glands are loaded with granules, at least at the resting stage. It would be interesting to compare the regulation of secretion in secretory cells of elapid venom glands with that known for other exocrine glands which have a substantial intracellular storage.

Acknowledgements. I wish to express my thanks to Prof. E. Kochva and Mr. U. Oron for valuable discussions, to Mrs. M. Wollberg and Miss L. Maman for help in preparing the photographs, to Mrs. R. Suzin for preparing the line drawings and to Mrs. R. Manneberg for preparing the manuscript.

References

Acton, H. W., Knowles, R.: The dose of venom given in nature by the *Echis carinatus* at a single bite. Indian J. med. Res. **1**, 414—424 (1914)

Allon, N.: Studies on venom synthesis and injection by *Vipera palaestinae*. M.Sc. Thesis, Tel-Aviv University, Israel (in Hebrew with English summary), 1973

Allon, N., Kochva, E.: The quantities of venom injected into prey of different size by *Vipera palaestinae* in a single bite. J. exp. Zool. **188**, 71—75 (1974)

Amsterdam, A., Ohad, I., Schramm, M.: Dynamic changes in the ultrastructure of acinar cell of the rat parotid gland during the secretory cycle. J. Cell Biol. **41**, 753—773 (1969)

Avrameas, S., Uriel, J.: Méthode de coloration des acides aminés à l'aide de la L-aminoacide-oxhydrase. C.R. Acad. Sc. (Paris) **261**, 584—586 (1965)

Bawa, S. R., Walia, R. P. S., Goyal, S., Kanwar, K. C.: Fine structure of the venom gland of Indian Krait (abstract). J. ultrastruct. Res. **37**, 257 (1971)

Ben-Shaul, Y., Lifshitz, S., Kochva, E.: Ultrastructural aspects of secretion in the venom glands of *Vipera palaestinae*. In: Toxins of Animal and Plant Origin, Vol. I, pp. 87—105. London: Gordon and Breach 1971

Bobeau, G.: Histo-physiologie normale et pathologique de la glande à venin du Cobra. Bull. Soc. Roy. Sci. Méd. Nat. (Bruxelles) **36**, 53—58 (1936)

Bücherl, W.: Über die Ermittlung von Durchschnitts- und Höchst-Giftmengen bei den häufigsten Giftschlangen Südamerikas. In: Die Giftschlangen der Erde, pp. 67—120. Marburg: Behringwerk-Mitteilungen 1963

Burns, B., Pickwell, G. V.: Cephalic glands in sea snakes (*Pelamis*, *Hydrophis*, and *Laticauda*). Copeia **1972 (3)**, 547—559 (1972)

Fairely, N. H., Splatt, B.: Venom yields in Australian poisonous snakes. Med. J. Aust. **1**, 336—348 (1929)

Fontana, F.: Treatise on the venom of the viper, Vol. 1. London 1787

Gans, C.: The feeding mechanism of snakes and its possible evolution. Amer. Zool. **1**, 217—227 (1961)

Gans, C., Elliott, W. B.: Snake venoms: production, injection, action. Advanc. Oral Biol. **3**, 45—81 (1968)

Gans, C., Kochva, E.: The accessory gland in the venom apparatus of viperid snakes. Toxicon **3**, 61—63 (1965)

Gennaro, J. F., Jr., Anton, A. H., Sayre, D. F.: The fine structure of pit viper venom and additional observations on the role of aromatic amines in the physiology of the pit viper. Comp. Biochem. Physiol. **25**, 285—293 (1968)

Gennaro, J. F., Jr., Callahan, W. P. III, Lorincz, A. F.: The anatomy and biochemistry of a mucus-secreting cell type present in the poison apparatus of the pit viper *Ancistrodon piscivorus piscivorus*. Ann. N.Y. Acad. Sci. **106**, 463—471 (1963)
Gennaro, J. F., Jr., Leopold, R. S., Merriam, T. W.: Observations on the actual quantity of venom introduced by several species of crotalid snakes in their bite. Anat. Rec. **139**, 303 (1961)
Gennaro, J. F., Jr., Squicciarini, P. J., Heisler, M., Hall, H. P.: The microscopic anatomy and histochemistry of the poison apparatus of the cottonmouth moccasin, *Ancistrodon p. piscivorus*. Anat. Rec. **136**, 196 (1960)
Kaiser, E., Michl, H.: Chemistry and pharmacology of the venoms of *Bothrops* and *Lachesis*. In: Venomous Animals and Their Venoms, Vol. II, pp. 307—318. New York-London: Academic Press 1971
Klauber, L. M.: Rattlesnakes. Berkeley-Los Angeles: Univ. of California Pr. 1956
Kochva, E.: A quantitative study of venom secretion by *Vipera palaestinae*. Amer. J. trop. Med. Hyg. **9**, 381—390 (1960)
Kochva, E.: Oral glands of the reptilia. In: Biology of the Reptilia, Vol. VIII. London-New York: Academic Press 1977 (in press)
Kochva, E., Gans, C.: The venom gland of *Vipera palaestinae* with comments on the glands of some other viperines. Acta Anat. (Basel) **62**, 365—401 (1965)
Kochva, E., Gans, C.: Histology and histochemistry of venom glands of some crotaline snakes. Copeia **1966**, 506—515 (1966)
Kochva, E., Gans, C.: The structure of the venom gland and secretion of venom in viperid snakes. In: Animal Toxins, pp. 195—203. Oxford-New York: Pergamon Press 1967
Kochva, E., Gans, C.: Salivary glands of snakes. Clin. Toxicol. **3**, 363—387 (1970)
Kochva, E., Oron, U., Bdolah, A., Allon, N.: Regulation of venom secretion and injection in viperid snakes (Abst.). Toxicon **13**, 104 (1975)
Kochva, E., Shayer-Wollberg, M., Sobol, R.: The special pattern of the venom gland in *Atractaspis* and its bearing on the taxonomic status of the genus. Copeia **1967**, 763—772 (1967)
Kondo, H., Kondo, S., Sadahiro, S., Yamauchi, K., Ohsaka, A., Murata, R., Hokama, Z., Yamakawa, M.: Estimation by a new method of the amount of venom ejected by a single bite of *Trimeresurus* species. Jap. J. med. Sci. Biol. **25**, 123—131 (1972)
Lifshitz, S.: Fine structure of the venom gland and venom secretion by *Vipera palaestinae*: possible seasonal variations. M.Sc. Thesis, Tel-Aviv University, Israel (in Hebrew, with English summary), 1977
Lucca, F. L. de, Haddad, A., Kochva, E., Rothschild, A. M., Valeri, V.: Protein synthesis and morphological changes in the secretory epithelium of the venom gland of *Crotalus durissus terrificus* at different times after manual extraction of venom. Toxicon **12**, 361—368 (1974)
Mays, C. E.: Comparative morphology and histochemistry of the venom apparatus of some proteroglyphous snakes, *Laticauda* and *Dendroaspis*. Wasmann J. Biol. **29**, 81—96 (1971)
Meldolesi, J.: Regulation of pancreatic exocrine secretion. Pharmacol. Res. Commun. **8**, 1—24 (1976)
Minton, S. A., Jr.: Common antigens in snake sera and venoms. In: Toxins of Animal and Plant Origin, Vol. III, pp. 905—917. London: Gordon and Breach 1973
Minton, S. A., Jr., Minton, M. R.: Venomous Reptiles. New York: Charles Scribner's Sons 1969
Odor, D. L.: The poison gland of the cottonmouth moccasin, *Ancistrodon p. piscivorus*, as observed with the electron microscope. J. Morph. **117**, 115—134 (1965)
Odor, D. L., Gennaro, J. F.: The poison gland of the cottonmouth moccasin, *Ancistrodon p. piscivorus*, as observed with the electron microscope. Anat. Rec. **136**, 343 (1960)
Oron, U., Bdolah, A.: Regulation of protein synthesis in the venom gland of viperid snakes. J. biol. Chem. **56**, 177—190 (1973)
Oron, U., Bdolah, A.: Intracellular transport of secretory proteins in the venom gland of the snake *Vipera palaestinae*. A radioautographic study. In: Electron Microscopy 1976, Vol. II. Jerusalem: Tal International 1976
Palade, G.: Intracellular aspects of the process of protein synthesis. Science **189**, 347—358 (1975)
Rosenberg, H. I.: Histology, histochemistry, and emptying mechanism of the venom glands of some elapid snakes. J. Morph. **123**, 133—156 (1967)
Rotenberg, D., Bamberger, E. S., Kochva, E.: Studies on ribonucleic acid synthesis in the venom glands of *Vipera palaestinae* (Ophidia, Reptilia). Biochem. J. **121**, 609—612 (1971)

Schaeffer, R. C., Jr., Bernick, S., Rosenquist, T. H., Russell, F. E.: The histochemistry of the venom glands of the rattlesnake *Crotalus viridis helleri*—I. Lipid and non-specific esterase. Toxicon **10**, 183—186 (1972a)
Schaeffer, R. C., Jr., Bernick, S., Rosenquist, T. H., Russell, F. E.: The histochemistry of the venom glands of the rattlesnake *Crotalus viridis helleri*—II. Monoamine oxidase, acid, and alkaline phosphatase. Toxicon **10**, 295—297 (1972b)
Schenberg, S., Pereira Lima, F. A., Nogueira-Schiripa, L. N., Nagamori, A.: Unparallel regeneration of snake venom components in successive milkings. Toxicon **8**, 152 (1970)
Shaham, N., Kochva, E.: Localization of venom antigens in the venom gland of *Vipera palaestinae*, using a fluorescent-antibody technique. Toxicon **6**, 263—268 (1969)
Shaham, N., Levy, Z., Kochva, E., Bdolah, A.: Localization of venom antigens in the venom gland of *Vipera palaestinae*. Histochem. J. **6**, 98 (1974)
Sierakowska, H., Shugar, D.: Cytochemical localization of phosphodiesterase by the azo dye simultaneous coupling method. Biochem. Biophys. Res. Commun. **11**, 70—74 (1963)
Sobol-Brown, R.: Localization of some enzymes in the main venom glands of viperid snakes. J. Morph. **143**, 247—258 (1974)
Sobol-Brown, R., Brown, M. B., Bdolah, A., Kochva, E.: Accumulation of some secretory enzymes in venom glands of *Vipera palaestinae*. Amer. J. Physiol. **229**, 1675—1679 (1975)
Velikii, V. N.: O nervnykh okonchaniyakh v zhelezakh yadovitykh zmei. Trudy S-Peterburgskogo Obshcheva estestvoispytatelei. Otdelenie zoologii i Fiziologii **21**, 16—17 (1890)
Warshawsky, H., Haddad, A., Goncalves, R. P., Valeri, V., Lucca, F. L. de: Protein synthesis and secretion by the venom gland of the rattle-snake *Crotalus durissus terrificus* as revealed by electron microscopic radioautography after ^{3}H-tyrosine injection. Anat. Rec. **172**, 422 (1972)
Warshawsky, H., Haddad, A., Goncalves, R. P., Valeri, V., Lucca, F. L. de: Fine structure of the venom gland epithelium of the South American rattlesnake and radioautographic studies of protein formation by the secretory cells. Amer. J. Anat. **138**, 79—120 (1973)
Wolter, M.: Die Giftdrüse von *Vipera berus* L. Jena Z. med. Naturw. **60**, 305—357 (1924)

Part II

Chemistry and Biochemistry of Snake Venoms

CHAPTER 4

Enzymes in Snake Venom

S. IWANAGA and T. SUZUKI

A. Introduction

A number of animal venoms including those of snakes, gila monsters, scorpions, spiders, and bees contain various enzymes in addition to toxic elements. These enzyme activities can not be ignored when considering the pathophysiologic action of the venom as a whole (MELDRUM, 1965). It is generally agreed that the enzymes in snake venoms act in the following ways: (a) effect local capillary damage and tissue necrosis by proteinases, phospholipases, arginine ester hydrolases, and hyaluronidase (SLOTTA, 1955; KAISER, 1958; SUZUKI and IWANAGA, 1970); (b) cause diverse coagulant and anticoagulant actions by various proteinases and phospholipase A (MEAUME, 1966); and (c) induce acute hypotension and pain due to release of vasoactive peptides by kinin-releasing enzyme (kininogenase) (SUZUKI and IWANAGA, 1970). The other enzymes proposed as toxic elements in snake venoms (BELLER, 1948) are 5′-nucleotidase, phosphodiesterase and related enzymes, cholinesterase, and L-amino acid oxidase. However, numerous studies, in which the venoms of many species have been fractionated by chromatography and electrophoresis and the enzyme activities of the separate fractions assessed, have demonstrated that none of these enzymes are responsible for the acute toxicity of snake venoms (MINTON, 1971).

It is well known that snake venoms, one of the most concentrated enzyme sources in nature are valuable expedients in biochemical research. L-amino acid oxidase, for example, has been widely used for identifying optical isomers of amino acids and for preparing α-keto acid (MEISTER, 1965); phosphodiesterase, for structural studies of nucleic acids and dinucleotide coenzymes (LASKOWSKI, 1966); proteinase, for the amino acid sequence studies of peptides and proteins (MELLA et al., 1967; VAN DER WALT and JOUBERT, 1972); and phospholipase A_2, for lipid research (VAN DEENEN and DE HAAS, 1966). Furthermore, some of the snake venom enzymes, e.g., thrombinlike enzymes (reptilase, ancrode, and batroxobin) and procoagulant (stypven), have certain applications in the clinical field. These biochemical and therapeutic uses of snake venom enzymes have led to intensive attempts to study the occurrence, purification, and characterization of the enzymes.

B. Distribution of Enzymes in Snake Venoms

At least 26 enzymes, most of them hydrolases, have been detected in snake venoms (Table 1). Of these enzymes, 12 are found in all venoms, although their contents differ significantly; the rest occur mainly in certain taxonomic groups or are characteristic of only a few species. Since immunologic studies of venoms generally show an

Table 1. Enzymes found in snake venoms

Enzymes found in all snake venoms
Phospholipase A_2 (3.1.1.4), L-Amino acid oxidase (1.4.3.2), Phosphodiesterase (3.1.4.1), 5'-Nucleotidase (3.1.3.5), Phosphomonoesterase (3.1.3.2), Deoxyribonuclease (3.1.4.6), Ribonuclease (2.7.7.16), Adenosine triphosphatase (3.6.1.8), Hyaluronidase (4.2.99.1), NAD-nucleosidase (3.2.2.5), Arylamidase, Peptidase
Enzymes found in crotalid and viperid venoms
Endopeptidase, Arginine ester hydrolase, Kininogenase (3.4.4.21), Thrombinlike enzyme, Factor X activator, Prothrombin activator
Enzymes found mainly in elapid venoms
Acetylcholinesterase (3.1.1.7), Phospholipase B (3.1.1.5), Glycerophosphatase
Enzymes found in some venoms
Glutamic-pyruvic transaminase (2.6.1.2), Catalase (1.11.1.6), Amylase (3.2.1.1), β-Glucosaminidase, Lactate dehydrogenase (1.1.1.27), Heparinaselike enzyme

absence of common antigens in venoms of remotely related species such as cobras and rattlesnakes, the widely distributed enzymes evidently differ between these taxa in molecular properties. Thus, comparative investigations of enzyme activities of the venoms confirm the large heterogeneity of this natural product. Certain enzymes are typical for venoms of certain snake families. The elapid venoms, for example, are characterized by acetylcholinesterase, which is never found in viperid and crotalid venoms (ZELLER, 1948). On the other hand, endopeptidase, arginine ester hydrolase, thrombinlike enzyme, kininogenase, and procoagulant, which are distributed in viperid and crotalid venoms, are not detected in the elapid venoms so far investigated (DEUTSCH and DINIZ, 1955). With very few exceptions, elapid venoms (*Ophiophagus hannah* and *Pseudechis collettii*) contain low proteolytic and arginine ester hydrolyzing activities (MEBS, 1970). When compared with viperid and crotalid venoms, no remarkable differences are found in the contents of phospholipase A_2, endopeptidase, phosphodiesterase, 5'-nucleotidase and hyaluronidase. However, the contents of procoagulant and thrombinlike enzyme differ significantly from each other, as will be described later. Therefore even closely related snake species show considerable quantitative differences in their enzyme activities. However, it is very difficult to explain the different contents of enzymes in closely related snake species, since the enzymes may be subjected to great variations depending on the condition of the snake (e.g., age, nutrition, sex, living space or circumstances) and the handling of the venom (vacuum dried, lyophilized) and its storage. Recently, BONILLA et al. (1973) compared several enzyme activities in the pooled venom samples from timber rattlesnakes *(C.horridus horridus)* at four stages of growth (3–6, 7–12, 13–18 months, and adults). The results suggest a continued increase in the total protein content of the crude venoms from birth to the adult stage (Table 2). The L-amino acid oxidase activity, likewise, increases with age, a finding previously reported by JIMENEZ-PORRAS (1964) and FIERO et al. (172). Moreover, the protease activity increases with age,

Table 2. Some properties of adult and juvenile *C. h. horridus* venoms (BONILLA et al., 1973)

	Months			
	3–6	7–12	13–18	Adults
Protein concentration[a] (mg/ml)	16,80	18,00	18,60	19,75
Phosphodiesterase (units/mg protein)	0.0067	0.0186	0.0145	0.0081
L-amino acid oxidase[b] (units/mg powder)	0.024	0.081	0.202	0.234
Prothrombin time[c] (s)	2.2	2.0	2.0	3.5
Thrombinlike activity (s)	6.6[e]	5.7[e]	6.1[e]	11.9[f]
Protease[d] (units/mg powder)	829	1100	1670	2876
Color	Colorless	Colorless	Yellow	Yellow

[a] Measured on 28 mg powder/ml solution.
[b] 1 unit = /μ mole of oxygen consumed/10 ml mixture/min.
[c] Control time = 12.3 s.
[d] Casein hydrolase activity.
[e] This activity corresponds to that observed when 0.625 units of thrombin were added to the test system.
[f] This activity corresponds approximately to that observed when 1.25 units of thrombin were added to the test system.

whereas the activities of phosphodiesterase and thrombinlike enzyme apparently decrease in the adult snakes. Hence, it is evident that the venoms can hardly be standardized and variations in composition, especially of enzyme activities, are to be expected.

Another difficulty to be considered in the comparative studies of enzyme activities of snake venoms is that the values obtained for the enzyme activities do not represent absolute values for the venom concerned. Factors in the venom itself can influence the activity of the enzyme, at least partially. For example, some of the venoms *(V. ammodytes)* contain an inhibitor that reduces the proteolytic activity of the crude venom (RAUDONAT, 1955) and a kinin-destroying enzyme, mainly endopeptidase, can interfere with the assay method of kininogenase activity (SUZUKI and IWANAGA, 1970). Moreover, snake venoms contain factors that potentiate the effect of released kinins on isolated smooth-muscle preparation (FERREIRA and ROCHA E SILVA, 1965).

Differences in the composition of snake venoms are not only restricted to their enzymes but also to their polypeptide toxins and biologically active substances. It is well known that elapid venoms contain toxins of molecular weight below 10000, which pass the dialysis membrane, whereas those of viperid and crotalid venoms are of higher molecular weights and nondialyzable. The experimental results are shown in Table 3. Of the venom amount of the elapids obtained, 30%–75% pass the dialysis membrane, whereas only comparatively small proportions of the viperid and crotalid venoms are dialyzable (5–17%). These results suggest the following characteristics for snake venoms: elapid venoms—small molecular substances and poor in enzymes; viperid and crotalid venoms—higher molecular proteins and rich in enzymes.

Table 4 summarizes some properties of snake venom enzymes which have been isolated and characterized. At least 19 different enzymes have been isolated in the

Table 3. Amount of non dialyzable and dialyzable components in elapid, viperid, and crotalid venoms[a] (MEBS, 1969)

	Initial venom amount (mg)	Nondialyzable amount (mg)	Percent dialyzed
Elapidae:			
Naja naja	100	65	35
Naja naja atra	80	20	75
Naja nigricollis	100	61	39
Naja haje	40	15	62
Naja nivea	100	60	40
Hemachatus haemachatus	50	22	56
Ophiophagus hannah	100	55	45
Dendroaspis angusticeps	70	29	59
Bungarus fasciatus	100	66	34
Pseudechis collettii	100	62	38
Viperidae:			
Vipera russellii	100	87	13
Bitis gabonica	40	38	5
Crotalidae:			
Crotalus atrox	100	90	10
Crotalus durissus terrificus	100	87	13
Bothrops jararaca	100	83	17

[a] The venoms dissolved in distilled water (100 mg in 5 ml) were dialyzed in a slowly rotating cellophane bag (Kalle, Wiesbaden, Germany) against a tenfold amount of distilled water at 4° C; the water was changed after 24 and 48 h. At the end of 48 h the residue of dialysis and the dialysate were lyophilized separately. The nondialyzable amount was subtracted from the initial venom weight to obtain the quantity of dialysis.

venoms. This is the minimum number of substantively different enzymes, since several enzymes must clearly exist which represent the activities of adenosine triphosphatase, glycerophosphatase, peptidases, glutamic-pyruvic transaminase, catalase, amylase, β-glucosaminidase, and heparinase. An interesting feature of enzymes in snake venom is their high stability when stored in a dry state. Rattlesnake venom, for example, when stored for ~50 years has approximately the same biologic activity as freshly extracted venom (RUSSELL and EVENTOV, 1964). Other venoms have also been shown to retain lethality and enzyme activities of phosphodiesterase, 5′-nucleotidase, phosphomonoesterase, phospholipase A_2, and cholinesterase, except for L-amino acid oxidase, during storage periods of 17–39 years at room temperature (SMITH and HINDLE, 1931; IWANAGA et al., 1958; SUGIURA et al., 1972). Thus, most of the properties of snake venoms seem to be well retained in promptly lyophilized material.

C. Methods for Purification, Isolation, and Crystallization of Snake Venom Enzymes

Many reports describing procedures for purifying snake venom enzymes have appeared since SLOTTA and FRAENKEL-CONRAT (1938) successfully separated a crystal-

Table 4. Some properties of enzymes found in snake venoms[a]

Trivial name	Typical substrate	Molecular weight	Characteristics
Phospholipase A_2	Phosphatidyl-choline	11000–15000	Simple protein, heat stable, histidine active site
L-amino acid oxidase	L-amino acid	100000–130000	Glycoprotein, 2 moles FAD per mole enzyme, heat unstable
Phosphodiesterase	Oligonucleotides	115000	Heat labile, EDTA sensitive, acid unstable, optimum at pH 9
5′-Nucleotidase	5′-Mononucleotides	100000	Heat labile, Zn^{2+} sensitive, EDTA sensitive, acid unstable, optimum at pH 8.5
Phosphomono-esterase	p-Nitrophenyl-phosphate	100000	Heat labile, Zn^{2+} sensitive, EDTA sensitive, acid unstable, optimum at pH 8.5–9
Deoxyribonuclease	DNA and RNA		Optimum at pH 5.0
Ribonuclease	RNA	15900	Optimum at pH 7–9, specific towards pyrimidine nucleotides
Hyaluronidase	Hyaluronic acid		Heat labile, optimum at pH 4.6, resembles testicular enzyme
NAD-nucleosidase	NAD	100000	Heat labile, optimum at pH 7.5, nicotinamide sensitive
Arylamidase	L-Leucine naphthylamide	100000	Heat labile, SH-enzyme, PCMB sensitive, optimum at pH 8.5
Endopeptidase	Casein, Hemoglobin	21400–95000	Glycoprotein, metal (Ca^{2+}, Zn^{2+}) protease, EDTA sensitive, heat labile, optimum at pH 8–9
Arginine ester hydrolase	BAEE, TAME	27000–30000	Glycoprotein, heat stable, DFP sensitive, optimum at pH 8–9
Kininogenase	Plasma kininogen, BAEE	33500	Heat stable, DFP sensitive, specific towards kininogen
Thrombinlike enzyme	Fibrinogen, BAEE	28000–33000	Glycoprotein, heat stable, DFP sensitive
Factor X activator	Factor X	78000	Glycoprotein, heat labile, DFP insensitive, EDTA sensitive, activates also Factor IX
Prothrombin activator	Prothrombin	56000	Glycoprotein, heat labile, DFP insensitive, EDTA sensitive
Factor V activator	Factor V, BAEE	20000	DFP sensitive, heat stable
Acetylcholin-esterase	Acetylcholine	126000	Heat labile, DFP sensitive, optimum at pH 8–8.5
Phospholipase B	Lysolecithin		Heat stable, optimum at pH 10

[a] DFP = Di*iso*propylphosphorofluoridate; PCMB = p-Chloromercuribenzoate; BAEE = Benzoyl-L-arginine ethyl ester; TAME = Tosyl-L-arginine methyl ester.

lizable protein, crotoxin, from the venom of *C. durissus terrificus*. However, not until the advent of various high resolution methods in the past 20 years has much progress been made toward isolating the venom constituents in a pure and biologically active form. The older methods, such as heat and pH treatments, alcohol fractionation, salting out, free-boundary electrophoresis, and ultracentrifugation, tend to be non-specific by present-day standards and thus inefficient. The newer methods usually employ mild conditions of pH, temperature, and solvent, and so favor the retention of biologic activity. However, no common method of systematically fractionating the venom constituents has been decided on, since experience accumulated during these years indicates that the behavior of the venom components in the purification procedures differ greatly from one venom to another, even in closely related snake species. Striking examples of these new methods are ordinary and recycling molecular-sieve chromatography, gradient elution on columns of ion exchangers and hydroxyapatite, preparative polyacrylamide gel electrophoresis, and isoelectric focusing. Moreover, nowadays more attractive techniques, e.g., affinity chromatography, hydrophobic chromatography, droplet countercurrent, and immunoabsorption, are available for the purification and isolation of venom constituents. Reviews of the theories and applications of these techniques have appeared in alternate years in Methods in Enzymology, edited by COLOWICK and KAPLAN (1956 to the present). The reader is also referred to the useful book on fractionation of specific snake venoms by HENRIQUES and HENRIQUES (1971).

I. Polyacrylamide Gel Electrophoresis

The electrophoretic method using starch gel (NEELIN, 1963; BERTKE et al., 1966) or polyacrylamide gel (DELORI and GILLO, 1968; BASU et al., 1969) has been widely utilized in the study of protein components of venoms from elapid and crotalid snakes. The method is very effective not only for identification of the venom components but also for comparative biochemical studies. Figure 1 shows polyacrylamide gel electrophoretic patterns of venoms from various species of North American snakes. The reproducibility of this technique is very high and more than ten protein bands stained with amido black can be detected.

Method (BONILLA and HORNER, 1969). Venoms are prepared for electrophoresis by dissolving 14–28 mg in 1.0 ml 0.1 M Tris- 0.1 M citric acid buffer, pH 2.9 containing 6 M urea and 10^{-4} M pyronine-Y dye as a marker. Insoluble material is removed by centrifugation at 27500 *g* for 30 min. Electrophoresis on polyacrylamide gels (12%) in 6 M urea, is carried out under the following experimental conditions: voltage, 250 V (constant); current, 100 mA; pre-run, 3.5 h; electrolyte, 0.37 M glycine-citric acid buffer, pH 3.0; load, 20–40 µl (~0.9 mg protein); separations are performed at room temperature for 4–5 h, but coolant (4° C) is circulated through the cooling plates at all times. The gels after electrophoresis are stained for 24 h with amido black and destained electrophoretically (40 min) with a mixture of methanol-acetic acid-water (5:1:5, v/v) or 7% acetic acid.

II. Isoelectric Focusing

Electrofocusing, developed by SVENSSON (1962), is now a well-known technique for separating multiple forms of proteins and enyzmes. This method was first applied by TOOM et al. (1969) to study the venom components of two snakes of distinctly dissimilar phylogenetic classification and habitat. Although electrofocusing is

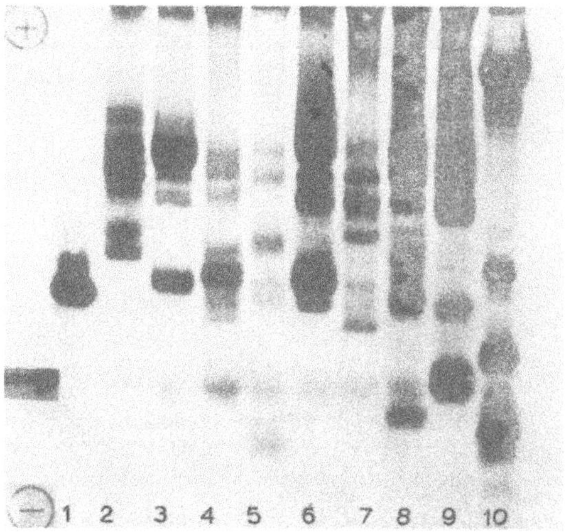

Fig. 1. A Comparative electropherogram of: *1*, lysozyme; *2*, *Heloderma suspectum*; *3*, *C. scutulatus*; *4*, *C. m. mollosus*; *5*, *C. basiliscus*; *6*, *C. v. helleri*; *7*, *C. v. cerberus*; *8*, *C. v. viridis*; *9*, *C. h. horridus*; *10*, human parotid fluid. Polyacrylamide gel (12%) electrophoresis in 6 M urea was carried out at pH 3.0 at 250 V for 6 h. The gels were stained with amido black and destained with methanol-acetic acid-water (5:1:5, v/v) (BONILLA et al., 1971)

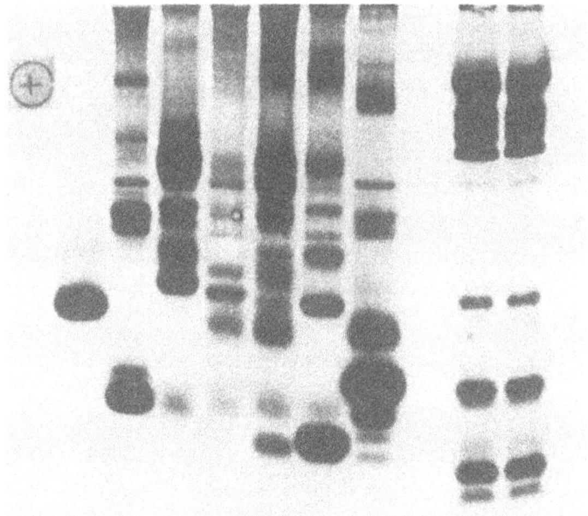

Fig. 1. B Comparative electropherogram of: *1*, lysozyme; *2*, *C. adamanteus*; *3*, *C. scutulatus*; *4*, *C. h. atricaudatus*; *5*, *C. v. viridis*; *6*, *C. d. terrificus*; *7*, *Naja naja*; *8*, Blank; *9* and *10*, human parotid fluid. The conditions were the same as those of Figure 1A (BONILLA et al., 1971)

usually applied as one of the last steps in the fractionation process due to its high resolving power, its direct application to a mixture is also useful for determining the isoelectric points of the various constituents.

Method (SIMON et al., 1969). The experiments are carried out in an LKB analatic column of 110 ml capacity; a density gradient is formed with sucrose solutions. The carrier ampholyte, Ampholine, at 1% concentration is used to form a pH gradient from 3–10. A sample of 5–10 mg

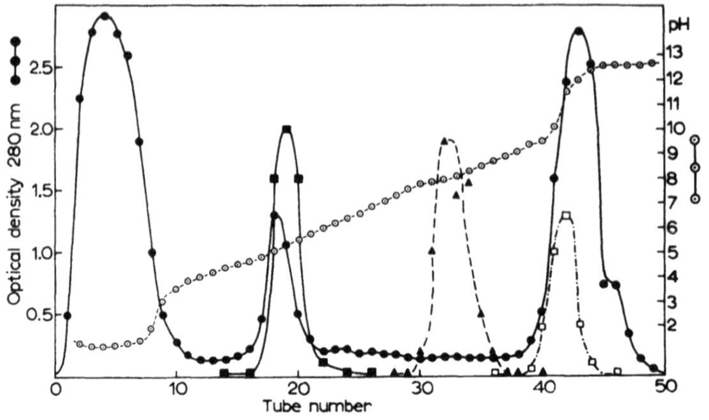

Fig. 2. Electrofocusing of *Naja naja atra* venom with pH range at 3–10. ●—●: absorbancy at 280 nm; ⊙—⊙: pH; □—□: toxicity. Arbitrary enzymatic activities are plotted as follows: ■—■: phospholipase A; ▲—▲: L-amino acid oxidase (SIMON et al., 1969)

venom in 2.0 ml less dense solution is allowed to replace the less dense solution in the middle fraction. The anode electrolyte solution is placed at the top. Focusing is performed at 4° C for 72 h; the voltage is initially adjusted to maintain a maximum input power of 2 V. After 24 h operation, the voltage is fixed at 750 V for the next 48 h; the current finally drops to less than 1 mA. At the end of the run, the column is emptied and 2 ml fractions are automatically collected. Absorbancies at 280 nm, pH and enzyme activities are determined on each tube withouth removing the ampholines and sucrose.

Figures 2 and 3 show the results of electrofocusing on the venoms of *Naja naja atra* and the Malayan pit viper *(Aghistrodon rhodostoma)*. Recovery of protein is nearly quantitative and the isoelectric point in each fraction is determined as part of the experiment. This technique is very useful both as a preliminary tool and as a separation method when only small amounts of protein are available for assay.

III. Molecular-Sieve Chromatography

So-called gel filtration is a liquid column chromatographic method of separating solute molecules according to differences in molecular size. The separation is achieved by percolating the sample through a bed of porous, uncharged gel particles. The wide acceptance of gel filtration is due to the method's simplicity, rapidity, and economy. It can be used whenever sufficient molecular size differences exist among sample substances and it yields highly reproducible results. Solute recoveries approach 100% and scale-up to large sample volumes is easily accomplished. Gel filtration is an extremely mild method, rarely causing denaturation of labile substances. Similarly to the xero gels, cross-linked dextran (Sephadex), polyacrylamide (Bio-Gel P), and agarose (Sepharose and Bio-Gel A) are produced and marketed in many particle sizes. Except for agarose they must be hydrated prior to use. Dextran and polyacrylamide gels have generally high resistance to chemical attack by reagents commonly used in biochemical experiments. Both are stable from pH 2 to pH 10; lengthy exposure of the gels to strongly acidic (<pH 1.0) or alkaline conditions (>pH 11) should be avoided, especially at high temperature. Separation by molecular-sieve chromatography can be qualitatively divided into two categories:

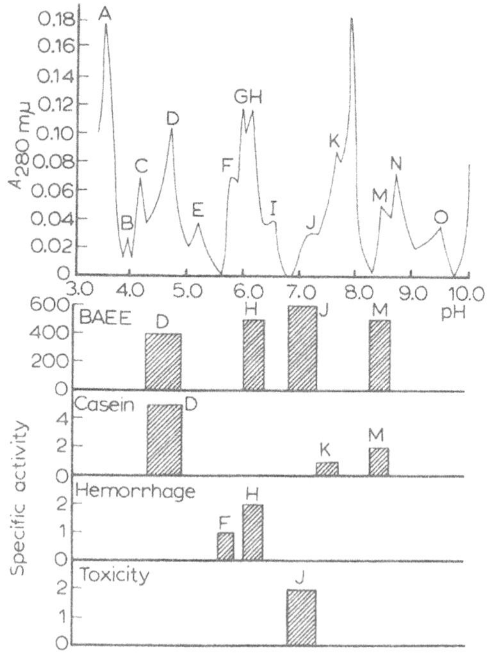

Fig. 3. Isoelectric focusing of the components of the Malayan pit viper (*A. rhodostoma*) venom. *Upper:* isoelectric point distribution of the ultraviolet-absorbing components. *Lower:* isoelectric point distribution of the esterase, protease, hemorrhagic, and toxic activities. Esterase and protease activities were calculated from the equation: 1000 × absorbancy change/min/mg venom. Hemorrhagic activity is expressed in terms of a scale from zero (no activity) to 3 (severe hemorrhage). Relative toxicity is the ratio of the LD_{50} of whole venom to that of the fraction. BAEE = Benzyol-L-arginine ethyl ester (TOOM et al., 1969)

group separation and fractionation. The gel, the bed dimensions, and the sample volumes depend on the category into which the separation falls.

In the studies on snake venom enzymes, group separation using Sephadex G-100 or G-150 has been generally applied, especially in the initial step of the purification procedures. By this method, enzymes with low molecular weight including phospholipase A_2, arginine ester hydrolases, kininogenases, and thrombinlike enzyme can be successfully separated from L-amino acid oxidase, all of which are known to have a high molecular weight, ~85000 (OSHIMA et al., 1972). Moreover, gel filtration is also very useful in separating polypeptide toxins including neurotoxins, cardiotoxins, cytotoxins, and proteinase inhibitors as well as various enzymes from elapid venoms (BOQUET et al., 1966; HOKAMA et al., 1976; TAKAHASHI and OHSAKA, 1970). The method has also been used to isolate a biologically active peptide such as bradykinin potentiators (KATO and SUZUKI, 1971).

Method (HOKAMA et al., 1976): Lyophilized *N. nivea* venom (2.43 g, lot 112c—0110, obtained from Sigma Chemical Co., St. Louis) is dissolved in 5 ml 0.1 M $(NH_4)HCO_3$ buffer, pH 7.9; the solution is applied to a column of Sephadex G-75 (5 × 138 cm) previously equilibrated with the same buffer. The column is eluted with the equilibration buffer at 4° C and fractions of 14 ml are collected at a flow rate of 42 ml/h. The elution profile is shown in Figure 4A. Six major peaks with absorption at 280 nm are obtained. The fractions indicated by the *solid bar* are combined, lyophilized and further fractionated by ion exchange chromatography (Fig. 4B).

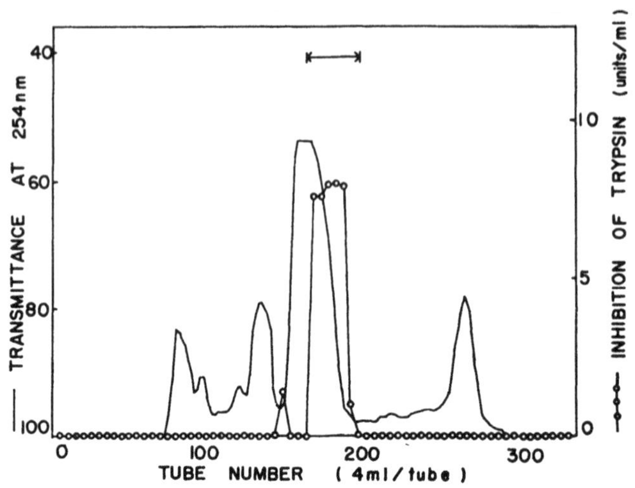

Fig. 4. A Gel-filtration of *Naja nivea* venom on a Sephadex G-75 column. The lyophilized venom (2.43 g) was applied to a 5 × 138 cm column of Sephadex G-75 previously equilibrated with 0.1 M ammonium carbonate buffer, pH 7.9. Elution was done at room temperature with the same buffer and fractions of 14 ml were collected at a flow rate of 42 ml (HOKAMA et al., 1976)

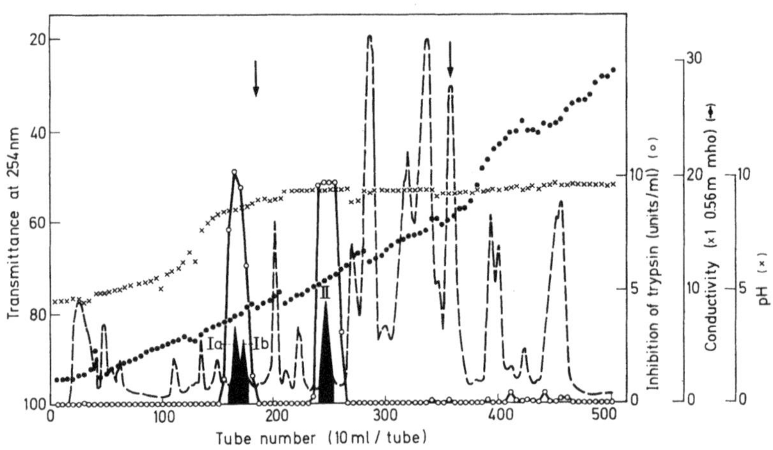

Fig. 4. B Further separation of polypeptide-containing fractions on an SE-Sephadex column. The pooled fraction (964 mg) obtained in Figure 4A was applied to a 2.5 × 63.5 cm column of SE-Sephadex equilibrated with 0.05 M ammonium acetate buffer, pH 4.7. A linear gradient elution was started at room temperature with 970 ml each equilibration buffer in the mixing vessel and 0.2 M ammonium acetate buffer, pH 9.5, in the reservoir. The buffer in the reservoir was replaced by 0.5 M and then 1.0 M, pH 9.5, as indicated by the *arrows*. The flow rate was adjusted at 30 ml/h (HOKAMA et al., 1976)

IV. Ion-Exchange Chromatography

Ion-exchange chromatography is one of the best methods for separating protein mixtures. Adsorption to ion exchangers primarily involves the formation of multiple ionic bands between charged groups on the protein and available groups of opposite charge on the absorbent. Thus, chromatographic separation depends on the different

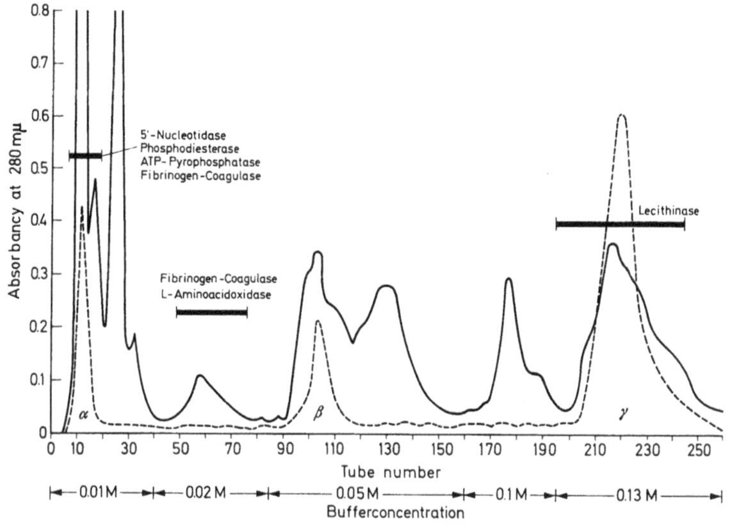

Fig. 5. Chromatogram of 200 mg venom from *C. atrox* on a 1.5 × 25 cm column of DEAE-cellulose. Eluting buffer was phosphate at pH 7.2 with stepwise changes in concentrations as indicated below the *abscissa*. Fractions of 3 ml were collected at a flow rate of ~0.2 ml/min. ——: Absorbancy at 280 nm; ---: the proteolytic activity expressed as the absorbancy at 280 nm given by 0.2 ml effluent under the conditions of the Kunitz test (PELEIDEPER and SUMYK, 1961)

elution of the adsorbed proteins by a variety of techniques based either on alteration of the charged state of the protein (pH) or on the use of agents capable of competing with the adsorbed protein for the charged sites on the adsorbent. The affinity and capacity of a particular pH and salt concentration must be accurately specified according to these parameters if data are to be significant. A number of ion exchangers in general use for separating protein mixtures are commercially available; these adsorbents may be classified into several large categories depending on the matrix to which the charged groups are attached, such as resin, cellulose, "Sephadex", and polyacrylamide (Biogel). For the fractionation of enzymes and toxins in snake venoms, cellulose or Sephadex anion exchangers with the diethylaminoethyl-(DEAE-) group and the cation exchangers with the carboxymethyl-(CM-) group or sulfoethyl-(SE-) group have been successfully used; some experimental examples are shown in Figures 5–9. This method is very useful for both initial separation of venom into as many discrete fractions as possible and large-scale preparative work. In general, DEAE-cellulose and CM-cellulose seem effective in fractionating crotalid and viperid venoms (PFLEIDERER and SUMYK, 1961; SATO et al., 1965). However, CM-Sephadex and Amberlite CG-50 appear most promising for separating cobra venom enzymes and toxins because of the basic nature of most protein constituents of the venom. The latter resin was especially chosen for separating several toxins of the venoms from the genera, *Naja*, *Hemachatus*, and *Dendroaspis* (STRYDOM and BOTES, 1970). The following two methods are general procedures for separating enzymes in crotalid and elapid venoms.

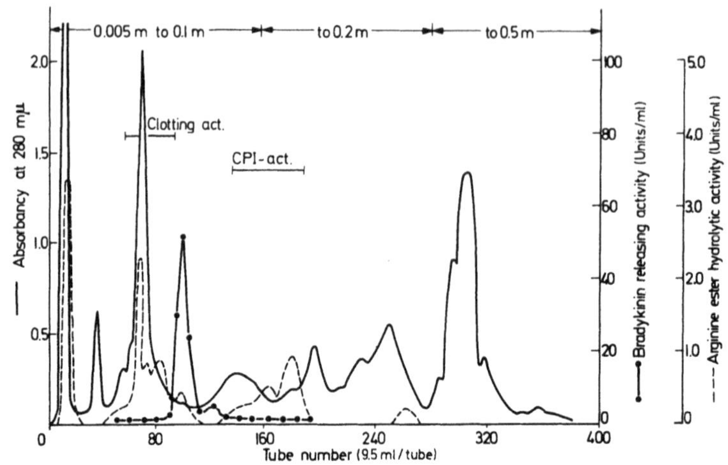

Fig. 6. Chromatogram of 1 g venom of *A. halys bomhoffii* on a 3 × 40 cm column of DEAE-cellulose (0.68 mEq./g). Eluting buffer was acetate at pH 7.0 with a concave gradient in concentration as indicated in *upper* figure (SATO et al., 1965)

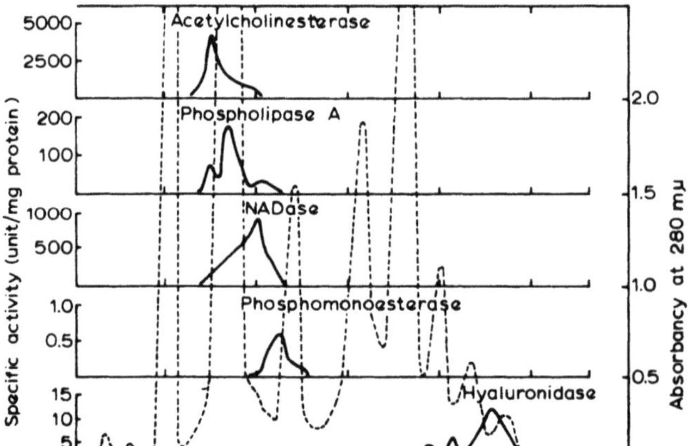

Fig. 7. Chromatography of *Bungarus multicinctus* venom on CM-Sephadex C-50 column (2.5 × 75 cm) by gradient elution with ammonium acetate buffer, from 0.05 M, pH 5.0 to 1.0 M, pH 6.8. Eluates of 3 ml each were collected at a flow rate of 15–18 ml/h. *Dotted line* indicates protein content estimated by absorbancy at 280 nm (LEE et al., 1972)

Method I (PFLEIDERER and SUMYK, 1961). The lyophilized *Crotalus atrox* venom (100 mg) is dissolved in 0.01 M Soerensen phosphate buffer, pH 7.2 and centrifuged to remove insoluble materials. The venom concentrations used do not exceed 3% and are not lower than 1%. A column is made with DEAE-cellulose (Serva Entwicklungslabor, Heidelberg) and the ion exchanger is packed under about 0.2 atom pressure in columns of varying sizes, depending on the amount of venom to be fractionated. Approximately 10 g dry exchanger with a capacity of 0.5–0.6 m Eq./g is sufficient for separating 100 mg crude venom. Before the venom solution is applied the columns are usually washed overnight with the starting buffer. They are regenerated by

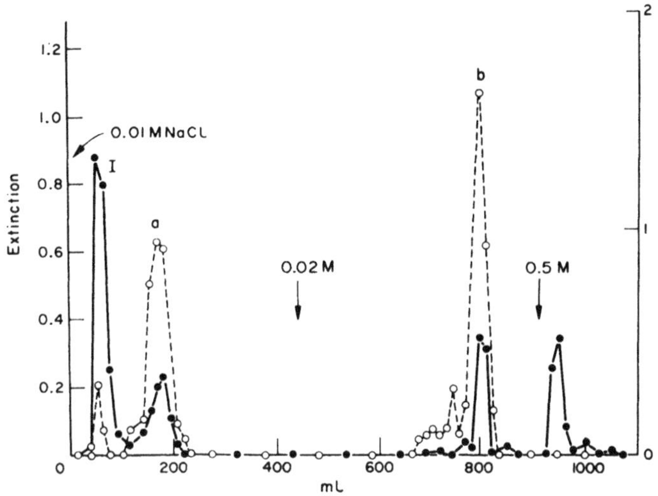

Fig. 8. CM-cellulose column chromatography of *Laticauda semifasciata* venom. The protein content of the eluate was determined by the absorbancy at 280 nm. Peaks *a* and *b* in the figure correspond to erabutoxins "*a*" and "*b*". —●—: $A_{1\,cm}$ at 280 nm; --○--: Toxicity expressed in terms of the body wt. of mice, 50% of which can be killed by 1 ml fraction (TAMIYA et al., 1967)

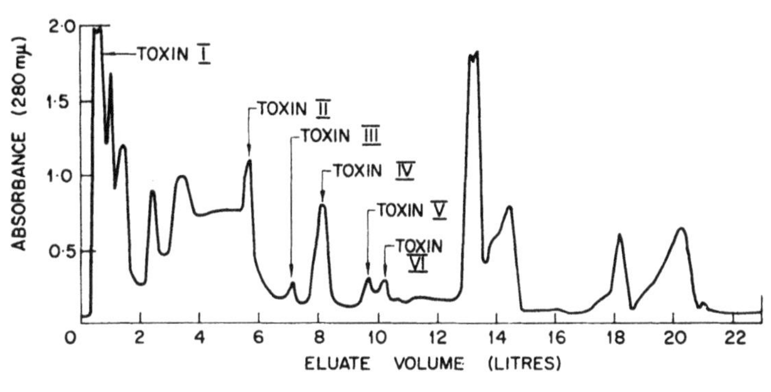

Fig. 9. Chromatography of *H. haemachatus* venom on Amberlite CG-50. Venom (20 g) was applied to a column (3.8 × 150 cm) of CG-50 and eluted with a 24 liter linear gradient of ammonium bicarbonate, pH 7.9, from 0.05 M to 0.6 M (STRYDOM and BOTES, 1971)

washing with 1% NaOH followed by the buffer until the effluent reaches the desired pH. The chromatograms are developed by a stepwise or simple gradient elution technique, using Soerensen phosphate buffer of pH 7.2. Linear gradient from 0.01 M to 0.2 M concentration is achieved by adding 0.33 M buffer to the mixing chamber containing 700 ml 0.01 M buffer. Flow rate is adjusted to 12 ml/h and fractions of 3 ml (for small column 20 × 1.0 cm) are collected at 4° C (Fig. 5).

Method II (STRYDOM and BOTES, 1971). Amberlite CG-50 resin (British Drug Houses, 200 mesh, type II), 500 g, is first suspended in 2 liters 2 N H_2SO_4 and heated at 80° C for 30 min and then washed two times with distilled water. The resin (H-form) is resuspended in 2 liters 2 N NH_4OH to convert the ammonium form and the upper portion is decanted. To the suspension 2 liters 2 N NH_4OH is added again and the resin is heated at 80° C for 10 min, then filtrated and washed with distilled water. The resin (NH_4-form) thus prepared is packed in a 1.9 × 150-cm

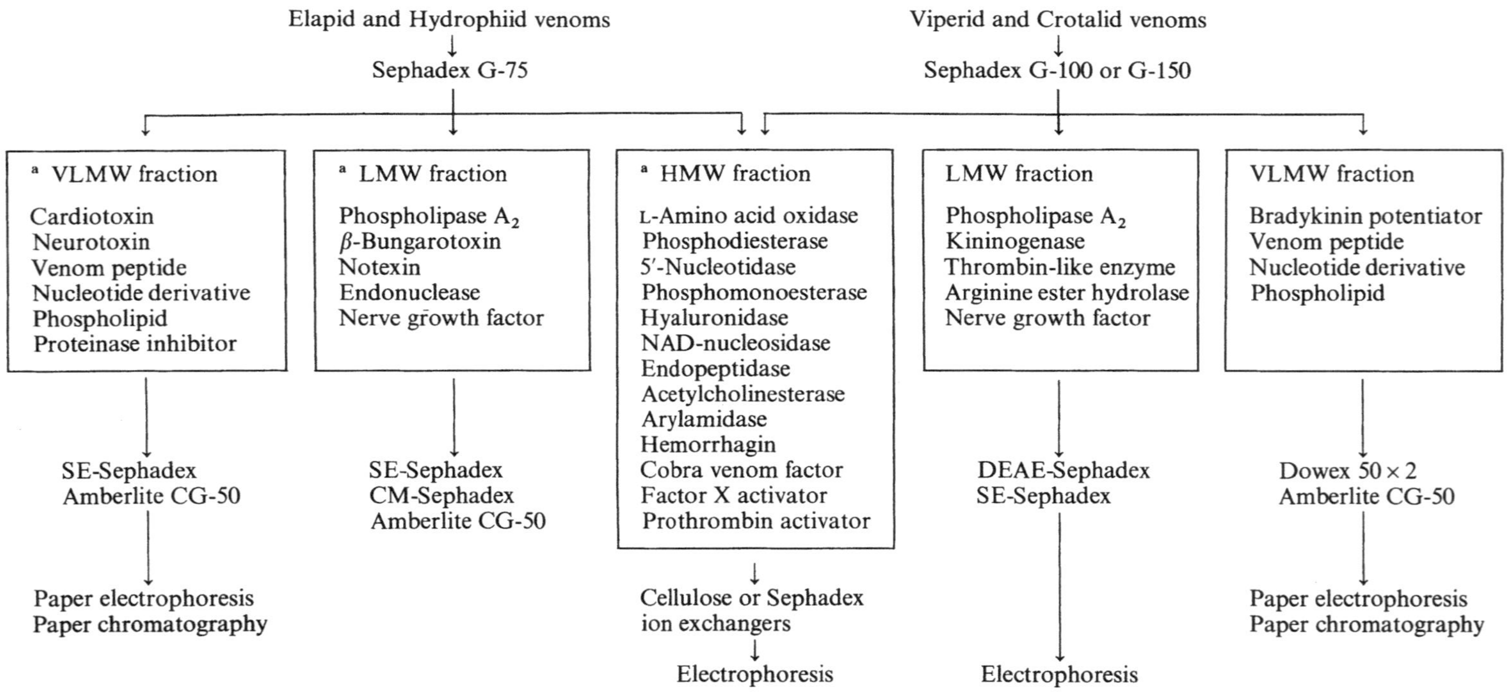

[a] VLMW, Very low molecular weight; LMW, Low molecular weight; HMW, High molecular weight.

Fig. 10. A systematic procedure for fractionation of the components from elapid, viperid, crotalid, and hydrophiid venoms column. The equilibration buffer is 0.05 M $(NH_4)HCO_3$, pH 8. Elapid venom (250 mg) is dissolved in 5 ml 0.02 M $(NH_4)HCO_3$ and clarified by centrifugation. The supernatant is applied to the column and a linear gradient of 3 liters from 0.05 M to 0.8 M $(NH_4)HCO_3$ is used to elute the fractions at a flow rate of 50 ml/h. The eluate is continuously monitored at 260 and 280 nm using a Beckman Spectrochrom, model 130.

At the end of this section we propose a systematic procedure for fractionation of the venom constituents, incorporating the results from the methods described here (Fig. 10).

D. Biochemical Properties of Snake Venom Enzymes

I. Oxidoreductases

1. L-Amino Acid Oxidase

All snake venoms contain a very active L-amino acid oxidase (ZELLER and MARITZ, 1944). When L-leucine is used as the substrate, a turnover number of the venom enzyme is about 400 times higher than that of mammalian L-amino acid oxidase. For this reason, the venom L-amino acid oxidase has been widely used in biochemical studies for identification of optical isomers of amino acid (PARIKH et al., 1958), laboratory preparation of α-keto acid from L-amino acid (MEISTER, 1952, 1954, 1965), and production of thyroxine from 3,5-diiodotyrosine (SHIBA and CAHNMANN, 1962a, 1962b). The enzyme catalyzes the following reaction accompanied with the reduction of FAD:

$$R-\underset{\displaystyle NH_2}{\underset{|}{CH}}-COOH + 1/2\,O_2 \rightarrow R-COCOOH + NH_3 \text{ (in the presence of catalase)} \quad (1)$$

$$R-\underset{\displaystyle NH_2}{\underset{|}{CH}}-COOH + H_2O + O_2 \rightarrow R-COOH + NH_3 + H_2O_2 \text{ (in the absence of catalase)} \quad (2)$$

$$R-\underset{\displaystyle NH_2}{\underset{|}{CH}}-COOH + FAD \rightleftarrows [R-\underset{\displaystyle NH}{\underset{|}{C}}-COOH] + FAD-H_2 \quad \text{(i)}$$

$$[R-\underset{\displaystyle NH}{\underset{|}{CH}}-COOH] + H_2O \rightleftarrows R-\underset{\displaystyle O}{\underset{\|}{C}}-COOH + NH_3$$

$$FAD-H_2 + O_2 \rightarrow FAD + H_2O_2\,. \quad \text{(ii)}$$

Thus, the reaction takes place in two steps [see schemes (i) and (ii)] and the intermediate imino acid is readily hydrolyzed to α-keto acid in the presence of water. In the absence of catalase, α-keto acid is decarboxylated and oxidized to the corresponding fatty acid by H_2O_2, which is produced during the enzyme reaction.

L-amino acid oxidase is responsible for the yellow color in snake venoms, because it contains FAD as the prosthetic group. As shown in Table 5, the enzyme activity is detected in all the venoms tested belonging to Elapidae, Viperidae and Crotalidae, except in white venoms of *Denisonia textilis*, *Bothrops itapetiningae* (ZELLER, 1948), and *Vipera ammodytes* (KORNALIK and MASTER, 1964). Nor has the activity been

Table 5. Oxidation of L-leucine by various snake venoms (ZELLER, 1948)

Venom	Q_{O_2}[a]	Venom	Q_{O_2}
Elapidae		Crotalidae	
Bungarus caeruleus	250	*Agkistrodon mokasen*	45
Bungarus fasciatus	230	*Agkistrodon piscivorus*	380
Dendroaspis angusticeps	50	*Agkistrodon halys blomhoffii*	165
Naja bungarus	380	*Bothrops alternatus*	340
Naja flava	60	*Bothrops atrox*	760
Naja haje	250	*Bothrops cotiara*	390
Naja melanoleuca	240	*Bothrops jararaca*	750
Naja naja	100	*Bothrops jararacussu*	400
Naja nigricollis	100	*Bothrops itapetiningae*	0
Notechis scutatus	40	*Bothrops neuwiedii*	590
Pseudechis australis	50	*Bothrops nummifera*	190
Pseudechis porphyriacus	190	*Crotalus adamanteus*	50
Sepedon haemachates	120	*Crotalus cinereus*	100
Viperidae		*Crotalus horridus*	70
Vipera ammodytes	310	*Crotalus lucasensis*	60
Vipera aspis	610	*Crotalus ruber*	10
Vipera aspis Hugyi	2440	*Crotalus terrificus terrificus*	10
Vipera berus	+	*Crotalus terrificus basilicus*	80
Vipera latastei	620	*Crotalus viridis*	270
Vipera lebetina	1570	*Crotalus viridis oregons*	250
Vipera russellii	760	*Trimeresurus flavoviridis*	163
Bitis arietans	380		
Bitis gavonica	320		
Cerastes vipera	420		
Echis carinatus	130		
Sistrurus catenatus	100		

[a] $Q_{O_2} = O_2$uptake, µl/h/mg venom.

found in the venom of the sea snakes (Hydrophiidae). It seems that the activity of elapid venoms is relatively low compared with viperid and crotalid venoms (MEBS, 1970). The enzyme content occupies $\sim 4\%$ (w/w) of the total proteins in crotalid venoms.

Assay method (WELLNER and LICHTENBERG, 1971). *Principle.* Phenylalanine is oxidized by the amino acid oxidase to phenylpyruvate; its enol form reacts with borate to give a complex with a high absorbancy at 300 nm. Catalase is added to prevent the α-keto acid from being destroyed by H_2O_2.

Reagents. Tris-HCl buffer, 0.4 M, pH 7.5 at 37° C (pH 7.8 at 25° C). Catalase, 1200 units ml. L-phenylalanine, 0.04 M. Trichloroacetic acid (TCA), 25%. Borate-arsenate solution: 1 mole of sodium arsenate and 1 mole of boric acid in final volume of 1 liter, adjusted to pH 6.5 with concentrated HCl, filtered if necessary.

Procedure. A reaction mixture containing Tris buffer (80 µmoles), catalase (60 units), and L-amino acid oxidase (2–30 units) in a volume of 0.7 ml is placed in an 18 × 150 mm test tube. The reaction is started by adding 0.1 ml 0.04 M L-phenylalanine and the test tube is immediately placed in a water bath at 37° C with shaking (about 200 cycles/min). After exactly 15 min the reaction is stopped by adding 0.2 ml TCA. The mixture is transferred to a conic centrifuge tube and centrifuged. A 0.5 ml aliquot of the supernatant is transferred to a test tube containing 2.5 ml borate-arsenate solution and mixed well. The solution is allowed to stand at least 30 min at room temperature (22°–26° C); then the absorbancy at 300 nm is measured using a blank in which the enzyme is omitted. The readings remain constant for several hours.

Definition of Units and Specific Activity. One unit of activity is the amount of enzyme required to give an absorbancy of 0.030 at 300 nm under the above conditions. This unit is equivalent to that defined earlier as the amount of enzyme required to catalyze the uptake of 1 μl oxygen in 30 min in a manometric assay, using L-leucine as substrate. The specific activity of the crystalline enzyme *(C. adamanteus)* usually ranges between 10,000 and 13,600 units/mg protein.

Comments. Many methods of determining the activity of L-amino acid oxidase are now available. They include the classic Warburg manometry (BENDER and KREBS, 1950), measurement of ammonia production utilizing microkjeldahl determination (BLANCHARD et al., 1944), colorimetric assay (NAGATSU and YAGI, 1966), and measurement of ammonia coupled with the NADH-dependent reductive amination of 2-oxoglutarate catalyzed by exogeneous glutamate dehydrogenase (HOLME and GOLDBERG, 1975). Of these methods, later is recommended because it is reasonably sensitive and precise and a linear relationship between activity and enzyme concentration prevails to an absorbance change of 0.050/min.

Purification. The enzyme was first purified from the venom of *A. piscivorus* by SINGER and KEARNEY (1950). Later WELLNER and MEISTER (1960) succeeded in isolating and crystallizing the L-amino acid oxidase from the venom of *C. adamanteus*. The enzyme preparations from other venoms such as *A. halys blomhoffii* (SUZUKI and IWANAGA, 1958 b), *Vipera palestinae* (SHAHAM and BDOLAH, 1973), *Vipera ammodytes* (KURTH and AURICH, 1973), and *A. caliginosus* (SUGIURA et al., 1975) have also been partially or highly purified. The procedure described below is for purifying the enzyme from the venom of the eastern diamondback rattlesnake *(C. adamanteus)*.

Procedure (WELLNER, 1971). *Step 1.* 1 g dried or lyophilized venom from *Crotalus adamanteus* is dissolved in 100 ml distilled water at room temperature (22°–26° C) in an Erlenmeyer flask. Then 10 ml 0.1 M L-leucine is added and the flask is immediately stoppered with a three-hole stopper fitted with a thermometer and glass tube through which nitrogen is passed. The solution (under nitrogen) is heated to 70° C by immersing the flask in a 90°–95° C water bath with stirring. A temperature of 70° C is reached within 3–4 min and maintained for 5 min. The solution is then cooled in an ice bath and the precipitated protein is removed by centrifugation (8000 *g* for 10 min) and discarded. All the subsequent steps are carried out between 0° and 5° C.

Step 2. The supernatant solution from step 1 (occasionally opalescent) is treated with a suspension of calcium phosphate gel[1] (dry wt., 405 mg) and the pH is adjusted to 5.5 by addition, with stirring, of ~5 ml 0.1 N HCl. After standing for 30 min at 0° C with occasional stirring, the suspension is centrifuged (4000 *g* for 10 min) and the supernatant solution is discarded. The gel is washed twice by resuspension in 120 ml cold distilled water followed by centrifugation at 4000 *g* for 10 min. The washings, which contain little or no enzyme, are discarded. The gel is resuspended thoroughly with a glass homogenizer in 35 ml 2.30 M $(NH_4)_2SO_4$ containing 0.08 M sodium acetate (pH 4.6). After standing for 1 h or longer with occasional stirring, the suspension is centrifuged (8000 *g* for 10 min), and the precipitate is discarded.

Step 3. Solid $(NH_4)_2SO_4$ (4.8 g) is dissolved in the clear yellow supernatant solution (34 ml) obtained in step 2. After standing for 15 min at 0° C, the enzyme is centrifuged (8000 *g* for 15 min) and the supernatant solution is discarded. The yellow precipitate is redissolved in 2–3 ml of cold distilled water.

---

[1] The calcium phosphate gel is prepared essentially as described (SINGER and KEARNEY, 1950); 2 liters 0.25 M $CaCl_2$ is added with vigorous stirring to 2 liters 0.167 M $Na_3PO_4 \cdot 12H_2O$. The gel is washed four times with distilled water (the gel is allowed to settle by gravity and the supernatant is siphoned off); it is then resuspended in water and neutralized with dilute HCl (phenolphthalein external indicator). The gel is then washed with distilled water until no chloride is detectable in the supernatant when tested with acidified silver nitrate. The dry weight is determined and adjusted to 20–30 mg/ml. No aging of the gel is neccessary.

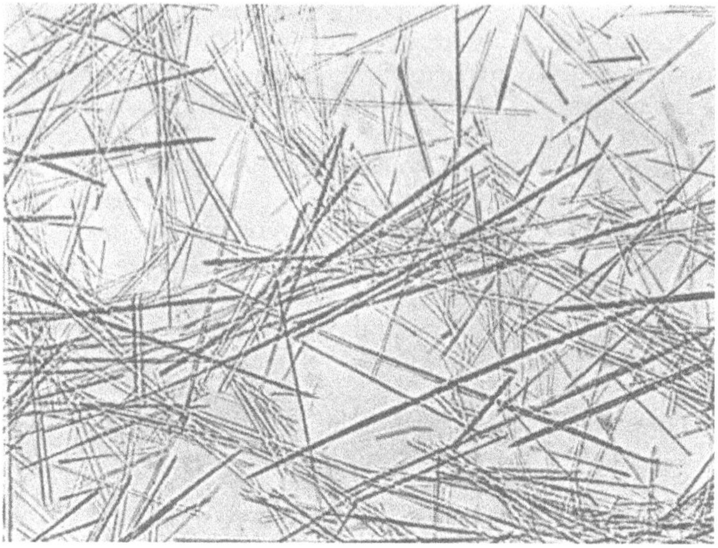

Fig. 11. Crystals of L-amino acid oxidase (*C. adamanteus* venom), ~x 500 t (WELLNER and MEISTER, 1960)

Step 4. The enzyme solution is placed in a cellophane dialysis sack and dialyzed against 6–7 liters of cold distilled water (5° C) with continuous stirring. The water is changed after 3 h of dialysis. Crystallization usually begins within 24 h and may be complete after 48 h. A higher yield of crystals is sometimes obtained after longer dialysis periods. Recrystallization is carried out as follows.

Step 5. The crystals are redissolved in 1–2 ml 0.1 M KCl. Insoluble material, occasionally noted at this stage, is removed by centrifugation and the solution is dialyzed against cold distilled water. Crystallization usually begins within 15 min and may be complete after 2–24 h. The crystals appear as thin yellow needles, easily visible under the low power of a standard microscope (Fig. 11).

A summary of the results obtained in two typical experiments is given in Table 6. Preparation I was made from 1 g pooled and dried venom and preparation II from 642 mg dried venom from a single snake. The values are given on the basis of 1 g venom.

The purification procedure may readily be brought to the dialysis step in one normal working day. If desired, the purification may be interrupted for about a day at the end of any step.

Physical and Chemical Properties. The purified enzyme is stable for several months at 0°–5° C as a crystalline suspension in water, as a concentrated solution in 0.1 M KCl, or in 0.1 M Tris-HCl buffer, pH 7.2. It loses its activity in frozen and lyophilized states. Table 7 summarizes the physicochemical properties of the enzyme isolated from *C. adamanteus* venom. The native enzyme with a molecular weight of 135000 is a noncovalent dimer consisting of two subunits with a molecular weight each of ~70000. It is a glycoprotein containing ~5% carbohydrate and 2 moles FAD/mole enzyme. Although the enzyme appears pure by several physical criteria, it can be resolved by both electrophoresis and ion-exchange chromatography into three major components with equal specific activity. The same phenomenon was also

Table 6. Purification of L-aminoacid oxidase from 1 g pooled and dried *Crotalus adamanteus* venom (preparation I) and from 642 mg dried venom from one snake (preparation II) (WELLNER, 1971)

Fraction	Preparation I			Preparation II		
	Total activity[a]	Specific activity[b]	Yield (%)	Total activity[a]	Specific activity[b]	Yield (%)
Original venom	350	270	(100)	471	360	(100)
Step 1	362	365	103	443	530	94
Step 2	244	3120	70	391	5070	83
Step 3	243	4430	69	388	6050	82
Step 4	144	6900	41	338	7630	72
Step 5	130	6900	37	304	7600	65

[a] Units $\times 10^{-2}$ (calculated on the basis of 1 g dried venom).
[b] Units/ml/absorbancy at 275 mμ.

Table 7. Physicochemical properties of L-amino acid oxidase isolated from *C. adamanteus* venom

Property	Value
Sedimentation coefficient, $S_{20,w}$	6.54 S
Diffusion coefficient $D_{20,w}$	4.52×10^{-7} cm^2/s
Partial specific volume ($\bar{v}$)	0.733 (ml/g)
Molecular weight[a]	135000
Electrophoretic mobility	-3.35×10^{-5} cm$^2 \cdot$s$^{-1} \cdot$V^{-1}
Frictional ratio (f/fo)	1.39
Isoelectric point (pI)[b]	5.2–8.4
Carbohydrate content	3–4%
NH_2-terminal residue	Alanine (Tyrosine)
Number of disulfide bond	6–7
Number of free SH-group	4
FAD content	2 mole/mole

[a] By sedimentation and diffusion (DEKOK and RAWITCH, 1969).
[b] Due to a microheterogeneity of the enzyme (WELLNER, 1971).

confirmed by SHAHAM and BDOLAH (1973) for the enzyme isolated from the venom of *Vipera palestinae*. Although the reason for such heterogeneity has not been fully understood, the three isozymes seem to result from the various combinations of the differing subunits and yield native dimer. In fact, two polypeptide chains with similar amino acid sequence but different mobilities and NH_2-terminal residues are found in the enzyme in unequal amounts (a ratio of 2.5:1). Moreover, HAYES and WELLNER (1969) have shown that the three major isozymes are separated further into multiple components, all possessing enzyme activity, by isoelectric fractionation in a pH gradient (Fig. 12). To explain this phenomenon, several possibilities may be considered on the analogy of other enzymes. One possibility is that the isozymes differ in the number or position of amide groups, as proposed for the multiple forms of cytochrome c (FLATMARK and VESTERBERG, 1966). Other possibilities are that the

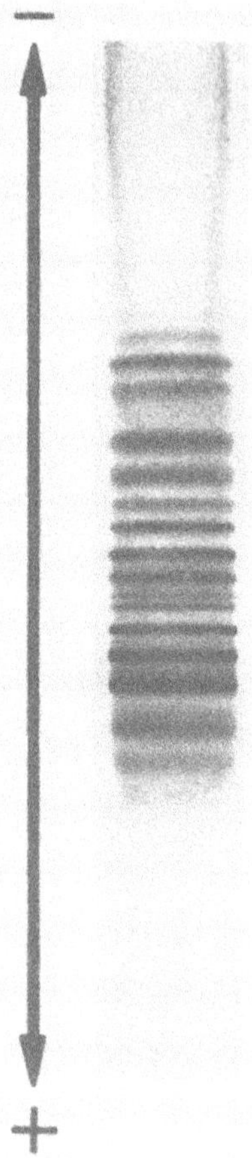

Fig. 12. Separation of L-amino acid oxidase (*C. adamanteus* venom) by electrofocusing in polyacrylamide gel. Stained for protein with Coomassie brilliant blue (HAYES and WELLNER, 1969)

isozymes differ in carbohydrate content, as revealed for the ribonuclease isozymes (PLUMMER, 1968), or in conformation, as suggested for mitochondrial malic dehydrogenase (KAPLAN, 1968). However, further studies are required to resolve the microheterogeneity observed.

Table 8 shows the amino acid and carbohydrate compositions of the mixture of L-amino acid oxidase isozymes A, B, and C. Although the composition of isozyme A differs slightly from that of the mixture of isozymes with respect to a few amino acids, the overall analyses are quite similar (DEKOK and RAWITCH, 1969). The absorption spectra of L-amino acid oxidase under different conditions are shown in Figure 13. The enzyme exhibits three maxima at 275, 390, and 462 nm. The absorbancy of a 0.1% solution at these wavelengths is 1.79, 0.178, and 0.171, respectively (WELLNER, 1971).

The purified enzyme from *C. adamanteus* venom is inactivated by storage in the frozen state of temperatures between $-5°$ and $-60°$ C, with maximal inactivation observed at $\sim -20°$ C (CURTI et al., 1968). The rate of inactivation is dependent on the pH of storage and on the ionic composition of the medium. The inactivation is

Table 8. The amino acid and carbohydrate composition of L-amino acid oxidase (*C. adamanteus* venom)

	Isozymes A–C	
	g/100 g of protein[a]	Residues/mole[b]
Lysine	7.5	7.57
Histidine	2.5	27.1
NH_2	1.0	81.0
Arginine	7.9	65.4
Aspartic acid	8.8	100.0
Threonine	5.2	67.2
Serine	4.0	59.3
Glutamic acid	10.0	100.5
Proline	3.3	44.3
Glycine	3.2	72.2
Alanine	4.1	75.6
Half-cystine[c]	1.3	16.5
Valine	4.1	53.7
Methionine[c]	2.0	15.9
Isoleucine	5.6	64.8
Leucine	6.1	69.8
Tyrosine	6.9	55.4
Phenylalanine	6.8	59.8
Tryptophan	2.0	14.2
N-Acetylglucosamine	1.7	11.1
Fucose	0.4	3.3
Mannose	1.6	12.7
Galactose	1.2	9.5
Sialic acid	0.4	2.0
FAD	1.2	2.0
Weight recovery	99.2	

[a] Averaged or extrapolated values of the data obtained from three hydrolysates with hydrolysis times of 22, 48, and 72 h. Values were corrected for moisture content of the sample.
[b] The molecular weight assumed was 135000.
[c] Determined as oxidized derivatives after performic acid oxidation in the case of the mixture of isozymes. Determined as half-cystine in the case of isozyme A (DEKOK and RAWITCH, 1969).

accompanied by changes in the visible absorption spectrum and by a decrease in the rate of photoreduction with ethylenediaminetetraacetate. The inactivated enzyme in most cases can be reactivated completely by heating at pH 5, with a full return of the spectrum of native enzyme. Thus, it seems that the inactivation is due to a limited conformational change of the enzyme structure, particularly in the vicinity of the flavin prosthetic group. A similar instability of the enzyme from *Vipera ammodytes* venom was also reported (KURTH and AURICH, 1976).

Enzymatic Properties. The pH optimum for the oxidation of L-leucine is 7.5. However, a different pH optimum may be obtained under other experimental conditions or with other substrates (PAGE and VANETTEN, 1969, 1971). For example, the enzyme does not oxidize lysine and ornithine at pH 7.5, but these substrates are easily oxidized at pH 9.4. As previously shown in schemes (i) and (ii), the oxidation of α-amino acid proceeds in two steps, forming imino acid as the intermediate product.

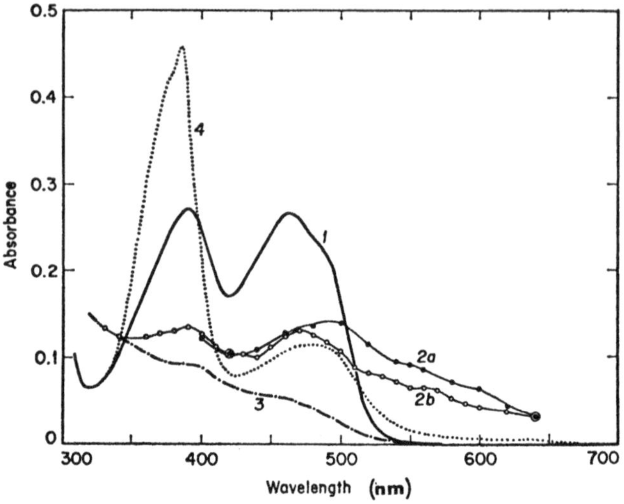

Fig. 13. Spectra of L-amino acid oxidase (*C. adamanteus* venom). *1*, Oxidized enzyme; *2a*, Intermediate produced in stopped-flow experiment with L-phenylalanine; *2b*, Intermediate produced in stopped-flow experiment with L-leucine; *3*, Reduced enzyme; *4*, Semiquinoid enzyme (MASSAY and CURTI, 1976)

However, it has never been demonstrated that imino acid is formed in the reaction catalyzed by this enzyme. HAFNER and WELLNER (1971) have evidence that the formation of imino acid is shown directly by allowing the amino acid oxidase reaction to proceed in the presence of $NaBH_4$, when the imino acid is reduced to the corresponding racemic amino acids. Thus, when $NaBH_4$ is added to a reaction mixture of L-amino acid oxidase and L-leucine, a significant amount of D-leucine is formed as follows:

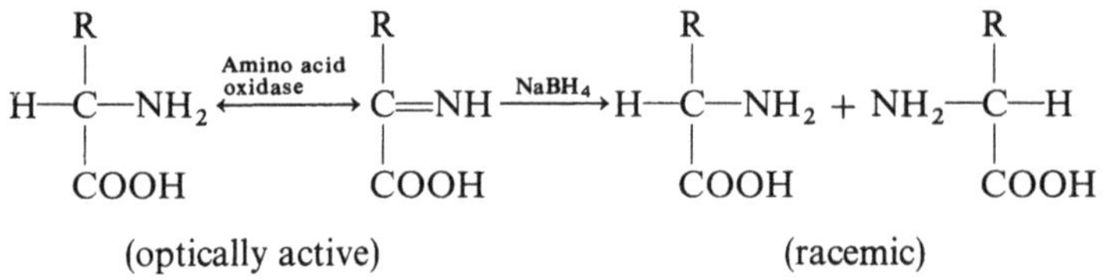

Although snake venom L-amino acid oxidase acts specifically on L-5-amino-carboxylic acids, the reaction rate of a number of amino acids differs significantly. As shown in Table 9 longer chained amino acids are more sensitive to the enzyme. Among the best substrates, the following L-amino acids may be listed: leucine, phenylalanine, tyrosine, tryptophan, and methionine. On the other hand, serine, threonine, aspartic acid, glutamic acid, asparagine, alanine, isoleucine, and valine are oxidized extremely slowly. There is no specificity towards the optical isomers except for α-carbon, since L-isoleucine, L-alloisoleucine and β-phenylserine are all susceptible to the enzyme. The Km values estimated by ZELLER et al. (1965) using the purified enzyme from *C. adamanteus* venom are 14.3 mM for L-leucine, 1.8 mM for L-phenylalanine, and 3.8 mM for L-tryptophan. The maximum velocity of the oxidation of L-phenylalanine

Table 9. Relative rate of oxidation of various aminoacids by snake venom L-aminoacid oxidase[a] (SUZUKI and IWANAGA, 1960)

Amino acids	*A. halys blomhoffii*	*T. flavoviridis*	*N. melanoleuca*
DL-Alanine	8	8	0
DL-β-Alanine	0	0	0
DL-2-Aminobutyric acid	121	63	0
DL-2-Aminovaleric acid	154	204	31
DL-2-Aminocaproic acid	127	133	74
DL-2-Aminolauric acid	0	0	0
DL-Valine	0	0	0
L-Leucine	165	163	77
DL-Isoleucine	21	76	0
DL-2-Aminoisobutyric acid	0	0	
DL-2-Aminoisoheptonic acid	132	98	
L-Glutamic acid	0	0	0
DL-Aspartic acid	0	0	0
L-Asparagine	7	42	
L-Tyrosine	218	228	246
DL-Bromotyrosine	109	121	
DL-Iodotyrosine	98	105	
DL-Phenylglycine	16	12	
DL-Phenylalanine	177	192	111
DL-Phenylserine	0	0	0
DL-Tryptophan	128	79	76
L-Histidine	12	12	0
L-Proline	0	0	0
DL-Serine	0	0	0
DL-Threonine	0	0	0
DL-Homoserine	44	56	
L-Arginine	77	165	32
L-Canavanine	96	122	
DL-Citrulline	119	145	
DL-Ornithine	0	0	0
DL-Lysine	0	0	0
DL-Homolysine	0	0	
DL-Diaminobutyric acid	0	0	
DL-Methionine	168	279	94
DL-Ethionine	14	24	
DL-Propionine	0	0	
DL-Buthionine	0	0	
L-Cysteine	143	136	
DL-Homocysteine	191	176	
L-Cystine	0	0	0
DL-Jienkolic acid	0	0	
DL-S-Methylcysteine	179	209	
DL-S-Ethylcysteine	157	157	
DL-S-Butylcysteine	12	0	
DL-S-Methylmethionine	0	0	

[a] Conditions: Reaction mixture contained 1 mg venom, 0.2 M Tris-buffer (pH 7.2), and 5×10^{-4} M L- or DL-amino acid in a total volume of 2.2 ml (37.5° C, air). The enzyme activity is expressed as O_2 uptake, µl/h/mg venom.

is not affected by the presence of 20 mM D-phenylalanine. The snake venom enzyme oxidizes many sulfur-containing amino acids, but shows no measurable activity with any of the sulfoxide derivatives, S-adenosyl-L-methionine, cysteic acid, homocysteic acid, lanthionine, or cystathionine (CHEN et al., 1971). The affinity for the various substrates at pH 7.5 in decreasing order is L-methionine ($Km = 0.35$ mM), L-homocystine (0.72 mM), L-homocysteine (1.3 mM), S-adenosyl-L-homocysteine (1.9 mM), S-ribosyl-L-homocysteine (2.2 mM), L-djenkolic acid (3.1 mM), L-cysteine (4.5 mM), and L-cystine (5.0 mM). The oxidation of L-cysteine proceeds as follows (CHEN et al., 1971; UBUKA et al., 1975; UBUKA and YAO, 1973):

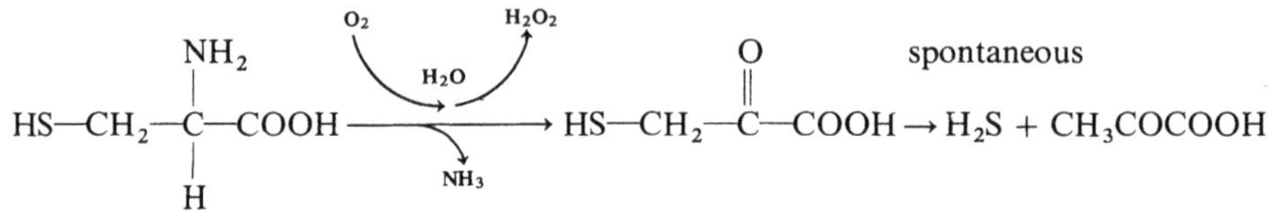

L-cysteine 2-mercaptopyruvate pyruvate

L-amino acid oxidase is inhibited by high concentration of good substrates, not by poor substrates. The extent of inhibition depends on the oxygen tension. At pH 7.5 with air as the gas phase, L-leucine, for example, inhibits the enzyme at concentrations higher than 5×10^{-3} M. Under similar conditions, L-valine does not appreciably inhibit at a concentration as high as 0.3 M. The enzyme activity is strongly inhibited competitively by benzoic, salicylic, mandelic, and iodoacetic acids (ZELLER, 1948).

2. Lactate Dehydrogenase

MCLEAN et al. (1971) reported that some snake venoms catalyzed the conversion of lactate to pyruvic acid. The presence of this enzyme was demonstrated in the following venoms: *N. naja*, *N. naja atra*, *N. nigricollis*, *N. melanoleuca*, *N. nivea*, *N. haje*, *Dendroaspis jamensoni*, *Dendroaspis polylepis*, and *Demansia textilis*. However, no report on purification of this enzyme has yet been published.

II. Enzymes Acting on Phosphate Esters

Snake venoms are known to contain at least four enzymes which act on the hydrolysis of phosphate esters. DELEZENNE and MOREL 1919 were the first to witness the disintegration of nucleic acids and the production of nucleosides in the presence of snake venoms. However, this and other phosphatases of the venoms were not fully investigated until almost 20 years later. Although TAKAHASHI (1932) and UZAWA (1932) provided the evidence that crotalid venoms contain phosphatases that hydrolyze synthetic phosphomonoester and phosphodiester compounds, the first systematic study on the occurrence of phosphodiesterase and 5′-nucleotidase in venom was made by GULLAND and JACKSON (1938). It is now well known that most venoms contain endonuclease, exonuclease, 5′-nucleotidase, and nonspecific phosphomonoesterase. The independent existence of adenosinetriphosphatase (ATPase) in

Table 10. Phosphodiesterase and ATPase distribution among venoms (PEREIRA et al., 1971)

Venoms	Rate		ATPase/ Phosphodiesterase ratio
	Phosphodiesterase[b]	ATPase[a]	
Vipera russellii	2.07	61.6	29.8
Trimeresurus flavoviridis	1.04	52.0	50.0
Bothrops jararaca	1.01	42.4	42.0
Bitis gavonica	0.94	38.0	40.0
Hemachatus haemachatus	0.94	16.4	17.4
Bothrops atrox	0.74	55.2	74.6
Bothrops asper	0.70	19.6	28.0
Crotalus adamanteus	0.62	37.6	60.6
Bothrops medusa	0.39	25.6	65.6
Naja nigricollis	0.38	10.4	27.4
Bitis arietans	0.14	4.0	28.6

[a] μmoles/h/mg venom.
[b] The activity of phosphodiesterase was measured using calcium bis-p-nitrophenylphosphate.

ophidian venoms has been reported (ZELLER, 1950a; JOHNSON et al., 1953; SCHIRIPA and SCHENBERG, 1964, 1974; BRISBOIS et al., 1968). Also, PEREIRA and LIMA (1971) reported that the well-known phosphodiesterase is biologically and biochemically differentiated from ATPase on the basis of a disproportional distribution among venoms (Table 10). However, the existence of ATPase in venom is still doubtful, because PFLEIDERER and ORTANDERL (1962) showed that during purification the ratio of the two activities of phosphodiesterase and ATPase remains constant and concluded that both activities are intrinsic properties of the same enzyme. Similar results have also been obtained by BOMAN (1959) and SUZUKI et al. (1960a).

For the purpose of isolating a particular enzyme, a venom must be found with a high concentration of that enzyme and a low concentration of the others. The levels and relative amounts of the four enzymes, endonuclease, phosphodiesterase, 5′-nucleotidase, and nonspecific phosphomonoesterase, in crotalid and elapid venoms are presented in Table 11 (RICHARDS et al., 1965). These data show that *N. nigricollis* venom is unusually high in the nonspecific phosphatase. Since this enzyme is extremely difficult to separate from phosphodiesterase, *Naja* venom can be ruled out as a source of the latter enzyme. This venom is also poor in 5′-nucleotidase and endonuclease. In the four remaining venoms, all obtained from members of the pit viper family, the levels of the different enzymes vary in roughly the same manner from venom to venom. *Bothrops atrox* and *C. adamanteus* are relatively rich in enzymes, whereas *A. piscivorus* and *C. atrox* are poor. Another example showing a different content of phosphatases is the *Bungarus multicinctus*. This venom contains little exonuclease, although 5′-nucleotidase and nonspecific phosphomonoesterase are normally present (SUZUKI and IWANAGA, 1960a). In summary, the differing quantities of the four enzymes contained in venoms must be considered when isolating a particular enzyme, for example, phosphodiesterase, an enzyme widely used for the structural studies of nucleic acid and its related substances.

Table 11. Levels of enzymes in five snake venoms[a] (RICHARDS et al., 1965)

Species of venom	Units of enzyme × 10^3 per mg dry venom				Ratio of enzymes: Phosphodiesterase = 1.0		
	Phosphodiesterase	Nonspecific phosphatase	5'-Nucleotidase	Endonuclease	Nonspecific phosphatase	5'-Nucleotidase	Endonuclease
Agkistrodon piscivorus	7.8	0.55	495	3.3	0.070	64	0.42
Bothrops atrox	36	1.8	1070	3.4	0.050	30	0.095
Crotalus adamanteus	25	1.3	1390	8.8	0.052	56	0.35
Crotalus atrox	8.7	0.39	860	2.8	0.045	99	0.32
Naja nigricollis	17	54	360	1.1	3.2	21	0.065

[a] The following substrates were used for enzyme assay; calcium bis-p-nitrophenyl phosphate for phosphodiesterase (unit = μmoles p-nitrophenol per min), sodium p-nitrophenyl phosphate (unit = μmoles p-nitrophenol per min), 5'-AMP for 5'-nucleotidase (unit = μmoles inorganic phosphate per min), and DNA for endonuclease (unit = amount of enzyme giving an increase in absorbancy at 260 nm of 1.0 per min.

1. Endonuclease

Although DELEZENNE and MOREL (1919) and TABORDA et al. (1952) described the presence of both ribonuclease and deoxyribonuclease in snake venom, little attention was paid to these enzymes until the purification of an endonuclease from *Bothrops atrox* by GEORGATSOS and LASKOWSKI (1962). It is now known that certain venoms contain an endonuclease with an optimum at pH 5.0 (HAESSLER and CUNNINGHAM, 1957) in addition to phosphodiesterase with an optimum at pH 8.9. These venoms are as follows: *A. piscivorus*, *Bothrops atrox*, *C. adamanteus*, *C. atrox*, *N. nigricollis* (GEORGATSOS and LASKOWSKI, 1962), *Vipera russelli* (MCLENNAN and LANE, 1968a), *Naja oxiana* (VASILENKO and RAIT, 1975), and *T. flavoviridis* (MAENO, 1962). Since the well-known venom phosphodiesterase also hydrolyzes both double- and single-stranded DNAs and ribosomal and transfer RNAs, the activity of endonuclease in crude venom must be carefully estimated under the following conditions (GEORGATSOS and LASKOWSKI, 1962): the substrate consists of calf thymus DNA, 0.04 mg/ml in 0.2 M sodium acetate buffer, pH 5.0; 3 ml substrate and 1 ml enzyme (about 20 μg of *C. adamanteus* venom) are mixed and transferred to a spectrophotometer cuvette, in which they are incubated at 37° C. Changes in A_{260} and A_{330} are followed against a blank of substrate and water until A_{330} begins to increase at a substantial rate. If this occurs before enough points have been recorded to determine a strainght line for A_{260} against time, the assay is repeated using a more diluted venom. Satisfactory results are obtained with dilutions of between 1:75 and 1:110, under which conditions A_{330} remains relatively stable for 1–2 h. A unit of endonuclease is defined as the amount of enzyme giving an increase in absorbance at 260 nm of 1.0 min.

An endonuclease of the venom of *Bothrops atrox* has been purified ~1000-fold from 42% acetone precipitate (WILLIAMS et al., 1961), a by-product of the preparation of venom phosphodiesterase. The purified enzyme can split both RNA and DNA at a similar rate and has an optimum activity at pH 5.0 and requires no magnesium. It is stable at pH 6.0 but loses more than half of its activity at pH 4.0 when boiled for 30 s or when it is left at 4° C for 72 h. The enzyme is most stable at pH 8.0. This endonuclease acts on DNA and produces predominantly tri or higher oligonucleotides, all of which terminate in 3′-monoesterified phosphate. At the early stages of digestion, dGpGp = deoxyguanylyl-(3′→5′)-deoxyguanylyl-(3′)-phosphate is the most susceptible bond. As the digestion progresses the specificity relative to the adjacent bases decreases and the length of the substrate chain becomes more significant. After digestion is completed, fragments are obtained in which all four bases occur in terminal positions in an almost random distribution. A ribonuclease that proved to be specific for RNA was purified from *N. oxiana* (VASILENKO and RAIT, 1975). The enzyme has a molecular weight of 15,900 and is activated by magnesium ions. It does not show any preference on base splitting. The products of RNA hydrolysis are 5′-phosphoric esters of oligonucleotides containing between two and six base residues.

2. Phosphodiesterase

Of the four phosphatases contained in snake venoms, phosphodiesterase is one of the most well-known enzymes. It has been studied to permit its use as a tool for sequencing or characterizing oligonucleotides and polynucleotides. This enzyme, also

Table 12. Phosphodiesterase activity in various venoms (Kocholaty et al., 1971)

Venom	Enzyme activity[a]	Venom	Enzyme activity[a]
Crotalidae		Viperidae	
A. bilineatus	82	*Bitis arietans*	12
A. c. mokeson	0	*Bitis gavonica*	18
A. p. piscivorus	47	*Echis carinatus*	16
A. rhodostoma	26	*V. r. formosensis*	78
B. atrox asper	50	*V. russellii*	59
C. adamanteus	84		
C. atrox	31	Elapidae	
C. d. durissus	52	*B. caeruleus*	0
C. d. terrificus	64	*B. fasciatus*	0
C. h. horridus	23	*B. multicinctus*	0
C. scutulatus	23	*Micrurus f. fulvius*	18
C. v. helleri	36	*N. melanoleuca*	19
C. u. viridus	52	*N. naja naja*	19
Sistrurus m. barbouri	2	*N. naja kaouthia*	29
T. flavoviridis	48	*Ophiophagus hannah*	35

[a] Determined using calcium bis-p-nitrophenyl phosphate as substrate and expressed in units per mg venom equal to ΔA_{440} min × 1000/mg protein.

termed venom exonuclease (Laskowski, 1966, 1971), is widely distributed in various venoms from all three families of venomous snakes (Table 12). Hydrophiid and colubrid venoms also possess this enzyme (Mebs, 1970; Setoguchi et al., 1968; Tu and Toom, 1971). However, the venoms of the *Bungarus* family show little or no phosphodiesterase activity. As described previously, Uzawa (1932) first found the enzyme in the venoms of *T. flavoviridis* and *A. halys blomhoffii* by using diphenylphosphate as the substrate. Later Gulland and Jackson (1938) detected phosphodiesterase activity in the venoms of 12 snakes. Venom phosphodiesterase is characterized by its successive removal of 5′-mononucleotide units from the polynucleotide chain in stepwise fashion from the end that bears a free 3′-hydroxyl-group; pN_2pN_1pN or N_2pN_1pN. Some snake venoms contain more than one exonuclease. The venom of *C. adamanteus* has three chromatographically separable enzymes with activities parallel to those of DNase (Boman and Kaletta, 1957). Similar findings were made in the venoms of *N. naja* (Suzuki and Iwanaga, 1958c) and *A. halys blomhoffii* (Suzuki et al., 1960a). The three enzymes from the latter venom exhibit a similar behavior to optimal pH, stability, and group reagents, but behave differently to magnesium ions. Their hydrolytic activity also differs somewhat from deoxyoligonucleotides and yeast RNA.

Assay Method I (Björk, 1963). *Principle.* The hydrolysis of calcium di-p-nitrophenylphosphate yiels p-nitrophenylphosphate and assumes a yellow color due to the liberation of p-nitrophenylate (400 nm = 16200) at alkaline pH.

Procedure. The reaction mixture contains 1.0 ml 0.1 M Tris-HCl buffer, pH 8.9, 1.2 ml 0.001 M calcium di-p-nitrophenylphosphate, 0.2 ml enzyme solution, and adjusted to 3 ml with water. The mixture is incubated at 37° C and the reaction is stopped by the addition of 3 ml 0.05 N NaOH. The absorbancy is determined at 400 nm against a blank containing all components but the enzyme solution. A unit of the enzyme is defined as the amount of enzyme liberating 1 μmole of p-nitrophenol/min.

Method II (RAZZELL, 1963). The principle is the same as that of Method I except that p-nitrophenyl thymidine-5′-phosphate is used as substrate. The assay is performed in a cuvette containing 100 μmoles Tris-HCl buffer, pH 8.9, and 0.5 μmole substrate in a total volume of 1.0 ml. Prior to the addition of enzyme, the cuvette is equilibrated at 37° C. On addition of enzyme the increase in absorbance is measured at 400 nm. An increase in absorbance of 1.2 units is equivalent to the hydrolysis of 1.0 μmole substrate.

Comments. Although the above two methods are used by many researchers to determine venom phosphodiesterase activity, the following assay methods are also available. Since venom phosphodiesterase hydrolizes NAD, its activity can be assayed by measuring the decrease of absorption at 340 nm after reduction of NAD with alcohol dehydrogenase (FUTAI and MIZUNO, 1967). Another method is based on the spectrophotometric determination of adenosine released from adenylyl-(3′,5′)-adenosine (ApA) ($Km = 83$ uM), guanylyl-(3′,5′)-adenosine (GpA), adenylyl-(3′,5′)-guanosine (ApG) ($Km = 23$ uM). Adenosine is liberated from the dinucleoside monophosphates used as substrates following the decrease in absorbance at 265 nm after addition of an excess of adenosine deaminase (IPATA and FELICIOLI, 1969). Furthermore, instead of p-nitrophenyl thymidine-5′-phosphate, thymidine 5′-(2,4-dinitrophenyl) phosphate has been used as substrate especially for the kinetic studies on venom phosphodiesterase, since the liberation of 2,4-dinitrophenol (ε 400 nm = 14450) follows directly under both acidic and alkaline conditions (VON TIGERSTROM and SMITH, 1969).

Purification. Venom phosphodiesterase has been isolated by many investigators, in particular LAKSOWSKI and co-workers. Several methods for preparing the purified enzyme have been described (BUTLER, 1955; RAZZELL, 1963; LASKOWSKI, 1966; PRIVAT DE GARILHE, 1964). The major goal of purification has been directed toward removing the contaminating 5′-nucleotidase and phosphomonoesterase. A successful and widely used step was introduced by SINSHEIMER and KOERNER (1952). Monophosphatases are precipitated at pH 4 with a low concentration of acetone and the remaining exonuclease is precipitated with a higher acetone concentration. Commercially available preparations essentially represent this stage and contain per unit of exonuclease: 10^{-4} unit of 5′-nucleotidase, 10^{-3} unit of nonspecific phosphomonoesterase and about the same amount of endonuclease. Further purification is required for removal of these contaminants when the enzyme preparation is used for sequence analysis of polynucleotides. Since the acetone precipitation step is not applicable to all venoms, the choice of method depends on the availability of the starting venom. The venoms applicable to the acetone precipitation are as follows: *C. adamanteus* (RICHARDS et al., 1967), *Bothrops atrox* (BJÖRK, 1963), *Hemachatus haemachatus* (BJÖRK, 1961), *Vipera lebetina* (NIKOL'SKAYA et al., 1963), *Vipera aspis* (BALLARIO et al., 1977), and *A. halys blomhoffii* (SUZUKI and IWANAGA, 1958c). It is important to note that the method developed for purifying phosphodiesterase in some venoms is not always applicable to other venoms. The following procedure is a conventional method for isolating the enzyme from *C. adamanteus* venom.

Procedure (DOLAPCHIEV et al., 1974). *Preliminary Inactivation of 5′-nucleotidase.* Suspension 5 g *C. adamanteus* venom (from the Miami Serpentarium, Miami, Florida) in 225 ml water is stirred for 1 h at room temperature. A small amount of insoluble material is removed by centrifugation at 5000 *g* for 15 min. To the solution 225 ml 0.2 M acetic acid is added with stirring. The mixture is incubated at 37° C for 3 h to inactivate 5′-nucleotidase; the mixture is then cooled to 2° C.

Table 13. Summary of purification procedure of *C. adamanteus* venom phosphodiesterase (DOLAPCHIEV et al., 1974)

Step of purification	Protein A_{280}	Total activity units	Specific activity U/A_{280}	Yield %
Pretreated venom	5900	157	0.027	100
Acetone	586	150	0.26	96
Con-A Sepharose	26.5	75	2.8	48
Bio-Gel P-2-0	9.8	69	7.0	44
QAE Sephadex A-50	5.7	58	10.2	37

Step 1. Acetone (362.5 ml) precooled to −17° C is added slowly to keep the temperature below 5° C. The mixture is stirred for 30 min in an ice bath and then centrifuged at 0° C at 13000 *g* for 30 min. After the supernatant is transferred to an alcohol bath (−17° C) and 6.5 ml 1 M sodium acetate is added to attain pH 4.0, 43.5 ml 1 M sodium acetate, pH 4.0, are added and stirred for 15 min. Acetone (22.5 ml) is added and the mixture is stirred at −17° C for 60 min. The mixture is then centrifuged at 13000 *g* for 30 min at −17° C. The supernatant is returned to the alcohol bath (−17° C) and 115 ml acetone (−17° C) is added. Stirring is continued for 30 min and the precipitate containing exonuclease is collected by centrifugation (13000 *g*, −17° C, 30 min). It is dissolved in 20 ml 0.2 M sodium acetate, pH 6.0, dialyzed overnight at 4° C against 1 liter 0.2 M sodium acetate, pH 6.0, and clarified by brief centrifugation at 4° C.

Step 2. The dialyzed solution (25–30 ml) is applied to a column (35 × 1.5 cm) of Concanavalin-A Sepharose (Pharmacia Fine Chemicals, Uppsala), previously equilibrated with 0.2 M sodium acetate, pH 6.0, at room temperature (22° C). The elution is first made by the original buffer at a flow rate of 20 ml/h, until the absorbance of the effluent at 280 nm falls to 0.05. At this time 0.05 M α-methyl-D-mannopyranoside in equilibrating buffer is added. (This elutes endonuclease and nonspecific phosphatase with about 10–12% of exonuclease.) When absorbance at 280 nm falls below 0.1, the buffer is changed to 0.05 M sodium phosphate, pH 7.2, containing 1 M NaCl and 0.3 M α-methyl-D-mannopyranoside. After 30 ml of this solution is passed through the column, the flow is stopped for 6 h, and is resumed again with a flow rate reduced to 10 ml/h. The fractions (∼ 120 ml) containing exonuclease are collected.

Step 3. The exonuclease eluted in step 2 is dialyzed at 4° C against Ficoll 400 (Pharmacia Fine Chemicals) almost to dryness. The dialysis tubing is washed with a total of 10 ml 0.2 M sodium acetate, pH 6.0, and clarified at 4° C by centrifugation at 4000 rpm for 10 min. The solution is charged on a column of Bio-Gel P-200 (80 × 2.5 cm), equilibrated with 0.2 M sodium acetate, pH 6.0, at room temperature. The elution is made with the equilibration buffer at a flow rate of 15 ml/h and 3 ml fractions are collected. The exonuclease is eluted quantitatively in the first large peak (tubes 40–65), the contents of which are pooled.

Step 4. The collected material from step 3 is concentrated to dryness on Ficoll at 4° C, dissolved in a minimal amount of 0.01 M Tris-HCl buffer, pH 8.5, and dialyzed at 4° C against the same buffer for 6–8 h. The dialyzed solution is applied to a column (30 × 1.1 cm) of QAE-Sephadex, equilibrated with 0.01 M Tris-HCl buffer, pH 8.5. The elution is made at 4° C with the same buffer at a flow rate of 20 ml/h. The exonuclease appears in the first fraction, showing a constant specific activity across the peak. The enzyme is divided for convenience into samples of 1 unit each and lyophilized or freezed. Lyophilization results in a loss of about 10% of activity; little loss occurs on further storage at −17° C.

Table 13 summarizes the purification procedure. An overall purification of the enzyme is about 350-fold with a yield of 37%. The preparation is homogeneous on disc polyacrylamide-gel electrophoresis at pH 4 without sodium dodecylsulfate (SDS) and at pH 7.0 with SDS.

Comments. New methods for the purification of venom phosphodiesterase include an affinity chromatography technique (FRISCHAUF and ECKSTEIN, 1973; TAT-

SUKI et al., 1975), preparative electrophoresis on a slab gel of polyacrylamide (BALLARIO et al., 1977), and DEAE-cellulose chromatography with an unusual alkaline condition (PHILIPPS, 1975). However, the desired affinity chromatography with 0-(4-nitrophenyl)-0′-phenylthiophosphate ester coupled to the CNBr-activated Sepharose 4B (CUATRECASAS, 1970) to purify exonuclease from *Bothrops atrox* venom does not result in complete purification. A method combined with phosphocellulose chromatography must be used. Furthermore, several methods have been proposed for removal of contaminating 5′-nucleotidase from a commercially available enzyme; for example, 5′-nucleotidase can be selectively inactivated with $ZnCl_2$, a method used for purifying exonuclease from viper venom (NIKOL'SKAYA et al., 1963). A method involving the use of a Dowex 50 column was devised by KELLER (1964) and SULKOWSKI and LASKOWSKI (1971). By these procedures, the contaminating 5′-nucleotidase activity is reduced by 100- to 1000-folds without loss of exonuclease.

Physicochemical Properties. Very little is known about the chemical and physical properties of venom phosphodiesterase. The enzyme is heat labile and inactivated at temperatures higher than 50° C. It is stable in the pH range of 6–9, but outside these pH limits activity rapidly decline (BJÖRK, 1963). The enzyme from *Bothrops atrox* venom seems to be a glycoprotein consisting of a single chain with a molecular weight of 130000 (FRISCHAUF and ECKSTEIN, 1973). The molecular weight of the enzyme isolated from *C. adamanteus* was estimated to be 115000 (PHILIPPS, 1975). It has a basic property showing the isoelectric point around pH 9.

Enzymatic Properties. Venom phosphodiesterase (calcium di-p-nitrophenylphosphate as substrate) is active in the pH range of 8–9.9 with a peak at pH 8.4–9.2. However, when deoxyoligonucleotides or RNA (yeast) is used as the substrate, its optimal pH is found at pH 10–11 (SUZUKI et al., 1960). The enzyme requires 15 mM magnesium ions to show optimal activity even with the synthetic substrates (PHILIPPS, 1975; SUZUKI et al., 1960; RAZZELL and KHORANA, 1959). Its activity is inhibited by reducing agents such as cysteine, GSH, thioglycolate, and ascorbic acid, 50% inhibition is observed at 7.5×10^{-3} M, 1.5×10^{-3} M, 1.5×10^{-3} M, and 4×10^{-3} M, respectively. EDTA is also a potent inhibitor and 50% inhibition occurs at ~8–12.5×10^{-5} M and is reversible by the addition of excess magnesium ions (RAZZELL and KHORANA, 1959; SUZUKI et al., 1960). Of a variety of cations tested, only copper inhibits the activity; this effect is easily demonstrated at 10^{-4} M. Although virtually nothing is known about the properties of the enzyme active site, BROWN and BOWLES (1965) showed that venom phosphodiesterase requires the following for activity: intact tryptophan and tyrosine residues, SH groups, and S-S bridges.

The synthetic substrates most rapidly hydrolyzed have been found to be p-nitrophenyl thymidine-5′-phosphate and thymidine 5′-(2,4-dinitrophenyl)phosphate. In general, diesters of deoxyribonucleotides are hydrolyzed faster than those of ribonucleotides. Other details of specificity toward various synthetic substrates are shown in Table 14 (RAZZELL, 1963). In addition, the enzyme hydrolyzes 3′,5′-cyclic AMP (SUZUKI et al., 1960), uridine-2′,3′-phosphate, and cyclo-pTpT, cyclo-pTpTpT, and cyclo-pTpTpTpT, which do not have any terminal group. This indicates that venom phosphodiesterase has an endonucleolytic activity in addition to the exonuclease activity. According to MCLENNAN and LANE (1968a), there is about one endonucleolytic cleavage for every 15 exonucleolytic cleavages during the 1st h of hydrolysis of wheat embryo ribosomal RNA by venom phosphodiesterase. More-

Table 14. Substrate specificity of venom (*C. adamenteus*) phosphodiesterase (RAZZELL and KHORANA, 1959)

Substrate	V_{max}	K_m
	µmoles/h/mg	M
p-Nitrophenyl-pT	36500	5.0×10^{-4}
pTpT	6840	2.1×10^{-4}
p-Nitrophenyl-pU	1275	5.4×10^{-4}
TpT	278	5.3×10^{-4}
Di-p-nitrophenyl phosphate	39	7.7×10^{-4}
Benzyl-p-nitrophenyl phosphate	315	6.8×10^{-3}
Methyl-p-nitrophenyl phosphate	714	1.2×10^{-2}

over, this enzyme digests poly(adenosine diphosphate ribose) endonucleolytically as shown in Figure 14 (MATSUBARA et al., 1970). Other compounds hydrolyzed by venom phosphodiesterase are ATP, ADP, adenosine-5′-tetraphosphate, dCDP-choline (SUGINO, 1957), TDP-rhamnose (OKAZAKI, 1959), UDP-glucose, GDP-mannose, dephosphocoenzyme A, NAD, NADP, FAD, di(thymidine-5′)-pyrophosphate, di (adenosine-5′)-pyrophosphate, and di(adenosine-5′)-triphosphate (RAZZELL, 1963); this indicates that it has the intrinsic property of the nucleotide pyrophosphatase activity (DOLAPCHIEV et al., 1974). Oligonucleotides bearing 3′-phosphate end groups are hydrolyzed even more slowly than di(p-nitrophenyl)-phosphate. No differences have been found between the purine or pyrimidine oligonucleotides. A 5′,5′-phosphodiester linkage appears to be equivalent to a 5′,3′ linkage. These observations suggest that the basic element to which the enzyme binds for hydrolytic action is a "nucleoside 5′-phosphoryl" group (Fig. 15).

Venom phosphodiesterase is capable of hydrolyzing both DNA and RNA (MILLER et al., 1970; HOLLEY et al., 1964). Double-strand DNA is a better substrate than denatured DNA. With native DNA a two-phase reaction is observed. The initial very rapid rate is independent of NaCl concentration. After about one-third of the linkages has been hydrolyzed, the rate slows down to that of denatured DNA and becomes salt dependent (WILLIAMS et al., 1961; BJÖRK, 1967). With RNA as substrate, native rRNA and sRNA are resistant to 60 µg/ml commercial enzyme (HADJIOLOV et al., 1967), but after heat denaturation rRNA is readily and sRNA partially digested (COUSIN, 1963). RICHARDS et al. (1967) and WECHTER (1967) showed that venom exonuclease is capable of hydrolyzing dinucleoside monophosphate with one or both nucleosides containing arabinose, indicating that it is totally blind to sugar, at least in a qualitative sense (OGILVIE and HRUSKA, 1976). However, oligonucleotide containing glucosylated hydroxymethyl cytosine found in T even phage DNA blocks the action of the enzyme. As to the more detailed base specificity of this enzyme, the reader is referred to the excellent review by LASKOWSKI (1971). Although venom phosphodiesterase shows a broad specificity towards a number of nucleotide derivatives as described above, its most characteristic mode of action is in the stepwise degradation from the end of the oligonucleotide chain bearing a 3′-hydroxyl group, resulting in the successive release of nucleoside-5′-phosphate units. Thus, the enzyme is very useful for determining the sequences of both ribo and deoxyribooligonucleotides and identifying α and ω terminal nucleotides.

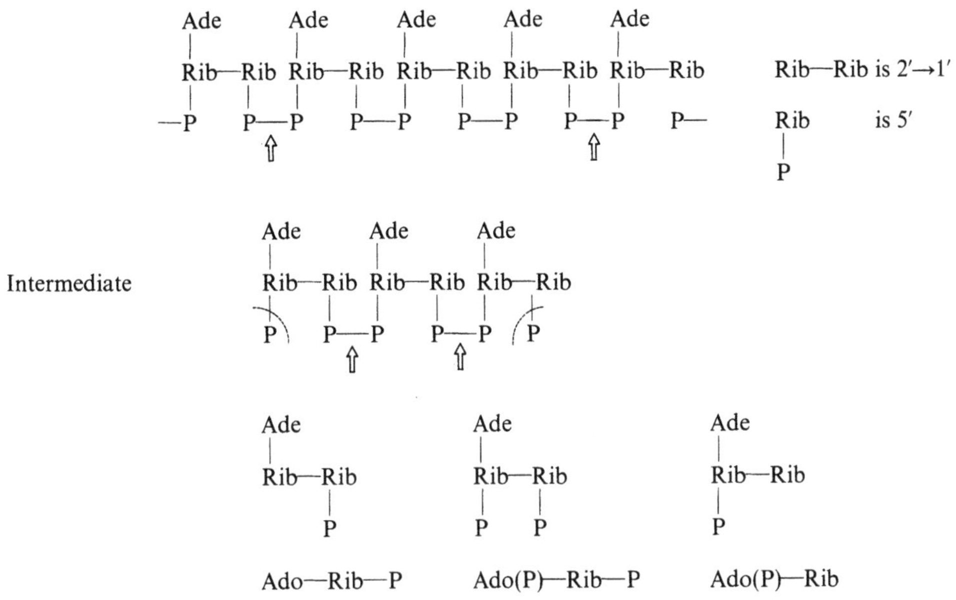

Fig. 14. Cleavage sites of poly (ADP-ribose) with venom phosphodiesterase (*C. adamanteus*). The *arrows* indicate cleavage at pyrophosphate. *Dotted lines* indicate release of terminal phosphate by alkaline phosphomonoesterase. Ade, adenine; Rib, ribose; P, phosphate; Ado, adenosine (MATSUBARA et al., 1970)

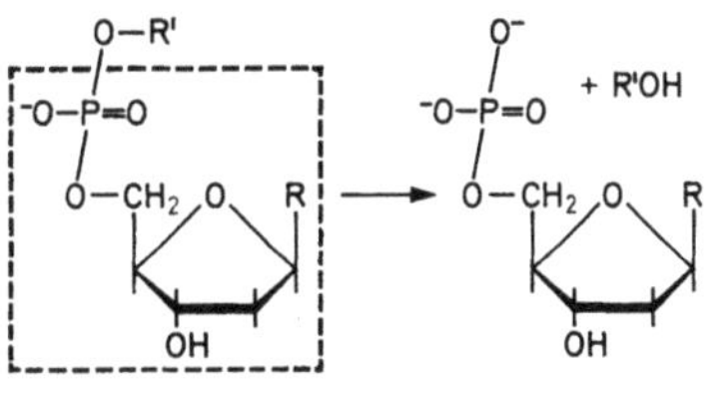

Fig. 15. A basic structural element to which venom phosphodiesterase binds for the hydrolysis of phosphodiester (RAZZELL and KHORANA, 1959)

3. 5'-Nucleotidase

A specific phosphomonoesterase, 5'-nucleotidase is found in all venoms so far examined. The enzyme activity of the elapid venoms is relatively low compared to viperid and crotalid venoms (MEBS, 1970). This enzyme was first noted by GULLAND and JACKSON in 1938. It hydrolyzes specifically phosphate monoester, which links with a 5'-position of DNA and RNA. On dialysis of crude venom (0.2–0.5%, w/w), the activity increases two or three times that of the nondialyzed sample, suggesting that some substance, probably zinc ions, which are abundant in crude venom, inhibits the activity (SUZUKI and IWANAGA, 1958). Compared to venom phosphodiesterase, this enzyme is relatively unstable on heat and acid treatments and thus has been applied to inactivate 5′-nucleotidase contaminated in the preparation of venom phosphodiesterase (SINSHEIMER and KOERNER, 1952; SUZUKI and IWANAGA, 1958; SULKOWSKI and LASKOWSKI, 1971; BJÖRK, 1964; NIKOL'SKAYA et al., 1963).

Assay Method (SUZUKI and IWANAGA, 1958). The reaction mixture, containing 4 μmoles 5′-AMP, 0.1 ml 0.3 M $MgCl_2$, 0.5 ml 0.2 M glycine-NaOH buffer, pH 8.5, and 0.2 ml enzyme solution in a total volume of 0.9 ml, is incubated at 37° C for 15 min. The liberated inorganic phosphate is estimated by the method of ALLEN (1940).

Comments. In addition to the above methods, the following microassays for 5′-nucleotidase have been developed: (a) measurement of radioactive adenosine separated from the substrate by paper chromatography (MURRAY and FRIEDRICHS, 1969); (b) spectrophotometric measurement of the rate of conversion of adenosine to inosine in the presence of adenosine deaminase (IPATA, 1967); (c) measurement of ammonia produced in the adenosine deaminase reaction (BELFIELD et al., 1970; BOOTSMA et al., 1972), and (d) microradioisotopic determination of the ^{14}C-adenosine produced with a small alumina column, which binds tightly the substrate under alkaline conditions (SURAN, 1973; GENTRY and OLSSON, 1975).

Purification. Venom 5′-nucleotidase has been purified from the venoms of *A. piscivorus* (HURST and BUTLER, 1951; HEPPEL and HILMOE, 1951), *A. halys blomhoffii* (SUZUKI and IWANAGA, 1958b), *C. adamanteus* (WILLIAMS et al., 1961; TATSUKI et al., 1975), *Hemachatus haemachatus* (BJÖLK, 1964), *Bothrops atrox* (SULKOWSKI et al., 1963), *Vipera lebetina* (NIKOL'SKAYA et al., 1964), and *N. naja atra* (CHEN and LO, 1968). The enzyme with highest purity was prepared from *Bothrops atrox* venom, using 30 g crude venom. However, the procedure is tedious and the method requires a large amount of expensive lyophilized venom. The affinity chromatography developed recently in our laboratory for the preparation of venom phosphodiesterase almost free from 5′-nucleotidase is also applicable to separate venom 5′-nucleotidase. The method is described below.

Procedure (TATSUKI et al., 1975). The lyophilized venom (10 mg) of *C. adamanteus* dissolved in 6 ml 0.05 M sodium acetate buffer, pH 7.0, is applied to a small column (1.8 × 3 cm) of NAD^+-Sepharose 4B (prepared exactly according to the method of MOSBACH et al., 1972), previously equilibrated with the same buffer. Stepwise elution is started with 100 ml 0.05 M sodium acetate buffer, pH 7.0; fractions of 3 ml per tube are collected at 4° C, at a flow rate of 25 ml/h. The elution buffer is successively replaced with 60 ml 0.1 M acetate buffer, pH 7.0, and finally with 80 ml 0.2 M sodium bicarbonate buffer, pH 8.9, containing 1 mM NADH. The elution pattern is shown in Figure 16. The first protein peak contains phosphodiesterase and 5′-nucleotidase is desorbed on elution with the buffer containing 1 mM NADH. A final washing with 1.0 N NH_4OH elutes no further activity. The used column can be regenerated by washing first with 0.5 M NaCl and then with the equilibration buffer. The yield of the 5′-nucleotidase preparation, using the affinity column, is not very great, 23–32% recovery of the total activity in the venom. Moreover, the preparation contains a small amount of phosphodiesterase. However, this method is very simple and rapid and also applicable for other venoms including *A. halys blomhoffii*, *Bothrops atrox*, and *A. contortrix mokasen*.

Comments. For the further removal of contaminating phosphodiesterase in the above preparation, DEAE-cellulose chromatography according to the method of BJÖRK (1964) is recommended.

Physicochemical Properties. Because of a very low content of the enzyme in snake venom and the high price of the starting material, no substantial preparation has so far been made. Thus, there is no information about the chemical nature and physical properties. CHEN and LO (1968) reported that 5′-nucleotidase isolated from *N. naja*

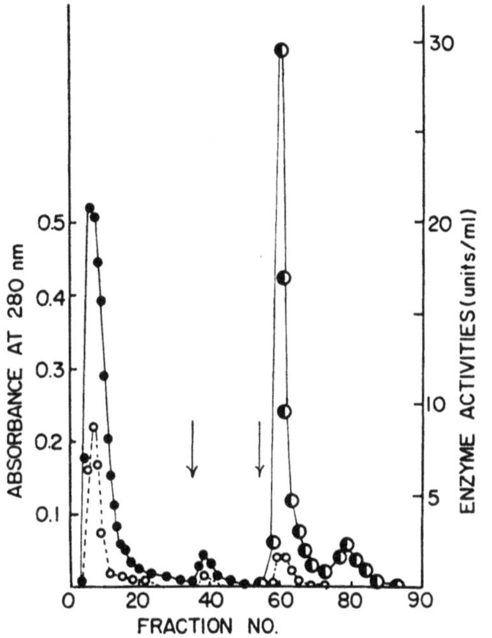

Fig. 16. Chromatography of *C. adamanteus* venom on an NAD^+-Sepharose 4B column. After equilibration with 0.05 M acetate buffer 10 mg venom was applied to the column (1.8 × 3 cm), pH 7.0. Stepwise elution was carried out with 100 ml equilibration buffer, 60 ml 0.1 M acetate buffer, pH 7.0, and 80 ml 0.2 M $NaHCO_3$ buffer, pH 8.7, containing 1 mM NADH. Fractions of 3 ml per tube were collected at 4° C and at a flow rate of 25 ml/h. Absorbance at 280 nm (●), phosphodiesterase (○), and 5′-nucleotidase (◐) (TATSUKI et al., 1975)

atra venom has a molecular weight of 100000. This value seems reasonable, because venom 5′-nucleotidase activity of *Bothrops atrox* (SULKOWSKI et al., 1963) and *A. halys blomhoffii* (SUZUKI and IWANAGA, 1960a) appears in the void volume fraction on a Sephadex G-100 column. The enzyme seems to consist of a glycoprotein (OSHIMA and IWANAGA, 1969).

Enzymatic Properties. The purified enzyme is unstable below pH 5.0 and on heat treatment at 55° C. It is stabilized in the presence of 1 mM 3′-AMP and 1 mM magnesium ions. The pH-optimum for 5′-nucleotidase from different snake species has not been fully agreed upon because of discrepancies probably due to differences in degree of purification and in assay conditions. A maximum activity is shown in pH range 7.8–9.5 and the enzyme does not require any metals to show this maximum activity. However, with EDTA (10^{-3} M) the enzyme is completely inactivated after less than 5 h at both pH 7.3 and 8.9. This inactivation seems to be reversible. The enzyme activity is also sensitive to zinc ions but is not influenced by oxidizing or reducing agents or by SH-reagents (BJÖRK, 1964; CAMPOS and YARLEQUE, 1974).

The substrate specificity of venom 5′-nucleotidase is summarized in Table 15. Different mononucleotides are hydrolyzed at different rates and 5′-AMP is found to be the most susceptible substrate. The Km values on 5′-AMP and nicotinamide mononucletide (NMN) are 10^{-4} M and 8×10^{-4} M, respectively (HEPPEL and HIL-

Table 15. Relative rate of hydrolysis of different mononucleotides by 5′-nucleotidase

Substrate	Venoms		
	B. atrox[a]	*T. flavoviridis*[b]	*A. halys blomhoffii*[c]
5′-AMP	100[d]	100[d]	100[d]
5′-IMP	41	–	65.3
5′-UMP	36	38.9	52.2
5′-CMP	89	54.8	90.2
5′-GMP	42	32	87.0
5′-dGMP	33	–	37.0
5′-dAMP	39	–	58.6
5′-dCMP	62	–	55.8
5′-dTMP	72	41.2	49.6
NMN	15	–	–
FMN	0	–	0
2′,3′-AMP	0	–	0
5′-hydroxy-UMP	–	70.9	–
5-dimethylamino-UMP	–	0	–
3-methyl-UMP	–	38.4	–
4-deoxy-UMP	–	0	–
4-dimethyl-CMP	–	88.0	–
6-methyl-AMP	–	16.5	–
6-dimethyl-AMP	–	24.1	–
Spongo-UMP	–	7.0	–
5-bromo-UMP	–	16.7	–
p-nitrophenyl phosphate	0	–	0
β-Glycerophosphate	–	–	0.5
Choline phosphate	–	–	0
Ribose-5-P	0	–	1.1
Glucose-1-P	–	–	0

[a] SULKOWSKI et al. (1963).
[b] MIZUNO et al. (1961).
[c] SUZUKI et al. (1961).
[d] Phosphate liberation with 5′-AMP is assumed to be 100.

MOE, 1951). The enzyme does not act on ribose-5′-phosphate, 3′-AMP, p-nitrophenyl phosphate, all of which are hydrolyzed by venom nonspecific phosphomonoesterase, and no release of inorganic phosphate from ATP, dpXp, dpXpXp by this enzyme has been observed.

4. Nonspecific Phosphomonoesterase

Snake venoms contain two nonspecific phosphomonoesterases, which show an optimal pH at 5.0 and at 8.5. They seem to be catalysts with a different enzyme entity, because some of the venoms contain both acid and alkaline phosphatases, whereas others contain only one type (TU and CHUA, 1966). *A. acutus* venom shows only acid phosphatase activity, whereas the venom of *Ophiophagus hannah*, only alkaline. Many venoms belonging to Elapidae, Hydrophiidae, Viperidae, and Crotalidae show both acid and alkaline phosphatase activities. The presence of phosphomonoesterase was first reported by YOSHIDA (1941) in the venom of *Trimeresurus flavoviridis* (Habu). Later many investigators found that the venom hydrolyzes a number of biologically important compounds such as ATP, glucose-l-phosphate, FMN, and NMN (ZELLER, 1950b; KORNBERG and PRICER, 1950). In spite of the common occurrence of the enzyme in snake venoms, it has not been completely purified and therefore little is known about its physicochemical properties.

Assay Methods for Alkaline Phosphatase (SULKOWSKI et al., 1963). The enzyme is routinely determined with the use of p-nitrophenylphosphate as substrate, which is not hydrolyzed by 5′-nucleotidase. The reaction mixture contains 1.0 ml 0.1 M glycine-NaOH buffer, pH 9.5, 1.2 ml 0.001 M p-nitrophenylphosphate, 0.3 ml $MgCl_2$, 0.1 ml enzyme solution, and water up to 3.0 ml. The mixture is incubated at 37° C for 15 min and the reaction is terminated by adding 3 ml 0.05 N NaOH. The absorbancy is measured at 400 nm against a blank that contains all reagents except the enzyme. One unit of activity is defined as the amount of enzyme which liberates 1 μmole of p-nitrophenol (ε400 nm = 16200) per min.

Assay Method for Acid Phosphatase (TU and CHUA, 1966). The method is based on the work of HOFSTEE (1954). One-half ml 0.0036 M 0-carboxyphenylphosphate is placed into both the blank and the test cuvettes. To the blank cuvette 2.0 ml 0.15 M sodium acetate, pH 5.0, and 0.5 ml deionized water are added to reach a final volume of 3.0 ml. Thus, the final concentration for the substrate is 0.6 mM in 0.1 M buffer solution. The same amount of buffer is added to the test cuvette. At zero time, 0.5 ml venom solution is introduced and mixed by inverting the cuvette. The initial rate of hydrolysis of the substrate at 25° C is determined from the increase in absorbancy at 300 nm due to the liberation of salicylic acid. Venom concentration is adjusted to give a straight line at least for 5 min. One unit of acid phosphatase activity is equivalent to 1 μmole of the substrate (300 nm = 3500) hydrolyzed per min.

Purification. Nonspecific alkaline phosphatase from the venom of *Bothrops atrox* has been purified by acetone precipitation followed by a CM-cellulose column, $Ca_3(PO_4)_2$ gel treatment, gel-filtration on Sephadex G-100, and chromatography on a DEAE-cellulose column (SULKOWSKI et al., 1963). Through these procedures ~ 7.4 mg purified enzyme is obtained from 10 g lyophilized venom and an ~200-fold purification is achieved. The enzyme has also been partially purified from the venoms of *A. halys blomhoffii* (SUZUKI and IWANAGA, 1958b) and *N. naja atra* (SUZUKI and IWANAGA, 1958c). Also acid phosphatase has been partially purified from the venom of sea snake, *Lacticauda semifasciata* (UWATOKO-SETOGUCHI, 1970).

Enzymatic Properties. The purified *Bothrops atrox* enzyme has an alkaline pH optimum at pH 9.5. It is unstable on treatment with heat (55° C) or acid (<pH 4.0). The enzyme is activated by either magnesium ions (10^{-3} M) or calcium ions (10^{-3} M) and strongly inhibited by EDTA (10^{-4} M), cysteine (10^{-3} M) and zinc ions (10^{-3} M) (SUZUKI and IWANAGA, 1958). As shown in Table 16, this enzyme is responsible for hydrolysis of mononucleoside 3′,5′-phosphate. Of the 12 substrates tested only inorganic phosphate and uridine 2′,3′-phosphate are not hydrolyzed. Although the exact molecular weight of this enzyme is not known, an approximate molecular weight of 90000–100000 daltons is estimated from the data of the gel-filtration experiment (SULKOWSKI et al., 1963; SUZUKI and IWANAGA, 1960).

Venom acid phosphatase has the highest activity at pH 4.5–5.0 (TU and CHUA, 1966). It is inhibited by potassium fluoride (10^{-2} M) and EDTA (10^{-2} M), but zinc ions do not influence its activity. The acid phosphatase purified from the sea snake venom hydrolyzes p-nitrophenylphosphate (km = .59 mM), 2′-AMP, 3′-AMP, 5′-AMP, and ATP, but glucose-1-phosphate, glucose-6-phosphate and glycerophosphate, which are very susceptible to venom alkaline phosphatase, are resistant to it.

Table 16. Action of venom nonspecific phosphomonoesterase on various substrates (SULKOWSKI et al., 1963)

Substrate	*B. atrox* venom (relative activity, %)
5′-AMP	100
5′-dAMP	100
3′-AMP	80
Ribose-3-P	48
ATP	40
dXpYp	58
dpGp	26
FMN	80
NMN	40
PRPP[a]	130
PPi	0

[a] PRPP = 5-Phosphorylribose l-pyrophosphate.

5. "Paraoxonase" (0,0-Diethyl 0-p-Nitrophenyl Phosphate 0-p-Nitrophenyl Hydrolase)

Enzymes hydrolyzing paraoxon (the structure is shown below) have been found in mammalian serum by ALDRIDGE (1953), who also reported the enzyme to be present in many other tissues with maximum concentrations in the liver.

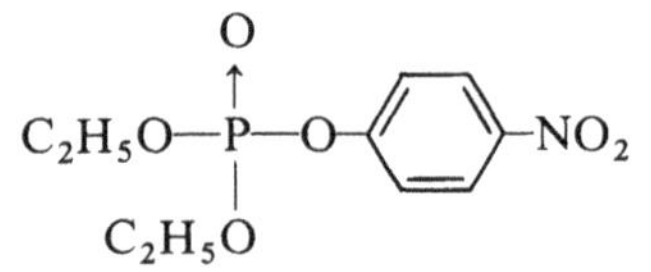

Diethyl p-nitrophenylphosphate (paraoxon)

This enzyme was first reported in snake venom by MENDE and MORENO (1975). Snake venoms seem to show marked species differences for the presence of "paraoxonase." Of four venoms (Russell's viper, *C. adamanteus*, *A. contortrix contortrix*, and *N. naja*) tested, only the venom of Russell's viper shows significant paraoxonase activity. *N. naja* venom exhibits the activity, but its level shows a specific activity of ~ 6% of Russell's viper venom.

Assay Method (MENDE and MORENO, 1975). The conditions for assay of "paraoxonase" are as follows: 0.1 ml enzyme solution, 50 μl 0.1 M paraoxon solution (dissolved in propylene glycol) and 0.85 ml 50 mM Tris-HCl buffer, pH 7.4, containing 5 mM $CaCl_2$. Hydrolysis rates are followed at 400 nm or at the isobestic wavelength of 348 nm (ARMSTRONG et al., 1966) in a Gilford 2000 spectrophotometer. One unit of activity is defined as the amount of enzyme which liberates 1 μmole of p-nitrophenol per min.

Purification (MENDE and MORENO, 1975). The separation of "paraoxonase" from the venom of Russell's viper can be done by gel filtration on Sephadex G-75 and chromatography on a phospho-cellulose column. Fractionation of the venom reveals separate phosphatase activities directed against p-nitrophenyl phosphate (phosphomonoesterase), bis-(p-nitrophenyl)phosphate (phosphodiesterase), 5′-AMP (5′-nucleotidase), and paraoxon. On gel filtration, the first three activities are eluted ahead of the latter. They could be resolved further by phospho-cellulose cation exchange chromatography. Although the purification of "paraoxonoase" has been performed, homogeneity of the isolated enzyme was not indicated.

Enzymatic Properties (MENDE and MORENO, 1975). The outstanding characteristic of venom "paraoxonase" is its extreme heat stability. This is in contrast to the phosphodiesterase, phosphomonoesterase, and 5′-nucleotidase reported to date in various snake venoms. The molecular weight of this enzyme is 9600, as estimated by gel filtration on Sephadex G-75. This enzyme, as all known enzymes of this type (MAZUR, 1946; MOUNTER, 1951; AUGUSTINSSON, 1954; ALDRIDGE, 1953), requires the presence of a divalent cation. Maximum activity is obtained in the presence of calcium ions (5 mM). In the presence of strontium ions (5 mM) the reaction rate is 50% of that of calcium ions; other divalent cations (Mg^{2+}, Zn^{2+}, Ba^{2+}, Ni^{2+}, Mn^{2+}, Cu^{2+}, Co^{2+}) effect slower activities. The enzyme activity is intact following incubation with iodoacetate (9 mM) or p-chloromercuribenzoate (5 mM). Only EDTA causes virtually total inhibition of the venom "paraoxonase" activity, which is fully restored on addition of excess calcium ions.

III. Enzymes Acting on Glycosyl Compounds

1. Hyaluronidase

Hyaluronidase is defined as an enzyme that catalyzes the cleavage of internal glycosidic bonds of certain acid mucopolysaccharides of animal connective tissues, e.g. sodium hyaluronic acid and sodium chondroitin sulfate A and C. This enzyme is widely distributed in mammalian testes, leech heads, many invasive bacteria, venoms of snakes, bees, scorpions, spiders, and poisonous fishes (MAYER et al., 1960). It is also referred to as the "spreading factor", because hydrolysis of hyaluronic acid facilitates toxin diffusion into the tissues of a victim (DURAN-REYNALS, 1936). All snake venoms so far examined contain hyaluronidase, but it is present in a relatively higher concentration in the viperid and crotalid venoms than in the elapid venom (DURAN-REYNALS, 1939; ZELLER, 1948; FAVILLI, 1956). Similar to testicular hyaluronidase, this venom enzyme is a typical endo-N-acetylhexosaminidase, which cleaves the bond between C-1 of hexosamine and the oxygen bridge and yields mainly tetrasaccharide units $(GlcUA\text{-}GlcNAc)_4$. Its action is also intensified by the action of transglycosidase. Table 17 shows the distribution of this enzyme in snake venoms (JAQUES, 1956).

Table 17. Hyaluronidase activity in various snake venoms (JAQUE, 1956)

Enzyme source	Viscosity-reducing activity (McClean-Hale units)	Relative activity
Standard testis	182000	1
V. aspis italica	45500	0.25
V. russellii	59000	0.325
Echis carinatus	61000	0.335
Bungarus caeruleus	1525000	8.37
N. tripudians	2780	0.015
N. nigricollis	2800	0.015

Assay Method (DI-FERRANTE, 1956). *Principle.* The turbidimetric method described here is based on the formation of relatively insoluble complexes between isolated acid mucopolysaccharides and cetyltrimethylammonium bromide. The amount of turbidity which develops upon addition of cetyltrimethylammonium bromide into a solution of acid mucopolysaccharide is proportional to the amount of acid mucopolysaccharide in the system; no turbidity develops when cetyltrimethylammonium bromide is added to chondroitin sulfate or hyaluronate that has been depolymerized by incubation with the enzyme. *Reagents.* Acetate buffer; 0.2 M sodium acetate-acetic acid, pH 6, to which NaCl is added to give a concentration of 0.15 M. Acid mucopolysaccharide solution; 50 mg sodium chondroitin sulfate or sodium hyaluronate are dissolved in 100 ml acetate buffer. Cetyltrimethylammonium bromide reagent; 2.5 g are dissolved in 100 ml 2% NaOH.

Procedure. An aliquot of enzyme dissolved in 0.6 ml 0.2 M acetate buffer, pH 6, is incubated at 37.5° C with 200 μg of either chondroitin sulfate or hyaluronate, dissolved in 0.4 ml acetate buffer. The incubation time is limited to 15 min. At the same time, standards containing 200, 100, 50, 25 μg substrate and one blank containing buffer alone and another with enzyme alone are prepared. At the end of the incubation period, addition of 2 ml cetyltrimethylammonium bromide reagent stops the reaction (bringing the pH to 12.5) and produces the turbidity. After mixing by inversion, the optical densities are determined within 10 min against the blank and readings are taken at 400 nm. The optical densities given by the standards, plotted against the amount of acid mucopolysaccharide present in each of them, constitute the calibration line to which are referred the optical densities of the tubes containing the enzyme. It is, therefore, possible to ascertain the amount of acid mucopolysaccharide depolymerized by each quantity of enzyme by subtracting the residual amount of substrate from that originally present in each tube. The unit of enzyme activity is expressed as the quantity of enzyme which produces a 50% reduction of the turbidity given by the initial quantity (200 μg) of substrate.

Comments. Several methods including a viscometric assay (HUMPHREY and JAQUES, 1953), a bioassay (JAQUES, 1953), a different turbidimetric assay (MATHEWS and INOUYE, 1961; BENCHETRIT et al., 1977), and colorimetric assay for N-acetylhexosamine released (ARONSON and DAVIDSON, 1967) are available for the determination of hyaluronidase activity. However, these appear rather tedious compared to the method described above.

Purification. The enzyme from *C. atrox* venom is precipitated with half-saturated $(NH_4)_2SO_4$ (MADINAVEITIA, 1941). CHIU (1960) and TURAKULOV et al. (1969) have partially purified the enzyme from the venoms of *N. naja atra* and *N. oxiana.* Except for these reports, no information is available on the purification of venom hyaluronidase.

Enzymatic Properties. The pH optimum of hyaluronidase in various snake venoms is practically at the same level: the enzyme of *V. russellii* venom has the optimum at pH 4.6 and its activity is considerably reduced outside the range of pH 4.6–6.5 (MCLEAN and HALE, 1940), whereas the enzyme from *Bothrops alternatus* and *C. terrificus* has its optimum pH at 5.5–7.0 (FAVILLI, 1940). The enzyme is almost completely destroyed when the venom solution is heated at 70° C for 30 min (FAVILLI, 1939). The enzyme in *N. haje* is also heat labile, partially inhibited by sodium gentisate, but not affected by EDTA. It hydrolyzes hyaluronate and chondroitin sulfate A or C but not heparin. In these properties, the venom enzyme resembles the testicular hyaluronidase.

2. Heparinaselike Enzyme

β-Heparin (chondroitin sulfate B) is well known for its powerful anticoagulant action, by interacting with antithrombin III contained in blood plasma. When heparin is incubated with 20 μg of *Bothrops atrox* venom for 60 min at 37° C, it loses most of its anticoagulant activity (DEVI and COPLEY, 1970). The anticoagulant action of heparin therefore appears to be mainly destroyed by a heparinase contained in the venom. The heparinaselike enzyme of *Bothrops atrox* venom is different from venom hyaluronidase, since β-heparin is not a substrate for the latter enzyme. DEVI and COPLEY (1970) have found that venom heparinase splits glycosidic bonds of polysaccharides other than those bonds degrated by enzymes of different origins. This enzyme is widely distributed in various clot-promoting venoms of crotalid snakes, e.g. *Crotalus* and different species of *Bothrops* (DEVI and COPLEY, 1971). It seems to be a heat-stable enzyme, but no further properties of venom heparinase are known.

3. NAD Nucleosidase

NAD nucleosidase catalyzes the hydrolysis of the nicotinamide N-ribosidic linkage of NAD and has been isolated from various mammalian tissues. The presence of an NAD-destroying enzyme in snake venom was first demonstrated by BHATTACHARYA (1953), who reported that nicotinamide was released when crude venom from *Bungarus fasciatus* was incubated with NAD. Later SUZUKI et al. (1960) examined venoms of nine Asian poisonous snakes and found similar activity in the venoms of *Trimeresurus gramineus* and *Bungarus multicinctus*. It is now known that the enzyme is found in the venoms of several members of the Crotalidae, and of the genus *Bungarus*. The venoms of all six members of *Agkistrodon* genus examined contain NAD nucleosidase activity. In contrast, with a few exceptions, venoms of *Crotalus*, *Bothrops*, *Bitis*, *Vipera*, and *Trimeresurus* show only a very weak activity. No NAD nucleosidase activity is detected in venoms of the *Naja* genus tested (TATSUKI et al., 1975). In general, the distribution of this enzyme in snake venoms seems more restricted than that of other enzymes, such as phosphodiesterase, 5'-nucleotidase, phospholipase A, hyaluronidase, and L-amino acid oxidase, which are found in all venoms (Table 18).

Assay Method (TATSUKI et al., 1975). Measurement of the enzyme activity is based on the determination of NAD^+ level with cyanide before and after incubation of β-NAD^+ with the enzyme, according to ZATMAN et al. (1953). The reaction mixture consists of 0.4 ml 0.1 M phosphate buffer, pH 6.0, 1.0 μmole β-NAD^+ and enzyme, in a total volume of 0.7 ml. After incubation at 37° C for 30 min, 2.3 ml 1.0 M KCN is added and absorbance is measured at 340 nm. One unit of enzyme is defined as the amount which cleaves 1 μmole β-NAD^+ per min.

Purification (TATSUKI et al., 1975). The method described here has been developed for the purification of NAD nucleosidase from the venom of *A. halys blomhoffii*.

Step 1. The lyophilized venom (3 g, total A_{280} units = 3200) dissolved in 20 ml 0.05 M sodium acetate buffer, pH 6.0, is applied to a column of Sephadex G-100 (4.0 × 126 cm), previously equilibrated with the same buffer and eluted at 4° C with the same buffer at a flow rate of 46 ml/h. The protein with NAD nucleosidase activity is concentrated in the first peak and the fractions are combined, concentrated to a final volume of 10 ml by freeze-drying, and dialyzed overnight at 4° C against 3 liters 0.05 M acetate buffer, pH 6.0.

Step 2. The dialyzed solution is applied to a DEAE-cellulose column (3.0 × 47.5 cm), equilibrated with 0.05 M acetate buffer, pH 7.5. A linear gradient elution is performed with 1 liter each of the equilibration buffer and 0.2 M acetate buffer, pH 6.0, at a flow rate of 30 ml/h. Most of the NAD nucleosidase appears in the first peak and the fractions are collected, concentrated, and desalted by a Sephadex G-25 column (3.5 × 120 cm).

Step 3. The material obtained from step 2 is chromatographed by a column of DEAE-Sephadex (3.0 × 52 cm), equilibrated with 0.005 M acetate, pH 7.0. A linear gradient elution is performed with 500 ml each of the equilibration buffer and 0.1 M acetate buffer, pH 7.0. The buffer in the reservoir is replaced by 0.2 M acetate buffer, pH 7.0, on emergence of tube 75. Fractions of 10.6 ml per tube are collected at a flow rate of 100 ml/h. The protein with NAD

Table 18. Distribution of NAD nucleosidase activity in various snake venoms (TATSUKI et al., 1975)

Species	NAD nucleosidase activity (units/mg venom)
Crotalidae	
A. halys blomhoffii	0.026
A. piscovorus piscivorus	0.11
A. contortrix contortrix	0.027
A. contortrix mokasen	0.139
A. acutus	0.024
Viperidae	
Causus rhombeatus	0.060
Elapidae	
B. multicinctus	0.293
B. fasciatus	0.235

[a] Incubation mixture contained 0.4 mg venom, 0.4 ml 0.1 M phosphate buffer, pH 6.0, and 1.0 µmole β-NAD^+ in a total volume of 0.7 ml. After incubation at 37° C for 30 min, activity was assayed by the cyanide method. The following venoms showed no NAD nucleosidase activity under the conditions described above: *C. adamanteus, C. atrox, C. durissus terrificus, C. viridis viridis, C. basiliscus, T. okinavensis, T. flavoviridis, T. mucrosquamatus, B. atrox, Bitis gavonica, Bitis arietans, V. russellii, V. palestinae, V. ammodytes, Echis carinatus, N. nivea, N. haje, N. naja atra, N. melanoleuca, N. hannah, N. naja samarensis, N. nigricollis, Ophiophagus hannah, Dendroaspis angusticeps, Dendroaspis polylepis*, and *Hemachatus haemachatus*.

nucleosidase activity is mainly obtained in tubes 116–172, and the fractions are combined, lyophilized, and desalted as mentioned in the preceeding step.

Step 4. Finally NAD nucleosidase is purified with a molecular sieving on a Sepharose 6B column (2.8 × 29 cm), equilibrated with 0.05 M acetate buffer, pH 6.0. Elution is made with the equilibration buffer and 5.8 ml fractions per tube are collected at a flow rate of 62 ml/h. The protein peak with a small shoulder appears in tubes 23–32. The final yield of enzyme activity through these procedures is ~21% and it results in 25-fold purification of the enzyme. The purified material gives a single major band of protein on disc polyacrylamide-gel electrophoresis in the presence of sodium dodecyl sulfate (SDS). However, without SDS, it shows two or three bands, indicating that the sample is not entirely pure.

Enzymatic Properties (TATSUKI et al., 1975). The venom NAD nucleosidase shows maxium activity at pH 7.5 and is stable in neutral pH range. The enzyme is stable at 40° C but loses its activity above 60° C. On storage of the purified enzyme in 0.1 M phosphate buffer, pH 6.0, for at least 6 months at −10° C, the catalytic activity decreases by less than 10%. The enzyme hydrolyzes β-NAD^+, $NADP^+$, and 3-acetylpyridine adenine dinucleotide. No hydrolysis is observed of α-NAD^+, NADH, NADPH, and NMN^+. The Km values for β-NAD^+, $NADP^+$, and 3-acetylpyridine adenine dinucleotide are 8.3×10^{-4} M, 5.7×10^{-4} M, and 7.4×10^{-4} M, respectively. Over 60% inhibition of β-NAD^+ hydrolysis is observed in the presence of 10^{-3} M $HgCl_2$ and cysteine. Iodoacetic acid, PCMB, and EDTA have no significant effect.

Comments. Most NAD nucleosidases from mammalian tissues have been found as insoluble protein bound to microsomal particles (WINDMUELLER and KAPLAN, 1962; GREEN and BODANSKY, 1965; STATHAKOS and WALLENFELS, 1966) and their activities are inhibited by nicotinamide and isonicotinic hydrazide (ZATMAN et al., 1954). In contrast, a soluble NAD nucleosidase purified from bull semen is not inhibited by nicotinamide and does not catalyze a pyridine base exchange (YUAN and ANDERSON, 1971). The venom enzyme described here is sensitive to pyridine derivatives and catalyzes a pyridine base exchange reaction (SUZUKI et al., 1960). Thus, the properties of venom NAD nucleosidase seem to be similar to those of the particle-bound NAD nucleosidases from pig brain and beef spleen.

IV. Enzymes Acting on Peptide Bonds

Snake venoms contain several proteases, including endopeptidases, peptidases, proteinases with a limited specificity such as thrombinlike enzyme, arginine ester hydrolase, prothrombin activator, Factor X activator, and kininogenase (kinin-releasing enzyme). Most of these proteases, with the exception of peptidases, are mainly found in crotalid and viperid venoms. In general, elapid and hydrophiid venoms do not show any proteolytic activities, whereas a strong peptidase activity is detected in some of the elapid venoms, such as *Bungarus multicinctus*. The distribution of the proteases with limited specificity appears to be more restricted than that of others; Factor X activator is specifically found in Russell's viper venom and prothrombin activator in *Echis carinatus* venom. These so-called procoagulants are described in Chapter 18 of this book. In the past, the existence of collagenaselike enzyme has been noted in snake venoms. However, it is now known that the enzyme, which acts directly and specifically on native collagen similarly to mammalian collagenase, does not exist in any of the snake venoms (OHSAKA, 1960). Moreover, a gelatinase activity previously found in the venoms of *Bothrops jararaca* and *Vipera palestinae* is explained by the action of the endopeptidases contained in these venoms. In fact, a highly purified endopeptidase isolated from the venom of *A. halys blomhoffii* digests not only casein and denatured hemoglobin but also gelatin (IWANAGA et al., 1976).

The first indication that snake venoms could dissolve meat was reported by DE LACERDA (1884). NOC (1904) later observed the digestion of gelatin and fibrin by some venoms. Although many investigators (SLOTTA, 1955; KAISER and MICHEL, 1958) subsequently reported on the proteolytic actions of snake venom components, a systematic study using 15 snake venoms and different substrates was first undertaken by DEUTSCH and DINIZ in 1955. They observed that the activity of the venoms on the synthetic substrate, α-N-benzoyl arginine ethylester (BAEE), which is one of the typical substrates for trypsin, is usually not related to their action on protein such as denatured hemoglobin. This indicates that the venom endopeptidase, long believed to have a trypsinlike activity, is distinct from trypsin. Subsequently venom endopeptidases have been purified from a number of crotalid and viperid venoms and it is now known that they differ from the well-characterized mammalian and plant endopeptidases, such as trypsin, α-chymotrypsin, elastase, papain, and bromelain.

Crotalid and viperid venoms hydrolyze BAEE, α-N-toluenesulfonly-L-arginine methylester (TAME), and α-N-acetyl tyrosine ethylester (ATEE), α-N-benzoyl-L-arginine p-nitroanilide (BAPA), well-known substrates for trypsin and α-chymotrypsin. However, the many studies performed so far indicate that the venom proteolytic enzymes having such hydrolytic activities differ from trypsin and α-chymotrypsin in their enzymatic properties; this will be described later. Some of these enzymes are known to be related to thrombinlike enzyme and kininogenase found in snake venoms. Table 5, 19, 20 and 21 show the distribution of several proteolytic activities in various snake venoms.

Table 19. Distribution of proteinase, arginine ester hydrolase, kininogenase, and thrombinlike enzyme in various snake venoms (OSHIMA et al., 1969)

	Proteinase activities[a]	Arginine ester hydrolase activity[b]	Bradykinin releasing activity[c]	Clotting activity[d]
Crotalidae:				
Agkistrodon halys blomhoffii	24.5	1.8	25.2	–
A. piscivorus piscivorus	35.3	4.6	28.0	±
A. contortrix contortrix	49.5	11.1	72.6	+
A. contortrix mokeson	46.5	10.2	38.6	+
A. acutus	25.5	2.9	0.5	++
Crotalus adamanteus	13.8	16.8	20.4	±
C. atrox	59.0	4.2	124.3	++
C. durissus terrificus	25.7	8.9	56.5	++
C. viridis viridis	27.5	9.1	233.5	±
C. basiliscus	77.0	4.0	24.5	±
Trimeresurus flavoviridis	22.5	1.5	3.0	±
T. okinavensis	19.0	2.2	4.3	–
T. mucrosquamatus	26.8	34.1	28.6	±
T. gramineus	11.5	8.0	54.4	++
Bothrops jararaca	7.8	2.3	10.4	++
B. atrox	17.8	3.8	5.0	++
Viperidae:				
Vipera russellii	2.6	0.4	1.3	–
V. palestinae	6.5	5.0	40.0	–
V. ammodytes	21.5	1.1	107.8	–
Echis carinatus	23.5	1.1	9.6	±
Causus rhombeatus	3.1	1.8	6.6	–
Bitis gavonica	11.3	2.7	215.0	±
B. arietans	10.0	1.0	6.57	–
Elapidae:				
Naja naja atra	0.9	–	3.92	–
Naja melanoleuca	1.5	–	Not detectable	–
Ophiophagus hannah	6.4	–	Not detectable	–
Naja naja samarensis	0.3	–	0.4	–
Naja nigricollis	0.5	–	0.3	±
Bungarus fasciatus	Not detectable	–	0.1	–
Bungarus multicinctus	Not detectable	–	Not detectable	–
Dendroaspis angusticeps	1.0	–	15.6	±
Hemachatus haemachatus	2.0	–	0.2	±

[a] The activity was defined as μg tyrosine equivalent of TCA-soluble product formed per min per mg protein.
[b] The activity was defined as μmoles TAME hydrolyzed per min per mg protein.
[c] The activity was defined as the amount of enzyme which releases kinin equivalent to 1 μg synthetic bradykinin per min per mg protein.
[d] The activity was determined from the time when fibrin-fibers appeared.
++ within 3 min; + within 20 min; ± within 2 h; – over 2 h.

1. Endopeptidases

As shown in Tables 19 and 21, endopeptidases are mainly found in crotalid and viperid venoms. Some elapid venoms, e.g., *Hemachatus haemachatus* and *Ophiophagus hannah*, contain caseinolytic enzyme but its activity is much lower than that estimated in many crotalid venoms. A common feature of venom endopeptidases is

Table 20. Esterolytic and proteolytic activities of snake venoms (GEIGER and KORTMANN, 1977)

Venom	Enzymatic activity on		
	BAEE (mUnits/mg toxin)[a]	BAPA (mUnits/mg toxin)[b]	HMW-kininogen (mUnits/mg toxin)[c]
Bothrops bilineatus	1520	1.0	0,44
B. neuwiedi	2900	2.0	0.44
B. jararacussu	680	2.2	0.13
B. jararaca	2500	2.0	2.22
B. lanceolatus	1680	0.5	1.8
B. alternata	1940	0.0	2.63
B. atrox (Maranhao)	2340	0.0	1.68
B. pradoi	1580	2.2	0.26
B. atrox moojeni	4040	1.0	2.2
B. cotiara	2360	0.0	1.48
B. atrox (Columbia)	1560	0.8	1.27
Cerastes cerastes	2640	5.1	1.69
Echis carinatus (Pakistan)	100	0.0	0.26
B. hypoprorus	160	0.0	0.42
B. atrox asper	680	2.0	0.66
Trimeresurus flavoviridis	740	0.6	0.66
Agkistrodon halys blomhoffii	680	0.0	1.4
Crotalus adamanteus	605	0.3	0.93
Agkistrodon rhodostoma	1100	0.0	0.98
Crotalus terrificus	3380	0.9	0.71
Naja naja	0	0.3	0.2
Vipera russellii	1010	0.3	0.68
Agkistrodon contortrix	810	—	0.15
A. c. mokasen	4170	1.9	2.4
Vipera lebetina	3180	1.0	1.4
Crotalus h. horridus	4440	28.5	0.46
Bitis gavonica	2660	1.4	0.91

[a] Alcohol dehydrogenase-linked kallikrein assay, substrate: BAEE (TRAUTSCHOLD et al., 1974).
[b] Trypsin assay, substrate: BAPA (FRITZ et al., 1974).
[c] mUnits kininogen activity is defined as nmol bradykinin/min.

that they seem to be metal proteases and they hydrolyze peptide bonds with amino groups contributed by leucine and phenylalanine residues. Another common characteristic point is that they are easily inactivated by EDTA and reducing agents such as cysteine. In these properties venom endopeptidases completely differ from the well-known mammalian proteases.

Assay Method (SATAKE et al., 1963a). *Principle.* The enzyme is assayed with 2.0% casein solution in Tris-HCl buffer, pH 8.5, at 37° C. Undigested casein is precipitated with trichloroacetic acid (TCA) and filtered or centrifuged. Digested casein in the supernatant is determined with the Folin-Ciocalteau reagent.

Reagents. 0.4 M Tris-HCl buffer, pH 8.5. Casein; 2 g casein (Hammersten quality) are suspended in 100 ml 0.4 M Tris-HCl buffer and heated for 15 min in a boiling bath to make a solution. 0.44 M TCA, 0.4 M sodium carbonate, Folin-Ciocalteau reagent; the commercially available reagent is diluted three times with distilled water before use. Standard tyrosine solution; the tyrosine standard is prepared by dissolving 18.10 mg pure, dry tyrosine in 1 liter 0.2 M HCl.

Table 21. Esterolytic and proteolytic activities of snake venoms (KOCHOLATY et al., 1971)

	% Protein (biuret)[a]	Proteinase (casein)[b]	TAME[c]	BAPNA[d]
Crotalidae				
A. billineatus	62	53	637	23
A. c. mokeson	65	131	1450	178
A. p. piscivorus	68	87	561	504
A. rhodostoma	75	750	892	17
B. atrox	75	66	230	94
C. adamanteus	73	20	4100	196
C. atrox	80	328	308	13
C. d. durissus	75	22	1098	264
C. d. terrificus	79	78	450	46
C. h. horridus	80	51	625	112
C. scutulatus	70	31	910	91
C. v. helleri	71	24	2567	44
C. v. viridus	75	120	1233	117
Sistrurus m. barbouri	74	83	375	32
T. flavoviridis	87	83	56	6
Viperidae				
B. arietans	65	20	80	0
B. gavonica	64	15	240	0
E. carinatus	74	141	193	53
V. formosensis	67	3	65	0
V. russellii	70	0	82	0
Elapidae				
B. caeruleus	87	6	0	0
B. fasciatus	91	9	0	0
B. multicinctus	75	4	0	0
Micrurus f. fulvius	90	0	0	0
N. melanoleuca	81	3	0	0
N. naja naja	80	2	0	0
N. naja kaouthia	80	6	0	0
Ophiophagus hannah	76	28	36	11

[a] Determined by a biuret method (GORNALL et al., 1949) and expressed in percent of the dried venom.
[b] Determined by the method of KUNITZ and expressed as the Kunitz unit.
[c] Determined by a spectrophotometric method and expressed in units of venom protein by the formula ΔA247 min × 1000/mg venom.
[d] Determined by a spectrophotometric method and expressed in units of venom protein by the formula ΔA440 min × 1000/mg venom.

Procedure. Casein solution, 0.5 ml, is digested for 15 min at 37° C with 0.5 ml suitably diluted enzyme solution. The reaction is terminated by adding 0.1 ml 0.44 M TCA; after standing 30 min, the mixture is filtered through Toyo or Whatman filter paper, No. 2. To 0.5 ml filtrate are added 2.5 ml 0.4 M Na_2CO_3 and 0.5 ml Folin-Ciocalteau reagent. After the mixture has stood for 20 min, the blue color is read at 660 nm and compared against a standard tyrosine solution.

Definition of Unit and Specific Activity. One unit of the enzyme, expressed as proteinase units (PU), is defined as the amount of enzyme yielding an increase in color equivalent to 1.0 μg tyrosine per min with Folin's reagent. Specific activity is expressed as unit per mg protein.

Comments. The above procedure was originally based on the KUNITZ method (1947). The Anson method (ANSON, 1938), which involves determining the increase in TCA-soluble products that result from digestion of urea-denatured hemoglobin, is also available. A convenient qualitative assay for locating the active fraction during enzyme purification is provided by the gelatin-digesting test (WILKES and PRESCOTT, 1976).

Purification. Venom endopeptidase has been highly purified from the venoms of *A. halys blomhoffii* (OSHIMA et al., 1968a), *A. piscivorus leucostoma* (WAGNER et al., 1968), *T. flavoviridis* (TAKAHASHI and OHSAKA, 1970), *Vipera russellii* (DIMITROV, 1971), *Bitis arietans* (VAN DER WALT and JOUBERT, 1971), and *C. atrox* (PFLEIDERER and SUMYK, 1961). Some of these venoms contain two or three endopeptidases that are chromatographically separable. Three enzymes, proteinase, a, b, and c, have been found in the venom of *A. halys blomhoffii*, three in *C. atrox*, two in *Vipera russellii*, three in *Bitis arietans*, and two or three in *T. flavoviridis*. Although their substrate specificities towards the insulin B-chain are similar, the physicochemical properties of the individual enzymes differ significantly. One explanation for the multiplicities of venom endopeptidases is their instability due to autodigestion. Another explanation is their glycoprotein nature due to a microheterogeneity of carbohydrate chains, at least in the isolated proteinases from *A. halys blomhoffii* venom. Moreover, venom endopeptidase tends to aggregate to higher molecular weight species at low pH, as revealed by VAN DER WALT and JOUBERT (1972). However, no detailed study on the multiplicities of these enzymes is available and further experiments are required. The method described below is the isolation procedure of endopeptidase from the venom of *A. piscivorus leucostoma*.

Procedures (PRESCOTT and WAGNER, 1976). All chromatographic procedures are carried out at 4–5° C to minimize loss of enzymic activity.

Step 1. Preparation of Venom for Chromatography. Lyophilized venom of *A. p. leucostoma* is purchased from Miami Serpentarium, Miami, Florida. Normally 1–5 g dried venom is used in an isolation experiment; the volume suggested below is suitable for a sample of ~2 g. The venom is dissolved in 20–50 ml 5 mM Tris-HCl buffer, pH 8.5, and dialyzed against this buffer overnight. The somewhat turbid solution is clarified by centrifugation at 5400 *g* for 5–10 min and the clear supernatant fluid is stored at 4° C until used.

Step 2. Chromatography on DEAE-Sephadex A-50. DEAE-Sephadex A-50 is suspended in distilled water and allowed to stand for several hours, after which the fine particles are decanted. The ion-exchange material is suspended in 0.5 N HCl, filtered immediately, resuspended in distilled water, then washed several times in distilled water. The DEAE-Sephadex is next suspended in 0.5 N NaOH, allowed to stand for 15–20 min, then filtered and again suspended in 0.5 N NaOH for a few minutes. After filtration the resin is washed in distilled water until the washings are neutral to pH paper. The hydroxide form of DEAE-Sephadex thus prepared is suspended in 5 mM Tris-HCl buffer, pH 8.5, and allowed to equilibrate before being poured in a 2.5 × 50 cm column which is thoroughly washed with the buffer at 5° C. The sample from step 1 is applied and the column is washed with the same buffer at a rate of 60 ml/h until the unadsorbed material emerges. The chromatogram is then developed by the application of a linear gradient from 0 to 0.1 M NaCl; the effluent is collected in 10-ml fractions at a flow rate of 50–60 ml/h. The first cylinder of the gradient-producing apparatus typically contains 1 liter 5 mM Tris-HCl buffer, pH 8.5, and the second contains an equal amount of the same buffer that is 0.1 M in NaCl. For experiments in which less than 1 g venom is used as the starting material, the total volume of the gradient is reduced to 600 ml; for samples over 5 g it should be increased correspondingly. In some experiments the column is washed sequentially with 0.2 M and then with 1.0 M NaCl as shown in Figure 7 to ensure elution of all proteolytic activity, but this step is not essential inasmuch as *leucostoma* peptidase A is eluted at about 0.05 M NaCl. This fraction always

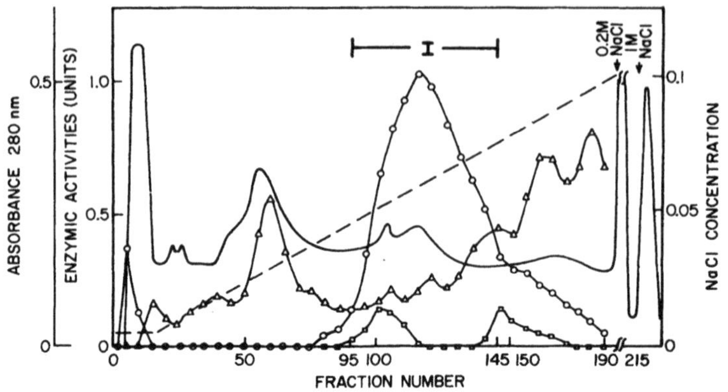

Fig. 17. Chromatography of crude, dialyzed *A. piscivorus leucostoma* venom on DEAE-Sephadex A-50 in 5 mM Tris-HCl, pH 8.5; 2 g venom was dialyzed then applied to a 2.5 × 50 cm column and eluted at ~50 ml/h into 12 ml fractions; ——, absorbance at 280 nm; ○, proteolytic activity toward denatured hemoglobin; △, esterase activity toward N-benzoyl-L-arginine ethylester; □, arylamidase activity toward L-leucyl-β-naphthylamide; – – –, NaCl gradient. Fraction I was selected for further purification (WAGNER et al., 1968)

contains the greatest amount of activity toward hemoglobin substrate, although a small amount of proteolytic activity emerges in the breakthrough fraction; some lots of the venom contain a third chromatographically distinct proteolytic peak.

Step 3. Rechromatography on DEAE-Sephadex A-50. The protease from step 2 (fraction I in Fig. 17) is dialyzed against 5 mM borate-NaOH buffer, pH 9.2, and applied to a 2.5 × 50 cm column of DEAE-Sephadex A-50 that has been equilibrated with this buffer. The chromatogram is developed with ~700 ml linear gradient of increasing NaCl concentration as in step 2 (0–0.1 M NaCl), with a flow rate of 60 ml/h. Fractions of 10 ml are collected in tubes containing 1 ml 0.1 M Na_2HPO_4, pH 8.0, to lower the pH of the eluate. Each tube is read at 280 nm, and every fifth fraction is assayed for the three types of enzymic activity. The proteolytic activity emerges in a prominent peak that is only partially separated from smaller protein fractions with esterase and arylamidase activities.

Step 4. Gel Filtration. The active material from step 3 is concentrated to ~5–10 ml by ultrafiltration with an Amicon UM-05 membrane under a nitrogen atmosphere of 50 psi. The concentrated sample is applied to a 2.5 × 50 cm column of Sephadex G-75 previously equilibrated with 5 mM Tris-HCl buffer, pH 8.5, which is 0.1 M in NaCl, and eluted at a flow rate of 15–20 ml/h until a total volume of 150–250 ml has been collected in fractions of 3–5 ml. The exact volume at which the chromatogram is considered fully developed should be ascertained by monitoring the column effluent at 280 nm, either manually or by a flow analyzer. The emergence of the proteolytic activity frequently is preceded by two relatively small components possessing esterase without protease activity. The third and largest fraction is highly proteolytic but also contains some BAEE activity. In some experiments, this fraction may also be contaminated by arylamidase (described in a later section); if this is the case, rechromatography under the same conditions is advisable.

Step 5. Rechromatography on DEAE-Sephadex. The protease fraction from step 4 is dialyzed for 18 h against 5 mM borate-NaOH buffer, pH 9.6, and applied to a 2.5 × 50 cm column of DEAE-Sephadex A-50, which has been equilibrated with the same buffer. The protease is eluted with 800–850 ml of a linear gradient of NaCl (20 mM–0.5 M) in the same buffer, with fractions of 6 ml collected at a rate of 15 ml/h in tubes containing 1 ml 0.1 M Tris-HCl buffer, pH 7.8. Three components are separated by this procedure; the second and most prominent is protease, uncontaminated by esterase, which emerges in the third peak. Those fractions that show protease activity without esterase are combined to form the final preparation. A summary of a purification experiment is shown in the Table 22.

Table 22. Summary of the purification of *Leucostoma* peptidase A (PRESCOTT and WAGNER, 1976)

Step	Treatment	Total protein (mg)	Total enzyme units[a]			Specific activity			% Recovery[b] of protease
			Protease	Esterase	Aryl-amidase	Protease	Esterase	Aryl-amidase	
1.	Dialysis	2568	3186	5100	3870	1,24	1,99	1.51	100
2	Chromatography (DEAE-Sephadex A-50, pH 8.5)	668	2022	528	429	3.03	0.79	0.64	64
3	Rechromatography (DEAE-Sephadex A-50, pH 9.2)	389	1702	229	132	4,38	0.59	0.34	53
4	Gel filtration (Sephadex G-75)	211	1260	23	0	5.97	0.11	0.0	40
5	Rechromatography (DEAE-Sephadex A-50, pH 9.6)	128	984	0	0	7.69	0.00	0.0	31

[a] See text for definition of units.
[b] Represents the cumulative recovery in the isolation procedure.

Comments. The purified preparation of *leucostoma* peptidase A described above has been found to be homogeneous by moving boundary electrophoresis at several pH values and by polyacrylamide gel electrophoresis at pH 9.5. Moreover, enzymic assays for activity toward BAEE and L-leucyl-β-naphthylamide show the absence of detectable amounts of esterase and arylamidase, respectively. The absence of arginine ester hydrolase is one of the criteria for functional purity of venom endopeptidase. Because most of the crotalid and viperid venoms contain the esterase, this enzyme has been considered a major proteolytic enzyme of the venoms. However, it is now clear that arginine ester hydrolyse does not hydrolyze both hemoglobin and casein.

Physicochemical Properties. The venom endopeptidase is stable for several weeks either frozen or at 4° C; however, prolonged storage accompanied by freezing and thawing results in some autolysis, which is manifest by the appearance of one or two new bands on gel electrophoresis, even when no appreciable loss in activity is evident. All the proteinases so far purified are inactivated by heating for 10 min at 80° C. Table 23 summarizes the physicochemical properties of venom endopeptidases isolated from crotalid and viperid venoms. With the exception of the enzymes from the venom of *A. halys blomhoffii*, their molecular weights are in the range of 21400–24000. The isoelectric points also differ significantly, indicating that some are acidic and others are basic. The amino acid compositions of the purified enzymes are shown in Table 24. Common features include similar compositions and high contents of aspartic acid and glutamic acid. All three proteinases from *A. halys blomhoffii* venom contain a large amount of carbohydrates. Attention has been paid to the metal content of venom endopeptidases. All enzymes examined so far contain 1–2 g atoms of calcium or 1 g atom of zinc per enzyme molecule; however, a proteinase isolated from the venom of *Vipera russellii* contains non-heme iron (DIMITROV, 1971).

Table 23. Physiochemical properties of snake venom proteinases

Property	*A. halys blomhoffii*[a]			*A. p. leucostoma*[b]	*T. flavoviridis*[c]	*Bitis arietans*[d]
	Proteinase a	Proteinase b	Proteinase c	Peptidase A	H_2-Proteinase	
Sedimentation coefficient, $S_{20,w}$ (S)	3.59	4.94	5.54	2.87	2.43	2.60
Diffusion coefficient $D_{20,w}$ (cm^2, s^{-1})	—	5.88	5.26	10.66	—	9.3
Partial specific volume, $\bar{v}$ (ml/g)	—	0.722	0.695	0.711	—	0.722
Intrinsic viscosity [η] (dl/g)	—	0.052	0.046	—	—	—
Molecular weight	50200	95500	72300	22400	—	—
Archibald procedure						
Sedimentation equilibrium	—	—	—	—	22400	21400
Sedimentation diffusion	—	92000	67000	22500	—	24300
Isoelectric point	6.00	4.16	3.85	6.5	10.6	5.0
Metal content	—	2 Ca/mole	—	2 Ca/mole 1 Zn/mole	1 Ca/mole 1 Zn/mole	—

[a] OSHIMA et al. (1968).
[b] WAGNER et al. (1968).
[c] TAKAHASHI and OHSAKA (1970).
[d] VAN DER WALT and JOUBERT (1971).

Table 24. Amino acid compositions of venom proteinases

Amino acid	*A. halys blomhoffii*[a]			*A. p. leucostoma*[b] Peptidase A	*Bitis arietans*[c] Protease A
	Proteinase a	Proteinase b	Proteinase c		
	g residues per 100 g protein			Mean nearest integer	
Lys	6.36	3.94	5.01	10	8
His	2.01	2.57	3.58	9	8
Arg	4.73	4.01	2.34	6	10
Asp	12.00	12.39	11.11	29	26
Thr	4.82	3.69	3.10	15	8
Ser	4.21	2.69	3.41	18	10
Glu	8.32	8.46	8.67	19	13
Pro	2.77	3.73	3.36	6	8
Gly	2.88	2.56	3.16	12	8
Ala	3.15	2.73	2.83	11	10
1/2 Cys	5.09	4.54	5.38	6	6
Val	3.91	4.27	3.75	15	11
Met	1.62	2.70	2.39	5	7
Ile	3.96	4.83	3.62	10	12
Leu	6.07	5.83	4.21	19	8
Tyr	4.05	3.51	6.06	5	10
Phe	3.18	2.48	2.59	6	7
Trp	1.84	1.69	1.90	4	6
Total	82.54%	78.84%	77.79%	205	176
Neutral sugars	8.15	7.6	3.91	—	—
Amino sugars	4.72	6.5	3.34	—	—
Sialic acid	0.81	3.1	1.21	—	—
Total (%)	3.68	17.1	8.46	—	—

[a] OSHIMA et al. (1968).
[b] WAGNER et al. (1968).
[c] VAN DER WALT and JOUBERT (1971).

The essential role of metal ions in catalysis is indicated by the fact that both EDTA and o-phenanthroline inhibit proteolysis. Removal of zinc ions by o-phenanthroline in the presence of calcium ions inhibits the action of *leucostoma* peptidase A, which can be reactivated by the addition of zinc ions (WAGNER et al., 1968). Thus, zinc is the catalytically essential metal; it is likely that calcium stabilizes the enzyme. In contrast, the removal of calcium ions of proteinase b (*A. halys blomhoffii* venom) by electrodialysis or EDTA results in conformational change of the enzyme protein, as judged from the blue shift in its ultraviolet difference spectra (OSHIMA et al., 1971). This conformational change of the protein with concomitant loss of proteolytic activity is irreversible; addition of calcium ions does not result in activation of the enzyme activity or reversal of the denaturation. The proteinase b seems to contain 1 mole free-SH group, which is titrable only in the presence of 8 M urea and EDTA (10^{-2} M). It appears, therefore, that the metal is probably involved in stabilizing the enzyme molecule and that the -SH groups are closely related to the activity of proteinase b.

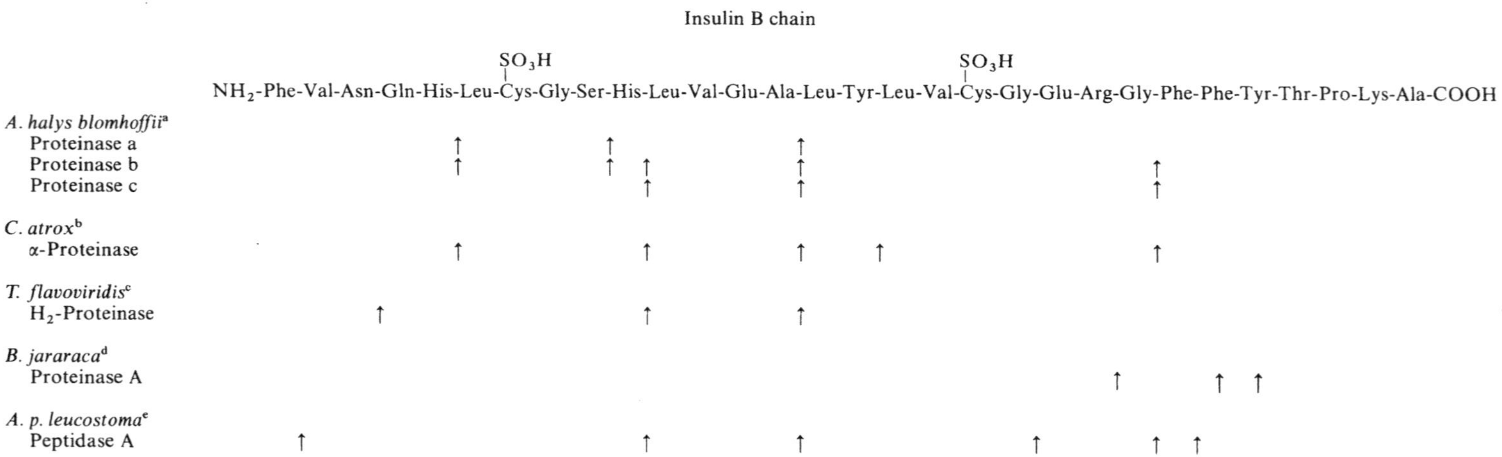

Fig. 18. Cleavage sites of venom proteinase on oxidized insulin B chain. [a] (OSHIMA et al., 1968), [b] (PELEIDERER and KRAUS, 1965), [c] (TAKAHASHI and OHSAKA, 1970), [d] (HENRIQUES et al., 1966), [e] (SPIEKERMAN et al., 1973)

Enzymatic Properties. Most of venom endopeptidases are active in the alkaline pH region, with the exception that one of two proteinases found in the venom of *Vipera russellii* show the optimum at pH 3.6 (DIMITROV, 1971). *Leucostoma* peptidase A (Table 23) exhibits maximal activity toward hemoglobin substrate at pH 8.5. The pH optimum of proteinases a, b, and c (Table 23) are 10.5, 9.8, and 8.9, respectively, when casein is used as substrate (SATAKE et al., 1963a). These three proteinases are irreversibly inactivated by 10^{-2} M EDTA and their activities are slightly inhibited by -SH reagents, including PCMB, monoiodoacetic acid, N-ethylmaleimide, and 5,5′-dithiobis(2-nitrobenzoic acid). On prolonged incubation with proteinase b (Table 23), PCMB (10^{-3} M) causes significant inhibition. Moreover, 2-mercaptoethylamine, cysteine, glutathione, and 2-mercaptoethanol strongly inactivate their caseinolytic activities. These properties, with the exception of the PCMB inhibition on proteinase b, seem to be common to all venom endopeptidases. Venom endopeptidases are not inhibited by DFP, TLCK, TPCK, soybean trypsin inhibitor, or pancreatic basic trypsin inhibitor, all of which are potent inhibitors of so-called pancreatic serine proteases.

Venom endopeptidase catalyzes the hydrolysis of peptide bonds of a wide variety of natural and synthetic substrates, including casein, hemoglobin, gelatin, elastin, collagen, fibrinogen, insulin, glucagon, bradykinin, polylysine, polytyrosine, polyphenylalanine, and polytryptophan (IWANAGA et al., 1976; PRESCOTT and WAGNER, 1976). The proteinase shows in general little activity toward small synthetic peptides such as di- and tri-peptides, although a number of NH_2-substituted and doubly substituted dipeptides are hydrolyzed slowly (SPIEKERMAN et al., 1973). It does not split ester and amide bonds of synthetic substrates, such as α-N-toluene-sulfonyl-L-arginine methyl ester, α-N-acetyltyrosine ethyl ester, leucineamide, L-leucyl-β-naphthyl amide, and N-benzoylarginine amide. Moreover, it exhibits no actvity against any exopeptidase substrates tested. Employing the general formula, R′-NH-CHR-CO-X, cleavage of the CO-X bond is demonstrated when R represents the side chain from phenylalanine, tyrosine, threonine, asparagine, aspartic acid, tryptophan, alanine, histidine, and glycine. The X component of substrate is derived mainly from hydrophobic amino acids including phenylalanine, leucine, and valine. Thus, it seems likely that venom endopeptidase hydrolyzes many kinds of substrates with a specificity that is directed toward bonds in which amino groups are contributed by the hydrophobic residues. The sites of hydrolysis of several polypeptides and proteins are shown in Figure 18 and Table 25.

2. Peptidases

Although elapid venoms do not contain appreciable endopeptidase activity, a powerful hydrolytic activity towards oligopeptides is observed in elapid venoms. GHOSH et al. (1939) first found that the venoms of *N. naja* and *Bungarus fasciatus* hydrolyze Leu-Gly and Leu-Gly-Gly. Later MURATA et al. (1963) reported that the peptides Carbobenzoxyl-Gly-Pro-Leu-Gly-Pro, Gly-Pro-Leu-Gly, Gly-Pro-Leu, Gly-Gly-Phe, and Gly-Gly-Gly are rapidly hydrolyzed by the venoms of *N. naja atra* and *Bungarus multicinctus*. When Gly-Pro-Leu-Gly is used as the substrate, hydrolysis occurs first in the bond between Pro and Leu, producing Gly-Pro and Leu-Gly, and the resulting Leu-Gly is slowly cleaved further. In particular, *B. multicinctus* venom

Table 25. The sites of hydrolysis of various polypeptides by venom protease

Substrate	Cleavages sites	Venom
Insulin A chain	8 9 12 13 14 15 15 16 Ala-Ser, Ser-Leu, Tyr-Gln, Gln-Leu	*C. atrox*[a] α-Protease
Glucagon	5 6 8 9 15 16 21 22 25 26 Thr-Phe, Thr-Ser, Asp-Ser, Asp-Phe, Tyr-Leu	*A. halys blomhoffii*[b] Proteinase c
Bradykinin	4 5 6 7 Gly-Phe, Phe-Ser	*A. halys blomhoffii*[c] Proteinase b
Mellitin	4 5 7 8 15 16 19 20 24 25 Ala-Val, Lys-Val, Ala-Leu, Trp-Ile, Arg-Gln	*C. atrox*[d] α-Protease
RSCM-toxin	3 4 4 5 11 12 21 22 22 23 Cys-Phe, Phe-Ile, Ser-Gln, Tyr-Thr, Thr-Lys 24 25 28 29 31 32 41 42 46 47 Met-Trp, Asn-Phe, Gly-Met, Cys-Ala, Pro-Lys 47 48 53 54 55 56 56 57 60 61 Lys-Val, Asn-Ile, Lys-Cys, Cys-Cys, Asp-Asn	*Bitis arietans*[e] Protease A
RSCM-ribonuclease	2 3 3 4 4 5 10 11 45 46 Glu-Thr, Thr-Ala, Ala-Ala, Arg-Gln, Thr-Phe 50 51 51 52 56 57 61 62 75 76 Ser-Leu, Leu-Ala, Ala-Val, Lys-Asn, Ser-Tyr 89 90 97 98 99 100 100 101 102 103 Ser-Ser, Tyr-Lys, Thr-Thr, Thr-Gln, Ala-Asn	*Bitis arietans*[e] Protease A
Cytochrome c	1 2 5 6 23 24 27 28 32 33 Gly-Asp, Lys-Gly, Gly-Gly, Lys-Thr, Leu-His 39 40 47 48 55 56 67 68 69 70 Lys-Thr, Thr-Tyr, Asn-Lys, Tyr-Leu, Glu-Asn 71 72 72 73 73 74 76 77 80 81 Pro-Lys, Lys-Lys, Lys-Tyr, Pro-Gly, Met-Ile 90 91 93 94 100 101 Glu-Arg, Asp-Leu, Lys-Ala	*Bitis arietans*[e] Protease A

[a] PFLEIDERER and KRAUSS (1965).
[b] SATAKE et al. (1963).
[c] SUZUKI and IWANAGA (1970).
[d] JENTSCH (1969).
[e] VAN DE WALT and JOUBERT (1972).

exhibits a very powerful peptidase activity towards such substrate. The hydrolysis of dipeptides by various snake venoms was also investigated by TU et al., (1965) and TU and TOOM (1967a, b, 1968). However, no studies are available on the purification and properties of the venom peptidases.

3. Arginine Ester Hydrolases

As described in the previous section, all the venoms belonging to Elapidae and Hydrophiidae examined so far do not show any arginine ester hydrolase activity. A notable exception is *Ophiophagus hannah* venom, which exhibits a weak activity towards arginine esters. This enzyme activity is widely detected in the venoms of

Crotalidae and Viperidae (Tables 19, 20, and 21). The first indication of the existence of this enzyme in snake venoms was made by DEUTSCH and DINIZ (1955), who found the activity in 15 crotalid and viperid venoms, using BAEE as the substrate. Later HAMBERG and ROCHA E SILVA (1957) and DEVI et al. (1959) reported that the "bradykinin releasing" and "clotting" activities in the venom of *B. jararaca* are associated with the arginine ester hydrolase but not with its caseinolytic activity. Since then many investigators have purified arginine ester hydrolases from the venoms of *B. jararaca* (HOLTZ et al., 1960; HABERMANN, 1961; HENRIQUES et al., 1960; HENRIQUES and EVSEEVA, 1969), *A. halys blomhoffii* (SATO et al., 1965), and *A. contortrix laticinctus* (TOOM et al., 1970). It is now known that crotalid venoms contain at least three arginine ester hydrolases that are chromatographically separable and that some of these enzymes are related to the kininogenase and thrombinlike enzyme (SUZUKI and IWANAGA, 1970). The substrate specificities of all these enzymes are strictly directed to the hydrolysis of ester or peptide linkages to which an arginine residue contributes the carbonyl group (SATO et al., 1965; TOOM et al., 1970).

Assay Method I (SATO et al., 1965). *Principle.* This method is based upon the quantitative reaction of esters, such as TAME, with hydroxylamine, yielding the hydroxamic acid derivative (HESTRIN, 1949).

Reagents. 0.4 M Tris-HCl buffer, pH 8.5; 0.1 M TAME; 3.5 N NaOH; 2 M $NH_2OH \cdot HCl$; 6% trichloroacetic acid (TCA) containing 4 N HCl; 0.11 M $FeCl_3$ containing 0.04 N HCl.

Procedure. The reaction mixture containing 0.8 ml 0.4 M Tris-HCl buffer, pH 8.5, 0.1 ml enzyme, and 0.1 ml 0.1 M TAME solution is incubated at 37° C for 15 min. At the conclusion of the incubation time, the concentration of remaining TAME is determined. The reaction is terminated by an alkaline hydroxylamine solution (prepared by mixing an equal volume of 3.5 N NaOH and 2 M NH_2OH) and the hydroxamate formation is complete after 30 min at room temperature. At this time, 0.5 ml 6% TCA-HCl solution is added, followed by 2.0 ml ferric chloride solution. The samples are deaerated under water-aspirator vacuum conditions with simultaneous vortexing. The absorbance at 500 nm is determined against the reference blank (minus enzyme). Nonenzymatic hydrolysis of TAME is negligible under these conditions.

Assay Method II (SATO et al., 1965). *Principle.* This method involves titration of the amount of acid, α-N-tosyl-L-arginine, liberated with time by utilizing a recording pH stat. *Procedure.* Assays are performed in a pH stat maintained at a constant temperature of 25° C. The cell should be supplied with a thermostat and be capable of continual stirring. The syringe is filled with carefully standardized NaOH at concentrations of 0.02 N. One ml substrate (15 μmoles TAME) is first placed in the pH stat vessel and the temperature equilibrated. The pH is then adjusted to 8.5 by automatic addition of base from the pH stat. The enzyme is added in 0.02 ml aliquots and the reaction rate is followed for at least 10 min on the recorder. The results are converted to μmoles TAME hydrolyzed per min.

Definition of a Unit and Specific Activity. One unit of the activity is defined as the amount of enzyme required to hydrolyze 1 μmole TAME per min.

Comments. For rapid scanning of arginine ester hydrolase, method I is available. However, the pH stat should also be used for accurate estimation of the activity, since the colorimetric method is a substractive method and only small changes between initial and final TAME concentrations are noted owing to the high levels of the substrate.

Purification. An arginine ester hydrolase from the venoms of *A. halys blomhoffii* and *A. contortrix laticinctus* has been highly purified to physicochemically homogeneous states (SATO et al., 1965; TOOM et al., 1970). The purified enzyme was prepared by repeated chromatographies on a DEAE-cellulose column and a hydroxylapatite column. Through these procedures, most of the venom kinonogenase and thrombin-

Table 26. Properties of kininogenase and nonproteolytic arginine ester hydrolase isolated from snake venoms

Property	*A. halys blomhoffii*[a]	*Bitis gavonica*[b]	*A. contortrix*[c] *laticinctus*
Sedimentation coefficient, $S_{20,w}$	—	—	2.7
Diffusion coefficient, $D_{20,w}$	—	—	8.3×10^{-7} cm^2·s
Molecular weight	—	33500[d]	31000[e]
Isoelectric point	—	—	9.1
Kininogenase activity	4.7[f]	30.3[f]	—
BAEE-esterase activity	3.9[g]	3.81[g]	3.72[h]
TAME-esterase activity	1.7	0.47	3.55
pH optimum	8.5–9.2	9.5	8.5
Inhibitors[i]			
DFB	Inhibition	Inhibition	Inhibition
PBTI	Inhibition	No inhibition	Inhibition
SBTI	No inhibition	No inhibition	Inhibition

[a] SATO et al. (1975).
[b] MEBS (1969).
[c] TOOM et al. (1970).
[d] Determined by gel-filtration.
[e] Determined by sedimentation-diffusion.
[f] Kinin equivalent (μg/min/mg protein).
[g] μmoles/min/mg protein.
[h] Moles/min/mole protein.
[i] PBTI = pancreatic basic trypsin inhibitor; SBTI = soy bean trypsin inhibitor.

like enzyme, which show also arginine ester hydrolyzing activity, were separated into other fractions. The preparations from both venoms did not contain any venom endopeptidases and had a high degree of purity as evidenced by at least four criteria: ultracentrifugation, polyacrylamide-gel electrophoresis, chromatography on Sephadex G-75 or DEAE-Sephadex A-25, and isoelectric focusing.

Physicochemical Properties. One characteristic of venom arginine ester hydrolase is its high stability to heat. The enzyme from *A. halys blomhoffii* retains about 60% of activity on heating for 20 min at 80° C. It does not lose the activity when freeze-thawed and the frozen preparation can be stored for at least 6 months without loss of activity.

The purified enzyme from the venom of *A. contortrix laticinctus* has a sedimentation coefficient of 2.7 S, a diffusion coefficient of 8.3×10^{-7} cm$^2 \cdot$s^{-1}, and a molecular weight of ~30000 (Table 26). The isoelectric point is 9.1, indicating that it is a basic protein. These molecular properties are very similar to those of the enzyme isolated from *A. halys blomhoffii*.

Enzymatic Properties. The enzyme exhibits a rather broad pH optimum from 7.0 to 9.0. Below pH 7 and above pH 9 the activity drops off rather rapidly. The rate of hydrolysis of BAEE by the purified enzyme is increased almost twofold by the addition of 1 mM Mn^{2+}, Zn^{2+}, and Co^{2+}, whereas Mg^{2+} has little effect (TOOM et al., 1970). The enzyme is completely inactivated by di*iso*propylphosphofluoridate (DFP), and phenylmethylsulfonyl fluoride, suggesting that it has an "active serine" residue as the catalytic site. However, inhibition of the enzyme activity by soybean,

Table 27. Hydrolysis of substrates by purified esterase (TOOME et al., 1970)

Substrate	Km	Moles per min per mole of enzyme[a]
N-Benzoyl-L-arginine ethyl ester	1.17×10^{-4}	3.72
N-Benzoyl-L-arginine methyl ester	4.50×10^{-5}	3.68
p-Toluenesulfonyl-L-arginine methyl ester	1.49×10^{-3}	3.55
p-Nitrophenyl acetate	5.0×10^{-3}	0.09
N-Benzoyl-L-alanine ethyl ester		0
Benzyloxycarbonyl lysine methyl ester		0
Benzyloxycarbonyl lysine benzyl ester		0
L-Lysine ethyl ester		0
L-Lysine-p-nitrophenyl ester		0
L-Lysine-p-nitroanilide		0
N-Benzoyl-L-arginine-p-nitroanilide		0
N-Benzoyl-L-arginine-p-naphthylamide		0
N-Benzoyl-L-arginine amide		0
α-N-p-Tosyl-L-arginine amide		0
N-Benzoyl-L-tyrosine ethyl ester		0
Acetyl-L-tyrosine ethyl ester		0
Indophenyl acetate		0
Fibrin		0
Casein		0
Hemoglobin		0
Congocoll		0
Azocoll		0

[a] Based on a molecular weight of 30000.

ovomucoid, and pancreatic basic trypsin inhibitors has not been observed (SATO et al., 1965; SUZUKI and IWANAGA, 1970). Furthermore, EDTA, 0-phenanthroline, cysteine, glutathione, and ascorbic acid, all of which are potent inhibitors of venom endopeptidases, do not affect the esterolytic activity.

As shown in Table 27, the purified enzyme from the venom of *A. contortrix laticinctus* hydrolyzes BAEE, BAME, TAME, and p-nitrophenyl acetate. When the arginine residue is replaced with alanine, lysine, or tyrosine, hydrolysis does not take place. Also no hydrolysis is detected on the amide bonds of L-lysine-p-nitroanilide, N-benzoyl-L-arginine amide, α-N-tosyl-L-arginine amide, or N-benzoyl-L-arginine p-nitroanilide, even with a hundredfold excess of enzyme. In like manner, none of the proteolytic enzyme substrates (casein, azocoll, hemoglobin, and fibrin) are hydrolyzed by the purified enzyme (TOOM et al., 1970). These substrate specificities are very similar to those of the enzyme isolated from the venom of *A. halys blomhoffii* by SATO et al. (1965). The Km values calculated for the substrates BAEE, BAME, and TAME are 1.17×10^{-4} M, 4.50×10^{-5} M, and 1.49×10^{-3} M, respectively.

A similar type of arginine ester hydrolase has been found in the venoms of *C. adamanteus* and *T. flavoviridis* (SUZUKI and IWANAGA, 1970). Although the biologic activities of this enzyme are largely unknown, it may be related to the hypotension and increase of capillary permeability observed after injection of crotalid venoms. In fact, the purified enzyme isolated from *A. halys blomhoffii* induced an increased capillary permeability when the sample was tested on skin from the back of albino rabbits in accordance with the method of MILES and WILHELM (1955), its potency was comparable with that of hog pancreatic kallikrein (SATO et al., 1965). Venom arginine ester hydrolase described in this section is differentiated in its enzymatic properties from the venom kininogenase and thrombinlike enzyme widely distributed in crotalid and viperid venoms. A natural protein substrate for this enzyme is still unknown.

4. Kininogenase

One of the most prominent physiologic findings resulting from the injection of crotalid venoms into the animal body is the lowering of blood pressure. ROCHA E SILVA et al. (1949) showed the liberation of a new physiologically active substance from euglobulin by the action of *Bothrops jararaca* venom and gave the name "bradykinin" to this substance, which lowered blood pressure. Since proteolytic activity was especially high in crotalid venoms, the kinin liberation from a precursor protein, called kininogen, was first thought to be due to venom endopeptidase. However, DEUTSCH and DINIZ (1955) later reported that no definite relationship was found between proteolytic and bradykinin-releasing activities. Furthermore, HAMBERG and ROCHA E SILVA (1957) found that bradykinin—releasing and -clotting activities remained even after *Bothrops jararaca* venom was heated at 100° C for 3–5 min. It is now known that all the crotalid and viperid venoms contain a kininogenase (previously named bradykinin-releasing enzyme), which specifically liberates a vasoactive nonapeptide, bradykinin, from plasma kininogens and that the enzyme is differentiated from the so-called arginine ester hydrolase and thrombinlike enzyme contained in the venoms. While the venom kininogenase is known to hydrolyze synthetic substrates, BAEE, BAME, and TAME, the activity is much weaker than that of thrombinlike enzyme and arginine ester hydrolase.

Assay Method (IWANAGA et al., 1965; YANO et al., 1971). *Principle.* This method utilizes the smooth muscle contraction elicited by bradykinin, which is released by the action of kininogenase on kininogen. For the bioassay the reader is referred to an article of WEBSTER and PRADO (1970).

Reagents. Plasma kininogen substrate; citrated blood (0.2 ml 20% sodium citrate/10 ml blood) is taken in silicon-coated tubes, the plasma separated and either used on the same day or frozen in the tubes. The plasma is heated at 60° C for 30 min. Following this treatment, it is dialyzed against running tap water at 4° C and used as substrate. Buffer: 0.0066 M sodium phosphate buffer, pH 8.0. Synthetic bradykinin is a product of Sandoz Co., Switzerland.

Procedure. The reaction mixture contains 0.5 ml plasma kininogen, 0.5 ml 0.0066 M phosphate buffer, pH 8.0, and 0.1 ml enzyme, in a total volume of 1.1 ml. After incubation at 37° C for 3–5 min, an aliquot of the reaction mixture is taken and assayed on the isolated guinea pig ileum or rat uterus. The amount of bradykinin liberated is calculated from the rate of contraction of the smooth muscle compared to the standard curve prepared with various amounts of synthetic bradykinin. One unit of kininogenase is defined tentatively as the amount of enzyme releasing bradykinin equivalent to 1 μg synthetic bradykinin per min.

Comments. The enzyme activity of kininogenase can be estimated either by measuring the quantity of kinin formed from kininogen or by measuring its ability to cleave synthetic ester substrates, e.g., BAEE. However, the latter method, although more precise, is not as specific, since other arginine ester hydrolases contained in the venom cleave the ester bonds. Either method can be used following the purification

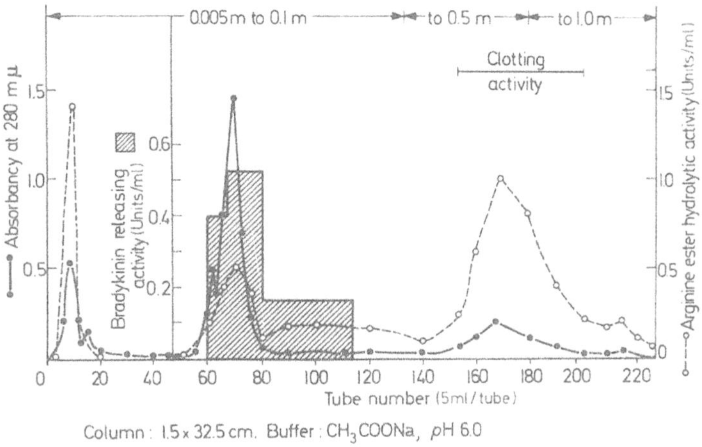

Fig. 19. Purification of kininogenase on a CM-cellulose column. The partially purified kininogenase from the venom of *A. halys blomhoffii* was applied to the column, 1 mg applied sample hydrolyzed 1.65 μmoles TAME per min and released from kininogen bradykinin corresponding to 4.7 μg synthetic bradykinin per min (SUZUKI et al., 1966)

of venom kininogenase, but the method based on formation of kinins should be employed when the enzyme is prepared, particularly during the early steps of the purification.

Purification. Venom kininogenase has been partially purified from the venoms of *B. jararaca* (HABERMANN, 1959; HOLTZ et al., 1960; RAUDONAT and ROCHA E SILVA, 1962), *C. atrox* (HOLTZ et al., 1960), *A. halys blomhoffii* (SATO et al., 1965; SUZUKI et al., 1966), *Echis carinatus* (COHEN et al., 1969; DE VRIES and COHEN, 1969), and *Bitis gavonica* (MEBS, 1969b). For separation of this enzyme, repeated chromatographies on a DEAE-cellulose column and chromatography on a CM-cellulose column or a hydroxylapatite column are required to remove a kininase (kinin-destroying enzyme) and other arginine ester hydrolases contained in the venoms. All venoms examined so far contain two kininogenases that are separable by gel filtration on a Sephadex G-75 column or by DEAE-cellulose chromatography. The difference between the two enzymes is still unclear, but one of the kininogenases seems to have a lower molecular weight (SUZUKI and IWANAGA, 1970). The purification procedure developed for the venom of *A. halys blomhoffii* is as follows:

Procedures (SUZUKI and IWANAGA, 1970). The lyophilized venom is dissolved at a concentration of 100 mg/ml in 0.005 M sodium acetate, pH 7.0, and centrifuged to remove insoluble materials. The clear venom solution is then applied to a column of DEAE-cellulose (3 × 40 cm), equilibrated with 0.005 M sodium acetate, pH 7.0. The concave gradient elution is started with 1 liter equilibration solvent in the mixing vessel and 0.1 M sodium acetate, pH 7.0, in the reservoir, the latter is replaced by 0.2 M and 0.5 M sodium acetate, pH 7.0, as descirbed in the footnote to Figure 6. The flow rate is adjusted to 25 ml/h, and 9.5 ml fractions are collected at 4° C. The fractions containing kininogenase activity (tubes 91–120) are combined, concentrated to ~ 10 ml by freeze-drying, and desalted by passage through a column of Sephadex G-25 (2.5 × 40 cm).

The desalted fraction thus obtained is further purified by chromatography on a CM-cellulose column (1.5 × 32.5 cm), equilibrated with 0.005 M sodium acetate, pH 6.0. A linear gradient elution under the conditions described in the footnote to Figure 19 is made from 0.005 M to

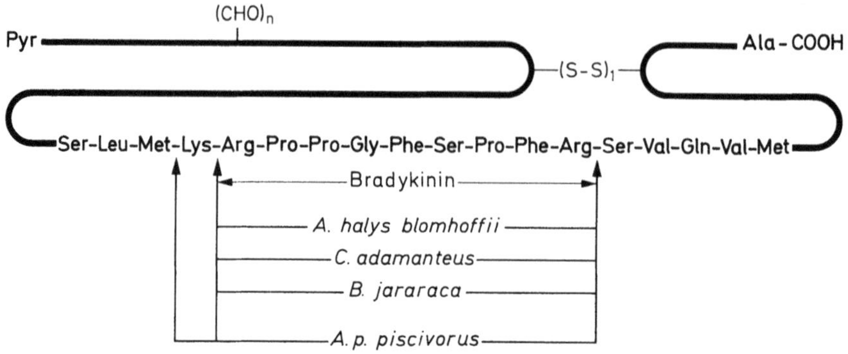

Fig. 20. Cleavage sites of venom kininogenase on bovine plasma low-molecular-weight kininogen. Pyr = pyroglutamic acid; CHO = carbohydrate chain (SUZUKI and IWANAGA, 1970)

0.1 M sodium acetate, pH 6.0. Through this procedure, a thrombinlike enzyme is freed from the kininogenase fractions (Fig. 19), and a functionally pure enzyme, which is not contaminated with endopeptidase, L-amino acid oxidase, phospholipase A_2, hyaluronidase, phosphodiesterase and NAD nucleotidase, is obtained. The arginine ester hydrolase activity in the purified kininogenase accounts for less than 10% of the total hydrolase present in the venom.

Comments. The kininogenase and thrombinlike enzyme of the venom can in general be separated by column chromatography on DEAE-cellulose column; the latter can be purified to an ultracentrifugally and electrophoretically homogeneous state. However, the former enzyme has not yet been obtained in a physicochemically pure form.

Physicochemical Properties. The purified enzyme is stable in the frozen state for at least 6 months and no loss of activity is observed when it is lyophilized. It is also known as a heat-stable enzyme, but activity is completely lost by heating the preparation for 20 min in a boiling water bath. Although no detailed study has been made of the molecular properties of venom kininogenase, the purified enzymes from the venoms of *Bitis gavonica* (MEBS, 1969) and *Echis carinatus* (COHEN et al., 1969) are known to have a molecular weight of 33500 and 22000, respectively.

Enzymatic Properties. The optimum activity of the enzyme is found at pH 8.5–9.0, and the same pH is optimal for the hydrolysis of BAEE and liberation of kinin from kininogen (IWANAGA, et al., 1965). Cations such as Ca^{2+}, Mg^{2+}, Mn^{2+}, Zn^{2+}, Cd^{2+}, and Fe^{3+} have no effect in tests using dialyzed kininogen and kininogenase. The enzyme from the venom of *A. halys blomhoffii* is inactivated by DFP and pancreatic basic trypsin inhibitor (Trasylol), whereas both inhibitors do not inactivate the kininogenase isolated from *Bitis gavonica* venom (MEBS, 1969). The release of kinin by the enzyme is inhibited by the synthetic substrates BAEE and TAEE the degree of inhibition depending on the ester concentration. L-Lysine ethyl ester and α-N-benzoylarginine amide, which are not hydrolyzed by kininogenase, do not inhibit the liberation of bradykinin (IWANAGA et al., 1965; MEBS, 1969). The kinin released from plasma kininogens has been identified as bradykinin with the use of enzymes from the venoms of *A. halys blomhoffii* (SUZUKI et al., 1966), *B. jararaca* (HAMBERG, 1962), and *C. adamanteus*. However WEBSTER and PIERCE (1963) found that the venom of *A. contortrix* might liberate kallidin (lysylbradykinin) in addition to bradykinin (Fig. 20).

V. Enzymes Acting on Carboxylic Ester Bonds

Snake venoms contain several enzymes that act on substrates with carboxylic ester bonds, e.g., phospholipids, acetylcholine, and arylacetate. Of these enzymes phospholipases and acetylcholinesterase have specific biologic functions and have been extensively studied. In addition to these enzymes, some snake venoms are known to exhibit a strong arylesterase activity the biologic functions of which are not yet defined. This enzyme hydrolyzes p-nitrophenylacetate, α- or β-naphthylacetate and indoxylacetate. However, it is still unclear whether the hydrolysis is due to a side reaction of some well-known enzyme or to a specific enzyme. Our experimental results have shown that no liberation of p-nitrophenol or β-naphthol results from incubation of p-nitrophenylacetate or β-napthylacetate with the venoms of *A. halys blomhoffii* and *T. flavoviridis*. On the contrary, these esters are hydrolyzed by the venoms of *N. naja atra* and *Bungarus multicinctus*, in an especially rapid manner by the latter venom (SATAKE et al., 1963). These elapid venoms are known to have a strong cholinesterase activity and it is possible that the hydrolysis of these substrates is mediated by the venom cholinsterase. In fact, MCLEAN et al. (1971) reported that most of the elapid venoms including *N. naja*, *N. nigricollis*, *N. melanoleuca*, *N. nivea*, *N. haje*, *Ophiophagus hannah*, *Bungarus fasciatus*, *B. caeruleus*, *Dendroaspis jamesoni*, *D. polyepsis*, and *D. angusticeps* hydrolyze indoxylacetate, α-naphthylacetate, and α-naphthylbutyrate.

It is also known that *C. adamanteus* venom has the ability to hydrolyze N-methylindoxylacetate, which has been used as a substrate for serum cholinesterase (ELLIOTT and PANAGIDES, 1972). However the venom does not show any cholinesterase activity, so this enzyme is not responsible for the hydrolysis. Thus, the results indicate the presence of an unknown esterase in the venom, which differs evidently from cholinesterase found in elapid venoms. To obtain further information on these esterases, isolation studies may be required in the future.

1. Phospholipase A_2

Phospholipases are important enzymes in lipid metabolism and in investigations of phospholipid structure and lipid-protein interactions, especially with regard to deciphering structure-function relationships of biologic membranes and lipoproteins. Of these enzymes, the phospholipase A_2, which hydrolyzes selectively the 2-acyl group from sn-3-phosphoglycerides, have been studied most extensively. This enzyme is widely found in the venoms of snakes, bees, and scorpions as well as in animal tissues. One of the richest sources of phospholipase A_2 is the venoms of snakes of the families Viperidae, Crotalidae, Elapidae, and Hydrophiidae. The content of the enzyme in various venoms differs somewhat from venom to venom; one venom *(C. h. horridus)* shows only a weak phospholipase activity (Table 28). The venom enzyme has been designated phospholipase A, phosphatidase A, lecithinase A, or hemolysin because of its ability to indirectly hemolyze red blood cells. In a thesis in 1905 LUDECKE suggested that snake venom produced a lytic compound by enzymatic action on lecithin and DELEZENNE and LEDEBT (1911) clearly demonstrated that an enzyme in cobra venom formed a hemolytic substance when it acted on horse serum or egg yolk. Hemolysis by snake venoms is due to the action of phospholipase A,

Table 28. Phospholipase A activity in various venoms (KOCHOLATY et al., 1971)

Venom	Enzyme activity[a]	Venom	Enzyme activity[a]
Crotalidae		Viperidae	
A. bilineatus	44	*Bitis arietans*	13
A. mokesen	35	*Bitis gavonica*	21
A. p. piscivorus	54	*Echis carinatus*	19
A. rhodostoma	27	*V. r. formosensis*	52
B. atrox	29	*V. russellii*	40
C. adamanteus	32	Elapidae	
C. atrox	25	*B. caeruleus*	34
C. d. durissus	9	*B. fasciatus*	11
C. d. terrificus	5	*B. multicinctus*	27
C. h. horridus	0.1	*Micrurus f. fulvius*	65
C. scutulatus	46	*N. melanoleuca*	68
C. v. helleri	18	*N. naja naja*	34
C. v. viridus	26	*N. naja kaouthia*	20
Sistrurus m. barbouri	32	*Ophiophagus hannah*	21
T. flavoviridis	42		

[a] Assayed at pH 7.0 using a 10% egg yolk suspension in 0.1 M Tris buffer as substrate and incubation time of 30 min at 37° C. Activity units are expressed in μ equiv. of fatty acid titrated using the average of the initial velocities measured with 5 and 10 μg venom protein.

either "indirectly" by producing lysophosphatides from serum or added lecithin, or "directly" by hydrolyzing phospholipids in the red cell membrane. It is now clear that in α-phosphatides the β-ester linkage is specifically attacked by venom phospholipase A_2 as shown below:

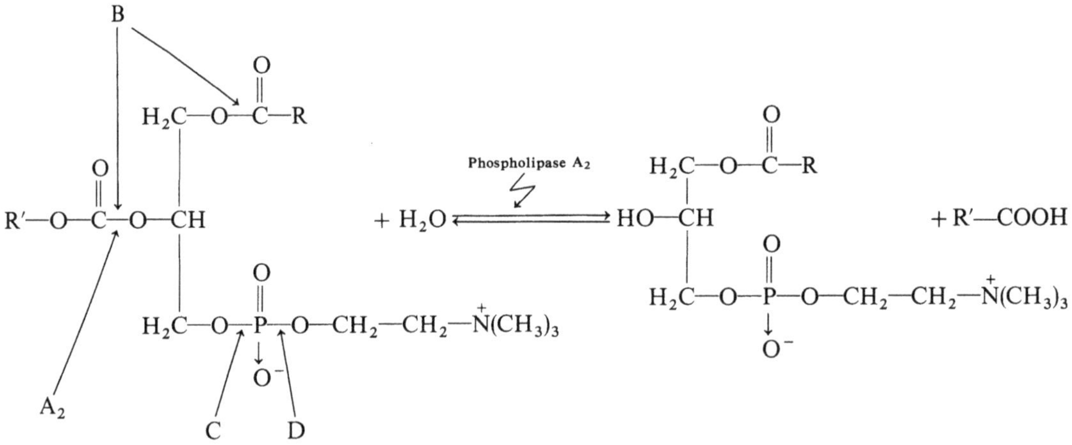

Thus, the positional specificity of this enzyme has made it an important tool in the structural analysis of phospholipids and triglycerides. More recently venom phospholipase A_2 has been widely used to probe lipid-protein interactions (SINGER, 1971). In addition, venom phospholipase A_2 possesses a number of interesting enzymatic properties, including an absolute requirement for Ca^{2+}, a remarkable heat stability, and a high degree of constraint in the tertiary structure imposed by numerous disulfide bridges. For these reasons, this enzyme has been extensively investigated by many researchers and it is one of the best characterized enzymes in snake venoms.

Assay Method I. (WELLS and HANAHAN, 1969). *Principle.* The hydrolysis of phospholipid can be followed by measuring titrimetrically the rate of release of fatty acid.

Reagents. A solution of phosphatidylcholine, 15 μmoles/ml, in 95% diethyl ether (peroxide free) and 5% methanol (anhydrous) is prepared fresh for each series of assays. No attempt is made to use a solution for more than 1 day. Even after storage for only a few days the solution turns yellow and becomes resistant to hydrolysis. All enzyme solutions are diluted at least 25-fold with a solution containing 0.22 M NaCl, 0.02 M $CaCl_2$, and 1 mM EDTA (pH 7.5). 0.02 N NaOH in 95% ethanol. Dilute stock 0.2 N aqueous NaOH 1:10 with 95% ethanol. This solution should be standardized each time it is used. Phenol red or cresol red indicators, 0.1% in water, 95% ethanol.

Procedure. The substrate solution (2.0 ml) is placed in a 5 ml volumetric flask and 25 μl enzyme preparation is added. After vigorous shaking for 30 s, the reaction is allowed to proceed for 10 min at 20–25° C. The reaction is terminated by the addition of 95% ethanol to a total volume of 5 ml. The fatty acids are immediately titrated with 0.02 N NaOH in 90% ethanol, using 1 drop of 0.1% cresol red as an indicator and an Ultraburet (Scientific Industries) to dispense the base. Zero-time reaction mixtures require 0.005–0.010 ml of base and the reproducibility of titration is 0.005 ml. To obtain data within an error of ~ 5%, the amount of enzyme is adjusted so that 0.100–0.150 ml base is required above the blank. This figure corresponds to 5%–10% hydrolysis. In numerous experiments zero-order kinetics are observed up to 25% hydrolysis or for 30 min.

Method II (KAWAUCHI et al., 1971a). The principle is essentially the same as that of Method I, but an automatic titrator (Radiometer TTTlc titrator equipped with a model SBR 2C recorder) is used to follow the rate of delivery of base.

Reagents. Substrate; about 650 mg phosphatidylcholine is dissolved in 6 ml ether and mixed with 20 ml water. The mixture is incubated at 60° C for 20 min and then diluted with water to a total volume of 40 ml. The solution is subjected to ultrasonication at 10 Kcycles for 25 min. 1.0 M NaCl; 0.01 M $CaCL_2$; sodium deoxycholate; 0.02 M KOH.

Procedure. 2 ml substrate solution, 1.0 ml 1.0 M NaCl, 1.0 ml 0.01 M $CaCl_2$, 1.0 ml sodium deoxycholate, and 0.4 ml water are put into a 10 ml volumetric flask in a bath with water circulating at 37° C. The flask is placed on a pH-stat titrator, and the mixture is adjusted to pH 8.2 with 0.02 M KOH. After preincubation for 5 min with stirring, 0.1 ml enzyme solution is added, and the fatty acids liberated are titrated with 0.02 M KOH using 0.5 ml glass micrometer syringe. A slow stream of nitrogen is added during the titration to maintain an atmosphere free of carbon dioxide. Under the above conditions, the reaction follows essentially zero-order kinetics.

Method III (MARINETTI, 1965). The decrease in turbidity of egg yolk suspension can be measured spectrophotometrically at 925 nm. This method is available for the measurement of the enzyme activity during the purification process because of its simplicity.

Procedure. The reaction mixture contains 0.5–0.8 ml egg yolk suspension (0.32 ± 0.03 μ-atom P per ml) in 0.15 M NaCl, adjusted to pH 6.8 with sodium barbital, plus 0.15 M NaCl solution to a volume of 2.8 ml. After thermal equilibration at 30° C, 0.2 ml enzyme solution in 0.15 M NaCl is added, and the same amount of saline is added to the control sample. The change in absorbance at 925 nm of the enzyme-treated sample, as compared with the control sample (adjusted to give $A_{925} = 0.600$), is measured spectrophotometrically. With this method one unit of activity is defined as the amount of enzyme that produces a decrease of 1.0 milliunit of absorbance per minute.

Definition of Units. Unit of phospholipase A_2 is defined as that amount of enzyme catalyzing the hydrolysis of 1 μmole phosphatidylcholine per minute.

Comments. Other methods are also employed for the assay of phospholipase A_2, the egg yolk coagulation method (HABERMANN and NEUMAN, 1954) and the erythrocyte hemolytic technique (BOMAN and KALETTA, 1957). These two simple methods are useful in the semiquantitative assay for the enzyme. Moreover, the hydroxylam-

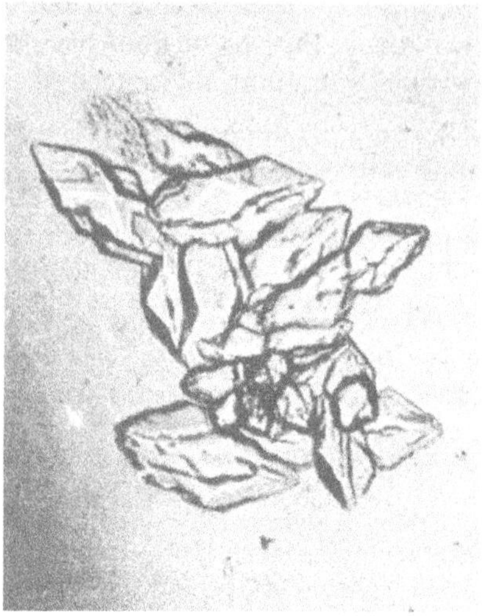

Fig. 21. Crystals of phospholipase A. Crystals were grown by dialysis in 2.2 M $(NH_4)_2SO_4$ (WELLS and HANAHAN, 1969)

ine method (MAGEE and THOMPSON, 1960; BROWN and BOWLES, 1966) for estimating loss of ester-linkage in phospholipids and the radioisotope method with 1,2-di[1-^{14}C] hexadecanoyl-*sn*-glycero-3-phosphocholine (Applied Science) (ROCK and SNYDER, 1975) are available.

Purification. Phospholipase A_2 has been highly purified from many venoms from snakes of the Hydrophiidae, Elapidae, Viperidae, and Crotalidae families. Some of the isolated enzymes from the venoms of *N. naja* (CURRIE et al., 1968), *N. naja atra* (SUZUKI et al., 1958), *C. adamanteus* (WELLS and HANAHAN, 1969; PASEK et al., 1975), and *C. atrox* (PASEK et al., 1975) have been crystallized (Fig. 21) and an X-ray crystallographic study is now in progress (PASEK et al., 1975). The isolation procedure of venom phospholipase A_2 is relatively simple, compared to those of other venom enzymes, such as phosphodiesterase, endopeptidase and L-amino acid oxidase. In many cases gel filtrations on Sephadex G-50 or Sephadex G-75 followed by ion-exchange chromatography on DEAE-cellulose or CM-cellulose yield an almost pure enzyme. During these procedures multiple forms of phospholipase A_2 can be found in most of the venoms used. SALACH et al. (1971 a) isolated 7–11 isoenzymes of the phospholipase in *N. naja* and *V. russellii* venoms, using the isoelectric focusing technique. Moreover, the existence of two or three isoenzymes with phospholipase A activity have been established from *C. adamanteus* (WELLS and HANAHAN, 1969), *A. halys blomhoffii* (IWANAGA and KAWAUCHI, 1959; KAWAUCHI et al., 1971 a), *N. nigricollis* (WAHLSTRÖM, 1971), *B. neuwieddii* (VIDAL et al., 1972 a), *V. palestinae* (SHILOAH et al., 1973 c), *V. berus* (DELORI, 1973), and *N. melanoleuca* (JOUBERT and VAN DER WALT, 1975). The properties of the isoenzymes will be described later. Although a number of the isolation procedures for venom phospholipase A_2 have been developed, an overall recovery of the enzyme is on the order of only 20%–30%. Two new methods for the purification of the enzyme have been recently devised. One involves

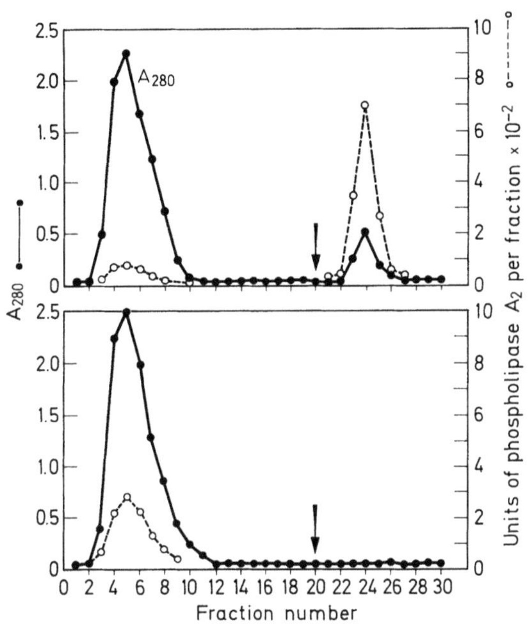

Fig. 22. *A* Total protein and phospholipase A_2 (*C. adamanteus* venom) activity elution profiles on PC-Sepharose 4B. Total venom proteins were loaded and run in Buffer I (see text) until A_{280} returned to baseline. *Arrow* indicates where elution with Buffer II (see text) is initiated. *B* The same as *A* except the $CaCl_2$ in Buffer I was replaced by NaCl (75 mM) (ROCK and SNYDER, 1975)

an affinity chromatography with rac-1-(9-carboxy)nonyl-2-hexadecylglycero-3-phosphocholine linked to AH-Sepharose 4B (Pharmacia, Uppsala) via the carboxyl group; the other, precipitation of the bulk of venom proteins with 50% isopropanol, precipitation of the enzymes from the isopropanol-soluble material with neodynium chloride, and final purification on DEAE-cellulose. Because of the simplicity of the methods and high recovery of the enzyme, these methods appear superior to the previous methods.

Affinity Chromatography (ROCK and SNYDER, 1975). All operations are carried out at 5° C. A column (0.9 x 15 cm) is packed with 5 ml PC-Sepharose and washed with 10 column volumes of Buffer I that contains Tris-HCl, pH 7.5 (50 mM), $CaCl_2$ (25 mM), NaCl (0.2 M), and EDTA (1 mM). The column is charged with 10 mg crude venom *(C. adamanteus)* made up in 2 ml Buffer I. This solution is allowed to pass into the column and is then followed by 0.5 ml Buffer I. The column is then plugged and allowed to stand for 2 h. At the end of this time five column volumes of Buffer I are passed through the column followed by five column volumes of Buffer II, consisting of Tris-HCl (50 mM) and EDTA (50 mM), pH 7.5. Fractions of 1 ml are collected at a flow rate of 15 ml/h (Fig. 22). Desired fractions are pooled, concentrated, and exchanged into a Tris-HCl (50 mM), $CaCl_2$ (25 mM), EDTA (1 mM) buffer, pH 7.5, for storage and assay using an Amicon ultrafiltration cell equipped with a PM-10 membrane. Further resolution of the two phospholipases present in this venom is achieved essentially as described by WELLS and HANAHAN (1969), using DEAE-cellulose (DE-52) column chromatography. The two enzymes isolated from this venom have a high yield (90%) and are homogeneous, as judged by polyacrylamide gel electrophoresis.

Isopropanol Precipitation Method (WELLS, 1975). 5 g *C. adamanteus* venom are dissolved in 250 ml 0.05 M acetate buffer, pH 5.25, containing 10 mM $CaCl_2$. To this solution is added

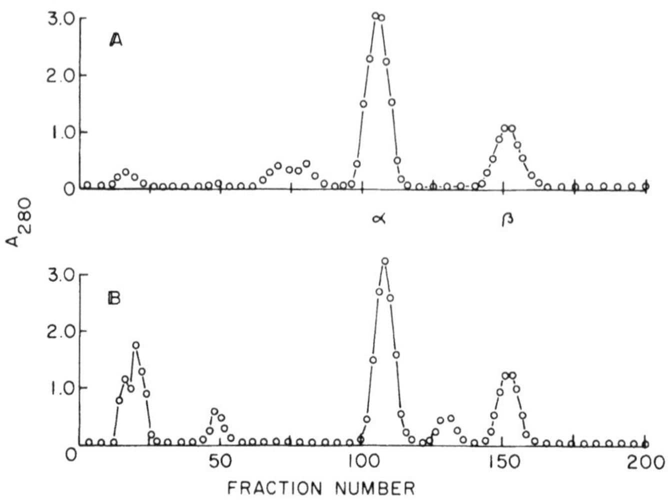

Fig. 23. DEAE-cellulose fractionation of phospholipase A_2 (*C. adamanteus* venom). Two different samples (*A* and *B*) were fractionated on a 1.8 × 100 cm column with an exponential gradient. The flow rate was 50 ml/h and 5 ml fractions were collected. α and β refer to the two forms of the enzyme (WELLS, 1975)

dropwise, in the course of 30 min and with rapid mixing at room temperature, 250 ml isopropanol. The suspension is stirred at room temperature for 30 min and then centrifuged in a Sorvall RC 2B, using a GSA head, at 5000 rpm/min for 30 min at 4° C. The slightly turbid supernatant solution is decanted and the precipitate discarded. To the supernatant solution is added 10 ml 0.5 M $NdCl_2$ in 0.05 M acetate buffer, pH 5.25. The suspension is mixed at room temperature for 30 min and centrifuged as described above. The supernatant solution is discarded and the precipitate dissolved in 50 ml 0.05 M Tris-HCl buffer, pH 8.0, containing 0.01 M EDTA. The solution is dialyzed in the cold for 48 h against 4 liters Tris-EDTA buffer. The dialysis buffer is changed twice at 18-h intervals. After dialysis. the protein solution is centrifuged and the supernatant solution concentrated with an Amicon Diaflo apparatus and a UM 10 membrane to 10 ml. This protein solution is applied to a 1.8 × 10 cm column of DEAE-cellulose (Whatman DE-52), that has been packed and equilibrated in 0.05 M Tris-HCl, pH 8.0, containing 1 mM EDTA. The column is eluted at room temperature with exponential gradient formed by using three chambers of a Buchler Varigrad. The first two chambers contain 400 ml each 0.05 M Tris-HCl, 1 mM EDTA, 0.02 M NaCl, pH 8.0 and the third chamber, an equal weight of 0.05 M Tris-HCl, 1 mM EDTA, 0.2 M NaCl, pH 8.0. A flow rate of 50 ml/h is maintained with a peristaltic pump and the eluate gradient is collected in 5-ml fractions. The elution profile is shown in Figure 23. The phospholipase $A_2\alpha$ and $A_2\beta$ isolated by this procedure are identical in all respects to enzymes isolated by the previous method (WELLS and HANAHAN, 1969). The obvious advantage of this procedure is the high yield of enzyme, ~80%, and the relative ease of the purification scheme.

Physicochemical Properties. The venom phospholipase A_2 exhibits considerable stability toward heat; the enzyme maintains full activity after being subjected to heating at 90° C for 15 min at pH 3.0. On storage of the enzyme preparation (*A. halys blomhoffii* venom) in 0.1 M acetate (pH 7.0) for 6 months, either at 4° C or at −10° C, the catalytic activity decreases by less than 10% (KAWAUCHI et al., 1971a). It also resists lyophilization, repeated thawings, urea (6 M), and acidic solvents such as 10% formic acid (BREITHAUPT, 1976). Table 29 summarizes the physicochemical proper-

Table 29. Physiochemical properties of venom phospholipase A_2

Property	*A. halys blomhoffii*[a]		*C. adamanteus*[b]		*Laticauda semifasciata*[c]	*N. melanoleuca*[d]		
	A-I	A-II	$A_2\alpha$	$A_2\beta$		DE-III	DE-II	DE-I
Sedimentation coefficient, $S_{20,w}$	1.80	1.90	3.11	3.11	1.93	1.88	1.93	1.79
Diffusion coefficient $D_{20,w}$ ($\times 10^{-7}$ cm^2/s)		13.35	9.02	9.02	0.141	10.8	10.3	10.4
Partial specific volume, $\bar{v}$ (ml/g)	0.730	0.712	0.718	0.718	0.71	0.704	0.703	0.708
Intrinsic viscosity, $[\eta]$	0.034	0.031	—	—	—	—	—	—
Frictional ratio (f/fo)	1.18	1.15	1.16	1.16	—	—	—	—
Molecular weight	13100[e]	13900[e]	29900[f]	31100[f]	11000[f]	14200[f]	13400[f]	12900[f]
Isoelectric point (pI)	10.0	4.0	4.55	4.40	6.60	—	—	—
Helix content	20%	27%	—	—	—	17.2%	19.3%	15.9%
Total amino acid residues	126	126	133[g]	—	108	119	119	118

[a] Kawauchi et al. (1971).
[b] Wells and Hanahan (1969).
[c] Tu et al. (1970).
[d] Joubert and van der Walt (1975).
[e] Calculated with Scherage-Mandelkern equation.
[f] From $S_{20,w}$, $D_{20,w}$, and $\bar{v}$.
[g] Tsao et al. (1975).

Table 30. Amino acid composition of phospholipase A_2

Amino acid	*C. adamanteus*			*A. halys blomhoffii*[c]		*C. atrox*[d]	*V. palestinae*[e]		*V. berus*[f]		
	$A_2\alpha$[a]	$A_2\beta$[a]	A_2[b]	A-I	A-II		F_1	F_2	P_1	P_2	P_4
Lys	16	16	7	17	8	14	10	9	19	13	8
His	5	5	2	2	1	4	3	3	4	5	2
Arg	12	12	5	6	4	10	3	3	10	10	4
Asp	30	30	16	14	17	34	18	18	40	34	11
Thr	13	13	7	6	5	16	7	7	12	13	5
Ser	13	13	7	5	4	16	7	7	17	16	4
Glu	24	24	13	6	13	28	12	12	22	19	6
Pro	16	16	9	5	5	18	4	4	12	14	4
Gly	24	24	13	10	13	30	14	15	35	27	8
Ala	15	15	8	5	7	18	7	7	13	13	4
Cys	30	30	14	14	14	28	12	12	27	17	10
Val	11	11	5	5	4	8	7	7	14	14	2
Met	2	2	1	3	2	4	4	4	11	8	2
Ile	11	11	5	7	7	14	4	4	16	16	4
Leu	11	11	5	5	5	14	9	9	15	15	5
Tyr	16	16	8	10	10	14	9	9	21	14	7
Phe	10	10	5	5	5	8	8	8	14	10	4
Trp	7	7	3	2	2	2	2	2	4	5	1
Total	266	266	133	126	126	280	140	140	298	259	91

[a] WELLS and HANAHAN (1969).
[b] TSAO et al. (1975).
[c] KAWAUCHI et al. (1971).
[d] HACHIMORI et al. (1971).
[e] SHILOAH et al. (1971).
[f] DELORI (1973).

Table 30 (continued)

Amino acid	*Bitis arietans*[g]	*Bitis gavonica*[h]	*N. naja naja*[i]	*N. naja atra*[j]	*N. nigricollis*[k]		*N. melanoleuca*[l]			*Laticauda semifasciata*[m]	*C. terrificus*[n]
					X	A_1	DE-I	DE-II	DE-III		
Lys	12	8	5	5	10	10	8	5	4	7	11
His	2	2	1	1	2–3	3	3	2	3	2	12
Arg	4	3	4	5	5	5	6	6	6	4	12
Asp	14	19	19	20	17	17	19	20	20	11	11
Thr	6	8	4	5	5	5	7	7	6	6	8
Ser	5	6	7	6	3	2–3	3	6	6	7	7
Glu	10	10	6	8	4	4–5	7	8	6	9	10
Pro	5	2	5	5	7	6	4	3	4	5	5
Gly	11	13	9	10	11	11	9	9	9	10	13
Ala	6	4	8	11	10	10	9	10	10	8	7
Cys	14	12	11	12	14	13	14	14	14	12	16
Val	3	3	4	4	4	4	4	4	4	4	2
Met	2	3	1	1	2	2	1	1	1	1	2
Ile	5	6	3	5	4	4	5	5	6	3	5
Leu	4	2	5	5	5	5	3	3	3	5	7
Tyr	8	10	6	9	8–9	9	9	9	9	10	12
Phe	5	5	3	4	5	5	4	4	4	3	7
Trp	1	2	1	3	2–3	1	3	3	3	1	3
Total	117	118	102	119	118–121	116–118	118	119	119	108	140

[g] HOWARD (1975).
[h] BOTES and VILJOEN (1974).
[i] DEEMS and DENNIS (1975).
[j] CHANG and LO (1972).
[k] DUMAREY et al. (1975).
[l] JOUBERT and VAN DER WALT (1975).
[m] TU et al. (1970).
[n] BREITHAUPT et al. (1974).

ties of phospholipase A_2 isolated from crotalid, elapid, and hydrophiid venoms. The molecular weight in the range 11000–31000 and the values reported in the literature for phospholipase A_2 from various sources are: pocine pancreatic, 15000 (DE HAAS et al., 1968); *N. naja*, 24000 (CURRIE et al., 1968); *C. atrox*, 14500 (WU and TINKER, 1969); *N. nigricollis*, two isozymes 13000 and 14500 (WAHLSTRÖM, 1971); *N. naja*, several isozymes ranging from 8500 to 20000 (SALACH et al., 1971a); *Bothrops neuwiedii*, two enzymes, 9500 and 20000 (VIDAL et al., 1972a); *Vipera palestinae*, 16000 (SHILOAH et al., 1973); and *N. naja atra*, 12500 (LO and CHANG, 1974). Although the molecular weight of the enzyme significantly differs from venom to venom, a dynamic equilibrium between dimer and monomer seems to exist which can shift towards either of the two forms depending on conditions, e.g., ionic strength and calcium ions in medium. Ultracentrifugal studies for *Bitis gavonica* enzyme for example, indicate the predominance of dimer under neutral conditions, whereas gel filtration studies, under similar conditions except for higher ionic strength, show that phospholipase A_2 is mainly in the monomer state. Addition of calcium ions shifts the equilibrium towards the dimer, this is reversed towards the monomer by addition of EDTA (BOTES and VILJOEN, 1974b). Thus, it is not inconceivable that the same might apply in the cases of *C. atrox* (WU and TINKER, 1969; HACHIMORI et al., 1971), *C. adamanteus* (WELLS and HANAHAN, 1969), and *B. neuwiedii* (VIDAL et al., 1972a), or that trace amounts of calcium ions might influence the equilibrium between dimer and monomer. However, another heterogeneity does not seem to be due to the monomer-dimer equilibrium, but rather to the charge difference of the enzyme. An example of this is *N. naja* venom, which has been shown to contain at least six phospholipases that are separable on ion exchange chromatography and polyacrylamide-gel electrophoresis (SHILOAH et al., 1973a).

The amino acid compositions of phospholipases A_2 isolated from various venoms are shown in Table 30. The comparison is limited to phospholipases A_2 containing 108–140 amino acid residues. High contents of aspartic acid, half-cystine, glycine, and tyrosine are common features of all phospholipases. The enzymes contain 12–14 half-cystine residues and consequently their cross-linking must be very similar. The number of basic amino acid residues reveals and interesting trend. Whereas the number of histidine residues range from 1 to 3 and that of arginine residues, from 3 to 6, the number of lysines of various phospholipases is quite variable, ranging from 4 to 17. No carbohydrate components nor free SH-groups have been found in the venom phospholipases. Circular dichroism (CD) studies of phospholipase A_2 monomer from the venom of *A. halys blomhoffii* indicate that it has α-helix content of 32%–37%. A negative trough at 233 nm in the CD spectra suggests the presence of a region with a right-handed α-helical structure. The α-helical contents of *C. adamanteus* phospholipase A_2 dimer (WELLS, 1971a) and *V. ammodytes* enzyme monomer (GUBENSEK and LAPANJE, 1974) have been estimated to be nearly 70% in the former and 24% in the latter. The CD spectra of three phospholipases A_2 from *N. melanoleuca* are very similar. The spectra show two negative maxima in the regions of 210 and 233 nm. The amount of α-helix are 28%, 27%, and 22% for DE-I, DE-II, and DE-III respectively (Table 29). The β-structure content is considered very small or nonexistent in these enzymes (JOUBERT and VAN DER WALT, 1975). Crystals of two venom phospholipases from *C. adamanteus* venom have recently been subjected to X-ray diffraction analysis (PASEK et al., 1975). The space group is $C222_1$, and a=108. 1 Å, b=79.4 Å, c=63.9 Å, with a dimer per asymmetric unit.

Primary Structure of Phospholipase A_2. Figure 24 shows the complete amino acid seuqences of the porcine pancreatic and three venom phospholipases A_2 so far established. To obtain the maximum degree of sequence homology, phospholipases A_2 are aligned with respect to the position of cysteine residues and a few deletions, arbitrarily assigned, are introduced. Whereas the enzymes of porcine pancreas and *Bitis gavonica* venom both contain six disulfide bridges, those from *N. melanoleuca* and *H. haemachatus* venoms are crosslinked by seven disulfide bridges. It is possible to position the 12 cysteinyl residues of the porcine pancreatic enzyme with the corresponding cysteinyl residues of the *N. melanoleuca* and *H. haemochatus* enzymes. The positions of invariant amino acid residues are given in Figure 24 in blocked regions. The high degree of homology between various phospholipases A_2 is immediately apparent. A comparison of all phospholipase A_2 structures shows that 30 residues including eight half-cystines are identical. Moreover, a very high sequence homology with the three isoenzymes of phospholipase A_2 from *N. melanoleuca* is found in the enzymes from the venoms of *H. haemochatus* and *Bitis gavonica* (JOUBERT, 1975).

Enzymatic Properties. Most of venom phospholipases A_2 are active in the alkaline pH region, pH 7.5–pH 8.5, and the enzyme activity decreases remarkably below pH 6 or above pH 10. The optimum temperature for enzyme activity is variable in various venoms (NAIR et al., 1976). Maximum enzyme activities with the venoms of *N. nigricollis, N. melanoleuca, N. n. siamensis, N. n. annulifera, N. naja* and *A. piscivorus* are observed at 65° C. *Bungarus fasciatus* and *Bitis gavonica* venoms show an optimum at 55° C and *Echis carinatus*, at 50° C. *C. scutulatus, C. scutulatus salvini*, and *C. adamanteus* venoms lose their phospholipase activity above 45° C. These variations in the rate of hydrolysis (dipalmitoyl lecithin as substrate) at elevated temperature may result from changes in the conformation of the enzyme molecules due to increased temperature (NAIR et al., 1976).

Venom phospholipase A_2 requires Ca^{2+} for catalytic activity. The activity of the enzyme is also enhanced by Na^+, K^+, Mg^{2+}, Mn^{2+}, and deoxycholate. Zn^{2+}, Cu^{2+}, Na_2-EDTA, phosphate, oxalate, sulfide, cyanide, citrate, fatty acids, and lysolecithin inhibit the enzyme. Especially long-chain fatty acids (palmitate, oleate, linoleate) cause inhibition at low concentration (less than 0.1 mM). This inhibition is prevented by addition of plasma albumin, which activates *N. naja* phospholipase A_2 activity in the absence of added fatty acid (SMITH et al., 1972). Low concentrations of Ba^{2+} increase the enzyme activity, whereas high concentrations inhibit the enzyme (BREITHAUPT, 1976). Phospholipase A_2 isolated from *B. neuwiedii* venom exhibits the same absolute requirement for divalent cations; it is maximally activated by Ca^{2+} and to a lesser degree by Co^{2+}, Mg^{2+}, and Cd^{2+}. Ba^{2+}, Mn^{2+}, and Sr^{2+} are inactive, but Fe^{2+}, Cu^{2+}, and Zn^{2+} are inhibitory (VIDAL et al., 1972a). This enzyme is inhibited by citrate and nitrate and inactivated after treatments with iodoacetic acid and 2-mercaptoethanol. There is no inhibition by 8 M urea and DFP.

The substrate specificity of venom phospholipase A_2 is now known in detail. This enzyme specifically cleaves the ester linkage at the 2-position of phosphoglycerides, giving rise to unsaturated fatty acids and 1-acylglycerophosphatides; the reaction

10 20

(a) H_2N-Asp-Leu-Thr-Gln-Phe-Gly-Asn-Met-Ile-Asn- - - - - - -Lys-Met-Gly-Glu-Ser-Val-Phe-
(b) H_2N-Ala-Leu-Trp-Gln-Phe-Arg-Ser-Met-Ile-Lys-Cys-Ala-Ile-Pro-Gly-Ser-His-Pro-Leu-Met-
(c) H_2N-Asn-Leu-Tyr-Gln-Phe-Lys-Asn-Met-Ile-His-Cys-Thr-Val-Pro-Asn-Arg- - -Pro-Trp-Trp-
(d) H_2N-Asn-Leu-Tyr-Gln-Phe-Lys-Asn-Met-Ile-Gln-Cys-Thr-Val-Pro-Asn-Arg- - -Ser-Trp-Trp-
(e) H_2N-Asn-Leu-Tyr-Gln-Phe-Lys-Asn-Met-Ile-His-Cys-Thr-Val-Pro-Asn-Arg- - -Ser-Trp-Trp-
(f) H_2N-Asn-Leu-Tyr-Gln-Phe-Lys-Asn-Met-Ile-Lys-Cys-Thr-Val-Pro-Ser-Arg- - -Ser-Trp-Trp-

30 40

Asp-Tyr-Ile-Tyr-Tyr-Gly-Cys-Tyr-Cys-Gly-Trp-Gly-Gly-Lys- - -Gly-Lys-Pro-Ile-Asp-
Asp-Phe-Asn-Asn-Tyr-Gly-Cys-Tyr-Cys-Gly-Leu-Gly-Gly- - -Ser-Gly-Thr-Pro-Val-Asn-
His-Phe-Ala-Asn-Tyr-Gly-Cys-Tyr-Cys-Gly-Arg-Gly-Gly-Lys- - -Gly-Thr-Pro-Val-Asp-
His-Phe-Ala-Asn-Tyr-Gly-Cys-Tyr-Cys-Gly-Arg-Gly-Gly- - -Ser-Gly-Thr-Pro-Val-Asp-
His-Phe-Ala-Asn-Tyr-Gly-Cys-Tyr-Cys-Gly-Arg-Gly-Gly- - -Ser-Gly-Thr-Pro-Val-Asp-
His-Phe-Ala-Asn-Tyr-Gly-Cys-Tyr-Cys-Gly-Arg-Gly-Gly- - -Ser-Gly-Thr-Pro-Val-Asp-

50 60

Ala-Thr-Asp-Arg-Cys-Cys-Phe-Val-His-Asp- - -Cys-Cys-Tyr-Gly-Lys-Met-Gly- - -Thr-
Glu-Leu-Asn-Arg-Cys- - -Gly-His-Thr-Asp-Asn-Cys- - -Tyr-Arg-Asp-Ala-Lys-Asn-Leu-
Asp-Leu-Asp-Arg-Cys-Cys-Gln-Ile-His-Asp-Lys-Cys- - -Tyr-Asp-Glu-Ala-Glu- - -Lys-
Asp-Leu-Asp-Arg-Cys-Cys-Gln-Ile-His-Asp-Asn-Cys- - -Tyr-Gly-Glu-Ala-Glu- - -Lys-
Asp-Leu-Asp-Arg-Cys-Cys-Gln-Ile-His-Asp-Asn-Cys- - -Tyr-Gly-Glu-Ala-Glu- - -Lys-
Asp-Leu-Asp-Arg-Cys-Cys-Gln-Thr-His-Asp-Asn-Cys- - -Tyr-Ser-Asp-Ala-Glu- - -Lys-

70 80

Tyr-Asp-Thr- - -Lys-Trp-Thr-Ser-Tyr-Asn- - -Tyr- - -Glu-Ile- - - - - - - -Gln-
Asn-Asp-Ser-Cys-Lys-Phe-Leu-Val-Asp-Asn-Pro-Tyr-Thr-Glu-Ser-Tyr-Ser-Tyr-Cys-Ser-
Ile-Ser-Gly-Cys-Trp-Pro-Tyr-Ile-Lys-Thr- - -Tyr-Thr- - - - -Tyr-Glu-Ser-Cys-Gln-
Ile-Ser-Gly-Cys-Trp-Pro-Tyr-Ile-Cys-Thr- - -Tyr-Thr- - - - -Tyr-Glu-Ser-Cys-Gln-
Ile-Ser-Gly-Cys-Trp-Pro-Tyr-Ile-Lys-Thr- - -Tyr-Thr- - - - -Tyr-Asp-Ser-Cys-Gln-
Ile-Ser-Gly-Cys-Arg-Pro-Tyr-Phe-Lys-Thr- - -Tyr-Ser- - - - -Tyr-Asp- - -Cys-Thr-

Fig. 24. Comparison of the amino acid sequences of various phospholipase A_2. (*a*) *Bitis gavonica* (BOTES and VILJON, 1974); (*b*) porcine pancreas (DE HAAS et al., 1970); (*c*) *N. melanoleuca* (fraction DE-I); (*d*) *N. melanoleuca* (fraction DE-II); (*e*) *N. melanoleuca* (fraction DE-III) (unpublished result courtest of JOUBERT); (*f*) *Hemachatus haemachatus* (fraction DE-I) (JOUBERT, 1975)

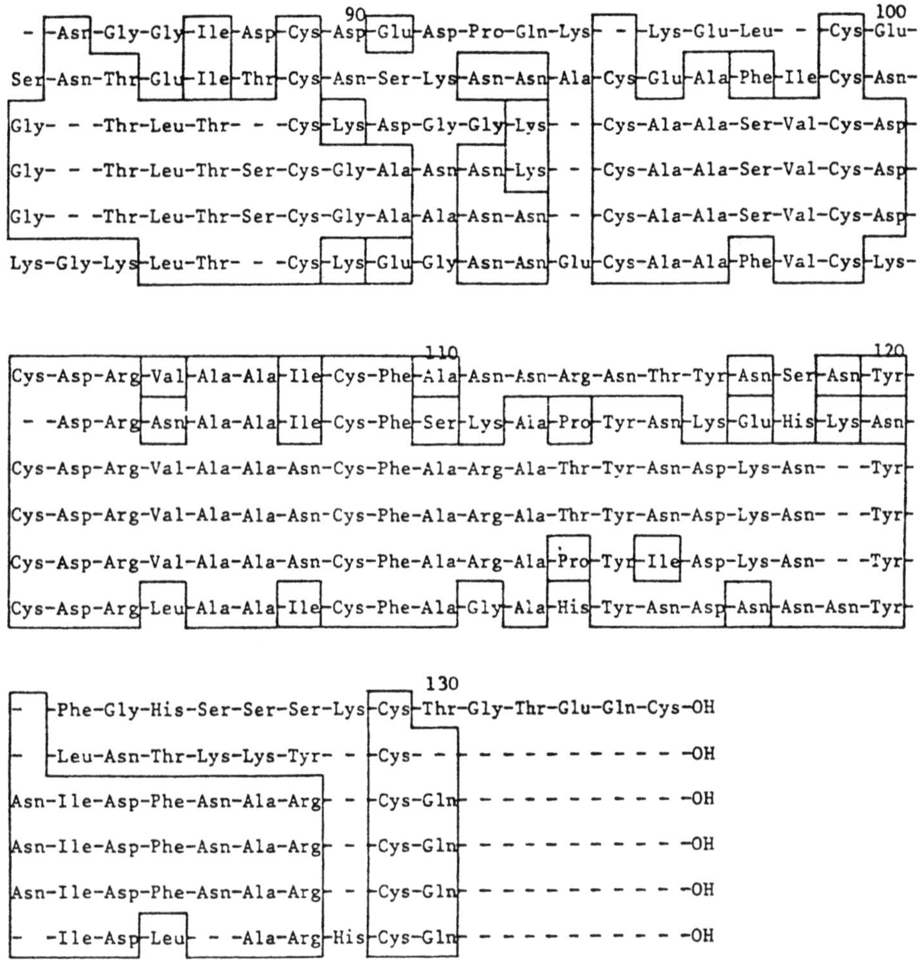

Fig. 24 (continued)

proceeds by 0-acyl cleavage, as evidenced by the enzymatic hydrolysis of 1,2-dipalmitoyl-*sn*-glycero-3-phosphorylcholine in the presence of $H_2{}^{18}O$ (WELLS, 1971c).

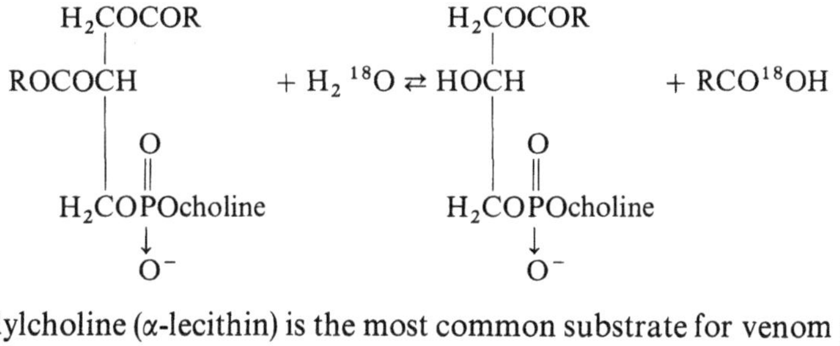

Phosphatidylcholine (α-lecithin) is the most common substrate for venom phospholipase A_2. The hydrolysis of this substrate can take place in free substrate form, in egg yolk, and in serum (TU et al., 1970; MARINETTI, 1961; CHINEN, 1972). Phospholipids

Table 31. Substrate specificity of venom phospholipase A_2[a] (VAN DEENEN and DE HAAS, 1963)

Hydrolysis	No hydrolysis
[I] 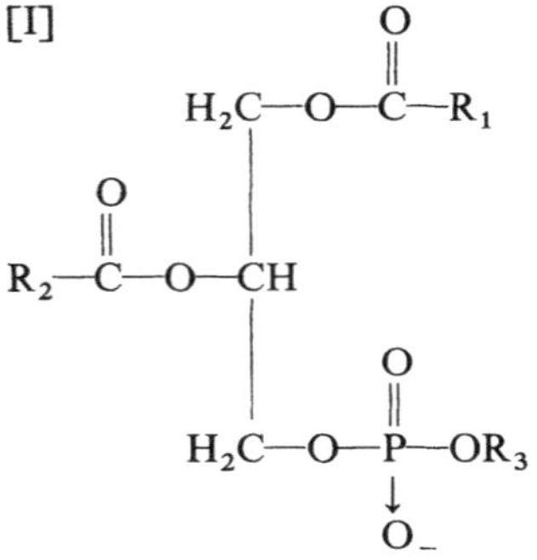 [I_a] $R_3{=}CH_2{-}CH_2{-}\overset{+}{N}(CH_3)_3$ [I_b] $R_3{=}CH_2{-}CH_2{-}NH_2$ [I_c] $R_3{=}CH_2{-}CH(NH_2){-}COOH$ [I_d] $R_3{=}H$ [I_e] $R_3{=}CH_2{-}CHOH{-}CH_2OH$	[VII] 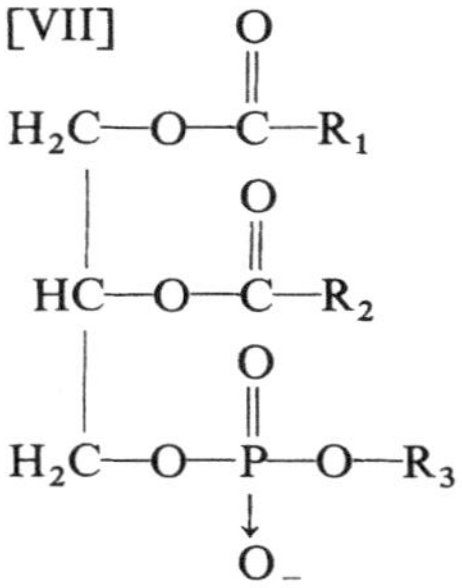 $R_3{=}CH_2{-}CH_2{-}\overset{+}{N}(CH_3)_3$
[II] 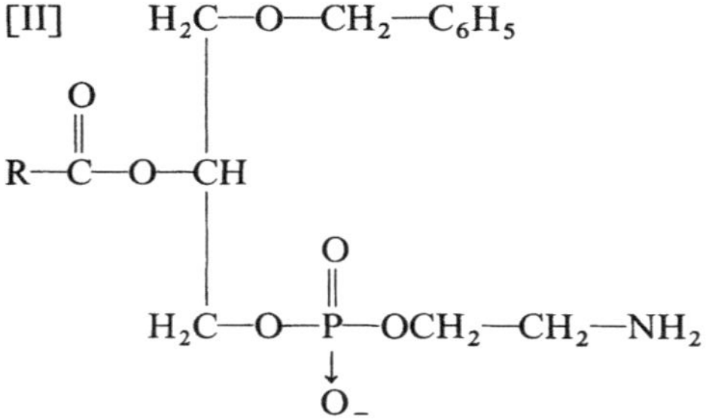	[VIII] 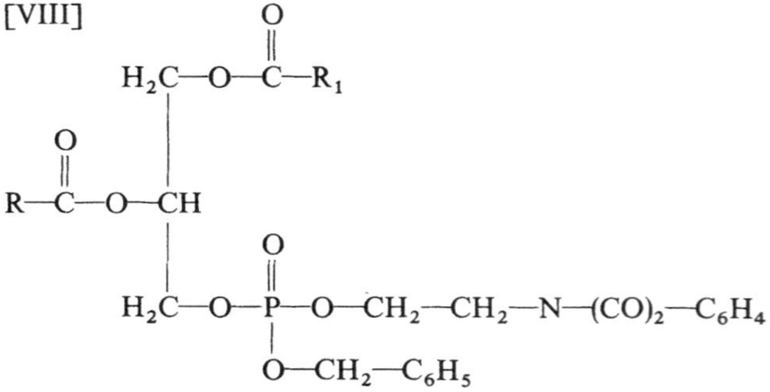
[III] 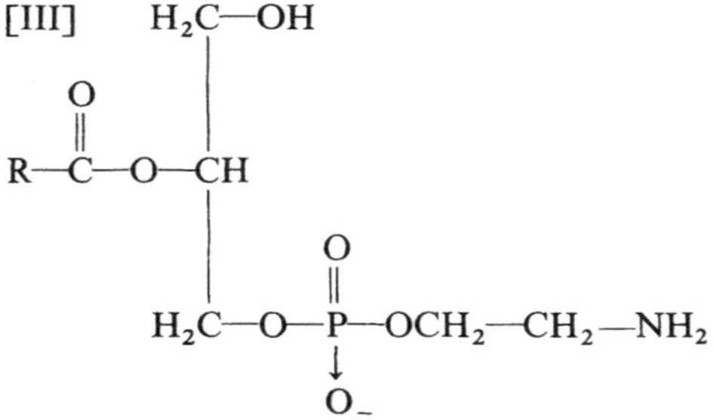	[IX] 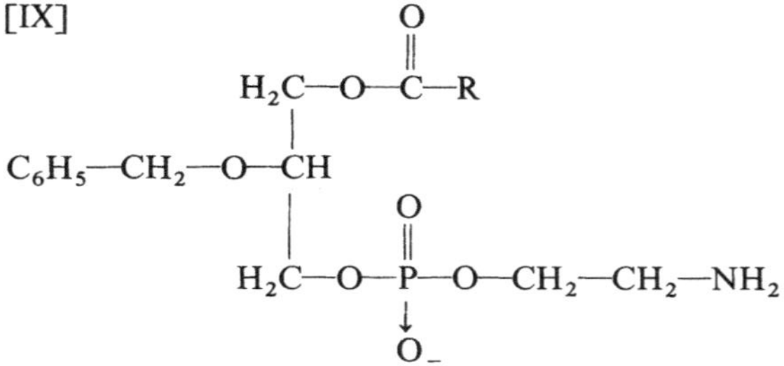

[IV]

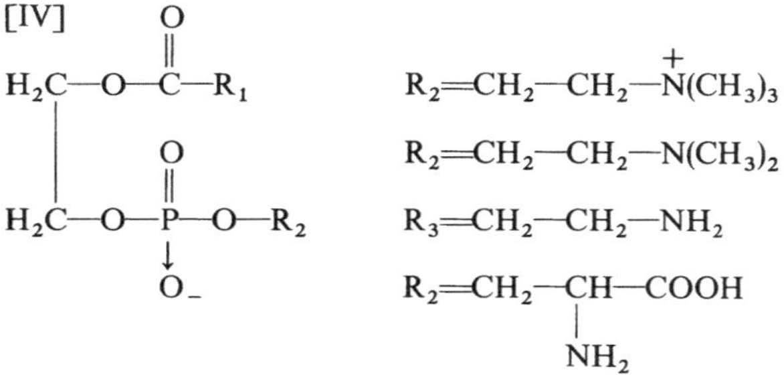

[V]

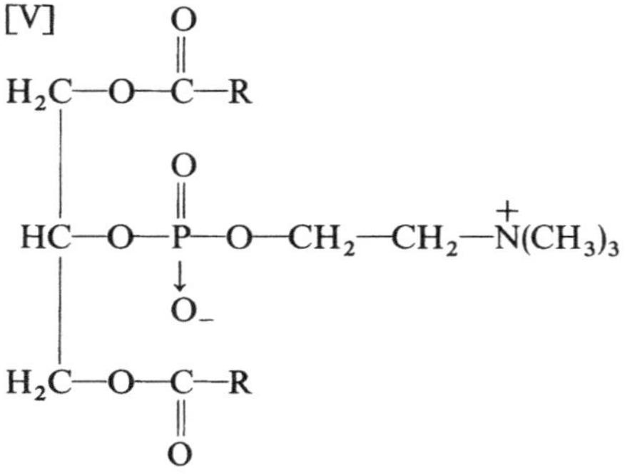

[VI]

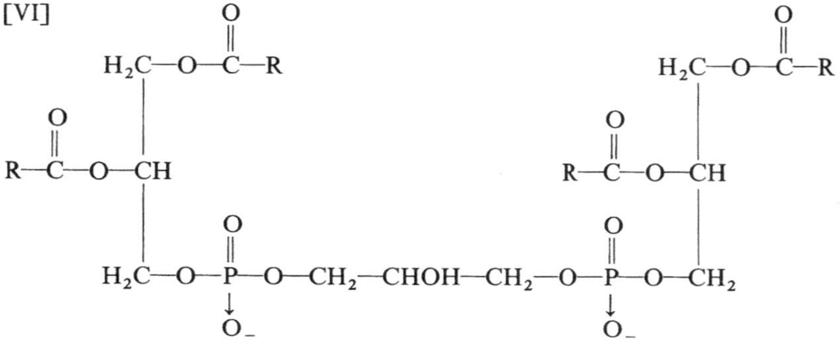

[X]

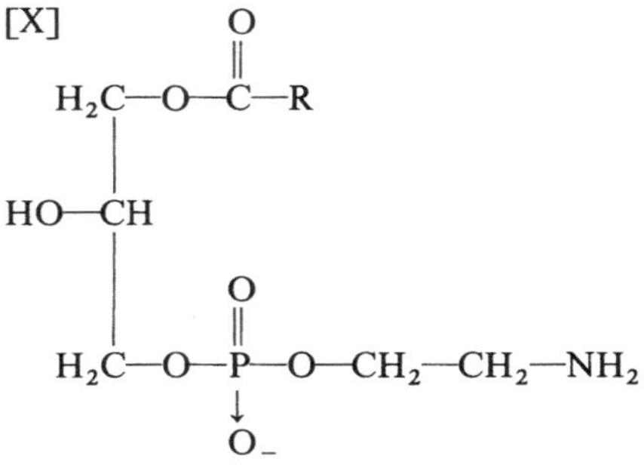

[XI]

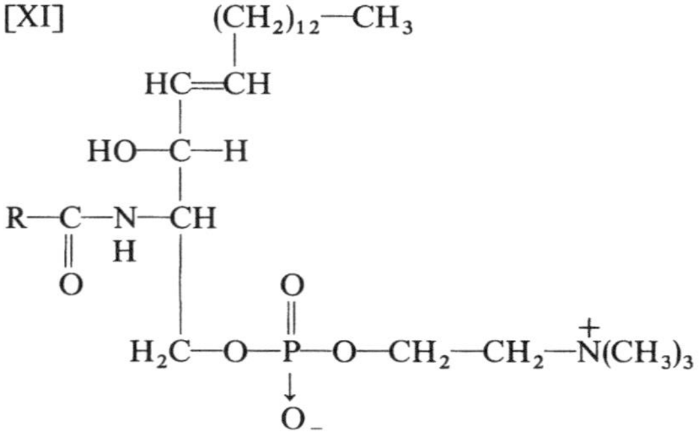

[a] [Ia]: L-α-lecithin; [Ib]: L-α-cepharin; [Ic]: L-α-phosphatidyl-serine; [IV]: Glycol derivatives; [V]: β-lecithin; [VI]: Cardiolipin; [VII]: D-α-lecithin; [XI]: Sphingomyelin.

of human serum high-density lipoprotein can also be hydrolyzed by the purified enzyme from *C. adamanteus* venom (PATTNAIK et al., 1976). VAN DEENEN and DE HAAS (1963) made detailed studies on substrate specificity of *C. adamanteus* phospholipase A_2, using various modified analogues of phospholipids and elucidated the following substrate characteristics for the enzyme (Table 31):

1. Within the class of α-phosphoglycerides, L-isomers are readily hydrolyzed, whereas D-α-phospholipids do not appear to be attacked.
2. L-α-lecithins containing fatty acids with greatly varying chain length are susceptible to phospholipase A_2 action; however, certain water-soluble short-chain compounds are hydrolyzed only at a very slow rate.
3. Aside from effects on the surface charge of the phosphoglyceride micelles, the nature of the polar headgroup esterified to the phosphoryl moiety does not form any prerequisite and its presence even appears to be dispensable.
4. Contrary to a blocking of the amino function, protection of the hydroxyl function of phosphatidylethanolamine causes inactivation of the substrate properties.
5. Both a γ-benzyl-β-acyl-α-phosphoglyceride and a β-acyllyso derivative are hydrolyzed, whereas the corresponding structural isomers carrying the fatty acid in γ-position appears unsusceptible to the enzyme action.
6. Glycol analogues are demonstrated to exhibit substrate activity.
7. Phospholipase A_2 catalyzes the hydrolysis of a symmetric β-lecithin into an optically active lysolecithin.

On the basis of these results, they postulated that the minimum structure which is required as substrates for venom phospholipase A_2 *(C. adamanteus)* may be illustrated as follows:

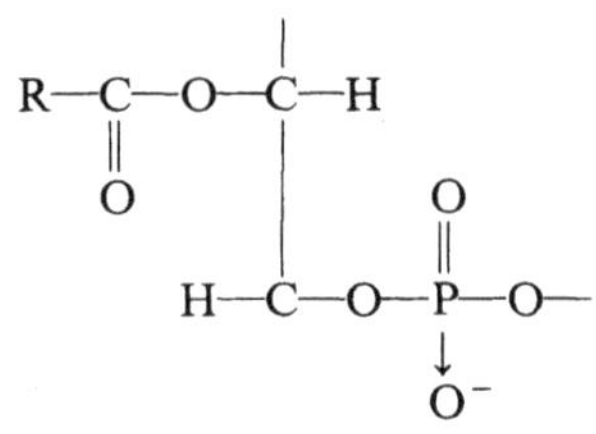

Kinetic investigations on the hydrolysis of various glycerophosphatides have also been made by WOELK and DEBUCH (1971) and COLES et al. (1974), using pure phospholipase A_2 isolated from *C. atrox*. In the diethyl ether medium, the relative rates of hydrolysis are phosphatidylcholine ($KM = 7.0 \times 10^{-3}$ M > phosphatidalcholine ≫ phosphatidylserine ≈ phosphatidalethanolamine > phosphatidylethanolamine ($Km = 26.7 \times 10^{-3}$ M), whereas in an aqueous medium, the relative rates are phosphatidylcholine phosphatidylethanolamine > phosphatidylserine > phosphatidalethanolamine ≈ phosphatidalcholine. The rate of hydrolysis of phosphatidylcholine is independent of the degree of desaturation of the fatty acids. Compared to 1,2-diacyl-sn-glycerol-3-phosphorylcholine and -ethanolamine, the corresponding 1-alk-1′-enyl-2-acyl-compounds (plasmalogens) are cleaved more slowly by the phospholipase A_2. The Km value for pure choline plasmalogen amounts to 96.0×10^{-3} M. Furthermore, WOELK and PEILER-ICHIKAWA (1974) found that acylalkenyl- and acylalkyl-phosphoglycerides are hydrolyzed at almost similar rates by the

Table 32. Hydrolysis of various glycerophosphatides, differing in the radical at the 1-position and in the fatty acid constituent at the 2-position, by purified phospholipase A_2 from *Crotalus atrox* venom (WOELK and PEILER-ICHIKAWA, 1974)

Substrate	Specific activity[a] (units/mg protein)
1-acyl-2-[^{14}C]linoleoyl-sn-glycero-3-phosphorylcholine	151.4 ± 10.2
1-alk-1'-enyl-2-[^{14}C]linoleoyl-sn-glycero-3-phosphorylcholine	25.6 ± 1.8
1-alk-1'-enyl-2-[^{14}C]linolenoyl-sn-glycero-3-phosphorylcholine	34.8 ± 2.0
1-alk-1'-enyl-2-[^{14}C]arachidonoyl-sn-glycero-3-phosphorylcholine	19.8 ± 1.5
1-alkyl-2-[^{14}C]linoleoyl-sn-glycero-3-phosphorylcholine	32.4 ± 1.1
1-alkyl-2-[^{14}C]linolenoyl-sn-glycero-3-phorphorylcholine	26.1 ± 2.0
1-alkyl-2-[^{14}C]arachidonoyl-sn-glycero-3-phosphorylcholine	18.2 ± 1.4

[a] One unit of enzyme activity is defined as the amount of enzyme which hydrolyzes 1 µmole of the substrate per min under conditions where zero-order kinetics apply. Specific activity is expressed in enzyme units per mg per protein.

Table 33. Hydrolytic indices of phospholipase A of various snake venoms for phosphatidylcholine analogues[a] (WAKU and NAKAZAWA, 1972)

Snake venoms	1-Acyl	1-O-Alkenyl-2-acyl-GPC	1-O-Alkyl-2-acyl-GPC
Crotalus adamanteus	100	5.0	2.7
Crotalus atrox	100	6.5	5.3
Crotalus basiliscus	100	4.5	0.0
Crotalus viridis viridis	100	8.0	5.7
Agkistrodon halys blomhoffii	100	28.2	67.5
Agkistrodon piscivorus piscivorus	100	28.8	21.7
Bothrops atrox	100	24.2	6.0
Vipera russellii	100	10.4	15.1
Trimeresurus flavoviridis	100	18.7	16.0
Naja naja atra	100	40.0	93.5
Naja naja	100	36.4	94.8

[a] The initial rates of hydrolysis of 1-O-alkenyl- and 1-O-alkyl-2-acyl-GPC by each venom are expressed as percentages of that of 1,2-diacyl-GPC.

enzyme (Table 32). Among phospholipases A_2 of snake venoms, the species of *Crotalus* mainly hydrolyze diacyl compound and the species of *N. naja* hydrolyze diacyl and 1-0-alkyl-2-acyl compounds at the same rates and 1-0-alkenyl-2-acyl compound at half this rate (Table 33) (WAKU and NAKAZAWA, 1972). In addition to the above phospholipids, a number of natural and synthetic derivatives are hydrolyzed by venom phospholipase A_2. They include α-lecithin, cardiolipin (diphosphatidylglycerol), egg yolk lipoprotein, membrane-bound phospholipids, and serum lipoproteins (TU, 1977).

The mode of action of venom phospholipase A_2 has been treated in a number of studies (WELLS, 1972, 1974a, b; RIBEIRO and DENNIS, 1973; ROBERTS et al., 1977a). RIBEIRO and DENNIS (1973) studied the colloidal states of dipalmitoylphosphatidylcholine at different temperatures in the presence of Triton X-100. They

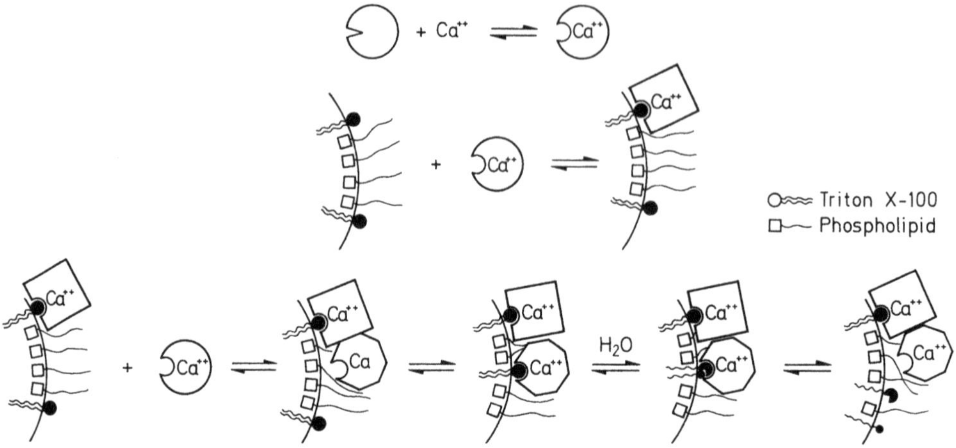

Fig. 25. "Dual-phospholipid" model for the action of venom phospholipase A_2 toward phospholipids contained in mixed micelles (ROBERTS et al., 1977)

found that at a higher temperatures the synthetic phospholipid in aqueous dispersion undergoes a thermotropic phase transition from bilayer to stable mixed micelles. Phospholipase A_2 activity *(N. naja naja)* towards the synthetic phospholipid at different temperatures showed a direct effect of the thermotropic phase transition of phospholipid on enzyme activity (DENNIS, 1973a). This result indicates that substrate must be in micellar form rather than either monomers or bilayers (DENNIS, 1973b; DEEMS et al., 1975). As described previously, phospholipase A_2 requires Ca^{2+} in its catalytic action. The attachment of Ca^{2+} induces a conformational change of the enzyme molecule, as shown in UV difference spectroscopy (VILJOEN et al., 1975). After the enzyme-Ca^{2+}-substrate complex is formed, the fatty acid is released from the enzyme, followed by the other product, lysophosphatidylcholine (WELLS, 1972; VILJOEN et al., 1974). The extensive kinetic and chemical studies along this line (ROBERTS et al., 1977a) have provided a possible mode of phospholipase A_2 action on mixed micelles (Fig. 25). The schematic diagram indicates that the enzyme must first bind Ca^{2+} (or inhibitory metals such as Ba^{2+} or Zn^{2+}) before it can bind phospholipid. Once Ca^{2+} is bound, the enzyme binds one phospholipid molecule at the interface. This binding causes a conformational change in the enzyme that leads to dimerization. A second phospholipid is then bound by the dimer at a functional active site and catalysis occurs. These two phospholipid sites are quite distinct, since they occur on different enzyme molecules. One would expect lateral diffusion of phospholipid in the mixed micelle to be quite rapid. This may be the primary means for bringing the second phospholipid in contact with the functional catalytic subunit. As the functional groups in the enzyme molecule, tyrosine, tryptophan, lysine, and histidine have been suggested (WELLS, 1971, 1973; VILJOEN et al., 1975; ROBERTS et al., 1977b).

2. Phospholipase B and Phospholipase C

As described in the previous section, all snake venoms so far investigated are known to possess a phospholipase of the type A_2. Several investigators have reported on the

Table 34. Phospholipase activity of some Australian snake venoms (DOERY and PEARSON, 1961, 1964)

Venom	Relative activity (%)		
	Phospholipase A[a]	Phospholipase B[b]	Direct hemolysin[c]
Pseudechis porphyriacus	100	100	100
Pseudechis australis	150	112	50
Pseudechis papuanus	150	–	100
Denisonia superba	50	112	50
Oxyuranus scutellatus	100	64	1
Notechis scutatus	50	57	2–3
Acanthophis antarticus	50	21	1
Demansia textilis textilis	20	–	12

[a] Determined by the method of NEUMAN and HABERMANN (1955).
[b] Determined using lysolecithin as substrate.
[c] Determined by the method of NEUMAN and HABERMANN (1954).

Table 35. 1-Monoacyl-sn-glycerophosphorylcholine (lysolecithin) hydrolysis by purified phospholipase A from *Vipera palestinae* (SHILOAH et al., 1972)

Source	Concentration (μg/ml)	Lysolecithin hydrolysis (%/h)	
		pH 7	pH 10
V. palestinae (purified)	25	15.6	80
C. adamanteus (crude venom)	450	6.5	90

additional ability of certain snake venoms and boiled venoms to hydrolyze lysophosphatides, i.e., to exhibit phospholipase B activity (VAN DEENEN and HAAS, 1963; DOERY and PEARSON, 1961; MOHAMED et al., 1968). However, it is now known that the latter enzyme is due to dual activity of the known phospholipase A_2. The first indication of phospholipase B activity in snake venoms was discovered by DOERY and PEARSON (1964), who demonstrated such an activity in Australian snake venoms (Table 34). In a later study, SHILOAH et al. (1973c) showed that a purified phospholipase A_2 from *V. palestinae* venom is able to hydrolyze lecithin at position 2 and lysolecithin at position 1. Thus, the enzyme displays both phospholipase A_2 and phospholipase B activities, the latter hydrolyzing the product of the first reaction (Table 35). *V. palestinae* venom phospholipase A_2 has a pH optimum at 9, but its B activity is low at this pH and increases steadily beyond pH 10.5. For the hydrolysis of lysolecithin the Lineweaver-Burk plot is found to be linear, giving $K_m = 1.1$ mM and $K_{cat} = 0.55\ s^{-1}$ at 37° C at pH 10.0. 2-Deoxy-lysolecithin is also hydrolyzed by this enzyme at pH 10, with $K_{cat} = 0.01\ s^{-1}$. For lecithin these constants can not be determined, but at 0.25 mM substrate the hydrolysis rate (at pH 9) of lecithin is about 1000 times of the hydrolysis rate of lysolecithin (at pH 10). An explanation for the great difference in A_2 and B activities of the purified phospholipase may lie, at least in part, in the difference between the physicochemical properties of lecithin and lysolecithin micelles in water. Whereas lecithin is known to form a laminar structure even at concentrations as low as 10^{-5} g/ml (about 0.012 mM), lysolecithin forms regular spherical micelles with a critical concentration for micelle formation of 10^{-4} g/ml (about 0.16 mM). Thus, the micellar size and shape may play a dominant role in the binding of the enzyme to the substrate. The fact that ether enhances phospholipase A_2 activity but inhibits phospholipase B activity may also be related to the physicochemical properties of the substances, since lecithin is ether-soluble whereas lysolecithin is not (SHILOAH et al., 1973c). In addition, the various phospholipase A_2 isozymes purified from *N. naja* venom have been shown to have phospholipase B activity and show the optimum pH at 9 for lecithin hydrolysis and above 10 for lysolecithin hydrolysis (SHILOAH et al., 1973b). These data indicate that phospholipase B activity found in the venoms is a dual action of the venom phospholipase A_2 itself.

BRAGANCA and KHANDEPARKAR (1966) indicated that a cytotoxic protein of *N. naja* venom exhibits phospholipase C activity, which releases phosphorycholine from α-lecithin. However, other authors were unable to detect it in the venom of *N. naja atra* (HSIEH and LEE, unpublished).

3. Acetylcholinesterase

An acetylcholine-hydrolyzing enzyme, so-called acetylcholinesterase, was first demonstrated in cobra venom by IYENGER et al. (1938). This enzyme is only found in the venoms of Elapidae and Hydrophiidae, not in those of Viperidae and Crotalidae. As indicated by MARNEY (1937) and NACHMANSOHN et al. (1942), cobra venom exhibits a hundred fold higher acetylcholinesterase activity than that of electroplax from the electric eel. Since the enzyme is involved in nerve transmission, venom acetylcholinesterase was at one time thought responsible for the neurotoxic action of elapid venoms (ZELLER, 1951). However, it is now definitely known that no relationship exists between the acetylcholinesterase and the venom neurotoxicity, because the enzyme activity in the venoms of *N. naja atra* and *Bungarus multicinctus* can be separated from the venom toxicity by employing electrophoretic methods (YANG et al., 1960a, b; CHANG and LEE, 1963).

The enzyme catalyzes the ester hydrolysis of acetylcholine as follows:

$$(CH_3)_3\overset{+}{N}-CH_2-CH_2-O-\underset{\underset{O}{\|}}{C}-CH_3 \rightarrow (CH_3)_3\overset{+}{N}-CH_2-CH_2-OH + CH_3COOH$$

Table 36 shows the distribution of acetylcholinesterase activity in the various elapid venoms (ZELLER, 1948). The activity is also found in the hydrophiid venom of *Enhydria schistosa* (TU and TOOM, 1971), but no activity is exhibited in any of the viperid and crotalid venoms.

Assay Method (YANG et al., 1960a). The method is based on the quantitative reaction of ester with hydroxylamine which yields the hydroxamic acid derivative (HESTRIN, 1949). The preparation of reagents used for the assay has been described in Sec. IV, 3. *Procedure.* A 0.5 ml 0.01% venom solution and 0.1 ml $MgCl_2$ are placed in a small test tube. After 3 min preincubation at

Table 36. Activity of acetylcholinesterase in various snake venoms (ZELLER, 1948)

Venom	Qche[a]	Venom	Qche[a]
Elapidae		Viperidae	
Acanthophis antarticus	9240	*Vipera russellii*	0
Bungarus caeruleus	24900	*Vipera aspis*	0
Bungarus fasciatus	18700	*Bitis arietans*	0
Demansia textilis	140	*Bitis gavonica*	0
Dendroaspis angusticeps	250	*Echis carinatus*	0
Denisonia superba	11000	Crotalidae	
Denisonia superba var.	3300	*Crotalus adamanteus*	0
Elaps corallinus	680	*Crotalus terrificus*	0
Naja bungarus	4800	*Agkistrodon halys blomhoffii*	0
Naja flava	7200	*Agkistrodon piscivorus*	0
Naja haje	1020	*Trimeresurus gramineus*	0
Naja melanoleuca	27900	*Trimeresurus flavoviridis*	0
Naja naja	13000	*Bothrops jararaca*	0
Naja nigricollis	40		
Notechis scutatus	3300		
Notechis scutatus var. *niger*	4260		
Notechis scutatus, white venom	3180		
Pseudechis australis	90		
Pseudechis porphyriacus	140		
Sepedon haemachates	6750		

[a] Qche = CO_2 μl/h/mg venom.

37° C, the reaction is initiated by addition of 1.0 ml 0.0064 M acetylcholine chloride. After 10 min, 4.0 ml alkaline hydroxylamine, which was prepared immediately before use by mixing equal volumes of 1.75 N NaOH and 1 M hydroxylamine-HCl, is added to terminate the reaction. Then 2.0 ml HCl (HCl, sp. gra. 1.18, diluted to 6 volumes) and 2.0 ml 0.185 M ferric chloride are added and the purple—brown color—which develops is determined spectrophotometrically at 540 nm. The quantity in μmole acetylcholine hydrolyzed per min is defined as one unit of enzyme activity.

Comment. The enzyme activity is also determined by the pH-stat method (refer to Sec. IV, 3) using the Radiometer titrator with automatic buret (ABU-12). The assay medium contains 0.1 M NaCl, 0.04 M $MgCl_2$ and 10 mM acetylcholine iodide; for determining the activity at low substrate concentrations, a dual syringe assembly for the ABU-12 is used.

Purification. In the past the acetylcholinesterase of *N. naja* and *Bungarus fasciatus* venoms was purified by fractional precipitation with Na_2SO_4 and $(NH)_2SO_4$ (CHAUDHURY, 1942, 1949). However, the reports did not show any purities of the isolated materials in the present sense. Recently, KUMAR and ELLIOTT (1973) have purified venom acetylcholinesterase, using affinity chromatography. The method is simple and only one component is observed in ultracentrifugation, immunodiffusion, immunoelectrophoresis, and disc-gel electrophoresis.

Procedure (KUMAR and ELLIOTT, 1973). The crude venom (300 mg) of *Bungarus fasciatus* is dissolved in 0.03 M Tris-HCl buffer, pH 8.2, and centrifuged at 10000 rpm/min (SS 34 head RC-2, Sorvall) for 15 min. The supernatant is placed on a Cellex-D (DEAE-cellulose, Bio-Rad Laboratory) column (2.5 × 40 cm), equilibrated with 0.03 M Tris-HCl buffer, pH 8.2. The column is eluted with the same buffer until the eluent absorption at 280 nm returns to the base line, followed by elution of the enzyme by using a continuous linear 0–0.5 M NaCl gradient (1 liter). The acetylcholinesterase fraction, concentrated by ultra-filtration (UM-10 Diaflow membrane), was placed on an affinity column of trimethyl-(m-aminophenyl)-ammonium chloride coupled to Sepharose 4 B (BERMAN and YOUNG, 1971). The column is then washed with 0.1 M NaCl containing 0.04 M $MgCl_2$ solution adjusted to pH 7.6 with $NaHCO_3$ until the eluate absorption at 280 nm returned to the base line. The retained enzyme is eluted by 10 mM edrophonium chloride [Tensilon, m-(trimethylamino)-phenylchloride]. About 4–5 column volumes are collected, excluding the void volume, and the eluent is dialyzed against the buffer and concentrated using a Diaflo UM-10 membrane. Through these procedures, a homogeneous enzyme expressing a specific activity of 220 mmoles acetylcholine hydrolyzed per h per mg is obtained with an overall yield of 59%.

Physicochemical Properties. N. naja venom acetylcholinesterase is inactivated by heating at 44° C for 1 h (CHAUDHURY, 1946). The purified enzyme from *Bungarus fasciatus* venom is stored at 2°–4° C for several weeks without loss in activity. The enzyme is stable when kept in frozen state at −16° C. The sedimentation coefficient of this enzyme is 5.82 S and its diffusion coefficient is 4.5×10^{-7} cm·s^{-1}. Thus, the molecular weight calculated by the Svedberg equation is 126000, assuming $\bar{v} = 0.75$. The value is in agreement with the molecular weight of 130000 ± 10000 estimated by the gel-filtration method. Furthermore, the frictional ratio as calculated from the sedimentation and diffusion data is 1.41 and the axial ratio 7.5. The *Bungarus fasciatus* enzyme is split into two apparently equal-sized subunits by 8 M urea-1 M NaCl, indicating that it consists of two subunits in the enzyme molecule. In agreement with this result, the number of active sites per molecule of acetylcholinesterase is titrated to be two, by using a carbamylating agent 0-nitrophenyl-dimethyl carbamate (KUMAR and ELLIOTT, 1973). Acethycholinesterase from *Bungarus fasciatus* has been viewed by electron microscopy, employing negative staining (NICKERSON and KUMAR, 1974). The basic monomeric unit is circular, with a diameter of 50 Å, and the association of subunits can form tetramers, but dimers are most frequently observed. The amino acid composition of the *Bungarus fasciatus* enzyme is shown in Table 37. Of interest is the similarity of the proportion of amino acid composition to that of electric eel acetycholinesterase.

Enzyme properties. Acetylcholinesterase of *Bungarus fasciatus* venom shows a maximum activity at pH 8.0 and the optimum temperature is 40° C, indicating instability at high temperature. The optimum pH for the venom of *N. naja atra* is 7.5 (CHANG and LEE, 1955). The purified enzyme not only hydrolyzes acetylcholine but also a number of ester substrates including acetylthiocholine ($K_m = 16.6$ µM), acetyl-β-methylcholine (516.6 µM), propionylcholine (33.1 µM), phenylacetate (1.14 mM), and indophenylacetate (1.41 mM) (KUMAR and ELLIOTT, 1973). The K_m value for acetylcholine iodide at pH 7.5 is 41.7 µM and the V is 8.6 mmole min^{-1}mg^{-1}. MOUNTER (1951) also showed that 3,3-dimethyl butyrate and triacetin are rapidly hydrolyzed by cobra venom, but tributyrin and benzoylcholine are not hydrolyzed at all. The enzyme exhibits substrate inhibition at high substrate concentrations, one of the characteristics of true cholinesterase. Also, the esterase activity is inhibited by di*iso*propylphosphofluoridate, eserine(physostigmine), caffein, and morphine (ZELLER, 1948). Trimethyl-(m-acetamidephenyl) ammonium iodide is a strong competitive inhibitor ($K_i = 76.6$ µM) to the *Bungarus fasciatus* enzyme (KUMAR and ELLIOTT, 1973). The enzyme is not inhibited by phenylmethylsulfonyl fluoride as is also the case with the electric eel enzyme, whereas human and rat acetylcholinesterase are inhibited.

Table 37. Amino acid composition of acetylcholinesterase from *Bungarus fasciatus* venom and *Electric eel*

Amino acid	Residues assuming four histidine residues	
	B. fasciatus[a]	*Electric eel*[b]
Lys	6	8
His	4	4
Arg	12	10
Asp	24	20
Thr	10	8
Ser	14	2
Glu	20	12
Pro	18	16
Gly	18	14
Ala	16	14
1/2Cys	2	2
Val	14	12
Met	4	5
Ile	6	6
Leu	22	16
Tyr	8	7
Phe	12	10

[a] KUMAR and ELLIOTT (1973).
[b] LEUZINGER and BAKER (1968).

An acetylcholinesterase inactivating factor was found in the venom of *N. naja atra* (CHANG and LEE, 1955; LEE et al., 1956). The ability of this venom to inactivate the enzyme activity is reversible blocked by various cations; Mg^{2+} at 0.06 M concentration is the most active. It is now known that the inactivating factor corresponds to one of cardiotoxins contained in the venom (LIN SHIAU et al., 1976). This factor is not effective against the acetylcholinesterase of mammalian tissue preparations.

VI. Enzyme Acting on Arylamides

Some snake venoms contain a leucyl-β-naphthylamide hydrolyzing enzyme, so-called arylamidase or amino acid naphthylamidase. The enzyme catalyzes the hydrolysis of L-leucyl-β-naphthylamide, yielding L-leucine and β-naphthylamin. This enzyme activity in snake venom was first discovered by MICHL and MOLZER (1965). They showed the presence of arylamidase in several elapid, viperid, and crotalid venoms. In 1967, TU and TOOM examined the distribution of arylamidase activity in 47 venoms from four venomous families, using L-leucyl-β-naphthylamide as substrate, and found that almost all of the venoms hydrolyze this substrate, although there are considerable species variations in the ability to split the substrate. Especially, the venoms of *Dendroaspis angusticeps*, *Oxyuranus scutellatus*, *Echis carinatus*, and *A. piscivorus piscivorus* were found to exhibit a significant activity. In general, elapid and viperid venoms exhibit relatively high activity, while those of hydrophiid show comparatively low activity. The overall activity of the crotalid venoms is quite low but the venoms of the genera *Agkistrodon* show considerably higher activity than the other members of the family.

Assay Method (TU and TOOM, 1976b). A solution consisting of 1 ml venom (1 mg/ml) is incubated at 37° C with 1 ml 0.02% L-leucyl-β-naphthylamide in 0.01 M phosphate buffer, pH 7.1, for 1 h. The reaction is stopped by the addition of 1 ml 25% trichloroacetic acid. Following centrifugation, 1 ml supernatant liquid is added to 1 ml 0.1% sodium nitrate. After standing 3 min, 1 ml 0.5% ammonium sulfamate is added and the mixture allowed to stand for 2 min. To this solution 2 ml 0.5% N-(1-naphthyl)-ethylenediamine alcoholic solution is added. After 30 min the absorbance at 580 nm is read and corrected with appropriate blanks.

Enzyme Properties. Up to date, no extensive purification of the enzyme from snake venoms has been achieved, with the exception of OSHIMA et al. (1968), who partially purified the enzyme from *A. halys blomhoffii* venom. According to their data, the venom arylamidase is relatively unstable and it is completely inactivated at 70° C for 30 min. The maximum activity is found at pH 8.5, and p-chloromercuribenzoate and Hg^{2+} strongly inhibit enzyme activity, suggesting that it is one of the thiol-active site enzymes. The enzyme resists EDTA and DFP and is activated in the presence of cyanide ions. The Km value to L-leucyl-β-naphthylamide is determined to be 1.5×10^{-3} M. The molecular weight of *A. halys blomhoffii* enzyme estimated by the gel-filtration method is ~128000.

E. Summary

Much research has been conducted on snake venom enzymes during the last two decades with many original and review publications on the subject. In recent years the research has focused on structural studies and mode of actions of certain venom enzymes, such as phospholipase A_2, thrombinlike enzyme, endopeptidase, and L-amino acid oxidase, which are abundant in various snake venoms. These results will not only stimulate extensive research on the relationship between structure and function of the enzyme but will also contribute to the use of snake venom enzyme in biochemical, pharmacologic, and clinical studies. There is as yet little knowledge as to why these enzymes are synthesized in the venomous gland or as to how enzyme production in the gland is controlled. These problems will be undertaken in the next decade.

References

Aldridge, W. N.: Serum esterases: I. Two types of esterase (A and B) hydrolysing p-nitrophenylacetate, propionate and butyrate, and a method for their determination. Biochem. J. **53**, 110—117 (1953)

Allen, R. J. L.: The estimation of phosphorus. Biochem. J. **34**, 858—865 (1940)

Anson, M. L.: The estimation of pepsin, trypsin, papain, and cathepsin with hemoglobin. J. gen. Physiol. **22**, 79—89 (1938)

Aronson, N. N. Jr., Davidson, E. A.: Lysosomal hyaluronidase from rat liver. I. Preparation. J. biol. Chem. **242**, 437—440 (1967)

Augustinsson, K. B.: Enzymatic hydrolysis of organophosphorus compounds. Acta chem. scand. **8**, 753—761 (1954)

Ballario, P., Bergami, M., Pedone, F.: A simple method for the purification of phosphodiesterase from *Vipera aspis* venom. Anal. Biochem. **80**, 646—651 (1977)

Banik, N. L., Gohil, K., Davison, A. N.: The action of snake venom, phospholipase A and trypsin on purified myelin in vitro. Biochem. J. **159**, 273—277 (1976)

Basu, A. S., Parker, R., O'Connor, R.: Disc electrophoresis of snake venoms. I. A qualitative comparison of the protein patterns from the species of Crotalidae and Elapidae. Canad. J. Biochem. **47**, 807—810 (1969)

Belfield, A., Ellis, G., Goldberg, D. M.: A specific colorimetric 5'-nucleotidase assay utilizing the Berthelot reaction. Clin. Chem. **16**, 396—401 (1970)

Benchetrit, L. C., Pahuja, S. L., Gray, E. D., Edstrom, R. D.: A sensitive method for the assay of hyaluronidase activity. Anal. Biochem. **79**, 431—437 (1977)

Bender, A. E., Krebs, H. A.: The oxidation of various synthetic α-amino acids by mammalian D-amino acid oxidase, L-amino acid oxidase of cobra venom and the L- and D-amino acid oxidase of *Neurospora crassa*. Biochem. J. **46**, 210—219 (1950)

Berman, J. D., Young, M.: Rapid and complete purification of acethylcholinesterases of electric eel and erythrocyte by affinity chromatography. Proc. nat. Acad. Sci. (Wash.) **68**, 395—398 (1971)

Bertke, E. M., Watt, D. D., Tu, T.: Electrophoretic patterns of venoms from species of Crotalidae and Elapidae snakes. Toxicon **4**, 73—76 (1966)

Bhattacharya, K. L.: Effect of snake venoms on coenzyme I. J. Indian chem. Soc. **30**, 685—688 (1953)

Björk, W.: Partial purification of phosphodiesterase, 5'-nucleotidase, lecithinase A, and acetylcholine esterase from Ringhals-cobra venom. Biochim. biophys. Acta (Amst.) **49**, 195—204 (1961)

Björk, W.: Purification of phosphodiesterase from *Bothrops atrox* venom, with special consideration of the elimination of monophosphatases. J. biol. Chem. **238**, 2487—2490 (1963)

Björk, W.: Activation and stabilization of snake venom 5'-nucleotidase. Biochim. biophys. Acta (Amst.) **89**, 483—494 (1964)

Björk, W.: Interactions of snake venom phosphodiesterase with DNA and RNA fragments. Ark. Kemi **27**, 515—537 (1967)

Blanchard, M., Green, D. E., Nocito, V., Ratner, S.: L-Amino acid oxidase of animal tissue. J. biol. Chem. **155**, 421—440 (1944)

Boman, H. G.: On the specificity of the snake venom phosphodiesterase. Ann. N. Y. Acad. Sci. **81**, 800—803 (1959)

Boman, H. G., Kaletta, U.: Chromatography of rattlesnake venom: a separation of three phosphodiesterases. Biochim. biophys. Acta (Amst.) **24**, 619—631 (1957)

Bonilla, C. A., Faith, M. R., Minton, S. A.: L-Amino acid oxidase, phosphodiesterase, total proteins and other properties of juvenile timber rattlesnake *(C. H. horridus)* venom at different stages of growth. Toxicon **11**, 301—303 (1973)

Bonilla, C. A., Fiero, M. K., Seifert, W.: Comparative biochemistry and pharmacology of salivary gland secretion. I. Electrophoreic analysis of the proteins in the secretions from human parotid and reptilian parotid (Duvernoy's) glands. J. Chromatog. **56**, 368—372 (1971)

Bonilla, C. A., Horner, N. V.: Comparative electrophoresis of *Crotalus* and *Agkistrodon* venoms from north American snakes. Toxicon **7**, 327—329 (1969)

Bootsma, J., Wolthers, B. G., Groen, A.: Determination of serum 5'-nucleotidase by means of a NADH-linked reaction. Clin. chim. Acta **41**, 219—222 (1972)

Boquet, P., Izard, Y., Jouannet, M., Meaume, J.: Recherches biochimiques et immunologiques sur le venin de serpents I. Essais de séparation des antigénes du venin de *Naja nigricollis* par filtration sur Sephadex. Ann. Inst. Pasteur (Lille) **111**, 719 (1966)

Botes, D. P., Viljoen, C. C.: *Bitis gavonica* venom. The amino acid sequence of phospholipase A. J. biol. Chem. **249**, 3827—3835 (1974 a)

Botes, D. P., Viljoen, C. C.: Purification of phospholipase A from *Bitis gavonica* venom. Toxicon **12**, 611—619 (1974 b)

Braganca, B. M., Khandeparkar, V. G.: Phospholipase C activity of cobra venom and lysis of Yoshida sarcoma cells. Life Sci. **5**, 1911—1920 (1966)

Breithaupt, H.: Enzymatic characteristics of *Crotalus* phospholipase A_2 and the crotoxin complex. Toxicon **14**, 221—233 (1976)

Breithaupt, H., Rübsamen, K., Habermann, E.: Biochemistry and pharmacology of the crotoxin complex. Biochemical analysis of crotapotin and the basic *Crotalus* phospholipase A. Europ. J. Biochem. **49**, 333—345 (1974)

Brisbois, L., Delori, P., Gillo, L.: Venins de serpents: Fractionnement d'un venin de cobra *(Naja naja atra)* par chromatographies sur gels de detrane. L'Ing. Chim. **50**, 45 (1968a)
Brisbois, L., Rabinovitch-Mahler, N., Delori, P., Gillo, L.: A study of the fractions of the venom *Naja naja atra* obtained by chromatography on sulphoethyl-Sephadex. J. Chromatog. **37**, 463—475 (1968b)
Brown, J.H., Bowles, M.E.: U.S. Army Med. Res. Lab., Fort Knox, Ky., Rept. **627**, 11 (1965)
Brown, J.H., Bowles, M.E.: Studies on the phospholipase A activity of *Crotalus atrox* venom. Toxicon **3**, 205—212 (1966)
Butler, G.C.: Phosphodiesterase from snake venoms. In: Colowick, S.P., Kaplan, N.O. (Eds.): Methods in Enzymology, Vol. 2, pp. 561—565. New York-London: Academic Press 1955
Campos, S., Yarleque, A.: 5'-Nucleotidasa en el veneno de la serpiente lachesis muta 1. Bol. Soc. Quimica Perú **XL**, 202—212 (1974)
Chang, C.C., Lee, C.Y.: Cholinesterase and anticholinesterase activities in snake venoms. J. Formosan med. Ass. **54**, 103—112 (1955)
Chang, C.C., Lee, C.Y.: Isolation of neurotoxins from the venom of *Bungarus multicinctus* and their modes of neuromuscular blocking action. Arch. Int. Pharmacodyn. **144**, 241—257 (1963)
Chaudhury, D.K.: Studies on cholinesterase. Isolation of cholinesterase from cobra venom *(Naja tripudians)*. Science Culture **8**, 238 (1942)
Chaudhury, D.K.: Studies on cholinesterase. III. Specificity of cholinesterase. Ann. Biochem. Exp. Med. **9**, 67—72 (1949)
Chen, S.S., Walgate, J.H., Duerre, J.A.: Oxidative deamination of sulfur amino acids by bacterial and snake venom L-amino acid oxidase. Arch. Biochem. Biophys. **146**, 54—63 (1971)
Chen, Y., Lo, T.B.: Chemical studies of Formosan cobra *(Naja naja atra)* venom. V. Properties of 5'-nucleotidase. J. clin. chem. Soc. **15**, 84 (1968)
Chinen, I.: Phospholipase A activity of habu snake venom by using chicken serum as a substrate. Ryuku Daigaku Nogakubu Gakujutsu Hokoku **19**, 259 (1972)
Chiu, W.C.: Studies on the snake venom enzyme. VII. On the hyaluronidase activity of Formosan snake venoms. J. Yamaguchi med. Ass. **9**, 1355—1360 (1960)
Cohen, I., Zur, M., Kaminsky, E., de Vries, A.: Isolation and characterization of kinin-releasing enzyme of *Echis coloratus* venom. Toxicon **7**, 3—4 (1969)
Coles, E., McIlwain, D.L., Rapport, M.M.: The activity of pure phospholipase A_2 from *Crotalus atrox* venom on myelin and on pure phospholipids. Biochim. biophys. Acta **337**, 68—78 (1974)
Cousin, M.: Influence de la structure secondaire des polytribonucleotides sur leur degradation par la phosphodiesterase de venin de serpent. Bull. Soc. chim. Biol. **45**, 1363—1368 (1963)
Cuatrecasas, P.: Protein purification by affinity chromatography. Derivatization of agarose and polyacrylamide beads. J. biol. Chem. **245**, 3059—3065 (1970)
Currie, B.T., Oakley, D.E., Broomfield, C.A.: Crystalline phospholipase A associated with a cobra venom toxin. Nature (Lond.) **220**, 371 (1968)
Curti, B., Massey, V., Zmudka, M.: Inactivation of snake venom L-amino acid oxidase by freezing. J. biol. Chem. **243**, 2306—2314 (1968)
Deems, R.A., Dennis, E.A.: Characterization and physical properties of the major form of phospholipase A_2 from cobra venom *(Naja naja naja)* that has a molecular weight of 11000. J. biol. Chem. **250**, 9008—9012 (1975)
Deems, R.A., Eaton, B.R., Dennis, E.A.: Kinetic analysis of phospholipase A_2 activity toward mixed micelles and its implications for the study of lipolytic enzymes. J. biol. Chem. **250**, 9013—9020 (1975)
de Haas, G.H., Postema, N.M., Nieuwenhuizen, W., van Deenen, L.L.M.: Purification and properties of phospholipase A from porcine pancreas. Biochim. biophys. Acta (Amst.) **159**, 103—117 (1968)
Dekok, A., Rawitch, A.B.: Studies on L-amino acid oxidase. II. Dissociation and characterization of its subunits. Biochemistry **8**, 1405—1411 (1969)
de Lacerda, J.B.: Lecons sur le Venin des Serpents du Bresil et sur la Methode de Traitement des Morsures Venimeuses par le Permaganate de Protease. Rio de Janeiro: Lombaerte 1884
Delezenne, C., Ledebt, S.: Formation de substances hémolytiques et du substances toxiques aux dépens du vitellus de l'oeuf soumis a l'action du cobra. C. R. Acad. Sci. [D] (Paris) **153**, 81—84 (1911)

Delezenne, C., Morel, H.: Action catalytique des venins des serpents sur les acids nucleiques. C. R. Acad. Sci. [D] (Paris) **168**, 244—246 (1919)

Delori, P.: Purification et propriétés physico-chimiques, chimiques et biologiques d'une phospholipase A_2 toxique isolée d'un venin de serpent Viperidae: *Vipera Berus*. Biochimie **55**, 1031—1045 (1973)

Delori, P., Gillo, L.: Separation of proteins of Elapidae snake venoms on polyacrylamide gel. J. Chromatog. **34**, 531—533 (1968)

Demel, R. A., Geurts van Dessel, W. S. M., Zwaal, R. F. A., Roelofsen, B., van Deenen, L. L. M.: Relation between various phospholipase actions on human red cell membranes and the interfacial phospholipid pressure in monolayers. Biochim. biophys. Acta (Amst.) **406**, 97—107 (1975)

Dennis, E. A.: Phospholipase A_2 activity towards phosphatidylcholine in mixed micelles: Surface dilution kinetics and the effect of thermotropic phase transitions. Arch. biochem. Biophys. **158**, 485—493 (1973a)

Dennis, E. A.: Kinetic dependence of phospholipase A_2 activity on the detergent triton X-100. J. Lipid Res. **14**, 152—159 (1973b)

Deutsch, H. F., Diniz, C. R.: Some proteolytic activities of snake venoms. J. biol. Chem. **216**, 17—26 (1955)

Devi, A., Banerjee, R., Saker, N.K.: Intern. Congr. Physiol. Sci. 21st. Buenos Aires Symp. Spec. Lectures, 1959

Devi, A., Copley, A. L.: Occurrence of heparinase-like enzyme in Viperidae group of snakes. Toxicon **8**, 129 (1970)

Devi, A., Copley, A. L.: Occurrence of heparinase-like enzyme in the venom of *Bothrops atrox*. In: de Vries, A., Kochva, E. (Eds.): Toxins of Animal and Plant Origin, pp. 471—481. New York-London-Paris: Gordon and Research Science 1971

de Vries, A., Cohen, I.: Hemorrhagic and blood coagulation disturbing action of snake venoms. In: Poller, L. (Ed.): Recent Advances in Blood Coagulation, pp. 277—297. London: J. & A. Churchill 1969

di Ferrante, N.: Turbidimetric measurement of acid mucopolysaccharides and hyaluronidase activity. J. biol. Chem. **220**, 303—306 (1956)

Dimitrov, G. D.: Purification and partial characterization of two proteolytic enzymes from the venom of *Vipera russelli*. Toxicon **9**, 33—44 (1971)

Doery, H. M., Pearson, J. E.: Haemolysins in venoms of Australian snakes. Observations on the haemolysins of the venoms of some Australian snakes and the separation of phospholipase A from the venom of *Pseudechis porphyriacus*. Biochem. J. **78**, 820—827 (1961)

Doery, H. M., Pearson, J. E.: Phospholipase B in snake venoms and bee venom. Biochem. J. **92**, 599—602 (1964)

Dolapchiev, L. B., Sulkowski, E., Laskowski, M., Sr.: Purification of exonuclease (phosphodiesterase) from the venom of *Crotalus adamanteus*. Biochem. Biophys. Res. Commun. **61**, 273—281 (1974)

Dumarey, C., Sket, M. D., Joseph, D., Boquet, P.: Etude d'une phospholipase basique du venin de *Naja nigricollis*. C. R. Acad. Sci. [D] (Paris) **280**, 1633—1635 (1975)

Dupont, J.: Catalytic properties of two phospholipase A from cobra *(Naja nigricollis)* venom. Toxicon **15**, 347—354 (1977)

Duran-Reynals, F.: The invasion of the body by animal poisons. Science. **83**, 286—287 (1936)

Duran-Reynals, F.: A spreading factor in certain snake venoms and its relation to their mode of action. J. exp. Med. **69**, 69—81 (1939)

Elliott, W. B., Panagides, K.: Hydrolysis of N-methylindoxyl acetate by a non-choline esterase type of esterase. Anal. Biochem. **45**, 345—348 (1972)

Favilli, G.: Nature of the diffusing factor of animal venoms. Arch. ital. med. sper. **4**, 929—938 (1939)

Favilli, G.: Mucolytic effect of several diffusing agents and of a diazotized compound. Nature **145**, 866—867 (1940)

Favilli, G.: Occurrence of spreading factors and some properties of hyaluronidases in animal parasites and venoms. In: Buckley, E. E., Porges, N., (Eds.), pp. 281—289. Washington, D.C.: Amer. Assoc. Adv. Sci. 1956

Ferreira, S. H., Rocha e Silva, M.: Potentiation of bradykinin and eledoisin by BPF (bradykinin factor) from *Bothrops jararaca* venom. Experientia (Basel) **21**, 347—349 (1965)

Fiero, M. K., Seifert, M., Weaver, W., Timothy, J., Bonilla, C. A.: Comparative study of juvenile and adult prairie rattlesnake (*Crotalus viridis viridis*) venoms. Toxicon **10**, 81—82 (1972)
Flatmark, T., Vesterberg, O.: On the heterogeneity of beef heart cytochrome c. I. Isoelectric fractionation by electrolysis in a natural pH-gradient. Acta chem. scand. **20**, 1497—1503 (1966)
Frischauf, A.-M., Eckstein, F.: Purification of a phosphodiesterase from *Bothrops atrox* venom by affinity chromatography. Europ. J. Biochem. **32**, 479—485 (1973)
Fritz, H., Trautschold, I., Werle, E.: Protease-inhibitoren. In: Bergmeyer, H. U. (Ed.): Methoden der enzymatischen Analyse, Vol. 2, pp. 1064—1077. Weinheim: Verlag Chemie 1974
Futai, M., Mizuno, D.: A new phosphodiesterase forming nucleoside 5′-monophosphate from rat liver. Its partial purification and substrate specificity for nicotinamide adenine dinucleotide and oligonucleotides. J. biol. Chem. **242**, 5301—5307 (1967)
Geiger, R., Kortmann, H.: Esterolytic and proteolytic activities of snake venoms and their inhibition by proteinase inhibitors. Toxicon **15**, 257—259 (1977)
Gentry, M. K., Olsson, R. A.: A simple, specific, radioisotopic assay for 5′-nucleotidase. Anal. Biochem. **64**, 624—627 (1975)
Georgatsos, J. G., Laskowski, M., Sr.: Purification of an endonuclease from the venom of *Bothrops atrox*. Biochemistry **1**, 288—295 (1962)
Ghosh, B. N., Dutt, P. K., Chowdhury, D. K.: Detection of dipeptidase, polypeptidase, carboxypeptidase and esterase in different snake venoms. J. Indian chem. Soc. **16**, 75 (1939)
Gornall, A., Bardavill, C. J., David, M. M.: Determination of serum protein concentration by means of the biuret reaction. J. biol. Chem. **177**, 751—766 (1949)
Green, S., Bodansky, O.: The solubilization, purification, and properties of nicotinamide adenine dinucleotide glycohydrolase from Ehrlich ascites cells. J. biol. Chem. **240**, 2574—2579 (1965)
Gubensek, F., Lapanje, S.: Circular dichroism of two phospholipase A from *Vipera ammodytes* venom. FEBS Letters **44**, 182—184 (1974)
Gul, S., Smith, A. D.: Haemolysis of washed human red cells by the combined action of *Naja naja* phospholipase A_2 and albumin. Biochim. biophys. Acta (Amst.) **288**, 237—240 (1972)
Gulland, J. M., Jackson, E. M.: Phosphoesterase of bone and snake venoms. Biochem. J. **32**, 590—596 (1938)
Habermann, E.: Über Zusammenhänge zwischen esterolytischen und pharmakologischen Wirkungen von Jararacagift, Kallikrein und Thrombin. Naunyn-Schmiedebergs Arch. exp. Path. Pharmak. **236**, 492—502 (1959)
Habermann, E.: Zuordnung pharmakologischer und enzymatischer Wirkungen von Kallikrein und Schlangengiften mittels Diisopropylfluorophosphat und Electrophorese. Naunyn-Schmiedebergs Arch. exp. Path. Pharmak. **240**, 552—572 (1961)
Habermann, E., Neuman, W. P.: Die Hemmung der Hitzekoagulation von Eigelb durch Bienengift. Ein Phospholipase-Effekt. Hoppe-Seylers Z. physiol. Chem. **297**, 174—193 (1954)
Hachimori, Y., Wells, M., Hanahan, D. J.: Observations on the phospholipase A_2 of *Crotalus atrox*: Molecular weight and other properties. Biochemistry **10**, 4084—4089 (1971)
Hadjiolov, A. A., Venkov, P. V., Dolapchiev, L. B., Genchev, D. D.: The action of snake venom phosphodiesterase on liver ribosomal ribonucleic acids. Biochim. biophys. Acta (Amst.) **142**, 111—127 (1967)
Haessler, H. A., Cunningham, L.: A comparison of several deoxyribonucleases of Type II. Exp. Cell Res. **3**, 304—311 (1957)
Hafner, E. W., Wellner, D.: Demonstration of amino acids as products of the reactions catalyzed by D- and L-amino acid oxidase. Proc. nat. Acad. Sci. (Wash.) **68**, 987—991 (1971)
Hamberg, U.: Isolation and molar activity of human bradykinin. Biochem. Biophys. Res. Commun. **7**, 95—100 (1962)
Hamberg, U., Rocha e Silva, M.: Release of bradykinin as related the esterase activity of trypsin and of the venom of *Bothrops jararaca*. Experientia (Basel) **13**, 489—490 (1957)
Hayes, M. B., Wellner, D.: Microheterogeneity of L-amino acid oxidase. Separation of multiple components by polyacrylamide gel electrofocusing. J. biol. Chem. **244**, 6636—6644 (1969)
Henriques, O. B., Evseeva, L.: Proteolytic, esterase, and kininreleasing activities of some Soviet snake venoms. Toxicon **6**, 205—209 (1969)
Henriques, O. B., Fichman, M., Beraldo, W. T.: Bradykinin releasing factor from *Bothrops jararaca* venom. Nature (Lond.) **187**, 414—415 (1960)

Henriques, S. B., Henriques, O. B.: Pharmacology and toxicology of snake venoms. In: Raskova, H. (Ed.): Pharmacology and Toxicology of Naturally occuring Toxins, Vol. 1, pp. 215—368. Oxford-New York: Pergamon Press 1971

Heppel, L. A., Hilmoe, R. J.: Purification and properties of 5'-nucleotidase. J. biol. Chem. **188**, 665—676 (1951)

Hestrin, S.: The reaction of acetylcholine and other carboxylic acid derivatives with hydroxylamine, and its analytical application. J. biol. Chem. **180**, 249—261 (1949)

Hofstee, B. H. J.: Direct and continuous spectrophotometric assay of phosphomonoesterase. Arch. Biochem. Biophys. **51**, 139—145 (1954)

Hokama, Y., Iwanaga, S., Tatsuki, T., Suzuki, T.: Snake venom proteinase inhibitors: Isolation of five polypeptide inhibitors from the venoms of *Hemachatus haemachatus* (Ringhal's cobra) and *Naja nivea* (Cape cobra) and the complete amino acid sequences of two of them. J. Biochem. **79**, 559—578 (1976)

Holley, R. W., Madison, J. T., Zamir, A.: A new method for sequence determination of large oligonucleotides. Biochem. Biophys. Res. Commun. **17**, 389—394 (1964)

Holme, D. J., Goldberg, D. M.: Coupled optical rate determination of amino acid oxidase activity. Biochim. biophys. Acta **377**, 61—70 (1975)

Holtz, P., Raudonat, H. W., Contzen, C.: Über das bradykininbildende Prinzip des Schlangengiftes. Naunyn-Schmiedebergs Arch. exp. Path. Pharmak. **239**, 54—67 (1960)

Howard, N. L.: Phospholipase A_2 from puff adder *(Bitis arietans)* venom. Toxicon **13**, 21—30 (1975)

Humphrey, J. H., Jaques, R.: Hyaluronidase: correlation between biological assay and other methods of assay. Biochem. J. **53**, 59—62 (1953)

Hurst, R. O., Butler, G. C.: The chromatographic separation of phosphatases in snake venoms. J. biol. Chem. **193**, 91—96 (1951)

Ipata, P. L.: A coupled optical enzyme assay for 5'-nucleotidase. Anal. Biochem. **20**, 30—36 (1967)

Ipata, P. L., Felicioli, R. A.: A convenient spectrophotometric assay for phosphodiesterase, using dinucleoside-monophosphates as substrates. Europ. J. Biochem. **8**, 174—179 (1969)

Iwanaga, S., Kawauchi, S.: Studies on snake venoms V. Column chromatography of lecithinase A in Japanese Mamushi venom (*Agkistrodon halys blomhoffii* BOIE). J. Pharm. Soc. Jpn. **79**, 582—586 (1959)

Iwanaga, S., Ohshima, G., Suzuki, T.: Proteinases from the venom of *Agkistrodon halys blomhoffii*. In: Lorand, L. (Ed.): Methods in Enzymology, Vol. XLVB, pp. 459—468. New York-San Francisco-London: Academic Press 1976

Iwanaga, S., Omori, T., Oshima, G., Suzuki, T.: Studies on snake venoms. XVI. Demonstration of a proteinase with hemorrhagic activity in the venom of *Agkistrodon halys blomhoffii*. J. Biochem. **57**, 392—401 (1965a)

Iwanaga, S., Sato, T., Mizushima, Y., Suzuki, T.: Studies on snake venoms. XVII. Properties of the bradykinin releasing enzyme in the venom of *Agkistrodon halys blomhoffii*. J. Biochem. **58**, 123—129 (1965b)

Iwanaga, S., Yang, C. C., Kawachi, S.: Some observation on the column chromatography of Formosan cobra venom. J. Pharm. Soc. Jpn. **78**, 791—794 (1958)

Iyenger, N. K., Sehra, H. B., Mukerji, B., Chopra, R. N.: Cholinesterase in cobra venom. Curr. Sci. India **7**, 51—53 (1938)

Jaques, R.: The hyaluronidase content of animal venoms. In: Buckley, E. E., Proges, N. (Eds.): Venoms, pp. 291—293. Washington D.C.: Amer. Ass. Advanc. Sci. 1956

Jentsch, J.: Weitere Untersuchungen zur Aminosäuresequenz des Melittins. II. Bevorzugte Spaltung der Valin-, Leucin- und Isoleucinbindungen durch α-Protease aus *Crotalus atrox* Gift. Z. Naturforsch. **24b**, 415—418 (1969a)

Jentsch, J.: Enzymatische Spaltung nativer cystinhaltiger Polypeptide durch Thermolysin II. Vergleich von Thermolysin mit α-protease aus *Crotalus* Gift und Subtilisin. Z. Naturforsch. 1290—1300 (1969b)

Jimenez-Porras, J. M.: Intraspecific variations in composition of venom of the jumping viper, *Bothrops nummifera*. Toxicon **2**, 187—196 (1964)

Johnson, M., Kaye, M. A. G., Hems, R., Krebs, H. A.: Enzymatic hydrolysis of adenosine phosphates by cobra venom. Biochem. J. **54**, 625—631 (1953)

Joubert, F. J.: *Hemachatus haemachatus* (Ringhals) venom. Purification, some properties and amino-acid sequence of phospholipase A (Fraction DE-I). Europ. J. Biochem. **52**, 539—554 (1975a)

Joubert, F. J.: *Naja melanoleuca* (Forest cobra) venom. The amino acid sequence of phospholipase A, Fraction DE-III. Biochim. biophys. Acta (Amst.) **379**, 329—359 (1975b)

Joubert, F. J., Van der Walt, S. J.: *Naja melanoleuca* (Forest cobra) venom. Purification and some properties of phospholipase A. Biochim. biophys. Acta (Amst.) **379**, 317—328 (1975)

Kaiser, E., Michel, H.: Die Biochemie der tierischen Gifte. Wien: Franz Deuticke 1958

Kaplan, N. O.: Nature of multiple molecular forms of enzymes. Ann. N. Y. Acad. Sci. **151**, 382—399 (1968)

Kato, H., Suzuki, T.: Bradykinin-potentiating peptides from the venom of *Agkistrodon halys blomhoffii*. Isolation of five bradykinin-potentiators and amino acid sequence of potentiator B and potentiator C. Biochemistry **10**, 972—980 (1971)

Kawauchi, S., Iwanaga, S., Samejima, Y., Suzuki, T.: Isolation and characterization of two phospholipase A's from the venom of *Agkistrodon halys blomhoffii*. Biochim. biophys. Acta (Amst.) **236**, 142—160 (1971a)

Kawauchi, S., Samejima, Y., Iwanaga, S., Suzuki, T.: Amino acid compositions of snake venom phospholipase A's. J. Biochem. **69**, 433—437 (1971b)

Keller, E. B.: The hydrolysis of "soluble" ribonucleic acid by snake venom phosphodiesterase. Biochem. Biophys. Res. Commun. **17**, 412—415 (1964)

Kocholaty, W. F., Ledford, E. B., Daly, J. G., Billings, T. A.: Toxicity and some enzymatic properties and activities in the venoms of Crotalidae, Elapidae and Viperidae. Toxicon **9**, 131—138 (1971)

Kornalik, F., Master, R. W. P.: A comparative examination of yellow and white venoms of *Vipera ammodytes*. Toxicon **2**, 109—111 (1964)

Kornberg, A., Pricer, W. E.: Nucleotide pyrophosphatase. J. biol. Chem. **182**, 763—778 (1950)

Kumar, V., Elliott, W. B.: The acetylcholinesterase of *Bungarus fasciatus* venom. Europ. J. Biochem. **34**, 586—592 (1973)

Kunitz, M.: Crystalline soybean trypsin inhibitor IIa. General properties. J. gen. Physiol. **30**, 291—310 (1947)

Kurth, J., Aurich, H.: Purification and some properties of L-amino acid oxidase from the venom of sand viper *(Vipera ammodytes)*. Acta biol. med. germ. **31**, 641 (1973)

Kurth, J., Aurich, H.: Einfluß von pH-Wert und Temperatur auf die Stabilität der L-Aminosäureoxydase aus dem Gift der Sandotter. Acta biol. med. germ. **35**, 175 (1976)

Laskowski, M., Sr.: Exonuclease (phosphodiesterase) and other nucleolytic enzymes from venom. In: Cantoni, G. L., Davies, D. R. (Eds.): Procedures in Nucleic Acid Research, Vol. 1, pp. 154—187, New York-Evanston-London: Harper-Row 1966

Laskowski, M., Sr.: DNase and their use in the studies of primary structure of nucleic acids. In: Nord, F. F. (Ed.): Advances in Enzymology, Vol. 29, pp. 165—220. New York: Interscience 1967

Laskowski, M., Sr.: Venom exonuclease. In: Boyer, P. D. (Ed.): Enzymes, Vol. 4, pp. 313—328. New York-London: Academic Press 1971

Lee, C. Y., Chang, C. C., Kamijo, K.: Cholinesterase inactivation by snake venoms. Biochem. J. **62**, 582—588 (1956)

Lee, C. Y., Chang, S. L., Kau, S. T., Luh, S.-H.: Chromatographic separation of the venom of *Bungarus multicinctus* and characterization of its components. J. Chromatog. **72**, 71—82 (1972)

Leuzinger, W., Baker, A. L.: Acetylcholinesterase. I. Large-scale purification, homogeneity, and amino acid analysis. Proc. nat. Acad. Sci. (Wash.) **57**, 446—450 (1968)

Lin Shiau, S. Y., Liao, C., Lee, C. Y.: Studies on anti-cholinesterase activity of cobra cardiotoxin. J. Formosan med. Ass. **75**, 440—448 (1976)

Lo, T. B., Chaung, W. C.: Symposium on snake venoms. J. Formosan med. Ass. **70**, 644 (1971)

Lo, T. B., Chang, W. C.: Phospholipase A from Formosan cobra *(Naja naja atra)* venom. In: Ohsaka, A., Hayashi, K., Sawai, Y. (Eds.): Animal, Plant and Microbial Toxins, Vol. 1, pp. 191—204. New York-London: Plenum Press 1974

Madinaveitia, J.: Diffusion factors. VII. Concentration of mucinase from testicular extracts and from *Crotalus atrox* venom. Biochem. J. **35**, 447—452 (1941)

Maeno, H.: Biochemical analysis of pathological lesions caused by Habu snake venom with special reference to haemorrhage. J. Biochem. **52**, 343—350 (1962)
Magee, W. L., Thompson, R. H. S.: The estimation of phospholipase A activity in aqueous systems. Biochem. J. **77**, 562—534 (1960)
Marinetti, G. V.: In vitro lipid transformations in serum. Biochim. biophys. Acta (Amst.) **46**, 468—478 (1961)
Marinetti, G. V.: The action of phospholipase A on lipoproteins. Biochim. biophys. Acta (Amst.) **98**, 554—565 (1965)
Marney, A.: C. R. Soc. Biol. (Paris) **126**, 573—574 (1937)
Mathews, M. B.: Animal mucopolysaccharidases. In: Neufeld, E. F., Ginsburg, V. (Eds.): Methods in Enzymology, Vol. 8, pp. 654—662. New York-London: Academic Press 1966
Mathews, M. B., Inouye, M.: The determination of chondroitin sulfate C-type polysaccharides in mixtures with other acid mucopolysaccharides. Biochim. biophys. Acta (Amst.) **53**, 509—513 (1961)
Matsubara, H., Hasegawa, S., Fujimura, S., Shima, T., Sugimura, T., Futai, M.: Studies on poly(adenosine diphosphate ribose) V. Mechanism of hydrolysis of poly(adenosine diphosphate ribose) by snake venom. J. biol. Chem. **245**, 3606—3611 (1970)
Mazur, A.: An enzyme in animal tissues capable of hydrolyzing the phosphorus-fluorine bond of alkyl fluorophosphates. J. biol. Chem. **164**, 271—289 (1946)
McLean, D., Hale, C. W.: Mucinase and tissue permeability. Nature (Lond.) **145**, 867—868 (1940)
McLean, R. L., Massaro, E. J., Elliot, W. B.: A comparative study of the homology of certain enzymes in elapid venoms. Comp. Biochem. Physiol. **39B**, 1023—1037 (1971)
McLennan, B. D., Lane, B. G.: The chain termini of polynucleotides formed by limited enzymic fragmentation of wheat embryo ribosomal RNA. II. Studies of a snake venom ribonuclease and pancreatic ribonuclease. Canad. J. Biochem. **46**, 93—107 (1968a)
McLennan, B. D., Lane, B. G.: The chain termini of polynucleotides formed by limited enzymic fragmentation of wheat embryo ribosomal RNA. I. Studies of snake venom phosphodiesterase. Canad. J. Biochem. **46**, 81—91 (1968b)
Meaume, J.: Les venins des serpents agents modificateurs de la coagulation sanguine. Toxicon **4**, 25—58 (1966)
Mebs, D.: Preliminary studies on small molecular toxic components of Elapid venoms. Toxicon **6**, 247—253 (1969)
Mebs, D.: Über Schlangengift-Kallikreine: Reinigung und Eigenschaften eines Kinin-freisetzenden Enzymes aus dem Gift der Viper *Bitis gavonica*. Hoppe-Seylers Z. physiol. Chem. **350**, 1563—1569 (1969a)
Mebs, D.: A comparative study of enzyme activities in snake venoms. Int. J. Biochem. **1**, 335—342 (1970)
Meister, A.: Enzymatic preparation of α-keto acids. J. biol. Chem. **197**, 309—317 (1952)
Meister, A.: The α-keto analogues of arginine, ornithine, and lysine. J. biol. Chem. **206**, 577—585 (1954)
Meister, A.: The use of snake venom L-amino acid oxidase for the preparation of α-keto acid. In: Buckley, E. E., Porges, N. (Eds.): Venoms, pp. 259—302, Washington D.C.: Amer. Ass. Adv. Sci. 1956
Meister, A.: Biochemistry of Amino Acid. New York-London: Academic Press 1965
Meldrum, B. S.: The actions of snake venom on nerve and muscle. The pharmacology of phospholipase A and polypeptide toxins. Pharmacol. Rev. **17**, 398—445 (1965)
Mella, K., Volz, M., Pfleiderer, G.: Application of *Crotalus atrox* venom α-protease for amino acid sequence determination. Anal. Biochem. **21**, 219—226 (1967)
Mende, T. J., Moreno, M.: A heat stable paraoxonase (0,0-Diethyl-0-p-Nitrophenyl phosphate 0-p-nitrophenyl hydrolase from *Russell's viper* venom. Biochemistry **14**, 3913—3916 (1975)
Meyer, K., Hoffmann, P., Linker, A.: Hyaluronidases. In: Boyer, P. D., Lardy, H., Myrbäck, K. (Eds.): The Enzymes, Vol. 4, pp. 447—460. New York-London: Academic Press 1960
Michl, H., Molzer, H.: The occurrence of L-leucyl-β-naphthylamide (LNA) splitting enzymes in some amphibia and reptile venoms. Toxicon **2**, 281—282 (1965)
Miles, A. A., Wilhelm, D. L.: Enzyme-like globulins from serum reproducing the vascular phenomena of inflammation. I. An activable permeability factor and its inhibitor in guinea-pig serum. Brit. J. exp. Path. **36**, 71—81 (1955)

Miller, J. P., Hirst-Bruns, M. E., Philipps, G. R.: Action of venom phosphodiesterase on transfer RNA from *Escherichia coli*. Biochim. biophys. Acta (Amst.) **217**, 176—188 (1970)
Minton, S. A.: Venom Diseases. Springfield (Ill.): Charles C. Thomas 1974
Misiorowski, R. L., Wells, M. A.: The activity of phospholipase A_2 in reversed micelles of phosphatidylcholine in diethyl ether: Effect of water and cations. Biochemistry **13**, 4921—4927 (1974)
Mizuno, Y., Ikehara, M., Ueda, T., Nomura, A., Ohtsuka, E., Ishikawa, F., Kanai, Y.: Interactions between synthetic nucleotide analogs and snake venom 5'-nucleotidase. Chem. Pharm. Bull. **9**, 338—340 (1961)
Mohamed, A. H., Kamel, A., Ayobe, M. H.: Studies of phospholipase A and B activities of Egyptian snake venoms and a scorpion toxin. Toxicon **6**, 293—298 (1968)
Mounter, L. A.: The specificity of cobra venom cholinesterase. Biochem. J. **50**, 122 (1951)
Mounter, L. A., Chanutin, A.: Dialkylfluorophosphatase of kidney. II. Studies of activation and inhibition by metals. J. biol. Chem. **204**, 837—846 (1953)
Murata, Y., Satake, M., Suzuki, T.: Studies on snake venom. XII. Distribution of proteinase activities among Japanese and Formosan snake venoms. J. Biochem. **53**, 431—437 (1963)
Murray, A. W., Friedrichs, B.: Inhibition of 5'-nucleotidase from Ehrlich ascites-tumor cells by nucleoside triphosphates. Biochem. J. **111**, 83—89 (1969)
Nachmansohn, D., Cox, R. T., Coates, C. W., Machado, A. L.: Action potential and enzyme activity in the electric organ of electrophorus electricus (Linnaeus). I. Cholineesterase and respiration. J. Neurophysiol. **5**, 499—515 (1942)
Nagatsu, T., Yagi, K.: A simple assay of monoamine oxidase and D-amino acid oxidase by measuring ammonia. J. Biochem. **60**, 219—221 (1966)
Nair, B. C., Nair, C., Elliott, W. B.: Temperature stability of phospholipase A activity. II. Variations in optimum temperature of phospholipase A_2 from various snake venoms. Toxicon **14**, 43—47 (1976)
Neelin, J. M.: Starch gel electrophoresis of cobra and rattlesnake venoms. Canad. J. Biochem. Physiol. **41**, 1073—1078 (1963)
Nickerson, P. A., Kumar, V.: Electron microscopic studies of acetylcholinesterase from *Bungarus fasciatus* venom. Toxicon **12**, 83—84 (1974)
Nikol'skaya, I. I., Kislina, O. S., Tikhonenko, T. I.: Separation of 5'-nucleotidase of *Vipera lebetina* venom from interfering enzyme. Dokl. Akad. Nauk. SSSR **157**, 475 (1964)
Nikol'skaya, I. I., Shalina, N. M., Budowski, E. I.: A method for the preparation of phosphodiesterase from viper venom. Biochemistry (U.S.S.R.) **28**, 759—763 (1963)
Noč, F.: Sur quelques propèrietés physiologiques des differents venins de serpents. Ann. Inst. Pasteur (Lille) **18**, 387—406 (1904)
Ogilvie, K. K., Hruska, F. H.: Affect of spleen and snake venom phosphodiesterases on nucleotides containing nucleosides in the *syn* conformation. Biochem. Biophys. Res. Commun. **68**, 375—378 (1976)
Ohsaka, A.: Biochemistry of Snake Venoms. Recent Advances in Medical Science and biology, Vol. 1, pp. 269—322. Tokyo: Nat. Inst. Health, Japan, 1960a
Ohaska, A.: Proteolytic activities of Haub snake venom and their separation from lethal toxicity. Jap. J. med. Sci. Biol. **13**, 33—41 (1960b)
Okazaki, R.: Isolation of a new deoxyribosidic compound, thymidine diphosphate rhamnose. Biochem. Biophys. Res. Commun. **1**, 34—38 (1959)
Omori, T., Iwanaga, S., Suzuki, T.: The relationship between the hemorrhagic and lethal activities of Japanese Mamushi *(Agkistrodon halys blomhoffii)* venom. Toxicon **2**, 1—4 (1964)
Oshima, G., Iwanaga, S.: Occurrence of glycoproteins in various snake venoms. Toxicon **7**, 235—238 (1969)
Oshima, G., Iwanaga, S., Suzuki, T.: Studies on snake venoms. XVIII. An improved method for purification of proteinase b from the venom of *Agkistrodon halys blomhoffii* and its physicochemical properties. J. Biochem. **64**, 215—225 (1968b)
Oshima, G., Iwanaga, S., Suzuki, T.: Some properties of proteinase b in the venom of *Agkistrodon halys blomhoffii*. Biochim. biophys. Acta (Amst.) **250**, 416—427 (1971)
Oshima, G., Matsuo, Y., Iwanaga, S., Suzuki, T.: Studies on snake venoms. XIX. Purification and some physicochemical properties of proteinases a and c from the venom of *Agkistrodon halys blomhoffii*. J. Biochem. **64**, 227—238 (1968a)

Oshima, G., Omori-Satoh, T., Iwanaga, S., Suzuki, T.: Studies on snake venom hemorrhagic factor I (HR-I) in the venom of *Agkistrodon halys blomhoffii*. Its purification and properties. J. Biochem. **72**, 1483—1444 (1972)

Oshima, G., Sato-Ohmori, T., Suzuki, T.: Proteinase, arginineester hydrolase and a kinin releasing enzyme in snake venoms. Toxicon **7**, 229—233 (1969)

Page, D. S., Vanetten, R. L.: L-amino acid oxidase. I. Effect of pH. Biochim. biophys. Acta (Amst.) **191**, 38—45 (1969)

Page, D. S., Vanetten, R. L.: L-amino acid oxidase. II. Deuterium isotope effects and the action mechanism for the reduction of L-amino acid oxidase by L-leucine. Biochim. biophys. Acta (Amst.) **227**, 16—31 (1971)

Parikh, J. R., Greenstein, J. P., Winitz, M., Birnbaum, S. M.: The use of amino acid oxidases for the small-scale preparation of the optical isomers of amino acids. J. Amer. chem. Soc. **80**, 953—958 (1958)

Pasek, M., Keith, C., Feldman, D., Singler, P. B.: Characterization of crystals of two venom phospholipase A_2. J. molec. Biol. **97**, 395—397 (1975)

Pattnaik, M. M., Kezdy, F. J., Scanu, A. M.: Kinetic study of the action of snake venom phospholipase A_2 on human serum high density lipoprotein 3. J. biol. Chem. **251**, 1984—1990 (1976)

Pfleiderer, G., Krauss, A.: Die Wirkungsspezifität von Schlangengift-Proteasen *(Crotalus atrox)*. Biochem. Z. **342**, 85—94 (1965)

Pfleiderer, G., Ortanderl, F.: Identität von phosphodiesterase und ATP-pyrophosphatase aus Schlangengift. Biochem. Z. **337**, 431—435 (1963)

Pfleiderer, G., Sumyk, G.: Investigation of snake venom enzymes. I. Separation of rattlesnake venom proteinases by cellulose ionexchange chromatography. Biochim. biophys. Acta (Amst.) **51**, 482—493 (1961)

Pereira Lima, R. A., Schenberg, S., Schiripa, L. N., Nagamori, A.: ATPase and phosphodiesterase differentiation in snake venoms. In: de Vries, A., Kochva, E. (Eds.): Toxins of Animal and Plant Origins, Vol. 1, pp. 464—470. New York: Gordon and Breach 1971

Plummer, T. H., Jr.: Glycoproteins of bovine pancreatic juice. Isolation of ribonuclease C and D. J. biol. Chem. **243**, 591—5966 (1968)

Prescott, J. M., Fredricks, K. K., Bingham, P. H.: Proteases of *Agkistrodon piscivorus leucostoma* venom. In: Ohsaka, A., Hayashi, K., Sawai, Y. (Eds.): Animal, Plant, and Microbial Toxins. Vol. 1, pp. 217—234. New York-London: Plenum Press 1974

Prescott, J. M., Wagner, F. W.: Leucostoma peptidase A. In: Lorand, L. (Ed.): Methods in Enzymology, Vol. **45B**, pp. 397—404. New York-San Francisco-London: Academic Press 1976

Privat de Garilhe, M.: Les Nuclease. Paris: Hermann 1964

Raudonat, H. W.: Papierchromatographische Abtrennung eines Proteasen-Hemmstoffes aus Schlangengiften. Naturwissenschaften **42**, 559—560 (1955)

Raudonat, H. W., Rocha e Silva, M.: Separation of the bradykinin releasing enzyme from the clotting factor in venom from *Bothrops jararaca*. Naunyn-Schmiedebergs Arch. exp. Path. Pharmak. **243**, 232—236 (1962)

Razzell, W. E.: Phosphodiesterases. In: Colowick, S. P., Kaplan, N. O. (Eds.): Methods in Enzymology, Vol. 6, pp. 236—245. New York-London: Academic Press 1963

Razzell, W. E., Khorana, H. G.: Studies on polypeptides III. Enzymic degradation. Substrate specificity and properties of snake venom phosphodiesterase. J. biol. Chem. **234**, 2105—2113 (1959)

Ribeiro, A. A., Dennis, E. A.: Effect of thermotropic phase transitions of dipalmitoyl phosphatidylcholine on the formation of mixed micelles with Triton X-100. Biochim. biophys. Acta (Amst.) **332**, 26—35 (1973)

Richards, G. M., du Vair, G., Laskowski, M., Sr.: Comparison of the levels of phosphodiesterase, endonuclease, and monophosphatases in several snake venoms. Biochemistry **4**, 501—503 (1965)

Richards, G. M., Tutas, D. J., Wechter, W. J., Laskowski, M., Sr.: Hydrolysis of dinucleoside monophosphates containing arabinose in various internucleotide linkage by exonuclease from the venom of *Crotalus adamanteus*. Biochemistry **6**, 2908—2914 (1967)

Roberts, M. F., Deems, R. A., Dennis, E. A.: Dual role of interfacial phospholipid in phospholipase A_2 catalysis. Proc. nat. Acad. Sci. (Wash.) **74**, 1950—1954 (1977a)

Roberts, M. F., Deems, R. A., Mincey, T. C., Dennis, E. A.: Chemical modification of the histidine residue in phospholipase A_2 *(Naja naja naja)*. A case of half-site reactivity. J. biol. Chem. **252**, 2405—2411 (1977 b)
Rocha e Silva, M., Beraldo, W. T., Rosenfeld, G.: Bradykinin, a hypotensive and smooth muscle stimulating factor released from plasma globulin by snake venoms and by trypsin. Amer. J. Physiol. **156**, 261—273 (1949)
Rock, C. O., Snyder, F.: Rapid purification of phospholipase A_2 from *Crotalus adamanteus* venom by affinity chromatography. J. biol. Chem. **250**, 6564—6566 (1975)
Russell, F. E., Eventov, R.: Lethality of crude and lyophilized *Crotalus* venom. Toxicon **2**, 81—82 (1964)
Salach, J. I., Seng, R., Tisdale, H., Singer, T. P.: Phospholipase A of snake venom. II. Catalytic properties of the enzyme from *Naja naja*. J. biol. Chem. **246**, 340—347 (1971 b)
Salach, J. I., Turini, P., Seng, R., Hauber, J., Singer, T. P.: Phospholipase A of snake venoms. I. Isolation and molecular properties of isoenzymes from *Naja naja* and *Vipera russellii* venoms. J. biol. Chem. 246, 331—339 (1971 a)
Samejima, Y., Iwanaga, S., Suzuki, T., Kawauchi, Y.: Partial amino acid sequence of snake venom phospholipase A. Biochim. biophys. Acta (Amst.) **221**, 417—420 (1970)
Satake, M., Murata, Y., Suzuki, T.: Studies on snake venoms. XIII. Chromatographic separation and properties of three proteinases from *Agkistrodon halys blomhoffii* venom. J. Biochem. **53**, 483—417 (1963 a)
Satake, M., Omori, T., Iwanaga, S., Suzuki, T.: Studies on snake venoms. XIV. Hydrolysis of insulin B chain and glucagon by proteinase c from *Agkistrodon halys blomhoffii* venom. J. Biochem. **54**, 8—16 (1963 b)
Sato, T., Iwanaga, S., Mizushima, Y., Suzuki, T.: Studies on snake venoms XV. Separation of arginine ester hydrolase of *Agkistrodon halys blomhoffii* venom into three enzymatic entities: "Bradykinin releasing", "Clotting", and "Permeability increasing". J. Biochem. **57**, 380—391 (1965)
Sato, S., Tamiya, N.: The amino acid sequences of erabutoxins, neurotoxic proteins of sea-snake *(Laticauda semifasciata)* venom. Biochem. J. **122**, 453—461 (1971)
Schenberg, S., Perira, Lima, F. A., Schiripa, L. N., Nagamori, A.: Snake venom ADPase. In: Ohsaka, A., Hayashi, K., Sawai, Y. (Eds.): Animal, Plant, and Microbial Toxins, Vol. 1, pp. 249—262. New York-London: Plenum Press 1974
Schiripa, L. N., Schenberg, S.: 'Etudo da ATPase, ADPase e 5'-Nucleotidase de venonos ofidicos. Ciencia e Cultura **16**, 194—195 (1964)
Setoguchi, Y., Morisawa, S., Obo, F.: Investigation of sea snake venom. III. Acid and alkaline phosphatases (phosphodiesterase, phosphomonoesterase, 5'-nucleotidase and ATPase) in sea snake *(Laticauda semifasciata)* venom. Acta Med. Univ. Kagoshima **10**, 53—60 (1968)
Shaham, N., Bdolah, A.: L-amino acid oxidase from *Vipera palestinae* venom: Purification and assay. Comp. Biochem. Physiol. **B46**, 691—698 (1973)
Shiba, T., Cahnmann, H. J.: Conversion of 3,5-diiodotyrosine to thyroxine by rattlesnake venom. Biochim. biophys. Acta (Amst.) **58**, 609—610 (1962 a)
Shiba, T., Cahnmann, H. J.: Synthesis of specifically iodine-131 and carbon-14-labeled Thyroxine. J. Org. Chem. **27**, 1773—1778 (1962 b)
Shiloah, J., Klibansky, C., de Vries, A.: Phospholipase isoenzymes from *Naja naja* venom II. Phospholipase A and B activities. Toxicon **11**, 491—497 (1973 a)
Shiloah, J., Klibansky, C., de Vries, A.: Phospholipase isozymes from *Naja naja* venom I. Purification and partial characterization. Toxicon **11**, 481—490 (1973 b)
Shiloah, J., Klibansky, C., de Vries, A., Berger, A.: Phospholipase B activity of a purified phospholipase A from *Vipera palstinae* venom. J. Lipid Res. **14**, 267—278 (1973 c)
Simon, J., Brisbois, L., Gillo, L.: Fractionation of cobra venom by electrofocusing. J. Chromatog. **44**, 209—211 (1969)
Singer, S. J.: The molecular organization of biological membranes. In: Rothfield, L. I. (Ed.): Structure and Function of Biological Membranes, pp. 146—222. New York-London: Academic Press 1971
Singer, T. P., Kearney, E. B.: The L-amino acid oxidases of snake venom. I. Prosthetic group of the L-amino acid oxidase of Moccasin venom. Arch. Biochem. **27**, 348—262 (1950)
Singer, T. P., Kearney, E. B.: The L-amino acid oxidases of snake venom. III. Reversible inactivation of L-amino acid oxidases. Arch. Biochem. Biophys. **33**, 377—413 (1951)

Sinsheimer, R. L., Koerner, J. F.: A purification of venom phosphodiesterase. J. biol. Chem. **198**, 293—296 (1952)

Slotta, K.: Chemistry and biochemistry of snake venoms. Prog. Chem. Org. Nat. Prod. **12**, 406—465 (1955)

Slotta, K. H., Fraenkel-Conrat, H.: Schlangengift. III. Mitteil. Reinigung und Krystallisation des Klapperschlangen-Giftes. Ber. Deut. **71**, 1076—1081 (1938)

Smith, A. D., Gul, S., Thompson, R. H. S.: The effect of fatty acids and of albumin on the action of a purified phospholipase A_2 from cobra venom on synthetic lecithins. Biochim. biophys. Acta (Amst.) **289**, 147—157 (1972)

Smith, M. A., Hindle, E.: Experiments with the venom of *Laticauda*, *Pseudechis* and *Trimeresurus* species. Trans. roy. Soc. trop. Med. Hyg. **25**, 115—120 (1931)

Spiekerman, A. M., Fredericks, K. K., Wagner, F. W., Prescott, J. M.: Leucostoma peptidase A: A metalloprotease from snake venom. Biochim. biophys. Acta (Amst.) **293**, 464—475 (1973)

Stathakos, D., Wallenfels, K.: Löslichmachen und Anreicherung der NAD-nucleosidase aus Rindermilz. Biochem. Z. **346**, 89—106 (1966)

Strydom, A. J. C., Botes, D. P.: Snake venom toxins. Purification, properties, and complete amino acid sequence of two toxins from Ringhals *(Hemachatus haemachatus)* venom. J. biol. Chem. **246**, 1341—1349 (1971)

Strydom, D. J., Botes, D. P.: Snake venom toxins-I. Preliminary studies on the separation of toxins of Elapidae venoms. Toxicon 203—209 (1970)

Sugino, Y.: Studies on deoxynucleosidic compounds. II. Deoxycytidine diphosphate choline in sea urchin eggs. Biochim. biophys. Acta (Amst.) **40**, 425—434 (1957)

Sugiura, M., Sasaki, M., Ito, Y., Akatsuka, M., Oikawa, T., Kakino, M.: Purification and properties of L-amino acid oxidase from the venom of Kankokumamushi *(Agkistrodon caliginosus)*. Snake **7**, 83—90 (1975)

Sulkowski, E., Björk, W., Laskowski, M., Sr.: A specific and nonspecific alkaline monophosphatase in the venom of *Bothrops atrox* and their occurrence in the purified venom phosphodiesterase. J. biol. Chem. **238**, 2477—2486 (1963)

Sulkowski, E., Laskowski, M., Sr.: Inactivation of 5′-nucleotidase in commercial preparations of venom exonuclease (phosphodiesterase). Biochim. biophys. Acta (Amst.) **240**, 443—447 (1971)

Suran, A. A.: A simple microradioisotopic assay for 5′-nucleotidase activity. Application to central nervous tissues. Anal. Biochem. **55**, 593—600 (1973)

Suzuki, T., Iizuka, K., Murata, Y.: Studies on snake venoms. IX. On the studies of diphosphopyridine nucleotidase in snake venom. J. Pharm. Soc. Jpn. **80**, 868—875 (1960d)

Suzuki, T., Iwanaga, S.: Studies on snake venom. II. Some observations on the alkaline phosphatases of Japanese and Formosan snake venoms. J. Pharm. Soc. Jpn. **78**, 354—361 (1958a)

Suzuki, T., Iwanaga, S.: Studies on snake venom. IV. Purification of alkaline phosphatases in cobra venoms. J. Pharm. Soc. Jpn. **78**, 368—375 (1958b)

Suzuki, T., Iwanaga, S.: Studies on snake venoms. III. Purification of some enzymes in Japanese Mamushi venom (*Agkistrodon halys blomhoffii*, Boie). J. Pharm. Soc. Jpn. **78**, 362—367 (1958c)

Suzuki, T., Iwanaga, S.: Studies on snake venom alkaline phosphatases. Protein Nucleic Acid Enzyme **6**, 265—279 (1960a)

Suzuki, T., Iwanaga, S.: Studies on snake venoms. VIII. Substrate specificity of L-amino acid oxidase in Mamushi (*Agkistrodon halys blomhoffii*, Boie) and Habu (*Trimeresurus flavoviridis*, Boulenger) venoms. J. Pharm. Soc. Jpn. **80**, 1002—1005 (1960b)

Suzuki, T., Iwanaga, S.: Snake venoms. In: Erdös, E. G. (Ed.): Bradykinin, Kallidin, and Kallikrein. Handbook of Experimental Pharmacology, Vol. 25, pp. 193—212, Springer, Berlin-Heidelberg-New York: Springer 1970

Suzuki, T., Iwanaga, S., Kawauchi, S.: Isolation of crystalline lecithinase A (hemolysin) from Formosan cobra venom (*Naja naja atra* Cantor). J. Pharm. Soc. Jpn. **78**, 568—569 (1958)

Suzuki, T., Iwanaga, S., Nagasawa, S., Sato, T.: Purification and properties of bradykininogen and of the bradykinin-releasing and -destroying enzymes in snake venom. In: Erdös, E. G., Back, N., Sicuteri, F. (Eds.): Hypotensive Peptides, pp. 149—160. Berlin-Heidelberg-New York: Springer 1966

Suzuki, T., Iwanaga, S., Nitta, K.: Studies on snake venom. XI. On the hydrolysis of cyclic mononucleotides by snake venom. J. Pharm. Soc. Jpn. **80**, 1040—1044 (1960c)

Suzuki, T., Iwanaga, S., Sasai, M.: Substrate specificities of snake venom 5'-nucleotidase. The 14th Congress on Jap. Pharm. Soc. (Abs.), p. 210 (1961)
Suzuki, T., Iwanaga, S., Satake, M.: Studies on snake venom. VI. Fractionation of three phosphodiesterases from venom of Mamushi (*Agkistrodon halys blomhoffii*, Boie). J. Pharm. Soc. Jpn. **80**, 857—861 (1960a)
Suzuki, T., Iwanaga, S., Satake, M.: Studies on snake venom. VII. On the properties of three phosphodiesterases obtained from Mamushi venom (*Agkistrodon halys blomhoffii*, Boie). J. Pharm. Soc. Jpn. **80**, 861—867 (1960b)
Svensson, H.: Isoelectric fractionation, analysis, and characterization of ampholytes in natural pH gradient. II. Buffering capacity and conductance of isoionic ampholytes. Acta chem. scand. **16**, 456—466 (1962)
Taborda, A. R., Taborda, L. C., Williams, J. N., Jr., Elvehjem, C. A.: A study of the deoxyribonuclease activity of snake venoms. J. biol. Chem. **195**, 207—226 (1952)
Takahashi, H.: Über Fermentative Dephosphorierung der Nukleinsäure. J. Biochem. **16**, 463—481 (1932)
Takahashi, T., Ohsaka, A.: Purification and characterization of a proteinase in the venom of *Trimeresurus flavoviridis*. Biochim. biophys. Acta (Amst.) **198**, 293—307 (1970)
Tatsuki, T., Iwanaga, S., Oshima, G., Suzuki, T.: Snake venom NAD nucleosidase: Its occurrence in the venoms from the genus *Agkistrodon* and purification and properties of the enzyme from the venom of *A. halys blomhoffii*. Toxicon **13**, 211—220 (1975)
Tatsuki, T., Iwanaga, S., Suzuki, T.: A simple method for preparation of snake venom phosphodiesterase almost free from 5'-nucleotidase. J. Biochem. **77**, 831—836 (1975)
Tigerstrom, R. G. von, Smith, M.: Preparation of the 2,4-dinitrophenyl esters of thymidine 3'- and thymidine 5'-phosphate and their use as substrates for phosphodiesterases. Biochemistry **8**, 3067—3070 (1969)
Toom, P. M., Squire, P. G., Tu, A. T.: Characterization of the enzymatic and biological activities of snake venoms by isoelectric focusing. Biochim. biophys. Acta (Amst.) **181**, 339—341 (1969)
Toom, P. M., Solie, T. N., Tu, A. T.: Characterization of a nonproteolytic arginine ester-hydrolyzing enzyme from snake venom. J. biol. Chem. **245**, 2549—2555 (1970)
Trautschold, I., Werle, E., Schweitzer, G.: Kallikrein. In: Bergmeyer, H. U. (Ed.): Methoden der enzymatischen Analyse, Vol. 2, pp. 1031—1040, Weinheim: Verlag Chemie 1974
Tsao, F. C., Keim, P. S., Heinrikson: *Crotalus adamanteus* phospholipase A_2-α: Subunit structure, NH_2-terminal sequence, and homology with other phospholipases. Arch. Biochem. Biophys. **167**, 706—717 (1975)
Tu, A. T.: Venoms. Chemistry and Molecular Biology, pp. 23—63. New York-London-Sydney-Toronto: John Wiley 1977
Tu, A. T., Chua, A.: Acid and alkaline phosphomonoesterase activities in snake venoms. Comp. Biochem. Physiol. **17**, 297—307 (1966)
Tu, A. T., Chua, A., James, G. P.: Peptidase activities of snake venoms. Comp. Biochem. Physiol. **15**, 517—523 (1965)
Tu, A. T., Hong, B.-S.: Purification and chemical studies of a toxin from the venom of *Lapemis hardwickii* (Hardwick's sea snake). J. biol. Chem. **296**, 2772—2779 (1971)
Tu, A. T., Passey, R. B., Toom, P. M.: Isolation and characterization of phospholipase A from sea snake, *Laticauda semifasciata* venom. Arch. Biochem. Biophys. **140**, 96—106 (1970)
Tu, A. T., Toom, P. M.: The presence of a L-leucyl-β-naphthylamide hydrolyzing enzyme in snake venoms. Experienta (Basel) **23**, 1—5 (1967a)
Tu, A. T., Toom, P. M.: Hydrolysis of peptides by snake venoms of Australia and New Guinea. Aust. J. exp. Biol. med. Sci. **45**, 561—567 (1967b)
Tu, A. T., Toom, P. M.: Hydrolysis of peptides by Crotalidae and Viperidae venoms. Toxicon **5**, 201—205 (1968)
Tu, A. T., Toom, P. M.: Isolation and characterization of the toxic component of *Enhydrina schistosa* (common sea snake) venom. J. biol. Chem. **246**, 1012—1016 (1971)
Turakulov, Y. K., Sakhibov, D. N., Sorokin, V. M., Yukel'son, L. Y.: Separation of central-Asian cobra venom by means of gel filtration through Sephadex and determination of biological activity of the resulting fractions. Biokhimiya **34**, 1119—1122 (1969)
Ubuka, T., Ishimoto, Y., Kasahara, K.: Determination of 3-mercaptopyruvate-cysteine disulfide, a product of oxidative deamination of L-cystine by L-amino acid oxidase. Anal. Biochem. **67**, 66—73 (1975)

Ubuka, T., Yao, K.: Oxidative deamination of L-cystine by L-amino acid oxidase from snake venom: Formation of S-(2-oxo-2-carboxyethylthio)cysteine and S-(carboxymethylthio)cysteine. Biochem. Biophys. Res. Commun. **55**, 1305—1310 (1973)

Uwatoko-Setoguchi, Y.: Studies on sea snake venom. VI. Pharmacological properties of *Laticauda semifasciata* venom and purification of toxic components, acid phosphomonoesterase and phospholipase A in the venom. Acta Med. Univ. Kagoshima **12**, 73—96 (1970)

Uzawa, T.: Über die Phosphomonoesterase und die Phosphodiesterase. J. Biochem. **15**, 19—28 (1932)

Van Deenen, L. L. M., de Haas, G. H.: The substrate specificity of phospholipase A. Biochim. biophys. Acta (Amst.) **70**, 538—553 (1963)

Van Deenen, L. L. M., de Haas, G. H.: Phosphoglycerides and phospholipases. Ann. Rev. Biochem. **35**, 157—194 (1966)

Van der Walt, S. J., Joubert, F. J.: Studies on puff adder *(Bitis arietans)* venom. I. Purification and properties of protease A. Toxicon **9** 153—161 (1971)

Van der Walt, S. J., Joubert, F. J.: Studies on puff adder *(Bitis arietans)* venom II. Specificity of protease A. Toxicon **10**, 341—349 (1972)

Vasilenko, S. K., Rait, V. K.: Isolation of highly purified ribonuclease from cobra *(Naja oxiana)* venom. Biokhimiya **40**, 578—583 (1975)

Vidal, C. A., Cattaneo, P., Stoppani, A. O. M.: Some characteristic properties of phospholipase A_2 from *Bothrops neuwiedii* venom. Arch. Biochem. Biophys. **151**, 168—179 (1972a)

Vidal, J. C., Molina, H., Stoppani, A. O. M.: A general procedure for the isolation and purification of phospholipase A isoenzymes from *Bothrops* venoms. Acta Physiol. latino amer. **23**, 91—109 (1972b)

Vidal, J. C., Stoppani, A. O. M.: Isolation and purification of two phospholipase A from *Bothrops* venoms. Arch. Biochem. Biophys. **145**, 543—556 (1971)

Viljoen, C. C., Botes, D. P., Schabort, J. C.: Spectral properties of *Bitis gavonica* venom phospholipase A_2 in the presence of divalent metal ion, substrate and hydrolysis products. Toxicon **13**, 343—351 (1975)

Viljoen, C. C., Schabort, J. C., Botes, D. P.: *Bitis gavonica* venom. A kinetic analysis of the hydrolysis by phospholipase A_2 of 1,2-dipalmitoyl-sn-glycero-3-phosphorylcholine. Biochim. biophys. Acta (Amst.) **360**, 156—165 (1974)

Viljoen, C. C., Visser, L., Botes, D. P.: Histidine and lysine residues and the activity of phospholipase A_2 from the venom of *Bitis gavonica.* Biochim. biophys. Acta (Amst.) **483**, 107—120 (1977)

Wagner, F. W., Spiekerman, A. M., Prescott, J. M.: Leucostoma peptidase A. Isolation and physical properties. J. biol. Chem. **243**, 4486—4493 (1968)

Wahlström, A.: Purification and characterization of phospholipase A from the venom of *Naja nigricollis.* Toxicon **9** 45—56 (1971)

Waku, K., Nakazawa, Y.: Hydrolyses of 1-0-alkyl-, 1-0-alkenyl-, and 1-acyl-2-[1-^{14}C]-linoleoyl-glycero-3-phosphorylcholine by various phospholipases. J. Biochem. **72**, 149—155 (1972)

Webster, M. E., Pierce, J. V.: The nature of the kallidins released from human plasma by kallikreins and other enzymes. Ann. N.Y. Acad. Sci. **104**, 91—107 (1963)

Webster, M. E., Prado, E. S.: Grandular kallikreins from horse and human urine and hog pancreas. In: Perlmann, G. E., Lorand, L. (Eds.): Methods in Enzymology, Vol. 19, pp. 681—699. New York-London: Academic Press 1970

Wechter, W. J.: Nucleic acids. I. The synthesis of nucleotides and dinucleoside phosphates containing *ara*-cytidine. J. med. Chem. **10**, 762—773 (1967)

Wellner, D.: L-amino acid oxidase (snake venom). In: Tabor, H., Tabor, C. W. (Eds.): Methods in Enzymology, Vol. 17, Part B, pp. 597—600. New York-London: Academic Press 1971

Wellner, D., Lichtenberg, L. A.: Assay of amino acid oxidase. In: Tabor, H., Tabor, C. W. (Eds.): Methods in Enzymology, Vol. 17, Part B, pp. 592—596. New York-London: Academic Press 1971

Wellner, D., Meister, A.: Crystalline L-amino acid oxidase of *Crotalus adamanteus*. J. biol. Chem. **235**, 2013—2018 (1960)

Wells, M. A.: Evidence that the phospholipases A_2 of *Crotalus adamanteus* are dimer. Biochemistry **10**, 4074—4078 (1971a)

Wells, M. A.: Spectral peculiarities of the monomer-dimer transition of the phospholipase A_2 of *Crotalus adamanteus* venom. Biochemistry **10**, 4078—4083 (1971b)

Wells, M. A.: Evidence for 0-acyl cleavage during hydrolysis of 1,2-diacyl-sn-glycero-3-phosphorylcholine by the phospholipase A_2 of *Crotalus adamanteus* venom. Biochim. biophys. Acta (Amst.) **248**, 80—86 (1971 c)

Wells, M. A.: A kinetic study of the phospholipase A_2 *(Crotalus adamanteus)* catalyzed hydrolysis of 1,2-dibutyryl-sn-glycero-3-phosphorylcholine. Biochemistry **11**, 1030—1041 (1972)

Wells, M. A.: The mechanism of interfacial activation of phospholipase A_2. Biochemistry **13**, 2248—2257 (1974 a)

Wells, M. A.: A phospholipase A_2 model system. Calcium enhancement of the amino-catalyzed methanolysis of phosphatidylcholine. Biochemistry **13**, 2258—2264 (1974 b)

Wells, M. A.: A simple and high yield purification of *Crotalus adamanteus* phospholipase A_2. Biochim. biophys. Acta (Amst.) **380**, 357—505 (1975)

Wells, M. A., Hanahan, D. J.: Studies on phospholipase A. I. Isolation and characterization of two enzymes from *Crotalus adamanteus* venom. Biochemistry **8**, 414—424 (1969)

Wilkes, S. H., Prescott, J. M.: Aeromonas neutral protease. In: Lorand, L., (Ed.): Methods in Enzymology, Vol. 45, pp. 404—415. New York-San Francisco-London: Academic Press 1976

Williams, E. J., Sung, S.-C., Laskowski, M., Sr.: Action of venom phosphodiesterase on deoxyribonucleic acid. J. biol. Chem. **236**, 1130—1134 (1961)

Windmueller, H. G., Kaplan, N. O.: Solubilization and purification of diphosphopyridine nucleotidase from pig brain. Biochim. biophys. Acta (Amst.) **56**, 388—391 (1962)

Woelk, H., Debuch, H.: Die Wirkung der Phospholipase A aus Schlangengift auf Phosphatidylcholin, Phosphatidyläthanolamin und auf die entsprechenden Plasmalogene. Hoppe-Seylers Z. physiol. Chem. **352**, 1275—1281 (1971)

Woelk, H., Peiler-Ichikawa, K.: The action of phospholipase A_2 purified from *Crotalus atrox* venom on specifically labeled 2-acyl-1-alk-1'-enyl- and 2-acyl-1-alkyl-sn-glycero-3-phosphorylcholine. Febs Letters **45**, 75—78 (1974)

Wu, T. W., Tinker, D. D.: Phospholipase A_2 from *Crotalus atrox* venom. I. Purification and some properties. Biochemistry **8**, 1558—1568 (1969)

Yang, C. C., Chiu, W. C., Kao, K. C.: Biochemical studies on snake venoms. VII. Isolation of venom cholinesterase by zone electrophoresis. J. Biochem. **48**, 706—713 (1960 b)

Yang, C. C., Iwanaga, S., Kawachi, S.: Biochemical studies on the Formosan snake venoms. II. Some observations on the column chromatography of cobra venom. J. Formosan med. Ass. **58**, 527—532 (1958)

Yang, C. C., Kao, K. C., Chiu, W. C.: Biochemical studies on the snake venoms. VIII. Electrophoretic studies on banded kreit *(Bungarus multicinctus)* venom and the relation of toxicity with enzyme activities. J. Biochem. **48**, 714—722 (1960 a)

Yano, M., Nagasawa, S., Suzuki, T.: Partial purification and some properties of high molecular weight kininogen, bovine kininogen-I. J. Biochem. **69**, 471—481 (1971)

Yoshida, S.: Studies über die Phosphodiesterase. J. Biochem. **34**, 23—37 (1941)

Yuan, J. H., Anderson, B. M.: Bull semen nictoinamide adenine dinucleotide nucleosidase. I. Purification and properties of the enzyme. J. biol. Chem. **246**, 2111—2115 (1971)

Zatman, L. J., Kaplan, N. O., Colowick, S. P.: Inhibition of spleen diphosphopyridine nucleotidase by nicotinamide, an exchange reaction. J. biol. Chem. **200**, 197—212 (1953)

Zatman, L. J., Kaplan, N. O., Colowick, S. P., Ciotti, M. M.: Effect of isonicotinic acid hydrazide on diphosphopyridine nucleotidases. J. biol. Chem. **209**, 453—466 (1954)

Zeller, E. A.: Enzymes of snake venoms and their biological significance. Ad. Enzymol. **8**, 459—495 (1948)

Zeller, E. A.: The formation of pyrophosphate from adenosine triphosphate in the presence of a snake venom. Arch. Biochem. **28**, 138—139 (1950 a)

Zeller, E. A.: Über Phosphatasen: Über eine neue Adenosine Triphosphatase. Helv. chim. Acta **33**, 821—833 (1950b)

Zeller, E. A.: Enzymes as essential components of toxins. In: Sumner, J. B., Myrback, K. (Eds.): Enzymes, Vol. 1, pp. 986—1013. New York: Academic Press 1951

Zeller, E. A., Maritz, A.: Über eine neue L-Aminosäure Oxidase. Helv. chim. Acta **27**, 1888—1902 (1944)

Zeller, E. A., Ramachander, G., Fleisher, A., Ishimaru, T., Zeller, V.: Ophidian L-amino acid oxidase. The nature of the enzyme-substrate complexes. Biochem. J. **95**, 262—269 (1965)

Zwaal, R. F. A., Roelofsen, B., Comfurius, P., Van Deenen, L. L. M: Organization of phospholipids in human red cell membranes as detected by the action of various purified phospholipases. Biochim. biophys. Acta (Amst.) **406**, 83—96 (1975)

CHAPTER 5

Chemistry of Protein Toxins in Snake Venoms

E. KARLSSON

A. Introduction

The main function of snake venoms lies in the procuring of food and its digestion. The death of the prey is due to respiratory or circulatory failure caused by various neurotoxins, cardiotoxins, coagulation factors, and other substances acting alone or synergistically. The various enzymes injected into the prey start the digestion of the tissues. The venoms thus contain substances designed to affect vital processes, such as the function of nerves and muscles, the action of the heart, the circulation of the blood, and the permeability of membranes. Snake venoms and other toxic secretions contain a large number of pharmacologically highly active substances with a specific mode of action. Since such compounds are of great value in the investigation of important physiologic processes, the research on venoms is not the esoteric activity that one might think it to be considering the exotic origin of many venoms.

Snake venoms are complex mixtures. Most of the constituents are proteins, but low molecular weight compounds, such as peptides, nucleosides, and metal ions are also present. The exact number of compounds a venom may contain is not known. Intensive fractionation of some cobra and sea snake venoms indicates that the number of different proteins present in amounts of 0.5% or higher may exceed 25, and that the number will increase if one also considers proteins present at the 0.1% level.

This article mainly concerns neurotoxins, which have during the last few years attracted the interest of many biochemists and pharmacologists. Several review articles on neurotoxins have appeared since 1970 (JIMENÉZ PORRAS, 1970; LEE, 1970, 1971, 1972; CHEYMOL et al., 1972; TU, 1973; KARLSSON, 1973; MEBS, 1973; ZLOTKIN, 1973; YANG, 1974; EAKER, 1975). The neurotoxins are the most toxic venom constituents and are divided into two pharmacologic classes on the basis of their sites of action: namely, postsynaptic, and presynaptic neurotoxins.

Like curare, the *postsynaptic neurotoxins* (Sect. B.I.) bind to the nicotinic acetylcholine receptors and thereby prevent the depolarizing action of acetylcholine. These toxins are usually referred to as *curaremimetic*, *curariform*, or *curare-like* toxins, or simply neurotoxins. They have been intensively investigated in the last decade following the purification of the first toxins. More than 40 such toxins have been sequenced, and a great many chemical modifications aimed at the identification of the active site have also been carried out. No other group of venom constituents has received so much attention.

Presynaptic neurotoxins (Sect. C.) inhibit the release of acetylcholine and their lethality is much higher than that of the postsynaptic toxins.

Snakes belonging to the families *Elapidae* (cobras, kraits, mambas, tiger snakes, coral snakes, etc.) and *Hydrophidae* (sea snakes) have typical neurotoxic venoms with a high neurotoxin content. Curaremimetic toxins have not been isolated from venoms of other families, which does not necessarily mean that such toxins are not present. Most venoms of *Viperidae* (vipers), *Crotalidae* (pit vipers such as rattle snakes, moccasins, habu, etc.), and *Colubridae* (boom slang) have not been fractionated as thoroughly as for instance cobra venoms, and small amounts of curariform toxins might have escaped detection. Negative immunologic tests may also reflect a new immunologic type rather than the absence of postsynaptic toxins.

Presynaptic neurotoxins are extremely lethal and structurally related to *phospholipase* A. Whether the inhibition of the transmitter release is due to the phospholipase activity is not yet known, but indirect evidence indicates that it might be so (Sect. C.VIII.).

Some of the presynaptic neurotoxins can also act as *myonecrotic toxins* producing necrosis of muscle fibers (Sects. C.V. and C.VII.3.).

Membrane toxins form another large group of toxins (Sect. B.II.). They change the permeability of membranes in a great variety of cells and tissues. Depending on the assay system used they are often referred to as cardiotoxins, lytic factors, cytotoxins, etc.—names which indicate the various types of membranes affected. Membrane toxins have been isolated only from elapid venoms.

Finally, under the title *other toxins* (Sect. D.), toxins, for which definite chemical and/or pharmacologic information in most cases is not yet available, will be briefly described. Considering the rapid development in toxin research, these "other toxins" will probably be familiar substances within a few years.

Despite the great variety of activities displayed by the toxins discussed in Section B, they are all clearly homologous with regard to structure, as are the presynaptic neurotoxins described in Section C. The two structural classes are defined as follows:

1. Molecules with a *postsynaptic neurotoxin-membrane toxin structure*. They have about 60–70 amino acid residues in a peptide chain cross-linked by four or five disulfides. Curaremimetic toxins, membrane toxins, and some proteins with an unknown function belong to this group, of which about 70 have been sequenced (Figs. 4 and 8). The different types of molecules probably have evolved from a common ancestor protein having about 60 residues. The evolution and phylogenetic relationships are discussed by Strydom in a separate review article in this volume of the Handbook.

2. Molecules with a *phospholipase structure* having about 120–140 amino acid residues and six to eight disulfides. Some toxins are complexes of two or three subunits, of which at least one is a phospholipase A. Presynaptic neurotoxins, myonecrotic toxins, basic phospholipases with high lethality or pathologic activity, and other proteins having phospholipase structure are referred to this group. Only three members of this group have been sequenced to date. The compositions of a few more are also known sufficiently well to show homology with the known sequences.

These venom toxins are very resistant molecules: most of them survive boiling in neutral or weakly acidic solutions and are only reversibly denatured by urea or guanidine hydrochloride. They are, however, rapidly inactivated by strong alkali as a result of desulfurization and/or disulfide interchange. It has also been known for a long time that the toxicity of cobra venom withstands boiling. This reflects the heat stability of neurotoxins, membrane toxins, and phospholipases.

The stable protein structures of the two classes of toxins probably have evolved first for some unknown reason, and the different activities have then arisen through mutations, with retention of the features responsible for the stability of the overall structure.

However, all of these toxins, except *crotoxin*, referred to in the two groups are from elapids or hydrophids. The two fundamental structures probably reflect only evolutionary solutions within these two families of snakes. Evolution among crotalids, viperids, and colubrids might have followed other lines based on structures different from the above two. In fact, the basic phospholipase constituents of crotoxin apparently show only a limited homology with the elapid phospholipases, since the disulfide pairing is different (Sect. C.III. and Fig. 11). Phospholipases in general from crotalid and viperid venoms also seem to have only a limited degree of sequential homology with the elapid phospholipases (SAMEJIMA et al., 1974).

Crotamine from *Crotalus durissus terrificus* variety *crotaminicus* is a basic protein containing only 42 amino acid residues. Its sequence has no apparent similarity with the sequences of any neurotoxins, membrane toxins, or phospholipases. Since many crotalid venoms contain basic proteins having approximately the same size as crotamine, some of these compounds might be structurally related to crotamine and form another fundamental structure group (Sect. D.I. and IV.).

B. Toxins with Postsynaptic Neurotoxin-Membrane Toxin Structure

I. Curaremimetic Toxins

1. Introduction

As the name implies, these toxins mimic the action of curare, but there are also differences between them. The onset of the action is slower but the duration longer with the venom toxins, which appear to be specific for the nicotinic cholinergic receptor, whereas curare also binds to mucopolysaccharides and other proteins, such as acethylcholinesterase (EHRENPREIS, 1960; HASSÓN, 1962). The isolation of the cholinergic receptor was greatly facilitated, if not made possible by the introduction of the venom toxins as specific markers in the assay for the receptor (CHANG and LEE, 1963; CHANGEUX et al., 1970; MILEDI et al., 1971). The venom toxins are bound much more strongly to the receptors than curare and they also are more potent. The intravenous LD_{50} for D-tubocurarine chloride (mol wt 682) is 200 μg/kg mouse and for the curaremimetic toxins (mol wts 7000–8000) is normally in the range of 50–150 μg/kg mouse. Compared on molar basis, the snake venom toxins are 15–40 times more potent. The intravenous and intraperitoneal lethal doses are practically the same for the venom toxins, but the subcutaneous dose can be slightly higher. It was for cobrotoxin 30% higher than the intraperitoneal dose (Sect. B.II.2) (LEE et al., 1968). The subcutaneous LD_{50} for curare is about six times higher than the intravenous dose.

The first investigation of a cobra *(Naja naja)* venom was made by BRUNTON and FAYRER (1873, 1874). The showed that the venom was both neurotoxic and cardiotoxic. Death of experimental animals was due to respiratory paralysis, and the symptoms of intoxication resembled those caused by curare. RAGOTZI (1890) demonstrated that the paralysis was peripheral, arising from an action on nerve endings similar to that of curare. The onset of paralysis was slower with the venom and was reversible only with extreme difficulty.

BRUNTON and FAYRER (1873) demonstrated that cobra venom was not inactivated by boiling. WOLFENDEN (1886) showed that the toxins are proteins which are slowly dialyzable, i.e., have a low molecular weight.

Many attempts have been made to isolate cobra toxins. The early workers relied mainly on fractional precipitation with various salts and organic solvents, but in the mid-1930s precipitation was combined with electrophoresis or adsorption to tungstic acid and batchwise elution with barium chloride. About 20–25 years later, paper and gel electrophoresis were used to fractionate cobra venoms. Starch gel electrophoresis revealed 14 components, but not even this comparatively good fractionation was sufficient to obtain a toxin preparation free of any direct activity against cardiac or skeletal muscle. The purification of toxins and other venom constituents was therefore, considered particularly difficult, an opinion still held at the beginning of the 1960s (MELDRUM, 1965). Snake venoms also contain many proteins which are similar in size, charge, and solubility, and it is difficult, often maybe even impossible, to purify toxins by means of any of the above methods. The work on neurotoxins up to the mid-1960s has been reviewed by many authors (SLOTTA, 1955; KAISER and MICHL, 1958; BOQUET, 1964, 1966; MELDRUM, 1965; DEVI, 1968; GHOSH and CHAUDHURI, 1968).

The early workers lacked to a great extent not only convenient isolation methods but also means to rapidly and accurately analyze the composition of proteins. The introduction of ion exchangers with a hydrophilic matrix, cellulose (SOBER and PETERSON, 1954; PETERSON and SOBER, 1956), and gel filtration (PORATH and FLODIN, 1959) led to the great breakthrough in protein chromatography. Amberlite IRC-50 (Bio-Rex 70) is older, but this resin does not have the same general importance as the cellulose ion exchangers, since it is mainly useful for chromatography of basic proteins. The development of the amino acid analysis method (MOORE et al., 1958; SPACKMAN et al., 1956, 1958) was to revolutionize protein chemistry. Within a few years these new methods became standard procedures in many laboratories and were soon applied to purification of snake toxins.

Then by the mid-1960s, independently in Taiwan (YANG, 1966), Japan (TAMIYA and ARAI, 1966), and Sweden (KARLSSON et al., 1966), neurotoxins were purified by using ion-exchange chromatography as the final purification step. The correct amino acid composition and the N- and C-terminal amino acids were also determined. The first amino acid sequences of neurotoxins were then elucidated a few years later (EAKER and PORATH, 1967; BOTES and STRYDOM, 1969; YANG et al., 1969). At the time of this writing, the sequences of more than 40 curaremimetic toxins have been determined by means of EDMAN degradation (EDMAN, 1950). At present, snake neurotoxins actually represent one of the largest families of sequenced proteins. The opinion about the isolation of venom constituents has also changed. The purification has to be regarded as easy when the appropriate methods are used. No homogenization, extraction, solubilization with detergents, or precipitation of the starting material is required. The components are soluble in aqueous buffers, and after centrifugation to remove small amounts of insoluble inactive material, the sample can be directly submitted to chromatographic fractionation. The toxins are also easy to assay and so robust that working in a cold room is usually not necessary.

2. Isolation of Curaremimetic Toxins

The purification can often be achieved directly by ion-exchange chromatography alone, but an initial gel filtration is usually desirable.

Various cation exchangers have been used. We have exclusively used Bio-Rex 70 or Amberlite IRC-50 (alternative commercial products), a copolymer of methacrylic acid with divinylbenzene and styrene. When properly used for chromatography of basic proteins, this resin has an unsurpassed resolving power, and I shall, therefore, describe some aspects of the chromatography of toxins which, although reported earlier in various connections, deserve to be collected and summarized here.

The particle size should be small, <400 mesh. The equilibration is more time-consuming than with other ion exchangers, since Bio-Rex 70 has the highest total capacity of all ion exchangers presently available. A very large number of carboxylic groups have to be titrated which should require the passage of tens of bed volumes of buffer through the column before equilibrium is attained. The situation is different with cellulose and Sephadex ion exchangers where only a few bed volumes of the new buffer are required for equilibration. We have adopted the practice of suspending the resin in five to ten volumes of ammonium acetate (0.20 M) and titrating to the desired pH (6.5 or 7.3) with ammonia or acetic acid (0.20 M). After settling and decanting, the same procedure is repeated (usually two or three times) until the changes is less than 0.05 pH-units after a new addition of acetate (KARLSSON et al., 1971; KARLSSON and EAKER, 1972a). This careful equilibration to an exactly defined starting condition is a requirement for reproducible experiments.

We have used unbuffered ammonium acetate as eluant, since the resin itself is a very strong buffer in the vicinity of pH 6.5, the approximate pK_a value. The pH of the effluent will be determined by the equilibrium condition of the resin and not by the pH of the eluant.

At pH below 6, the curaremimetic toxins adsorb practically irreversibly to Bio-Rex 70. Ammonium acetate is volatile, which facilitates the recovery by lyophilization. Ammonium acetate also improves the resolution. Isotoxins differing only by a single amino acid replacement, such as Ile→Ser (KARLSSON et al., 1971) or Pro→Ser (KARLSSON et al., 1972a), are separated in ammonium acetate but not in sodium phosphate buffers.

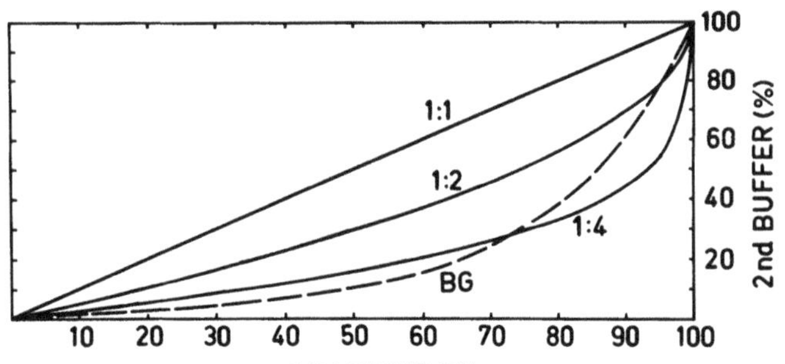

Fig. 1. Gradient profiles: BG, the Beckman gradient used in the isolation of neurotoxins compared to gradients obtainable by a simple device of two connected cylinders having the cross-sectional areas in ratio 1:1, 1:2, and 1:4, respectively

We have used gradient elution to isolate the toxins and the Beckman gradient pump Model 131 (Beckman Inc., Palo Alto, California, USA) with a special program cam (Part No. 324812) to form the gradient. Since this instrument is not a common one, the gradient profile is shown in Figure 1. The Beckman gradient can be satisfactorily approximated by a simple device consisting of two connected cylinders with cross-sectional areas in the ratio 1:4 and with the output from the larger vessel (BOCK and LING, 1954).

The purification of the main curaremimetic toxins of some Asian *Naja naja* subspecies has been described (KARLSSON et al., 1971; KARLSSON and EAKER, 1972a). A single chromatography on Bio-Rex 70 gives the toxins in pure or nearly pure ($\leqq 3\%$ contaminants) form.

The Indian cobra *Naja naja naja* has two almost identical toxins accounting for up to 30% of the venom protein. They differ only by an Ile→Ser replacement and are obtained cross-contaminated to a very low degree which is insignificant for most purposes (KARLSSON et al., 1971).

The main neurotoxin of *Naja naja siamensis* (*siamensis* toxin or toxin *siamensis* 3) accounts for 20–30% of the weight of the lyophilized venom. This is the highest content of an individual neurotoxin found in the venom of any terrestrial snake, and as described in the original communication (KARLSSON et al., 1971), it is obtained from the Bio-Rex 70 column contaminated to about 3% with another toxin, which can be removed by gel filtration on Sephadex G-50. A more convenient method of purifying this important toxin directly from the crude venom by simple chromatography on Bio-Rex 70 by a stepwise change of the eluant has also been described (KARLSSON and SUNDELIN, 1976). An alternative procedure using successively phosphocellulose, Sephadex G-50, and carboxymethyl cellulose has been described by COOPER and REICH (1972).

The isolation of toxins of only one particular type, e.g. curaremimetic toxins, can often be done by ion-exchange chromatography alone, as exemplified above. However, to purify several types of toxins from the same batch of venom, a combination of separation methods, such as gel filtration and ion-exchange chromatography, appears to be the rational approach. Gel filtration fractionates the venom mainly according to size into groups, such as curaremimetic toxins/membrane toxins, phospholipases, and larger enzymes. The appropriate fraction is then submitted to ion-exchange chromatography, where the separation depends to a great extent on differences in charge and the distribution of charged groups.

3. Characteristics of Curaremimetic Toxins

The curaremimetic toxins are low molecular weight basic proteins with isoelectric points in the vicinity of pH 9–10. The covalent structures of toxins sequenced to date are shown in Figure 4.

The toxins belong to two distinct size groups, usually called *short* and *long neurotoxins*. The name refers initially to the peptide chain length, but a more stringent classification considers the number of disulfides and sequential similarities. A numeric designation, such as 61-4 type toxin refers to the number of amino acid residues and disulfides, respectively.

Short neurotoxins contain 60–62 amino acids and four disulfides (mol wt ca. 7000), whereas the long ones usually have 71–74 residues and five disulfides (mol wt ca. 8000), but recently a "long" toxin with only 66 residues but five disulfides was isolated (MAEDA and TAMIYA, 1974; sequence 18, Fig. 4). Not only the number of disulfides but also particular sequences, such as the stretch Ala-Ala-Thr between the disulfides 2 and 3 in long neurotoxins, are typical.

A toxin from *Pelamis platurus* supposed to have 55 residues (TU et al., 1975) is not homogeneous, since the deviations from integral values for the molar ratios of several amino acids are too large. The toxin probably is a homologue to *pelamitoxin* A (sequence 36: schistosa 5, Fig. 4) from the same venom (WANG et al., 1976).

Three toxins from *Naja nigricollis mossambica* Peters were reported to have 63 residues each. The sequence for two of the toxins up to position 47 and the C-terminal sequence Cys-Asn-Asn were established (ROCHAT et al., 1974), but no extra amino acid residue was found as compared to a 62-residue toxin. The remaining part of the molecules comprises the loops 3 (Cys 49–Cys 61) and 4 (Cys 62–Cys 68) (homology numbering according to Fig. 4), which are invariably of the same length in all of the neurotoxins and membrane toxins sequenced to date (Fig. 4 and sequences 1–18 in Fig. 8). It is therefore unlikely that this region of the molecules should accomodate the extra residue. The toxins probably have one residue less of proline than reported. The proline values observed in the analyses can be too high, since during acid hydrolysis some cystine can be converted to cysteine, which co-elutes with proline (KARLSSON et al., 1972a).

The pairing of four disulfides is apparently the same in all neurotoxins and membrane toxins (Figs. 4 and 8). The fifth disulfide in the long neurotoxins pinches off a stretch of sequence which is partly deleted in the short toxins, thereby shortening the second disulfide loop to about the same length as in the short neurotoxins (Figs. 5 and 6). The common disulfide pairing and the common pharmacologic properties might lead one to expect that the three-dimensional structures of the neurotoxins should be similar, but there is in fact a considerable amount of evidence that the structures of the long and short toxins in solution and in the absence of the target might be quite different.

The two classes of toxins differ in the following respects:

a) *Immunology:* antiserum against any toxin apparently neutralizes all other toxins of the same (e.g., long or short) group, but none of the other group. The nonneurotoxins (cardiotoxins, cytotoxins, lytic factors, etc.) are also immunologically different from the neurotoxins (BOQUET et al., 1973). Each toxin probably has at least three antigenic sites (see Chap. 19 by BOQUET in this volume of the Handbook) and apparently none of them is common to all of the toxins.

b) *Circular dichroism* spectra are considerably different for the two groups of neurotoxins (TSETLIN et al., 1975). The spectra (Fig. 2) are atypical for proteins and the contents of α-helix, β-structure, and random coil are difficult to estimate.

c) *Stability:* although both types are heat resistant and only reversibly denaturated by urea or guanidine hydrochloride, they differ in sensitivity toward other treatments, such as lyophilization and a number of chemical modifications.

α) *Freeze-drying* of a monomeric form of a long neurotoxin leaves traces of trimers, maximally 5% dimers, and the rest remains in monomeric form, whereas lyophilization of short toxins can produce considerable amounts of dimers, trimers, and higher aggregates.

β) *Chemical modifications* tend to have a more serious effect on the activity of a short toxin than on that of a long one. The converse has not yet been observed.

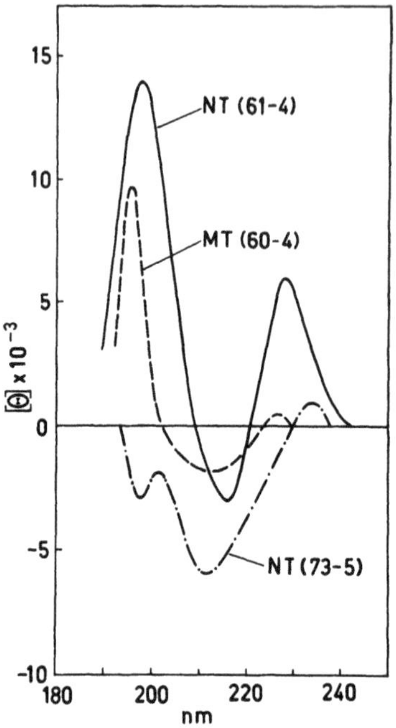

Fig. 2. Circular dichroism spectra of *Naja naja oxiana* toxins (redrawn after TSETLIN et al., 1975). NT (73-5): the 73-5 type neurotoxin oxiana I (sequence 4, Fig. 4), NT (61-4): the 61-4 type neurotoxin oxiana II (No. 31), and MT (60-4): the membrane toxin cytotoxin I (No. 16, Fig. 8)

d) *Binding to the receptor*: the dissociation constants for the receptor-toxin complex are about the same for all toxins ($5.7–8.2 \times 10^{-10}$ M at pH 7.4 and 20°). The kinetics of the complex formation and dissociation are, however, very different. Short toxins associate with the receptor about six to seven times faster and dissociate five to nine times faster than the long neurotoxins (CHICHEPORTICHE et al., 1975).

This great difference in the dissociation rates probably explains the observation that a neuromuscular block caused by a short neurotoxin can be reversed by washing with neostigmine (TAZIEFF-DEPIERRE and PIERRE, 1966; SU et al., 1967; LEE et al., 1972a), whereas the block by a long neurotoxin is irreversible in similar experiments (CHANG and LEE, 1963; LEE et al., 1972a).

Since the dissociation constants are about the same, that may imply that all toxins expose a similar surface to the same binding area on the receptor. To expose that surface the toxins have to undergo conformational changes, which according to the kinetic data requires more time in the case of the long neurotoxins. The structure of the bound toxins might be very different from that of the free ones. Amino acids situated in the interior of the free toxin might then even get into contact with the receptor.

There also are some striking differences among toxins of the same group. Short toxins of the type 62-4 crystallize relatively easily. Crystals have also been obtained of 60-4 type toxins, but despite great efforts in several laboratories, no one has yet succeeded in crystallizing a 61-4 toxin or any long neurotoxin.

Erabutoxin b (62-4) and toxin α (61-4) of *Naja nigricollis* have identical circular dichroism spectra in water and similar to the short toxin spectrum shown in

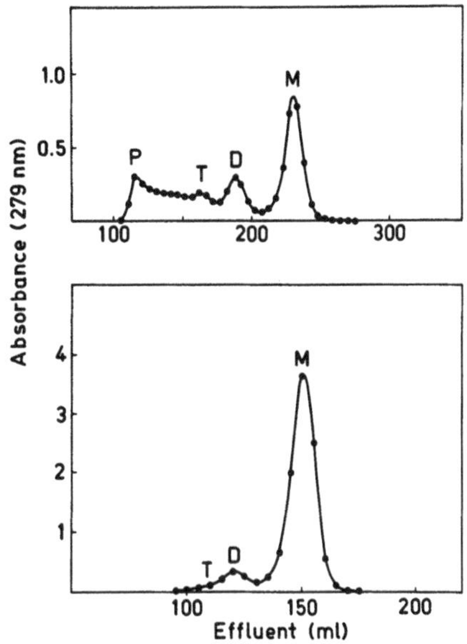

Fig. 3. Gel filtration on Sephadex G-50 of *badly* freeze-dried neurotoxins. Upper figure: *Enhydrina schistosa* toxin 5 (type 60-4). P, T, D, and M denote polymers, trimers, dimers, and monomers, respectively. The diagram shows an extreme case in which thawing occurred during lyophilization from 0.2 M ammonium acetate resulting in a pH drop. Similar aggregation will invariably occur if the freeze-drying is done from acidic media of low ionic strength, e.g., 0.1 M acetic acid. Lyophilization from neutral ammonium acetate (0.2 M or less) is generally harmless without any extensive aggregation if the sample remains frozen throughout. Lower figure: *Siamensis* toxin (type 71-5). A similar chromatogram with the same relative amounts of monomers, dimers, and trimers is obtained whether the lyophilization is done badly or not. Freeze-drying from acidic media will not increase the aggregation of the *siamensis* toxin, thus indicating the more robust character of the long neurotoxins

Figure 2. However, trifluoroethanol has very little effect on the spectrum of toxin α, but changes drastically that of erabutoxin b, inducing two negative peaks at 222 and 207 nm (MENEZ et al., 1976).

Most of the toxins have LD_{50} (i.v.) in the range of 50–150 µg/kg mouse. The difference is partly due to the lack of uniformity among toxicity assays done in different laboratories. In some cases even the use of different strains of mice might be responsible for the difference. But there are conspicuous differences which must in some way depend on the structure. Toxin I (type 73-5) of *Dendroaspis viridis* has an LD_{50} of 45 µg/kg mouse, and toxin V (type 72-5) from the same venom is only about half as toxic, 80 µg/kg (Sequences 4 and 5, Fig. 4). The two toxins have exactly the same sequences except that the longer toxin I has its extra amino acid glycine as the C-terminal residue (BECHIS et al., 1976). It is presently not possible to explain how the absence of this extra glycine can have such a large effect on the lethality.

There are also toxins which have much higher lethal doses ranging from about 500 and up to 60000 µg/kg mouse. In these cases mutations have occurred in apparently critical positions in the molecules and reduced the toxicity. These compounds will be discussed further in Sections B.I.5. and 6a.

4. Interaction with the Acetylcholine Receptor

The binding between the neurotoxins and their target is evidently very strong, since dissociation constants in the range of 10^{-10}–10^{-11} M have been obtained in experiments which appear to mimic physiologic conditions rather well; toxin binding in the absence of detergents to membrane fragments of electric organs of electric fishes with the receptors still incorporated in the membrane (WEBER and CHANGEUX, 1974; CHICHEPORTICHE et al., 1975). The strong binding should mainly be due to hydrophobic forces and hydrogen bonding. As shown by chemical modifications (Sect. B.I.6f.), the toxins are not covalently bound to the receptor by any disulfide interchange reactions. The binding to the solubilized receptor is not prevented by 1.5 M NaCl, indicating that the interaction is not primarily electrostatic (unpublished observation). As already mentioned (Sect. B.I.3.), the dissociation constants are about the same for both short and long neurotoxin complexes with the receptor, but the complex with a short toxin is both formed and dissociated much more rapidly.

It has been shown that the affinity of a long neurotoxin (siamensis toxin) for the receptor is temperature dependent and decreases rapidly below 11° C (LESTER, 1971). This might partly be due to decreased hydrophobic interaction, but also to the fact that the rate of association of the toxin with the receptor diminishes rapidly with decreasing temperature, whereas the rate of dissociation of the toxin-receptor complex is hardly affected (KLETT et al., 1973). The thermal energy requirement suggests that the binding involves a large conformational change in the toxin, the target, or both. At low temperature, the siamensis toxin cannot assume the conformation required for the binding. This temperature dependence has a practical consequence in the isolation of the receptor by affinity chromatography on matrix-bound siamensis toxin; the adsorption of the receptor has to be done at room temperature instead of in a cold room (KARLSSON et al., 1972b).

One mole of neurotoxin binds 90000 g of receptor protein (KLETT et al., 1973; KARLSSON, unpublished), but higher values have also been reported. Whether the toxin forms a 1:1 complex with the receptor is not known. The receptor itself has not been properly characterized with respect to molecular weight and quaternary structure.

5. Structural Information

If the half-cystines are aligned so that they correspond in position and deletions and/or insertions are arranged, it can be seen that there is close homology between the neurotoxins (Fig. 4) and the non-neurotoxins (Fig. 8).

Under the assumption that the active site, e.g. the surface exposed to the receptor in the receptor-toxin complex is similar in long and short neurotoxins, I will attempt to deduce structure-function relationships from comparative sequence data. If not stated otherwise, the numbering of amino acid residues throughout the Sections B.I.5–7 and B.II. will be the homology numbering used in Figures 4 and 8.

Trp 29, Arg 37, and Gly 38 are invariant in both groups of neurotoxins but not in non-neurotoxins. They are classified as *functionally invariant* and are assumed to be important for the neurotoxicity.

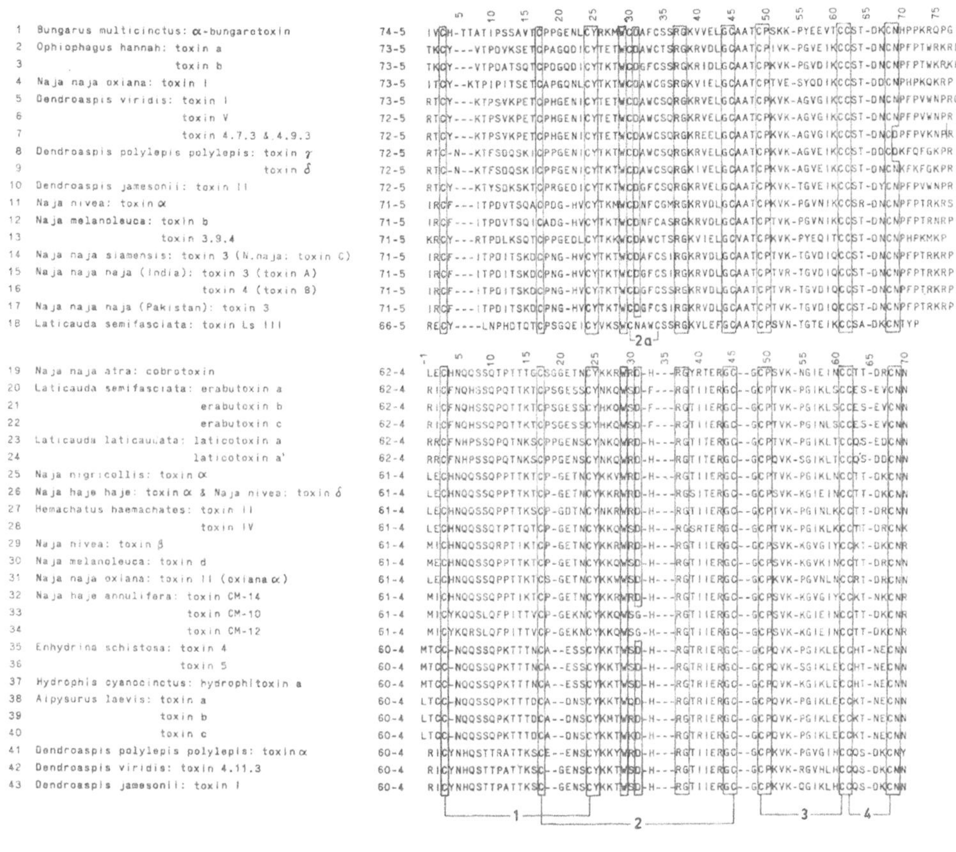

Fig. 4. Amino acid sequences of postsynaptic neurotoxins aligned for maximal homology with the sequences of non-neurotoxins shown in Fig. 8. Invariant amino acids are placed within frames. Aspartic acid at position 69 of the sequences 7 and 8 is probably due to deamidation during the sequence determination. One letter codes for the amino acids are used: A, Ala; B, Asx; C, Cys; D, Asp; E, Glu; F, Phe; G, Gly; H, His; I, Ile; K, Lys; L, Leu; M, Met; N, Asn; P, Pro; Q, Gln; R, Arg; S, Ser; T, Thr; V, Val; Y, Tyr; W, Trp; Z, Glx. The notations 74-5, 73-5, etc. in the column ahead of the sequences denote the number of amino acid residues and disulfides. The disulfides are: 1) Cys 3–Cys 24, 2) Cys 17–Cys 45, 3) Cys 49–Cys 61, and 4) Cys 62–Cys 68. The extra disulfide 2a of the long toxins connects Cys 30 to Cys 34. The sequences are compiled from: 1) Mebs et al. (1972). 2) and 3) Joubert (1973). 4) Grishin et al. (1974a). 5) and 6) Bechis et al. (1976). 7) Banks et al. (1974). 8) Strydom (1972). 9) Strydom (1973). 10) Strydom and Botes *unpublished* quoted by Strydom (1973). 11) Botes (1971). 12) Botes (1972). 13) Shipolini et al. (1974). 14)–17) Arnberg et al. (1977). 14) Hayashi *unpublished* quoted by Maeda and Tamiya (1974)*. 15) Nakai et al. (1971)*. 16) Ohta and Hayashi (1973)*. 18) Maeda and Tamiya (1974). 19) Yang et al. (1969, 1970). 20) and 21) Sato and Tamiya (1971). 22) Tamiya and Abe (1972). 23) and 24) Sato *unpublished* quoted by Maeda and Tamiya (1974). 22)–24) Maeda and Tamiya (1977). 25) Eaker and Porath (1967). 26) Botes and Strydom (1969); Botes et al. (1971). 27) and 28) Strydom and Botes (1971). 29) Botes (1971). 30) Botes (1972). 31) Grishin et al. (1973); Arnberg et al. (1974). 32)–34) Joubert (1975a). 35) and 36) Fryklund et al. (1972). Toxin 36, schistosa 5, is the same as pelamitoxin A of *Pelamis platurus* (Wang et al. (1976) and hydrophitoxin b of *Hydrophis cyanocinctus* (Liu and Blackwell (1974). 37) Liu and Blackwell (1974). 38)–40) Maeda and Tamiya (1976). 41) Strydom (1972). 42) Banks et al. (1974). 43) Strydom and Botes *unpublished* quoted by Strydom (1973)

* Toxins A, B, and C have Asp instead of Asn at positions 67 and 69 indicating a probable deamidation during sequence determination.

Position 31 is usually occupied by aspartic acid, except in the long toxin Ls III (Sequence 18) where it is replaced by asparagine and in the short toxins CM-10 and CM-12 (Sequences 33 and 34) by glycine. All of these three toxins have a low toxicity. Toxin Ls III has an LD_{50} (i.v.) of 1200 (MAEDA et al., 1974) and CM-10 and CM-12 of 5000 and 60000 μg/kg mouse, respectively (JOUBERT, 1975a). But it is not possible to ascribe the drop in activity only to the replacement of Asp 31, since other mutations have also occurred and the cumulative effect of all these changes accounts for the large decrease in lethality. Modification of the highly conserved Asp 31 can be done without inactivation (Sect. B.I.6c). Toxin Ls III will be discussed further in Sections B.I.6a, b, and c, the discussion here will be confined to the other two toxins lacking Asp 31.

Toxin CM-10 has a residual activity of 2% and CM-12 of only 0.2% when compared to the third *Naja haje annulifera* toxin CM-14 which has a normal LD_{50} of 120 μg/kg mouse. The residual toxicity of at least CM-10 appears to be significant and not due to contamination. Both toxins belong serologically to the short toxins indicating that the reduced toxicity is not due to great changes in the overall structure of the molecules. Except the replacement of aspartic acid to glycine at position 31, other changes have also occurred in the stretch between Cys 3 and Cys 17. The usual Asn 5 has been replaced by Lys and Ser/Thr 9 by Leu and both changes result in loss of hydrogen binding capability. The additional mutation to Phe at position 11 occurs in a place where *radical mutations* are observed, i.e. changes to residues with a very different character. Position 11 can be occupied by Thr, Pro, Arg, or Phe. CM-10 has a glutamine residue at position 7 and this is replaced by arginine in CM-12 with a devastating effect on the activity. This change occurs not only at the expense of hydrogen bonding, but it also introduces a second positive charge to this part of the molecule, where no other toxin has more than one.

Lys 27 and Lys/Arg 53 are highly conserved, but the positive charge can be neutralized without inactivation. The short neurotoxins are, however, comparatively more sensitive to modifications at these positions (Sect. B.I.6a).

A comparison of the sequences of neurotoxins and non-neurotoxins shows that ten positions are identical; Cys 3, 17, 24, 45, 49, 61, 62, 68, Gly 44, and Pro 50. Residue 69, which is Asn in all sequences except 7 and 8, will also be regarded as invariant. The amide group was probably lost at some stage of the sequence determination of the toxins 7 and 8. These amino acids will be called *structurally invariant*.

Residue 25 is invariantly Tyr in all neurotoxins, apparently for structural reasons, since residue 25 is either Tyr or *conservatively* replaced by another hydrophobic residue, Phe, in all of the membrane toxins and other non-neurotoxic proteins listed in Figure 8. However, whether a mutation can be regarded as conservative depends ultimately on the role of the particular residue, for instance serine at the active site of serine-histidine esterases and proteases cannot be replaced by threonine. If the phenolic hydroxyl of the tyrosine residue was involved in a hydrogen bond, substitution by phenylalanine would not be conservative from the functional point of view.

The structurally invariant or conserved amino acids are assumed to be essential for the general folding and the disulfide pairing. It is interesting to note that each disulfide has an invariant or conserved residue (Phe 25 in sequences 17, 18, and 23, Fig. 8) at one or the other end of the bridge. Considering other possibilities; one or more disulfides without any such amino acids, or with invariant (conserved) amino acids at both ends of the bridge, the probability for the observed distribution is rather low. Therefore, these amino acids probably have some important role, and that might be to regulate the disulfide pairing.

There are also positions which are invariant only in short (Ser 8, Glu 42, Arg 43, Gly 48, Val 52, Lys 53, and Gly 56) or long neurotoxins (Gly 20, Cys 30, 34, Lys 39, Ala 47, Thr 48, Ser 63, and Asp 66). Of these invariants Gly 20 and Arg 43 are also found in membrane toxins and are therefore regarded as structurally invariant. The remaining invariants are apparently not required for the neurotoxicity, since they are confined only to one or the other group of neurotoxins. These probably have predominantly a structural role and will be classified as *structurally invariant in short or long neurotoxins*.

The disulfides are invariant, but that is hardly surprising since a mutation should change the disulfide pairing and the overall structure of the molecule.

Glycine residues also are frequently invariant. Gly 38 is preserved in neurotoxins and Gly 44 in neurotoxins and non-neurotoxins. Additional glycine residues are invariant in one or two types of molecules. Long neurotoxins and membrane toxins have conserved Gly 20 and short toxins Gly 48 and 56. Replacement of glycine by any other amino acid will always introduce a side chain and that is often not allowed for sterical reasons. The short neurotoxins have an invariant glycine at position 48 between the disulfides 2 and 3; apparently there is no room there for a side chain. The long toxins and the membrane toxins have three residues in the corresponding place.

The neurotoxins have totally 22 or 23 invariant amino acids only three of them are considered to be preserved for functional reasons. Twenty amino acids should then be required to obtain the configuration in which the three functionally invariant amino acids are placed in their proper positions. The active site of an enzyme also consists of only few amino acids, and the role of the remaining part of the molecule should be to provide the proper environment and position for the catalytically active amino acid residues.

There are several so far inexplicable pecularities in the sequences. The short neurotoxins, for instance, have five to ten homodipeptides. They are especially frequent in the stretch from Cys 3 to Cys 17; Gln-Gln, Ser-Ser, and Thr-Thr are the most common pairs, even the tripeptide Thr-Thr-Thr is often present in that part of the sequence. The only long neurotoxin with many pairs is α-bungarotoxin, which has 10, other long toxins usually have two or three, only one (No. 8) has four.

The short neurotoxins always have two residues, usually Asn-Asn, at the C-terminus following the eighth half-cystine, whereas the membrane toxins (Nos. 1–18, Fig. 8) invariably terminate in a single asparagine residue. One can wonder why no short neurotoxin has only one residue after the last disulfide, or why no membrane toxin has two.

Loop 1 (Cys 3–Cys 24) is variable in length in all neurotoxins and contains, except Cys 17, only one additional structurally invariant amino acid, Ser 8 in the short toxins and Gly 20 in the long ones. The parts outside the disulfide bridges can also vary. Usually two residues precede the first disulfide, but six 60-4 type toxins (Nos. 35–40) have three, among them a cysteine which can be alkylated without loss of activity (FRYKLUND et al., 1972; KARLSSON et al., 1972a). In the long neurotoxins the tail after the last disulfide is variable by as much as six residues.

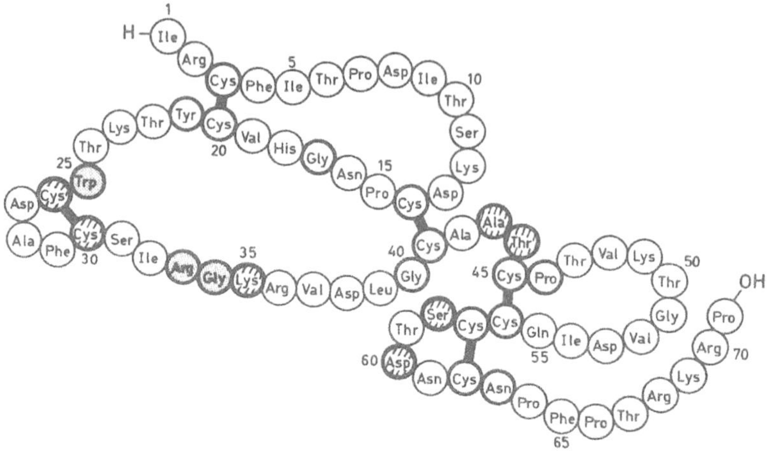

Fig. 5. The covalent structure of a long postsynaptic neurotoxin, the *siamensis* toxin of *Naja naja siamensis*. The toxin comprises 20–30% of the weight of the dried venom. Considering the price and availability of the venom and its toxin content, the *siamensis* toxin is one of the easiest available of all snake venom neurotoxins. Heavy circles, such as Cys 3, denote structurally invariant amino acids; hatched circles, such as Cys 30, amino acids invariant only in long neurotoxins; and stippled circles, such as Trp 25, functionally invariant amino acids. The stretch between Cys 20 and Cys 41 probably forms a protrusion similar to the corresponding region of erabutoxin b (Figs. 7a and b)

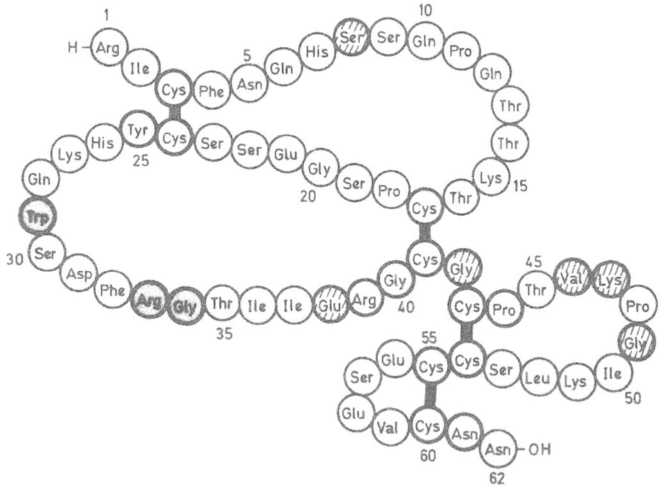

Fig. 6. The covalent structure of a short neurotoxin, *erabutoxin* b of *Laticauda semifasciata*, the first postsynaptic toxin for which the three-dimensional structure was determined. The symbols are the same as in Figure 5. The stretch between Cys 24 and Cys 41 forms a very pronounced protrusion (Figs. 7a and b) and is believed to have a vital role

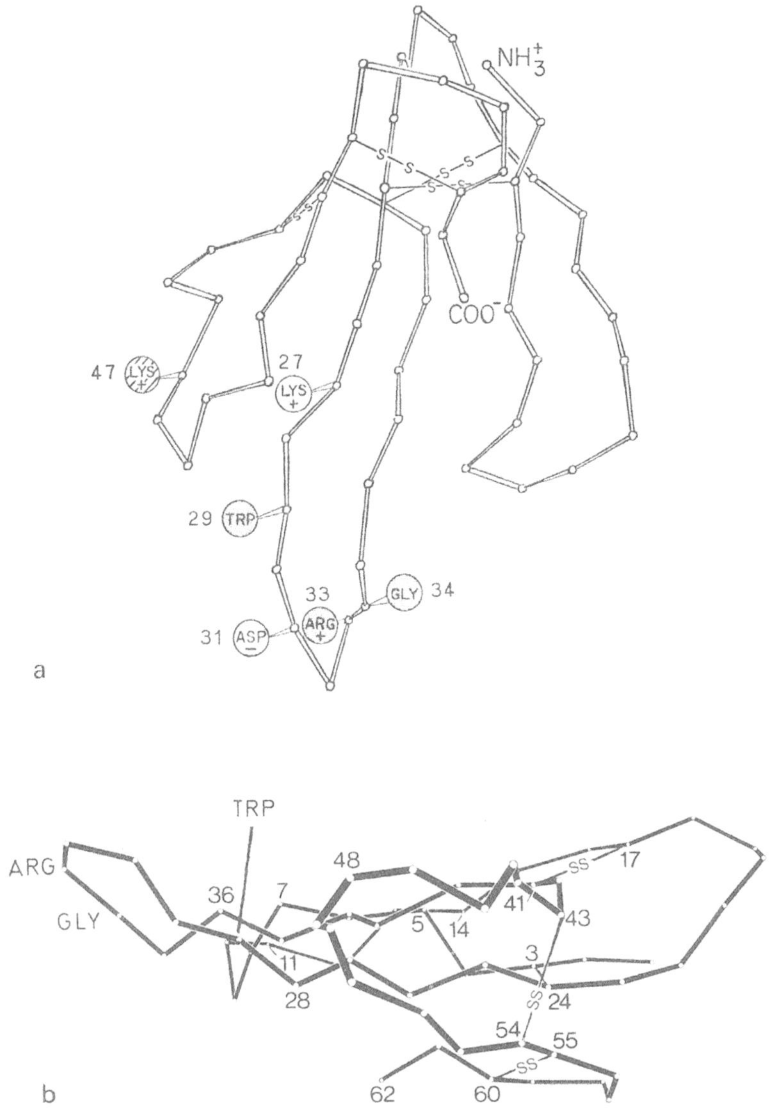

Fig. 7a and b. Three-dimensional structure of *erabutoxin* b. (a) "Front" view showing the extended loop with the functionally invariant Trp 29, Arg 33, and Gly 38. Lys 47 is invariant only in short neurotoxins (Arg 37, Gly 38, and Lys 53 according to the homology numbering in Fig. 4). Acetylation of Lys 27 or Lys 47 decreased the lethality by 83 and 92%, respectively (Sect. B.I.6 a). Trp 29 and Asp 31 have been modified in other homologous toxins without full detoxification. Ozonization of Trp 29 decreased the lethality by 92% (B.I.6 c), and modification of Asp 31 with glycine methyl ester after activation with water soluble carbodiimide had no effect on the activity (B.I.6 d). (After TSERNOGLOU and PETSKO, 1976; reproduced by permission of the authors.) (b) "Side" view showing the molecule as "an elongated saucer with a footed stand formed by the six-membered ring (loop 4) at the C-terminal end." (After LOW et al., 1976, reproduced by permission of the authors)

The loops 3 (Cys 49–Cys 61) and 4 (Cys 62–Cys 68) in neurotoxins and membrane toxins invariably have 12 and 6 residues, respectively. Loop 3 contains five or six hydrophobic residues and is one of the most hydrophobic regions in all molecules.

Loop 2 (Cys 24–Cys 45) always has 16 residues in the short and 20 in the long neurotoxins. It contains all of the functionally invariant amino acids and almost certainly the recognition site for the receptor. The guanidino group of the invariant Arg 37 (Arg 33 in Figs. 5 and 6) probably is a counterpart to the quaternary ammonium group of acetylcholine and binds to the same site on the receptor, but the final strong binding must involve multipoint contacts between the toxin and its target (Sect. B.I.7).

This speculation regarding a possible functional role for the stretch between Cys 24 and Cys 45 is supported by the recent elucidation in two laboratories of the three-dimensional structure of *erabutoxin* b[1] (type 62-4) (LOW et al., 1976; TSERNOGLOU and PETSKO, 1976).

The toxin is an extended molecule with a protrusion formed by loop 2, bearing all of the functionally invariant amino acids. The central core is assembled about the four disulfide bridges (Figs. 7a and b). It is suggested that the central protrusion fits into a cleft in the acetylcholine receptor.

A more thorough discussion of the three-dimensional structure is given by LOW in Chapter 6 of this Handbook.

Indirect information on the three-dimensional structure of long toxins mainly concerning the position of the C terminal tail is available. Spectral data on toxin I of *Naja naja oxiana* (sequence 4) show that the tryptophan fluorescence is very effectively quenched by anions (I^-) and much less so by cations (Cs^+). This indicates that a number of cationic groups are in the neighborhood of the tryptophan residues, and it is suggested that the C terminal heptapeptide containing three cationic residues (one arginine, two lysines) is folded into a close proximity of the invariant Trp 29 and/or the variant Trp 33 (BUKOLOVA-ORLOVA et al., 1976).

The corresponding stretch in the long neurotoxins with the functionally invariant amino acids also contains many polar residues and radical mutations, such as Pro-Ser-Asp-Arg 19, Val-Arg 40, etc., which preferably occur at the surface of the molecules. Studies of the siamensis toxin (sequence 14) show that Lys 27 has the most reactive amino group, Trp 29 reacts easily (Lys 23 and Trp 25 in Fig. 5), Tyr 21 exposed as indicated by its apparent pK_a of 10.5–11.0 (Sect. B.I.6a, d, and e). The occurrence of polar residues and radical mutations, the chemical data, and the general pharmacologic similarity between the two types of toxins strongly indicate that the stretch with the functionally invariant amino acids has an exposed position and that it forms a similar protrusion in the long neurotoxins as in the short ones. The extra disulfide should, however, alter the shape of the protrusion in the long toxins substantially as compared to that of the short toxins. But the size of the protrusion does not appear to be critical, since very drastic modification are allowed in this part of the toxin molecules (Sect. B.I.7).

[1] TSERNOGLOU and PETSKO (1976) probably also determined the structure of erabutoxin b, since they write in their article (p. 2) "our toxin is very similar, or perhaps identical to erabutoxin b."

6. Chemical Modifications

Chemical modifications are used in attempts to deduce structure-function relationships, but this approach has the limitation that only amino acids with reactive side chain groups can be investigated. There are presently no methods to modify amino acids such as proline, phenylalanine, valine, glycine, etc. Peptide synthesis offers a possibility to study the role of all amino acids, and although cobrotoxin has been synthesized in 20% yield by the Merrifield method, no synthetic homologues have been described (AOYAGI et al., 1972).

a) Amino Groups

Acetylcholine, D-tubocurarine, decamethonium, and other cholinergic agonists and antagonists are cations, and it is, therefore, logical to assume that cationic groups might be essential for the function of the curaremimetic toxins.

Amino groups have been modified by several means. The modifications have implied: 1. a change to a negative charge (reaction with pyridoxal phosphate followed by reduction of the Schiff's base with sodium borohydride), 2. a change to an uncharged group (acetylation, carbamylation, trinitrophenylation, dansylation), and 3. preservation of the positive charge (guanidination).

Reaction with pyridoxal phosphate followed by reduction with sodium borohydride preserved 50% of the toxicity of the siamensis toxin and the pharmacologic properties of the native toxin. Several derivatives were probably obtained. This method was used to prepare highly radioactive derivatives for the assay of the cholinergic receptor (COOPER and REICH, 1972).

All neurotoxins have a free N terminal amino group.

Lys 27 and Lys/Arg 53 are highly conserved. Lys 53 is even invariant in short toxins (Fig. 4).

Five toxins have Lys 27 replaced by either glutamic acid (Nos. 2 and 5–7) or methionine (No. 39), but all of them appear to have a normal lethality. Selective acetylation of Lys 27 or 53 has a comparatively large effect on a short but not on a long neurotoxin. This will be discussed further below.

There are two long toxins which do not preserve a positive charge at position 53. Toxin I of *Naja naja oxiana* (No. 4) has glutamic acid, thereby introducing a negative charge, and the 66-5 type toxin Ls III of *Laticauda semifasciata* has an asparagine. Both toxins have a much diminished lethality. Toxin I has an LD_{50} (i.v.) of 560 and Ls III of 1200 µg/kg mouse. In the case of toxin I, the reduced toxicity might mainly be due to this single mutation, since other positions in the molecule do not differ significantly from those of other long toxins. The decreased lethality of Ls III is certainly also due to other simultaneous mutations, such as the replacement Asp→Asn at position 31 (Sect. B.I.5). The toxin also lacks a part of the C terminal tail that in all other long toxins contains one to three cationic residues. Shortening of this tail will decrease the activity as discussed in Section B.I.6 b.

Extensive modifications of the amino groups in the siamensis toxin—LD_{100} (i.v.) 100 µg/kg mouse—have been done by carabamylation, acetylation, and guanidination (KARLSSON et al., 1972c; KARLSSON and EAKER, 1972b). In the subsequent discussion, the modified residues will be referred to by their numbers in the sequence in Figure 5.

The toxin has six amino groups. Mono-, di-, and up to hexacarbamyl derivatives have been investigated. All derivatives, except of course the fully substituted toxin, have several isomers. The only class of isomeric derivatives completely resolved into individual components was the monoacetyl toxins. All of the six isomers were isolated by a single chromatography on Bio-Rex 70, which is a good illustration of the excellent resolving power of this resin.

Complete carbamylation changes the net charge at neutral pH from about +4 to about −2 and the lethality to 3000 μg/kg mouse. This low residual activity of only 3% was not due to any contaminants, since amino acid analysis following the purification on carboxymethyl cellulose did not indicate any inhomogeneity. However, the hexacarbamyl toxin is still highly potent; its lethality expressed on a molar basis is 0.37 and that of D-tubocurarine chloride 0.29 μmol/kg mouse. It also is one of the very few anionic compounds with affinity for the acetylcholine receptor.

The lethality of the carbamylated toxins decreases with increasing derivatization. Sublethal doses of modified toxins produce respiratory distress lasting for much shorter time than that caused by the native toxin. The symptom recession time is only about 30 min for the fully (hexa-)carbamylated toxin and can be as long as 6 h for the monomeric native toxin. The modified toxins are obviously more reversible. They also kill more rapidly. The survival time for mice given a lethal dose of the fully carbamylated toxin is only about 30 min and can be 6 h for the native toxin. These toxins are excreted rather rapidly, and a more reversibly bound toxin will not kill an animal unless the dose is sufficiently high to cause death quickly (a case of decreased reversibility is described in Sect. B.I.6 h).

All of the six monoacetyl toxins have a lethal dose of 150 μg/kg mouse, two-thirds of the initial lethality, and their binding to the extra junctional receptors of chronically denervated muscles appear to be identic to that of the native toxin (LIBELIUS, 1974 and personal communication). Lys 23 has the most reactive and Lys 49 the least reactive amino group (unpublished observation), corresponding to residues 27 and 53 according to the homology table in Figure 4.

The closely homologous toxin naja 3 of *Naja naja naja* (sequence 15) has the same lethal dose as the siamensis toxin. It has only five amino groups with an arginine residue rather than lysine at position 49. The pentacarbamyl naja 3 has the same net charge as the pentacarbamyl siamensis toxin, but it is three times more lethal. The residual activities were 20 and 7%, respectively, but the pentacarbamyl siamensis toxin was actually a mixture containing in varying amounts probably all of the six possible isomers of which only one still had an unmodified lysine 49.

The results indicate that the removal of the positive charge from the highly conservative cationic residue 53 in the long toxins has a large effect only in combination with several other changes in the molecule. But a neutralization of only a single charge has the same effect irrespective of the position as shown by the identity of the monoacetyl toxins.

The five possible monoacetyl derivatives of the 62-4 type erabutoxin b—LD_{50} (i.v.) 120 μg/kg mouse—have been isolated. Chromatography on Bio-Rex 70 was used for the final purification. Acetylation of lysine 27 or lysine 47 had a great effect, reducing the toxicity by 83 and 92%, respectively, whereas selective acetylation of any of the other three amino groups did not affect the lethality. Lys 27 has the most reactive and Lys 47 the least reactive amino group, which are in homologous positions to the lysine residues with corresponding reactivities in the siamensis toxin (HORI and TAMIYA, 1976). The numbers 27 and 47 refer to the sequence in Figure 6, the corresponding homology numbers being 27 and 53.

The great difference in lethality between the various monoacetyl derivatives of erabutoxin b indicates that a short toxin often is more vulnerable to modifications of some apparently critical amino acids. The same vulnerability does not always exist in a long toxin as is evident from a comparison of the monoacetyl derivatives and from the modification of the invariant tryptophan (Sect. B.I.6 d).

Modification of amino groups in other short toxins have also been carried out. Trinitrophenylation of lysine 27 in the 62-4 type *cobrotoxin*—sequence 19, LD_{50} (i.p.) 55 μg/kg mouse—had no effect, but after modification also of lysine 53 the lethality was lost "almost completely" (CHANG et al., 1971 a). From a diagram in the original article showing the lethality as a function of the number of modified amino groups, it can be estimated that the residual activity approaches 2% when the four amino groups of cobrotoxin are trinitrophenylated. The modification of the two lysine residues 27 and 53 was also followed by loss of reactivity toward antiserum against the native toxin, indicating that the serious drop in lethality was a consequence of great conformational disturbances rather than being due to modification of lysine 53 per se. The corresponding amino group in the homologous erabutoxin b, can be selectively acetylated although with a considerable reduction of lethality. A simultaneous modification of the two apparently critical lysine residues 27 and 53 should have a very drastic effect on the activity of a short neurotoxin.

Dansylation of the corresponding lysine residues in the 61-4 type toxin α or I of *Naja haje haje*—sequence 26, LD_{50} (s.c.) 55 μg/kg mouse—reduced the activity by 92% (CHICHEPORTICHE et al., 1972). The higher residual lethality of toxin α as compared to that of cobrotoxin indicates that the 61-4 type toxins probably are less sensitive than the 62-4 toxins to modifications of the highly conserved cationic residues at positions 27 and 53.

Guanidination has a rather small effect on the toxicity, probably owing to the preservation of the positive charge. Guanidination of all of the five lysine residues in siamensis toxin reduced the lethality by 50% (KARLSSON et al., 1972c). Guanidination of the three lysine residues of cobrotoxin had no effect, and after trinitrophenylation of the remaining free N terminal amino group, the activity was still unaltered (CHANG et al., 1971 a).

The three erabutoxins a, b, and c have practically the same lethal doses and their sequences are very similar. The distribution of amino groups in toxin b is shown in Figure 6. Toxin a has the same distribution, but toxin c has one less; lysine 51 (homology number 58) is missing. Guanidination of the five amino groups, or only of the four ε-amino groups of toxins a and b reduced the lethality by 50%. One should expect that guanidination of toxin c, which has one amino group less, should at most have the same effect, but it had instead a greater effect and reduced the lethality by 85% (HORI and TAMIYA, 1976). It is presently not possible to explain this paradox.

All these experiments with different types of toxins clearly show that amino groups are not essential for the function of the curaremimetic toxins, but the preservation of the charge at positions 27 and 53 is of some importance, especially in toxins of the type 62-4.

I will remark here that there exists a less stringent use of the word *essential*, the definition of which is *absolutely necessary*, and a modification of an essential residue should abolish the activity altogether. If a modification leaves a very low residual activity, it is difficult to decide whether the modified residue(s) is (are) essential or not. In such a case, another design of the experiment should be tried including the use of milder reagents and efficient fractionation methods to remove inactive dimers (Sect. B.I.6d) and all traces of native toxin.

b) Arginine Residues

The neurotoxins have an invariant arginine residue at position 37. Apart from the N-terminal α-amino group Arg 37 is the only cationic group common to all curaremimetic toxins. It has been assumed that Arg 37 should be essential for the activity, being the counterpart to the cationic group of all other cholinergic ligands. Experimental evidence or counterevidence for this assumption does not yet exist. Cobrotoxin (sequence 19) with six arginine residues has been treated with phenylglyoxal (YANG et al., 1974). The reactivity of the different arginine residues was pH-dependent. At pH 6.0 Arg 28 reacted most rapidly and full toxicity of 55 μg/kg mouse was retained. At pH 6.7 Arg 28 and the invariant Arg 37 were modified and the activity dropped by 75%. At pH 7.5 Arg 28, Arg 30, and Arg 37 reacted and 3% of the lethality remained. Finally at pH 8.0 Arg 40 was also modified leaving 2% of the toxicity. Arg 43 and Arg 67 did not react.

The experiment clearly shows that the modification of the invariant Arg 37 has a great effect on the toxicity, but the results could be interpreted to mean that Arg 37 is non-essential, since 25% of the lethality remained after the modification. However, following objections can be raised against this interpretation:

1. Although the rate of the modification of the various arginine residues is pH-dependent it seems unlikely that at pH 6.7, reaction occurred exclusively at Arg 28 and 37. The other two reactive argines 30 and 43 probably also reacted to a minor extent. After one hour at 27° C using a 100-fold molar excess of phenylglyoxal to cobrotoxin amino acid analysis indicated that 1.9 residues of arginine had been modified, which could mean that a substantial fraction of the invariant Arg 37 was still unmodified. The remaining intact Arg 37 would also react at pH 7.5 and 8.0 and the low residual activities could then as a matter of fact depend on the reduction of the unmodified Arg 37.

2. The reaction with phenylglyoxal is slowly reversible at neutral pH (TAKAHASHI, 1968). The residual activity of the di-, tri-, and tetrasubstituted cobrotoxin might therefore, also depend on a reversal of the derivatization in vivo or prior to assay.

Enzymic digestion by a protease from the soil bacterium *Arthrobacter* (HOFSTEN et al., 1965) can successively remove a di-, tri-, and tetrapeptide from the C terminal end of the siamensis toxin. When the tetrapeptide Arg-Lys-Arg-Pro (residues 68–71, Fig. 5) was removed, the lethality changed from 100 to 200 μg/kg mouse. The removal of a di- or tripeptide has less effect and reduced the toxicity to 150 μg/kg.

Accidental removal of the C terminal tripeptide has also occurred. A sample of 200 mg of siamensis toxin lost the peptide Lys-Arg-Pro upon passage in 0.20 M ammonium acetate (pH 6.9) through a column of Sephadex G-50 that had been used repeatedly for several years. This was apparently due to microorganisms having evolved a highly specific enzyme to metabolize the minute amounts of toxin adsorbed to the gel in each experiment (unpublished observation).

It is not surprising that the two arginine residues contained in the C terminal tail are not essential, since the tail is present only in the long neurotoxins and can hardly be required for the neurotoxocity. The "defective" 66-5 toxin (sequence 18) also lacks the basic part of the tail.

c) *Carboxyl Groups*

Six out of seven carboxyl groups in cobrotoxin were amidated with glycine methyl ester after activation with water soluble carbodiimide and the lethality dropped by 25%. The modification included the highly conserved Asp 31 (Sect. B.I.5). The seventh carboxyl, the variant Glu 21 could not be modified until the molecule was unfolded with 6 M guanidine hydrochloride. This modification was accompanied by inactivation, probably as a consequence of conformational changes, since the reactivity towards antiserum was also lost (CHANG et al., 1971 a).

d) *Tryptophan*

The invariant tryptophan has attracted considerable attention and experimental effort. Ozonization in formic acid of the long neurotoxins siamensis toxin and the closely homologous toxin B, or naja 4 (sequences 14 and 16) has been done with retention of 50–80% of the initial activity of 100 μg/kg mouse (KARLSSON et al., 1973; OHTA and HAYASHI, 1974a). A large fraction of the toxicity was also retained after treatment with 2-hydroxy-5-nitrobenzyl bromide (Koshland's reagent) or 2-nitro-5-carboxyphenyl-sulphenyl chloride. After treatment of the siamensis toxin with Koshland's reagent three toxic derivatives were isolated by a combination of gel filtration and ion-exchange chromatography. Two of the derivatives had two substituents each and residual activities of 20 and 33%, whereas the third derivative with only one substituent was half as toxic as the native toxin (KARLSSON et al., 1973).

Toxin 7C of *Naja naja siamensis*—type 62-4, LD_{100} (i.v.) 150 μg/kg mouse (KARLSSON et al., 1971)—was also ozonized and the isolated N-formylkynurenine derivative was 8% as toxic as the native toxin (KARLSSON et al., 1973). The closely homologous cobrotoxin differing probably only by an Lys/Arg replacement was treated with several reagents (2-hydroxy-5-nitrobenzyl) bromide, 2-nitrophenyl-sulphenyl chloride, N-bromosuccinimide, or ozone), and the toxicity dropped by 94–98% (CHANG and YANG, 1973), thus supporting the observation from the study with toxin 7C that the modification of the invariant tryptophan affects the 62-4 type toxins more seriously than the long toxins. Similar observations have also been made with other 62-4 toxins; one example is erabutoxin b, which lost about 90% of the lethality after treatment with an 80-fold molar excess of Koshland's reagent (SETO et al., 1970). The residual activity of 8% obtained for the isolated N-formylkynurenine derivative of toxin 7C is significant, allowing the conclusion that the invariant tryptophan is not essential for the function. In the other cases, no particular derivatives of short toxins were isolated, but the use of a large excess of reagents ensured that no native toxin was left to account for the low residual toxicity.

Formylation of tryptophan in the 61-4 type toxin α or I of *Naja haje haje*—sequence 26, LD_{50} (s.c.) 55 μg/kg mouse—reduced the lethality by only 50% as tested on the unfractionated reaction mixture (CHICHEPORTICHE et al., 1972). This might indicate that formylation is less disruptive than other tryptophan modifications in short toxins or that 61-4 type toxins have a greater structural stability than the 62-4 type toxins mentioned above.

Aggregation of both short and long neurotoxins has often been observed following the modification of tryptophan, tyrosine, or arginine (KARLSSON et al., 1973; KARLSSON and SUNDELIN, 1976; KARLSSON, unpublished). The aggregation is promoted by high protein concentration and substitution of large aromatic groups into the molecule. Dimers and higher aggregates of the toxin derivatives are often inactive, and it is, therefore, advisable to test the activity of monomeric derivatives, easily obtainable by gel filtration.

e) Tyrosine

Position 25 is occupied by tyrosine in all neurotoxins and in most nonneurotoxins (Figs. 4 and 8). Only in a few nonneurotoxins has it been conservatively replaced by phenylalanine. This seems to imply that tyrosine has some connection with a feature common to neurotoxins and nonneurotoxins, such as the disulfide pairing (Sect. B.I.5).

Nitration of the invariant tyrosine in the two long neurotoxins toxin B (naja 4) and siamensis toxin (sequences 16 and 14) reduced the activity only by 20–30% (OHTA and HAYASHI, 1974b; KARLSSON and SUNDELIN, 1976). Nitration of tyrosine 25 in the 61-4 type toxin α of *Naja nigricollis*—sequence 25, LD_{100} (i.v.) 90 μg/kg mouse—also gave a high residual activity of 60% (KARLSSON and SUNDELIN, 1976). Nitration of the invariant tyrosine in toxins containing two residues of tyrosine, such as cobrotoxin (sequence 19) and the closely homologous toxin 7C of *Naja naja siamensis*, has not been done without simultaneous modification of the other tyrosine residue as well, which in both cases caused great conformational changes leading to complete inactivation (CHANG et al., 1971b; KARLSSON and SUNDELIN, 1976). Iodination of both tyrosines in cobrotoxin has been accomplished without affecting the lethality (HUANG et al., 1973). This probably indicates that iodination is a milder method than nitration.

The invariant tyrosine is evidently not essential for the function of any neurotoxin. The reactivity and titration data indicate environmental differences for this tyrosine in the two types of toxins. In long neurotoxins, it is accessible and reacts without unfolding the molecule. A tenfold molar excess of tetranitromethane was sufficient for complete reaction (OHTA and HAYASHI, 1974b). The apparent pK_a of the tyrosine is in the range of 10.5–11.0. In short neurotoxins, the invariant tyrosine does not react or reacts very slowly even at a 10000-fold molar excess of tetranitromethane in the absence of denaturating agents (RAYMOND and TU, 1972). The apparent pK_a is in the range of 11.6–12.0, which is another indication that the invariant tyrosine is much less exposed than in the long neurotoxins.

f) Disulfide Bridges

The extra disulfide in the long neurotoxins can be selectively reduced and alkylated with high retention of the activity. Two 71-5 type toxins have been modified in that way, viz. toxin α of *Naja nivea*—sequence 11, LD_{50} (i.v.) 70 μg/kg mouse—and toxin III of *Naja haje*—LD_{50} (s.c.) 65 μg/kg mouse. The alkylation of toxin α was done with iodoacetate introducing two negative charges and the lethality dropped by 91% (BOTES, 1974), but upon alkylation of toxin III with uncharged iodoacetamide, the toxicity was reduced only by 8% (CHICHEPORTICHE et al., 1975). Complete reduction and alkylation destroys the native structure of cobrotoxin and consequently also its activity. The reduction can, however, be reversed by gentle air oxidation to reform the proper disulfide pairing, thereby restoring the toxicity (YANG, 1966).

Treatment of the purified acetylcholine receptor with a 1600-fold molar excess of dithiothreitol for 1 h at room temperature followed by treatment with iodoacetate reduces the toxin-binding capacity only by 19%, whereas treatment with a high excess of iodoacetate alone has no effect. This indicates that the toxin is not bound by an interchange reaction involving a disulfide in the toxin and a sulfhydryl group in the receptor, or a sulfhydryl group obtained by reduction of a reactive disulfide in the receptor (KARLSSON et al., 1976). The disulfides obviously have only a structural role.

g) Histidine

Histidine is clearly not an essential amino acid, since there are toxins, such as toxin a of *Ophiophagus hannah* (No. 2), which have no histidine. Iodination of erabutoxin b (type 62-4) introduced two iodine atoms into His 26 without affecting the activity (SATO and TAMIYA, 1970). His/Phe 33 in the short toxins probably is a conservative mutation. If the pK_a of the imidazole is sufficiently low, His 33 has no charge and becomes like phenylalanine exclusively a hydrophobic, aromatic amino acid.

Iodination of histidine followed by catalytic reduction with pure tritium gas has been used to prepare highly radioactive derivatives of toxin α of *Naja nigricollis* (MENEZ et al., 1971).

h) Modifications Involving a Large Increase in Size

Two different types of dimers, which can be separated by chromatography on CM cellulose, are obtained by freeze-drying the siamensis toxin. They are equally lethal with LD_{100} (i.v.) doses about 500 μg/kg mouse, corresponding to a 40% activity as compared on a molar basis with the monomeric native toxin. The assay behavior is different. They penetrate much more slowly to the receptors, since the latent period before development of symptoms can be as long as 12 h for a lethal dose of a dimer and is less than 3 h for a monomer. But the dimers are bound much more irreversibly, since they can give rise to very long-lasting respiratory distress. Symptoms have been observed for 48 h, whereas a monomer produces respiratory distress for maximally 6 h (KARLSSON et al., 1971). Despite the increased irreversibility, the dimers have a diminished molar lethality (Sect. B.I.6a), but the penetration to the target is probably so slow that a large fraction of the dimers is being excreted before reaching the site of action.

Treatment of the siamensis toxin with N-carboxy-DL-alanine anhydride introduced about 70 alanine residues into the molecule distributed in three to four polypeptide chains with an average length of about 20 residues. This alaninated toxin retained the reactivity toward antiserum and apparently also the neurotoxicity, since it could inhibit the binding of ^{125}I-labeled toxin to the acetylcholine receptor (AHARONOV et al., 1974).

7. Discussion

In every case where a modification has inactivated a toxin, the inactivation has been due to serious conformational disturbances and not to the modification of the affected amino acid per se. By another design of the experiment, it has been possible to modify the corresponding amino acids in another neurotoxin with retention of considerable lethality. It has in fact not yet been possible to identify a functionally essential amino acid by any chemical modification, but the guanidino group of the invariant Arg 37 might be an essential cationic group, a counterpart to the quaternary ammonium group of acetylcholine.

Of the three amino acids classified as functionally invariant, Trp 29 is evidently not essential, since it can be modified without causing inactivation. Why is it then invariant? The evolution of toxins to their present efficiency has probably been attained by the preservation of some particular amino acids, which are not essential in the rigorous meaning of the word. They can be modified, and it should be possible to have toxins without one or more of these amino acids, but the neurotoxicity should be lower. I think that the invariant Trp 29 and Gly 38 as well as the highly conserved Asp 31 and Lys/Arg 53 are such *effectors* which are not essential but increase the activity and the specificity of the neurotoxins. However, another hypothesis refers to the preservation of an amino acid not only to functional and structural features of the molecule itself, but also to the DNA level, such as the conformation of the gene requires a constant base sequence, which then codes for the invariant amino acid (NORTH, 1972).

Of the many amino acids which have been modified, at least one of them should normally come into contact with the receptor. The strong binding is certainly the sum of interactions between many sites in the toxins and the receptor. It is, therefore, not surprising that at least one of the interacting amino acids can be modified without abolishing the activity, since the interaction between the remaining intact sites should be sufficient to hold the toxin-receptor complex together. Such a modification would result in a weaker binding and increased reversibility, manifested by a shorter symptom recession time and a higher lethal dose (Sect. B.I.6a).

However, it is surprising that the most drastic modifications have been done in the region which contains all of the functionally invariant amino acids. It forms a protrusion in the short, and most likely also in the long neurotoxins, and is believed to have a functionally vital role by fitting into a cleft in the acetylcholine receptor (Sect. B.I.5). The activity is retained even after substitution of two bulky 2-hydroxy-5-nitrobenzyl groups into the invariant tryptophan residue, which leads to about a threefold increase of its size. The charge of the highly conserved Lys 27 and Asp 31 can be neutralized. The central protrusion in the long neurotoxins with its extra disulfide should already in its native state be rather different from that in the short toxins. After reduction and alkylation of the extra disulfide, the difference should be even more pronounced. Large variations are evidently allowed in the region which probably is the functionally essential one.

II. Membrane Toxins

1. Introduction

In addition to the curaremimetic toxins, many other basic proteins of low molecular weight have been isolated from elapid venoms. Most of these compounds act on various membranes increasing their permeability, and owing to the use of different assay systems, various functional names have been invented, such as cardiotoxin, cytotoxin, and direct lytic factor (DLF). Trivial names such as cobramine indicate the origin and basic character of such compounds, while some other names (toxin γ, toxin 12B, toxin F_8, etc.) are based on elution order in some chromatographic system.

The isolation procedure is similar to that used for postsynaptic neurotoxins. In fact, the purification of membrane toxins is often achieved simultaneously with the purification of the curaremimetic toxins in the same gradient elution chromatogram.

CONDREA (1974) suggested the common name *membrane-active polypeptides* for these toxins, but in analogy with the neurotoxins, the name *membrane toxins* will be used here.

2. Mode of Action

The sequences 1–18 in Figure 8 are those of membrane toxins. The lethal dose depends on the type of administration and the relation LD (i.v.) < LD(i.p.) ≪ LD (s.c.) is probably true for each toxin, but a toxin can be more potent intraperitonially than another one intravenously. Lethality data for all of the toxins in Figure 8 are not available. The LD_{50} (i.v.) for the toxins 3, and 8–15 and probably also for most other membrane toxins are in the range of 750–2000 μg/kg mouse. The toxins 17 and 18 are, however, much less potent and have LD_{50} (i.v.) as high as 7500 μg/kg. For some of the toxins, two lethal doses have been determined: toxins 8 and 11 each have and LD_{50} (i.v.) of 750 μg/kg and an LD_{50} (i.p.) of 2000-2500 μg/kg (FRYKLUND and EAKER, 1975a, b); toxin 4 has an LD_{50} (i.p.) of 1500 μg/kg and an LD_{50} (s.c.) as high as 18000 μg/kg (LEE et al., 1968).

Death is due to the cardiotoxic effects, is of rapid onset, and can occur within 10 min following an intravenous injection of an LD_{100} (FRYKLUND and EAKER, 1975a). The lethality is greatly increased in the presence of phospholipase A, which also has a potentiating effect on other activities displayed by these toxins. One of the factors contributing to the increased lethality is massive hemolysis caused by the toxins in the presence of phospholipase A. Death by "shock" follows quickly hastened by K^+ relased from the lysed red cells stopping the heart. Phospholipase A alone does not have the same effects.

The function, if any, of the remaining proteins (Nos. 19–23) is unknown. Number 21 might act synergistically with other constituents of the venom (VILJOEN and BOTES, 1974). Number 19 is neither hemolytic nor cardiotoxic (CHEYMOL et al.,

1974). They are much less toxic than the membrane toxins. Numbers 20, 21, and 23 are not lethal at a dose level of 20000 μg/kg mouse, nor are 19 and 22 at 3000 μg/kg (not tested for higher doses).

An electrostatic interaction between the positively charged toxin and the negatively charged surface of the membrane is presumed to be involved in the initial binding. For the further process, two hypotheses have been proposed.

According to the first view, the hydrophobic parts of the toxin then penetrate into the hydrophobic layer of the membrane and disrupt its structure (KLIBANSKY et al., 1968). This resulting disorder and leakiness should then render the membrane phospholipids accessible to be attacked by phospholipase A. The hydrolysis products, lysophosphatides, are lytic and will further increase the damage.

According to the second hypothesis, the membrane is disrupted by an interchange reaction between disulfides in the toxin and sulfhydryl groups in the membrane (VOGT et al., 1970). Such a mechanism should probably require a particularly reactive disulfide in the toxin, but all the disulfides appear to have the same reactivity. Reduction of a membrane toxin, toxin γ (No. 11), with an equimolar amount of dithiotreitol reduces all disulfides to about the same extent (FRYKLUND and EAKER, 1975b). Another indirect evidence against the disulfide interchange mechanism is that the lytic action of melittin, a basic polypeptide from bee venom, which is devoid of disulfides, is also potentiated by phospholipase A (VOGT et al., 1970; MOLLAY and KREIL, 1974).

The toxin-induced permeability change has many biochemical, pharmacologic, and pathologic consequences:

hemolysis, species-dependent with red cells from different animals showing great differences in susceptibility;

cytotoxicity causing lysis of a number of cells, such as Yoshida sarcoma cells, human leukocytes, rat lymphocytes and rat bone marrow cells;

depolarization of excitable membranes with such effects as block of axonal conduction in peripheral nerves, contracture and paralysis of skeletal muscle, and ventricular fibrillation and systolic arrest of heart muscle;

transport effects, such as inhibition of accumulation of anions, amino acids, glucose, etc. of tissues (thyroid, kidney, small intestines, etc.) and cells;

effects on membranal enzymes, increase of the activities of glyceraldehyde-3-phosphate dehydrogenase, adenylate kinase, 3-phosphoglycerate kinase, and aldolase presumably owing to some disorganization of the membrane which exposes previously unavailable sites; *inactivation* of Mg^{2+}-dependent, Na^{+}-K^{+}-activated ATPase which requires an intact membrane in order to function properly.

More thorough presentations of the various effects of the membrane toxins are found in several review articles (JIMENEZ PORRAS, 1968, 1970; LEE, 1971, 1972; TU, 1973; CONDREA, 1974) and in Chapter 13 by CONDREA in the present Volume of this Handbook by CONDREA.

Toxin γ (Fig. 9) liberates calcium from muscle fibres (TAZIEFF-DEPIERRE et al., 1969). Since all membrane toxins qualitatively appear to have the same effect on different membranes, it is likely that they also liberate calcium from all membranes susceptible to their action. Consequently, calcium antagonizes the action of membrane toxins. For instance, injection of $CaCl_2$ into rats can completely suppress the cardiotoxicity of toxin γ (TAZIEFF-DEPIERRE et al., 1969). As shown for axonal membranes, the protective effect of calcium is due to inhibition of toxin binding (VINCENT et al., 1976). This might be a result of calcium-induced phase transitions of phospholipids into a state such that the toxins cannot bind to the membranes (LEUNG et al., 1976).

It is interesting to note that low molecular weight basic proteins apparently with the same mode of action as membrane toxins have been found in plants. Several toxins from mistletoes, parasitic plants of the family *Loranthaceae*, have been isolated and sequenced. The *mistletoe toxins* are very basic with isoelectric points about pH 11. They are very stable and heating of an aqueous solution at 100° C for 30 min has no influence on the toxicity. The LD_{50} (i.p.) is 500 μg/kg mouse. The toxins consist of 46 amino acids in a peptide chain cross-linked by three disulfides (SAMUELSSON, 1973). No sequence homology with membrane toxins or crotamine (Sect. D.I) is apparent. The toxins in low concentrations (1–10 μg/ml) produce depolarization and contracture in rabbit papillary and frog skeletal muscle, and the effects can be reversed by calcium (12 m*M*). It is suggested that the toxins by binding to the cell membrane displace calcium (ANDERSSON and JÓHANNSSON, 1973).

3. Structural Information

The membrane toxins (Nos. 1–18, Fig. 8) have about 25 residues of the hydrophobic amino acids (Pro, Ala, Val, Met, Ile, Leu, Tyr, Phe, and Trp), whereas the short neurotoxins have less than 20. They also have exceptionally many lysines, few carboxylic groups, and very few arginine residues. The net charge at neutral pH is high, between +6 and +10, compared to +3 to +4 for the short neurotoxins. Probably the membrane toxins have a tensid character with a basic hydrophilic and a hydrophobic part, but they are certainly more than mere cationic detergents.

The space between the disulfides 2 and 3 is occupied by a tripeptide as in the long neurotoxins and in contrast to the short toxins where the corresponding place is invariably occupied by a single glycine residue. The membrane toxins, like the long neurotoxins, also have few homodipeptides, except toxins 17 and 18 which have seven pairs each.

The typical "neurotoxic" invariances Trp 29, Arg 37, and Gly 38 are absent.

Structurally invariant are eight half-cystines, Gly 20 (also in long neurotoxins), Arg 43 (also in short neurotoxins), Gly 44, Pro 50, and Asn 69. Tyr/Phe 25 is regarded as structurally conserved. Further invariances are Pro 11, Lys 15, Thr 16, Pro 18, Asn 22, Leu 23, and Lys 51, some of which might play a role in determining the specific toxin structure while others might play a predominantly functional role.

The total number of invariant amino acids is 20 as compared to 22 or 23 in the neurotoxins, but the number of conservative mutations appears to be higher. Conservative replacements occur for instance at Leu/Ile-1, in the stretch 9–13, at Tyr/Phe-25, in the stretch 52–57, and at Lys/Arg-67. The point mutations are restricted to about the same extent as in the neurotoxins. Considering other features, the restrictions imposed on membrane toxins are even more severe. The evolution has not produced any "long" membrane toxins. The stretch between Cys 3 and Cys 17 has either ten or 11 residues and is the only one which can vary in length. The same stretch varies in the long neurotoxins with as much as three residues, and the following stretch between Cys 17 and Cys 24 is variable in both long and short toxins.

1	Hemachatus haemachates: toxin 11	61-4	LKCHN--KLVPFLSKTCPDGKNLCYKMSMQV-T---PMIPIKRGCTDTCPKSS-LLVKVVCCKT-DKCN
2	toxin 12A	61-4	LKCHN--KVVPFLSKTCPEGKNLCYKMTLKK-V---PKIPIKRGCTDACPKSS-LLVNVMCCKT-DKCN
3	toxin 12B (lytic factor)	61-4	LKCHN--KLVPFLSKTCPEGKNLCYKMTMLK-M---PKIPIKRGCTDACPKSS-LLVKVVCCNK-DKCN
4	Naja naja atra: cardiotoxin	60-4	LKC-N--KLVPLFYKTCPAGKNLCYKMFMVA-T---PKVPVKRGCIDVCPKSS-LVLKYVCCNT-DRCN
5	cardiotoxin analogue I	60-4	LKC-N--KLIPIASKTCPAGKNLCYKMFMMS-D---LTIPVKRGCIDVCPKSN-LLVKYVCCNT-DRCN
6	Naja naja (India): cytotoxin I	60-4	LKC-N--KLIPLAYKTCPAGKNLCYKMYMVS-N---KTVPVKRGCIDVCPKNS-LVLKYECCNT-DRCN
7	cytotoxin II	60-4	LKC-N--KLVPLFYKTCPAGKNLCYKMYMVA-T---PKVPVKRGCIDVCPKSS-LVLKYVCCNT-DRCN
8	Naja naja (Cambodia): cardiotoxin (toxin F_8)	60-4	LKC-N--KLIPIASKTCPAGKNLCYKMFMMS-D---LTIPVKRGCIDVCPKNS-LLVKYVCCNT-DRCN
9	Naja melanoleuca: cytotoxin V^{II}_1	60-4	LEC-N--KLVPIAHKTCPAGKNLCYQMYMVS-K---STIPVKRGCIDVCPKSS-LLVKYVCCNT-DRCN
10	cytotoxin $V^{II}_{1}{}'$	60-4	IEC-N--KLVPIAHKTCPAGKNLCYQMYMVS-K---STIPVKRGCIDVCPKSS-LLVKYVCCNT-DRCN
11	Naja mossambica pallida: toxin γ	60-4	LKC-N--QLIPPFWKTCPKGKNLCYKMTMRA-A---PMVPVKRGCIDVCPKSS-LLIKYMCCNT-DKCN
12	Naja mossambica mossambica: cytotoxin V^{II}_1	60-4	LKC-N--QLIPPFWKTCPKGKNLCYKMTMRA-A---PMVPVKRGCIDVCPKSS-LLIKYMCCNT-NKCN
13	cytotoxin V^{II}_2	60-4	LKC-N--QLIPPFWKTCPKGKNLCYKMTMRG-A---SKVPVKRGCIDVCPKSS-LLIKYMCCNT-DKCN
14	cytotoxin V^{II}_3	60-4	LKC-N--RLIPPFWKTCPEGKNLCYKMTMRL-A---PKVPVKRGCIDVCPKSS-LLIKYMCCNT-NKCN
15	cytotoxin V^{II}_4	60-4	LKC-N--KLIPIAYKTCPEGKNLCYKMMLAS-K---KMVPVKRGCINVCPKNS-ALVKYVCCST-DRCN
16	Naja naja oxiana: cytotoxin I	60-4	LKC-K--KLVPLFSKTCPAGKNLCYKMFMVA-A---PHVPVKRGCIDVCPKSS-LLVKYVCCNT-DKCN
17	Naja melanoleuca: cytotoxin homologue V^{II}_2	61-4	IKCHN--TLLPFIYKTCPEGQNLCFKGTLKF-P---KKTTYNRGCAATCPKSS-LLVKYVCCNT-NKCN
18	cytotoxin homologue V^{II}_3	61-4	IKCHN--TLLPFIYKTCPEGQNLCFKGTLKF-P---KKTTYKRGCAATCPKSS-LLVKYVCCNT-NKCN
19	Hemachatus haemachates: toxin 9B	63-4	LICHN--RPLPFLHKTCPEGENICYKMTLKKTP---MKLSVKRGCTEACPSAR-PLVQVECCKT-DKCNW
20	Dendroaspis angusticeps: toxin Ta1 (F_{VII})	61-4	TMCYSHTTTSRAILTNC--GENSCYRKSRRH-P---PKMVLGRGC--GCPPGD-DNLEVKCCTSPDKCNY
21	Dendroaspis viridis: toxin Ta2	60-4	MICYSHKTPQPSATITC--EEKTCYKKSVRK-L---PAVVAGRGC--GCPSKE-MLVAIHCCRS-DKCNE
22	toxin 4.9.6	60-4	MICYSHKTPQNSATITC--EEKTCYK-FVTK-L---PGVILARGC--GCPKKEIFRKSIHCCRS-DKCNE
23	Naja melanoleuca: protein S_4C_{11}	66-5	LTCLICPEKYCNKVHTCRNGENICFKRFY-E--GNLLGKRYPRGCAATCPEAK-PREIVECCST-DKCNH

Fig. 8. Amino acid sequences of nonneurotoxins aligned for maximal homology with the sequences of the curaremimetic neurotoxins in Figure 4. Numbers 1–18 are membrane toxins. Numbers 19–23 are proteins with a very low lethality. The i.v. lethal doses are probably higher than 20000 μg/kg mouse. Protein S_4C_{11} produces in mice hypersensitivity to sound and touch, but any other observations on the mode of action of the four compounds are not available. The sequences are compiled from: 1) and 2) JOUBERT (personal communication). 3) FRYKLUND and EAKER (1973). 4) NARITA and LEE (1970). 5) HAYASHI et al. (1975). 6) HAYASHI et al. (1971). 7) TAKECHI et al. (1972). 8) FRYKLUND and EAKER (1975a). 9) and 10) CARLSSON and JOUBERT (1974). 11) FRYKLUND and EAKER (1975b). (The snake having this toxin was formerly called *Naja nigricollis* but has been reclassified as *Naja mossambica pallida* (BROADLEY, 1968). The curaremimetic *toxin α* is found in both *nigricollis* and *pallida* subspecies.) 12)–14) LOUW (1974b). 15) LOUW (1974c). 16) GRISHIN et al. (1974b). 17) and 18) CARLSSON (1974). 19) JOUBERT (personal communication). 20) VILJOEN and BOTES (1973). 21) VILJOEN and BOTES (1974). 22) SHIPOLINI and BANKS (1974). 23) CARLSSON (1975)

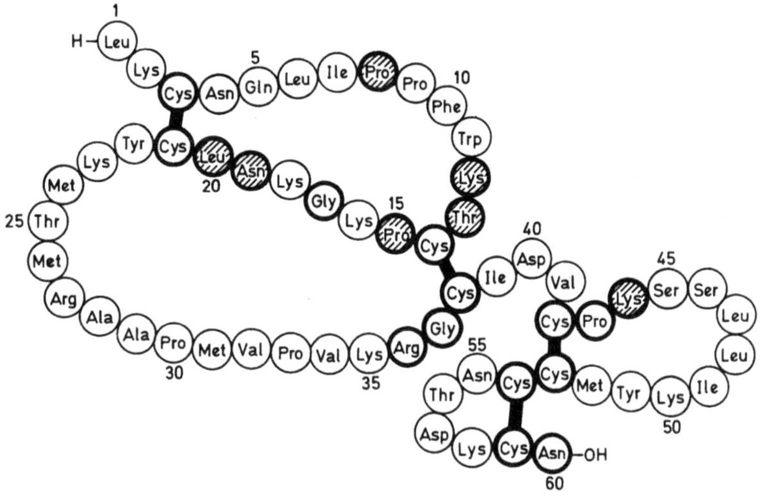

Fig. 9. The covalent structure of a membrane toxin, *toxin* γ of *Naja mossambica pallida*. The heavy circles symbolize structurally invariant amino acids common to both membrane toxins and neurotoxins. The hatched circles denote amino acids invariant in membrane toxins; some of these invariances should have a predominantly functional and others a structural role

The target of the membrane toxins enforces apparently structural requirements of at least the same severity as does the nicotinic receptor in the case of the neurotoxins. The target should then also be a very specific one. The great number of various cell membranes affected is not an indication of any lack of specificity on molecular level, but rather indicates that the target is a constituent of many different membranes.

The distribution of the typical invariant amino acids in membrane toxins is markedly different from that in neurotoxins as is evident from a direct comparison of Figure 9 with Figures 5 and 6. The stretch between Cys 3 and Cys 17 (numbering according to Fig. 8) contains three invariant amino acids, and the only neurotoxic invariant in that region is Ser 8 in the short toxins. A very hydrophobic pentapeptide sequence 9–13, containing the invariant Pro 10, is part of that stretch. The stretch between Cys 17 and Cys 24 has six residues, not less than four of them are invariant. Gly 20 is preserved also in the long neurotoxins. The stretch between Cys 24 and Cys 45, where all of the functionally invariant amino acids are located in the neurotoxins, contains in the membrane toxins only two structurally invariant amino acids Arg 43 and Gly 44. The majority of the amino acids are polar and radical mutations are frequent and the length of the stretch is the same as in the short neurotoxins. Both loop 3 (Cys 49–Cys 61) and loop 4 (Cys 62–Cys 68) are similar to the corresponding regions in the neurotoxins. The total number of amino acids is the same and loop 3 is as hydrophobic as in the neurotoxins. Both loops might therefore have a similar structural role in membrane toxins as in neurotoxins.

If the proposed mode of action—an initial electrostatic binding followed by penetration of a hydrophobic wedge into the membrane—is correct, then the necessary cationic group(s) in toxin γ (Fig. 9) should be provided by the invariant Lys 12 and/or Lys 44 and the wedge by the hydrophobic pentapeptide around Pro 8 (Lys 15, Lys 51, and Pro 11 according to the homology numbering).

4. Chemical Modifications

To date very few experiments with membrane toxins have been done, only a cardiotoxin from the Chinese cobra *Naja naja* Linn. has been modified. This toxin is a close homologue to the cardiotoxin of *Naja naja atra* (No.4, Fig.8) (KEUNG et al., 1975a).

Reduction of the disulfide bonds and alkylation with acrylonitrile abolished both the immunologic and biologic activity. This is not surprising since such a drastic treatment completely destroys the native conformation.

Treatment with a fourfold molar excess of tetranitromethane in the absence of denaturating agents led to nitration of two tyrosine residues. The third tyrosine, apparently a less exposed one, reacted in 5 M guanidine hydrochloride. Both the di- and trinitrated toxins retained the ability to precipitate the anticardiotoxin serum. The cytotoxic activity, lysis of Ehrlich ascites tumor cells, was slightly affected. The trinitrated toxin produced 25%, the dinitrated toxin 37%, and the native toxin 50% cytolysis at 10 μg/ml for 80 min (KEUNG et al., 1975b). One of the tyrosine residues certainly is the structurally invariant one in position 25 and the other two tyrosines are variant. A modification without serious conformational disturbances, as indicated by the retention of the immunologic activity, should not abolish the activity. This cardiotoxin is also more resistant than the 62-4 type neurotoxins, which do not withstand nitration of two residues of tyrosine.

C. Toxins with Phospholipase Structure

Several of the most potent venom toxins are either basic phospholipases A or contain a subunit which is a basic phospholipase A. To this group belong presynaptic toxins, myonecrotic toxins, and toxic phospholipases.

The presynaptic toxins inhibit the release of acetylcholine and intoxicated animals die from respiratory paralysis. Myonecrotic toxins damage muscle fibers and can give rise to myoglobinuria. Basic phospholipases can cause bleeding from the nose and bloody sputum in test animals.

Many of the toxins display both neurotoxicity and myotoxicity and the classification of such molecules as neurotoxins or myonecrotic toxins indicates only their most conspicuous characteristic.

I. Notexin and its Homologues

The Australian tiger snake *Notechis scutatus scutatus* has both curaremimetic and presynaptic toxins. Three homologous proteins have been isolated from the tiger snake venom. Two of them, *notexin* (*not*echis tox*in*) and *notechis* II-5, have a presynaptic effect whereas the third one, *notechis* II-1, shows neither toxicity nor enzymic activity.

Both notexin and notechis II-5 can be purified directly from the crude venom by a single run on Bio-Rex 70 at pH 6.50 using the Beckman gradient of 0.09 M ammonium acetate vs. 1.40 M. However, an initial fractionation of the venom by gel filtration on Sephadex G-75 facilitates the purification of notechis II-5 and the postsynaptic toxins. Notexin and notechis II-5 elute from the ion exchanger at ammonium ion concentrations of 0.5 M and 0.8 M, respectively. Before lyophilization, the samples are dialyzed against 0.01 M ammonium acetate, since freeze-drying from an ammonium acetate concentration above 0.2 M can lead to formation of insoluble aggregates. Freeze-drying from the 0.01 M ammonium acetate yields readily soluble monomeric products.

The LD_{50} (i.v.) of notexin and notechis II-5 are 17 and 45 μg/kg mouse, respectively. Both toxins are single-chain proteins containing 119 amino acid residues and seven disulfides. The molecular weights are about 13500 (KARLSSON et al., 1972d; HALPERT and EAKER, 1975, 1976).

Both toxins display a weak phospholipase A activity when assayed against egg yolk (KARLSSON, 1973). However, the enzymatic activity is greatly enhanced in the presence of the emulsifying agent, sodium deoxycholate (HALPERT et al., 1976), a phenomenon observed also with β-bungarotoxin (STRONG et al., 1976) and with other phospholipases A such as the porcine pancreatic enzyme (HAAS et al., 1968) and *Crotalus adamanteus* phospholipase A_2 (UTHE and MAGEE, 1971).

Upon treatment with p-bromophenacyl bromide (VOLWERK et al., 1974) notexin loses practically all (99.8%) of its lethality, phospholipase A activity, and myotoxicity. The modified notexin was chromatographed on Bio-Rex 70 under conditions where it was well separated from the native toxin. Neither the residual toxicity (LD_{100} (i.v.) = 10 mg/kg mouse) nor the residual enzymatic activity were due to contamination with unmodified toxin, since they were not diminished by rechromatography. The reagent modifies histidine-48. At neutral pH both native and modified notexins bind calcium at a 1:1 molar ratio. The dissocation constant for the native toxin-calcium complex is 1.4×10^{-4} M and that of the modified toxin-calcium complex 2.5×10^{-2} M (HALPERT et al., 1976).

Notechis II-5 also binds calcium and is inactivated by p-bromophenacyl bromide. There seems to be only quantitative differences between notechis II-5 and notexin. Notechis II-5 is less toxic but has higher phospholipase A activity (Table 3).

Notechis II-1 also has 119 amino acid residues and seven disulfides. Although it is neither a toxin nor a phospholipase, it does bind calcium and has a histidine-48 residue which reacts with p-bromophenacyl bromide.

Notexin and notechis II-5 show great homology with porcine pancreatic phospholipases A_2 and phospholipases from other elapids. When the sequences are aligned for maximal homology (Fig. 10), 43 out of 129 (33%) are identical. The sequence of notechis II-1 is not completely known, but its N terminal half is clearly homologous to those of the phospholipases A listed in Figure 11.

II. Taipoxin

The Australian taipan *Oxyuranus scutellatus scutellatus* has an extremely potent venom. The i.v. LD_{50} is only 12 μg/kg mouse, which is even lower than that of notexin. The toxin *taipoxin* (*taip*an *toxin*) which is mainly responsible for this extreme lethality accounts for about 16% of the dry weight of the venom and has an i.v. LD_{50} of only 2.1 μg/kg mouse. The content of curaremimetic toxins is low, less than 5%.

Taipoxin is obtained practically pure (>97%) simply by gel filtration of the crude venom on Sephadex G-75 in neutral 0.10 M ammonium acetate and can be

Homology alignment of pancreatic and snake venom phospholipases A

```
1             5               10             15                20                25                  30
Ala-Leu-Trp-  -   -Arg-Ser-Met-   -Lys-   -Ala-Ile-Pro-Gly-Ser-His-Pro-Leu-Met-Asp-Phe-Asn-Asn-  -   -   -   -   -   -
Ala-Val-Trp-  -   -Arg-Ser-Met-   -Gln-   -Thr-Ile-Pro-Asn-Ser-Lys-Pro-Tyr-Leu-Glu-Phe-Asn-Asp-  -   -   -   -   -   -
Asn-Leu-Tyr-  -   -Lys-Asn-Met-   -His-   -Thr-Val-Pro-----Asn-Arg-Pro-Trp-Trp-His-Phe-Ala-Asn-  -   -   -   -   -   -
Asn-Leu-Tyr-  -   -Lys-Asn-Met-   -Gln-   -Thr-Val-Pro-----Asn-Arg-Ser-Trp-Trp-His-Phe-Ala-Asn-  -   -   -   -   -   -
Asn-Leu-Tyr-GLN-PHE-Lys-Asn-Met-ILE-His-CYS-Thr-Val-Pro-----Asn-Arg-Ser-Trp-Trp-His-Phe-Ala-Asn-TYR-GLY-CYS-TYR-CYS-GLY-
Asn-Leu-Tyr-  -   -Lys-Asn-Met-   -Lys-   -Thr-Val-Pro-----Ser-Arg-Ser-Trp-Trp-His-Phe-Ala-Asn-  -   -   -   -   -   -
Asn-Leu-Tyr-  -   -Lys-Asn-Met-   -His-   -Thr-Val-Pro-----Ser-Arg-Pro-Trp-Trp-His-Phe-Ala-Asp-  -   -   -   -   -   -
Asn-Leu-Val-  -   -Ser-Tyr-Leu-   -Gln-   -Ala-Asn-His-Gly-Arg-Arg-Pro-Thr-Arg-His-Tyr-Met-Asp-  -   -   -   -   -   -
Asn-Leu-Val-  -   -Ser-Tyr-Leu-   -Gln-   -Ala-Asn-His-Gly-Lys-Arg-Pro-Thr-Trp-His-Tyr-Met-Asp-  -   -   -   -   -   -

31            35                  40                45                50                55                60
Leu-  -  -Ser-  -   -   -   -   -Glu-  -  -Arg-  -  -Glu-Thr-  -  -Asn-  -  -Arg-Asp-  -Lys-Asn-Leu-Asp-Ser-
Leu-  -  -Ser-  -   -   -   -   -Glu-  -  -Ala-  -  -Gln-Val-  -  -Asn-  -  -Thr-Gln-  -Lys-Glu-Leu-Ser-Ser-
Arg-  -  -Lys-  -   -   -   -   -Asp-  -  -Arg-  -  -Gln-Ile-  -  -Lys-  -  -Asp-Glu-  -Glu-Lys-Ile-Ser-Gly-
Arg-  -  -Ser-  -   -   -   -   -Asp-  -  -Arg-  -  -Gln-Ile-  -  -Asn-  -  -Gly-Glu-  -Glu-Lys-Ile-Ser-Gly-
Arg-GLY-GLY-Ser-GLY-THR-PRO-VAL-ASP-Asp-LEU-ASP-Arg-CYS-CYS-Gln-Ile-HIS-ASP-Asn-CYS-TYR-Gly-Glu-ALA-Glu-Lys-Ile-Ser-Gly-
Arg-  -  -Ser-  -   -   -   -   -Asp-  -  -Arg-  -  -Gln-Thr-  -  -Asn-  -  -Ser-Asp-  -Glu-Lys-Ile-Ser-Gly-
Arg-  -  -Lys-  -   -   -   -   -Asp-  -  -Arg-  -  -Gln-Val-  -  -Asn-  -  -Glu-Lys-  -Gly-Lys-Met-----Gly-
Trp-  -  -Ser-  -   -   -   -   -Glu-  -  -Arg-  -  -Lys-Ile-  -  -Asp-  -  -Ser-Asp-  -Glu-Lys-Lys-----Gly-
Ala-  -  -Ser-  -   -   -   -   -Glu-  -  -Arg-  -  -Lys-Ile-  -  -Asp-  -  -Asp-Glu-  -Gly-Lys-Lys-----Gly-

61               65                  70                 75                 80                  85               90
   -Lys-Phe-Leu-Val-Asp-Asn-   -Tyr-Thr-Glu-Ser-   -Ser-Tyr-----Ser-   -----Ser-Asn-Thr-Glu-Ile-Thr-   -Asn-Ser-Lys-Asn-
   -Arg-Phe-Leu-Val-Asp-Asn-   -Tyr-Thr-Glu-Ser-   -Lys-Phe-----Ser-   -----Ser-Gly-Thr-Glu-Val-Thr-   -Ser-Asp-Lys-Asn-
   ---------------------Trp-   -Tyr-Ile-Lys-Thr-   -Thr-Tyr-Glu-Ser-   -----Gln-Gly-Thr-Leu-Thr-----   -Lys-Asp-Gly-Gly-
   ---------------------Trp-   -Tyr-Ile-Lys-Thr-   -Thr-Tyr-Glu-Ser-   -----Gln-Gly-Thr-Leu-Thr-Ser-   -Gly-Ala-Asn-Asn-
CYS---------------------Trp-PRO-Tyr-Ile-Lys-Thr-TYR-Thr-Tyr-Asp-Ser-CYS-----Gln-Gly-Thr-Leu-Thr-Ser-CYS-Gly-Ala-Ala-Asn-
   ---------------------Arg-   -Tyr-Phe-Lys-Thr-   -Ser-Tyr-Asp-----   -Thr-Lys-Gly-Lys-Leu-Thr-----   -Lys-Glu-Gly-Asn-
   ---------------------Trp-   -Tyr-Leu-Thr-Leu-   -Lys-Tyr-Lys-----   -Ser-Gln-Gly-Lys-Leu-Thr-----   -Ser-Gly-Gly-Asn-
   ---------------------Ser-   -Lys-Met-Ser-Ala-   -Asp-Tyr-Tyr-----   -Gly-Glu-Asn-Gly-Pro-Tyr-----   -Arg-Asn-Ile-Lys-
   ---------------------Phe-   -Lys-Met-Ser-Ala-   -Asp-Tyr-Tyr-----   -Gly-Glu-Asn-Gly-Pro-Tyr-----   -Arg-Asn-Ile-Lys-

91               95                 100              105              110              115                120
Asn-Ala-   -Glu-Ala-Phe-Ile-   -Asn-   -   -Arg-Asn-   -   -Ile-   -   -Ser-Lys-   -Pro-   -Asn-Lys-Glu-His-Lys-----   -
Asn-Ala-   -Glu-Ala-Phe-Ile-   -Asn-   -   -Arg-Asn-   -   -Ile-   -   -Ser-Lys-   -Pro-   -Asn-Pro-Glu-Asn-Lys-----   -
Lys-----   -Ala-Ala-Ser-Val-   -Asp-   -   -Arg-Val-   -   -Asn-   -   -Ala-Arg-   -Thr-   -Asn-Asp-Lys-Asn-----Tyr-   -
Lys-----   -Ala-Ala-Ser-Val-   -Asp-   -   -Arg-Val-   -   -Asn-   -   -Ala-Arg-   -Thr-   -Asn-Asp-Lys-Asn-----Tyr-   -
Asn-----CYS-Ala-Ala-Ser-Val-CYS-Asp-CYS-ASP-Arg-Val-ALA-ALA-Asn-CYS-PHE-Ala-Arg-ALA-Pro-TYR-Ile-Asp-Lys-Asn-----Tyr-ASN-
Asn-Glu-   -Ala-Ala-Phe-Val-   -Lys-   -   -Arg-Leu-   -   -Ile-   -   -Ala-Gly-   -His-   -Asn-Asp-Asn-Asn-Asn-Tyr-----
Ser-Lys-   -Gly-Ala-Ala-Val-   -Asn-   -   -Leu-Val-   -   -Asn-   -   -Ala-Gly-   -Arg-   -Ile-Asp-Ala-Asn-----Tyr-   -
Lys-Lys-   -Leu-Arg-Phe-Val-   -Asp-   -   -Val-Glu-   -   -Phe-   -   -Ala-Lys-   -Pro-   -Asn-Asn-Ala-Asn-----Trp-   -
Lys-Lys-   -Leu-Arg-Phe-Val-   -Asp-   -   -Val-Glu-   -   -Phe-   -   -Ala-Lys-   -Pro-   -Asn-Asn-Ala-Asn-----Trp-   -

121            125               129
Leu-Asp-Thr-Lys-Lys-Tyr-----     ----       Porcine A2
Leu-Asp-Ser-Lys-Arg-Lys-Ala-     ----       Horse A2
Ile-Asp-Phe-Asn-Ala-Arg-----     -Gln       N. melanoleuca DE-I
Ile-Asp-Phe-Asn-Ala-Arg-----     -Gln       N. melanoleuca DE-II
Ile-Asp-Phe-Asn-Ala-Arg-----CYS-Gln         N. melanoleuca DE-III
Ile-Asp-Leu-----Ala-Arg-His-     -Gln       H. haemachatus DE-I
Ile-Asn-Phe-Lys-Lys-Arg-----     -Gln       N. nigricollis basic
Ile-Asp-Thr-Lys-Lys-Arg-----     -Gln       Notechis II-5
Ile-Asp-Thr-Lys-Lys-Arg-----     -Gln       Notexin
```

Fig. 10. The amino acid sequences of seven phospholipases A and two presynaptic toxins, notechis II-5 and notexin. The nine sequences are identical in not less than 43 (33%) out of 129 positions. The disulfide pairing as determined from the three-dimensional structure of the pork pancreatic enzyme is: 1) Cys 11–Cys 78, 2) Cys 27–Cys 128, 3) Cys 29–Cys 45, 4) Cys 44–Cys 100, 5) Cys 51–Cys 107, 6) Cys 61–Cys 93, 7) Cys 86–Cys 98 (DRENTH et al., 1976). The disulfide bridges of the curaremimetic neurotoxins always have an adjacent invariant amino acid (Sect. B.4). The phospholipases have invariant residues adjacent to the pairs 2, 3, 4, and 5 and conservative mutations at the pairs 1 (?) (Ala/Thr) and 7 (Ile/Val). The sequences are compiled from: Porcine A_2: HAAS et al. (1970), VERHEIJ, personal communication. Horse A_2: EVENBERG et al. (1977). *Naja melanoleuca* De-I and DE-II: JOUBERT (1975b). *Naja melanoleuca* DE-III: JOUBERT (1975c). *Hemachatus haemachatus* DE-I: JOUBERT (1975d). *Naja nigricollis* basic: OBIDAIRO et al. (1977). Notechis II-5: HALPERT and EAKER (1976b). Notexin: HALPERT and EAKER (1975)

Table 1. Taipoxin and its subunits

	Taipoxin	α	β	γ
Number of amino acid residues by amino acid analysis	372	119	120	135
Number of disulfides		7	7	8
Molecular weight by ultracentrifugation	46.800			
Carbohydrate residues				Fuc[a] 1 Man 2 NAGA 5 Gal 4 NANA 4
Formula weight	45.600	13.750	13.457[b] 13.473	18.354
Isoelectric point	~ 5	≧10	~ 7	<2.5
LD_{50} (i.v.) μg/kg mouse	2.1	300	>2000	>2000

[a] Fuc=fucose, Man=mannose, NAGA=N-acetyl-D-glucosamine, Gal=galactose, NANA=N-acetylneuraminic acid.
[b] consists of two very similar isoforms present in about equal amounts.

lyophilized directly from this medium. Some remaining impurities are removed by zone electrophoresis on a cellulose column at pH 7.5. Taipoxin cannot be isolated by ion-exchange chromatography, since ion exchangers tend to dissociate the active toxin complex.

Taipoxin is a noncovalent ternary complex of three different subunits which can be dissociated at neutral pH by 6 M guanidine hydrochloride, but not by 8 M urea. Dissociation also occurs at low pH and is virtually complete at pH 1.9. The three subunits have widely different isoelectric points (<2.5~7, ≧10, Table 1) and electrostatic forces seem to be important for holding the complex together. The dissociation at neutral pH is reversible: the complex re-forms and full toxicity is restored upon removal of the guanidine hydrochloride by dialysis. The dissociation at pH 1.9 seems to be irreversible, apparently owing to some effect of the low pH on the carbohydrate moiety of the γ-subunit.

Some data for taipoxin and its subunits are given in Table 1. The very basic α-subunit is the only one which has any appreciable toxicity alone, showing some resemblance to notexin. The γ-subunit is very acidic, owing at least in part to its four sialic acid residues. The β-subunit is poorly soluble at neutral pH and exists in at least two iso-forms which appear to be completely interchangeable in the complex.

The α-subunit exhibits low phospholipase A activity, but taipoxin shows essentially no enzymic activity even in the presence of deoxycholate (Table 3). Treatment of the taipoxin complex with p-bromophenacyl bromide can modify two histidine residues, one on the α- and the other on the β-subunit. The γ-subunit also has a histidine residue in a position corresponding to that in the other subunits, but it does not react, even when the free γ-subunit is treated with the reagent. Taipoxin is inactivated when the reactive histidine of the very basic α-subunit is modified. The modification of the β-subunit decreases the lethality to 10 μg/kg mouse, 20% residual activity (FOHLMAN, unpublished).

When the three subunits combine the enzymatic activity of the α-subunit is suppressed and the lethality compared on a molar basis is increased about 500-fold (FOHLMAN et al., 1976). No explanation can be given yet for this phenomenon. Similar effects have been observed with crotoxin (Sect. C.III).

The γ-subunit is clearly homologous to phospholipases but has an extra N-terminal octapeptide which is homologous to the activation peptide of the porcine prophospholipase A_2 (Fig. 11).

III. Crotoxin

Crotoxin, the main neurotoxin of the South American rattlesnake *Crotalus durissus terrificus*, was isolated in a crystalline form as early as 1938 by SLOTTA and FRAENKEL-CONRAT. The original isolation method is still used. The venom is dissolved in dilute (0.013–0.016 M) HCl, heated for 10 min at 70° C, and the coagulated protein is centrifuged off. Crotoxin is then precipitated at its isolectric point pH 4.7–4.8 (HENDON and FRAENKEL-CONRAT, 1976; BREITHAUPT, 1976a). The amorphous toxin can be crystallized from pyridine acetate at pH 4.4 upon slow cooling from 55° C (SLOTTA and FRAENKEL-CONRAT, 1938; SLOTTA, 1955).

Crystalline crotoxin was homogeneous in ultracentrifugation (GRALÉN and SVEDBERG, 1938) and in moving boundary electrophoresis (LI and FRAENKEL-CONRAT, 1942), but crotoxin obtained after isoelectric precipitation seems to be a non stoichiometric complex of several components, the proportions of which can also vary from one preparation to another (BREITHAUPT et al., 1975). This variation probably explains the varying lethal doses and some other divergent data shown in Table 2. The high toxicity is due to a complex between a basic phospholipase A, also called *crotoxin* B (basic), and an acidic protein, *crotoxin* A (acidic) or *crotapotin* (HENDON and FRAENKEL-CONRAT, 1971; RÜBSAMEN et al., 1971).

Crotoxin can be dissociated by ion exchangers. BREITHAUPT et al. (1975) adsorbed it to CM cellulose at pH 3.5 and separated the constituents by gradient chromatography. Two basic phospholipases accounted for 48% of the protein, two crotapotins accounted for 31% (the later eluting crotapotin peak might be a chromatographic artifact; see also RÜBSAMEN et al., 1971), and minor constituents (an acidic phospholipase A, crotamine, and other proteins) accounted for 8.4%. The recovery was 87.4%, which is normal in chromatography of proteins after adsorption to cellulose ion exchangers.

The basic phospholipase is moderately lethal (540 μg/kg mouse, Table 2) but upon recombination with crotapotin, practically full lethality can be restored (HENDON and FRAENKEL-CONRAT, 1971; RÜBSAMEN et al., 1971; BREITHAUPT et al., 1975). Both phospholipases isolated by BREITHAUPT et al. (1975) combine with crotapotin. The lethality of the basic phospholipase can also be potentiated by molecules other than crotoxin A or crotapotin. The nonlethal *volvatoxin* A2 (mol wt 25000, isoelectric point 4.5), a component of a mushroom cardiotoxin (LIN et al., 1973) forms a complex with the basic phospholipase and augments its toxicity significantly (JENG and FRAENKEL-CONRAT, 1976).

Crotapotin not only increases the toxicity of the basic phospholipase but also suppresses its enzyme activity by as much as 90% (BREITHAUPT, 1976a). A contrary result has, however, been obtained by FRAENKEL-CONRAT et al. (1976) who reported that crotoxin and crotoxin B have equal catalytic activities.

Table 2. Crotoxin and its subunits

	LD_{50} µg/kg mouse	Molecular weight	Isoelectric point
Crotoxin	i.p. 35[a] s.c. 370[d] i.p. 60[a] s.c. 500[c] i.v. 110[c]	30.000[e] 21.000[f] ~25.000[j]	4.7[k] 4.8–5.1[l]
Basic subunit phospholipase A (crotoxin B[a])	i.v. 540[c]	14.500[m] 15.800[n] 16.300[o] 13.000[b] 11.300[g]	9.5–9.8[l] 8.6[i]
Acidic subunit (crotoxin A[a] or crotapotin[c])	Nontoxic i.v. >50.000[c]	9.500[o] 8.400[b] 9.300[h]	3.4[l] 3.7[i]

[a] HENDON and FRAENKEL-CONRAT (1971), two preparations of toxin.
[b] HENDON and FRAENKEL-CONRAT (1971), amino acid composition.
[c] RÜBSAMEN et al. (1971).
[d] SLOTTA and FRAENKEL-CONRAT (1938).
[e] GRALÉN and SVEDBERG (1938) ultracentrifugation.
[f] HORST et al. (1972) elutes in gel filtration slightly after chymotrypsinogen A (mol. wt. 25.200).
[g] HORST et al. (1972) gel filtration in 6 M GuHCl of reduced and alkylated molecule.
[h] HORST et al. (1972) gel filtration in 6 M GuHCl of unreduced molecule.
[i] HORST et al. (1972) isoelectric focusing.
[j] RODRÍGUEZ and SCANNONE (1976) gel filtration.
[k] LI and FRAENKEL-CONRAT (1942) moving boundary electrophoresis.
[l] BREITHAUPT et al. (1974) isoelectric focusing.
[m] BREITHAUPT et al. (1974) gel filtration in 6 M GuHCl of reduced and alkylated molecule.
[n] BREITHAUPT et al. (1974) ultracentrifugation and dodecylsulfate-gel electrophoresis.
[o] BREITHAUPT et al. (1974) amino acid composition.

From the yields of the basic phospholipases (48%) and crotapotin(s) (31%) obtained by BREITHAUPT et al. (1975), and using the molecular weights determined in the same laboratory, the molar ratio phospholipase-crotapotin can be calculated. It varies between 0.90 and 1.02. The classic crotoxin thus appears to be a 1:1 complex of phospholipase-crotapotin. Since there are at least two homologues of the phospholipase, there should be at least two different neurotoxic complexes, coprecipitated with varying amounts of other proteins which do not contribute significantly to the toxicity.

Electrostatic interaction is probably decisive for holding crotoxin together. Like taipoxin it is dissociated by interaction with ion exchangers but can survive gel filtration (HENDON and FRAENKEL-CONRAT, 1976; RODRÍGUEZ and SCANNONE, 1976) and electrophoresis in a pH interval at least 4–7 (LI and FRAENKEL-CONRAT, 1942). The stability of the complex depends on the pH, i.e., the charge of the two constituents. At low or high pH values, when the two components have the same charge, the complex probably dissociates. A chromatographic isolation method based on a combination of gel filtration and electrophoresis analogous to that used for taipoxin might be an alternative to the procedure presently used, which historically belongs to the prechromatographic period of protein chemistry.

Crotoxin B has one histidine residue which reacts with p-bromophenacyl bromide. The modified enzyme is devoid of both lethality and catalytic activity. It can still combine with crotoxin A, but the complex is inactive. The crotoxin complex does not react with the reagent, nor does crotoxin A (FRAENKEL-CONRAT et al., 1976).

The two basic phospholipases isolated from the crotoxin complex by BREITHAUPT et al. (1975) have a phenylalanine residue at position 11, whereas the other phospholipases and toxin constituents have half-cystine (Fig. 11). The crotoxin components obviously have a different disulfide pairing, and they might, therefore, be homologous only to a limited extent with the other proteins.

Crotapotin consists of three peptide chains containing 40, 34, and 14 residues and joined by disulfide bonds (BREITHAUPT et al., 1974). This unusual structure might be the result of proteolytic fragmentation of a single-chain precursor molecule or an artifact due to hydrolysis of particularly susceptible peptide bonds, such as Asp-Pro bonds, during the heat coagulation of the venom at low pH.

IV. β-Bungarotoxin

The venom of *Bungarus multicinctus* was initially fractionated by zone electrophoresis in a starch block into three neurotoxic fractions called *α-*, *β-*, and *γ-bungarotoxin.* A postsynaptic type of neuromuscular blocking action was found in the α-fraction, whereas the action of the β- and γ-fractions appeared to be exclusively presynaptic (CHANG and LEE, 1963). Chromatography on CM-Sephadex G-50 resolved the venom into a great number of components and there seem to be at least six toxins with presynaptic activity (LEE et al., 1972; ETEROVIC et al., 1975). The somewhat different chromatographic patterns obtained in the two laboratories may reflect differences between the venom samples. The LD_{50} (i.p.) varied greatly for the different toxins. The lowest were in the range 10–20, the intermediate ones about 50, and the highest ones about 300 up to as high as 2000 μg/kg mouse.

Since the venom contains a great number of components, gel filtration should be suitable for an initial fractionation. It should at least separate presynaptic toxins from the postsynaptic ones and facilitate further purification by ion exchangers.

One toxin, LD_{50} (i.p.) 14 μg/kg mouse (LEE et al., 1972), consists of two subunits of molecular weight 8800 and 12400 held together by disulfide bonds (KELLY and BROWN, 1974).

V. Enhydrina schistosa Myonecrotic Toxins

The postsynaptic neurotoxins account for about 60% of the protein of *Enhydrina schistosa* (common sea snake) venom (KARLSSON et al., 1972a); nevertheless the clinical picture of poisoning is myotoxic rather than neurotoxic. Muscle-movement pains and myoglobinuria are the most characteristic symptoms in human snake bite victims (REID, 1961).

A toxin which produces myoglobinuria in mice upon intravenous injection has recently been purified by gel filtration on Sephadex G-75 and ion-exchange chromatography on Bio-Rex 70 (FOHLMAN and EAKER, 1977). This toxin, like notexin, is preferentially freeze-dried from 0.01 M ammonium acetate. It is a basic protein containing 120 residues and seven disulfides and has a molecular weight of 13500.

At doses above 100 μg/kg, the mice die rather rapidly as a result of respiratory failure, the syndrome resembling that caused by the presynaptic toxins notexin and

	-8	-7	-6	-5	-4	-3	-2	-1	1	2	3	4	5	6	7	8	9	10	11
Notexin									Asn	Leu	Val	Gln	Phe	Ser	Tyr	Leu	Ile	Gln	Cys
Notechis II-5									Asn	Leu	Val	Gln	Phe	Ser	Tyr	Leu	Ile	Gln	Cys
Notechis II-1									Asn	Leu	Val	Gln	Phe	Ser	Asn	Met	Ile	Gln	Cys
Naja nigricollis basic phospholipase A_2									Asn	Leu	Tyr	Gln	Phe	Lys	Asn	Met	Ile	His	Cys
Taipoxin α									Asn	Leu	Leu	Gln	Phe	Gly	Phe	Met	Ile	Arg	Cys
Taipoxin β									Asn	Leu	Val	Gln	Phe	Gly	Phe	Met	Ile	Gln	Cys
Taipoxin γ	Ser	Glu	Leu	Pro	Gln	Pro	Ser	Ile	Asp	Phe	Glu	Gln	Phe	Ser	Asn	Met	Ile	Gln	Cys
Pork pancreatic prophospholipase A_2		Glu	Glu	Gly	Ile	Ser	Ser	Arg	Ala	Leu	Trp	Gln	Phe	Arg	Ser	Met	Ile	Lys	Cys
Enhydrina schistosa myotoxin									Asn	Leu	Val	Gln	Phe	Ser	Tyr	Val	Ile	Gln	Cys
Crotalus durissus terrificus V									Ser	Leu	Leu	Gln	Phe	Asn	Lys	Met			
Crotalus durissus terrificus VI									His	Leu	Leu	Gln	Phe	Asn	Lys	Met	Lys	Leu	Phe

Fig. 11. Alignment showing homology among the amino-terminal sequences of porcine pancreatic prophospholipase A_2 and various toxins and toxin subunits discussed in the text. *Crotalus durissus terrificus* V and VI are basic phospholipases isolated from the crotoxin complex (BREITHAUPT et el., 1975)

taipoxin. If the mice do not die within 12 h, they either recover or go into a state of catabolism, apparently using up all energy stores. They lose weight, move about shakily, and die on the 4th or 5th day in an emaciated state. The toxicity thus involves two symptoms which are due to different pharmacologic and pathogenic mechanisms. LD_{50} (i.v.) for the fast-ensuing paralytic death is 110 μg/kg (neurotoxic lethal dose) and for the wasting death about 40 μg/kg (myotoxic lethal dose). Myoglobinuria appears at 30 μg/kg, which means that the toxin is extremely toxic for skeletal muscle. The myotoxin is not lethal and does not produce myoglobinuria at 500 μg/kg when injected intraperitoneally. This is in contrast to β-bungarotoxins which are also very lethal when administered intraperitoneally.

The toxin shows phospholipase A activity in the presence of deoxycholate. After modification of a single histidine residue with p-bromophenacyl bromide, no myoglobinuria or any other symptoms were observed in mice at a dose level of 5000 μg/kg and the residual enzymic activity was 0.5%.

The N terminal region is homologous to those of other phospholipases A (Fig. 11). The molecule lacks tryptophan, which proves that this amino acid has no essential functional role either in this toxin or in any of its homologues (FOHLMAN and EAKER, 1977).

VI. Some Other Toxic Phospholipases A

Basic phospholipases A in general appear to be toxic, having lethal doses of about 500 μg/kg mouse or even considerably less as exemplified by the presynaptic neurotoxins and myonecrotic toxins. Many of the acidic phospholipases A, however, are much less toxic and not lethal even at a dose level of 2000 μg/kg, although there are exceptions. An acidic phospholipase A (isoelectric point 5.1) from *Naja nigricollis* has a lethality of 800 μg/kg mouse (WAHLSTRÖM, 1971).

Table 3. Activities of snake venom phospholipases A and phospholipase toxins

Substance	LD_{50} (i.v.) µg/kg mouse	Phospholipase A activity µmol fatty acid/min/mg
Taipoxin	2.1	1
α-subunit	300	15
β-subunit	>2000	1
γ-subunit	>2000	1
Notexin	17	600
Notexin modified with *p*-bromophenacyl bromide	10,000	1
Notechis II-5	45	1000
Notechis II-1	>10,000	1
Enhydrina schistosa myonecrotic toxin	40[a] 110[b]	200
Naja nigricollis basic phospholipase A_2	500	200
β-bungarotoxin[c]	10[d]	130

Enzyme assay, except for β-bungarotoxin: substrate 1 part egg. yolk, 1 part 18 mM $CaCl_2$, and 1 part 8.1 mM sodium deoxycholate (pH 8.0, 25°). β-bungarotoxin: substrate 2 mM phosphatidylcholine, 1.9 mM sodium deoxycholate, 10 mM $CaCl_2$, 100 mM NaCl, and 0.05 mM EDTA (pH 8.0, 37°). Linear kinetics were observed during the first minutes. The enzyme activity was calculated from the initial slope of the curve liberated fatty acids vs. time. The titration was carried out in a pH-stat.

[a] Myotoxic lethal dose.
[b] Neurotoxic lethal dose.
[c] Data on β-bungarotoxin are from STRONG et al. (1976).
[d] Minimum lethal dose (i.p.).

The basic phospholipase A of *Naja nigricollis* consists of 118 amino acid residues and seven disulfides and is homologous to notexin and other phospholipases A (Fig. 10) (OBIDAIRO et al., 1976). The LD_{50} (i.v.) is about 500 µg/kg mouse. The final stages of intoxication in mice are characterized by bleeding from the nose and bloody sputum (unpublished observation).

DELORI (1971) isolated from the venom of *Vipera berus* a phospholipase A_2 with an apparent molecular weight of 12000 and LD_{50} (i.v.) of 500 µg/kg mouse.

SKET et al. (1973) described two basic phospholipases A_2 from *Vipera ammodytes* having lethal doses of 640 and 190 µg/kg mouse respectively.

A very toxic basic phospholipase A_2 with an LD_{100} (i.v.) of 50–150 µg/kg mouse has been isolated from the venom of *Vipera ammodytes ammodytes* (ALEKSIEV and TCHORBANOV, 1976, quoting ALEKSIEV and SHIPOLINI).

VII. Pharmacologic and Biochemical Effects

The pharmacologic and biochemical research on phospholipase toxins is just beginning to advance, and results from different laboratories are, therefore, sometimes difficult to reconcile. Any attempt to summarize a conclusion is also hazardous, but a short summary is nevertheless included here to complement the section on chemistry.

1. Presynaptic Neurotoxicity

A recent comparative study (CHANG et al., 1977) shows that taipoxin, β-bungarotoxin (the most lethal), and crotoxin inhibit the release of acetylcholine in a similar way. Earlier investigations indicated that notexin (HARRIS et al., 1973) and taipoxin (KAMENSKAYA and THESLEFF, 1974) produced the same type of neuromuscular block. All of these toxins eventually lead to depletion of the store of acetylcholine, since application of high K^+ to completely blocked nerves does not cause any further release of transmitter. Electronmicroscopic studies (CHEN and LEE, 1970; CULL-CANDY et al., 1976) also showed that the number of vesicles in the poisoned nerve terminals was considerably reduced. The axolemma was covered with omegashaped indentations having the appearance of vesicles frozen in a state of fusion with the terminal membrane. Thus, it appears as if the toxins do not interfere with the release mechanism itself, since the release of acetylcholine appears to proceed in rather normal fashion until the supply of vesicles has been depleted. However, more recent investigations, summarized by CHANG in a separate chapter in this volume of the Handbook, appear to contradict this interpretation. The reader should consult this chapter for a more thorough discussion on the relationship between the inhibition of the transmitter release by these toxins and the ultrastructural changes.

The relative potencies of the toxins are different in different species of animals. As compared on a weight basis, taipoxin is three times more potent than β-bungarotoxin and five times more potent than crotoxin in blocking the mouse diaphragm preparation, but is 30 and 100 times less potent, respectively, than crotoxin and β-bungarotoxin in the chick muscle. Compared with the mouse diaphragm, the rat diaphragm is about ten times more resistant to crotoxin and taipoxin but more sensitive to β-bungarotoxin (CHANG et al., 1977).

2. Inhibition of High Affinity Choline Uptake

β-bungarotoxin (LD_{50} i.p., 14 μg/kg mouse) (SEN et al., 1976) and taipoxin (DOWDALL, personal communication) inhibit the high affinity choline uptake by synaptosomes involved in the synthesis of acetylcholine. An inhibition of this uptake should then eventually lead to a depletion of the store of acetylcholine.

3. Postsynaptic Effects and Myotoxicity

Notexin causes depolarization in muscle fibers of mice inducing a small decrease of the resting membrane potential (HARRIS et al., 1973). Chick biventer cervicis muscle is more susceptible than rat diaphragm. One μg/ml (0.07 μM) notexin induces contracture of chick muscle. Pretreatment with curare does not prevent contracture. The twitch response and the response to acetylcholine are significantly decreased in chicks even at 0.1 μg/ml of notexin (LEE et al., 1976a).

Taipoxin, β-bungarotoxin, and crotoxin apparently do not affect the acetylcholine sensitivity or twitch response of muscles at all or very slightly (KAMENSKAYA and THESLEFF, 1974; LEE et al., 1976a; CHANG et al., 1977). Crotoxin induces the effects at much higher doses of 1 μM, ca. 25 μg/ml (BREITHAUPT, 1976b).

Upon local application notexin is a potent myonecrotic toxin causing necrosis of muscle fibres with oedema and infiltration of lymphocytes within 12–24 h. After three days the oedema has diminished and the necrotic fibres have been completely destroyed by lymphocytes. At this stage the regeneration starts and is complete within three weeks following the injection, by which time the muscle fibres of the proper type have been re-formed. Mitochondria-rich muscle fibres are preferentially damaged by notexin (HARRIS et al., 1975). The above effects have been observed in vivo but not yet in vitro. The modified notexin shows a week myotoxic effect, less than 1% of that of the native toxin.

Taipoxin when applied locally has the same kind of myotoxic effect in vivo as notexin but is about one-tenth as potent (HARRIS, personal communication).

4. Antagonism by High Mg^{2+}, Ca^{2+}, and Low Ca^{2+}

High Mg^{2+} (12 mM) or Ca^{2+} ($\geqq$9 mM) considerably delay the onset of the neuromuscular block as tested with β-bungarotoxin, crotoxin, and taipoxin. Low Ca^{2+} ($\leqq$0.5 mM) has a similar effect (CHANG et al., 1973, 1977). The delaying effect of high Ca^{2+} might depend on calcium-induced phase transitions of phospholipids in the nerve membrane into a state which obstructs the binding or action of the toxins. The inhibitory effect of high Ca^{2+} on the action of membrane toxins has been explained as due to such phase transitions (Sect. B.II.2). Ca^{2+} is indispensable for phospholipase A activity and the delaying effect of low Ca^{2+} can be ascribed to effects on the enzyme activity (Sect. C.VIII).

VIII. Phospholipase A Activity and Presynaptic Neurotoxicity

All of the presynaptic snake venom toxins or at least one of their subunits are phospholipases A. However, all organisms contain phospholipase A and it is plausible to assume that the enzymes arose first and evolved later to toxins. The catalytic activity associated with the toxins might, therefore, only be an evolutionary vestige.

Notechis II-1 may provide an evolutionary argument for the involvement of the catalytic activity in the neurotoxicity. The molecule binds calcium and has a reactive histidine residue but is devoid of all activity. If the two activities do not have the same basis, it seems surprising that both should be abolished by one or a few mutations.

The formation of the taipoxin complex and the suppression of the phospholipase activity of its α-subunit does not necessarily indicate that the neurotoxicity is not due to the enzyme activity. It might rather imply that a reduction of the phospholipase activity en route to the target is preferable, but if the enzyme activity is responsible for the neurotoxicity, it should also mean that taipoxin dissociates at the target, although the complex is strong and not dissociated by 8 M urea at neutral pH.

There are also some experiments which at least indirectly indicate the importance of the catalytic activity for neurotoxicity.

WERNICKE et al. (1974) showed that fatty acids liberated by the phospholipolytic action of β-bungarotoxin (LD_{50} i.p., 50–100 μg/kg mouse) were able to depress oxidative phosphorylation in the mitochondria of synaptosomes, thereby abolishing their energy store. They proposed, therefore, that the phopholipase A activity was responsible for the neurotoxic effects, and that the toxin would be able to enter the nerve terminal by endocytosis assumed to occur during synaptic transmission.

Another indirect evidence for the enzymic origin of the neurotoxicity is provided by the simultaneous inhibition of phospholipase activity, calcium binding, and toxicity either by modification with p-bromophenacyl bromide or by replacement of calcium with strontium. The calcium requirement for synaptic transmission at the myoneural junction can be satisfied by strontium, whereas the calcium requirement for the phospholipase A activity cannot. STRONG et al. (1976) were able to show that β-bungarotoxin (LD_{50} i.p., 10 µg/kg mouse) had no effect on the acetylcholine release at the myoneural junction in a calcium-free medium containing strontium, i.e., in the absence of catalytic activity. However, the loss of catalytic activity attending absence of calcium binding may only be a consequence of serious structural disturbances, since calcium apparently stabilizes the conformation. Notexin is less accessible to modification in 1 mM Ca^{2+} indicating that calcium holds the part of the molecule containing the reactive histidine in a more compact form.

SEN et al. (1976) demonstrated that the inhibitory action of 0.1 µM (ca. 2 µg/ml) β-bungarotoxin on the high affinity uptake of choline by synaptosomal preparations was not affected by a large excess (0.8 mM) of D,L-2,3-distearoyloxypropyl(dimethyl)-β-hydroxyethylammonium acetate, a competitive inhibitor of phospholipase A. But it is possible that the inhibition might not be effective for the specific substrates in synaptosomes. However, the inhibition of the choline uptake seems to be an enzymic effect, since other phospholipases (bee venom, pork pancreatic, *Naja nigricollis* basic) are also inhibitory when tested on synaptosomal preparations (DOWDALL, personal communication).

The discussion on the phospholipase activity and neurotoxicity can be summarized as follows: 1) so far, phospholipase activity is always associated with presynaptic toxins or at least with one of their subunits, 2) some of the effects can be produced by "ordinary" phospholipases, and 3) clearly demonstrated inhibition of catalytic activity has also implied abolition of toxicity.

All evidence is still indirect, but at present it seems very likely that the phospholipase activity plays a direct role in the presynaptic neurotoxicity.

IX. Concluding Remarks

Many of the substances described in this section display a broad spectrum of activities. They are to a varying degree phospholipases, presynaptic neurotoxins, and myonecrotic toxins. Notexin has all three activities in good measure. That does probably imply that its specific target is distributed both in nerve terminals and muscle membranes. This is a parallel to membrane toxins, which have their apparently specific target distributed in many different types of cells.

Concerning the structure of the toxins, the paradoxic situation exists that toxins with identical or very similar types of action have the most dissimilar quaternary structures, whereas molecules having apparently very homologous structures have very different activities.

Notexin, taipoxin, crotoxin, and β-bungarotoxin(s) are dissimilar molecules with a very similar type of presynaptic action. However, it appears to be possible to attain structural similarity by dissociation of the complex molecules and release of a notexin homologue.

Similar molecules with very different activities are exemplified by notexin (119 residues) and the basic phospholipase A of *Naja nigricollis* (118 residues). Their amino acid sequences are identical to 55% (65 positions) and conservative mutations (Sect. B.I.4) are frequent (Fig. 10). Despite this apparent similarity, the *nigricollis* enzyme is about 30 times less lethal, and the symptoms suggest that its lethality is due neither to myotoxicity nor neurotoxicity. It appears as though comparatively few mutations can give molecules with quite different specificities.

In some cases, the charge seems somehow to be important. Notexin and notechis II-5 have net charges of +2 and +3, respectively, at neutral pH. The very basic phospholipase of *Naja nigricollis* with a charge of +6 has on the other hand a much lower lethality, and acidic phospholipases are in general non-lethal. The properties are clearly not attributed to charge alone, since molecules like taipoxin and crotoxin are anions at neutral pH. But both of them have a very basic subunit and all phospholipase toxins should therefore have basic regions in their molecules. These regions might in some way be essential for the toxicity.

D. Other Toxins

I. Crotamine

Crotamine from *Crotalus durissus terrificus* var. *crotaminicus* is a basic polypeptide containing 42 amino acid residues and three disulfides. The molecular weight is 4880. The charge at neutral pH is +7 and the isoelectric point is pH 10.3.

The sequence (LAURE, 1975) shows no apparent similarities with the sequences of neurotoxins, membrane toxins, or phospholipases (Figs. 4, 8, and 10):

1 5 10 15 20
Tyr-Lys-Gln-Cys-His-Lys-Lys-Gly-Gly-His-Cys-Phe-Pro-Lys-Glu-Lys-Ile-Cys-Leu-Pro-Pro-
25 30 35 40
Ser-Ser-Asp-Phe-Gly-Lys-Met-Asp-Cys-Arg-Trp-Arg-Trp-Lys-Cys-Cys-Lys-Lys-Gly-Ser-Gly

The LD_{50} (i.v.) is 3400 µg/kg mouse. On the rat diaphragm, crotamine produces an immediate contracture followed by spontaneous and irregular twitchings (CHEYMOL et al., 1971a, b). The sensitivity of chick nerve-muscle preparations to crotamine decreases with the age of the chicken and eventually disappears (Sect. D.IV) (LEE et al., 1972c). The action of crotamine on rat diaphragm is prevented by tetrodotoxin, Ca^{2+}, Mg^{2+}, and K^+, but only partly by denervation or previous treatment with curare (CHEYMOL et al., 1971a, b; BRAZIL, 1971). Crotamine is suggested to act on mammalian muscle membranes by changing the Ca^{2+} or Na^+ permeability (Sect. D.IV). (CHEYMOL et al., 1971a, b).

II. Convulxin and Gyroxin

Convulxin and *gyroxin* are acidic, nondialyzable proteins from the venom of *Crotalus durissus terrificus*. Rapidly after injection into mice, convulxin produces convulsions and gyroxin fast-rolling movements of the body along its longitudinal axis (BRAZIL, 1972; LEE, 1972). Convulxin is said to be twice as lethal as crotamine (JIMÉNÉZ PORRAS, 1970 quoting BRAZIL et al.). Very little is known about the chemistry and pharmacology of the two toxins.

III. Mojave Toxin

The Mojave rattlesnake *Crotalus scutulatus scutulatus* has one of the most potent of all rattlesnake venoms, and recently attempts have been made to characterize its main toxic constituent (BIEBER et al., 1975; PATTABHIRAMAN and RUSSELL, 1975; HENDON, 1975). The toxin called *Mojave toxin* has an LD_{50} (i.v.) of only 28 μg/kg mouse. It is an acidic protein with an isoelectric point of 4.7. The molecular weight by gel filtration is 22000 and the toxin apparently consists of two subunits of an approximate size of 12000 each. The Mojave toxin is claimed to be cardiotoxic rather than neurotoxic (BIEBER et al., 1975), but its lethality is in the range observed with presynaptic toxins other than taipoxin. The subunits also appear to be in the same size range as the phospholipase constituents of the presynaptic toxins. One might, therefore, expect that the Mojave toxin be related to the phospholipase toxins.

IV. Other Crotalid Toxins

Low molecular weight basic toxins with isoelectric points above pH 10.8 have been isolated from the venoms of three North American rattlesnakes. The formula weights were: 6300–7000 (toxin from *Crotalus viridis viridis*), 6300–6800 (*Crotalus horridus atricaudatus*), and 4800–5200 (*Crotalus horridus horridus*). The last one appears to have an amino acid composition similar to that of crotamine and they are probably members of another fundamental toxin structure group (Sect. A).

The s.c. LD_{50} were between 32 and 43 mg/kg mouse, but the i.v. doses might be much lower. The onset of the symptoms was rapid. Mice showed ptosis, were ataxic, and had jerky body movements with a stiff-legged shuffling gait. Sublethal doses caused extreme tonic hyperextension of the hind limbs, often accompanied by rigidity of the tail for more than 6 h. Gasping respiration was observed. Convulsions generally preceded death, which was of rapid onset (BONILLA and FIERO, 1971).

The pharmacologic effects have been studied on chick biventer nerve-muscle preparations. Muscles from chicken older than five weeks are no longer sensitive (Sect. D.I). The toxins increase the contractile response to indirect stimulation and induce irregular spontaneous twitchings, and they appear to have a mode of action similar to that of crotamine. It is suggested that they have a presynaptic action in chicks, since pretreatment with β-bungarotoxin prevents the effects without abolishing the acetylcholine response of the muscle. The action on mammalian muscles appears to be mainly on the muscle membrane as suggested for crotamine. D-tubocurarine, tetrodotoxin, low (0.1 mM) Ca^{2+}, high (12 mM) Ca^{2+}, and high (10 mM) Mg^{2+} also prevent the action of the toxins on chick muscles (LEE et al., 1972b).

A protein called *myocardial depressor protein* has recently been isolated from the venom of *Crotalus atrox*, the Western diamondback rattlesnake. It produces severe myocardial depression in anesthetized animals. The effect is noticeable within seconds after intravenous administration and is primarily a drastic decrease in cardiac output and the left ventricular and arterial pressure, which depending on the dose can last for 2 h or longer. It is probably an acidic protein (adsorbed to DEAE cellulose at pH 8) and contains approximately 70 amino acid residues. It is devoid of the phospholipase A and the proteolytic and esterolytic activities known to exist in the crude venom (BONILLA and RAMMEL, 1976).

A potent hypotensive peptide, *hypotensin*, also from the venom of *Crotalus atrox* consists of approximately 20 amino acid residues and probably one disulfide. It induces a rapid decrease in systemic arterial pressure which lasts for 2 h or longer as studied in anesthetized dogs (BONILLA, 1976).

V. Viperotoxin

Viperotoxin from *Vipera palestinae* is a single-chain basic protein containing 108 amino acid residues (mol wt 12200) and three disulfides. The toxicity is potentiated by lipids but is still low: the LD_{50} (i.v.) is about 3000 μg/kg mouse in the presence of lipids and is about four times higher without them (MOROZ et al., 1966). The toxin causes circulatory failure (JIMÉNÉZ PORRAS, 1970; LEE, 1972 quoting BICHER et al.).

VI. Toxins from Bungarus caeruleus Venom

1. Ceruleotoxin

Ceruleotoxin is an acidic protein with an apparent molecular weight of 38000 ± 4000 as estimated by gel filtration and consists of two or three subunits with an apparent size of 15000 ± 2000. The LD_{100} (i.v.) is 50 μg/kg mouse. Death occurs after a long delay of up to 48 h. Ceruleotoxin has a postsynaptic type of action. It blocks the postsynaptic response to acetylcholine but does not bind significantly to the cholinergic receptor site, since it does not compete with the binding of a curaremimetic toxin (BON and CHANGEUX, 1975).

Ceruleotoxin is apparently composed of subunits having about the same size as the phospholipase constituents of the presynaptic toxins. A death time up to 48 h or even longer has also been observed with notexin. It has also been shown that notexin has a postsynaptic effect, decreasing the sensitivity of the motor end plate for acetylcholine (Sect. C.VII.3). Ceruleotoxin might, therefore, be another member of the phospholipase toxin group.

2. Post- and Presynaptic Neurotoxins

Two toxins of each type have recently been isolated. The most potent of the presynaptic toxins has an LD_{50} (i.p.) as low as 7.5 μg/kg mouse (LEE et al., 1976b).

E. Conclusion

Many curaremimetic toxins have been sequenced, and although there are many more which have not yet been characterized, the probability of detecting in elapid and hydrophid venoms toxins having sequences greatly different from those already known with amino acid replacements in positions presently considered as invariant seems rather low. But there might be inactive homologues which may give information of structurally or functionally important sites in the neurotoxins.

The situation is, however, quite different in the case of toxic phospholipases, myotoxins, and presynaptic toxins. Such toxins are certainly present in most snake venoms from Australia, a continent which has many elapids with extremely potent venoms. To date, only notexin and its homologues and taipoxin have been characterized chemically, but their biochemical and pharmacologic characterization is still far from complete. Neither crotoxin nor any of the β-bungarotoxins have been completely characterized.

The crystallographic work has begun, but the obvious future goals are the elucidation of the three-dimensional structures of a long neurotoxin and a presynaptic toxin.

Many viperids and crotalids also have very potent toxins, but only crotamine has been defined with regard to amino acid sequence. Many viperid and crotalid venoms have not been investigated at all. The high lethality of some of these venoms may depend on synergistically acting components or on easily dissociable complexes. In such a case, individual fractions obtained by some fractionation method may be nonlethal, whereas lethality is restored upon pooling. That seems to be the case with the venom of *Vipera russellii* (MASTER and RAO, 1961).

The greatest interest has been directed toward the most lethal venom constituents. It is also quite natural that the most dramatic components interest many investigators, but even many less lethal substances are well worth a greater interest. One such group of comparatively neglected compounds is hypotensin and analogous hypotensive peptides.

Obviously a great deal of work remains within the "easy" part of the toxin research; the isolation and structural characterization of toxins.

The difficult part, the elucidation at the molecular level of the basis for the toxin action, has hardly begun. This goal will not be achieved before the physiologic process which is being affected also is explained to some extent. Research on the mechanism of action of a toxin must necessarily develop in parallel with the progress in the understanding of the molecular mechanism of the particular function being affected by the toxin, which will thus serve as a tool for investigating the process. Toxin research will, therefore, inevitably lead into research on physiologic processes.

Acknowledgements. I thank Drs. DAVID EAKER, JAN FOHLMAN, JAMES HALPERT, GUNNAR SAMUELSSON and INGVAR SJÖHOLM for discussions, valuable suggestions, and criticism during the writing of this article.

The preparation of this review was supported by the Swedish Natural Science Research Council, dnr 220-036 and 2859-011.

References

Aharonov, A., Gurari, D., Fuchs, S.: Immunochemical characterization of *Naja naja siamensis* toxin and of a chemically modified toxin. Europ. J. Biochem. **45**, 297—303 (1974)

Aleksiev, B., Tchorbanov, B.: Action on phosphatidylcholine of the toxic phospholipase A_2 from the venom of Bulgarian viper *(Vipera ammodytes ammodytes)*. Toxicon **14**, 477—485 (1976)

Andersson, K. E., Jóhannsson, M.: Effects of viscotoxin on rabbit heart and aorta, and on frog skeletal muscle. Europ. J. Pharmacol. **23**, 223—231 (1973)

Aoyagi, H., Yonezawa, H., Takahashi, N., Kato, T., Izumiya, N., Yang, C. C.: Synthesis of a peptide with cobrotoxin activity. Biochim. biophys. Acta (Amst.) **263**, 823—826 (1972)

Arnberg, H., Eaker, D., Fryklund, L., Karlsson, E.: Amino acid sequence of oxiana α, the main neurotoxin of the venom of *Naja naja oxiana*. Biochim. biophys. Acta (Amst.) **359**, 222—232 (1974)

Arnberg, H., Eaker, D., Karlsson, E.: Amino acid sequences of the cobra venom neurotoxins *siamensis* 3, *naja* 3, *naja* 4, and *naja* 3P. (unpublished) (1977)

Banks, B. E. C., Miledi, R., Shipolini, R. A.: The primary sequences and neuromuscular effects of three neurotoxic polypeptides from the venom of *Dendroaspis viridis*. Europ. J. Biochem. **45**, 457—468 (1974)

Bechis, G., Rietschoten, J. Van, Granier, C., Jover, E., Rochat, H., Miranda, F.: On the characterization of two long toxins from *Dendroaspis viridis*. Bull. Inst. Pasteur Lille **74**, 35—39 (1976)

Bieber, A. L., Tu, T., Tu, A. T.: Studies of an acidic cardiotoxin isolated from the venom of Mojave rattlesnake *(Crotalus scutulatus)*. Biochim. biophys. Acta (Amst.) **400**, 178—188 (1975)

Bock, R. M., Ling, N. S.: Devices for gradient elution in chromatography. Anal. Chem. **26**, 1543—1546 (1954)

Bon, C., Changeux, J. P.: Ceruleotoxin: an acidic neurotoxin from the venom of *Bungarus caeruleus* which blocks the response to a cholinergic agonist without binding to the cholinergic receptor site. FEBS Letters **59**, 212—216 (1975)

Bonilla, C. A.: Hypotensin—A hypotensive peptide isolated from *Crotalus atrox* venom: Purification, amino acid composition and terminal amino acid residues. FEBS Letters **68**, 297—302 (1976)

Bonilla, C. A., Fiero, M. K.: Comparative biochemistry and pharmacology of salivary gland secretions. II. Chromatographic separation of the basic proteins from some North American rattlesnake venoms. J. Chromatog. **56**, 253—263 (1971)

Bonilla, C. A., Rammel, O. J.: Comparative biochemistry and pharmacology of salivary gland secretions. III. Chromatographic isolation of a myocardial depressor protein (MDP) from the venom of *Crotalus atrox*. J. Chromatog. **124**, 303—314 (1976)

Boquet, P.: Venins de serpents (1ère partie). Physio-pathologie de l'envenimation et propriétés biologiques des venins. Toxicon **2**, 5—41 (1964)

Boquet, P.: Venins de serpents (2ème partie). Constitution chimique des venins de serpents et immunité antivenimeuse. Toxicon **3**, 243—279 (1966)

Boquet, P., Poilleux, G., Dumarey, C., Izard, Y., Ronsseray, A. M.: An attempt to classify the toxic proteins of Elapidae and Hydrophidae venoms. Toxicon **11**, 333—340 (1973)

Botes, D. P.: Snake venom toxins. The amino acid sequences of toxins α and β from *Naja nivea* venom and the disulfide bonds of toxin α. J. biol. Chem. **246**, 7383—7391 (1971)

Botes, D. P.: Snake venom toxins. The amino acid sequences of toxins b and d from *Naja melanoleuca* venom. J. biol. Chem. **247**, 2866—2871 (1972)

Botes, D. P.: Snake venom toxins. The reactivity of the disulphide bonds of *Naja nivea* toxin α. Biochim. biophys. Acta (Amst.) **359**, 242—247 (1974)

Botes, D. P., Strydom, D. J.: A neurotoxin, toxin α, from Egyptian cobra *(Naja haje haje)* venom. J. biol. Chem. **244**, 4147—4157 (1969)

Botes, D. P., Strydom, D. J., Anderson, C. G., Christensen, P. A.: Snake venom toxins. Purification and properties of three toxins from *Naja nivea* (Linnaeus) (Cape cobra) venom and the amino acid sequence of toxin δ. J. biol. Chem. **246**, 3132—3139 (1971)

Brazil, O. V.: Neurotoxins from the South American rattle snake venom. J. Formosan med. Ass. **71**, 394—400 (1972)

Brazil, O. V., Excell, B. J.: Action of crotoxin and crotactin from the venom of *Crotalus durissus terrificus* (South American rattlesnake) on the frog neuromuscular junction. J. Physiol. (Lond.) **212**, 34—35P (1971)

Brazil, O. V., Excell, B. J., Sanatana, S. de Sa.: The importance of phospholipase A in the action of the crotoxin complex at the frog neuromuscular junction. J. Physiol. (Lond.) **234**, 63—64 P (1973)
Breithaupt, H.: Enzymatic characteristics of *Crotalus* phospholipase A_2 and the crotoxin complex. Toxicon **14**, 221—233 (1976 a)
Breithaupt, H.: Neurotoxic and myotoxic effects of Crotalus phospholipase A and its complex with crotapotin. Naunyn-Schmiedebergs Arch. Pharmacol. **292**, 271—278 (1976 b)
Breithaupt, H., Omori-Satoh, T., Lang, J.: Isolation and characterization of three phospholipases A from the crotoxin complex. Biochim. biophys. Acta (Amst.) **403**, 355—369 (1975)
Breithaupt, H., Rübsamen, K., Habermann, E.: Biochemistry and pharmacology of the crotoxin complex. Biochemical analysis of crotapotin and the basic phospholipase A. Europ. J. Biochem. **49**, 333—345 (1974)
Breithaupt, H., Rübsamen, K., Walsch, P., Habermann, E.: In vitro and in vivo interactions between phospholipase A and a novel potentiator isolated from so-called crotoxin complex. Naunyn-Schmiedebergs Arch. Pharmak. **269**, 403—404 (1971)
Broadley, D. G.: A review of the African cobras of the genus *Naja* (Serpentes: *Elapinae*). Arnoldia **3**, 1—14 (1968)
Brunton, T. L., Fayrer, J.: On the nature and physiological action of the poison of *Naja tripudians* and other Indian venomous snakes. Part I. Proc. roy. Soc. [B] **21**, 358—374 (1873). Part II. Ibid. **22**, 68—133 (1874)
Bukolova-Orlova, T. G., Permyakov, E. A., Burstein, E. A., Yukelson, L. Ya.: Reinterpretation of luminiscence properties of neurotoxins from the venom of Middle-Asian cobra *Naja oxiana* eichw. Biochim. biophys. Acta (Amst.) **439**, 426—431 (1976)
Carlsson, F. H. H.: Snake venom toxins. The primary structure of two novel cytotoxin homologues from the venom of forest cobra *(Naja melanoleuca)*. Biochem. Biophys. Res. Commun. **59**, 269—276 (1974)
Carlsson, F. H. H.: Snake venom toxins. The primary structure of protein S_4C_{11} a neurotoxin homologue from the venom of forest cobra *(Naja melanoleuca)*. Biochim. biophys. Acta (Amst.) **400**, 310—321 (1975)
Carlsson, F. H. H., Joubert, F. J.: Snake venom toxins. The isolation and purification of three cytotoxin homologues from the venom of the forest cobra *(Naja melanoleuca)* and the complete amino acid sequence of toxin $V^{II}1$. Biochim. biophys. Acta (Amst.) **336**, 453—469 (1974)
Chang, C. C., Chen, T. F., Lee, C. Y.: Studies of the presynaptic effect of β-bungarotoxin on neuromuscular transmission. J. Pharmacol. exp. Ther. **184**, 339—345 (1973)
Chang, C. C., Lee, C. Y.: Isolation of neurotoxins from the venom of *Bungarus multicinctus* and their modes of neuromuscular blocking action. Arch. int. Pharmacodyn. **144**, 241—257 (1963)
Chang, C. C., Lee, J. D., Eaker, D., Fohlman, J.: The presynaptic neuromuscular blocking action of taipoxin. A comparison with β-bungarotoxin and crotoxin. Toxicon **15**, 571—576 (1977)
Chang, C. C., Yang, C. C.: Immunochemical studies on the tryptophan-modified cobrotoxin. Biochim. biophys. Acta (Amst.) **295**, 595—604 (1973)
Chang, C. C., Yang, C. C., Hamaguchi, K., Nakai, K., Hayashi, K.: Studies on the status of tyrosyl residues in cobrotoxin. Biochim. biophys. Acta (Amst.) **236**, 164—173 (1971 b)
Chang, C. C., Yang, C. C., Nakai, K., Hayashi, K.: Studies on the status of free amino and carboxyl groups in cobrotoxin. Biochim. biophys. Acta (Amst.) **251**, 334—344 (1971 a)
Changeux, J. P., Kasai, M., Lee, C. Y.: Use of a snake venom toxin to characterize the cholinergic receptor protein of *Torpedo* electric tissue. Proc. nat. Acad. Sci. (Wash.) **67**, 1241—1247 (1970)
Chen, I. L., Lee, C. Y.: Ultrastructural changes in the motor nerve terminals caused by β-bungarotoxin. Virchows Arch. Abt. B. Zellpath. **6**, 318—325 (1970)
Cheymol, J., Bourillet, F., Roch-Arveiller, M.: Venins et toxines de serpents. Effets neuromusculaire. Actualités pharmacol. **25**, 179—240 (1972)
Cheymol, J., Goncalves, J. M., Bourillet, F., Roch-Arveiller, M.: Action neuromusculaire comparée de la crotamine et du venin de *Crotalus durissus terrificus* var. *crotaminicus*. I. Sur préparations neuromusculaire in situ. Toxicon **9**, 279—286 (1971 a). II. Sur préparations isolées. Toxicon **9**, 287—289 (1971 b)
Cheymol, J., Karlsson, E., Bourillet, F., Roch-Arveiller, M.: Activités biologiques des diverses fractions isolées du venin d'*Hemachatus haemachates*. Arch. int. Pharmacodyn. **208**, 81—93 (1974)

Chicheportiche, R., Rochat, C., Sampieri, F., Lazdunski, M.: Structure-function relationships of neurotoxins isolated from *Naja haje* venom. Physicochemical properties and identification of the active site. Biochemistry **11**, 1681—1691 (1972)

Chicheportiche, R., Vincent, J. P., Kopeyan, C., Schweitz, H., Lazdunski, M.: Structure-function relationship in the binding of snake neurotoxins to the *Torpedo* membrane receptor. Biochemistry **14**, 2081—2091 (1975)

Condrea, E.: Membrane-active polypeptides from snake venom: Cardiotoxins and haemocytotoxins. Experientia (Basel) **30**, 121—129 (1974)

Cooper, D., Reich, E.: Neurotoxin from the venom of the cobra, *Naja naja siamensis*. Purification and radioactive labelling. J. biol. Chem. **247**, 3008—3013 (1972)

Cull-Candy, S. G., Fohlman, J., Gustavsson, D., Lüllman-Rauch, R., Theseleff, S.: The effects of taipoxin and notexin on the function and fine structure of the murine neuromuscular junction. Neuroscience **1**, 175—180 (1976)

Delori, P. J.: Isolement, purification et étude d'une phospholipase A_2 toxique du venin de *Vipera berus*. Biochimie **53**, 941—942 (1971)

Devi, A.: The protein and nonprotein constituents of snake venoms. In: Bucherl, W., Buckley, E., Deulofeu, V. (Eds.): Venomous Animals and Their Venoms, Vol. I, pp. 119—165. New York-London: Academic Press 1968

Drenth, J., Enzing, C., Kalk, K., Vessies, J.: The three dimensional structure of pancreatic phospholipase A_2. Abstracts 04-6-353, 10th Int. Congr. Biochemistry, Hamburg, Germany, July 25—31, 1976

Eaker, D.: Structure and function of snake venom toxins. In: Walter, R., Meienhofer, J. (Eds.): Peptides: Chemistry, Structure and Biology. Proc. 4th American Peptide Symposium, pp. 17—30. Ann Arbor (Michigan): Ann Arbor-Science Publisher's 1975

Eaker, D., Porath, J.: The amino acid sequence of a neurotoxin from *Naja nigricollis* venom. 7th Int. Congress Biochem., Tokyo 1967. Col. VIII-3, Abstracts III, p. 499. Tokyo: The Science Council of Japan 1967

Edman, P.: Method for determination of the amino acid sequence in peptides. Acta Chem. Scand. **4**, 283—293 (1950)

Ehrenpreis, S., Fishmann, M. M.: The interaction of quaternary ammonium compounds with chondroitin sulfate. Biochim. biophys. Acta (Amst.) **44**, 577—585 (1960)

Eterovic, V. A., Hebert, M. S., Hanley, M. R., Bennett, E. L.: The lethality and spectroscopic properties of toxins from *Bungarus multicinctus* (Blyth) venom. Toxicon **13**, 37—48 (1975)

Evenberg, A., Meyer, H., Gaastra, W., Verheij, H. M., Haas de G. H.: Amino acid sequence of phospholipase A_2 from horse pancreas. J. biol. Chem. **252**, 1189—1196 (1977).

Fohlman, J., Eaker, D.: Isolation and characterization of a lethal myotoxic phospholipase A from the venom of the common sea snake *Enhydrina schistosa* causing myoglobinuria in mice. Toxicon **15**, 385—393 (1977)

Fohlman, J., Eaker, D., Karlsson, E., Thesleff, S.: Taipoxin, an extremely potent presynaptic neurotoxin from the venom of the Australian snake taipan *(Oxyuranus s. scutellatus)*. Isolation, characterization, quaternary structure and pharmacological properties. Europ. J. Biochem. **68**, 457—469 (1976)

Fraenkel-Conrat, H., Jeng, T. W., Hendon, R. A.: New studies on crotoxin, the dual neurotoxin of *Crotalus durissus terrificus*. Report at 10th Int. Congr. Biochemistry, Hamburg, Germany, July 25—31, 1976

Fryklund, L., Eaker, D.: Complete amino acid sequence of a nonneurotoxic hemolytic protein from the venom of *Hemachatus haemachatus* (African ringhals cobra). Biochemistry **12**, 661—667 (1973)

Fryklund, L., Eaker, D.: The complete amino acid sequence of a cardiotoxin from the venom of *Naja naja* (Cambodian cobra). Biochemistry **14**, 2860—2865 (1975a)

Fryklund, L., Eaker, D.: The complete covalent structure of a cardiotoxin from the venom of *Naja nigricollis* (African black-necked spitting cobra). Biochemistry **14**, 2865—2871 (1975b)

Fryklund, L., Eaker, D., Karlsson, E.: Amino acid sequences of the two principal neurotoxins of *Enhydrina schistosa* venom. Biochemistry **11**, 4633—4640 (1972)

Ghosh, B. N., Chaudhuri, D. K.: Venoms of Asiatic snakes. In: Bucherl, W., Buckley, E., Deulofeu, V. (Eds.): Venomous Animals and Their Venoms, Vol. I, pp. 577—610. New York-London: Academic Press 1968

Gralén, N., Svedbeg, T.: The molecular weight of crotoxin. Biochem. J. **32**, 1375—1377 (1938)

Grishin, E. V., Sukhikh, A. P., Adamovich, T. B., Ovchinnikov, Yu. A., Yukelson, L. Ya.: The isolation and sequence determination of a cytotoxin from the venom of the Middle-Asian cobra *Naja naja oxiana*. FEBS Letters **48**, 179—183 (1974b)
Grishin, E. V., Sukhikh, A. P., Lukyanchuk, N. N., Slobodyan, L. N., Lipkin, V. M., Ovchinnikov, Yu. A., Sorokin, V. M.: Amino acid sequence of neurotoxin II from *Naja naja oxiana* venom. FEBS Letters **36**, 77—78 (1973)
Grishin, E. V., Sukhikh, A. P., Slobodyan, L. N., Ovchinnikov, Yu. A., Sorokin, V. M.: Amino acid sequence of neurotoxin I from *Naja naja oxiana* venom. FEBS Letters **45**, 118—121 (1974a)
Haas, G. H. de, Postema, N. H., Nieuwenhausen, W., Deenen, L. L. M. de: Purification and properties of phospholipase A from porcine pancreas. Biochim. biophys. Acta (Amst.) **159**, 103—117 (1968)
Haas, G. H. de, Sloboom, A. J., Bonsen, P. P. M., Deenen, L. L. M. Van, Maroux, S., Puigserver, A., Desnuelle, P.: Studies on phospholipase A and its zymogen from porcine pancreas. I. The complete amino acid sequence. Biochim. biophys. Acta (Amst.) **221**, 31—53 (1970)
Halpert, J., Eaker, D.: Amino acid sequence of a presynaptic neurotoxin from the venom of *Notechis scutatus scutatus* (Australian tiger snake). J. biol. Chem. **250**, 6990—6997 (1975)
Halpert, J., Eaker, D.: Isolation and the amino acid sequence of a neurotoxic phospholipase A from the venom of the Australian tiger snake *Notechis scutatus scutatus*. J. biol. Chem. **251**, 7343—7347 (1976)
Halpert, J., Eaker, D., Karlsson, E.: The role of phospholipase activity in the action of a presynaptic neurotoxin from the venom of *Notechis scutatus scutatus* (Australian tiger snake). FEBS Letters **61**, 72—76 (1976)
Harris, J. B., Johnson, M. A., Karlsson, E.: Pathological responses of rat skeletal muscle to a single subcutaneous injection of a toxin isolated from the venom of the Australian tiger snake, *Notechis scutatus scutatus*. Clin. exp. Pharmacol. Physiol. **2**, 383—404 (1975)
Harris, J. B., Karlsson, E., Thesleff, S.: Effects of an isolated toxin from Australian tiger snake *(Notechis scutatus scutatus)* venom at the mammalian neuromuscular junction. Brit. J. Pharmacol. **47**, 141—146 (1973)
Hassón, A.: Interaction of quaternary ammonium bases with a purified acid polysaccharide and other macromolecules from the electric organ of electric eel. Biochim. biophys. Acta (Amst.) **56**, 275—292 (1962)
Hayashi, K., Takechi, M., Sasaki, T.: Amino acid sequence of cytotoxin I from the venom of the Indian cobra *(Naja naja)*. Biochem. Biophys. Res. Commun. **45**, 1357—1362 (1971)
Hayashi, K., Takechi, M., Sasaki, T., Lee, C. Y.: Amino acid sequence of cardiotoxin-analogue I from the venom of *Naja naja atra*. Biochem. Biophys. Res. Commun. **64**, 360—366 (1975)
Hendon, R. A.: Preliminary studies on the neurotoxin in the venom of *Crotalus scutulatus* (Mojave rattlesnake). Toxicon **13**, 477—482 (1975)
Hendon, R. A., Fraenkel-Conrat, H.: Biological role of the two components of crotoxin. Proc. natl. Acad. Sci. (Wash.) **68**, 1560—1563 (1971)
Hendon, R. A., Fraenkel-Conrat, H.: The role of complex formation in the neurotoxicity of crotoxin components A and B. Toxicon **14**, 283—289 (1976)
Hofsten, B. von, Kley, H. van, Eaker, D.: An extracellular enzyme from a strain of *Arthrobacter*. Biochim. biophys. Acta (Amst.) **110**, 585—598 (1965)
Hori, H., Tamiya, N.: Preparation and activity of guanidinated or acetylated erabutoxins. Biochem. J. **153**, 217—222 (1976)
Horst, J., Hendon, R. A., Fraenkel-Conrat, H.: The active components of crotoxin. Biochem. Biophys. Res. Commun. **46**, 1042—1047 (1972)
Howard, B. D.: Effects of β-bungarotoxin on mitochondrial respiration are caused by associated phospholipase A activity. Biochem. Biophys. Res. Commun. **67**, 58—65 (1975)
Huang, J. S., Liu, S. S., Ling, K. H., Chang, C. C., Yang, C. C.: Iodination of cobrotoxin. Toxicon **11**, 39—45 (1973)
Jeng, T. W., Fraenkel-Conrat, H.: Activation of crotoxin B by volvatoxin A2. Biochem. Biophys. Res. Commun. **70**, 1324—1329 (1976)
Jiménez Porras, J. M.: Pharmacology of peptides and proteins in snake venoms. Ann. Rev. Pharmacol. **8**, 299—318 (1968)
Jiménez Porras, J. M.: Biochemistry of snake venoms (a review). Clin. Toxicol. **3**, 389—431 (1970)
Joubert, F. J.: Snake venom toxins. The amino acid sequences of two toxins from Ophiophagus hannah *(King cobra)* venom. Biochim. biophys. Acta (Amst.) **317**, 85—98 (1973)

Joubert, F. J.: Snake venom toxins. The amino acid sequences of three toxins (CM-10, CM-12, and CM-14) from *Naja haje annulifera* (Egyptian cobra) venom. Hoppe Seylers Z. physiol. Chem. **356**, 53—72 (1975a)

Joubert, F. J.: *Naja melanoleuca* (Forest cobra) venom. The amino acid sequence of phospholipase A, fractions DE-I and DE-II. Biochim. biophys. Acta (Amst.) **379**, 345—359 (1975b)

Joubert, F. J.: *Naja melanoleuca* (Forest cobra) venom. The amino acid sequence of phospholipase A, fraction DE-III. Biochim. biophys. Acta (Amst.) **379**, 329—344 (1975c)

Joubert, F. J.: *Hemachatus haemachatus* (Ringhals) venom. Purification, some properties and amino acid sequence of phospholipase A (Fraction DE-I). Europ. J. Biochem. **52**, 539—554 (1975d)

Kaiser, E., Michl, H.: Die Biochemie der tierischen Gifte. Wien: Franz Deuticke 1958

Kamenskaya, M. A., Thesleff, S.: The neuromuscular blocking action of an isolated toxin from the elapid *(Oxyuranus scutellatus)*. Acta physiol. scand. **90**, 716—724 (1974)

Karlsson, E.: Chemistry of some potent animal toxins. Experientia (Basel) **29**, 1319—1327 (1973)

Karlsson, E., Arnberg, H., Eaker, D.: Isolation of the principal neurotoxins of two *Naja naja* subspecies. Europ. J. Biochem. **21**, 1—16 (1971)

Karlsson, E., Eaker, D.: Isolation of the principal neurotoxins of *Naja naja* subspecies from the Asian mainland. Toxicon **10**, 217—225 (1972a)

Karlsson, E., Eaker, D.: Chemical modifications of the postsynaptic *Naja naja* neurotoxins. J. Formosan med. Ass. **71**, 358—371 (1972b)

Karlsson, E., Eaker, D., Drevin, H.: Modification of the invariant tryptophan of two *Naja naja* neurotoxins. Biochim. biophys. Acta (Amst.) **328**, 510—519 (1973)

Karlsson, E., Eaker, D., Fryklund, L., Kadin, S.: Chromatographic separation of *Enhydrina schistosa* (common sea snake) venom and the characterization of two principal neurotoxins. Biochemistry **11**, 4628—4633 (1972a)

Karlsson, E., Eaker, D., Ponterius, G.: Modification of amino groups in *Naja naja* neurotoxins and the preparation of radioactive derivatives. Biochim. biophys. Acta (Amst.) **257**, 235—248 (1972c)

Karlsson, E., Eaker, D., Porath, J.: Purification of a neurotoxin from the venom of *Naja nigricollis*. Biochim. biophys. Acta (Amst.) **127**, 505—520 (1966)

Karlsson, E., Eaker, D., Rydén, L.: Purification of a presynaptic neurotoxin from the venom of the Australian tiger snake *Notechis scutatus scutatus*. Toxicon **10**, 405—413 (1972d)

Karlsson, E., Fohlman, J., Groth, M.: Purification of the acetylcholine receptor from the electric organ of *Torpedo marmorata*. Bull. Inst. Pasteur Lille **74**, 11—22 (1976)

Karlsson, E., Heilbronn, E., Widlund, L.: Isolation of the nicotinic acetylcholine receptor by biospecific chromatography on insolubilized *Naja naja* neurotoxin. FEBS Letters **28**, 107—111 (1972b)

Karlsson, E., Sundelin, J.: Nitration of tyrosine in three cobra neurotoxins. Toxicon **14**, 295—306 (1976)

Kelly, R. B., Brown, III, F. R.: Biochemical and physiological properties of a purified snake venom neurotoxin which acts presynaptically. J. Neurobiol. **5**, 135—150 (1974)

Keung, W. M., Leung, W. W., Kong, Y. C.: Studies of the status of disulfide linkages and tyrosine residues in cardiotoxin. Biochem. Biophys. Res. Commun. **66**, 383—392 (1975b)

Keung, W. M., Yip, T. T., Kong, Y. C.: The chemistry and biological effects of cardiotoxin from the Chinese cobra (*N. naja* Linn.) on hormonal responses in isolated cell systems. Toxicon **13**, 239—251 (1975a)

Klett, R. P., Fulpius, B. W., Cooper, D., Smith, M., Reich, E., Possani, L. D.: The acetylcholine receptor. Purification and characterization of a macromolecule isolated from *Electrophorus electricus*. J. biol. Chem. **248**, 6841—6853 (1973)

Klibansky, C., London, Y., Frenkel, A., Vries, A. de: Enhancing action of synthetic and natural basic polypeptides on erythrocyte-ghost phospholipid hydrolysis by phospholipase A. Biochim. biophys. Acta (Amst.) **150**, 15—23 (1968)

Laure, C. J.: Die Primärstruktur des Crotamins. Hoppe Seylers Z. physiol. Chem. **356**, 213—215 (1975)

Lee, C. Y.: Elapid neurotoxins and their mode of action. Clin. Toxicol. **3**, 457—472 (1970)

Lee, C. Y.: Mode of action of cobra venom and its purified toxins. In: Simpson, L. L. (Ed.): Neuropoisons: Their Pathophysiological Actions, Vol. I, pp. 21—70. New York: Plenum Press 1971

Lee, C. Y.: Chemistry and pharmacology of polypeptide toxins in snake venoms. Ann. Rev. Pharmacol. **12**, 265—286 (1972)
Lee, C. Y., Chang, C. C., Chen, Y. M.: Reversibility of neuromuscular blockade by neurotoxins from elapid and sea snake venoms. J. Formosan med. Ass. **71**, 344—349 (1972a)
Lee, C. Y., Chang, C. C., Chiu, T. H., Chiu, P. J. S., Tseng, T. C., Lee, S. Y.: Pharmacological properties of cardiotoxin isolated from Formosan cobra venom. Naunyn Schmiedebergs Arch. Pharmak. **259**, 360—374 (1968)
Lee, C. Y., Chang, S. L., Kau, S. T., Luh, S. H.: Chromatographic separation of the venom of *Bungarus multicinctus* and characterization of its components. J. Chromatog. **72**, 71—82 (1972b)
Lee, C. Y., Chen, Y. M., Karlsson, E.: Postsynaptic and musculotropic effects of notexin, a presynaptic neurotoxin from the venom of *Notechis scutatus scutatus* (Australian tiger snake). Toxicon **14**, 493—494 (1976a)
Lee, C. Y., Chen, Y. M., Mebs, D.: Chromatographic separation of the venom of *Bungarus caeruleus* and pharmacological characterization of its components. Toxicon **14**, 451—457 (1976b)
Lee, C. Y., Huang, M. C., Bonilla, C. A.: Mode of action of purified basic proteins from three rattlesnake venoms on neuromuscular junctions of the chick biventer cervicis muscle. In: Kaiser, E. (Ed.): Animal and Plant Toxins, pp. 173—178. München: Wilhelm Goldmann Verlag 1972c
Lester, H.: Dissertation, Rockefeller University, New York 1971
Leung, W. W., Keung, W. M., Kong, Y. C.: The cytolytic effect of cobra cardiotoxin on Ehrlich ascites tumor cells and its inhibition by Ca^{2+}. Naunyn Schmiedebergs Arch. Pharmacol. **292**, 193—198 (1976)
Li, C. H., Fraenkel-Conrat, H.: Electrophoresis of crotoxin. J. Amer. chem. Soc. **64**, 1586—1588 (1942)
Libelius, R.: Binding of ^{3}H-labelled cobra neurotoxin to cholinergic receptors in fast and slow mammalian muscles. J. Neural. Trans. **35**, 137—149 (1974)
Lin, J. Y., Jeng, T. W., Chen, C. C., Shi, G. Y., Tung, T. C.: Isolation of a new cardiotoxic protein from the edible mushroom, *Volvariella volvacea*. Nature (Lond.) New Biol. **246**, 524—525 (1973)
Liu, C. S., Blackwell, R. Q.: Hydrophitoxin b from *Hydrophis cyanocinctus* venom. Toxicon **12**, 543—546 (1974)
Louw, A. I.: Snake venom toxins. The purification and properties of five non-neurotoxic polypeptides from *Naja mossambica mossambica* venom. Biochim. biophys. Acta (Amst.) **336**, 470—480 (1974a)
Louw, A. I.: Snake venom toxins. The amino acid sequences of three cytotoxin homologues from *Naja mossambica mossambica* venom. Biochim. biophys. Acta (Amst.) **336**, 481—495 (1974b)
Louw, A. I.: Snake venom toxins. The complete amino acid sequence of cytotoxin V^{II}4 from the venom of *Naja naja mossambica*. Biochem. Biophys. Res. Commun. **58**, 1022—1029 (1974c)
Low, B. W., Preston, H. S., Sato, A., Rosen, L. S., Searl, J. E., Rudko, A. D., Richardson, J. S.: Three dimensional structure of erabutoxin b neurotoxic protein: Inhibitor of acetylcholine receptor. Proc. nat. Acad. Sci. (Wash.) **73**, 2991—2994 (1976)
Maeda, N., Takagi, K., Tamiya, N., Chen, Y. M., Lee, C. Y.: The isolation of an easily reversible post-synaptic toxin from the venom of a sea snake, *Laticauda semifasciata*. Biochem. J. **141**, 383—387 (1974)
Maeda, N., Tamiya, N.: The primary structure of the toxin Laticauda semifasciata III, a weak and reversibly acting neurotoxin from the venom of a sea snake, *Laticauda semifasciata*. Biochem. J. **141**, 389—400 (1974)
Maeda, N., Tamiya, N.: Isolation, properties and amino acid sequences of three neurotoxins from the venom of a sea snake, *Aipysyrus laevis*. Biochem. J. **153**, 79—87 (1976)
Maeda, N., Tamiya, N.: Correction of partial amino acid sequence of erabutoxins. Biochem. J. **167**, 289—291 (1977)
Master, R. W. P., Rao, S. S.: Identification of enzymes and toxins in venoms of Indian cobra and Russell's viper after starch gel electrophoresis. J. biol. Chem. **236**, 1986—1990 (1961)
Mebs, D.: Chemistry of animal venoms, poisons, and toxins. Experientia (Basel) **29**, 1328—1334 (1973)
Mebs, D., Narita, K., Iwanaga, S., Samejima, Y., Lee, C. Y.: Purification, properties and amino acid sequence of α-bungarotoxin from the venom of *Bungarus multicinctus*. Hoppe Seylers Z. physiol. Chem. **353**, 243—262 (1972)

Meldrum, B. S.: The actions of snake venoms on nerve and muscle. The pharmacology of phospholipase A and of polypeptide toxins. Pharmacol. Rev. **17**, 393—445 (1965)
Menez, A., Boquet, P., Fromageot, P., Tamiya, N.: On the role of tyrosyl and tryptophanyl residues in the conformation of two snake neurotoxins. Bull. Inst. Pasteur Lille **74**, 57—64 (1976)
Menez, A., Morgat, J. L., Fromageot, P., Ronsseray, A. M., Boquet, P., Changeux, J. P.: Tritium labelling of the α-neurotoxin of *Naja nigricollis*. FEBS Letters **17**, 333—335 (1971)
Miledi, R., Molinoff, P., Potter, L. T.: Isolation of the cholinergic receptor protein of *Torpedo* electric tissue. Nature (Lond.) New Biol. **229**, 554—557 (1971)
Mollay, C., Kreil, G.: Enhancement of bee venom phospholipase A_2 activity by melittin, direct lytic factor from cobra venom and polymyxin B. FEBS Letters **46**, 141—144 (1974)
Moore, S., Spackman, D. H., Stein, W. H.: Chromatography of amino acids on sulfonated polystyrene resins. An improved system. Anal. Chem. **30**, 1185—1190 (1958)
Moroz, C., Vries, A. de, Sela, M.: Isolation and characterization of a neurotoxin from *Vipera palestinae* venom. Biochim. biophys. Acta (Amst.) **124**, 136—146 (1966)
Nakai, K., Sasaki, T., Hayashi, K.: Amino acid sequence of toxin A from the venom of the Indian cobra *(Naja naja)*. Biochem. Biophys. Res. Commun. **44**, 893—897 (1971)
Narita, K., Lee, C. Y.: The amino acid sequence of cardiotoxin from Formosan cobra *(Naja naja atra)*. Biochem. Biophys. Res. Commun. **41**, 339—343 (1970)
Narita, K., Mebs, D., Iwanaga, S., Samejima, Y., Lee, C. Y.: Primary structure of α-bungarotoxin from *Bungarus multicinctus* venom. J. Formosan med. Ass. **71**, 336—343 (1972)
North, A. C. T.: Amino acid sequence and the genetic code. Nature (Lond.) New Biol. **239**, 76—77 (1972)
Obidairo, T. K., Tampitag, S., Eaker, D.: Isolation and determination of the amino acid sequence of a toxic basic phospholipase A from the venom of *Naja nigricollis*. (unpublished) (1976)
Ohta, M., Hayashi, K.: Localization of the five disulfide bridges in toxin B from the venom of the Indian cobra *(Naja naja)*. Biochem. Biophys. Res. Commun. **55**, 431—438 (1973)
Ohta, M., Hayashi, K.: Chemical modification of the tryptophan residue in toxin B from the venom of the Indian cobra. Biochem. Biophys. Res. Commun. **57**, 973—979 (1974a)
Ohta, M., Hayashi, K.: Chemical modification of the tyrosine residue in toxin B from the venom of the Indian cobra *Naja naja*. Biochem. Biophys. Res. Commun. **56**, 981—987 (1974b)
Pattabhiraman, T. R., Russell, F. E.: Isolation and purification of the toxic fraction of Mojave rattlesnake venom. Toxicon **13**, 291—294 (1975)
Peterson, E. A., Sober, H. A.: Chromatography of proteins. I. Cellulose ion-exchange adsorbents. J. Amer. chem. Soc. **78**, 751—755 (1956)
Porath, J., Flodin, P.: Gel filtration: A method for desalting and group separation. Nature (Lond.) **183**, 1657—1659 (1959)
Ragotzi, V.: Über die Wirkung des Giftes der *Naja tripudians*. Arch. path. Anat. Physiol. **122** 201—234 (1890)
Raymond, M. L., Tu, A. T.: Role of tyrosine in sea snake neurotoxin. Biochim. biophys. Acta (Amst.) **285**, 498—502 (1972)
Reid, H. A.: Myoglobinuria and sea-snake poisoning. Brit. med. J. **1**, 1284—1289 (1961)
Rochat, H., Gregoire, J., Martin-Moutot, N., Menashe, M., Kopeyan, C., Miranda, F.: Purification of animal neurotoxins: Isolation and characterization of three neurotoxins from the venom of *Naja nigricollis mossambica* Peters. FEBS Letters **42**, 335—339 (1974)
Rodríguez, O. G., Scannone, H. R.: Fractionation of *Crotalus durissus cumanensis* venom by gel filtration. Toxicon **14**, 400—403 (1976)
Rübsamen, K., Breithaupt, H., Habermann, E.: Biochemistry and pharmacology of the crotoxin complex. I. Subfractionation and recombination of the crotoxin complex. Naunyn Schmiedebergs Arch. Parmak. **270**, 274—288 (1971)
Samejima, Y., Iwanaga, S., Suzuki, T.: Complete amino acid sequence of phospholipase A_2-II isolated from *Agkistrodon halys blomhoffii* venom. FEBS Letters **47**, 348—351 (1974)
Samuelsson, G.: Mistletoe toxins. Systematic Zoology **22**, 566—569 (1973)
Sato, S., Tamiya, N.: Iodination of erabutoxin b: Diiodohistidine formation. J. Biochem. (Tokyo) **68**, 867—872 (1970)
Sato, S., Tamiya, N.: The amino acid sequences of erabutoxins, neurotoxic proteins of sea-snake *(Laticauda semifasciata)* venom. Biochem. J. **122**, 453—461 (1971)
Sen, I., Grantham, P. A., Cooper, J. R.: Mechanism of action of β-bungarotoxin on synaptosomal preparations. Proc. nat. Acad. Sci. **73**, 2664—2668 (1976)

Seto, A., Sato, S., Tamiya, N.: The properties and modification of tryptophan in sea snake toxin, erabutoxin b. Biochim. biophys. Acta (Amst.) **214**, 483—489 (1970)

Shipolini, R. A., Bailey, G. S., Banks, B. E. C.: The separation of a neurotoxin from the venom of *Naja melanoleuca* and the primary sequence determination. Europ. J. Biochem. **42**, 203—211 (1974)

Shipolini, R. A., Banks, B. E. C.: The amino acid sequence of a polypeptide from the venom of *Dendroaspis viridis*. Europ. J. Biochem. **49**, 399—405 (1974)

Sket, D., Gubenšek, F., Adamič, Š., Lebez, D.: Action of a partially purified basic protein fraction from *Vipera ammodytes* venom. Toxicon **11**, 47—53 (1973)

Slotta, K.: Chemistry and biochemistry of snake venoms. Fortschr. Chem. org. Naturst. **12**, 406—465 (1955)

Slotta, K. H., Fraenkel-Conrat, H. L.: Schlangengifte. III. Mitteil.: Reinigung und Krystallisation des Klapperschlangengiftes. Ber. dtsch. chem. Ges. **71**, 1076—1081 (1938)

Sober, H. A., Peterson, E. A.: Chromatography of proteins on cellulose ion-exchangers. J. Amer. chem. Soc. **76**, 1711—1712 (1954)

Spackman, D. H., Stein, W. H., Moore, S.: Automatic recording apparatus for use in chromatography of amino acids. Fed. Proc. **15**, 358 (1956), Anal. Chem. **30**, 1190—1206 (1958)

Strong, P. N., Goerke, J., Oberg, S. G., Kelly, R. B.: β-bungarotoxin, a pre-synaptic toxin with enzymatic activity. Proc. nat. Acad. Sci. (Wash.) **73**, 178—182 (1976)

Strydom, D. J.: Snake venom toxins. The amino acid sequences of two toxins from *Dendroaspis polylepis polylepis* (Black mamba) venom. J. biol. Chem. **247**, 4029—4042 (1972)

Strydom, D. J.: Studies on the toxins of *Dendroaspis polylepis* (Black mamba) venom. Dissertation, University of South Africa, Pretoria, 1973

Strydom, A. J. C., Botes, D. P.: Snake venom toxins. Purification, properties, and complete amino acid sequence of two toxins from ringhals *(Hemachatus haemachates)* venom. J. biol. Chem. **246**, 1341—1349 (1971)

Su, C., Chang, C. C., Lee, C. Y.: Pharmacological properties of the neurotoxin of cobra venom. In: Russell, F. E., Saunders, P. R. (Eds.): Animal Toxins, pp. 259—267. Oxford-New York: Pergamon 1967

Takahashi, K.: The reaction of phenylglyoxal with arginine residues in proteins. J. biol. Chem. **243**, 6171—6179 (1968)

Takechi, M., Hayashi, K., Sasaki, T.: The amino acid sequence of cytotoxin II from the venom of the Indian cobra *(Naja naja)*. Mol. Pharmacol. **8**, 446—451 (1972)

Tamiya, N.: Erabutoxins a, b, and c in sea snake *Laticauda semifasciata* venom. Toxicon **11**, 95—97 (1973)

Tamiya, N., Abe, H.: The isolation, properties, and amino acid sequence of erabutoxin c, a minor neurotoxic component of the venom of a sea snake *Laticauda semifasciata*. Biochem. J. **130**, 547—555 (1972)

Tamiya, N., Arai, H.: Studies on sea-snake venoms. Crystallization of erabutoxins a and b from *Laticauda semifasciata* venom. Biochem. J. **99**, 624—630 (1966)

Tazieff-Depierre, F., Czajka, M., Lowagie, C.: Action pharmacologique des fractions pures de venin de *Naja nigricollis* et liberation de calcium dans les muscles striés. C.R. Acad. Sci. [D] (Paris) **268**, 2511—2514 (1969)

Tazieff-Depierre, F., Pierre, J.: Action curarisante de la toxine α de *Naja nigricollis*. C.R. Acad. Sci. [D] (Paris) **263**, 1785—1788 (1966)

Tsernoglou, D., Petsko, G. A.: The crystal structure of a post-synaptic neurotoxin from sea snake at 2.2 Å resolution. FEBS Letters **68**, 1—4 (1976)

Tsetlin, V. I., Mikhaleva, I. I., Myagkova, M. A., Senyavina, L. B., Arseniev, A. S., Ivanov, V. T., Ovchinnikov, Yü. A.: Synthetic and conformational studies of the neurotoxins and cytotoxins of snake venom. In: Walter, R., Meienhofer, J. (Eds.): Peptides: Chemistry, Structure, and Biology. Proc. 4th American Peptide Symposium, pp. 935—941. Ann Arbor (Michigan): Ann Arbor Science Publ. 1975

Tu, A. T.: Neurotoxins of animal venoms: snakes. Ann. Rev. Biochem. **42**, 235—258 (1973)

Tu, A. T., Lin, T. S., Bieber, A. L.: Purification and chemical characterization of the major neurotoxin from the venom of *Pelamis platurus*. Biochemistry **14**, 3408—3413 (1975)

Uthe, J. F., Magee, W. L.: Phospholipase A_2: Action on purified phospholipids as affected by deoxycholate and divalent cations. Canad. J. Biochem. **49**, 776—784 (1971)

Viljoen, C. C., Botes, D. P.: Snake venom toxins. The purification and amino acid sequence of toxin F_{VII} from *Dendroaspis angusticeps* venom. J. biol. Chem. **248**, 4915—4919 (1973)
Viljoen, C. C., Botes, D. P.: Snake venom toxins. The purification and amino acid sequence of toxin Ta2 from *Dendroaspis angusticeps* venom. J. biol. Chem. **249**, 366—372 (1974)
Vincent, J. P., Schweitz, H., Chicheportiche, R., Fosset, M., Balerna, M., Lenoir, M. C., Lazdunski, M.: Molecular mechanism of cardiotoxin action on axonal membranes. Biochemistry **15**, 3171—3175 (1976)
Vogt, W., Patzer, P., Lege, L., Oldings, H. D., Wille, G.: Synergism between phospholipase A and various peptides and SH-reagents in causing haemolysis. Naunyn Schmiedebergs Arch. Pharmak. **265**, 442—454 (1970)
Volwerk, J. J., Pieterson, W. A., Haas, G. H. de: Histidine at the active site of phospholipase A_2. Biochemistry **13**, 1446—1454 (1974)
Wahlström, A.: Purification and characterization of phospholipase A from the venom of *Naja nigricollis*. Toxicon **9**, 45—56 (1971)
Wang, C. L., Liu, C. S., Hung, Y. O., Blackwell, R. Q.: Amino acid sequence of pelamitoxin a, the main neurotoxin of the sea snake *Pelamis platurus*. Toxicon **14**, 459—466 (1976)
Weber, M., Changeux, J. P.: Binding of *Naja nigricollis* (^{3}H)α-toxin to membrane fragments from *Electrophorus* and *Torpedo* electric organs. I. Binding of the tritiated α-neurotoxin in the absence of effector. Mol. Pharmacol. **10**, 1—14 (1974)
Wernicke, J. F., Oberjat, T., Howard, B. D.: The mechanism of action of β-bungarotoxin. J. Neurochem. **22**, 781—788 (1974)
Wolfenden, R. N.: On the nature and action of the venom of poisonous snakes. I. The venom of the Indian cobra *(Naja tripudians)*. J. Physiol. (Lond.) **7**, 327—356 (1886)
Yang, C. C.: Crystallization and properties of cobrotoxin from Formosan cobra venom. J. biol. Chem. **240**, 1616—1618 (1965)
Yang, C. C.: The disulfide bonds of cobrotoxin and their relationship to lethality. Biochim. biophys. Acta (Amst.) **133**, 346—355 (1966)
Yang, C. C.: Chemistry and evolution of toxins in snake venoms. Toxicon **12**, 1—43 (1974)
Yang, C. C., Yang, H. J., Chiu, R. H. C.: The position of disulfide bonds in cobrotoxin. Biochim. biophys. Acta (Amst.) **214**, 355—363 (1970)
Yang, C. C., Yang, H. J., Huang, J. S.: The amino acid sequence of cobrotoxin. Biochim. biophys. Acta (Amst.) **188**, 65—77 (1969)
Yang, C. C., Chang, C. C., Liou, I. F.: Studies on the status of arginine residues in cobrotoxin. Biochim. biophys. Acta (Amst.) **365**, 1—14 (1974)
Zlotkin, E.: Chemistry of animal venoms. Experientia (Basel) **29**, 1453—1466 (1973)

CHAPTER 6

The Three-Dimensional Structure of Postsynaptic Snake Neurotoxins: Consideration of Structure and Function

BARBARA W. LOW

A. Introduction

The structural expression of function in biological systems is three-dimensional at all levels of resolutions. In interactions between single molecules, for examples, between deoxyhemoglobin and oxygen, or between enzymes and their substrates, the relative geometric positioning of the specific groups of atoms and their distances from each other is critical as measured in Ångstroms (10^{-8} cm; 0.10 nm) or tenths of an Ångstrom. The proper articulation of the wrist depends on the size, shape, orientation, and placement of more gross segments, but the principle holds. Furthermore, interactions at all levels from macroscopic to molecular are recognized as frequently involving favorable geometric repositioning; that is, in molecular interactions, shifts from inactive to active conformations as, for example, the 12 Å shift of the phenolic OH which accompanies the flip-over swing of Tyr 248 in carboxypeptidase A when substrate binds to enzyme (QUIOCHO and LIPSCOMB, 1971). These shifts may be induced in one molecule by the proximity of another with which it interacts.

The three-dimensional structure of erabutoxin b, a postsynaptic neurotoxin in the venom of the sea snake *Laticauda semifasciata* (ARAI et al., 1964; TAMIYA and ARAI, 1966; SATO and TAMIYA, 1971; MAEDA and TAMIYA, 1977), has recently been established (LOW et al., 1976a, b; LOW, 1976a, b). This is the first detailed information about the stereochemistry of a protein involved in neurological function. It provides a basis for prime questions about function to be asked in three-dimensional terms, even though these cannot yet be completely answered, nor plausible mechanisms proposed, until the structure of the receptor protein/neurotoxin complex, or at least of the receptor protein alone, has been determined.

If the structure of only one neurotoxin, erabutoxin b, had been established in isolation, the significant features of the three-dimensional arrangement would have been essentially concealed. Fortunately, erabutoxin b may be considered a prototype postsynaptic snake neurotoxin. The findings from extensive chemical (sequence) studies of almost 50 different neurotoxins with a common mode of action from the venoms of both land and sea snakes in the families *Elapidae* and *Hydrophiidae* have established multiple sequence homologies. Indeed these postsynaptic neurotoxins constitute the largest homologous series of nonpathological proteins of common function yet studied. Physicochemical studies of toxins in solution [using optical rotatory dispersion (ORD), circular dichroism (CD), and laser-Raman techniques] have suggested common features of backbone chain conformation. Once the common features of many members of one class are identified, attention can be appropriately focused. Thus, one or more side chain group(s) identified as invariant or conservatively substituted are either absent on occasion or have been studied by chemical modification and the consequent effects on toxicity, immunological characteristics, and the in vitro conformation determined. We are now in a position to correlate chemical and stereochemical information.

The postsynaptic snake venom neurotoxins produce a nondepolarizing neuromuscular block. These single-chain basic proteins are thus curare-like in mode of action; they bind to nicotinic receptor in the postsynaptic membrane; acetylcholine release into the synapse is not inhibited but its binding to the receptor is blocked (CHANG and LEE, 1963; TAMIYA and ARAI, 1966; SATO et al., 1970; CHANGEUX et al., 1970, 1971; MILEDI et al., 1971; RAFTERY et al., 1971; HALL, 1972; LEE, 1972). These neurotoxins, as competitive binding studies have shown (WEBER and CHANGEUX, 1974), must at least make inaccessible, and probably occupy, the normal acetylcholine binding sites. The dissociation constant for acetylcholine binding is approximately 10^{-7} M; the dissociation constants of the neurotoxins lie within the range $5.7–8.2 \times 10^{-10}$ M (see KARLSSON, p. 116) to 2×10^{-11} M (WEBER and CHANGEUX, 1974). Acetylcholine produces depolarization of the postsynaptic membrane, a brief change in permeability which permits ion diffusion through the membrane. Following this transient effect, acetylcholine is then de-esterified by acetylcholine esterase. If, therefore, acetylcholine binding permits ion transport by inducing a conformational change in the receptor which opens channels in the membrane, then binding by nondepolarizing neurotoxins either inhibits such conformational changes or blocks any channels which may be opened.

Acetylcholine receptor is an oligomeric protein and extensive studies have been made of its subunit composition (KARLIN et al., 1975; KLETT et al., 1973; BIESECKER, 1973; RAFTERY et al., 1975; WEILL et al., 1974; ELDEFRAWI et al., 1975). Depending on the source, it has been shown that there are three or four different kinds of subunits (KARLIN et al., 1975; KARLIN, A., 1977). KARLIN has estimated that there are from two to four toxin-binding sites per receptor molecule. The models which have been invoked in discussing the function of cholinergic receptor, both in response to agonist and to antagonist (CHANGEUX et al., 1975; MAELICKE and REICH, 1975), consider the equilibria between different states of receptor as characterized by conformational changes either in receptor or toxin or both. No experimental findings require conformational flexibility of the toxins, although this is clearly not ruled out.

In order to discuss structure-function relationships in these neurotoxins we shall (Sect. B) describe first the three-dimensional structure of erabutoxin b considered as a protein without special emphasis on its functional role. This preliminary account will include discussion of the primary sequence of erabutoxin b and of other short chain toxins. The common and divergent features of the sequences of both classes of snake venom neurotoxins will then be presented. An account of the chemistry and chemical modification studies of neurotoxins will follow, principally directed towards the identification of those common residues which are implicated in neurotoxic activity either: a) because they play an essentially structural role, that is, they maintain the necessary and appropriate spatial relationships within the molecule (disulfide linkages are a prime example of this group); or b) because they appear to be directly involved in binding to the receptor, i.e., the toxic activity is reduced when they are modified even though the modification is not accompanied by gross structural (i.e., conformational) change.

Physicochemical studies which provide evidence concerning backbone chain conformation and the results of theoretical and model structures in the neurotoxins will be briefly considered. Other X-ray crystallographic studies of neurotoxins will be described.

In Section C the three-dimensional structure of erabutoxin b will be reexamined in terms of all information pertinent to the questions: 1. How appropriate is it to consider the erabutoxin b structure as a prototype model for both classes of neurotoxins? 2. Do the sequence homologies and chemical studies permit the reactive site to be recognized and its properties explored?

Section D will provide a summary and we shall there consider those questions which this new knowledge permits us to ask, and the ways in which these questions might be explored and answers sought.

B. The Postsynaptic Neurotoxins; Survey of Three-Dimensional Prototype Structure; Deviant Toxins, Chemical Modification Studies Preliminary Review

Erabutoxin b is one of three postsynaptic neurotoxins in the venom of the sea snake *Laticauda semifasciata*. It has 62 amino acid residues and four disulfide linkages, and thus belongs to the short chain class of snake toxins (62-4 in the KARLSSON terminology). The erabutoxins a and c are respectively Asn 26 and Asn 51 single residue substituted variants of erabutoxin b. The three toxins are found in the venom in the average approximate ratios 9:10:1 (TAMIYA, 1973). The isoelectric points are all above pH 9.2, and the molecular weights are 6838(a), 6861(b), and 6847(c).

I. Primary Sequence of Erabutoxin b

The residue sequence[1] of erabutoxin b (SATO and TAMIYA, 1971) is shown in Figure 1. The toxin belongs to the short chain toxin series 60↔62-4 to which, with one exception, all sea snake venom toxins so far isolated belong. The drawing shows the four invariant disulfide bridges in positions 3-24, 17-41, 43-54, and 55-60 (using the erabutoxin sequence enumeration). These positions correspond to 3-24, 17-45, 49-61, and 62-68 using the KARLSSON sequence enumeration[2], which orders all neurotoxin sequence alignments by putting the half cystines in register and thus preserving maximum homology in both short chain 60↔62-4 and long chain 66-5 and 71↔74-5 series.

[1] The sequence 21, 22 has been corrected to Glu.Ser to conform with results of further chemical studies (MAEDA and TAMIYA, 1977). The side chain order of the present revised sequence fits much better with the electron density distribution. The correction was not made when the results were first published (LOW et al., 1976a) because of the possibility of local map error.

[2] This enumeration unfortunately fails to assert the correct invariant length of the two closed loops 43-54 (49-61) and 55-60 (62-68). None of the toxins has residues at either KARLSSON position 54 or 65. These were left open to accomodate insertions in two non-neurotoxin venom proteins which in disulfide linkage placements and other features are, together with the membrane toxins, homologous with the postsynaptic neurotoxins (KARLSSON, p. 169 and p. 189).

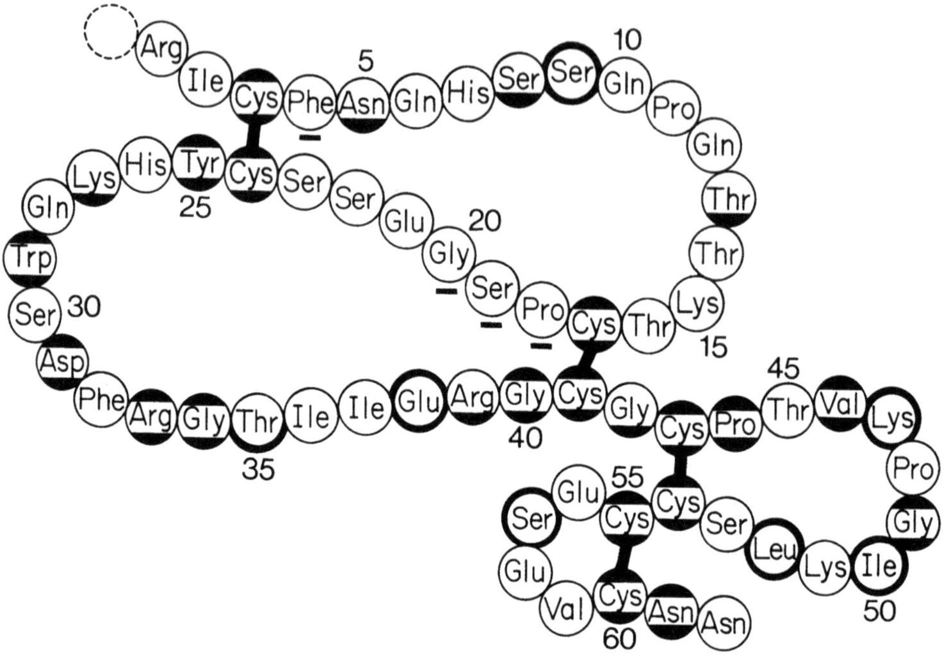

Fig. 1. Amino acid residue sequence of erabutoxin b[1] (SATO and TAMIYA, 1971), a short chain neurotoxin. The invariant residue positions found in both series of toxins are shown, emphasized by black caps top and bottom. The short chain invariants are emphasized by a black cap in the lower segment. Positions of conservative substitution in both series of toxins are shown with a heavy broader outline. Conservative substitution in the short chain series is shown with a heavy lower semicircular outline. Horizontal lines under residues indicate observed deletion positions *in the short chain series only*. The position of the N terminal extension in some 60–4 toxins is shown by a broken circle. [After Figure 1 of Low et al. Three-dimensional structure of erabutoxin b neurotoxic protein: Inhibitor of acetylcholine receptor. Proc. nat. Acad. Sci. (Wash.) **73**, 2991 (1976). The sequence 21.22 has been corrected to conform to further chemical studies (MAEDA and TAMIYA, 1977). The side chain fit of the revised sequence accords better with the electron density map]

II. Three-Dimensional Structure of Erabutoxin b

1. Molecular Size and Shape

Early studies (Low et al., 1971) of erabutoxin b crystals suggested that the molecule was disk shaped. It is an elongated concave disk or, more precisely, shallow saucer with footed stand, and fits into an ellipsoidal envelope approximately 38 Å × 28 Å × 15 Å. The molecular outline in projection is shown in Fig. 2, the intermolecular packing diagram for erabutoxin b projected down the c axis in the crystal structure. The inset drawings show the peptide chain wrap-up of the molecule: In the left-hand inset this is represented schematically as a continuous line, while in the right-hand inset the chain is outlined through the positions of adjacent α carbon atoms. The projected outlines emphasize the presence of a central core cluster of disulfide linkages from which emerge the three chain loops, residues 3-17, 24-41, and

[1] The Karlsson sequence enumeration is not used in this drawing.

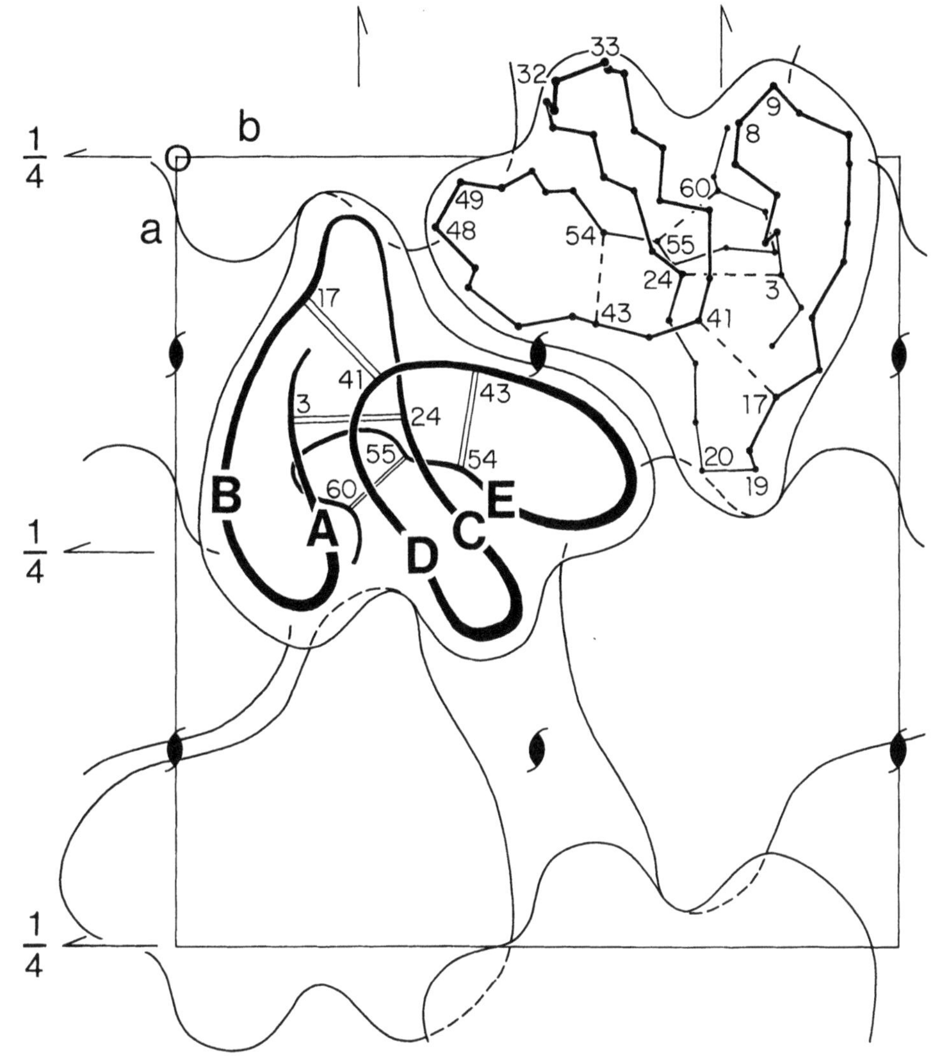

Fig. 2. Intermolecular packing diagram for erabutoxin b seen projected down the c axis. The left-hand inset drawing shows schematically the chain conformation and the disulfide bridge positions. The five β strands of the antiparallel pleated sheet are identified by the letters A, B, C, D, and E, following chain sequence order. The right-hand inset drawing shows the projected skeletal structure of a second erabutoxin b molecule related by a twofold screw axis parallel to c. Only α-carbon positions and disulfide bridges are shown. The erabutoxin enumeration of some positions, including the two central residue positions of four of the β turns are inserted. [Modified drawing after Figure 2 of Low et al. Three-dimensional structure of erabutoxin b neurotoxic protein: Inhibitor of acetylcholine receptor. Proc. nat. Acad. Sci. (Wash.) **73**, 2991 (1976)]

43-54, to form the broad lobes of the molecular outline. A short turn 17-23 forms the tapered neck region of the molecule. The long central loop is markedly foreshortened in this projection; all three loops emerge as broad fronds from the disulfide core. The projection drawings show that the molecule is unusually open, the neck and saucer regions being the thickness of only one peptide chain which loops back on itself in

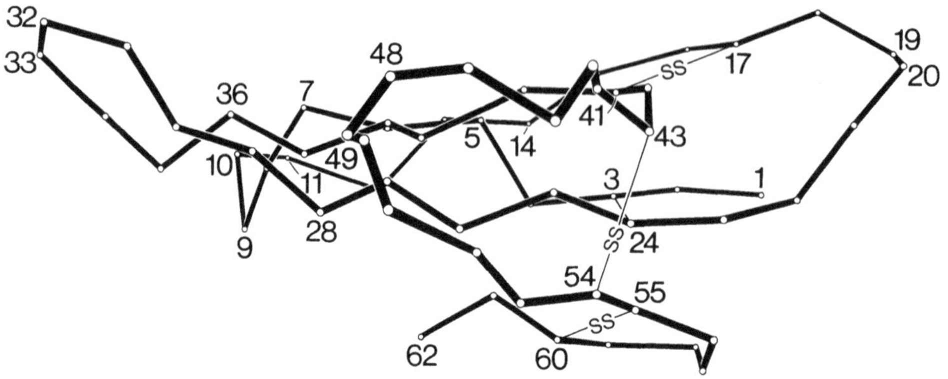

Fig. 3. The structure of erabutoxin b. Only α-carbon positions and disulfide bridges are shown. The residue positions enumerated are either half-cystines or indicate chain continuity and/or β turns. [After Figure 3 of Low et al. Three-dimensional structure of erabutoxin b neurotoxic protein: Inhibitor of acetylcholine receptor. Proc. nat. Acad. Sci. (Wash.) **73**, 2991 (1976)]

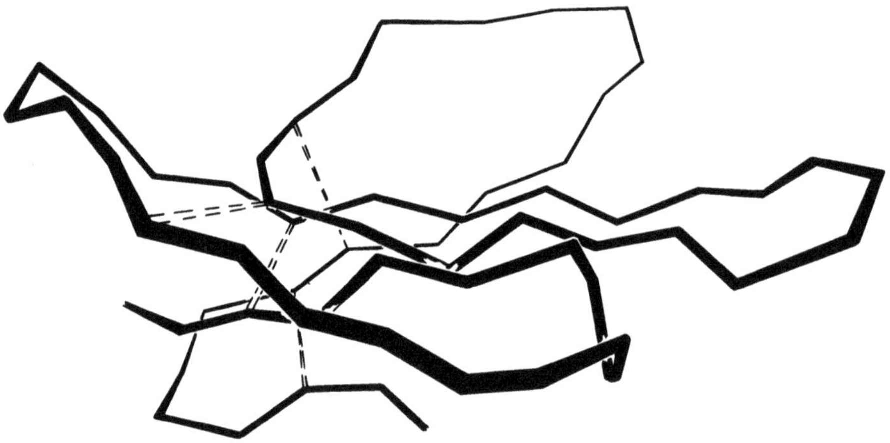

Fig. 4. Freehand sketch of erabutoxin b structure drawn from wire model bent at alpha carbon positions. Double broken lines indicate the disulfide linkages. The tapered neck region lies to the left of the disulfide core. The two lobes of the reactive site are the long central loop and the background ring. The drawing shows the shallow curve of the β sheet B.A.D.C.E. (front to back) and the steeply banked rim of the reactive site. The "stand" formed by the terminal six-membered ring lies under the disulfide core

the saucer to form a shell with residues bristling out. There is little "interior" in this molecule where side chain groups are completely buried and inaccessible to solvent. Chemical studies have shown relative inaccessibility of some side chains, e.g., Tyr 25 which lies deep in the hollow concavity of the molecule.

Peptide chain overlap occurs in the disulfide core region and near the termini where the six-membered ring 55-60 lies under the N-terminal segment. A side view of the molecular skeleton (Fig. 3) illustrates the molecular shape although it distorts into prominence the short tapered neck region of the molecule occupied by residues 17-23. It also fails to show clearly the sweep of the longest chain loop of residues 24-

41 and the "barrelling" curve of all three loops which sweeps down toward the β strand 54-49 and is sharply banked by the rim of segment 42-48. This can be seen in the freehand sketch (Fig. 4) made from a wire model of the molecule bent at the α carbon atom positions.

2. Backbone Chain Conformation in the Erabutoxin Molecule

The two principle backbone chain conformations found in globular proteins are the α helix and β pleated sheet. The reader is reminded that in both α helix and β pleated sheet the amide NH and carbonyl C=O of each peptide unit are hydrogen bonded to other peptide groups so that the maximum possible number of equivalent–C=O ···H–N– hydrogen bonds are formed. Whereas in the α helix hydrogen bonds are near neighbor and intrachain, in the β pleated sheet they may be inter- or intrachain. If the latter, they may be between intrachain regions which are close together or far removed in sequence.

There are no regions of α helix in erabutoxin b. There is an extensive twisted antiparallel β pleated sheet of five strands with alternate strands pointing in opposite directions (the forward direction points along the sequence from the N terminal end in the usual convention). The chain regions marked in Fig. 2, B, A, D, C, and E, form the strands of the sheet which is the curved surface of the saucer. In the extended parallel and antiparallel pleated sheet arrays found in fibrous proteins and proposed theoretically (see DICKERSON and GEIS, 1969), the sheet is essentially planar. In globular proteins the sheets are usually twisted and curve into a barrel. The orientation of the strands A, D, and C is clearly β pleated sheet even as seen in projection. The loop which forms the crossover connection joining βD and βE strands is right-handed (RICHARDSON, 1976). The β sheet emerges from the core disulfide region and hangs from it as a cupped hand from the wrist.

There are 31[1] residues, i.e., 50% of the structure in this sheet, with strand lengths βB 11-15, βA 3-8, βD 34-40, βC 24-31, and βE 51-55 (KARLSSON 11-15, 3-8, 38-44, 24-31, and 58-62). A schematic representation of the antiparallel β pleated sheet structure in this molecule is shown in Fig. 5, and Fig. 6 shows the hydrogen bonding in some regions of the sheet (LOW et al., 1976 b). The side chain groups along the β sheet strands point alternatively up and above, or down and below the sheet surface. Because of the interstrand hydrogen bonds the sheet is essentially a carapace. Side chains which point down are accessible to solvent or solute from below, those which point up into the concavity of the saucer are accessible from above. The sheet is truly a continuum and not penetrable by water even in those regions where hydrogen bonding is weak. This property of the sheet is one to which we shall return later in the discussion of function (LOW, 1976 b).

There are five turns in the erabutoxin b molecule where the peptide chain abruptly changes direction: between β strands A and B, β strands C and D, β strand E and the chain segment 42-48, in the tapered neck region 17-23, and finally through the closed six-membered ring Cys 55-Cys 60. These are between residues 7-10 (A→B), 31-34 (C→D), 47-50, 18-21, and 57-60 (LOW et al., 1976 a, b). The chain

---

[1] Some of the β strand lengths as reported here are slightly longer than the earlier minimal values (LOW et al., 1976 a, b).

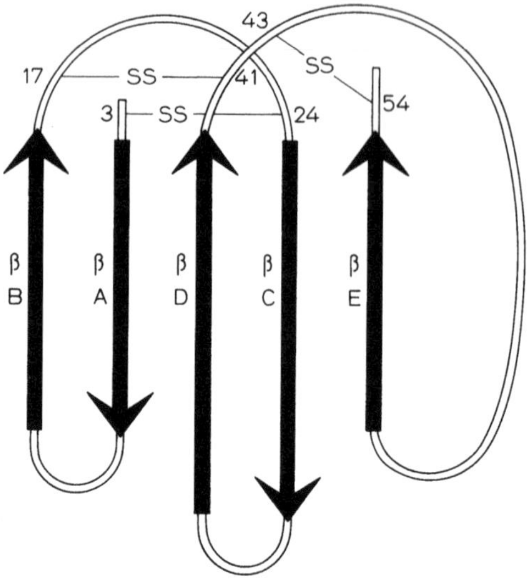

Fig. 5. Schematic representation of the antiparallel β pleated sheet structure in erabutoxin b. The strands are joined by disulfide bridges as shown. [Modified drawing after Figure 4, Low et al. Three-dimensional structure of erabutoxin b neurotoxic protein: Inhibitor of acetylcholine receptor. Proc. nat. Acad. Sci. (Wash.) **73**, 2991 (1976)]

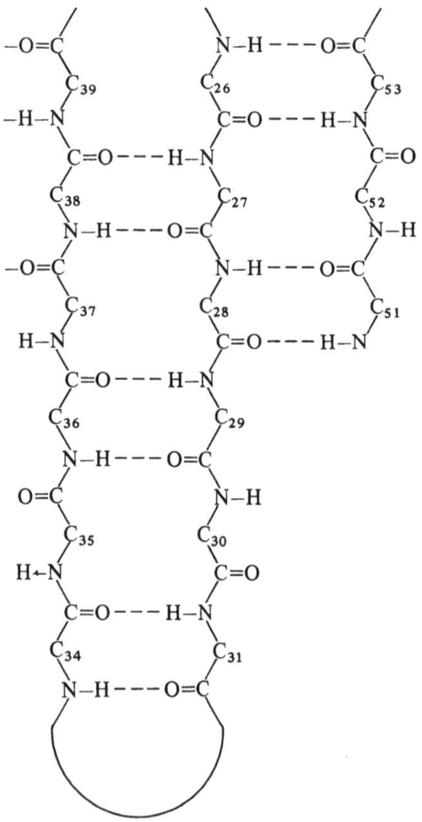

Fig. 6. A part of the hydrogen bonding between D.C.E. β strands of the reactive site (erabutoxin b) (Low et al. 1976b)

loops back on itself in all these regions through β turns; a four residue conformation with a hydrogen bond linking the carbonyl C=O of the first and the amide NH of the fourth residue (VENKATACHALAM, 1968).

III. Residue Sequences: Invariant and Conservative Substitutions in the Long and Short Chain Series of Neurotoxins

In both long and short chain series of neurotoxins (see Table 1) there are: a) positions of absolute residue invariance, the eight half-cystine positions providing prime examples of this group; b) positions of residue invariance with deviations in a few toxins which may or may not be accompanied by reduced levels of toxicity (e.g., Asp 31 or Val 52); c) positions of complete conservative substitution, e.g., position 59 (i.e., erabutoxin b 52) always occupied by a bulky hydrophobic (aliphatic) residue; and d) positions of conservative substitution with occasional deviations which may or may not be accompanied by reduced toxicity (e.g., Ser/Thr 9 or Val/Ile 57). We emphasize that the expression "conservative substitution" is used here to describe conservation of residue type which may or may not have functional significance. (In the serine proteases it is not simply an aliphatic hydroxyl group, but serine which is necessary). The short chain toxins considered separately also show special positions listed in Table 1b; they all have a two residue tail. The 61-4 and 60-4 toxins are

Table 1. [a]Neurotoxins: Invariant Residues and Conservative Substitutions[b]

a) Both Long and Short Series

3	9**	17	24	25	29*	31*	37	38
.. Cys	Ser/Thr	Cys	Cys	Tyr ...	Trp .	Asp	Arg	Gly ...

42	44	45	49	50	52*	53**	56*	57**	59
Glu/Asp .	Gly	Cys ...	Cys	Pro .	Val	Lys/Arg ..	Gly	Val/Ile .	Ile/Leu Val

61	62	64**	68	69*
. Cys	Cys .	Thr/Ser ...	Cys	Asn .... —

* Deviations from invariance (maximum 3)	Toxicity LD_{50}
29 a) Oxidized Trp in *Dendroaspis viridis*: toxin 4.7.3	900 µg/kg
31 a) Asn in *Laticauda semifasciata*: toxin Ls III	850 µg/kg
b) Gly in *Naja haje annulifera*: toxin CM-10	5000 µg/kg
c) Gly in *Naja haje annulifera*: toxin CM-12	62500 µg/kg
52 a) Lys in *Bungarus multicinctus*: α-bungarotoxin	
56 a) Tyr in *Bungarus multicinctus*: α-bungarotoxin	
b) Tyr in *Naja naja oxiana*: toxin I	560 µg/kg
c) Tyr in *Naja melanoleuca*: toxin 3.9.4	
69 a) Asp in *Dendroaspis viridis*: toxin 4.7.3	900 µg/kg
b) Asp in *Dendroaspis viridis*: toxin 4.9.3	160 µg/kg
c) Asp in *Dendroaspis polylepis polylepis*: toxin γ	

[a] Wherever toxicities are not cited they fall within the normal range.
[b] Karlsson enumeration employed throughout.

Table 1 cont.

** Deviations from conservative substitutions (maximum 4)

9 a) Pro in *Naja naja oxiana*: toxin I . . . . 560 μg/kg
b) Leu in *Laticauda semifasciata*: toxin Ls III . . . . 850 μg/kg
c) Leu in *Naja haje annulifera*: toxin CM-10 . . . . 5000 μg/kg
d) Leu in *Naja haje annulifera*: toxin CM-12 . . . . 62500 μg/kg
53 a) Asn in *Laticauda semifasciata*: toxin Ls III . . . . 850 μg/kg
b) Glu in *Naja naja oxiana*: toxin I . . . . 560 μg/kg
57 a) Glu in *Bungarus multicinctus*: α-bungarotoxin
b) Gln in *Naja naja oxiana*: toxin I . . . . 560 μg/kg
c) Glu in *Naja melanoleuca*: toxin 3.9.4
d) Thr in *Laticauda semifasciata*: toxin Ls III . . . . 850 μg/kg
64 a) Arg in *Naja nivea*: toxin α
b) Ala in *Laticauda semifasciata*: toxin Ls III . . . . 850 μg/kg

b) Short Neurotoxins Only

5* 8 13* 21 27* 39** 43 48

.... [Asn] .. [Ser] .... [Thr] ... (Glu/Asp) ... [Lys] ... (Thr/Ser) ... [Arg] .... [Gly] ...... —

* Deviations from invariance (maximum 2) Toxicity LD_{50}

5 a) Lys in *Naja haje annulifera*: toxin CM-10 . . . . 5000 μg/kg
b) Lys in *Naja haje annulifera*: toxin CM-12 . . . . 62500 μg/kg
13 a) Ile in *Naja haje annulifera*: toxin CM-10 . . . . 5000 μg/kg
b) Ile in *Naja haje annulifera*: toxin CM-12 . . . . .625000 μg/kg
27 a) Met in *Aipysurus laevis*: toxin b

** Deviation from conservative substitutions (maximum 2).

39 a) Tyr in *Naja naja atra*: cobrotoxin

c) Long Neurotoxins Only

18* 20 23 26* 30 34 39 41** 43*

—.... [Pro] . [Gly] .. (Ile/Val Leu) .. [Thr] ... [Cys] ... [Cys] .... [Lys] . (Val/Ile Leu) . [Leu]

46* 47 48 63 66 72*

.. [Ala] [Ala] [Thr] .... [Ser] .. [Asp] ..... [Pro] ......

* Deviations from invariance (maximum 2)

18 a) Ala in *Naja naja oxiana*: toxin I . . . . 560 μg/kg
b) Ala in *Naja melanoleuca*: toxin b
26 a) Arg in *Bungarus multicinctus*: α-bungarotoxin
b) Val in *Laticauda semifasciata*: toxin Ls III . . . . 850 μg/kg
43 a) Phe in *Laticauda semifasciata*: toxin Ls III . . . . 850 μg/kg
46 a) Val in *Naja melanoleuca*: toxin 3.9.4
72 a) Gln in *Dendroaspis polylepis polylepis*: toxin γ
b) Lys in *Dendroaspis polylepis polylepis*: toxin δ

** Deviation from conservative substitutions (maximum 2)

41 a) Glu in *Dendroaspis viridis*: toxin 4.7.3 . . . . 900 μg/kg
b) Glu in *Dendroaspis viridis*: toxin 4.9.3 . . . . 160 μg/kg

---

[ ] Invariant Residue. ( ) Conservative Substitution.

Normal toxicity range . . . . .50–150 μg/kg.

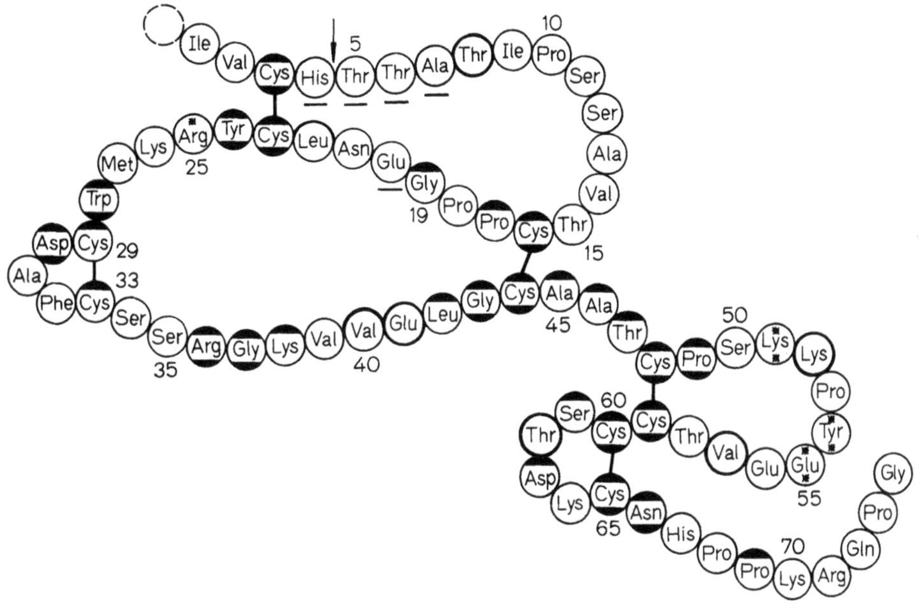

Fig. 7. Amino acid residue sequence of α bungarotoxin[1] (Mebs et al., 1971, 1972). The invariant residue positions found in both series of toxins are shown emphasized by black caps top and bottom. The long chain invariants are emphasized by a black cap in the upper segment. Positions of conservative substitution in both series of toxins are shown with a heavy broader outline. Conservative substitutions in the long chain series are shown with a heavy upper semicircular outline. Horizontal lines under residues indicate observed deletion positions in the long chain series only. The single possible insertion position is shown with an arrow ↓. The deviation (Arg 25) from the normal long chain invariant Thr 26 (listed in Table 1c) is shown with an asterisk in the upper segment. The deviations (Lys 51, Tyr 54, and Glu 55) from the normal (Karlsson) invariants Val 52 and Gly 56 and conservative substitution Val/Ile 57 (see Table 1a) are shown with asterisks top and bottom.

related to the 62-4 toxins by deletion of one or more residues in positions 4, 18, 19, and 20, or by a single extension at the N terminal end in some 60-4 toxins. All special positions common to both classes of neurotoxins and to short chain toxins alone are shown in Figure 1.

The most striking features of the long chain series are: a) the presence of a fifth invariant disulfide linkage Cys 30–Cys 34 which forms a pentapeptide loop, and b) a long tail segment of eight, nine (most common), or ten residues following the last disulfide linkage which contrasts with the two residue tail of the short chain toxins. The primary sequence of one long chain toxin, *α-bungarotoxin*, is shown in Figure 7 where the positions of residue invariants and conservative substitutions in all neurotoxins and in the long chain series alone are identified.

The sequences of fewer long chain (19) than short chain (26) toxins have been determined. This may be partially responsible for the greater number of invariant residues or residue types found in the former. Some special positions in long chain toxins (see Table 1c) are conserved in at least a majority of short chain toxins and

[1] The Karlsson sequence enumeration is not used in this drawing.

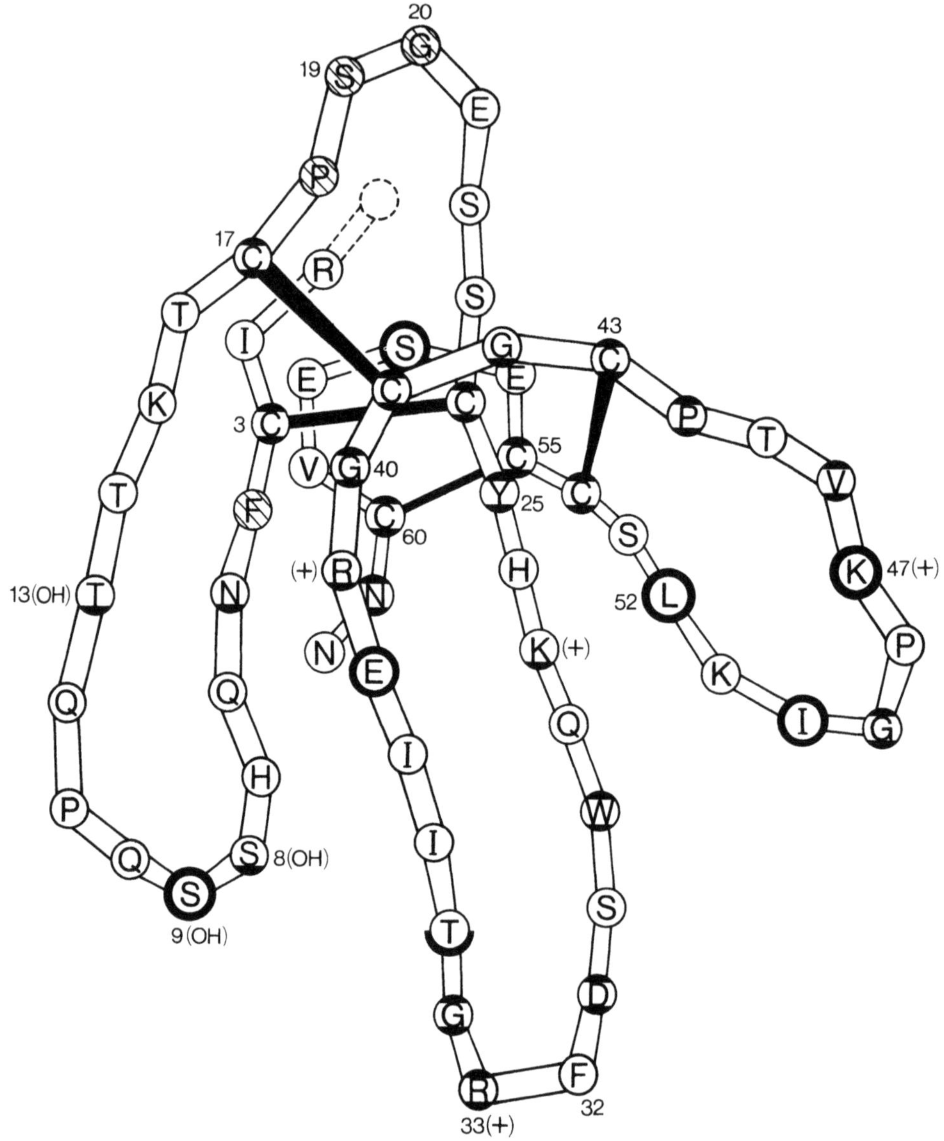

Fig. 8a. View (partially schematic) of the erabutoxin b[1] molecule shown looking down into the concavity. The invariant residue positions found in both series of toxins are shown emphasized by black caps top and bottom. The short chain invariants are emphasized by a black cap in the lower segment. Positions of conservative substitution in both series of toxins are shown with a heavy broader outline. Conservative substitutions in the short chain series are shown with a heavy lower semicircular outline. Deletion positions found in the short chain toxins are shown hatched. The position of the N terminal extension in some 60–4 toxins is shown by a broken circle. In either both or short chain series alone, the Ser and/or Ser/Thr special positions are shown as (OH); the Arg, Lys, and/or Lys/Arg are shown as (+)

[1] The Karlsson sequence enumeration is not used in this drawing.

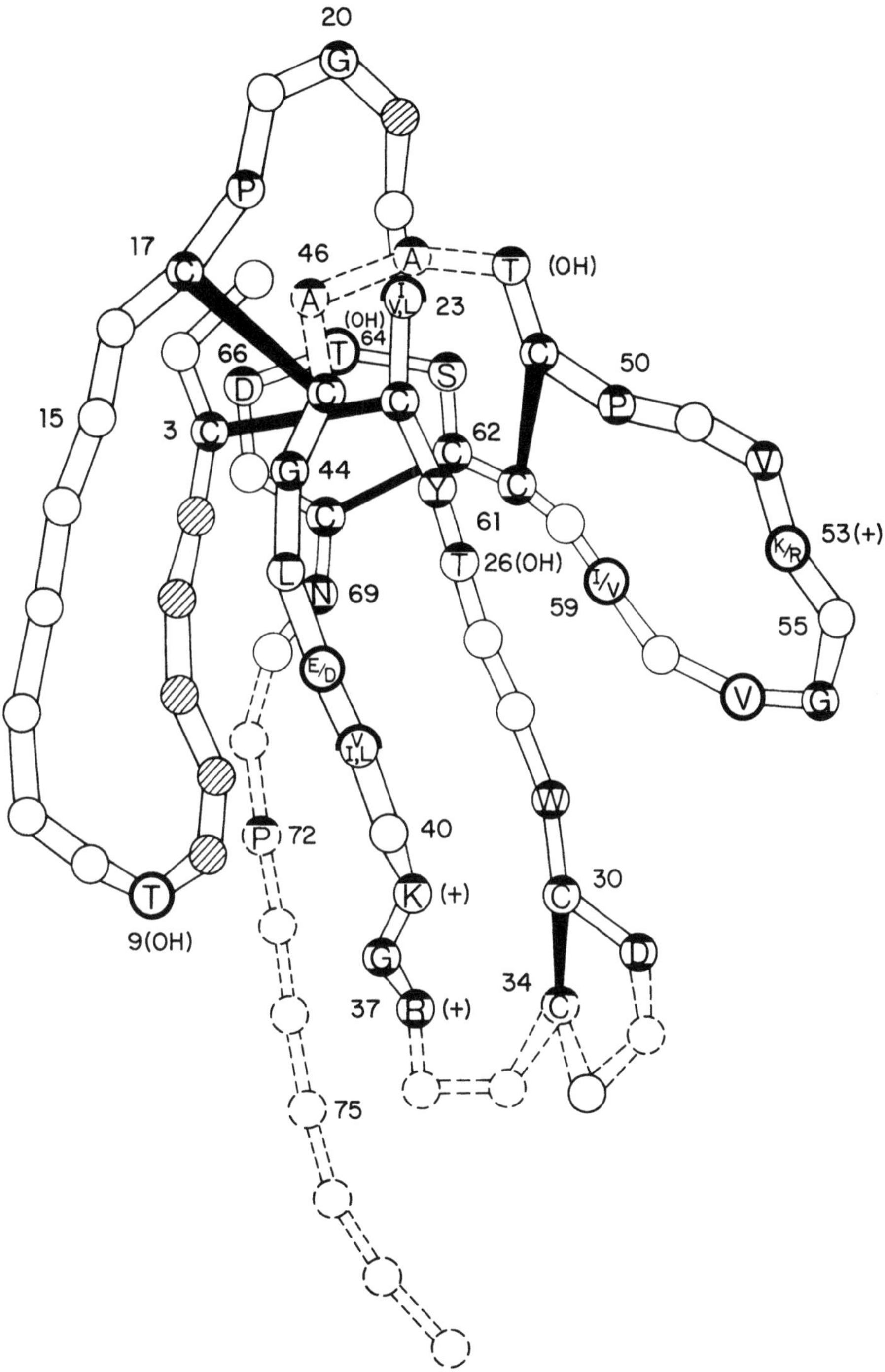

Fig. 8 b. (Legend see page 226)

vice versa. Thus in the short chain series position 18 is usually Pro; position 20 always Gly (when present), position 41 usually Ile, and position 66 often Asp. Similarly, the short chain near invariant (Table 1b) Lys 27 is, with only four exceptions, usually Lys in the long chain series. On the other hand, in the short chain series position 23 is usually Ser/Asn, position 26 usually Lys, and position 63 highly variable. The matched sites 39, 43, and 48 also show very different patterns of invariance between the two toxins. Short chain sites 8 and 13 are nonconservative in the long toxins.

Some substitution positions are radically nonconservative in both series, e.g., site 60 which may be Thr, Lys, or Gln in the long chain series and Asn, Ser, Thr, Lys, Tyr, Glu, or His in the short chain series, i.e, aliphatic or aromatic, cationic or anionic, with amide, imidazole or hydroxyl group. In the long chain series deletions occur usually as three together in positions 5–7, though they do occur in the region 4–8 and also, rarely, at position 21. Four residue insertions occur only and uniformly in positions 32, 34, 35, and 36 (the fifth disulfide is 30–34). The extension at the C terminal end has already been considered.

The toxin LsIII from *Laticauda semifasciata* with 66 amino acid residues (MAEDA et al., 1974; MAEDA and TAMIYA, 1974) is listed by KARLSSON as a long toxin. It has the characteristic fifth disulfide linkage of the long toxins but not the equally characteristic long tail.

In Figure 8a residue invariant and conservative substitution positions are shown looking down into the concavity of the erabutoxin b molecule. In Figure 8b the insertion, deletion, and extension positions in the long toxins are shown superposed on the erabutoxin b structure. A tentative model drawing of the fifth loop has been included.[1]

The "normal" range of toxicity for these neurotoxins expressed as LD_{50} and determined variously by different techniques and using different animals is 50–150 μg/kg body wt. When the overall patterns of deviation (Table 1) from maximum sequence homology are considered, deviations in one residue invariant Asp 31 and

[1] The erabutoxin b positions shown in Figures 8a and b both correspond to α carbon positions taken from the electron density map shortly after the structure was solved.

Fig. 8b. View (partially schematic) of the erabutoxin b molecule shown looking down into the concavity and modified to correspond to the long chain series model. All the residues are enumerated in the KARLSSON sequence. Residue positions identified ◒ are invariants common to both long and short chain series. Common conservatively substituted positions are shown with a heavy broader outline **O**. The order of the residue type variations in these positions reflects the distribution in the long chain series only. In some instances conservative substitution of both series appears as an invariant in one series alone. Positions found only in the long chain series are shown as ◠ or ◠ with the appropriate long chain series residues identified. This identification is also employed in the insertion positions shown sketched in - - -( )- - - with broken bonds. Residue extensions at the –COOH terminal end found in the long chain series are shown as ◌ and ◓. Deletion positions in the long chain series relative to the short chain series are shown hatched ▧.

Residue positions are shown using the one letter code: A = Ala; C = Cys; D = Asp; E = Glu; F = Phe; G = Gly; H = His; I = Ile; K = Lys; L = Leu; N = Asn; P = Pro; Q = Gln; R = Arg; S = Ser; T = Thr; V = Val; W = Trp; Y = Tyr two type-conserved positions Ser/Thr 9(OH) and Lys/Arg 53 are seen as consistently associated with reduced toxicity:

	LD_{50}	Deviations		
		9	31	53
Naja naja oxiana Toxin I	560 μg/kg	+		+
Laticauda semifasciata Toxin Ls III	850 μg/kg	+	+	+
Naja haje annulifera CM 10	5000 μg/kg	+	+	
Naja haje annulifera CM 12	62000 μg/kg	+	+	

Both CM 10 and CM 12 show further identical deviations in the short chain invariants Asn 5 and Thr 13. The order of magnitude of their difference in toxicity is associated with a single residue in position 7. In CM 12 this is Arg, a positively charged residue; in CM 10 it is Gln. There are only a few other deviations from Gln 7 in the short toxins and these are either His or Pro. It is clear that a long positively charged group in position 7 reduces toxicity. Tryptophan 29 (see Table 1a) of *Dendroaspis viridis* 4.7.3. is oxidized (BANKS et al., 1974) and the toxicity (LD_{50} = 900 μg/kg) greatly reduced compared to the otherwise identical *Dendroaspis viridis* 4.9.3. (LD_{50} = 160 μg/kg) (SHIPOLINI et al., 1973). Apart from these two examples the progression of reduced toxicity cannot be precisely identified as the sum of individual effects because there is no one toxin with only one deviation in 9, 31, 53, or in the short chain positions 5 and 13. Further, in *Lauticauda semifasciata* III for example, the abnormally short tail rather than a deviant 31 may be responsible in whole or in part for the magnitude of the reduction when *Naja naja oxiana* toxin I and *Laticauda semifasciata* III are compared.

The positions enumerated (including 7 and 29) are clearly implicated in toxic potency. Recent studies (ISHIKAWA et al., 1977) have shown that in twelve toxins toxicity is a linear function of the binding constant. If this be generally true then these positions are evidently involved in binding.

IV. Chemistry and Chemical Modification Studies

It is customary, and we have elsewhere (LOW et al., 1976a) followed this procedure, to consider the invariant residues in the neurotoxins as falling into two categories of functional and structural invariance based on the RYDÉN et al. (1973) classification. This classification depends on the assumption that certain residues are essential for folding of the peptide chain and thus for establishing and maintaining the three-dimensional conformation. Such residues defined as structurally invariant may be found in the closely related venom membrane toxins. Functional invariance in the RYDÉN classification resides by definition in those amino acid residues which are unique to the neurotoxins and are thus presumed to be directly related to the expression of neurotoxic function. The review by EAKER (1975) provides a more recent and extensive consideration of invariant and type-conserved residues. EAKER also designates positions as functionally invariant or conserved when they are found in the toxins with receptor-blocking function and not in the nonneurotoxic homologs. In this review we shall set aside these assumptions as possibly restrictive, though they may be correct, and will consider de novo the role of invariant and conservatively substituted residues.

1. Residues not Subject to Study by Group-Specific Reagents

The residues Ser/Thr(OH), Gly(H), Pro, Asn, Ala, and Leu/Ile/Val are found invariant or conservatively substituted in both long- and short-chain series of neurotoxins. These residues cannot be investigated by group specific reagents as a means of determining their contributions to toxicity.

a) Serine-Threonine

Information from deviant toxins about the possible role of the type-conserved hydroxyl group Ser/Thr 9 and the short chain invariant Thr 13 has been discussed. There is no information about most other members of the class, i.e., 64 (Table 1 a); 8 and 39 (Table 1 b); 26, 48, and 63 (Table 1 c), except that 64 and 39 can be substituted without reduction in toxicity. It would be interesting to study the effects of the reagent diisopropyl fluorophosphate (DFP) on a pure toxin [1] in order to determine whether any one of the serine residues might be unusually nucleophilic and react, for example, as does serine 195 in the active site of chymotrypsin (BALLS and JANSEN, 1952).

b) Glycine

Conformational (structural) roles can be assigned to all invariant glycines. They appear at positions of close approach of two chains, in constrained loops, or in the β turns which characterize the way in which the erabutoxin b chain usually folds back on itself. Thus (Table 1 a) Gly 44 (Gly 40 erabutoxin b) is in a tightly constrained region where a larger group would probably impede the Tyr 25 residue, and Gly 48 (Eb 42) in the short toxins is in a close-packed single residue loop between Cys 45 and Cys 49 (Eb 41, 43). The three β turn glycine positions are Gly 38 and 56, and for the long toxins (by analogy with erabutoxin) Gly 20 (Figs. 8 a and b). The β turn potential of glycine is high in any one of the four β turn positions (CHOU and FASMAN, 1974 b).

It is not known how insertion of the fifth disulfide-mediated loop affects conformation in the region 30–39 (Fig. 8 b). It is compatible (from model studies) with a β turn as shown in the drawing. The three nonglycine residues in position 56 are all Tyr (Table 1 a) which has a relatively high β turn potential in the third position. The deviation is not associated with reduced toxicity. Position 20 is, when present, as in erabutoxin, also invariant in the short toxins and forms the third residue of a β turn.

c) Proline

Proline is a corner-turning residue and therefore essentially structural in role. Proline 50 (Eb 44) appears to be in an important conformation-directing position in the closed loop 49-61 (12 residues) which in erabutoxin b is held rigid in the region 58-61 (Eb 51-54) as the βE strand of antiparallel-pleated sheet and as β turn

[1] DFP has been used to study thrombinlike activity in snake venom (SHEU, 1962) but has not been used to study the activity of pure neurotoxins.

region 53-57 (Eb 47-50). The spatial conformation of this whole ring appears to be important; its outer segment is the banked rim of the saucer. In the long chain series the high β turn potential of Pro at 18, together with Gly 20, probably maintains the β turn observed in the erabutoxins in the tapered neck region. The precise structural role of Pro 72 (Table 1c) is not evident; it probably controls in part the position of the long-tail region (see later).

d) Asparagine

Asparagine 69 is the first residue of the tail peptides in both short and long toxins. We assign a structure role to it not simply because it is also invariant in the venom non-neurotoxins, but because the whole six-membered ring and the length of the terminal tail peptides, whether short or long, are constant broad features of these neurotoxins and appear conformation related. We noted earlier the effect of variation in Asn 69 in the short toxin series.

e) Alanine, Leucine, Isoleucine, and Valine

In studies of the assembly of supramolecular structures, thermodynamic measurements have established the importance of hydrophobic interactions in the formation of ordered arrays. KARLSSON's studies (see p. 168) suggest the prime importance of these interactions in toxin binding and receptor. Some of the hydrophobic invariants and conservatively substituted residues appear essentially functional, i.e., involved in binding to the receptor. This may include Val 52, Val/Ile 57, and Ile/Leu/Val 59. There is a second group of hydrophobic residues in the long toxins Ile/Val/Leu 23, Val/Ile/Leu 41, Leu 43, Ala 46, and Ala 47, probably of structural significance, an opinion which stems from our hypothesis concerning the reactive site. The roles of all the residue types will be considered again later.

2. Invariant and Conservatively Substituted Residues as Studied by Chemical Modification

The residues which may be modified and are common to both series include four invariant disulfide linkages, i.e., residues Cys 3–Cys 24, Cys 17–Cys 45, Cys 49–Cys 61, Cys 62–Cys 68, Tyr 25, Trp 29, Asp 31, and Arg 37, together with the conservative substitutions Asp/Glu 42 and Lys/Arg 53. In the long chain series such invariants include Cys 30–Cys 34, Lys 39, and Asp 66, and in the short chain series Lys 27 and Arg 43. All of these residue positions have been modified in one or more neurotoxins, although rarely selectively. With the exception of the four disulfide linkages present in both classes of neurotoxins, no one invariant residue or conservative substitution has been shown to be "essential," using this term in the KARLSSON definition of essential to mean that total loss of toxicity accompanies modification. It will be evident that, with the exception of modifications which destroy conformation such as the reduction of the disulfide bridges, structure-function relationships are not defined in this all-or-none fashion. On the other hand, with few exceptions, the modification of invariant and conservatively substituted residues leads to reduction of toxicity. Thus invariance is evidently function related. However, there are differences between different neurotoxins in the effects of modification on "identical" residues. The reagent used in modification is also relevant. Furthermore toxicity may be affected by modification of noninvariant residues, e.g., Arg 30 in cobrotoxin (YANG et al., 1973).

We shall review briefly here the studies described in detail by KARLSSON (Ch. 5) and by YANG (1974) to provide a background for later detailed discussion of the three-dimensional structure.

a) Disulfide Linkages

A characteristic of the neurotoxins is the unusual resistance of their disulfide linkages toward enzyme cleavage, denaturing conditions at neutral pH and heat; they are also acid stable (CHRISTENSEN, 1955; HOMMA et al., 1964; YANG, 1965; CHICHEPORTICHE et al., 1972). When the four disulfide linkages of cobrotoxin are reduced, eight SH groups are established and there is total loss of toxicity (YANG, 1967), accompanied by complete loss of native conformation which is restored when the reduced toxin is reoxidized. The role of the disulfide linkages is clearly structural. Studies show that reduction of disulfide linkages in the receptor does not prevent reaction with neurotoxin (BARTELS and ROSENBERRY, 1971; KARLSSON et al., 1976). This certainly rules out the possibility that disulfide linkages might be involved in sulfhydryl-disulfide interchange.

The fifth disulfide linkage in the long neurotoxins can be selectively reduced and the molecule retains a large percentage of activity unless reduction is carried out by a procedure which introduces negative charges (BOTES, 1974).

b) Tyrosine

The invariant Tyr 25 in two long and one short neurotoxins has been nitrated with limited loss of toxicity (OHTA and HAYASHI, 1974; KARLSSON and SUNDELIN, 1976). However, in toxins with two tyrosine residues simultaneous nitration of both groups causes gross conformational changes and concomitant loss of toxicity (CHANG et al., 1971a; KARLSSON and SUNDELIN, 1976). The iodination of both tyrosines in cobrotoxin has no effect on activity (SHÜ et al., 1968; HUANG et al., 1973). The role of tyrosine is therefore difficult to characterize and is perhaps poised on the distinction between "functional" and "structural."

c) Tryptophan

In both long and short toxins (see KARLSSON, p. 179), modification of Trp 29 is accompanied by a loss of toxicity that is never complete; as little as 20% or as much as 98% being lost. Residual toxicity is dependent both on the toxin studied and the particular reagent employed. In spite of these variations in degree, the role of tryptophan is clearly functional.

d) Aspartic Acid, Glutamic Acid

Modification studies of carboxyl groups in the neurotoxins have been limited to one short chain toxin, cobrotoxin (CHANG et al., 1971b). All the carboxyl groups with the exception of Glu 21 have been modified without loss of toxicity. This is perhaps unexpected. Three toxins of low toxicity—Ls III, CM 10, and CM 12—show deviations in position Asp 31, and it is tempting to attribute this in part to the absence of a carboxyl group. The apparent anomaly of cobrotoxin can be explained if the invariant grouping required be the carbonyl group (SATO, 1977). The derivatives of cobrotoxin prepared by CHANG et al. (1971b) retain this group. Such an explanation would demand that the lowered toxicity of Ls III (where 31 is Asn) compared with *Naja naja oxiana* toxin I depends on the abnormally short tail and not on a deviant 31.

e) Arginine

Effects of chemical modification of arginine in one short chain toxin, cobrotoxin, have been studied. There are six arginines and these are modified sequentially as the pH is increased. Modification of invariant Arg 37 results in 75% loss of activity (followed by further reduction in toxicity as more arginines are modified). This is a large drop which might be even greater if, following the reaction (shown to be reversible), a free arginyl residue is released either in vivo or prior to assay (see KARLSSON, p. 178).

f) Amino Groups

The KARLSSON survey of chemical modification studies of amino groups in both long and short toxins has established that Lys/Arg 53 is important for optimal toxic activity. The studies of HORI and TAMIYA (1976) show greatly reduced toxicity, $LD_{50} = 1500$ μg/kg, when Lys 47 (KARLSSON, 53) of erabutoxin b is selectively acetylated. The prime functional role of Lys/Arg 53 is also evident from studies of the deviant toxins. In addition, Lys 27 is required for optimal toxicity in some short toxins although it can be exchanged for Met without a reduction in toxicity (Table 1 b).

3. Toxin Modification by Deletion or by Size Increase

a) Carboxyl-Terminal Deletion of a Long Chain Toxin

KARLSSON and EAKER (1972) have shown that removal of the –COOH terminal residues Arg-Lys-Arg-Pro of the long chain siamensis toxin by a protease reduces the toxicity by 50%. It appears significant here that toxin Ls III of low toxicity has only a two residue tail. The possible importance of a long C terminal tail segment in the long chain toxins which all have deletions in the region 4–8 (usually 5–7) appears evident on structural grounds and will be discussed later.

b) Polymerization

Freeze drying of the monomeric forms of both toxins leads to considerable polymerization of the short toxins and only limited polymerization of the long toxins, largely (~ 5%) as dimers. Dimers of the long chain siamensis toxin show 25% toxicity of the monomeric toxin (KARLSSON et al., 1971). The probable site of dimerization is not discussed, nor is dimer stability. The structural significance of this interaction is therefore in question.

4. Summary

1. The role of the four invariant disulfide bridges is established as structural. These linkages maintain the three-dimensional molecular stereochemistry.
2. On the assumption that erabutoxin b provides a prototype three-dimensional model, the invariant glycine and proline residues are also characterized as structural.

3. The following residues are characterized as functional in role:

a) On the basis of study of deviant toxins: 9 Ser/Thr OH, 29 Trp, 31 Asp, and 53 Lys/Arg. We add to this in a special category 5 Asn and/or 13 Thr in the short toxins, and note the restrictive character of residue 7. These residues may be of functional importance in so far as inappropriate substitutions disrupt structure (see later).

b) On the basis of chemical modification studies 29 Trp, 31 Asp, 37 Arg, 53 Lys/Arg, and in some instances 27 Lys (short series).

c) Without direct identification, but on the basis of the evidence for dependence of binding on nonelectrostatic interaction, some hydrophobic groups, perhaps 52 Val, 57 Val/Ile, and 59 Ile/Leu/Val; positions 57 and 59 are also hydrophobic in the membrane toxins. This does not, in our view, rule out their possible importance in neurotoxin binding.

The role of Tyr 25 is difficult to define. From the present studies we cannot determine the roles of all invariant residues and type-conserved positions. In assigning "functional" roles to certain residues we do so in much broader terms than is usual, e.g., in discussing the function of an enzyme. There attention is focused on the "active site" which has proved discrete and definable, often involving the reactive groups of a relatively few amino acid residues. Tyr 25 may be functional, but not in the sense that the hydroxyl OH is implicated in binding. Neurotoxin functional requirements may be more comparable to those of a multisubunit allosteric enzyme complex. Further, to express optimal function (i.e., toxicity) the toxin molecule must cross, in appropriate concentration, the synapse and bind to the receptor. Chemical modifications which affect its survival or transmission time will affect toxicity measurement. Similarly, modifications of one group which stereochemically blocks the binding or distorts the correct orientation of other groups will diminish toxicity.

When acetylcholine binds to the receptor a conformational change opens the ionic channel and provides transient membrane permeability (depolarization). Some antagonists (e.g., decamethonium) are depolarizing and toxic because depolarization is nontransient. Not only is acetylcholine binding competitively inhibited by these neurotoxins but depolarization is prevented.

If we focus attention simply on binding interactions, at least two types of interaction and residues appear to be involved. The neurotoxin most probably inhibits by binding directly to the acetylcholine binding site. We expect a positive charged group (quaternary nitrogen) to be involved as well as a carboxyl group. Arg 37 or Lys/Arg 53 are potential candidates for the former (studies of the detailed three-dimensional structure favor Arg 37, see later), while Asp 31 is a candidate for the latter. Other binding sites must be associated with the very low dissociation constant.

Other residues and interactions must also either inhibit that conformational change in the receptor which normally provides permeability or, if channels do open, they must block them by insertion or by capping. The binding site(s) of the neurotoxins as nondepolarizing antagonists are very probably different from the acetylcholine binding sites, yet they must be closely related. It appears possible that some toxins bind to more sites than is necessary for optimal function, that one or more peripheral groups may be lost without significantly reducing toxicity, and that these may be different for different toxins. This view is compatible with the assumption of a limited set of necessary and nonreplacable binding groups which form the "core" of functional competence. The findings of ISHIKAWA et al. (1977) that toxicity is a linear function of binding constants when essential functional groups are absent or modified underscores this conclusion.

V. Physicochemical Studies of Neurotoxins and Their Derivatives

1. Spectroscopic Studies of Native Toxin Conformation in Aqueous and Aqueous-Organic Solvent

a) Optical Rotatory Dispersion (ORD) and Circular Dichroism (CD) Spectra

The ORD studies of cobrotoxin initially gave spectra which differed so markedly from the spectra of right-handed α helix found in many proteins studied that interpretation was essentially speculative (YANG et al., 1967). Subsequently the presence of considerable regions of β structure in a postsynaptic neurotoxin was proposed from ORD and CD studies of the long chain α bungarotoxin by HAMAGUCHI et al. (1968), who noted the similarity between the CD spectra of α bungarotoxin and of the short chain cobrotoxin. The CD spectra of several short chain toxins: cobrotoxin (YANG et al., 1968), erabutoxin a and b (SATO et al., 1968; MENEZ et al., 1976a, b), *Naja nigricollis* α toxin (MENEZ et al., 1976a, b), toxin A (i.e., *Naja naja naja*), and toxin III (NAKAI et al., 1971), all resemble each other very closely. These studies establish a common conformational feature—antiparallel β pleated sheet—in both short and long toxins.

The CD spectra of α bungarotoxin have also been studied (HAMAGUCHI et al., 1968) as a function of pH and aqueous-organic solvent transitions. A shift to more characteristic α helix features was observed at very high pH and in 50% 2-chloroethanol. The CD and ORD spectra of *Naja haje* toxin α (61-4) and toxin III (71-5) have been studied as a function of pH and temperature. The long chain toxin is more resistant to conformational change (CHICHEPORTICHE et al., 1972). CD measurements have also been made to probe the conformational stabilities of one long and one short toxin from *Naja naja oxiana* as a function of pH, temperature, and solvent change (TSETLIN et al., 1975). In this study, the short chain toxin however has, under comparable conditions, higher conformational stability than the long chain toxin. The CD spectra of two short chain toxins, erabutoxin b and *Naja nigricollis* α toxin, studied as a function of increasing trifluoroethanol concentration, show the conformational stability of α toxin and relative instability of erabutoxin b. The latter change to spectra suggesting some α helical content (MENEZ et al., 1976b) as the trifluoroethanol content is increased. Therefore in the physicochemical studies, as in the chemical studies, after modification (in this instance of solvent environment) toxins display differences in response and their similarities become less marked: generalizations prove dangerous.

b) Laser-Raman Spectra

Studies of laser-Raman spectra of two sea snake neurotoxins isolated from *Lapemis hardwickii* and *Enhydrina schistosa* both indicate the presence of antiparallel β pleated sheet (YÜ et al., 1975). Further evidence for this conformation and the presence of random coil was found in studies of the short chain erabutoxins a and b, the atypical *Laticauda semifasciata* Ls III, (66-5) and *Naja naja naja* toxin 4 (toxin B)

(HARADA et al., 1976; TAKAMATSU et al., 1977). In Ls III random coil appears to predominate; there is some indication of α helix.

2. Spectroscopic Studies of Chemically Modified and/or Denatured Neurotoxins

a) Disulfide Linkages

Loss of native conformation in cobrotoxin after the –S–S– bridges are broken (YANG et al., 1968) has characterized disulfide linkages as structural. When the disulfide linkages are broken (HARADA et al., 1976) laser-Ramam spectra of the erabutoxins a and b and of Ls III also show loss of β pleated sheet structure and enhancement of random coil.

b) Tyrosine

The accessiblity and environment of tyrosine has been probed in four different studies: α) by spectrophotometric titration and UV perturbation spectroscopy (CHICHEPORTICHE et al., 1972; TSETLIN et al., 1975), β) by UV differential spectroscopy study of iodination in different solvents (MENEZ et al., 1976a, b), γ) by proton NMR study (ARSENIEV et al., 1977), and δ) by laser-Raman spectroscopy (HARADA et al., 1976; TAKAMATSU et al., 1977). It was concluded that in all the different toxins studied, except toxin B (TAKAMATSU et al., 1977), residue Tyr 25 is relatively inaccessible and located in a hydrophobic environment, although differences do exist between different neurotoxins.

c) Tryptophan

The environment and accessibility of tryptophan was probed by similar techniques in parallel studies. The common conclusion was that tryptophan is "buried" or "partially buried." MENEZ et al. (1976a, b) consider that both Trp 29 and Tyr 25 are in an isolated region of the molecule, relatively unsusceptible to conformational perturbation by solvent.

VI. Theoretical and Model Studies of Neurotoxin Conformation and Three-Dimensional Structure

Predictive studies of structure in the neurotoxins have been of two kinds. The first involves prediction of chain conformation—α helix, β pleated sheet, or β turn—and is based essentially on the evaluation of conformation-forming tendencies of single residues or of dipeptides. The second, more extensive approach, involves an effort to predict, not simply the presence and location of regions of particular conformation (secondary structure), but the three-dimensional (tertiary) structure of the whole molecule.

1. Prediction of Conformation in the Neurotoxins

a) α Helix

Initial restraints on α helical content of the neurotoxin structures arise from the stereochemical restrictions implied by the presence of four intrachain disulfide linkages, although it is formally possible to construct a model with α helix in the regions 53–61 (KARLSSON) and in the two long intrachain loops bridged by the disulfide linkages 3–24 and 17–45. Predictive studies (LOW et al., 1971) suggested one turn of α helix in erabutoxin b (Eb 36–39). More recently TSETLIN et al. (1975) have used the procedure of CHOU and FASMAN (1974b) to predict conformation in 26 toxins: a single α helical region 1–7 was predicted in *Naja naja oxiana* toxin II. These predictions conflict with the structural finding in erabutoxin b and the assumption of common toxin stereochemistry.

b) β Pleated Sheet

TSETLIN and his colleagues (1975) also predicted β pleated sheet structure and have reported regions of β structure at 13–17 and 53–57 (Eb 54–58 and KARLSSON 61–66) for *Naja naja oxiana* toxin II. Prediction of β sheet for toxin II in the 53–57 region would conflict with the necessity for closing the last disulfide-bonded loop. LOW and her colleagues (1976a) proposed somewhat different predictions for erabutoxin b based on the CHOU and FASMAN (1974a, b) procedure.

c) β Turns

In their study of potential β turn regions, TSETLIN and his colleagues (1975) predicted β turns for both toxin II (61-4) and toxin I (73-5) in several positions, i.e., toxin I 4–9, 18–21, 25–28, 34–37, 36–39, 66–69, and 69–72, and toxin II 33–39, 43–48, 53–57, and 66–69 (KARLSSON enumeration). The β turns found in erabutoxin b are at 7–10, 18–21, 31–34 (KARLSSON 31–38), 47–50 (KARLSSON 53–57), and 57–60 (KARLSSON 64–68). The complete β turn predictions of LOW et al. (1976b) for erabutoxin b (using CHOU and FASMAN) are 17–20, 18–21, 43–48, and 53–57. The correct prediction 18–21 has a totally acceptable but considerably lower potential than the adjacent prediction 17–20.

2. Predictions of Three-Dimensional Structure in the Neurotoxin Series

a) Model Structure Studies

The three-dimensional structure of the neurotoxins predicted from consideration of chemical observations and model-building principles (RYDÉN et al., 1973) is considerably different from the structure of erabutoxin b established by X-ray crystal structure analysis: it is a very much more compact and globular array. A correct and near-correct prediction of two β turn regions were made. The study illustrates the large number of variables in a structure of this size, and the difficulty of limiting possible models by the use of chemical, physicochemical, and space-filling requirements.

b) Energy Minimization Studies

The proposed models compatible with energy minimization studies proposed by GABEL et al. (1976) do not show the essential features of the erabutoxin b structure either in shape or in the presence of extensive β sheet. Correct or near-correct predictions of several β turns were made in this study.

c) Theoretical Chemical Models

The models proposed by SMYTHIES et al. (1975) are more difficult to consider in detail as they are based on proposed specific regions of receptor-toxin interaction rather than on the overall restrictions of peptide chain continuity. A β pleated sheet is however a fundamental feature of the structural model proposed.

VII. X-ray Crystal Structure Studies of Other Neurotoxins

The topology of sequence invariance and conservative substitutions has so far been explored in the neurotoxins in terms of the erabutoxin b structure and a plausible long chain modification of it. In the next section a possible reactive site region will be described; it is a region surprisingly little perturbed by the range and scale of the deletions, insertions, and extensions which characterize the homologous neurotoxins compared to erabutoxin b as prototype. Direct evidence that common function is associated with common structure (conformation) in many neurotoxins comes largely from limited solution studies.

Detailed information is needed to confirm the assumption of structural invariance in the reactive site. Ideally X-ray crystal structure analyses should be made of at least: a) one short chain toxin which differs markedly from erabutoxin b (e.g., *Aipysurus laevis* toxin a), b) one long chain toxin, and c) one of the deviant neurotoxins of abnormally low toxicity, e.g., *Laticauda semifasciata* III. Unfortunately, because of difficulties in crystallization there is now information only about toxins which are closely related to erabutoxin b and all therefore in the short chain series.

1. Erabutoxin a (Asn 26 Erabutoxin b)

When the structure of erabutoxin b was established by X-ray crystal structure analysis, the structure of erabutoxin a was essentially established by analogy (Low et al., 1971). The X-ray diffraction maxima obtained from crystals of this second toxic component in the venom of *Laticauda semifasciata* are almost identical with those from erabutoxin b. The near identity of the structures is evident also from the electron density maps: The three dimensional difference-Fourier map shows only one major peak at position 26 where histidine in erabutoxin b is replaced by asparagine erabutoxin a (Low et al., 1976b).

2. Neurotoxin b from Laticauda semifasciata (Philippines)

The three-dimensional structure of neurotoxin b from the Philippines sea snake *Laticauda semifasciata* has recently been determined by Tsernoglou and Petsko (1976) at 2.2 Å resolution. The sequence of this toxin has not been determined, but the reported amino-acid composition (Tu et al., 1971) differs in lysine (1), histidine (1), arginine (1), serine (2), glycine (1), and valine (1) content from that of erabutoxin b isolated from the venom of *Laticauda semifasciata* found in the Ryuku Islands (Tamiya and Arai, 1966). Furthermore, neurotoxin b was reported as having only 61 amino residues, yet Tsernoglou and Petsko (1976) used the erabutoxin b sequence (Sato and Tamiya, 1971) with 62 residues in order to fit the peptide chain to their electron density map. If, therefore, the two toxins do differ and come from different subspecies, the three-dimensional structures are virtually identical. Tamiya and Takasaki (1978) have analyzed venom of the sea snake *Laticauda semifasciata* from the Philippines. They showed that the main neurotoxic components of the venom are erabutoxin a and b. It appears therefore that the reported (Tu et al., 1971) presence of two different neurotoxins in venom of the Philippines sea snake *Laticauda semifasiata* is erroneous. There is no subspecies.

3. Erabutoxin c

Erabutoxin c (Asn 51 erabutoxin b, TAMIYA and ABE, 1972), the third (62-4) minor component from the venom of *Laticauda semifasciata*, crystallizes in a form different from that common to the normal erabutoxins a and b, but identical with an unusual form of erabutoxin b (PRESTON et al., 1975). Furthermore, the two-dimensional data from the crystals of erabutoxin c are virtually identical with those of the alternative erabutoxin b form. It appears, therefore, that these two erabutoxins b and c also have a common three-dimensional structure.

4. Laticotoxin a and Cobrotoxin

Laticotoxin a (SATO et al., 1969) is a neurotoxin found in the venom of the sea snake *Laticauda laticaudata*. Preliminary crystallographic measurements (SEARLE et al., 1973) suggest a possible close relationship between the structure of this toxin and that of cobrotoxin (WONG et al., 1972), even though there are a significant number of residue differences between them. Nonetheless, close similarity between crystal structures (both are 62-4 toxins) suggests a common three-dimensional structure.

C. Structure-Function Relationship in the Postsynaptic Neurotoxins. The Three-Dimensional Structure of Erabutoxin b as Prototype in both Long and Short Toxins

I. Erabutoxin b and the Short Toxins: The Reactive Site

Consider erabutoxin b as the appropriate model structure for the snake venom postsynaptic neurotoxins. The reactive site then asserts itself. Most of the invariant and type-conserved positions common to both long and short chain toxins are found in the right-hand wing of the molecule (Figs. 8a and b and Fig. 9) below the disulfide core in that shallow depression (which banks sharply to a steep rim) encompassed by an imaginary line drawn round the loop 32–49 ... 32 (KARLSSON 32–56 ... 32). Not only are most (all but three) of the residues common to both series found within this loop, but all but one of those found there which appear directly implicated in function, point into, or up from, the concavity (i.e., towards the reader) (Fig. 10). That is, their Cα–Cβ bonds lie on the upper surface of the D.C.E. sweep of the β pleated sheet, or point up above the backbone chain rim in the region 43–49. These, in detail, are the residues Trp 29, Asp 31, Arg 33 (KARLSSON 37), Lys 47 (Lys/Arg KARLSSON 53), Ile 50 (Val/Ile KARLSSON 57), Leu 52 (Ile/Leu/Val KARLSSON 59), as well as Tyr 25. Within this region and also pointing up are all the common glycine residues Gly 34 (KARLSSON 38), Gly 40 (KARLSSON 44), Gly 49 (KARLSSON 56), the common proline Pro 44 (KARLSSON 50), as well as Glu 38 (Asp/Glu KARLSSON 42) and Val 46 (KARLSSON 52) which points down, but also into the closed ring, and forms a part of its surface.

Apart from the consequent focus of interest in the functional role of this segment of structure, the presence of so many structure invariants suggests the very close relationship between structure and function which has, for some residues, bedevilled

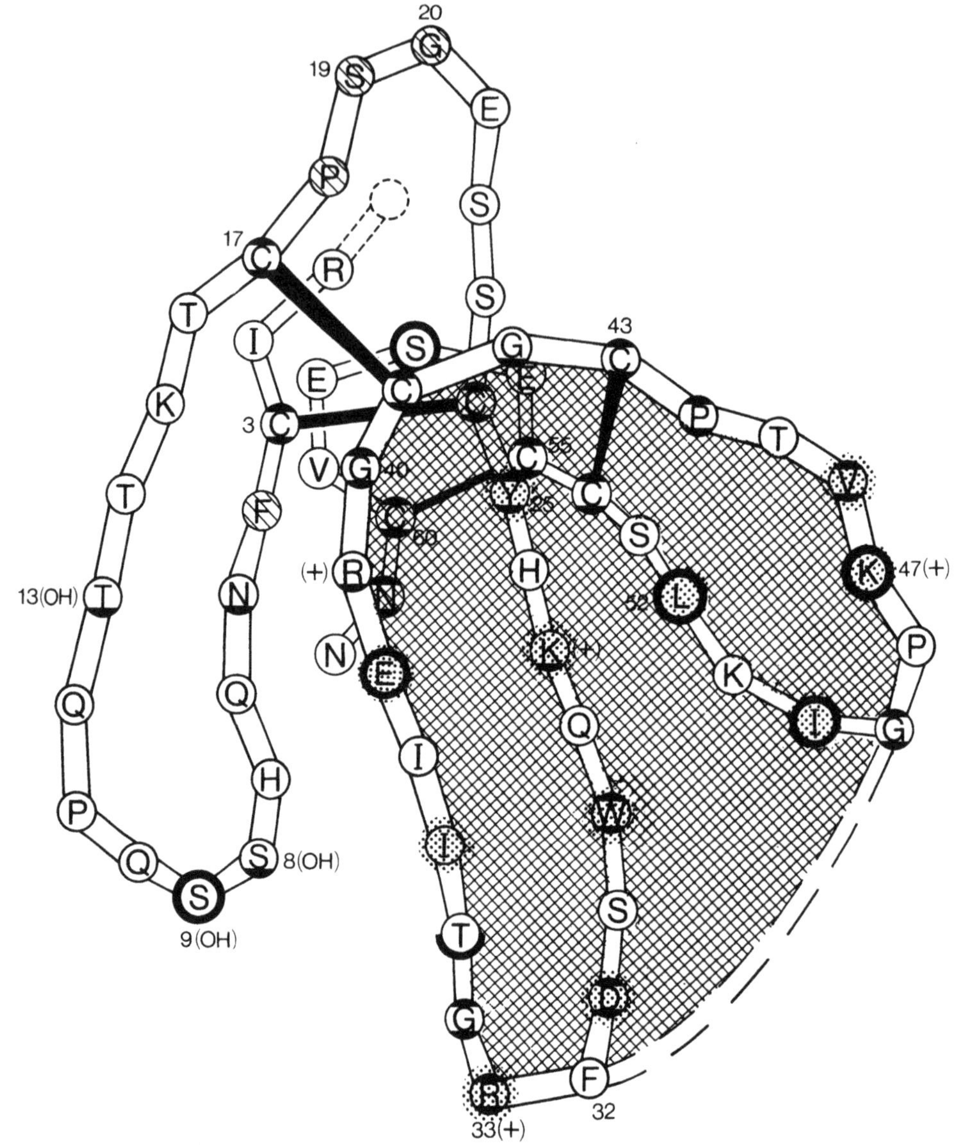

Fig. 9. View (partially schematic) of the erabutoxin b[1] molecule shown looking down into the concavity. The invariant and conservatively substituted residues are shown as in Figure 8a. The reactive site region 32–49···32 is shown cross-hatched. Those invariant or conservatively substituted residues which appear to have primarily a functional role are shown dotted. Other symbols are those used earlier

efforts to define and distinguish these two roles. The implication of conformational specificity is unmistakable.

There is no doubt concerning the structural (stabilizing) role of the disulfide linkages. The cupped reactive site is secured directly to two of the four disulfide

[1] Karlsson sequence enumeration is not used in this drawing.

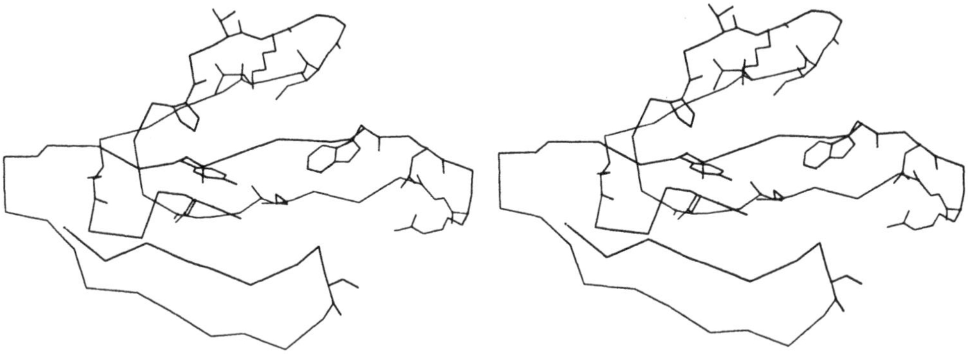

Fig. 10. Stereopair drawings of the structure of erabutoxin b showing common invariant and type-conserved positions for long and short chain toxins combined. The Cys positions are omitted (see Table 1). Ser 9, Ser 57, and Asn 61 are the three residues outside the reactive site. To see the figure in stereo, most readers will need to use a stereoscopic viewer. Inexpensive stereo viewers may be obtained from Taylor-Merchant Corporation, 25 West 45 Street, New York, N.Y. 10036. If a stereo viewer is not available, it is recommended that the drawing be held at arms length and the eyes focused at infinity. Some time may be required to relax the eye muscles so that each eye is focused on one half of the stereo pair. As the multiple images as first seen merge, concentrate on the central image and bring it slowly into focus. Once the drawing appears as three dimensional, it may be moved slowly toward the viewer. Viewing without the aid of a viewer may prove extremely difficult. Figure 10 was produced by the GRIP-75 molecular graphics system built by the University of North Carolina, Department of Computer Science, with the help of many users.

linkages: to Cys 41–Cys 17 (KARLSSON 45–17) and to Cys 24–Cys 3 which hold the two distal ends of one segment of this region, the central long looping frond of erabutoxin b 41–24 (largely βD βC strands). Attached to it, through Cys 41–Gly 42–Cys 43 (short series), is the second segment of the reactive site, the closed ring 43–54 (KARLSSON 49–61) formed and internally constrained by the Cys 43–Cys 54 bond.

Finally, the reactive site appears protected on its undersurface by the six-membered ring Cys 55–Cys 60 and the two residue tail. At its upper end, therefore, as viewed in the drawings, the conformational restraints which hold and maintain the reactive site are seen to be extensive.

The loop region of the reactive site 41–24 with its long curved tonguelike protrusion includes, besides the half-cystines, six residue invariants common to both short and long toxins (Tyr 25, Trp 29, Asp 31, Arg 33, Gly 34, and Gly 40, Fig. 8a) and one type conserved position, Glu/Asp 38. In the short toxins there are, in addition, two more invariants, Lys 27 and Arg 38 (KARLSSON 43), and one type-conserved position Thr/Ser 35 (KARLSSON 39). Most of the invariants which appear "functional" are in this loop (see p. 232). Later detailed consideration of interactions will emphasize the relationships between structural and functional roles.

In the second half of the reactive site, the ring of invariant length Cys 43–Cys 54 (KARLSSON 49–61), are three common invariants, Pro 44 (KARLSSON 50), Val 46 (KARLSSON 52), and Gly 49 (KARLSSON 56), and three common type-conserved positions, Lys/Arg 47, Ile/Val 50, and Ile/Leu/Val 52: This is a highly constrained conformation.

There are only three common special positions outside the proposed reactive site region: a) Ser/Thr 9, b) Ser 57 (Thr/Ser KARLSSON 64) in the β turn region of the terminal six-membered ring, and c) position Asn 61 (KARLSSON 69) in the tail peptide.

These observations emphasize the remarkable conformational inflexibility of the reactive site as a function of sequence. They further suggest that the reactive site is generally unperturbed by the differences between nondeviant members of the short toxin series, a view strengthened in detail when specific interactions are considered.

II. Erabutoxin b and the Short Toxins: Nonreactive Site Regions

To the left of the reactive site is the 3–17 loop with A and B β strands joined by β turn 7–10 and lying alongside the D β strand to form the five-stranded β sheet continuum. This loop is attached to the reactive site through the disulfide core (Cys 3–Cys 24; Cys 17–Cys 41) and held rigid at its upper end.

In the short chain series a deletion may possibly occur at position 4 in the loop. The effect of such a deletion on the loop structure itself and on the reactive site is not easy to estimate. This loop includes Ser/Thr/(OH)9, one of the three common special positions not found in the reactive site. Furthermore, from a study of the deviant toxins, it is apparently implicated in function. This is the only such residue which lies outside the reactive site. A deletion at 4 must affect the spatial relationship between Ser/Thr 9 and the reactive site. Ser 9 points downwards, is in the 7–10 β turn, and on the edge of the loop. There are no insertion positions in the short chain with respect to erabutoxin. There is an N-terminal extension position of one residue in six toxins (see KARLSSON, p. 169), which has no evident effect on toxic activity. This extension is a consequence of the deletion at position 4.

The single deletion at position 4 and the consequent N-terminal extension cited here in six toxins result from the Karlsson view that the disulfide linkage in these toxins is formed by the second (cystinyl) residue in the sequence – 1,1,Cys 2, Cys 3. If the linkage is formed by the first Cys residue then no perturbation of Ser/Thr(OH)9 is expected and no extension position exists.

In erabutoxin b the βB strand lies alongside the βD strand and is hydrogen bonded to it (although the end of the D C loop sticks out). The βB strand thus prevents both lateral access to the reactive site along part (37–40) of its left edge as well as access from beneath. From a different viewpoint one could argue that it defines the left-hand limit on the open protruding tongue, and stabilizes the three stranded β pleated sheet of the reactive site.

In the tapered neck region of erabutoxin Cys 17–Cys 24, there is a β turn Pro/Ser/Gly/Glu which is strongly dependent on Pro 18/Gly 20 (residues usually found in the short toxins when positions 18 and 20 are filled). The β turn directs the loop away from the disulfide core. Deletion may occur in the neck region of the short toxins, shortening it by a one or two residue section from positions 18, 19, and 20. Although these deletions must produce a large local change in the neck region, this should not affect the reactive site, well protected as it is by the disulfide barrier. Direct involvement of this region in function can be excluded.

There are no toxins which lack the short hexapeptide ring near the C terminal end. It underlies the upper end of the reactive site and includes the special position Thr/Ser 64. A structural role associated with the protection of the reactive site appears probable. The uniform occurrence of a two residue C terminal tail following the hexapeptide ring suggests a strong if undetermined structural role of this segment.

From the viewpoint of the short chain series, the only apparent anomaly in the designation of the loop 32–49 ... 32 as a well-defined and unperturbed reactive site region lies, therefore, in the presence of the supposed "functional" residue Ser 9 (OH) not only outside this region and pointing downwards, but subject to change when position 4 is deleted. This anomaly is most usefully explored when we examine the long toxin series which show deletions, usually (two exceptions) three residues long, in the 4–8 region. Such deletions must even more radically alter the architecture of the whole 3–17 loop and thus in particular modify the Thr/Ser 9 position. A simple resolution of this dilemma would be to characterize the 9(OH) position as a coincidental absence in the deviant toxins of low toxicity. This seems to us however to skirt the most remarkable feature of the reduced toxicity of Ls III, CM 10, and CM 12, which is the involvement (see p. 227) of residues in the 3–17 loop. The role of this whole loop and the Thr/Ser 9 position will be reconsidered later.

III. Erabutoxin and the Long Toxins: Reactive Site

One section of the reactive site in the long toxins Cys 49–Cys 61 remains totally unchanged while the other is radically different from its short toxin equivalent. The loop 24–41 (Karlsson 24–45) of eighteen residues in the short toxins is replaced in the long toxins by a loop of 22 residues with a five-membered ring formed by the fifth disulfide bond, through the invariant Cys 30–Cys 34. Asp 31 lies within this ring which can form a β turn.

When models are made of the long toxin loop, many structural features of the short toxin region can be maintained. The extra (fifth) disulfide bridge, Cys 30–Cys 34, can be fitted into the structure with surprisingly little overall distortion, as shown in Figure 8b. The ring stands high above the edge of the β turn and, for example, the Asp 31–Arg 37 interaction can be maintained as it is found in erabutoxin b. The sequence Cys 34, 35, 36, Arg 37 will also form a β turn. With the exception of an exaggerated pleat along the chain near 38, 39, and 40, the overall structure of the loop need not be perturbed by the extension. The long toxin protrusion is broader at its termination than the narrow tongue of the short toxins.

In the long, as in the short toxins, the basic features in this region are not subject to extensive modification among members of the series. Not only are there four further long toxin special positions 26, 39, 41, and 43 (exclusive of the two half cystines) as shown in Figure 8b, but if the limits (Table 1c) had been eased to admit four rather than two deviations, positions 27, 28, and 35 would also have been included as special positions.

IV. Erabutoxin and the Long Toxins: Nonreactive Site Regions

In the long toxins, the tapered neck region has one occasional deletion at position 21; there are no other differences between the region in the two series. The invariant three residue (46 Ala, 47 Ala, and 48 Thr) insertion between Cys 45 and Cys 49 appears to be without functional significance.

We have noted the significant differences between the 3–17 loop in the short and long toxins. The loop in the long toxins (with the exception of that in α bungarotoxin) is inadequate to provide lateral protection for part of the 37–44 strand. The long toxins are not less toxic than the short toxins. If, therefore, the 3–17 loop be protective, an alternative must be found. This leads us to consideration of the role of the C terminal extension, which is important for toxicity, even though in *Laticauda semifasciata* III, which has an abnormally short tail of six residues, this is not unambiguously evident. Toxicity is however reduced by 50% when the four terminal residue peptide Arg/Lys/Arg/Pro is lopped off from the long chain siamensis toxin by a protease. Finally, as KARLSSON has noted (p. 167), toxin I of *Dendroaspis viridis* has a toxicity almost twice that of toxin 5 from the same venom although the sequences are precisely the same except that toxin I has one more residue, glycine, at the C-terminal end.

In our view, the C-terminal tail peptide in the long toxins displaces the 3–17 loop of the short toxins both spatially and in its protective role. It appears probable that the tail peptide forms a β strand roughly in the position of the A β strand in the short toxins, and in this position protects the 37–44 edge of the reactive site. That is, specifically, it prevents access to this site both laterally and from below. Obviously such a view implies that the 3–17 loop in the long toxins is not immutable and fixed with respect to the whole three-dimensional array, and particularly not with respect to the reactive site. It further demands that the functional role of the serine 9 residue, if this does indeed have such a role, be expressed not in a fixed spatial relationship to the main reactive site, but rather in some flexible mode. The differences between the three-dimensional structures of the short toxins and of the long toxins would then reside, not only in one segment of the reactive site region, but in a totally different arrangements of the 3–17 loops, and in the involvement for the long toxins of the long C-terminal tail in hydrogen bonding with the reactive site.

V. Long and Short Toxins: Biochemical and Biological Differences

We have discussed the overall structural differences between the short and long toxins. Even if the particular model structure proposed for the long toxins proves wrong, large differences must exist in the 3–17 and 24–45 loops, and in the C-terminal region.

a) It is not then surprising that the two classes are immunologically different nor that the polymerization patterns at low temperatures differ (KARLSSON, p. 165).

b) The differences in the circular dichroism spectra between the two groups could arise because of structural differences in the variant segments and need not imply gross structural differences in the reactive site regions.

c) Slower association and dissociation rates for the long compared to the short toxins is certainly compatible, as KARLSSON suggests, with more extensive conformational change associated with long toxin binding to the reactive site. These changes could occur in adjacent regions, or there may be differences between the conformational changes in receptor as long or short toxins bind.

d) KARLSSON remarks that chemical modification has, in general, a more serious effect on toxic activity in the short series. We see no obvious explanation of this effect. Studies of the details of intramolecular binding in erabutoxin b do show that some short-toxin invariants are involved. Such intramolecular bonds maintain conformation; they may be more numerous and provide more extensive stabilizing interactions in the long toxins. The 24–45 loop has many long toxin invariants or near-invariant, type-conserved positions as we discussed earlier.

e) The most remarkable difference between the two series of toxins is the observation that the neuromuscular block caused by a short neurotoxin can be reversed by washing with neostigmine, whereas the block caused by a long neurotoxin is irreversible under similar conditions (see KARLSSON, p. 166).

VI. Erabutoxin b and the Short Toxin Series: Detailed Intramolecular Packing

1. β Pleated Sheet and β Turns

In the earlier description of the β pleated sheet (p. 219), we observed the formal definition of hydrogen bonds in determining the length of the β strands. More recent studies have modified and lengthened some strands (SATO et al., 1977). The details are not important, it is the extent of lateral close packing between adjacent strands which provides an inpenetrable sheet and makes the residues within the barrelling curve of the β sheet inaccessible from beneath.

The whole of the 1–17 loop is close packed and reverses direction with a well-defined β turn. The deviant changes in positions 5 and 13 (CM 10 and 12) are not of the kind to disrupt main chain–main chain interaction.

We have hitherto considered Ser/Thr(OH)9 as probably "functional." However, in the 7–10 β turn the replacements Leu and Pro (Table 1c) could, in the third position (CHOU and FASMAN, 1974b), disrupt this structure. All the replacements are associated with lowered toxicity. Replacement of a rigid β turn by a flexible loop could either interfere with the reactive site or fail to protect it adequately. With this view of disruptive effects the reduction in toxicity of CM 12 versus CM 10 could then be associated with the added effects of a charged Arginyl (Arg 7) group in flexible regions which could prevent toxin binding in the normal mode. The A strand of the 1–17 loop is close packed to the βD strand of reactive site along the length 37–40. The D and C strands are hydrogen bonded throughout the whole length of the loop 41–24 (KARLSSON 45–24), which includes the β turn 31–34 (KARLSSON 31–37) where the chain reverses direction. None of the deviations in this reactive site loop appear particularly likely to break either β structure or β turn. This first region of the reactive site is hydrogen bonded to the second segment through the span C–E along the length C 24–28 to E 55–51. There are no deviant positions in this strand nor in the whole of the second segment of the reactive site. The cross packing is invariant and the β turn unmodified.

2. Intramolecular Interactions: Particularly Those Involving Invariant and Type-Conserved Residues

a) *Main Chain–Main Chain and Main Chain–Side Chain Hydrogen Bonds*

There is only one main chain–main chain hydrogen bond which is not involved in the β structure. It is between the C=O of residue 2 and the NH group of residue 59. A series of hydrogen bonds between main chain peptide and amino and carbonyl side chain groups (in some instances bifurcated) bind the molecule together. Thus, within the loop 1–17 there are bonds between the main chain positions 3, 5, 6, and 10 and the side chains 14(OH), 13(OH), 10(γNH_2), and 6(γNH_2), respectively. Although only one of the side chains involved (13) is a formal short series invariant, positions 14, 10, and 6 are usually Thr, Gln, and Gln respectively in the short series. Furthermore, the deviant changes in 13(CM 10 and 12) would eliminate the interactions observed, reduce structural rigidity, and in this way affect toxicity. A main chain–side chain hydrogen bond between main chain positions 37 and the hydroxyl cf Ser 8, links the 1–17 loop to the adjacent reactive site. This 1–17 loop is also hydrogen-bonded through the amino terminal group of Arg 1 to the carboxyl group of Glu 58 (KARLSSON 66) and through position 4 to the carbonyl group of Asn 61 (KARLSSON 69). Thus two further invariants are involved in binding the 1–17 loop to other regions of the molecule.

Within the reactive site the 24–41 loop is crosslinked to the rest of the structure by main chain–side chain interactions: 1. between the carbonyl of position 25 and the amide nitrogen of Asn 61; 2. between the side chain nitrogen of His 26 and the carbonyl group of residue 60. This is mediated through a solvent molecule; and 3. between the carbonyl of position 60 and the side chain nitrogen of Asn 62. Finally, there is a charge–charge interaction between the terminal carboxyl group and Arg 39. This latter interaction provides a particularly obvious comment on the differences between the long and short chain toxins. Position 39 (KARLSSON 43) is an invariant leucine in the long chain toxins. As the C terminal residue is not near position 39 in the long chain toxins, clearly such an invariant as Arg would be inappropriate.

b) *Side Chain–Side Chain Interactions*

Most of the side chain–side chain interactions observed involve invariant or type-conserved residues implicated directly in function or structure, although there is 1. a hydrogen bond between the carbonyl group of Glu 28 and the ε amino group of Lys 51; 2. a solvent mediated hydrogen bond between the side chain nitrogen of His 7 and Ser 8(OH), and 3. a charge–charge interaction between Arg 1 and the Glu 58 carboxyl group.

Both residue 31 Asp and residue 37 Arg have been implicated in function; they are joined together by charge–charge interaction. These two residues may bind to the acetylcholine binding site; the distance between the charged nitrogen of arginine and the carbonyl group of aspartic acid is similar to that found between the acetyl and quaternary amino groups of acetylcholine. The contribution of Gly 34 (KARLSSON 38) to the structural rigidity in this region has been noted. It has also a quasi-functional role, since if the side chain were larger than hydrogen it would interfere with the Asp-Arg charge–charge interactions.

Tryptophan 29 has also been implicated in function. It forms hydrophobic bonds with Ile 50 (KARLSSON 57) a general conservative position (Val/Ile), as well as with Ile 36 (KARLSSON 40). When this latter residue is not isoleucyl, it is either valyl or arginyl. We have not listed this position as type-conserved in both series because Arg/Ile/Val are not usually considered common types. However, the hydrocarbon chain region of arginyl residue can form hydrophobic interactions and could thus replace Ile/Val[1]. These X-ray crystallographic observations confirm the findings of MENEZ et al. (1976a, b) that the tryptophan residue is relatively inaccessible. We know that hydrophobic toxin receptor binding is implicated in function and may consider this whole grouping of positions 29, 50 (KARLSSON 57), and 36 (KARLSSON 40) as forming a hydrophobic region. On this basis, position KARLSSON 40 ought to be considered as type conserved. Two further residues have been considered as probably functional, these, 46 (KARLSSON 52) and 52 (KARLSSON 59), show hydrophobic interactions in erabutoxin b. This might be considered the site of a second probable hydrophobic functional grouping, although this could be a structural interaction providing a further source of rigidity in the closed turn 43–54 (KARLSSON 49–51). The whole of this loop 43–54 (KARLSSON 49–61) is highly constrained and there are many hydrophobic interactions across it.

The role of Tyr 25 is frequently considered structural. It forms a hydrogen bond with another type-conserved position, Asp/Glu 38 (KARLSSON 42). The chain region of Lys 27 (a short toxin series invariant) appears to form hydrophobic bonds with the chain region of Glu 38. If Glu 38 be considered a functional residue, then we may assign a structural role to Tyr 25, considering it as positioning the glutamic acid residue. Lysine 27 would also, in these terms, be structural in the short as well as most of the long toxins. Furthermore, if Glu 38 be considered the functional residue then perhaps the devastating effect of Arg 7 in CM 12 toxin can be explained in terms of its possible interaction with Glu 38. A charge–charge bond between Arg 7 and Glu 38 could well destroy any functional role of the glutamic acid carboxyl group. It is, of course, possible to turn the argument around and consider Glu 38 and Lys 27 as positioning groups in this region and assign a functional role to Tyr 25, even though this may not involve the hydroxyl group. At present the ambiguity cannot by resolved. The observations on the tyrosine environment confirm the conclusion of TAKAMATSU et al. (1977) concerning the hydrophobic environment and relative inaccessibility of the tyrosine residue.

In this discussion we note that one of the functional residues, Lys-Arg 53, is completely independent and forms no intramolecular bonds; it lies on the periphery of the molecule on the edge of the closed loop of the reactive site. Its function appears independent of intramolecular interaction with other residues.

D. Conclusions

I. The Present View

The determination of the three-dimensional structure of one neurotoxin, erabutoxin b, has proved the "Rosetta Stone," the key to the interpretation of a wealth of chemical, physicochemical, and toxicological information about more than 40 different postsynaptic neurotoxins in both land and sea snake *(Elapidae, Hydrophiidae)* venoms. From this cross-study a broad understanding of the structure-function

[1] Professor David C. Richardson (Duke University) with whom I have discussed this question tells me that in several proteins the hydrocarbon chain of arginyl does form hydrophobic interactions to other hydrophobic side chain groups.

Table 2. [a]Neurotoxins: Sequence of Invariant Conservatively Substituted Residues with Probable Assignment of Role

a) Long and Short Series Combined.

Position	3	9	17	24	25	29	31	37	38
Residue	[Cys]	(Ser/Thr)	[Cys]	[Cys]	[Tyr]	[Trp]	[Asp]	[Arg]	[Gly]
Role	S	S/F	S	S	F/S	F	F	F	S

Position	40	42	44	45	49	50	52	53	56	57
Residue	(Arg/Ile Val)	(Glu/Asp)	[Gly]	[Cys]	[Cys]	[Pro]	[Val]	(Lys/Arg)	[Gly]	(Val/Ile)
Role	F?	F/S	S	S	S	S	F?	F	S	F?

Position	59	61	62	64	68	69
Residue	(Ile/Leu Val)	[Cys]	[Cys]	(Thr/Ser)	[Cys]	[Asn]
Role	F?	S	S	S/F	S	S

b) Short Neurotoxins Only

Position	5	8	13	21	27	39	43	48
Residue	[Asn]	[Ser]	[Thr]	(Glu/Asp)	[Lys]	(Thr/Ser)	[Arg]	[Gly]
Role	S/F	S	S/F		S/F		S	S

c) Long Neurotoxins Only

Position	18	20	23	26	30	34	39	41	43
Residue	[Pro]	[Gly]	(Ile/Val Leu)	[Thr]	[Cys]	[Cys]	[Lys]	(Val/Ile Leu)	[Leu]
Role	S	S	S		S	S		S	S

Position	46	47	48	63	66	72
Residue	[Ala]	[Ala]	[Thr]	[Ser]	[Asp]	[Pro]
Role	S	S	S			S

[ ] Invariant Residue. ( ) Conservative Substitution.

F Functional residue; S Structural residue; F/S or S/F Role uncertain, the first letter corresponds to the tentative primary assignment.
A question mark after the letter implies a tentative assignment to one role even though the alternative is possible.

[a] Karlsson enumeration employed throughout.

relationships has developed and the reactive site of the molecule persuasively defined. There are (see Table 1) 18 residue invariants and six (possibly seven, see Table 2) conservatively substituted positions common to both series of toxins. Of these at least 13 appear to be wholly structural in role. Because the sequence homologies in the neurotoxins appear to define and describe both structural stability and functional invariance, the detailed interpretation seems generally appropriate for the whole class, which includes α-bungarotoxin and cobrotoxin as well as other elapid and hydrophid toxins.

The structural information about erabutoxin b and the essentially identical erabutoxins a and c characterizes the short toxin series in most precise detail. The long toxin series are almost equally well characterized; structural differences need not affect the proposed functional groupings in the reactive site. Furthermore, where differences in sequence length outside the reactive site region must affect the structure of the long toxins, the changes offer plausible alternative means of maintaining structural integrity and providing protection for the reactive site region.

1. Structure: General

The molecular shape is that of a shallow saucer with footed stand. Six short peptide strands, five in antiparallel β structure, form the saucer from three loops of peptides; the central loop section (left-hand segment) of the reactive site region (Fig. 9) is longer and protrudes, curling upwards like a tongue. The remarkable rigidity of the neurotoxin structure hinges not only on the central core of four disulfide bridges but equally on the five-stranded β structure, the β turns where the chain changes direction, as well as very many main chain–side chain, side chain–side chain cross-linking interactions. These are particularly evident in the closed ring 49–61 (here and elsewhere the KARLSSON enumeration is used consistently) segment of the reactive site which is formed from one outer E strand of the barrelling β pleated sheet and from the curved rim 49–56. The ring is too open for hydrogen bonding; it is held and maintained by cross-linking interaction involving side chain groups which also serve to block access from below. The hydrophobic residue 59 is a particularly significant cross-linking group.

Except where the terminal ring (the foot) underlies the disulfide core, the structure is only one peptide chain thick. The whole saucerlike depression of the molecule is a scooped out shell or carapace through which even water molecules cannot pass. The two surfaces thus formed appear to have characteristic roles. Within the concave reactive site region (32–45 ... 49–56 ... 32) functionally important residues point into the concavity and protrude from the inner surface of the shell. On the outer convex surface and pointing downwards are the two common hydroxyl positions 9(OH), 64(OH), and the "stand," the six-membered ring.

The short toxin molecule may be divided into five segments.

a) The 1–17 antiparallel ABβ strands and β turn. The A strand of this region is strongly bonded to the left-hand edge of the reactive site (strand D).

b) The tapered neck region of variable length which is apparently structurally insignificant.

c) and d) The two reactive site loops 24–45 and 49–56, wholly invariant in length and highly crosslinked to each other and to segments a and e.

e) The terminal hexapeptide disulfide bridged loop and two residue tail.

2. Comparison of Short and Long Toxins

The first 1–17 loop of the long toxins is considerably shortened by deletion. On the other hand (with one exception, a deviant of low toxicity) all long toxins have a long

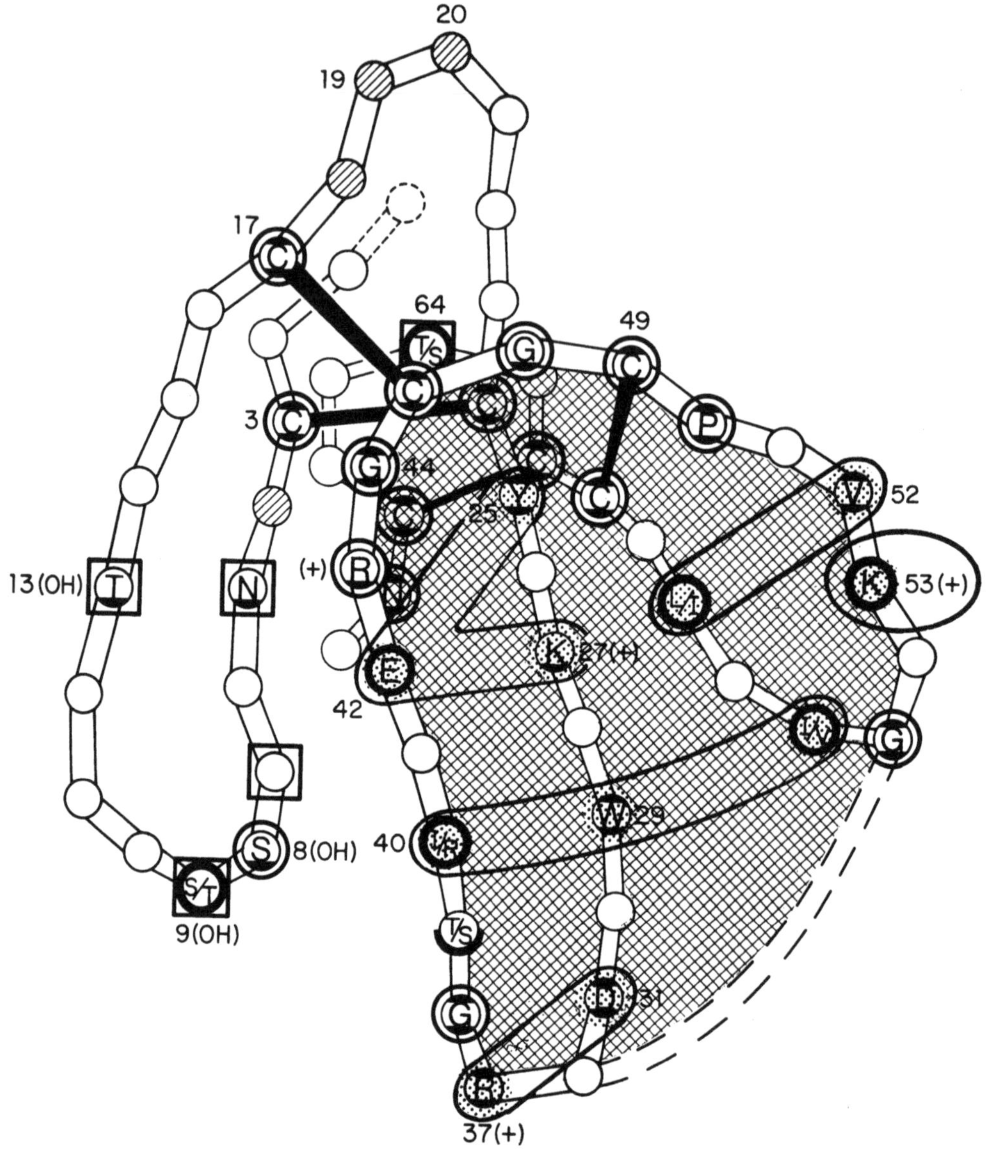

Fig. 11a. View (partially schematic) of the structure of the erabutoxin b molecule shown looking down into the concavity. In this figure the only residue positions indicated are those which correspond to invariant and conservative substitutions. The structure is thus a prototype of the short toxin series. The invariant residue positions found in both series of toxins are shown emphasized by black caps top and bottom. The short chain invariants are emphasized by a black cap in the lower segment. Positions of conservative substitution in both series of toxins are shown with a heavy broader outline. Conservative substitutions in the short chain series are shown with a heavy lower semicircular outline. Deletion positions found in the short chain toxins are shown hatched. The position of the N terminal extension in some 60–4 toxins is shown by a broken circle. All the residues are enumerated in the KARLSSON sequence. As in Figure 9, the reactive site region is shown cross-hatched. Those invariant or conservatively substituted residues which appear to have primarily a functional role are shown dotted. Those residues to which a structural function has been assigned are shown enclosed in a large circle. In this drawing the conservative substitution observed in position 40 is also indicated. The residues which are shown enclosed in square boxes lie outside the reactive site region and appear implicated in function, although the description structural or functional is uncertain and ill defined. Heavy lines enclose those residues which form part of each of the five functional groupings

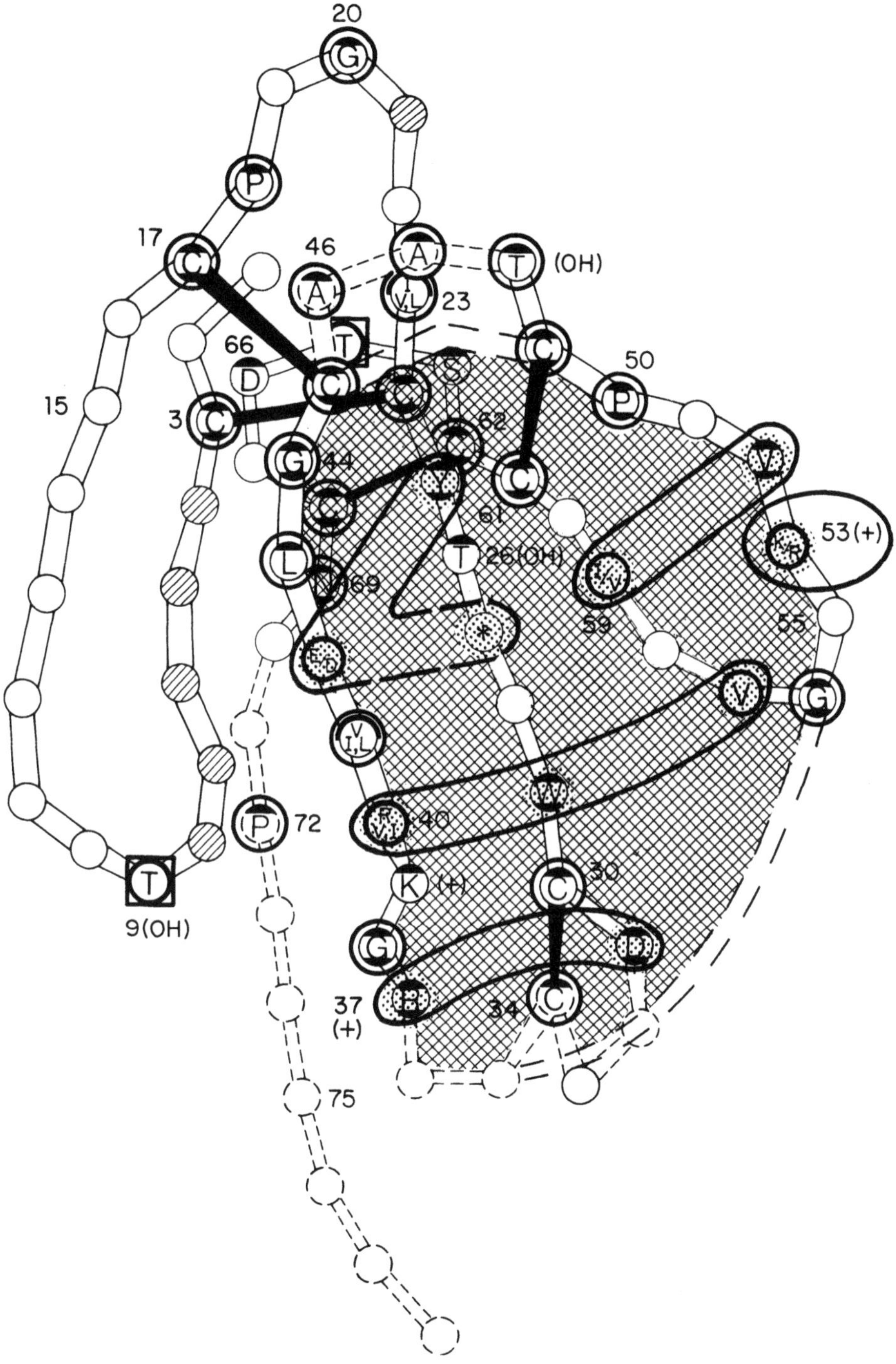

Fig. 11 b. (Legend see page 250)

C terminal tail. This suggests the essential and interchangeable roles of loop and tail peptide. In the short series the Aβ strand prevents access to the reactive site; it helps maintain its structural integrity by crosslinking. When shortened by deletion, it cannot properly do this. The long C terminal tail could easily loop around, and, lying longside the edge of the reactive site, both protect it from lateral access and, by crosslinking, maintain structural rigidity.

The tapered neck region is not substantially different between the two series nor does this part of the molecule appear to play any significant role.

The reactive site of these neurotoxins (Figs. 11a and b) is thus defined and characterized. In both series it is formed by two lobes of the molecule, the loop 24–45 and the closed ring 49–61. The outer edge of the closed ring banks up steeply to form the rim, the other edge is the central D strand of the five-stranded β structure. The closed ring 49–61 in both series is of common length. Extensive crosslinking interactions and constant length suggest a common invariant conformation. The first lobe of the reactive site, the loop 24–45, is constant within each series, but in the long series includes the broadening extension of the pentapeptide fifth disulfide bridged ring. Structurally this ring need not, from model studies, affect the detailed stereochemistry of the rest of the loop. In particular it need not disturb the interaction between the functional groupings of the site. There are, therefore, certain regions of the molecule which might be described as structural "segments" with a protective role: in the short toxins the Aβ strand, in the long toxins the C terminal tail, and perhaps in both series the hexapeptide loop 62–68.

3. Structural and Functional Residues

In Table 2 the invariant and conservatively substituted residues are shown with the assignment functional (F), structural (S), or uncertain (F/S or S/F). The proposed role assignments in the long series must be more tentative.

Fig. 11b. View (partially schematic) of the structure of the erabutoxin b molecule looking down into the concavity and modified to correspond to the long toxin series model. The invariant residue positions found in both series of toxins are shown emphasized by black caps top and bottom ◓. Common conservatively substituted positions are shown with a heavy broader outline **O**. The order of the residue type variations in these positions reflects the distribution in the long chain series only. In some instances conservative substitution of both series appears as an invariant in one series alone. Positions found only in the long chain series are shown as ◓ or ○ with the appropriate long chain series residues identified. This identification is also employed in the insertion positions shown sketched in with broken bonds. Residue extensions at the –COOH terminal end found in the long chain series are shown ◌ and ◓. Deletion positions in the long chain series relative to the short chain series are shown hatched ▨. All the residues are enumerated in the Karlsson sequence. As in Figure 11a the reactive site region is shown cross-hatched. Those invariant or conservatively substituted residues which appear to have primarily a functional role are shown dotted ◍. Those residues to which a structural function has been assigned are shown enclosed in a large circle ◯. In this drawing the conservative substitution observed in position 40 is also indicated. The residues which are shown enclosed in square boxes lie outside the reactive site region and appear implicated in function, although the description structural or functional is uncertain and ill defined. Heavy lines enclose those residues which form part of each of the five functional groupings. Position 27 has been shown as part of one functional grouping. There is an asterisk in this position which is usually Lys in the long chain toxins (see text)

a) Structural Residues

These have been discussed in detail earlier. They serve to establish and define the structural integrity which is maintained by multiple cross linking interactions between variable and invariable regions of residues. The molecule is remarkably formed and held with a precision unexpected in so open a structure.

The residues defined as structural are:

1. The eight disulfide bridge residues (Cys 3, 17, 24, 45, 49, 61, 62, and 68) common to all toxins and almost certainly the residues of the fifth disulfide bridge (Cys 30, Cys 34) which close the pentapeptide loop in the long toxins.
2. Ser 8 (short series) and Thr 48 (long series).
3. Gly 38, Gly 44, and Gly 56. In the long series Gly 20, and in the short series Gly 48.
4. Pro 50 and in the long series Pro 18 and Pro 72.
5. Asn 69.
6. In the long series probably Ile/Val/Leu 23, Val/Ile/Leu 41, Leu 43, Ala 46, and Ala 47.
7. Arg 43 in the short series.

b) Functional Groupings

The description functional implies direct involvement in binding to receptor. There appear to be five such groupings:

1. Arg 37–Asp 31: These are linked by a charge–charge interaction and are both at the extreme protruding end of the reactive site. Gly 38 could be considered a part of this group and therefore quasi-functional since a larger residue would impede the Arg-Asp interaction. We have chosen to describe Gly 38 as structural; Arg 37 and Gly 38 are absolute invariants. In deviant toxins where 31 is no longer Asp, toxicity is reduced. Chemical studies are consistent with this view if it be assumed that the carbonyl is the functional part of the carboxyl group. This first grouping probably occupies the binding site for acetylcholine on the receptor. This grouping is the only functional site on the molecule (compare Figs. 11a and 11b) which could be affected by local changes in the long toxin series. However, model-building studies have shown that the Arg-Asp interaction need not be affected by the presence of the adjacent disulfide bridged ring. The distance between the charges is appropriate for acetylcholine.

2. Arg/Ile/Val 40–Trp 29–Val/Ile 57; The core of this group is Trp 29. Toxicity is substantially lowered or essentially lost when it is modified (the tryptophan residue probably interacts directly with the receptor). All three residues point upwards into the concavity. Arg/Ile/Val 40 was not tabulated as a conservatively substituted position in Table 1, but if, as is proposed, we consider the hydrocarbon region of Arg as a hydrophobic alternative, then there are no deviations in position 40. Deviations in position 57 do not always affect toxicity. The two residues 40 and 57 both provide positioning hydrophobic interactions with Trp 29 and are possible sites of hydrophobic interactions with the receptor.

3. Lys/Arg 53: This is a second site of presumed charge–charge interaction with the receptor. Deviant toxins show reduced toxicity and chemical modifications emphasize the need for a charged group here for optimal toxicity. Unlike the other

positions of functional importance, this residue is isolated on the edge of the reactive site and is not involved in intramolecular interactions.

4. Val 52–Ile/Leu/Val 59: There are hydrophobic interactions between the residues in these positions which could be maintained even in the presence of deviant Lys 52. I have listed this as a functional grouping because thermodynamic studies and the magnitude of the binding constant suggest that there are multiple-binding sites and that some of them are hydrophobic. It is possible to consider this grouping as part of the complex which by bonding interactions maintains the impressive structural rigidity of the closed loop 49–61.

5. Glu/Asp 42–Tyr 25
‖ ‖
Lys 27 Pro 50 : – (The short chain near-invariant Lys 27 is usually Lys in the long chain toxins.) This grouping is perhaps the most controversial and tentative of our five assignments. The carboxyl of Glu 42 forms a hydrogen bond with the Tyr OH and there are hydrophobic interactions between the chain regions of Lys 27 and Glu 42. Tyrosine 25 packs against Pro 50. As we discussed, Tyr 25 thus could be considered the functional group positioned by Glu/Asp 42, Lys 27, and Pro 50, or alternatively Glu/Asp 42 could be considered the functional group positioned by Tyr 25 and Lys 27. Interactions with receptor may not in either case involve the reactive groups of the side chain hydroxyl and carboxyl. The assignment as functional may be in error, it is possible that this group of interactions is wholly concerned with structural integrity; possible, but in my view less probable.

c) Residues of Uncertain Role

Some of the residues designated F/S, S/F or F? in Table 2 have been discussed earlier, i.e., Tyr 25, Lys 27 (short series), Glu/Asp 42, Val 52, Val/Ile 57, and Ile/Leu/Val 59. Other residues designated S/F are important to maintain full toxic competence, i.e., Ser/Thr 9, Asn 5, and Thr 13 (the latter two short series).

The question of the range of acceptable substitutions (not affecting toxicity) in any one position, whether invariant, conservatively substituted, or apparently variant, cannot be explored exhaustively. Inappropriate substitutions may: 1. perturb the stereochemistry, e.g., by disrupting the β structure; or 2. perturb the stereochemistry by interacting with another residue or group of residues of functional or structural importance (see p. 243 for the rationale of the effect of Arg 7 in *Naja haje annulifera* CM 12 toxin) as well as simply replace residues, functionally important per se, e.g., Asp 31 or Lys/Arg 53. Perturbations can thus be introduced in structural and functional groupings by inappropriate substitutions of variant residues.

II. Future Studies—New Questions and Their Resolution

A description of the reactive site and of the functional groupings has been presented. It is plausible, the evidence available is necessary, but not sufficient: nevertheless it appears a persuasive model. The identity and arrangement of functional groups which interact with the acetylcholine receptor can be established experimentally only by the determination of the detailed three-dimensional structure of the toxin-receptor complex.

If the Asp-Arg grouping does bind to the acetylcholine site of the receptor molecule as is proposed, then the other functional groupings must lead both to tighter binding and also to inhibition or blocking of that conformational change which permits ionophoresis.

The determination of the structure of the receptor alone would permit some questions to be answered by model studies "fitting" toxin to receptor, but both these studies must wait on the isolation of receptor and the preparation of good crystals.

The isolation, purification, and crystallization of receptor presents a formidable task. Indeed, only a few (short) toxins have been crystallized. Although an understanding of the probable mechanism of action depends on studies of the complex, some useful further investigations of toxins should be made. Key studies to be carried out if the toxins can be crystallized are:

a) Determination of the structure of a short toxin of normal toxicity with a large number of sequence differences in the variable regions (e.g., *Naja nigricollis* toxin α). Such a study would confirm or refute the conclusion of structural invariance within the series.

b) Determination of the structure of one or two long toxins of normal toxicity in order to test the theory of limited structural modification of the short toxin prototype, and also to provide a check on the role assigned here to the C terminal tail peptide.

c) Determination of the structure of as many deviant toxins as possible, in particular *Naja naja oxiana* toxin I, *Laticauda semifasciata* toxin Ls III, *Naja haje annulifera* CM 10, *Naja haje annulifera* CM 12, and *Dendroaspis viridis* 4.7.3.

If a residue be wholly "functional" (replacement leads to lower toxicity) then the structural integrity of the molecule should not be distorted when it is replaced. However, if it be quasi-functional an exchange may perturb the structure either locally or more generally. It would be particularly interesting in this regard to study the CM 10, CM 12 toxins where short chain invariants and a non-type conserved residue Arg 7 are involved in reduced toxicity.

d) Determination of three or more closely related cardiotoxin (cytotoxin) structures with evident structural similarity but without neurotoxic activity.

Once studies of this kind have resolved the questions we can now ask, we shall be able to ask new questions and seek even more illuminating answers.

Acknowledgements. I thank Professor NOBUO TAMIYA who first stimulated my interest in the postsynaptic neurotoxins of snake venoms, for his generous cooperation and stimulating insights. I am grateful to Professor CHEN-YUAN LEE who has provided a viewpoint and outlook which informs the whole field and influenced the writing of this chapter. I am grateful also to my colleague, Mrs. JANE S. RICHARDSON for many lively and provocative discussions of protein structure, as well as my colleague, Dr. LAWRENCE S. ROSEN, who read and criticized the manuscript. This work was supported by Grant NS-07747 from the National Institutes of Health and by the Columbia University Center for Computing Activities which made generous grants of computer time. The 2.5-Å electron density map discussed here was interpreted using the GRIP-75 molecular graphics system build by the Universiy of North Carolina, Department of Computer Science with the help of many users.

References

Arai,H., Tamiya,N., Toshioka,S., Shinonaga,S., Kano,R.: Studies on Sea-Snake Venoms. I. Protein nature of the neurotoxin component. J. Biochem. (Tokyo) **56**, 568—571 (1964)

Arseniev,A.S., Balashova,T.A., Utkin,Y.N., Tsetlin,V.I., Bystrov,V.F., Ivanov,V.T., Ovchinnikov,Y.A.: Proton NMR study of the conformation of neurotoxin II from middleasian cobra *Naja naja oxiana* venom. Europ. J. Biochem. **71**, 595—606 (1976)

Balls,A.K., Jansen,E.F.: Stoichiometric inhibition of chymotrypsin. Advanc. Enzymol. **13**, 321—343 (1952)

Banks,B.C.E., Miledi,R., Shipolini,R.A.: The primary sequences and neuromuscular effects of three neurotoxic polypeptides from the venom of *Dendroaspis viridis*. Europ. J. Biochem. **45**, 457—468 (1974)

Bartels,E., Rosenberry,T.L.: Snake neurotoxins: effect of disulfide reduction on interaction with electroplax. Science **174**, 1236—1237 (1971)

Biesecker,G.: Molecular properties of the cholinergic receptor purified from *Electrophorus electricus*. Biochemistry **12**, 4403—4409 (1973)

Botes,D.P.: Snake venom toxins. The reactivity of the disulphide bonds of *Naja nivea* toxin α. Biochim. biophys. Acta (Amst.) **359**, 242—247 (1974)

Chang,C.C., Lee,C.Y.: Isolation of neurotoxins from the venom of *Bungarus multicinctus* and their modes of neuromuscular blocking action. Arch. int. Pharmacodyn. **144**, 241—257 (1963)

Chang,C.C., Yang,C.C., Hamaguchi,K., Nakai,K., Hayashi,K.: Studies on the status of tyrosyl residues in cobrotoxin. Biochim. biophys. Acta (Amst.) **236**, 164—173 (1971 a)

Chang,C.C., Yang,C.C., Nakai,K., Hayashi,K.: Studies on the status of free amino and carboxyl groups in cobrotoxin. Biochim. biophys. Acta (Amst.) **251**, 334—344 (1971 b)

Changeux,J.-P., Kasai,M., Lee,C.Y.: Use of a snake venom toxin to characterize the cholinergic receptor protein. Proc. nat. Acad. Sci. (Wash.) **67**, 1241—1247 (1970)

Changeux,J.-P., Benedetti,L., Bourgeois,J.-P., Brisson,A., Cartaud,J., Devaux,P., Grunhagen,H., Moreau,M., Popot,J.-L., Sobel,A., Weber,M.: Some structural properties of the cholinergic receptor protein in its membrane environment relevant to its function as a pharmacological receptor. In: Cold Spring Harbor Symposia on Quantitative Biology, The Synapse, Vol. XI, pp. 211—230. Pub. Cold Spring Harbor, N.Y.: Cold Spring Harbor Lab. 1975

Changeux,J.-P., Meunier,J.C., Huchet,M.: Studies on the cholinergic receptor protein of *Electrophorus Electricus*. I. An assay in vitro for the cholinergic receptor site and solubilization of the receptor protein from electric tissue. J. molec. Pharmacol. **7**, 538—553 (1971)

Chicheportiche,R., Rochat,C., Sampieri,F., Lazdunski,M.: Structure-function relationships of neurotoxins isolated from *Naja haje* venom. Physicochemical properties and identification of the active site. Biochemistry **11**, 1681—1691 (1972)

Chou,P.Y., Fasman,G.D.: Conformational parameters for amino acids in helical, β-sheet, and random coil regions calculated from proteins. Biochemistry **13**, 211—222 (1974 a)

Chou,P.Y., Fasman,G.D.: Prediction of protein conformation. Biochemistry **13**, 222—245 (1974 b)

Christensen,P.A.: South African Snake Venoms and Antivenoms. Johannesburg: The South African Inst. Med. Res. 1955

Crane,G.A., Rosen,L.S., Low,B.W.: Unpublished studies (1977)

Dickerson,R.E., Geis,I.: The Structure and Action of Proteins. New York: Harper & Row 1969

Eaker,D.: Structure and Function of Snake Venom toxins. In: Walter,R., Meienhofer,J. (Eds.): Peptides: Chemistry, Structure and Biology. Proc. 4th Am. Peptide Symposium, pp. 17—30. Ann Arbor, Michigan: Ann Arbor—Science Publisher's Inc. 1975

Eldefrawi,M.E., Eldefrawi,A.T., Shamoo,A.E.: Molecular and functional properties of the acetylcholine-receptor. Ann. N.Y. Acad. Sci. **264**, 183—202 (1975)

Gabel,D., Rasse, D., Scheraga,H.A.: Search for low-energy conformations of a neurotoxic protein by means of predictive rules, tests for hard-sphere overlaps, and energy minimization. Int. J. Peptide Res. **8**, (3), 237—252 (1976)

Hall,Z.W.: Release of neurotransmitters and their interaction with receptors. Ann. Rev. Biochem. **41**, 925—952 (1972)

Hamaguchi,K., Ikeda,K., Lee,C.Y.: Optical rotatory dispersion and circular dichroism of neurotoxins isolated from the venom of *Bungarus multicinctus*. J. Biochem. (Tokyo) **64**, 503—506 (1968)

Harada, I., Takamatsu, T., Shimanouchi, T., Miyazawa, T., Tamiya, N.: Raman spectra of some neurotoxins and denatured neurotoxins in relation to structure and toxicities. J. Phys. Chem. **80**, 1153—1156 (1976)
Homma, M., Okonogi, T., Mishima, S.: Studies on sea snake venoms. I. Biological toxicities of venoms possessed by three species of sea snake captured in coastal water of Amami Oshima. Gunma J. med. Sci. **13**, 283—296 (1964)
Hori, H., Tamiya, N.: Preparation and activity of guanidinated or acetylated erabutoxins. Biochem. J. **153**, 217—222 (1976)
Huang, J. S., Liu, S. S., Ling, K. H., Chang, C. C., Yang, C. C.: Iodination of cobrotoxin. Toxicon **11**, 39—45 (1973)
Ishikawa, Y., Menez, A., Hori, H., Yoshida, H., Tamiya, N.: Structure of snake toxins and their affinity to the acetylcholine receptor of fish electric organ. Toxicon **15**, 477—488 (1977)
Karlin, A.: Current Problems in Acetylcholine Receptor Research. In: Rowland, L. F.: Pathogenesis of Human Muscular Dystrophies. Amsterdam: Excerpta Medica, 1977, pp. 73—84
Karlin, A., Weill, C., McNamee, M., Valderrama, R.: Facets of the structures of acetylcholine receptors from *Electrophorus* and *Torpedo*. In: Cold Spring Harbor Symposia on Quantitative Biology. The Synapse. Vol. XL, pp. 203—210. N.Y. Cold Spring Harbor Lab.: Pub. Cold Spring Harbor, 1975
Karlsson, E., Arnberg, H., Eaker, D.: Isolation of the principal neurotoxins of two *Naja naja* subspecies. Europ. J. Biochem. **21**, 1—16 (1971)
Karlsson, E., Eaker, D.: Chemical modifications of the postsynaptic *Naja naja* neurotoxins. J. Formosan med. Ass. **71**, 358—371 (1972)
Karlsson, E., Fohlman, J., Groth, M.: Purification of the acetylcholine receptor from the electric organ of *Torpedo marmorata*. Bull. Inst. Pasteur **74**, 11—22 (1976)
Karlsson, E., Sundelin, J.: Nitration of tyrosine in three cobra neurotoxins. Toxicon **14**, 295—306 (1976)
Klett, R. P., Fulpius, B. W., Cooper, D., Smith, M., Reich, E., Possani, L. D.: The acetylcholine receptor. J. biol. Chem. **248**, 6841—6853 (1973)
Lee, C. Y.: Chemistry and pharmacology of polypeptide toxins in snake venoms. Ann. Rev. Pharmacol. **12**, 265—286 (1972)
Low, B. W.: The three dimensional structure of erabutoxin b neurotoxic protein. The Fifth International Symposium of Animal, Plant, and Microbial Toxins of the International Society on Toxinology in San Jose, Costa Rica 1976a.
Low, B. W.: Unpublished studies (1976b)
Low, B. W., Potter, R., Jackson, R. B., Tamiya, N., Sato, S.: X-ray crystallographic study of the erabutoxins and of a diiodo derivative. J. biol. Chem. **246**, 4366—4368 (1971)
Low, B. W., Preston, H. S., Sato, A., Rosen, L. S., Searl, J. E., Rudko, A. D., Richardson, J. S.: Three dimensional structure of erabutoxin b neurotoxic protein: Inhibitor of acetylcholine receptor. Proc. nat. Acad. Sci. (Wash.) **73**, 2991—2994 (1976a)
Low, B. W., Preston, H. S., Sato, A., Rosen, L., Richardson, J. S.: Unpublished studies (1976b)
Maeda, N., Takagi, K., Tamiya, N., Chen, Y.-M., Lee, C. Y.: The isolation of an easily reversible post-synaptic toxin from the venom of a sea snake, *Laticauda semifasciata*. Biochem. J. **141**, 383—387 (1974)
Maeda, N., Tamiya, N.: The primary structure of the toxin Laticauda semifasciata III, a weak and reversible acting neurotoxin from the venom of a sea snake, *Laticauda semifasciata*. Biochem. J. **141**, 389—400 (1974)
Maeda, N., Tamiya, N.: Correction of partial amino acid sequence of erabutoxins. Biochem. J. **167**, 289—291 (1977)
Maelicke, A., Reich, E.: On the interaction between cobra α-neurotoxin and the acetylcholine receptor. In: Cold Spring Harbor Symposia on Quantitative Biology, The Synapse, Vol. XL, pp. 231—235. N.Y. Cold Spring Harbor Lab.: Pub. Cold Spring Harbor 1975
Mebs, D., Narita, K., Iwanaga, S., Samejima, Y., Lee, C. Y.: Purification, properties, and amino acid sequence of α-bungarotoxin from the venom of *Bungarus multicinctus*. Hoppe-Seylers Z. physiol. Chem. **353**, 243—262 (1972)
Mebs, D., Narita, K., Lee, C. Y.: Amino acid sequence of α-bungarotoxin from the venom of *Bungarus multicinctus*. Biochem. Biophys. Res. Commun. **44**, 711—716 (1971)
Menez, A., Bouet, F., Fromageot, P., Tamiya, N.: On the role of tyrosyl and tryptophanyl residues in the conformation of two snake neurotoxins. Bull. Inst. Pasteur **74**, 57—64 (1976a)

Menez, A., Boquet, P., Tamiya, N., Fromageot, P.: Conformational changes in two neurotoxic proteins from snake venoms. Biochim. biophys. Acta (Amst.) **453**, 121—132 (1976b)

Meunier, J.-C., Sealock, R., Olsen, R., Changeux, J.-P.: Purification and properties of the cholinergic receptor protein from *Electrophorus electricus* electric tissue. Europ. J. Biochem. **45**, 371—394 (1974)

Miledi, R., Molinof, P., Potter, L. T.: Isolation of the cholinergic receptor protein of Torpedo electric tissue. Nature (Lond.) **229**, 554—557 (1971)

Nakai, K., Sasaki, T., Hayashi, K.: Amino acid sequence of toxin A from the venom of the Indian cobra *(Naja naja)*. Biochem. Biophys. Res. Commun. **41**, 893—897 (1971)

Ohta, M., Hayashi, K.: Chemical modification of the tyrosine residue in toxin B from the venom of the Indian cobra *Naja naja*. Biochem. Biophys. Res. Commun. **56**, 981—987 (1974)

Preston, H. S., Kay, J., Sato, A., Low, B. W., Tamiya, N.: Crystalline erabutoxin c. Toxicon **13**, 273—275 (1975)

Quiocho, F. A., Lipscomb, W. W.: Carboxypeptidase A: a protein and an enzyme. Advanc. Protein Chem. **25**, 1—59 (1971)

Raftery, M. A., Schmidt, J., Clark, D. G., Wolcott, R. G.: Demonstration of a specific α-bungarotoxin binding component in *Electrophorus electricus* electroplax membranes. Biochem. biophys. Res. Commun. **45**, 1622—1629 (1971)

Raftery, M. A., Vandlen, R. L., Reed, K. L., Lee, T.: Characterization of *Torpedo californica* acetylcholine receptor: Its subunit composition and ligand-binding properties. In: Cold Spring Harbor Symposia on Quantitative Biology, The Synapse, Vol. XL, pp. 193—202. N.Y.: Cold Spring Harbor Lab., Pub. Cold Spring Harbor 1975

Richardson, J. S.: Handedness of crossover connections in β sheets. Proc. nat. Acad. Sci. (Wash.) **73**, 2619—2623 (1976)

Rydén, L., Gabel, D., Eaker, D.: A model of the three-dimensional structure of snake venom neurotoxins based on chemical evidence. Int. J. Peptide Protein Res. **5**, 261—273 (1973)

Sato, A.: The X-Ray Crystallographic Studies on Sea Snake Neurotoxins. Ph.D. Thesis, Dept. of Chemistry, Tohoku Univ. Jpn 1977

Sato, A., Rosen, L. S., Richardson, J. S., Low, B. W.: Unpublished studies (1977)

Sato, N., Tamiya, N., Ikeda, K., Hamaguchi, K.: Unpublished studies (1968)

Sato, S., Abe, T., Tamiya, N.: Binding of iodinated erabutoxin b; A sea snake toxin to the endplates of the mouse diaphragm. Toxicon **8**, 313—314 (1970)

Sato, S., Tamiya, N.: Iodination of erabutoxin b: Diiodohistidine formation. J. Biochem. (Tokyo) **68**, 867—872 (1970)

Sato, S., Tamiya, N.: The amino acid sequences of erabutoxins, neurotoxic proteins of sea-snake *(Laticauda semifasciata)* venom. Biochem. J. **122**, 453—461 (1971)

Sato, S., Yoshida, H., Abe, H., Tamiya, N.: Properties and biosynthesis of a neurotoxic protein of the venoms of sea snakes *Laticauda laticaudata* and *Laticauda colubrina*. Biochem. J. **115**, 85—90 (1969)

Searl, J. E., Fullerton, W. W., Low, B. W.: X-ray crystallographic study of laticotoxin a. J. biol. Chem. **248**, 6057—6058 (1973)

Sheu, Y. S.: Influence of diisopropylfluorophosphate on the thrombinlike action of snake venoms. J. Formosan med. Ass. **61**, 245—250 (1962)

Shipolini, R. A., Bailey, G. S., Edwardson, J. A., Banks, B. E. C.: Separation and characterization of polypeptide from the venom of *Dendroaspis viridis*. Europ. J. Biochem. **40**, 337—344 (1973)

Shü, I. C., Ling, K. H., Yang, C. C.: Study on I^{131} labeled cobrotoxin. Toxicon **5**, 295—301 (1968)

Smythies, J. R., Bennington, F., Bradley, R. J., Bridgers, W. F., Morin, R. D., Romine, W. O.: The molecular structure of the receptor-ionophore complex at the neuromuscular junction. J. theor. Biol. **51** (1), 111—126 (1975)

Takamatsu, T., Harada, I., Shimanouchi, T., Ohta, M., Hayashi, K.: Raman spectrum of toxin B in relation to structure and toxicity. FEBS Letters **72**, (2) 291—294 (1976)

Tamiya, N.: Erabutoxins a, b, and c in sea snake *Laticauda semifasciata* venom. Toxicon **11**, 95—97 (1973)

Tamiya, N., Abe, H.: The isolation, properties and amino acid sequence of erabutoxin c, a minor neurotoxic component of the venom of a sea snake *Laticauda semifasciata* venom. Biochem. J. **130**, 547—555 (1972)

Tamiya, N., Arai, H.: Studies on sea-snake venoms. Crystallization of erabutoxins a and b from *Laticauda semifasciata* venom. Biochem. J. **99**, 624—630 (1966)

Tamiya, N., Takasaki, C.: Detection of erabutoxins in the venom of sea snake *Laticauda semifasciata* from the Philippines. Biochim. biophys. Acta (Amst.) **532**, 199—201 (1978)
Tsernoglou, D., Petsko, G. A.: The crystal structure of a postsynaptic neurotoxin from sea snake at 2.2 Å resolution. FEBS Letters **68** (1), 1—4 (1976)
Tsetlin, V. I., Mikhaleva, I. I., Myagkova, M. A., Senyavina, L. B., Arseniev, A. S., Ivanov, V. T., Ovchinnikov, Y. A.: Synthetic and conformational studies of the neurotoxins and cytotoxins of snake venom. In: Walter, R., Meienhofer, J. (Eds.): Peptides: Chemistry, Structure and Biology. Proc. 4th Am. Peptide Symposium, pp. 935—941. Ann Arbor, Michigan: Ann Arbor-Science Publisher's Inc., 1975
Tu, A. T., Hong, B., Solie, T. N.: Characterization and chemical modifications of toxins isolated from the venoms of the sea snake *Laticauda semifasciata*, from Philippines. Biochemistry **10** (8), 1295—1304 (1971)
Venkatachalam, C. M.: Stereochemical criteria for polypeptides and proteins. V. Conformation of a system of three linked peptide units. Biopolymers **6**, 1425—1436 (1968)
Weber, M., Changeux, J.-P.: Binding of *Naja nigricollis* [^{3}H] α-toxin to membrane fragments from *Electrophorus* and *Torpedo* electric organs. II. Effect of cholinergic agonists and antagonists on the binding of the tritiated α-neurotoxin. J. molec. Pharmacol. **10**, 15—34 (1974)
Weill, C. L., McNamee, M. G., Karlin, A.: Affinity-labeling of purified acetylcholine receptor from *Torpedo californica*. Biochem. Biophys. Res. Commun. **61**, 997—1003 (1974)
Wong, C., Chang, T. W., Lee, T. J., Yang, C. C.: X-ray crystallographic study of cobrotoxin. J. biol. Chem. **247**, 608 (1972)
Yang, C. C.: Enzymic hydrolysis and chemical modification of cobrotoxin. Toxicon **3**, 19—22 (1964)
Yang, C. C.: Crystallization and properties of cobrotoxin from Formosan cobra venom. J. biol. Chem. **240**, 1616—1618 (1965)
Yang, C. C.: The disulfide bonds of cobrotoxin and their relationship to lethality. Biochim. biophys. Acta (Amst.) **133**, 346—355 (1967)
Yang, C. C.: Chemistry and evolution of toxins in snake venoms. Toxicon **12**, 1—43 (1974)
Yang, C. C., Chang, C. C., Hamaguchi, K., Ikeda, K., Hayashi, K., Suzuki, T.: Optical rotatory dispersion of cobrotoxin. J. Biochem. (Tokyo) **61**, 272—274 (1967)
Yang, C. C., Chang, C. C., Hayashi, K., Suzuki, T., Ideka, K., Hamaguchi, K.: Optical rotatory dispersion and circular dichoism of cobrotoxin. Biochim. biophys. Acta (Amst.) **168**, 373—376 (1968)
Yang, C. C., Chang, C. C., Liu, I. F.: Studies on the Status of Arginine Residues in Cobrotoxin. 9th Int. Congr. Biochem. Stockholm. Colloquium D, Abs. p. 455, 1973
Yü, N. T., Lin, T. S., Tu, A. T.: Laser raman scattering of neurotoxins isolated from the venoms of sea snakes *Lapemis hardwickii* and *Enhydrina schistosa*. J. biol. Chem. **250**, 1782—1785 (1975)

CHAPTER 7

The Evolution of Toxins Found in Snake Venoms

D. J. STRYDOM

A. Introduction

The past decade has seen both the beginnings of knowledge on the chemical structure of snake venom toxins and the subsequent explosion in the amount of available data on this subject. The chemistry of these proteins has been dealt with by KARLSSON in Chapter 5. One of the possible types of information that can be gleaned from such a mass of data on protein structures is the evolutionary history of the genes coding for those proteins, as well as information on the biologic classification of the organisms possessing these genes.

This chapter will show how thoughts on the evolution of snake venom toxins have developed as more and more data were obtained during the last few years. To this end, we will first give a brief resumé of the types of toxins found in venoms and discuss a few methods which have been used to investigate phylogenetic relationships of proteins before going on to the subject of toxin phylogenetics.

I. The Toxin-Types of Snake Venoms

The toxic proteins of snake venoms can at present be grouped into more than ten categories on the basis of their chemical structures and pharmacologic properties. For the sake of simplicity, we will adhere to the classification of four broad groups by KARLSSON (Chap. 5 in this volume of the Handbook).

1. Curaremimetic postsynaptic neurotoxins (consisting of both "short" and "long" neurotoxins).
2. Membrane toxins (cardiotoxins, cytotoxins, direct lytic factors, *angusticeps*-type toxins, *melanoleuca*-type toxins, etc.).
3. Toxins with phospholipase structure.
4. Other toxins (crotamine, etc.).

To facilitate following the different types of reasoning used later in this chapter, we present an example of how groups 1 and 2 are aligned with each other to show maximum homology (Fig. 1). Most of these alignments were checked by program ALIGN (STRYDOM, 1973a), and in all cases we can say that these proteins are mutually homologous.

The introduction of deletions/insertions has been minimized, causing some minor differences from other published alignments (KARLSSON, 1973; CARLSSON, 1975; JOUBERT, 1973; DAYHOFF, 1972; MAEDA and TAMIYA, 1974; RYDÉN et al., 1973; LOUW, 1974a). A popular alignment of Asn 4 of most cardiotoxins with Asn 5 of *Hemachatus* direct lytic factor seems unnecessary in that an extra deletion has to be

```
   1        10        20        30        40        50        60        70    76
 1 LECHNQQSSQPPTTKTCP-GETNCYKKRWRDH----RGSITERGCG--CPSVKKGIEINCCTTDKCNN--------
 2 RICYNHQSSTRATTKSCE--ENSCYKKYWRDH----RGTIIERGCG--CPKVKPGVGIHCCQSDKCNY--------
 3 RICFNQHSSQPQTTKTCPSGSESCYNKQWSDF----RGTIIERGCG--CPTVKPGIKLSCCESEVCNN--------
 4 MICYKQQSLQFPITTVCP-GEKNCYKKQWSGH----RGTIIERGCG--CPSVKKGIEINCCTTDKCNR--------
 5 MICYSHKTPQPSATITCE--EKTCYKKSVRKL----PAVVAGRGCG--CPSKEMLVAIHCCRSDKCNE--------
 6 LTCLICPEKYCNKVHTCRNGENICFKRFYEGN---LLGKRYPRGCAATCPEAKPREIVECCSTDKCNH--------
 7 TKCY---VTPDATSQTCPDGQDICYTKTWCDGFCSSRGKRVDLGCAATCPIVKPGVEIKCCSTDNCNPFPTWRKRP
 8 RTCN---KTFSDQSKICPPGENICYTKTWCDAWCSQRGKRVELGCAATCPKVKAGVEIKCCSTDDCDKFQFGKPR-
 9 IVCH-TTATIPSSAVTCPPGENLCYRKMWCDAFCSSRGKVVELGCAATCPSKKPYEEVTCCSTDKCNHPPKRQPG-
10 LKCHN--KLVPFLSKTCPEGKNLCYKMTMLKM----PKIPIKRGCTDACPKSSLLDKVVCCNKDKCN---------
11 LKCH---KLVPPVWKTCPEGKNLCYKMFMVST----STVPVKRGCIDVCPKNSALVKYVCCSTDKCN---------
12 LKCN---KLIPLAYKTCPAGKNLCYKMYMVSN----KTVPVKRGCIDVCPKNSLVLKYECCNTDRCN---------
```

Fig. 1. Alignment of sequences of a few selected toxins from groups 1 and 2 of snake toxins. The IUPAC one-letter amino acid code is used in this and the subsequent figures.

1 = *Naja haje annulifera* α (BOTES and STRYDOM, 1969)
2 = *Dendroaspis polylepis* α (STRYDOM, 1972a)
3 = Erabutoxin a (SATO and TAMIYA, 1971)
4 = *Naja haje* CM-10 (JOUBERT, 1975e)
5 = *Dendroaspis angusticeps* F8 (VILJOEN and BOTES, 1974)
6 = *Naja melanoleuca* S_4C_{11} (CARLSSON, 1975)
7 = *Ophiophogus hannah* A (JOUBERT, 1973)
8 = *Dendroaspis polylepis* γ (STRYDOM, 1972a)
9 = α-bungarotoxin (MEBS et al., 1972)
10 = *Hemachatus haemachatus* DLF (FRYKLUND and EAKER, 1973)
11 = *Naja haje annulifera* $V^{11}1$ (WEISE et al., 1973)
12 = *Naja naja* cytotoxin I (HAYASHI et al., 1971)

postulated. Alignment of Asn 4 (and His 4) of cardiotoxins with the His 4 of the *Hemachatus* protein is compatible with, e.g., His 4 of many short neurotoxins and Asn 4 of *D. polylepis* long neurotoxins. Likewise, the popular alignment of the His 32 (or Phe 32) of short neurotoxins with Phe 33 (or Trp 33) of long neurotoxins is unneccessarily forced since it would also introduce an extra deletion, as well as forcing a horrific alignment of cardiotoxins with neurotoxins in this position. The carboxylterminal part of *O. hannah* toxins also does not need a deletion for alignment—it is well-aligned with, e.g., *D. polylepis* long toxins and having one amino acid aligning beyond all other long neurotoxins is in harmony with, e.g., the shorter length of *L. semifasciata* LS III. The current alignment of the *melanoleuca*-type toxin, S_4C_{11}, especially with Gly 31 aligning with the constant Asp 31 of neurotoxins (which is Gly 31 in the neurotoxin homologues CM−10 and CM−12 of *N. haje annulifera* venom!), only needs a repetition of Leu 33 to insert the one extra amino acid with reference to short neurotoxins, cardiotoxins, and *angusticeps*-types.

II. Methods Used in Studying Protein Phylogenetics

Since ZUCKERKANDL and PAULING'S (1965) classic paper, a number of approaches have been developed to extract phylogenetic information from protein sequences. I will not attempt an extensive review of this subject, which is in itself a very broad field of study, but will only touch on a few aspects.

It is convenient to subdivide the different approaches to molecular phylogenetics (and especially *protein* phylogenetics) into four divisions, although combinations of these methods are often used.

1. Matrix Methods

These methods are exemplified by the FITCH and MARGOLIASH (1967) method. A matrix of differences between individual proteins in a set of homologous proteins is set up. This matrix is used to generate a tree relationship of the proteins by clustering techniques. Alternate trees are set up on a trial and error basis and each tree is evaluated as to the distances between every possible pair of proteins via the branches of the tree. A "standard deviation" of these values from the actual data is calculated. The tree with a minimum "standard deviation" is taken to represent the best phylogeny.

The clustering method works well provided the mutation rates of all the proteins in such a set are constant. In practice this proviso is usually not met. Varying mutation rates are usually discerned when negative branch lengths are generated during clustering procedures. FARRIS (1972) has shown that difference matrices can, however, be used even in cases where mutation rates are different by the Distance Wagner Procedure. This method has not yet been put into widespread use.

2. Ancestor Sequence Method

DAYHOFF and PARK (1969) have been the major proponents of the ancestor sequence method. In brief, this method starts off with a tree generated by a matrix method and calculates ancestral sequences for the nodes in the tree. From these ancestral sequences are calculated the minimum number of amino acid changes which have occurred in the set of proteins. Alternate trees are created by systematic swopping around of branches of the first tree and the tree with the lowest minimum number of amino acid changes is taken as the "best" tree. This method is very tricky to program.

3. Maximum Parsimony Method

This method was introduced by BARNABAS et al. (1972). It is basically a matrix method but also makes use of the actual sequences of the proteins. A mathematic method constructs maximum parsimony ancestral codon residues, i.e., residues which minimize mutational change over the network (a network depiction of trees is used to facilitate computations). A network "length" is calculated from these ancestral codon sequences and the network systematically changed to search for a minimization of network length. Computing time is quite lengthy for this method.

4. Subjective Methods

Here I group methods which are usually used to modify phylogenies obtained by matrix methods by subjectively deciding that certain features of the amino acid sequence of a number of proteins from an homologous set are more important than numbers from the matrix method. It can for example, be decided that half-cystinyl residues which are conserved (or not conserved) place certain proteins closer together (or further apart) in a phylogenetic relationship than numeric methods would allow. The reasoning could be: half-cystinyl residues are usually very important for protein structure and selection will usually be against any changes in the protein that impair the formation of the correct disulfide bridges. Convergent or divergent changes in other parts of the proteins could then lead to "wrong" mutational distances being found between such proteins. It is obvious that this type of subjective reasoning will find a place in the construction of phylogenies wherever widely variable mutation rates are to be found, since in such cases the numeric methods have difficulties.

Data other than actual sequences can also be brought to bear on phylogenies. An example would be the naming of snake short neurotoxins as the most primitive snake toxins since only *that* type was at that stage known to be present in the venom of the most primitive front-fanged snakes, the sea snakes (LEE, 1972).

All these methods have their weaknesses, but it should still be possible to use these methods, or combinations of them, in studying most homologous protein families. PEACOCK and BOULTER (1975) recently evaluated methods 2 and 3 and concluded that where a low number of amino acid substitutions were concerned, the ancestral amino acid sequence method yielded more accurate results, and when there were great differences (more than 30%) in sequences, the matrix and maximum parsimony methods were slightly more accurate. It is conceivable that with the additional judicious application of some subjective considerations, most protein groups should be amenable to phylogenetic study.

B. Historic Development of Snake Toxin Phylogenetics

The first amino acid sequence of a snake venom toxin, that of *N. nigricollis* toxin α, was completed in 1967 (EAKER and PORATH, 1967) and was followed 2 years later by the sequences of *N. haje* toxin α (BOTES and STRYDOM, 1969) and cobrotoxin (YANG et al., 1969). By 1971, sequences of 11 snake toxins were known—two long neurotoxins, two hydrophid short neurotoxins, and seven elapid short neurotoxins. STRYDOM (1972b) applied the matrix method of FITCH and MARGOLIASH (1967) to these sequences to show that the divergence of long and short neurotoxins occurred *before* the divergence of elapid and hydrophid snakes. This method of constructing phylogenies depends on constant mutation rates of the genes coding for the relevant proteins. We have since then noticed that long neurotoxins mutated faster than short neurotoxins did (STRYDOM, 1973a). This is especially seen when comparing the mutation distances between the long toxins of *Dendroaspis polylepis* and *Dendroaspis jamesonii* venoms (18) with the mutation distance found between the short toxins of the same species (11), although the pairs *Naja nivea–Naja melanoleuca* also show the same effect (11–8). The possibility, therefore, still existed that, on the data then available, the short hydrophid toxins could be ancestral to both short and long elapid neurotoxins, although an experimental attempt to normalize the mutation rates through manipulation of the difference matrices (STRYDOM, unpublished) did not change the earlier conclusion (STRYDOM, 1972b).

With the advent of the first amino acid sequence of a cardiotoxin (NARITA and LEE, 1970), LEE and co-workers (LEE, 1972; NARITA et al., 1972) looked at this other possibility and speculated that, since the composition of sea snake venoms is seemingly much simpler than that of land snake venoms (at that stage only short neurotoxins were known from sea snake venoms), the hydrophid short neurotoxins were the ancient form of snake toxins. They reasoned that the elapid short neurotoxins evolved from the hydrophid short neurotoxins and that the former then later gave rise to two separate lines—the one being the cardiotoxins, the other being the cobra long neurotoxins. From the cobra long neurotoxins then would have arisen α-bungarotoxin.

This is an example of the subjective reasoning method for constructing phylogenies. Here too, subsequent data has cast doubt on the validity of the arguments. Some cardiotoxins and the long neurotoxins have, for example, common structural features—a similar length between half-cystinyl residues 1 and 2 and a common ancestral sequence—Cys-Ala-Ala-Thr-Cys—between half-cystines 4 and 5 of the cardiotoxins (corresponding to half-cystines 6 and 7 of the long neurotoxins). It is, therefore, unlikely that long neurotoxins and cardiotoxins independently evolved out of short neurotoxins.

When more long neurotoxin sequences became known, a plausible mechanism for the evolution of long neurotoxins from short neurotoxins became apparent (STRYDOM, 1972a). Near the middle of the polypeptide chain, the short neurotoxins have the sequence type: Cys-Tyr-Thr-Lys-X-Trp-Ser/Arg-Asp-His-Arg-Gly. If in one case the seryl residue mutated to a cysteinyl residue (one nucleotide base change in the gene), it could conceivably be nondeleterious because of similar steric properties. If then an homologous unequal crossing over event inserted 12 nucleotide bases into this gene, the resultant sequence would be: Cys-Tyr-Thr-Lys-X-*Trp-Cys-Asp-His-Trp-Cys-Asp-His*-Arg-Gly. The two cysteinyl residues might then form a disulfide bridge—as is in fact found for the long neurotoxin of *Naja nivea* venom (BOTES, 1971). Compare this hypothetic sequence with that of the long neurotoxin of *D. polylepis* venom (STRYDOM, 1972a): Cys-Tyr-Thr-Lys-Thr-Trp-Cys-Asp-Ala-Trp-Cys-Ser-Gln-Arg-Gly, and this mechanism is indeed plausible. Furthermore, this extra disulfide bridge can be reduced with little effect on the structure and activity of the toxins (BOTES, 1974), and from this follows that it is more probably a later development in the structure of these proteins. The chain elongation found for long neurotoxins can be explained by a single base change in the chain terminating codon. See, for example, the mechanism advanced for the chain elongation of hemoglobin Constant Spring (CLEGG et al., 1971) and the additional proof for this from hemoglobin Cranston (BUNN et al., 1975).

TU (1973) seemed to agree with this mechanism for evolving a long neurotoxin from a shorter toxin with his scheme whereby cardiotoxins evolved from short neurotoxins and in turn gave rise to long neurotoxins. It is, however, unlikely that a short neurotoxin could have lost its neurotoxicity (and therefore specific structural features) to give rise to a cardiotoxin and then have long neurotoxins evolve from a cardiotoxin and regain neurotoxicity and the same specific structural features as the short neurotoxins have.

BARKER and DAYHOFF (1972) agreed with the findings that the three types of toxins were homologous and calculated a tree for 14 toxins including two long neurotoxins and three cardiotoxins by the ancestral sequence method. They did not voice any opinion on which protein was the more primitive. Their arrangement of the short neurotoxins indicates a wide variation in mutation rates for the cobra neurotoxins and differs somewhat from that of STRYDOM (1973b). Their arrangement was programmed into program PHYMOD and no improvement in "standard deviation" over that with the published schemes was found. Resolution of these discrepancies will have to await studies making use of many more toxin amino acid sequences.

Application of a slightly more sophisticated matrix method when more cardiotoxin sequences became known (STRYDOM, 1973b) led to a suggested evolutionary scheme where cardiotoxins were seen as the ancient form of snake venom toxins, with short and long neurotoxins evolving separately from a common neurotoxic protein which has evolved from the cardiotoxin ancestor. With yet a further doubling in the number of toxin sequences known (to 43) and the discovery of *angusticeps*-type toxins, doubts were raised as to the validity of *this* toxin evolution scheme (STRYDOM, 1973a).

STRYDOM (1973a) showed that application of matrix methods on the three better known groups of toxins (long and short neurotoxins and cardiotoxins) cannot *objectively* discriminate between consideration of any of the three types as ancestral types of toxin. Subjectively, the long neurotoxins seem "younger" as per the argument above, but no choice can be made between the other groups when the effect of variable mutation rates are taken into account. Adding the *angusticeps*-type toxins to the tree does not remove the dilemma—either a cardiotoxin or a short neurotoxin could still be the ancestral form of toxin. When ancestral amino acid sequences were constructed on the basis of the two alternative schemes, the ancestral sequence for the tree having the short neurotoxin as most primitive toxin was more easily constructed, with less ambiguities than the ancestral sequence for the tree depicting cardiotoxin as the most primitive toxin. This would seem to favor the short neurotoxin as being the most primitive toxin. STRYDOM (1973a) also showed that there is a possibility of homology between a short region of bovine ribonuclease and a short neurotoxin, cobrotoxin, because of the following remarkable correspondence in sequences. Ribonuclease, residues 65–73 (SMYTH et al., 1963), has the sequence: Cys-Lys-Asn-Gly-Gln-Thr-Asn-Cys-Tyr, while residues 17–25 of cobrotoxin have the sequence Cys-Ser-Gly-Gly-Glu-Thr-Asn-Cys-Tyr. The rest of the sequences did not have a visible correspondence. Application of computer program ALIGN (STRYDOM, 1973a), which is used to test for homology of proteins, showed a faint, but definite internal duplication in the sequences of snake toxins, which would suggest that either snake toxins or their evolutionary precursors had evolved through gene elongation via a gene-doubling event. The evolutionary scheme for snake toxins was consequently that an ancestral ribonuclease underwent gene duplication which yielded the lines that led on the one hand to the modern ribonuclease and on the other to snake venom toxins. The short neurotoxin form was, according to this, the first of the snake venom toxins to evolve and the long neurotoxin and cardiotoxin types derived from this in turn through further gene duplication. The proposed ancestor of the neuro- and cardiotoxins was probably already a ribonuclease because the divergence of mammals and reptiles before the acquiring of a toxic secretion by snakes was deemed more plausible. The separate and parallel development of ribonuclease activity in snakes and mammals was furthermore thought improbable. The ancestral ribonuclease would, therefore, in the light of the internal duplication of its homologue, snake toxin, also exhibit such an internal homology. It is still possible to argue against this study's relegation of the short neurotoxin to "primitive" status. There exists the possibility that precisely the placing of short neurotoxins and *angusticeps* types on two different lines leading from the ancestral toxin in the model (which makes the short neurotoxin the most ancient toxin) is the factor that causes a more facile generation of ancestral amino acid sequence. Further, if it can be argued that the mutation rate of *angusticeps* toxins is an order of magnitude higher than the rate for short neurotoxins (unpublished), it is possible to place the *angusticeps* type and short neurotoxins on the same line leading from the ancestral protein. The ancestral sequence is then just as difficult to generate as in the case where the cardiotoxin is taken as being more primitive, and we would be back to square one.

No phylogenies have as yet been reported for the other groups of toxins from snake venoms—the protease inhibitors (TAKAHASHI et al., 1974a, b; STRYDOM, 1973c, 1976) and phospholipase A (presynaptic neurotoxins).

In conclusion, we can sum up the development of thoughts on the evolution of snake toxins up to this stage as showing that, solely looking at the sequences of snake toxins, it is not possible to make a clear-cut choice among the different possibilities of grouping the major types of toxins. The arguments are quite strong that long neurotoxins are relative newcomers on the scene, but we cannot say whether a short neurotoxin type or cardiotoxin type was the ancestral protein. The position (if any) of the toxins which are homologous to protease inhibitors or phospholipases A, in a possible evolutionary scheme, is also unknown.

C. Current Views on the Evolution of Snake Toxins

As we have seen in the previous section, the snake toxins themselves do not promise to yield enough information on their origin. A new line of reasoning has now given new arguments toward making a choice.

Since snake toxin homologues have not yet been found in mammalian exocrine secretions, it is possible that the evolutionary precursors of these toxins will be found among the other proteins in snake venoms. One possible source of information is the recent data on the structures of snake venom phospholipases A (JOUBERT, 1975a, b, c; HALPERT and EAKER, 1975; BOTES and VILJOEN, 1974b; SAMESJIMA et al., 1974).

The action of cardiotoxins on membranes is potentiated by phospholipase A (see a review by CONDREA, 1974). Further, both cardiotoxins (BRAGANCA et al., 1967) and phospholipase A (WELLS, 1971; VAN DER WALT et al., BOTES and VILJOEN, 1974a) readily undergo dimerization—in the case of phospholipase with concomitant allosteric effects (either inhibition of activity or actual generation of activity). Comparing the phospholipase A of *N. melanoleuca* venom (DE.I) and a cardiotoxin (V^{11}-2) from the same venom (Fig. 2), there is a number of correspondences in sequences from the region 58–118 of the phospholipase and the full sequence of the cardiotoxin—e.g., cystinyl residues 3, 15, 22, 43, and 60, tyrosyl residues 12 and 52, the alanyl-alanyl sequence at positions 40–41, a leucyl residue at position 7, glycyls at positions 18 and 25, lysyl at position 28, and arginyl at 59, all numbers referring to the cardiotoxin sequence. The sequences of one of the most primitive-long neurotoxins (α-bungaro-

```
1 ..... K G C F P K M S A Y D Y Y - C G E N G P Y C R N I K K K C L R
        58
2 ..... S G C W P Y I K T Y T Y E S C - Q G T L T C K D G G - K C A A
        1               10                 20                 30
3       I K C H N T L L P F I Y K T C P E G Q N L C F K G T L K F P K

4       L K C H - K L V P P V W K T C P E G K N L C Y K M F M V S T S

5       I V C H* T A T I P S S A V T C P P G E N L C Y R K M W C* S S R


1       F V C D C D V E A A F C F A K A P Y N N A N W N I D T K K R C Q - OH
                                                                  118
2       S V C D C D R V A A N C F A R A T Y N D K N Y N I D F N A R C Q - OH
                        40                 50                  60
3       K T T Y N R G C A A T C P K S S L L V K - - Y V C C N T D R C N - OH

4       T V P V K R G C I D V C P K N S A L V K - - Y V C C S T D K C N - OH

5       G K V V E L G C A A T C P S K K P Y Q E - - V T C C S T D K C N*
```

Fig. 2. Comparison of the amino acid sequences of phospholipases A and toxins of snake venoms.
1 = Notexin (HALPERT and EAKER, 1975)
2 = *Naja melanoleuca* phospholipase DE-I (JOUBERT, 1975b)
3 = *Naja melanoleuca* $V^{11}2$ (CARLSSON, 1974)
4 = *Naja haje annulifera* $V^{11}1$ (WEISE et al., 1973)
5 = α-bungarotoxin (MEBS et al., 1972)
Areas of identity between the groups are indicated. All of the deletions except that at position 51–52 (cardiotoxin numbering) are introduced to align the proteins within their respective groups
* = One or more amino acids are left out to align long neurotoxins (see Fig. 1)

toxin), another phospholipase, notexin, and another cardiotoxin is shown for comparison and to vindicate some of the deletions which had to be introduced to achieve maximum alignment. Only one deletion (of two residues) is introduced into the toxin sequences at position 51–52 without precedent from previous alignments of toxins. It is obvious that there is homology between the toxins and phospholipases.

Another possible source of information on the origin of snake venom toxins is the weak homology previously seen for a region of bovine ribonuclease and cobrotoxin (see above, STRYDOM, 1973a). The recent elucidation of the amino acid sequence of a rattlesnake toxin, crotamine, from *Crotalus durissus terrificus* (LAURE, 1975) also bears on this resemblance.

Crotamine and ribonuclease seem to be homologous (Fig. 3). Comparing region 55–95 of ribonuclease with the sequence of crotamine, it is seen that four of the six half-cystinyl residues of crotamine align perfectly with four out of five half-cystinyl residues in that region of ribonuclease. Furthermore, the same Asp-Cys-Arg sequence is found for both proteins around position 30 of crotamine.

Although crotamine does not immediately seem homologous to the elapid toxins, the fact that homology of a small region of ribonuclease and cobrotoxin had been indicated prompted alignment of ribonuclease with phospholipase A and snake toxins. As Figure 4 shows, a weak but definite homology can be seen. The homology is

```
        1                   10                  20
1.      Y K Q C H K K G G H C F P K E K I C L P
        55
2.      Q A I C S Q G Q V T C K N G Q T N C Y Q

        21                  30                  40
1.      P S S D F G K M D C R W R K C C K K G S G

2.      S Y S T M S I T D C R E T G S S K V P N C .....
```

Fig. 3. Homology of bovine ribonuclease and crotamine of the rattlesnake, *Crotalus durissus terrificus*.

1 = Crotamine (LAURE, 1975)
2 = Bovine ribonuclease (SMYTH et al., 1963)

```
          1                 10                  20                  30                  40                  50                  60
1.        . . . V A K R S G L L W Y S A Y G C Y C G W G G G R P Q B A T S R C C F V H B C C Y G K A...
2....F L R Q H V D Y P K S S A P D S R T Y C N Q M M ...
3....F E R Q H M D S S T S A A S S S - N Y C N Q M M K S R N L T - K D R C K P V - - N T F V H E S L A D - V Q A V C S Q K N
4.        . . . . K M G E S V F D Y I Y Y G C Y C G W G G K G K P I D A T D R C C F V H D C C Y G K M G T Y D - T K W T S Y N Y E
5.... Q C A N H G K R P T W H Y M D Y G C Y C G A G G S G T P V N E L D R C C K I H D D C Y D E A G K K G - C F P K M S A Y D
6....H C T V P N R - P W W H F A N Y G C Y C G R G G K G T P V D D L D R C C Q I H D K C Y D E A E K I S G C W P Y I K T Y T
7.                                                                                                      I K C H N T L L P F I

                          70          80          90          100         110
3.        V - A C K N G Q T N C Y Q S Y S T M S I T D C R E T G S S K Y P N C A Y K T T Q A N K H I I V A C E G N P ...
4.        I - - - Q N G G I D C D E D P Q K K E L - - C E C D R V A A I C F A N N R N T Y N S N Y F G H S S S K C ...
5.        Y - Y C G E N G P Y C R N I K K K C - L R F C D C D V E A A F C F A K A P Y N N A N W N I D T K K R C Q
6.        Y E S C Q - G T L T C K - D G G K C A A S V C D C D R V A A N C F A R A T Y N D K N Y N I D F N A R C Q
7.        Y K T C P E G Q N L C F K G T L K F P K K T T Y N R G C A A T C P K S S L L V K Y V C C N T D R C N
```

Fig. 4. Comparison of structure of ribonucleases with phospholipases and snake toxins.

1 = *Crotalus adamanteus* phospholipase A (TSAO et al., 1975)
2 = *Chelydra serpentina* (turtle) ribonuclease (BARNARD et al., 1972)
3 = Bovine ribonuclease (SMYTH et al., 1963)
4 = *Bitis gabonica* phospholipase A (BOTES and VILJOEN, 1974)
5 = *Notexin* (HALPERT and EAKER, 1975)
6 = *Naja melanoleuca* phospholipase DE-I (JOUBERT, 1975 b)
7 = *Naja melanoleuca* cardiotoxin V[11]2 (CARLSSON, 1974)

Areas of identities between ribonucleases and any one of the snake venom proteins are indicated

mostly apparent in the tyrosyl-cystinyl sequence (alignment positions 19–20), aspartyl-arginyl-cystinyl sequence (33–35), and the cystinyl residues at positions 64, 71, and 83. A number of other similarities are indicated in Figure 4. It is important to note that the same regions of ribonuclease and cobrotoxin which were previously found to be homologous are aligned in this alignment.

The major conclusion to come from these homologies is that, as the cardiotoxins seem to be more similar than other toxins to phospholipase A (the short neurotoxins, for example, need a deletion of three amino acids in the region 50–70 of phospholipase to effect alignment), the cardiotoxins are the ancient form of snake toxins. This could have arisen as follows, bearing in mind the properties of phospholipase A and cardiotoxins as discussed above.

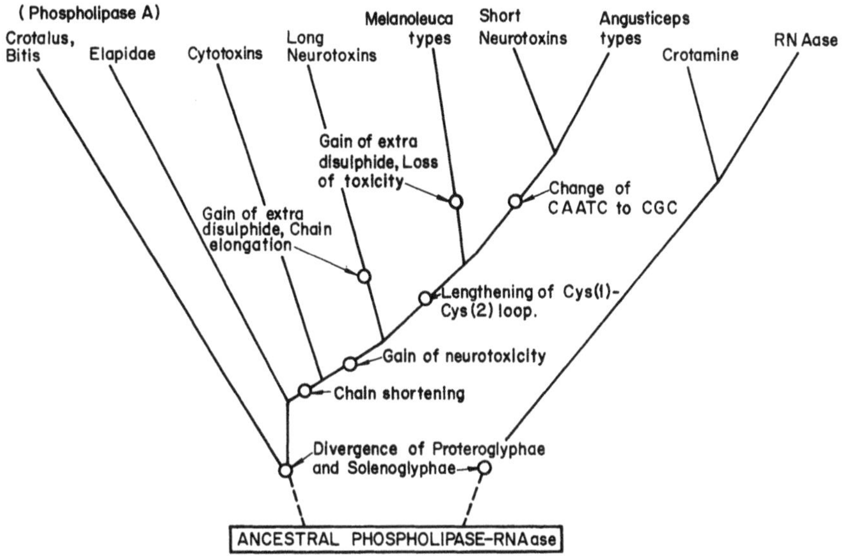

Fig. 5. Phylogeny of ribonuclease, phospholipase A, and snake venom toxins

A dimer of phospholipase in an elapid ancestor developed direct lytic activity on blood cells (or other cells) mostly through one partner of the dimer. This changed protein shortened through loss of the amino terminal half of the protein but could still associate with phospholipase A. Thereby it became the direct precursor of the cardiotoxins.

The following scheme for evolution of snake venom toxins can now be set up in the light of the above discussions (Fig. 5). Starting off from an ancestral protein, a phospholipase-ribonuclease, which was the ancestor of both modern phospholipase and ribonuclease, we follow the ribonuclease line to find that in the *Crotalidae*, at least, a "toxin" developed from ribonuclease. Following the phospholipase A line, we reach the divergence point of the *Proteroglyphae* and *Solenoglyphae*. This divergence gives rise to the *Crotalus* and *Bitis* phospholipases which seem to be more remotely related to the cardio- or cytotoxins than the elapid phospholipases are. On the *Proteroglyphae* line, the divergence point of phospholipases A and "phospholipase-cardiotoxin" is found. Relatively recently the phospholipase A line gave rise to presynaptic neurotoxins. The relatively recent development of presynaptic neurotoxins, such as notexin, is inferred from the close similarity of the notexin sequence to that of cobra phospholipases (HALPERT and EAKER, 1975). The "cardiotoxin-phospholipase" changed chain size to that of the modern cardiotoxins. This line leads on the one hand to the cytotoxins (cardiotoxins) found today in cobra venoms, and on the other hand to a protein which gains neurotoxicity through acquisition of residues such as the constant tryptophan, the Arg-Gly "active site" sequence, and a few correctly placed basic residues (KARLSSON, Chap. 5). This precursor of modern neurotoxins has not yet been found in venoms. It gave rise to the line of long neurotoxins and to a line which led on one side to the proteins classed as "*melanoleuca*-type" and on the other side to the short neurotoxins. It is possible that the "*angusticeps*-type" toxins then evolved from short neurotoxins, but it is also, to a lesser extent, possible that both short neurotoxins and *angusticeps*-types could have shared a different ancestor.

One difficulty with this classification is the position of the *melanoleuca*-type toxins. It is possible to argue that they are evolved from the neurotoxin precursor mentioned above and that they should, therefore, be placed in the scheme as diverging *before* the divergence point of the long neurotoxins. The main argument against this and for the stated classification is that it has precisely the same number of amino acid residues between the first and second half-cystines (short neurotoxin numbering) in the peptide chain as the short neurotoxins have. It is unlikely that two separate lengthening events would have given rise to the same number of amino acid residues being incorporated in a polypeptide chain.

Another possible difficulty with this classification is the divergence point of *Proteroglyphae* and *Solenoglyphae*. The known sequences of the phospholipases from the genera *Bitis* and *Agkistrodon* (BOTES and VILJOEN, 1974b; SAMESJIMA et al., 1974) are much more different from that of cardiotoxins than the sequences of the elapid phospholipases are. These *solenoglyph* phospholipases are relatively nontoxic, but the phospholipase A_2 of *Vipera russellii* (SALACH et al., 1971) is a highly toxic protein (STRONG et al., 1976), as some of the elapid phospholipases are, e.g., *Naja nigricollis* phospholipase (EAKER, 1975). Other *solenoglyph* phospholipases which are of comparable toxicity are those from *Crotalus durissus terrificus* venom (BREITHAUPT et al., 1975). The current scheme where the *Viperidae* and *Crotalidae* seem to have diverged from the *Elapidae* and *Hydrophiidae* before the lytic action of phospholipase-cardiotoxin evolved might, therefore, be changed if the sequences of highly toxic *solenoglyph* phospholipases prove to be close to those of the elapid phospholipases. On the other hand, the current scheme predicts that these *solenoglyph* toxic phospholipases will have either a different active site grouping for the toxicity, or even have a different *type* of toxicity. BREITHAUPT et al. (1975) consider the toxic *Crotalus* phospholipases as "connecting links in the molecular evolution of presynaptic neurotoxins derived from the class of phospholipases."

To enable a look at the finer detail of the evolution of snake toxins, a computer-derived phylogeny for the cardiotoxins, long and short neurotoxins, *angusticeps* types, and *melanoleuca* types is given in Figure 6. Program PHYMOD (STRYDOM, 1973b) was used for the main part of the derivation, while subjective reasoning as detailed above was applied to reach the final arrangement of the five main groups. No attempt was made to generate phylogenies for protease inhibitors or for phospholipases A and presynaptic neurotoxins since too few sequences are at present known for meaningful results to be obtained.

The main impression that this tree makes is that even within the main groups of toxins there are a number of subgroups. Sometimes these subgroups are associated with only a limited number of species, such as the sea snakes, but other subgroups contain quite a variety of species. This multitude of subgroups, with in some cases one species of snake producing toxins in nearly every subgroup, points to a danger in using snake toxin sequences to assist in classifying those species. Such a phylogeny is in the first place a phylogeny of the *genes* coding for these proteins and not a phylogeny of species. Until every toxin in a specific snake venom has been sequenced, and many snake venoms used for such studies, one cannot with any measure of confidence say that protein A from species X and protein B from species Y are

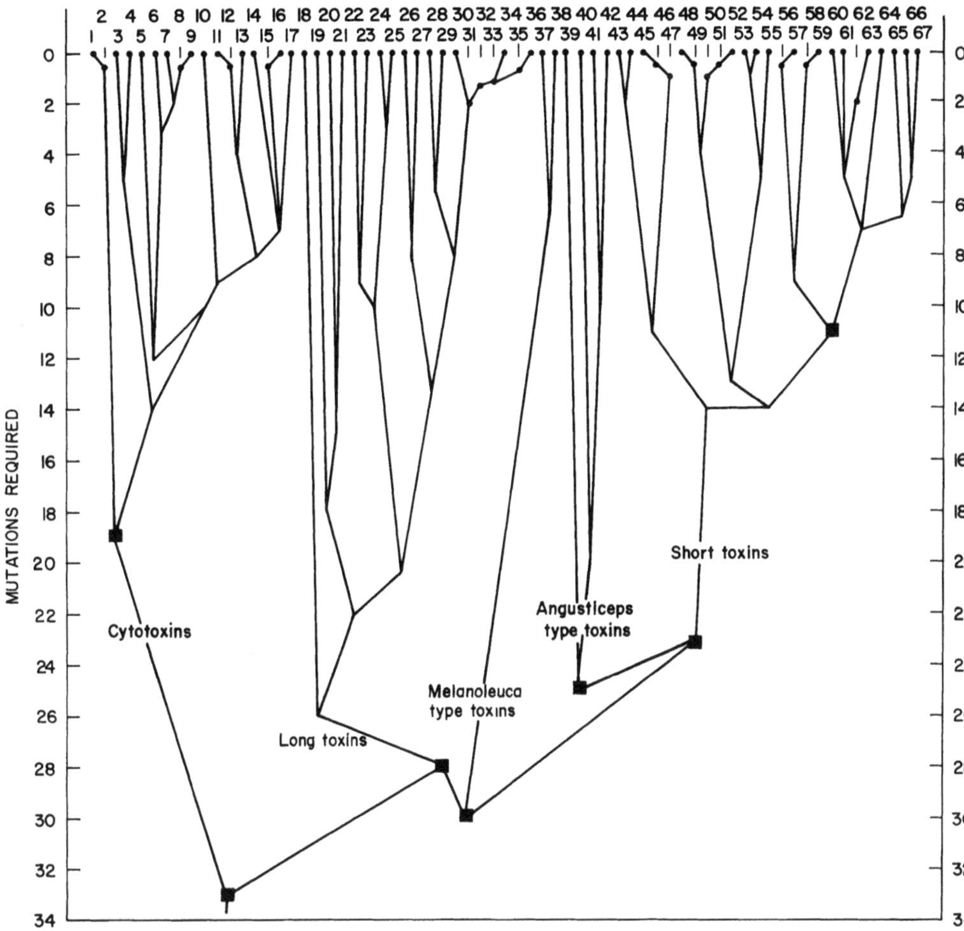

Fig. 6. Gene phylogeny of toxins from *proteroglyphae* venoms. The nodal positions in this tree indicate the average distance of those nodes from the branch tips in mutations required to effect an interchange of a hypothetic ancestral sequence at the nodal position to the actual sequences found for the toxins at the branch tips. Branch lengths are not related to actual mutational distances. The numbers at the top of the tree refer to toxins as follows:

1 = *Naja melanoleuca* V^{11}-2 (CARLSSON, 1974)
2 = *Naja melanoleuca* V^{11}-3 (CARLSSON, 1974)
3 = *Hemachatus haemachatus* 12B (FRYKLUND and EAKER, 1973)
4 = *Hemachatus haemachatus* XX (JOUBERT, F. J., unpublished)
5 = *Naja mossambica mossambica* V^{11}-4 (LOUW, 1974b)
6 = *Naja mossambica mossambica* V^{11}-3 (LOUW, 1974a)
7 = *Naja mossambica mossambica* V^{11}-2 (LOUW, 1974a)
8 = *Naja mossambica pallida* V^{11}-1 (FRYKLUND and EAKER, 1975a)
9 = *Naja mossambica mossambica* V^{11}-1 (LOUW, 1974a)
10 = *Naja haje annulifera* V^{11}-1 (WEISE et al., 1973)
11 = *Naja naja atra* cardiotoxin (NARITA and LEE, 1970)
12 = *Naja naja* cobramine B (TAKECHI et al., 1972)
13 = *Naja naja oxiana* Cytotoxin (GRISHIN et al., 1974a)
14 = *Naja naja* F8 (Cambodia) (FRYKLUND and EAKER, 1975b)

15 = *Naja melanoleuca* V^{11}1-iso-1 (CARLSSON and JOUBERT, 1974)
16 = *Naja melanoleuca* V^{11}1-iso-2 (CARLSSON and JOUBERT, 1974)
17 = *Naja naja* cobramine A (HAYASHI et al., 1971)
18 = *Laticauda semifasciata* LS III (MAEDA and TAMIYA, 1974)
19 = *Bungarus multicinctus* α-bungarotoxin (MEBS et al., 1972)
20 = *Naja naja oxiana* I (GRISHIN et al., 1974b)
21 = *Naja melanoleuca* 3.9.4 (SHIPOLINI et al., 1974)
22 = *Dendroaspis jamesonii kaimosae* II (STRYDOM, 1973d)
23 = *Dendroaspis viridis* 4.7.3 (BANKS et al., 1974)
24 = *Dendroaspis polylepis* γ (STRYDOM, 1972a)
25 = *Dendroaspis polylepis* δ (STRYDOM, 1972c)
26 = *Ophiophagus hannah* A (JOUBERT, 1973)
27 = *Ophiophagus hannah* B (JOUBERT, 1973)
28 = *Naja nivea* d (BOTES, 1971)
29 = *Naja melanoleuca* b (BOTES, 1972)
30 = *Naja naja* C (HAYASHI, 1974)
31 = *Naja naja siamensis* 3 (ARNBERG et al., 1973)
32 = *Naja naja naja* 3 (West Pakistan) (ARNBERG et al., 1973)
33 = *Naja naja naja* 3 (ARNBERG et al., 1973)
34 = *Naja naja* A (NAKAI et al., 1971)
35 = *Naja naja naja* 4 (ARNBERG et al., 1973)
36 = *Naja naja* B (HAYASHI, 1974)
37 = *Naja melanoleuca* S_4C_{11} (CARLSSON, 1975)
38 = *Naja haje annulifera* CM 13b (JOUBERT, 1975d)
39 = *Dendroaspis angusticeps* F 7 (VILJOEN and BOTES, 1973)
40 = *Dendroaspis polylepis* FS_2 (STRYDOM, 1972c)
41 = *Dendroaspis angusticeps* F 8 (VILJOEN and BOTES, 1974)
42 = *Dendroaspis viridis* 4.9.6. (SHIPOLINI and BANKS, 1974)
43 = *Laticauda laticaudata* A (SATO, 1974)
44 = *Laticauda laticaudata* A^1 (SATO, 1974)
45 = *Laticauda semifasciata* c (TAMIYA and ABE, 1972)
46 = *Laticauda semifasciata* b (SATO and TAMIYA, 1971)
47 = *Laticauda semifasciata* a (SATO and TAMIYA, 1971)
48 = *Enhydrina schistosa* 5 (FRYKLUND et al., 1972)
49 = *Enhydrina schistosa* 4 (FRYKLUND et al., 1972)
50 = *Aipysurus laevis* C (MAEDA and TAMIYA, 1976)
51 = *Aipysurus laevis* b (MAEDA and TAMIYA, 1976)
52 = *Aipysurus laevis* a (MAEDA and TAMIYA, 1976)
53 = *Dendroaspis jamesonii* I (STRYDOM, 1973d)
54 = *Dendroaspis viridis* 4.11.3 (BANKS et al., 1974)
55 = *Dendroaspis polylepis* α (STRYDOM, 1972a)
56 = *Naja haje annulifera* C 10 (JOUBERT, 1975e)
57 = *Naja haje annulifera* C 12 (JOUBERT, 1975e)
58 = *Naja haje annulifera* C 14 (JOUBERT, 1975e)
59 = *Naja nivea* β (BOTES, 1971)
60 = *Hemachatus haemachatus* IV (STRYDOM and BOTES, 1971)
61 = *Naja naja oxiana* II, α (ARNBERG et al., 1974; GRISHIN et al., 1973)
62 = *Naja mossambica pallida* α-2 (FRYKLUND and EAKER, 1975a)
63 = *Naja mossambica pallida* α (EAKER, personal communication; EAKER and PORATH, 1967)
64 = *Hemachatus haemachatus* II (STRYDOM and BOTES, 1971)
65 = *Naja melanoleuca* d (BOTES, 1972)
66 = *Naja naja atra* cobrotoxin (YANG et al., 1969)
67 = *Naja haje annulifera* α (BOTES and STRYDOM, 1969)

from orthologous genes in the two species and, therefore, that the difference between proteins A and B is due to species divergence and not gene divergence at an earlier point in time. In any case, the broad picture of this tree is still that a measure of correspondence between species classification and protein classification is to be found. Such a tree will give a much better reflection of species classification once more of the minor (and major!) constituents of snake venoms are studied in detail.

In summary, therefore, these schemes allow the visualization of the molecular mechanism by which nonvenomous salivary gland secretions evolved into the venomous secretion of *Elapidae* and *Hydrophidae* snakes. The molecular pathway to the toxic secretions of *Viperidae* and *Crotalidae* is unfortunately still only hinted at.

D. Future Possibilities

As more and more chemical structures of, and biologic data on, other hitherto neglected components of snake venoms become known, we can expect yet more types of proteins to come to light. Therefore, we should expect soon to have information on, for example, the reasons why some phospholipases are toxic and others not and what the distribution of phospholipases and presynaptic neurotoxins is among different families of snakes. Sequence studies on phospholipases and ribonucleases of reptilian origin (from other sources than venom) should also help to illuminate the differentiation of these enzymes into toxins.

With increasing knowledge of the pharmacologic properties of snake venom toxins, especially the effects of those compounds on biologic systems of natural prey of snakes, the interrelationships of these proteins will stand out much clearer. Furthermore, application of more sophisticated numeric and pattern recognition techniques should be of great help in understanding the data we already have on these proteins.

Finally, it is clear that studies on the evolution of snake venom toxins will not only answer questions on the origin and development of these enigmatic secretions but will also shed light on the molecular history of vertebrate enterosecretory proteins.

Acknowledgements. I gratefully acknowledge many discussions on the subject matter with Drs. D.P. Botes, F.J. Joubert, A.I. Louw, and L. Visser and Messrs F.H.H. Carlsson and D. Parris.

References

Arnberg, H., Eaker, D., Fryklund, L., Karlsson, E.: Amino acid sequence of oxiana α, the main neurotoxin of the venom of *Naja naja oxiana*. Biochim. biophys. Acta (Amst.) **359**, 222—232 (1974)

Arnberg, H., Eaker, D., Karlsson, E.: To be published, quoted by Karlsson (1973)

Banks, B.E.C., Miledi, R., Shipolini, R.A.: The primary sequences and neuromuscular effects of three neurotoxic polypeptides from the venom of *Dendroaspis viridis*. Europ. J. Biochem. **45**, 457—468 (1974)

Barker, W.C., Dayhoff, M.O.: Detecting distant relationship: Computer methods and results. In: Dayhoff, M.O. (Ed.): Atlas of protein sequence and structure, Vol. 5, pp. 101—110. Washington, D.C.: National Biomedical Research Foundation 1972

Barnabas, J., Goodman, M., Moore, G. W.: Descent of mammalian alpha globin chain sequences investigated by the maximum parsimony method. J. molec. Biol. **69**, 249—278 (1972)

Barnard, E. A., Cohen, M. S., Gold, M. H., Kim, J. K.: Evolution of ribonuclease in relation to polypeptide folding mechanisms. Nature (Lond.) New Biol. **240**, 395—398 (1972)

Botes, D. P.: Snake venom toxins. The amino acid sequences of toxins α and β from N. nivea venom and the disulfide bonds of toxin α. J. biol. Chem. **246**, 7383—7391 (1971)

Botes, D. P.: Snake venom toxins. The amino acid sequences of toxins b and d from *Naja melanoleuca* venom. J. biol. Chem. **247**, 2866—2871 (1972)

Botes, D. P.: Snake venom toxins. The reactivity of the disulphide bonds of *Naja nivea* toxin α. Biochim. biophys. Acta (Amst.) **359**, 242—247 (1974)

Botes, D. P., Strydom, D. J.: A neurotoxin, toxin α, from Egyptian cobra *(Naja haje haje)* venom I. Purification, properties and complete amino acid sequence. J. biol. Chem. **244**, 4147—4157 (1969)

Botes, D. P., Viljoen, C. C.: Purification of phospholipase A from *Bitis gabonica* venom. Toxicon **12**, 611—619 (1974a)

Botes, D. P., Viljoen, C. C.: *Bitis gabonica* venom. The amino acid sequence of phospholipase A. J. biol. Chem. **249**, 3827—3835 (1974b)

Braganca, B. M., Patel, N. T., Badrinath, P. G.: Isolation and properties of a cobra venom factor selectively cytotoxic to Yoshida sarcoma cells. Biochim. biophys. Acta (Amst.) **136**, 508—520 (1967)

Breithaupt, H., Omori-Satoh, T., Lang, J.: Isolation and characterization of three phospholipases A from the crotoxin complex. Biochim. biophys. Acta (Amst.) **403**, 355—369 (1975)

Bunn, H. F., Schmidt, G. J., Haney, D. N., Dluhy, R. G.: Haemoglobin Cranston, an unstable variant having an elongated β chain due to non-homologous crossover between two normal β chains. Proc. nat. Acad. Sci. (Wash.) **72**, 3609—3613 (1975)

Carlsson, F. H. H.: Snake venom toxins. The primary structures of two novel cytotoxin homologues from the venom of forest cobra *Naja melanoleuca)*. Biochem. Biophys. Res. Commun. **59**, 269—276 (1974)

Carlsson, F. H. H.: Snake venom toxins. The primary structure of protein S_4C_{11}, a neurotoxin homologue from the venom of forest cobra *(Naja melanoleuca)*. Biochim. biophys. Acta (Amst.) **400**, 310—321 (1975)

Carlsson, F. H. H., Joubert, F. J.: Snake venom toxins. The isolation and purification of three cytotoxin homologues from the venom of the forest cobra *(Naja melanoleuca)* and the complete amino acid sequence of toxin $V^{11}1$. Biochim. biophys. Acta (Amst.) **336**, 453—469 (1974)

Clegg, J. B., Weatherall, D. J., Milner, P. F.: Haemoglobin Constant Spring—chain termination mutant? Nature (Lond.) New Biol. **234**, 337—340 (1971)

Condrea, E.: Membrane-active polypeptides from snake venom: cardiotoxins and haemocytotoxins. Experientia (Basel) **30**, 121—129 (1974).

Dayhoff, M. O.: Atlas of Protein Sequence and Structure, Vol. V. Washington, D.C.: National Biomedical Research Foundation 1972

Dayhoff, M. O., Park, C. M.: Cytochrome C: building a phylogenetic tree. In: Dayhoff, M. O. (Ed.): Atlas of Protein Sequence and Structure, Vol. IV, pp. 7—16. Silver Spring: National Biomedical Research Foundation 1969

Eaker, D.: Structural nature of pre-synaptic neurotoxins from Australian elapid venoms. Toxicon **13**, 90—91 (1975)

Eaker, D. L., Porath, J.: The amino acid sequence of a neurotoxin from *Naja nigricollis* venom. Jap. J. Microbiol. **11**, 353—355 (1967)

Farris, J. S.: Estimating phylogenetic trees from distance matrices. Amer. Naturalist **106**, 645—668 (1972)

Fitch, W. M., Margoliash, E.: Construction of phylogenetic trees. Science **155**, 279—284 (1967)

Fryklund, L., Eaker, D.: Complete amino acid sequence of a non-neurotoxic hemolytic protein from the venom of *Hemachatus haemachatus* (African Ringhals cobra). Biochemistry **12**, 661—667 (1973)

Fryklund, L., Eaker, D.: The complete covalent structure of a cardiotoxin from the venom of *Naja nigricollis* (African black-necked spitting cobra). Biochemistry **14**, 2865—2871 (1975a)

Fryklund, L., Eaker, D.: The complete amino acid sequence of a cardiotoxin from the venom of *Naja naja* (Cambodian cobra). Biochemistry **14**, 2860—2865 (1975b)

Fryklund, L., Eaker, D., Karlsson, E.: Amino acid sequences of the two principal neurotoxins of *Enhydrina schistosa* venom. Biochemistry **11**, 4633—4640 (1972)

Grishin, E. V., Sukhikh, A. P., Adamovich, T. B., Ovchinnikov, Y. A., Yukelson, L. Y.: The isolation and sequence determination of a cytotoxin from the venom of the middle-asian cobra *Naja naja oxiana*. FEBS Letters **48**, 179—183 (1974a)

Grishin, E. V., Sukhikh, A. P., Lukyanchuk, N. N., Slobodyan, L. N., Lipkin, V. M., Ovchinnikov, Y. A., Sorokin, V. M.: Amino acid sequence of neurotoxin II from *Naja naja oxiana* venom. FEBS Letters **36**, 77—78 (1973)

Grishin, E. V., Sukhikh, A. P., Slobodyan, L. N., Ovchinnikov, Y. A., Sorokin, V. M.: Amino acid sequence of neurotoxin I from *Naja naja oxiana* venom. FEBS Letters **45**, 118—121 (1974b)

Halpert, J., Eaker, D.: Amino acid sequence of a pre-synaptic neurotoxin from the venom of *Notechis scutatus scutatus* (Australian tiger snake). J. biol. Chem. **250**, 6990—6997 (1975)

Hayashi, K.: Personal communication with Maeda and Tamiya (1974)

Hayashi, K., Takechi, M., Sasaki, T.: Amino acid sequence of cytotoxin I from the venom of the Indian cobra *(Naja naja)*. Biochem. Biophys. Res. Commun. **45**, 1357—1362 (1971)

Joubert, F. J.: Snake venom toxins. The amino acid sequences of two toxins from *Ophiophagus hannah* (King cobra) venom. Biochim. biophys. Acta (Amst.) **317**, 85—98 (1973)

Joubert, F. J.: *Naja melanoleuca* (forest cobra) venom. The amino acid sequence of phospholipase A, fraction DE-III. Biochim. biophys. Acta (Amst.) **379**, 329—344 (1975a)

Joubert, F. J.: *Naja melanoleuca* (forest cobra) venom. The amino acid sequence of phospholipase A, fractions DE-I and DE-II. Biochim. biophys. Acta (Amst.) **379**, 345—359 (1975b)

Joubert, F. J.: *Hemachatus haemachatus* (Ringhals) venom. Purification, some properties and amino acid sequence of phospholipase A (Fraction DE-I). Europ. J. Biochem. **52**, 539—554 (1975c)

Joubert, F. J.: Snake venom toxins. The purification and amino acid sequence of toxin CM-13b from *Naja haje annulifera* (Egyptian cobra) venom. Hoppe Seylers Z. physiol. Chem. **356**, 1901—1908 (1975d)

Joubert, F. J.: Snake venom toxins. The amino acid sequences of three toxins (CM-10, CM-12, and CM-14) from *Naja haje annulifera* (Egyptian cobra) venom. Hoppe Seylers Z. physiol. Chem. **356**, 53—72 (1975e)

Karlsson, E.: Chemistry of some potent animal toxins. Experientia (Basel) **29**, 1319—1327 (1973)

Laure, C. J.: Die Primärstruktur des Crotamins. Hoppe Seylers Z. physiol. Chem. **356**, 213—215 (1975)

Lee, C. Y.: Chemistry and pharmacology of polypeptide toxins in snake venoms. Ann. Rev. Pharmacol. **12**, 265—286 (1972)

Louw, A. I.: Snake venom toxins. The amino acid sequences of three cytotoxin homologues from *Naja mossambica mossambica* venom. Biochim. biophys. Acta (Amst.) **336**, 481—495 (1974a)

Louw, A. I.: Snake venom toxins. The complete amino acid sequence of cytotoxin $V^{11}4$ from the venom of *Naja mossambica mossambica*. Biochem. Biophys. Res. Commun. **58**, 1022—1029 (1974b)

Maeda, N., Tamiya, N.: The primary structure of the toxin *Laticauda semifasciata* III, a weak and reversibly acting neurotoxin from the venom of a sea-snake, *Laticauda semifasciata*. Biochem. J. **141**, 389—400 (1974)

Maeda, N., Tamiya, N.: Isolation, properties and amino acid sequences of three neurotoxins from the venom of a sea-snake, *Aipysurus laevis*. Biochem. J. **153**, 79—87 (1976)

Mebs, D., Narita, K., Iwanaga, S., Samejima, Y., Lee, C. Y.: Purification, properties, and amino acid sequence of α-bungarotoxin from the venom of *Bungarus multicinctus*. Hoppe Seylers Z. physiol. Chem. **353**, 243—262 (1972)

Nakai, K., Sasaki, T., Hayashi, K.: Amino acid sequence of toxin A from the venom of the Indian cobra *(Naja naja)*. Biochem. Biophys. Res. Commun. **44**, 893—897 (1971)

Narita, K., Lee, C. Y.: The amino acid sequence of cardiotoxin from Formosan cobra *(Naja naja atra)* venom. Biochem. Biophys. Res. Commun. **41**, 339—343 (1970)

Narita, K., Mebs, D., Iwanaga, S., Samejina, Y., Lee, C. Y.: Primary structure of α-Bungarotoxin from *Bungarus multicinctus* venom. J. Formosan med. Ass. **71**, 336—343 (1972)

Peacock, D., Boulter, D.: Use of amino acid sequence data in phylogeny and evaluation of methods using computer simulation. J. molec. Biol. **95**, 513—527 (1975)

Rydén, L., Gabel, D., Eaker, D.: A model of the three-dimensional structure of snake venom neurotoxins based on chemical evidence. Int. J. Pept. Protein Res. **5**, 261—273 (1973)

Salach, J. I., Turini, P., Seng, R., Hauber, J., Singer, T. P.: Phospholipase A of snake venoms. I. Isolation and molecular properties of isoenzymes from *Naja naja* and *Vipera russellii* venoms. J. biol. Chem. **246**, 331—339 (1971)

Samejima, Y., Iwanaga, S., Suzuki, T.: Complete amino acid sequence of phospholipase A_2-II isolated from *Akistrodon halys blomhoffii* venom. FEBS Letters **47**, 348—351 (1974)

Sato, S.: Personal communication with Maeda and Tamiya (1974)

Sato, S., Tamiya, N.: The amino acid sequences of erabutoxins, neurotoxic proteins of sea-snake *(Laticauda semifasciata)* venom. Biochem. J. **122**, 453—461 (1971)

Shipolini, R. A., Bailey, G. S., Banks, B. E. C.: The separation of a neurotoxin from the venom of *Naja melanoleuca* and the primary sequence determination. Europ. J. Biochem. **42**, 203—211 (1974)

Shipolini, R. A., Banks, B. E. C.: The amino acid sequence of a polypeptide from the venom of *Dendroaspis viridis*. Europ. J. Biochem. **49**, 399—405 (1974)

Smyth, D. G., Stein, W. H., Moore, S.: The sequence of amino acid residues in bovine pancreatic ribonuclease: revisions and confirmations. J. biol. Chem. **238**, 227—234 (1963)

Strong, P. N., Goerke, J., Oberg, S. G., Kelly, R. B.: β-Bungarotoxin, a pre-synaptic toxin with enzymatic activity. Proc. nat. Acad. Sci. (Wash.) **73**, 178—182 (1976)

Strydom, A. J. C.: Snake venom toxins. The amino acid sequences of two toxins from *Dendroaspis jamesonii kaimosae* (Jameson's mamba) venom. Biochim. biophys. Acta (Amst.) **328**, 491—509 (1973d)

Strydom, A. J. C., Botes, D. P.: Snake venom toxins. Purification, properties, and complete amino acid sequence of two toxins from Ringhals *(Hemachatus haemachatus)* venom. J. biol. Chem. **246**, 1341—1349 (1971)

Strydom, D. J.: Snake venom toxins. The amino acid sequence of two toxins from *Dendroaspis polylepis polylepis* (Black mamba) venom. J. biol. Chem. **247**, 4029—4042 (1972a)

Strydom, D. J.: Phylogenetic relationships of proteroglyphae toxins. Toxicon **10**, 39—45 (1972b)

Strydom, D. J.: Studies on the toxins of *Dendroaspis polylepis* (Black mamba) venom. Ph.D. Thesis: University of South Africa, Pretoria, 1972c

Strydom, D. J.: Snake venom toxins: The evolution of some of the toxins found in snake venoms. Systematic Zoology **22**, 596—608 (1973a)

Strydom, D. J.: Snake venom toxins. Structure-function relationships and phylogenetics. Comp. Biochem. Physiol. [B] **44**, 269—281 (1973b)

Strydom, D. J.: Protease inhibitors as snake venom toxins. Nature (Lond.) New Biol. **243**, 88—89 (1973c)

Strydom, D. J.: Snake venom toxins. Purification and properties of low molecular weight polypeptides of *Dendroaspis polylepis polylepis* (Black mamba) venom. Europ. J. Biochem. **69**, 169—176 (1976)

Takahashi, H., Iwanaga, S., Suzuki, T.: Distribution of proteinase inhibitors in snake venoms. Toxicon **12**, 193—197 (1974a)

Takahashi, H., Iwanaga, S., Suzuki, T.: Snake venom proteinase inhibitors. I. Isolation and properties of two inhibitors of kallikrein, trypsin, plasmin, and α-chymotrypsin from the venom of Russel's viper. *(Vipera russelli)*. J. Biochem. (Tokyo) **76**, 709—719 (1974b)

Takechi, M., Hayashi, K., Sasaki, T.: The amino acid sequence of cytotoxin II from the venom of the Indian cobra *(Naja naja)*. Mol. Pharmacol. **8**, 446—451 (1972)

Tamiya, N., Abe, H.: The isolation, properties, and amino acid sequence of erabutoxin C, a minor neurotoxic component of the venom of a sea-snake *Laticauda semifasciata*. Biochem. J. **130**, 547—555 (1972)

Tsao, F. H. C., Keim, P. S., Heinrikson, R. L.: *Crotalus adamanteus* phospholipase A_2-α: subunit structure, NH_2-terminal sequence, and homology with other phospholipases. Arch. Biochem. Biophys. **167**, 706—717 (1975)

Tu, A. T.: Neurotoxins of animal venoms: snakes. Annu. Rev. Biochem. **42**, 235—258 (1973)

Viljoen, C. C., Botes, D. P.: Snake venom toxins. The purification and amino acid sequence of toxin FVII from *Dendroaspis angusticeps* venom. J. biol. Chem. **248**, 4915—4919 (1973)

Viljoen, C. C., Botes, D. P.: Snake venom toxins. The purification and amino acid sequence of toxin Ta_2 from *Dendroaspis angusticeps* venom. J. biol. Chem. **249**, 366—372 (1974)
Walt, S. J. Van der, Botes, D. P., Viljoen, C. C.: (unpublished 1977)
Weise, K. H. K., Carlsson, F. H. H., Joubert, F. J., Strydom, D. J.: Snake venom toxins. The purification of toxins $V^{11}1$ and $V^{11}2$, two cytotoxin homologues from banded Egyptian cobra *(Naja haje annulifera)* venom, and the complete amino acid sequence of toxin V^{11} 1. Hoppe Seylers Z. physiol. Chem. **354**, 1317—1326 (1973)
Wells, M. A.: Evidence that the phospholipases A_2 of *Crotalus adamanteus* venom are dimers. Biochemistry **10**, 4074—4083 (1971)
Yang, C. C., Yang, H. J., Huang, J. S.: The amino acid sequence of cobrotoxin. Biochim. biophys. Acta (Amst.) **188**, 65—77 (1969)
Zuckerkandl, E., Pauling, L.: Molecules as documents of evolutionary history. J. Theor. Biol. **8**, 357—366 (1965)

CHAPTER 8

Nerve Growth Factors in Snake Venoms

R. A. HOGUE-ANGELETTI and R. A. BRADSHAW

A. Introduction

Among the wide variety of biologic substances present in snake venoms, nerve growth factor (NGF) is one of the most curious. As it is presently understood, NGF is an agent that regulates the growth and differentiation of neurons of sympathetic and, in some cases, sensory neural tissue (LEVI-MONTALCINI and ANGELETTI, 1968). There are three principal characteristic biologic effects of NGF:
1. Halo fiber outgrowth from explanted dorsal root or sympathetic ganglia (chick embryo) in culture;
2. Sympathetic ganglion enlargement in vivo in neonatal mice, characterized by both hyperplasia and hypertrophy;
3. Immunosympathectomy, the destruction of sympathetic chain ganglia by the in vivo injection of antiserum to NGF. There is however, no known exocrine function for NGF.

The unlikely existence of NGF in snake venom made its discovery all the more remarkable. Following the identification of NGF as a diffusable entity responsible for the neurite proliferation observed from host neural tissue as the result of the transplantation of sarcomas 37 and 180 (LEVI-MONTALCINI, 1952), COHEN et al. (1954) attempted to obtain a homogeneous preparation of this growth-promoting factor. However, considerable difficulty with nucleic acid contamination was encountered. Crude snake venom, as a source of phosphodiesterase, was used as a reagent to remove this contaminent. However, control bioassays revealed that the venom itself contained as much activity as the treated sarcoma sample. The ultimate identification of NGF as an apparently ubiquitous component of poisonous snake venoms was the end result of these initial observations (COHEN and LEVI-MONTALCINI, 1956). Equally as important, they also pointed the way to the discovery of the richest source of NGF known today (COHEN, 1960), the adult male mouse submandibular gland, the tissue from which the NGF for most chemical and biologic studies, both past and present, has been obtained.

This review details the information presently available for the different venom NGFs and compares these NGFs to that of mouse submandibular gland.

B. Distribution

NGF is widespread and has, in fact, been found in a variety of tissues in all vertebrates examined, albeit in rather low concentrations (LEVI-MONTALCINI and ANGELETTI, 1968). In addition to the male mouse submandibular gland *(vide infra)*, the

Table 1. Snake venoms identified to contain NGF

Viperidae	
Bitis gabonica	COHEN (1959); MAY and GUIMARD (1959)
Echis carinatus	MAY and GUIMARD (1959)
Echis coloratus	MOHAMED et al. (1971)
Vipera ammodytes ammodytes	BAILEY et al. (1975); BANKS et al. (1968); COHEN (1959)
Vipera aspis	COHEN (1959); MAY and GUIMARD (1959)
Vipera russellii	ANGELETTI (1968a); BANKS et al. (1968); COHEN (1959); PEARCE et al. (1972)
Crotalidae	
Agkistrodon piscivorus	BANKS et al. (1968); COHEN and LEVI-MONTALCINI (1956); COHEN (1959)
Ancistrodon contortrix lactocinctus	ANGELETTI (1968a)
Ancistrodon rhodostoma	BAILEY et al. (1975)
Bothrops atrox	COHEN (1959); GLASS and BANTHROPE (1975)
Bothrops jararaca	ANGELETTI (1968a, 1968b); COHEN (1959)
Crotalus adamanteus	ANGELETTI (1968a, 1968b); COHEN (1959); PEREZ-POLO (1974)
Crotalus atrox	ANGELETTI (1968a)
Crotalus horridus	COHEN (1959)
Crotalus terrificus	ANGELETTI (1968a)
Elapidae	
Dendroaspis viridis	BAILEY et al. (1975)
Naja melanoleuca	BAILEY et al. (1975)
Naja naja	ANGELETTI (1968a, 1969, 1970a, 1970b); COHEN (1959); HOGUE-ANGELETTI et al. (1976); MAY and GUIMARD (1959); SERVER et al. (1976)
Naja nigrocollis	BAILEY et al. (1975); MOHAMED et al. (1971)
Sepedon haemachatus	COHEN (1959)

only exceptions to this observation are the venom (and presumably also the venom glands) of the three principal families of poisonous snakes, i.e., *Elapidae*, *Crotalidae*, and *Viperidae*. As detailed in Table 1, a number of species in each family have been examined and, in each case, NGF has been identified by its unique biologic activity of inducing neurite proliferation from explanted embryonic chick dorsal root ganglia. As with mouse NGF (LEVI-MONTALCINI, 1966), the characteristic metabolic effects that accompany these morphologic changes, which may be collectively described as "pleiotypic activation" (HERSHKO et al., 1971), were also observed (COHEN, 1959). However, it is also clear that these entities maintain both species and family character. As detailed below, distinct immunologic specificity is observed among the different venom NGFs examined and between the snake NGFs and the mouse protein. This is clearly understood by the observation that anticobra venom NGF (*N. naja*) is unable to induce the striking immunosympathectomy in newborn mice that is characteristic of antimouse NGF (ANGELETTI, 1969; BAILEY et al., 1976). However, it is unknown whether anticobra NGF is effective in causing such an event in the homologous host, i.e., the cobra itself.

The relative amounts or potencies of the various snake venom NGFs are difficult to determine with accuracy. COHEN (1959) assayed the crude venom of a number of species from all three families using chick embryonic dorsal root ganglia and concluded that the venoms of the *Elapidae* and *Viperidae* were two to four times as potent as those the *Crotalidae*. However, the yield and specific activity of *Crotalus adamanteus* NGF (PEREZ-POLO, J. R., personal communication) appears to be analogous to that of the homogeneous elapid *(N. naja)* NGF (HOGUE-ANGELETTI et al., 1976). Thus, measurements of the amount and potency of NGF in the unpurified state may reflect a number of parameters such as inhibitors or toxins to the assay tissue and should not be taken as definitive evidence that the NGF of any tissue is less effective as a growth-regulating agent than any other NGF, particularly with respect to its physiologic role in the host organism.

C. Properties

I. Elapidae

The venom of five different species of elapids have been examined with respect to their NGF content (see Table 1). One of these, the NGF from the Indian cobra *Naja naja*, represents the most well-characterized NGF isolated from a snake venom. As such, it may be tentatively taken as a model to which other less well-characterized snake NGF molecules can be compared. This discussion will be presented (Sect. IV) following a description of the properties of NGFs from the various families.

1. Naja naja

Naja naja venom contains one of the highest concentrations of NGF of any venom and is relatively easy to purify, partly because of the well-known stability of NGF to extremes of pH and denaturing conditions (ANGELETTI, 1969). The initial procedure reported (ANGELETTI, 1970a) utilized gel filtration as well as ion-exchange chromatography on CM and DEAE cellulose. This was subsequently modified to omit the DEAE step (HOGUE-ANGELETTI et al., 1976). The elution profile of the initial gel filtration of the crude venom on a column of Sephadex G-100 in 1 M acetic acid is shown in Figure 1. The NGF activity is found in pool III. It is noteworthy that the NGF activity in any venom is extremely difficult to measure, not only in the crude state but also during purification as well, because the toxic compounds in these fractions override the stimulating effect of NGF on nerve cells in culture, the basis for the bioassay. The compounds thereby render localization of NGF in impure preparations uncertain. However, after these components are removed [in this case at the next stage in the purification, i.e., CM-cellulose chromatography (Fig. 2)], the bioassay becomes very clear. As a result of this difficulty, the absolute recovery of NGF from the crude venom cannot be calculated, but approximately 1.5 mg pure NGF/g lyophilized venom can be obtained. The material obtained from the CM-cellulose chromatography was usually homogeneous. However, in some preparations, it was necessary to use preparative disk gel electrophoresis which severely lowered the yield. Some NGF was also found in fraction II of the gel filtration step (Fig. 1) and this material was recovered following CM-cellulose chromatography as well.

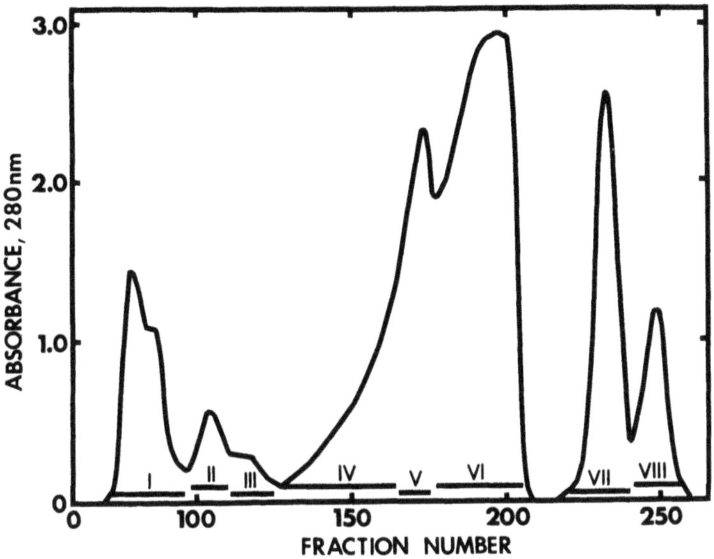

Fig. 1. Gel filtration of crude *Naja naja* venom on Sephadex G-50 at 4°. Bars and Roman numerals indicate the pools made from the 30 ml fractions. Taken from HOGUE-ANGELETTI et al. (1976)

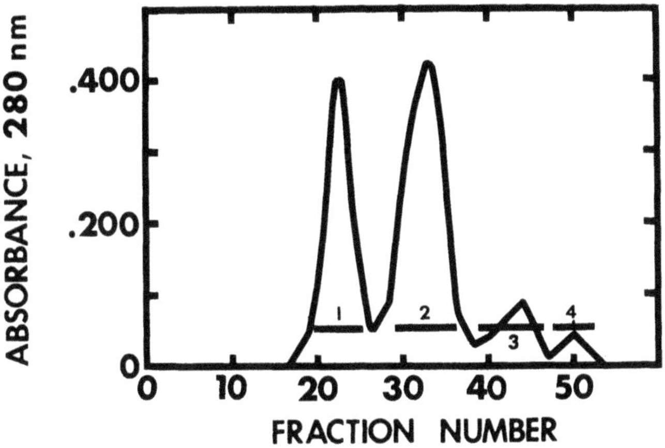

Fig. 2. Chromatography of Sephadex G-50 pool III on CM cellulose at 4°. Bars and Arabic numerals show the pool made of the 10 ml fractions. Taken from HOGUE-ANGELETTI et al. (1976)

The homogeneous *N. naja* NGF possesses a native molecular weight of 28000 as determined by sedimentation equilibrium and a minimum molecular weight of about 13000, as judged by sodium dodecyl sulfate (SDS) polyacrylamide gel electrophoresis, suggesting a dimeric structure of similar or identical polypeptide chains analogous to that found for the β-subunit of the mouse 7 S complex (ANGELETTI et al., 1971; GREENE et al., 1971). This hypothesis was confirmed by a tryptic peptide map of protein reduced and carboxymethylated with iodo-[^{14}C]-acetic acid. The elution profile of the acid soluble tryptic peptides on a column of Dowex 50×8 is shown in Figure 3. As seen from the amino acid composition (see Table 2), a total of 15 tryptic

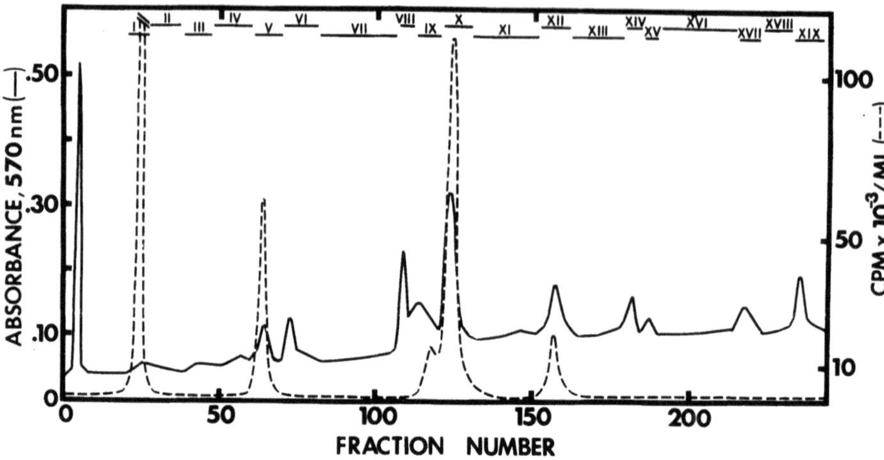

Fig. 3. Elution profile of soluble tryptic peptides of S-[^{14}C]carboxymethyl *Naja naja* NGF on a 0.9 x 20 cm column of Dowex 50 x 8 at 55°. The column was developed at 30 ml/h with a double linear gradient of pyridine acetate and monitored automatically by ninhydrin analysis (—) after alkaline hydrolysis. Fractions of 3.0 ml were collected. Radioactivity (---) was counted on 50 μl aliquots taken from alternate fractions. Fractions were pooled as indicated by the bars and corresponding Roman numerals. Taken from HOGUE-ANGELETTI et al. (1976). See original article for details

Table 2. Amino acid composition of mouse (β) and cobra (*Naja naja*) NGFs

Residue	*Naja naja*[a]	Mouse (β)[b]
Aspartic acid	16	11
Threonine	12	14
Serine	8	11
Glutamic acid	10	8
Proline	5	2
Glycine	7	5
Alanine	5	8
Half-cystine	6	6
Valine	10	13
Methionine	2	1
Isoleucine	6	5
Leucine	3	3
Tyrosine	3	2
Phenylalanine	4	7
Tryptophan	3	3
Lysine	9	8
Histidine	4	4
Arginine	3	7
Total	116	118

[a] Taken from HOGUE-ANGELETTI et al. (1976).
[b] Taken from ANGELETTI and BRADSHAW (1971).

peptides containing six S-[^{14}C]-carboxymethylcysteinyl residues would be expected if the native dimer possessed two identical subunits. Eleven were, in fact, detected, four of which contained a total of six cysteinyl residues, thus demonstrating the presence of the two identical chains in the 28000 molecular weight unit (HOGUE-ANGELETTI et al., 1976).

The partial amino acid sequence of *N. naja* NGF was determined from analyses of the soluble tryptic peptides and the fragments generated by BrCN (HOGUE-ANGELETTI et al., 1976). The tryptic peptides, as well as thermolytic peptides derived from the BrCN fragments, were sequenced by manual methods. Of the three BrCN fragments produced, the two largest (amino terminal and middle positions) were also partially structured by means of the automatic protein sequenator. The tentative sequence obtained is shown in Figure 4. The *N. naja* NGF structure contains 116 amino acids, with fewer basic and more potential acidic residues than the mouse protein, accounting for its lower pI (6.75 vs. 9.1). The six half-cystinyl residues occur in the same positions in the sequence as found for mouse NGF. Since *N. naja* NGF is devoid of sulfhydryl groups, these residues must occur as disulfides, probably in the same pattern as the mouse protein (ANGELETTI and BRADSHAW, 1971).

It is of interest to note that the first preparation of *N. naja* NGF (ANGELETTI, 1970a) was reported to contain 6% hexose. However, the material used for sequence analysis (HOGUE-ANGELETTI et al., 1976) was devoid of carbohydrate. That this material was homogeneous was established by several criteria including the observation that the amino terminal sequence Glu-Asp was the only sequence observed on analysis of the whole protein in the sequenator.

The biologic properties of the homogeneous *N. naja* NGF (ANGELETTI, 1969) are not notably different from those observed for impure preparations of the crotalid NGFs (LEVI-MONTALCINI and COHEN, 1956). Most importantly, this NGF elicited the outgrowth of neurites from explanted 8-day chick dorsal root ganglia, the principal bioassay (LEVI-MONTALCINI, 1966), with a specific activity of 1–10 ng/biological unit (BU) (ANGELETTI, 1970a; SERVER et al., 1976). In addition, injections of the purified NGF resulted in a marked increase in the volume of the sympathetic chain ganglia. A threefold increase in volume was achieved using 3×10^4 BU/g body weight/day in contrast to mouse NGF which elicited the same effect at 10^4 BU/g/day (ANGELETTI, 1969).

The effect of *N. naja* NGF on the metabolism of responsive neurons appears to be entirely similar to that reported for mouse NGF (LEVI-MONTALCINI and ANGELETTI, 1968; ANGELETTI, 1969). As first shown by COHEN (1959) with crotalid NGF, the presence of potent glycolytic inhibitors such as fluoride or cyanide does not prevent the growth effect of cobra NGF. This finding has otherwise been accounted for by the ability of embryonic ganglia to utilize a direct oxidative pathway to derive energy from carbohydrate sources. On the other hand, inhibition of protein synthesis caused by puromycin blocks the outgrowth of nerve fibers induced by NGF. Net protein synthesis appears to be required for the production of neurites in the NGF-stimulated ganglion cultures. Experiments with mitomycin, a potent inhibitor of DNA synthesis, seem to indicate that the growth effect elicited by NGF can take place without stimulation of new DNA synthesis. Inhibition of ribonucleic acid synthesis with actinomycin D, however, does not completely eliminate fiber outgrowth.

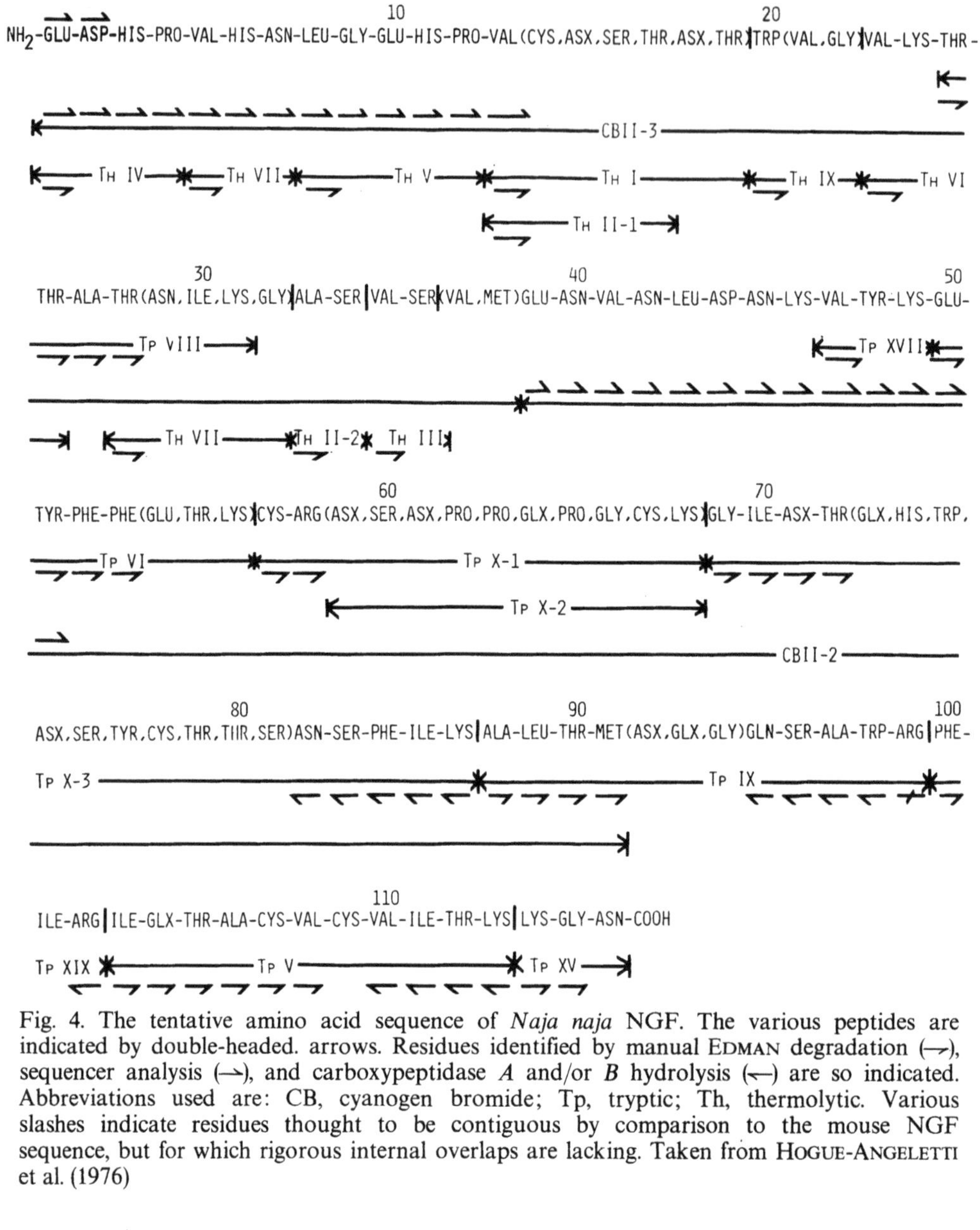

Fig. 4. The tentative amino acid sequence of *Naja naja* NGF. The various peptides are indicated by double-headed. arrows. Residues identified by manual Edman degradation (⇀), sequencer analysis (⇀), and carboxypeptidase *A* and/or *B* hydrolysis (↽) are so indicated. Abbreviations used are: CB, cyanogen bromide; Tp, tryptic; Th, thermolytic. Various slashes indicate residues thought to be contiguous by comparison to the mouse NGF sequence, but for which rigorous internal overlaps are lacking. Taken from Hogue-Angeletti et al. (1976)

2. Other Elapids

The NGFs from three other elapid species, *Naja nigricollis*, *Naja melanoleuca*, and *Dendroaspis viridis*, have been isolated in highly purified form (Bailey et al., 1975). In each case, the lyophilized venom was processed by gel filtration on Sephadex G-50 followed by chromatography of the active fraction on a column of SP-Sephadex C-25. In the case of *N. nigricollis*, a further fractionation on Sephadex G-100 was carried out. As judged by the criteria of electrophoresis, immunodiffusion, or amino end group analysis, none of the NGF preparations were homogeneous. The NGFs from *N. melanoleuca* and *N. nigricollis* were estimated to have molecular weights of 21000 and 22000 with pI values of 8.0 and 9.0, respectively. The NGF from *D. viridis* was found to have a molecular weight of 34000 with a pI of 10.0. Interestingly, all three preparations contained less than 2% carbohydrate and were unaffected electrophoretically by neuraminidase.

II. Crotalidae

As with the other families, all species of the crotalid family examined to date contain NGF. Two species of *Crotalidae* have been examined in detail, *Agkistrodon piscivorus* and *Crotalus adamanteus*, although some information from other species has also been reported. As with the *Viperidae*, some discrepancies in physical and chemical properties of the NGF isolated from these sources exist, which will be discussed in Section IV.

1. Agkistrodon piscivorus

The NGF from *A. piscivorus* was the first snake venom NGF to be highly purified (COHEN and LEVI-MONTALCINI, 1956; COHEN, 1959). The procedure employed ammonium sulfate precipitation and chromatography on columns of DEAE and CM cellulose. The most unusual aspect of this preparation was the initial step in which the venom was dissolved in a solution of ~7.5 M urea, 0.01 N NaOH, and allowed to stand for 90 min at 0° prior to the $(NH_4)_2SO_4$ precipitation. In the absence of this treatment, considerable biologic activity was lost during the subsequent fractionation. However, such conditions are known to favor carbamylation of protein amino groups from reaction with contaminating cyanate in the urea and, thus, the properties of the NGF prepared by this procedure may have been tempered by such modifications.

Although rigorous criteria of homogeneity were not established, this NGF was clearly highly purified. It behaved as a single component in the analytic ultracentrifuge with an S_{20} of 2.2 S, yielding an estimated molecular weight of about 20000 (COHEN, 1959). It possessed an absorbance ratio (280/260 nm) of 1.3 with an $E^{1\%}_{280\,nm} = 10.3$ and contained 1.6% hexose by the orcinol procedure. The biologic activity was completely destroyed by the action of proteolytic enzymes but was unaffected by RNase or DNase. Finally, of the variety of enzymic activities present in the crude venom, only RNase and protease activities were present in significant amounts in the purified sample. On the basis of specific activity and stability in 0.1 M NaOH, these activities could be discounted as contaminants. The nerve growth-promoting activity of *A. piscivorus* has also been isolated by BANKS et al. (1968) by a different procedure. Based on the few properties reported, this material is indistinguishable from that isolated by COHEN (1959).

2. Crotalus adamanteus

The NGF from *C. adamanteus* was originally isolated and characterized by ANGELETTI (1968a, b). When the lyophilized venom was dissolved in 0.05 M Tris-HCl buffer, pH 7.4 containing 0.1 M NaCl, and fractionated on a column of Sephadex G-100, the biologic activity was found in a rather broad band corresponding to a molecular weight range of 20000–40000 (ANGELETTI, 1968a). Further purification of this material on DEAE cellulose, Sephadex G-75, and CM cellulose yielded apparently homogeneous protein with respect to biologic activity (ANGELETTI, 1968b). However, it exhibited somewhat unusual behavior on columns of Sephadex. When the NGF obtained from the CM cellulose column was lyophilized and applied to Sephadex G-100 in 50 mM acetate buffer, pH 5.0, it showed a major peak with a poorly resolved minor peak eluting later. The two peaks gave $S_{20\,\omega}$ values of 2.53 and 1.56, corresponding to approximate molecular values of 20000–30000 and 12000, respectively. The lower molecular weight fraction was further separated on Sephadex G-25 into two components, both apparently containing NGF activity. Neither a sedimentation coefficient nor molecular weight estimate was made on the new component, labeled C, although on electrophoretic analysis it appeared indistinguishable from the 12000 mol wt species identified in the first separation.

In a similar but separate preparation, fractionation on Sephadex G-100 gave three distinct peaks. In addition to the major peak, which eluted in the intermediate position and had a $S_{20\,\omega}=2.56$, there was a high molecular weight component (estimated to be greater than 100000) and low molecular weight species (labeled D and estimated to be about 5000) (ANGELETTI, 1968b). The origin of the low weight species (D), which was electrophoretically distinct from the other components, cannot be ascertained with certainty, but it appears probable that it represents either an active proteolytic fragment of the parent molecule or a non-NGF species contaminated with small amounts of the active material. In view of the fact that no active fragments of mouse NGF have been found despite directed efforts (BRADSHAW et al., 1976), the latter explanation seems most likely.

The other major components clearly represent the dimeric (2.5 S) and monomeric (1.6 S) species corresponding to the active form (subunit) of mouse (ANGELETTI et al., 1971; GREENE et al., 1971) and cobra venom (HOGUE-ANGELETTI et al., 1976) NGFs. These results are in agreement with those of PEREZ-POLO (1974, personal communication) who has obtained *C. adamanteus* NGF in homogeneous form by a procedure utilizing gel filtration and ion-exchange chromatography. This material migrates on SDS gel electrophoresis as a single species with a molecular weight of 14100–14450, consistent with a polypeptide chain containing approximately ten more residues than the corresponding subunits of mouse (ANGELETTI and BRADSHAW, 1971) or *N. naja* (HOGUE-ANGELETTI et al., 1976) NGF.

PEREZ-POLO (1974; personal communication) has also obtained evidence for a higher molecular weight complex with a sedimentation coefficient of 4.5 S. Further, the components of this complex were found to freely interchange with $\alpha\beta$-subunits of mouse NGF (PEREZ-POLO, 1974). It seems probable that the higher molecular weight complex noted by ANGELETTI (1968b) *(vide supra)* represents the same material.

3. Bothrops jararaca

The NGF of this venom was purified to apparent homogeneity by ANGELETTI (1968b, 1969), using a procedure similar to that employed for the isolation of the *C. adamanteus* protein. The *B. jararaca* NGF also showed a size heterogeneity on Sephadex G-100, but the principal component possessed a molecular weight of about 30000.

4. Other Crotalids

In addition to the species already described, NGF has been identified in, or partially purified from, the venoms of *Crotalus atrox* (ANGELETTI, 1968a), *Crotalus terrificus* (ANGELETTI, 1968a), *Ancistrodon contortrix lactocinctus* (ANGELETTI, 1968a), *Ancistrodon rhodostoma* (BAILEY et al., 1975), and *Bothrops atrox* (GLASS and BANTHROPE, 1975). The first three species were examined only by analytic gel filtration on Sephadex G-100. Although the protein profiles, as judged by absorbance at 280 nm, were quite different in each case, the NGF activity was always found in a position corresponding to a molecular weight of 20000–40000, suggesting that the NGF of these snakes will not be significantly different from that isolated from the other crotalids.

The NGF from *A. rhodostoma* was isolated from venom that had already been partially purified by chromatography on TEAE cellulose (BAILEY et al., 1975). It was further purified on columns of Sephadex G-100 and Sephadex QAE A-25. However, the final product was impure as judged by polyacrylamide gel electrophoresis (three to four bands) and dansyl amino terminal analysis (glycine and serine). The active component possessed an apparent molecular weight (determined by gel filtration) of 34000 and a pI (determined by polyacrylamide electrofocusing) of 10.5. Most interestingly, when the sample was treated with neuraminidase, a change in the electrophoretic mobility of all bands of about 30% was observed. This result is consistent with the removal of sialic acid and suggests *A. rhodostoma* NGF is a glycoprotein. Insufficient material was available to test this hypothesis by direct carbohydrate analysis.

The NGF from *Bothrops atrox* was purified by chromatography on QAE A-25 and SP C-25 Sephadex and gel filtration on Sephadex G-100. This material was also heterogeneous on polyacrylamide gel electrophoresis (two main components with pI values of 8.0 and 9.0). As was found for *A. rhodostoma*, this NGF contained some 12% (wt/wt) carbohydrate, made up of N-acetylglucosamine, glucose, mannose, and galactose, and gave a molecular weight on gel filtration of 35000. SDS gel electrophoresis gave a value of 19000, suggesting the presence of a dimeric structure (GLASS and BANTHROPE, 1975).

III. Viperidae

NGF has been specifically identified in five species of *Viperidae* (Table 1). Of these, the NGF of *Vipera russellii* (Russell's viper) has been examined in greatest detail.

1. Vipera russellii

Initial studies on the NGF from this venom indicated that it possessed a molecular weight similar to that of *N. naja* (i.e., 20000–25000) (ANGELETTI, 1968a). Subsequently, this material was purified to homogeneity by PEARCE et al. (1972). In an initial report from this group (BANKS et al., 1968), they used a three-step procedure involving Sephadex G-150, G-75, and Cellex T which was later modified to include QAE A-25, SP C-25, and G-100 Sephadex in place of the Cellex T step (PEARCE et al., 1972). The NGF isolated by the latter modification gave a single diffuse band on disk electrophoresis at pH 3.8 and 5.2. It also migrated as a single component in gel electrofocusing with an isoelectric point of 10.5. However, the experimental error of this measurement was in the range of ± 1.0.

The molecular weight of *V. russellii* NGF was determined by both ultracentrifugal and gel filtration analyses. Values of 37000 and 34000 were obtained, respectively. No indication of dissociation at lower concentrations was observed by either method and no indication of a higher molecular weight complex, in agreement with the report of ANGELETTI (1968a), was obtained from gel filtration analyses of samples taken at intermediate steps.

The most striking feature of this preparation is the presence of 20% (wt/wt) carbohydrate including fucose, mannose, galactose, N-acetylglucosamine, and N-acetylneuraminic acid. The molecule also contains a high proportion of potentially acidic residues (59 of 274) which must occur largely in the amide form to account for the basic isoelectric point.

In marked contrast to the results of PEARCE et al. (1972), PEREZ-POLO (personal communication) has obtained a preparation of *V. russellii* NGF that is devoid of carbohydrate. This procedure also utilizes gel filtration on Sephadex G-100 and G-150 but uses DEAE and CM celluloses for the ion-exchange media. This material displays a sedimentation coefficient of 2.5 S and gives a molecular weight of 12900 on SDS gel electrophoresis suggesting a dimeric structure composed of subunits the same size as are found in mouse or *N. naja* NGF. No indication of a higher molecular weight complex was observed, and, unlike *C. adamanteus* NGF, this material would not recombine with any of the subunits of mouse 7 S NGF.

2. Other Viperids

The NGF of *Vipera ammodytes ammodytes* has been highly purified by BAILEY et al. (1975) using a three-step procedure with preparative isoelectric focusing as the final step. Although this material appeared to be relatively homogeneous on polyacrylamide gel electrophoresis, it produced a large number of amino terminal residues, the predominant one being isoleucine. As with the *V. russellii* NGF isolated by this laboratory, this material contained 32% carbohydrate. It gave an isoelectric point of 8.5 and a molecular weight (by gel filtration) of 34000.

MAY and GUIMARD (1959) and MOHAMED et al. (1971) examined the venoms of *V. aspis*, *E. carinatus*, and *E. coloratus*. The NGF of the last two venoms appeared highly active while that of *V. aspis* was considerably less potent (MAY and GUIMARD, 1959).

D. Comparison of Nerve Growth Factors

I. Relationship of Venom NGFs

1. Intrafamily

a) Elapidae

Among the reports describing the properties of elapid NGFs, there seems to be general agreement that these molecules possess a molecular weight of about 25000 and are composed of two very similar or identical polypeptide chains. Only the molecular weight of 34000 reported for *Dendroaspis viridis* (BAILEY et al., 1975) is at variance with this conclusion. However, the isoelectric points vary from 6.75 (*N. naja*, ANGELETTI, 1970a) to 10.0 (*D. viridis*, BAILEY et al., 1975). No elapid NGF has been isolated that contains significant carbohydrate.

b) Crotalidae

Homogeneous or highly purified NGF has been obtained from five crotalid species. Three of these, *A. piscivorus*, (COHEN, 1959), *C. adamanteus* (ANGELETTI, 1968b; PEREZ-POLO, 1974), and *B. jararaca* (ANGELETTI, 1968b) appear to be dimers of about 25000 molecular weight. In contrast, the NGFs isolated from *A. rhodostoma* (BAILEY et al., 1975) and *B. atrox* (GLASS and BANTHROPE, 1975) behave as higher molecular weight entities (ca. 35000) with significant carbohydrate contents. It is noteworthy, perhaps, that the yield of the latter two preparations was very low relative to the amounts obtained from *C. adamanteus* and *B. jararaca* venoms. All crotalid NGFs behaved as basic proteins with pI values ranging from 8.0 to 10.5.

c) Viperidae

Two viperid NGFs (*V. russelli* and *V. ammodytes ammodytes*) have been isolated. As prepared by PEARCE and co-workers (PEARCE et al., 1972; BAILEY et al., 1975), the NGF from this family is a glycoprotein of about 35000 molecular weight. No evidence for a quaternary structure was observed although definitive experiments to establish this point were not reported. However, NGF prepared from the same source (*V. russellii*) by PEREZ-POLO (personal communication) possesses a dimeric structure with a native molecular weight of ca. 25000. This material is devoid of carbohydrate. The overall yields were comparable, PEARCE et al. (1972) reporting 1.5 mg/g venom and PEREZ-POLO, 2.8 mg/g venom.

2. Interfamily

Although it would be surprising if proteins isolated from different species of the same snake family and possessing essentially identical biologic activity were not homologous, i.e., not related evolutionarily to a common ancestral precursor, such a relationship might not be found for interfamily representatives, particularly when the biologic activity in question is as general as the induction of nerve fiber growth. In lieu of primary structure information, immunochemical analyses are the most meaningful way to detect such relationships.

The first such study was reported by ANGELETTI (1971). Utilizing antiserum against *N. naja* NGF, immunologic cross-reactivity between NGFs purified from the three classes of snake venoms was detected. In the double diffusion test, precipitin bands of partial identity were found toward NGF from *C. adamanteus*, *B. jararaca*, and *V. russellii* venoms, although at higher antigen concentrations than the homologous antigen. To achieve a more quantitative estimate of the extent of cross-reactivity, the inhibition of in vitro biologic activity was measured. In this assay, a series of two-fold dilutions of antisera were first incubated for 1 h at 20° with 1 BU of NGF, and then cultured with responsive ganglia in vitro. The reciprocal of the highest dilution of the antiserum still giving inhibition of NGF activity is a measure of the extent of cross-reaction. *V. russellii* NGF was only 6% cross-reactive with anti-*N. naja* NGF, while *C. adamanteus* and *B. jararaca* NGFs were over 12% cross-reactive. Although these titers appear relatively low, it should be noted that mouse and *Naja naja* NGF show only a 1% cross-reaction, even though 65% of their amino acid residues are identical *(vide infra)*. These results have been confirmed by BAILEY et al. (1976), who, despite the heterogeneity of most of their antigen preparations, demonstrated slightly higher levels of cross-reactivity. Antisera against five venom NGFs from all three families showed levels of cross-reaction ranging from 5% to 50%, with the majority about 20–25% cross-reactive. Thus, by immunochemical criteria it may be concluded that all snake venom NGFs possess homologous structures although, not surprisingly, major antigenic determinants differ from family to family and probably even from species to species within a family.

In view of the clear demonstration that NGF from the three snake families are homologous, it is of interest to note that the various NGFs isolated can be subdivided into two apparent classes. On the one hand, NGFs isolated from *A. piscivorus*, *C. adamanteus*, *B. jararaca*, *N. naja*, *N. nigricollis*, *N. melanoleuca*, and *V. russellii* (in one laboratory) possess a molecular weight of about 25000, are composed of two identical or very similar subunits of about 13000 mol wt, and are devoid of carbohydrate. The β-subunit of mouse NGF may also be included in this description *(vide infra)*. On the other hand, the NGFs isolated from *B. atrox*, *A. rhodostoma*, *V. ammodytes ammodytes*, and *V. russellii* (in another laboratory) are somewhat larger (ca. 35000) and contains 10–20% carbohydrate. In some cases, a dimeric structure is indicated, while in others, this aspect of the molecule is unclear. It has been pointed out that the protein portion of this group of NGFs is about the same size as the first group (PEARCE et al., 1972), which may indicate that these two classes of venom NGF differ only in the presence of the carbohydrate. However, it should also be noted that all of the NGFs containing carbohydrate, except the single report on *V. russellii* NGF (PEARCE et al., 1972), have not been obtained in homogeneous form. In view of the conflicting reports for *V. russellii* NGF and the fact that several early preparations of venom NGF were reported to contain carbohydrate (ANGELETTI, 1970a; ANGELETTI, 1969; COHEN, 1959) before they were ultimately purified to homogeneity, there seems to be a strong possibility that there exists only a single class of NGF proteins throughout the vertebrate kingdom that are entirely proteinoid in character.

II. Relationship of Venom and Mouse NGFs

In addition to the snake venoms, the only other source of NGF rich enough to provide protein in large quantities is the male mouse submaxillary gland. The structural and functional properties of this protein have been extensively reviewed (LEVI-MONTALCINI, 1966; LEVI-MONTALCINI and ANGELETTI, 1968; BRADSHAW and YOUNG, 1976; BRADSHAW et al., 1976), and only the most salient features will be iterated here.

Mouse submaxillary NGF occurs and can be isolated as a high molecular weight complex (designated 7 S) (VARON et al., 1970). Of the three unique polypeptide chains found in 7 S NGF, only the β-subunit, which can also be isolated directly from gland homogenates (designated as 2.5 S NGF, BOCCHINI and ANGELETTI, 1969), contains biologic activity. β-(or 2.5 S) NGF contains two identical subunits (ANGELETTI et al.,

```
                                         10                                       20
NH2-SER-SER-THR-HIS-PRO-VAL-PHE-HIS-MET-GLY-GLU-PHE-SER-VAL-CYS-ASP-SER-VAL-SER-VAL-

    NH2-GLU-ASP-           -HIS-ASN-LEU-       -HIS-PRO-               -THR-ASX-THR-

                                         30                                       40
    TRP-VAL-GLY-ASP-LYS-THR-THR-ALA-THR-ASN-ILE-LYS-GLY-LYS-GLU-VAL-THR-VAL-LEU-ALA-

               -VAL-                                   -ALA-SER-   -SER-   -MET-GLU-

                                         50                                       60
    GLU-VAL-ASN-ILE-ASN-ASN-SER-VAL-PHE-ARG-GLN-TYR-PHE-PHE-GLU-THR-LYS-CYS-ARG-ALA-

    ASN-       -LEU-ASP-   -LYS-   -TYR-LYS-                                   -ASX-

                                         70                                       80
    SER-ASN-PRO-VAL-GLU-SER-GLY-CYS-ARG-GLY-ILE-ASP-SER-LYS-HIS-TRP-ASN-SER-TYR-CYS-

               -PRO-   -PRO-       -LYS-           -THR-GLX-

                                         90                                      100
    THR-THR-THR-HIS-THR-PHE-VAL-LYS-ALA-LEU-THR-THR-ASP-GLU-LYS-GLN-ALA-ALA-TRP-ARG-

           -SER-ASN-SER-  -ILE-                -MET-       -GLY-   -SER-

                                         110
    PHE-ILE-ARG-ILE-ASP-THR-ALA-CYS-VAL-CYS-VAL-LEU-SER-ARG-LYS-ALA-THR-ARG-COOH

                   -GLX-                       -ILE-THR-LYS-  -GLY-ASN-COOH
```

Fig. 5. Comparison of the amino acid sequences of the NGFs of cobra (*Naja naja*) venom and mouse submaxillary glands. The completed segments (top) correspond to mouse NGF and the incomplete segments (bottom) to cobra NGF. Only those residues of cobra NGF which *differ* from the mouse protein are shown

1971; GREENE et al., 1971), which, if they are not partially shortened by proteolysis during isolation (ANGELETTI et al., 1973; MOORE et al., 1974), contain 118 amino acids each. The amino acid sequence has been determined (ANGELETTI and BRADSHAW, 1971) (see Fig. 5), yielding a subunit molecular weight of 13259 (dimer mol wt 26518).

The most direct evidence that mouse and venom NGFs are related is provided by a comparison of the partial amino acid sequence of *N. naja* NGF with the established mouse structure. As shown in Figure 5, when the undetermined regions of *N. naja* NGF are optimized, there is a 64% identity of mammalian and reptilian proteins (HOGUE-ANGELETTI et al., 1976). It is clear that the two are structurally similar to a degree indicative of the close genetic relatedness found amoung members of functionally related families of proteins. It is also of interest to compare the cobra sequence to the proinsulin family since it has been established that a statistically significant relationship of the type associated with proteins that have evolved from a common precursor exists for mouse NGF and the proinsulin family (FRAZIER et al., 1972). Interestingly, the percentage of identical amino acid residues of cobra NGF as compared to proinsulin is the same as that observed for mouse, i.e., 20%. It appears, therefore, that the NGF and proinsulins are more closely related to themselves than to each other. Thus, the divergence of the NGF and insulin families probably occurred very early in vertebrate evolution, and that selective pressure has conserved the structure of NGF as strictly as that of the proinsulins.

Although the crystal structure of mouse NGF has not been completed (WLODAWER et al., 1975) and, therefore, very little is known about the three-dimensional structure of either mouse or *N. naja* NGF, there are some indications that the spatial relationships of both are similar. Studies on the solution topography of mouse NGF have shown that of the three tryptophan residues present, one is fully exposed on the surface of the molecule, one is completely buried, while the third is partially exposed (FRAZIER et al., 1973a). Since the titration curves of the reaction of the tryptophan residues with N-bromosuccinimide are very similar with the two proteins, the topographical location of the tryptophan residues in *N. naja* NGF are probably the same (ANGELETTI, 1970b). It has also been shown that *N. naja* NGF does not recombine with either the α- or γ-subunits of mouse NGF to form a higher molecular weight complex (SERVER et al., 1976). This may be a reflection of the absence of the carboxyl terminal arginine residue, present in mouse NGF, that has been shown to be required for the reformation of the mouse 7 S complex (MOORE et al., 1974).

Although the biologic properties of the cobra and mouse proteins are grossly similar, there are some differences. The two factors show an identical dose-response curve, but the extent of the response elicited by *N. naja* NGF is only about 50% that of mouse NGF (SERVER et al., 1976). In vivo, about three times as much *N. naja* NGF is needed to produce the same effect in neonatal mice. However, the hyperplastic and hypertrophic effects appear to be the same under histologic examination (ANGELETTI, 1969).

The interaction of NGF with plasma membrane receptors of responsive neurons has been shown to be the primary event in the stimulation of neurite proliferation in embryonic tissue (FRAZIER et al., 1973b). This recognitive entity or receptor provides, therefore, an additional assay for relatedness of the cobra and mouse proteins. When *N. naja* NGF was competed with bound mouse ^{125}I-NGF, it was found that about 80% of the labeled material was displaced as effectively with the cobra protein as with unlabeled mouse NGF (SERVER et al., 1976). Although these data show that some differences exist, they also clearly establish a high degree of structural identity in the portions of the molecule that are responsible for binding to the receptor.

Although detailed structural data for other snake venom NGFs is unavailable, immunochemical data establishing a relationship between the other venom NGFs and the mouse protein have been obtained.

In immunodiffusion tests, antiserum to mouse NGF was detected as a precipitin band merging in a line of identity with that of mouse NGF at concentrations of protein 50-fold greater. No precipitin lines were found for NGF from *C. adamanteus* and *B. jaracaca*. Complement fixation tests showed cross-reaction of both *N. naja* NGF and *B. jararaca* NGF when tested with antimouse NGF serum at ten-fold and

50-fold ratios of antiserum, respectively (ANGELETTI, 1971). Radioimmunoassay confirmed these observations for the cobra venom. Furthermore, antimouse serum inhibited the in vitro biologic activity of *N. naja*, *Crotalus adamanteus*, *Bothrops jararaca*, and *Vipera russellii* NGFs at levels of 6%, 6%, 12%, and 12%, respectively (ANGELETTI, 1969). On the contrary, antiserum to *N. naja* NGF did not detect cross-reaction with mouse NGF in either the immunodiffusion assay or the complement fixation test. However, a 1% cross-reaction was detected using the bioassay inhibition test. These data are clear evidence of a structural relationships between mouse NGF and the NGFs from snake venoms. BAILEY et al. (1976) confirmed the presence of a relationship between venom NGFs and mouse NGF, although they found that the antivenom NGF sera detected more cross-reaction than the antimouse NGF serum.

The clearly established evolutionary relationship between venom and mouse NGFs is also supported by a consideration of the tissue of origin of these proteins. The venom gland in snakes is a highly developed parotid gland. The principal secretory part is in the posterior section. The epithelial cells lining the secretory tubules contain secretory granules of size and density comparable to those found in the epithelial cells lining the convoluted tubules in the male mouse submandibular gland. In this regard, it is of interest to note that the mouse salivary secretion resembles the snake venom not only for its content of digestive and hydrolytic enzymes, but also for its poisonous properties (LIUZZI and ANGELETTI, 1968). Indeed, the mouse submaxillary gland represents almost the only toxin-secreting organ known among the mammals. Thus, the structural and functional relationships found for the snake and mouse NGFs appear to be manifestations of evolutionary events that can also be traced at the morphological level.

E. Role of NGF in Snake Venom

The question of the role of NGF in snake venoms is closely related to the question regarding the role of NGF in mouse submaxillary glands. In all the animal species examined, low levels of NGF are found in this type of structure, similar to the levels in serum and other tissues (LEVI-MONTALCINI, 1966). The sex difference found in mouse submaxillary gland, tenfold higher in males than females, is not found in other species, although this has not been examined in snakes.

Evidence continues to accumulate that for the developmental and maintenance functions that NGF exerts on the nervous system the low levels found in tissues other than the submaxillary gland are sufficient. Furthermore, based on sialectomy experiments, it also follows that some secondary source usually supplies the NGF in vivo (HENDRY and IVERSON, 1973). Realizing that there is no clear explanation for the presence of high concentrations of NGF in the submaxillary or venom glands (and their excretions), one can advance several hypotheses. For example, it has been suggested (MELDRUN, 1965) that the venom gland may play a role in removing excess NGF from the circulation. Alternatively, it is an equally attractive hypothesis that NGF may potentiate poisonous effects of venom (and mouse saliva) by stimulating responsive cells, and thus rendering them more vulnerable. However, it may also be that the NGF found in venom and saliva simply represents the manner in which excess material, otherwise synthesized for endocrine functions, is removed from the gland. If the venom or salivary gland is viewed as one of many sympathetic end organs that synthesize NGF as part of the regulation of that portion of the peripheral nervous system, this hypothesis becomes attractive indeed.

F. Concluding Remarks

This review has described the isolation and characterization of the NGFs from the three principal families of poisonous snakes. By comparison with each other and with the well-defined mouse NGF, it may be taken as established that the entities referred to in this review by the general name NGF are a group of proteins related by evolution from a common ancestral gene. It would be entirely inconsistent with a vast collection of data (DAYHOFF, 1972) to expect, as has been suggested (BAILEY et al., 1975), that the NGFs of snakes and the mouse would be identical in toto. Rather, they show as much "relatedness" as other proteins of the same function isolated from reptiles and rodents, i.e., they may be estimated to have 50–75% of their residues identical. However, even this extent of identity in sequence provides a basis for only limited immunochemical cross-reactivity (PRAGER and WILSON, 1971). Thus, there appears to be no compelling reason to adopt the suggestion of BAILEY et al. (1975) to use the term NGF "to define a specific type of biologic activity rather than to imply the existence of a unique chemical agent." On the contrary, within the limits of evolutionary change, this activity is associated with a unique factor and the description *nerve growth factor* should be reserved solely for use with it.

Acknowledgement. The authors would like to express their appreciation to Dr. Regino PEREZ-POLO, University of Texas, Austin, for providing them with data prior to publication. Portions of this work were supported by NIH research grant NS 10229.

References

Angeletti, R. H.: Studies on the nerve growth factor (NGF) from snake venom. Gel filtration patterns of crude venoms. J. Chromatog. **36**, 535—537 (1968 a)

Angeletti, R. H.: Studies on the nerve growth factor (NGF) from snake venom. Molecular heterogeneity. J. Chromatog. **37**, 62—69 (1968 b)

Angeletti, R. H.: Snake venom nerve growth factor. Ph.D. Thesis: Washington University, St. Louis 1969

Angeletti, R. H.: Nerve growth factor from cobra venom. Proc. nat. Acad. Sci. (Wash.) **65**, 668—674 (1970 a)

Angeletti, R. H.: The role of the tryptophan residues in the activity of the nerve growth factor. Biochim. biophys. Acta (Amst.) **214**, 478—482 (1970 b)

Angeletti, R. H.: Immunological relatedness of nerve growth factors. Brain Res. **25**, 424—427 (1971)

Angeletti, R. H., Bradshaw, R. A.: Nerve growth factor from mouse submaxillary gland: amino acid sequence. Proc. nat. Acad. Sci. (Wash.) **68**, 2417—2420 (1971)

Angeletti, R. H., Bradshaw, R. A., Wade, R. D.: Subunit structure and amino acid composition of mouse submaxillary gland nerve growth factor. Biochemistry **10**, 463—469 (1971)

Angeletti, R. H., Hermodson, M. A., Bradshaw, R. A.: Amino acid sequence of mouse 2.5 S nerve growth factor. II. Isolation and characterization of the thermolytic and peptic peptides and the complete covalent structure. Biochemistry **12**, 100—115 (1973)

Bailey, G. S., Banks, B. E. C., Carstairs, J. R., Edwards, D. C., Pearce, F. L., Vernon, C. A.: Immunological properties of nerve growth factors. Biochim. biophys. Acta (Amst.) **437**, 259—263 (1976)

Bailey, G. S., Banks, B. E. C., Pearce, F. L., Shipolini, R. A.: A comparative study of nerve growth factors from snake venoms. Comp. Biochem. Physiol. [B] **51**, 429—438 (1975)

Banks, B. E. C., Banthorpe, D. V., Berry, A. R., Davies, H. ff. S., Doonan, S., Lamont, D. M., Shipolini, R., Vernon, C. A.: The preparation of nerve growth factors from snake venoms. Biochem. J. **108**, 157—158 (1968)

Bocchini, V., Angeletti, P. U.: The nerve growth factor: purification as a 30000 molecular weight protein. Proc. nat. Acad. Sci. (Wash.) **64**, 787—794 (1969)

Bradshaw, R. A., Jeng, I., Andres, R. Y., Pulliam, M. W., Silverman, R. E., Rubin, J., Jacobs, J. W.: The structure and function of nerve growth factor. Proc. of the VIth Int. Congr. of Endocrinology, Vol. II, pp. 231—238. Amsterdam: Excerpta Medica 1976

Bradshaw, R. A., Young, M.: Nerve growth factor—recent developments and perspectives. Biochem. Pharmacol. **25**, 1445—1449 (1976)

Cohen, S.: Purification and metabolic effects of a nerve growth-promoting protein from snake venom. J. biol. Chem. **234**, 1129—1137 (1959)

Cohen, S.: Purification of a nerve growth promoting protein from the mouse salivary gland and its neurotoxic antiserum. Proc. nat. Acad. Sci. (Wash.) **46**, 303—311 (1960)

Cohen, S., Levi-Montalcini, R.: A nerve growth-stimulating factor isolated from snake venom. Proc. nat. Acad. Sci. (Wash.) **42**, 571—574 (1956)

Cohen, S., Levi-Montalcini, R., Hamburger, V.: A nerve growth stimulating factor from Sarcomas 37 and 180. Proc. nat. Acad. Sci. (Wash.) **40**, 1014—1018 (1954)

Dayhoff, M. O.: Atlas of Protein Sequence and Structure, Vol. V. Washington, D.C.: National Biomedical Research Foundation 1972

Frazier, W. A., Angeletti, R. H., Bradshaw, R. A.: Nerve growth factor and insulin. Science **176**, 482—488 (1972)

Frazier, W. A., Boyd, L. F., Bradshaw, R. A.: Interaction of nerve growth factor with surface membranes: biological competence of insolubilized nerve growth factor. Proc. nat. Acad. Sci. (Wash.) **70**, 2931—2935 (1973 b)

Frazier, W. A., Hogue-Angeletti, R. A., Sherman, R., Bradshaw, R. A.: Topography of mouse 2.5 S nerve growth factor. Reactivity of tyrosine and tryptophan. Biochemistry **12**, 3281—3293 (1973 a)

Glass, R. E., Banthorpe, D. V.: Properties of nerve growth factor from the venom of *Bothrops atrox*. Biochim. biophys. Acta (Amst.) **405**, 23—26 (1975)

Greene, L. A., Varon, S., Piltch, A., Shooter, E. M.: Substructure of the β subunit of mouse 7 S nerve growth factor. Neurobiology **1**, 37—48 (1971)

Hendry, I. A., Iversen, L. L.: Reduction in the concentration of nerve growth factor in mice after sialectomy and castration. Nature (Lond.) New Biol. **243**, 500—504 (1973)

Hershko, A., Mamont, P., Shields, R., Tomkins, G. M.: Pleiotypic response. Nature (Lond.) New Biol. **232**, 206—211 (1971)

Hogue-Angeletti, R. A., Frazier, W. A., Jacobs, J. W., Niall, H. D., Bradshaw, R. A.: Purification, characterization, and partial amino acid sequence of nerve growth factor from cobra venom. Biochemistry **15**, 26—34 (1976)

Levi-Montalcini, R.: Effects of mouse tumor transplantation on the nervous system. Ann. N.Y. Acad. Sci. **55**, 330—343 (1952)

Levi-Montalcini, R.: The nerve growth factor: its mode of action on sensory and sympathetic nerve cells. Harvey Lect. **60**, 217—259 (1966)

Levi-Montalcini, R., Angeletti, P. U.: Nerve growth factor. Physiol. Rev. **48**, 534—569 (1968)

Levi-Montalcini, R., Cohen, S.: In vitro and in vivo effects of a nerve growth-stimulating agent isolated from snake venom. Proc. nat. Acad. Sci. (Wash.) **42**, 695—699 (1956)

Liuzzi, A., Angeletti, P. U.: Studies on the toxic effects of mouse submaxillary gland extracts. Experentia (Basel) **24**, 1034—1035 (1968)

May, R. M., Guimard, J.: L'action stimulante des venins des serpents *Vipera*, *Naja*, *Bitis*, *Echis* sur la croissance des fibres medullaires de l'embryon de poulet in vitro. C.R. Acad. Sci. (Paris) **248**, 2657—2659 (1959)

Meldrun, B. S.: The actions of snake venoms on nerve and muscle. The pharmacology of phospholipase A and of polypeptide toxins. Pharmacol. Rev. **17**, 393—445 (1965)
Mohamed, A. H., Saleh, A. M., Ahmed, F.: Nerve growth factor from Egyptian snake venoms. Toxicon **9**, 201—204 (1971)
Moore, J. B. Jr., Mobley, W. C., Shooter, E. M.: Proteolytic modification of the β nerve growth factor protein. Biochemistry **13**, 833—840 (1974)
Pearce, E. L., Banks, B. E. C., Banthorpe, D. V., Berry, A. R., Davies, H. ff. S., Vernon, C. A.: The isolation and characterization of nerve growth factor from the venom of *Vipera russellii* Europ. J. Biochem. **29**, 417—425 (1972)
Perez-Polo, J. R.: *Crotalus adamanteus* snake venom nerve growth factor purification. Absts. Neurosci. Meetings (St. Louis), 371 (1974)
Prager, E. M., Wilson, A. C.: The dependence of immunological cross-reactivity upon sequence resemblance among lysozymes. I. Microcomplement fixation studies. J. biol. Chem. **246**, 5978—5989 (1971)
Server, A. C., Herrup, K., Shooter, E. M., Hogue-Angeletti, R. A., Frazier, W. A., Bradshaw, R. A.: Comparison of the nerve growth factor proteins from cobra venom *(Naja naja)* and mouse submaxillary gland. Biochemistry **15**, 35—39 (1976)
Varon, S., Nomura, J., Shooter, E. M.: The isolation of the mouse nerve growth factor protein in a high molecular weight form. Biochemistry **6**, 2202—2209 (1967)
Wlodawer, A., Hodgson, K. O., Shooter, E. M.: Crystallization of nerve growth factor from mouse submaxillary glands. Proc. nat. Acad. Sci. (Wash.) **72**, 777—779 (1975)

CHAPTER 9

Metal and Nonprotein Constituents in Snake Venoms

A. L. BIEBER

A. Introduction

Snake venoms have been extensively studied in the past and, in general, their gross composition has been quite well-established. Approximately 90% of the dry weight of most venoms consists of protein material. Most of the toxic and biologically active components of the venom are proteins from this major fraction of the dry weight. The nonprotein portion of the venom is a much smaller amount of material and, in general, is biologically less active. Included in the nonprotein fraction are metal ions, inorganic anions, and some small organic molecules including peptides, lipids, nucleosides, carbohydrates, and amines. DEVI (1968) in a review entitled "The protein and nonprotein constituents of snake venoms" has covered the literature pertaining to nonprotein constituents up to that time reasonably well. The review also contains substantial amounts of data from the laboratory of DEVI that does not appear to be published in the primary literature. In this review, I shall limit citations primarily to those that have appeared since the review by DEVI (1968) except where older literature citations are important for direct comparison or are very pertinent for discussion purposes.

B. Inorganic Constituents

I. Metal Content

The venoms from all species of snakes that have been examined contain metal ions as part of their overall composition. DEVI (1968) reported that work in her laboratory and in the laboratories of others showed that sodium, potassium, zinc, calcium, magnesium, iron, and cobalt were present, while attempts to detect manganese were uniformly unsuccessful. The most systematic study of metal composition in recent years is that of FRIEDRICH and TU (1971). The distribution of metals in venoms from 17 snake species including *Crotalidae*, *Viperidae*, and *Elapidae* was determined by atomic absorption analysis. Analyses for 15 metals were carried out on the venom before and after exhaustive dialysis. None of the venoms contained molybdenum, bismuth, selenium, platinum, palladium, silver, iron, or gold. Calcium, zinc, magnesium, sodium, potassium, copper, and manganese were detected in some but not all venoms tested. Sodium and potassium were found in the highest concentrations while magnesium, calcium, and zinc were the most prevalent divalent cations in the venoms. Much of the metal ion content was firmly bound to the nondialyzable fraction since high values were obtained after 48 h of dialysis against distilled water.

Copper was reported to be present in venoms from two species, both *Crotalidae*, while manganese was found in venoms from two species of *Elapidae* and from one *Viperidae*. The results were obtained with venoms from a limited number of individual snakes, two to five, in most cases. Thus, it is difficult to assess whether these results are general for the type of venoms examined or whether they are a reflection of the environment and history of the individual snakes from which the venom was obtained. Hemorrhagic and proteolytic activity decreased markedly after dialysis, suggesting that metal ions may play a role in these activities. In fact, hemorrhagic activity was shown to be partially restored by addition of magnesium ion to the dialyzed fraction. Neutron activation analysis of snake venoms from four species showed copper to be present in all four venoms and zinc was detected in one (GITTER et al., 1963). MOAV et al. (1964) demonstrated that copper and zinc were present in *V. palestinae* venom. Copper was at a high concentration in the neurotoxic fraction and zinc was at high levels in the hemorrhagic fraction. Recent studies of venoms from *Cerastes* by EL-HAWARY and HASSAN (1974a) showed water as the major component (75%) with sodium and potassium as the cations at highest concentrations exceeding the concentration of calcium by approximately tenfold. HIRAKAWA (1974) showed that venoms from *Trimeresurus* species had potassium, zinc, sodium, calcium, magnesium, and copper in order of decreasing concentrations.

II. Nonmetal Inorganic Content

The amount of information on nonmetal inorganic constituents in venom is rather limited. DEVI (1968) presented the results of studies on the phosphorus content of whole venoms from several species. The total phosphorus content varied from 9.36/100 to 14.0/100 mg but the units were not specified. Thus, interpretation of the data is difficult in terms of absolute values, but the data does allow comparison of amounts of different forms of phosphorus in venoms from different species. Total inorganic phosphorus ranged from 5.46 to 5.71/100 mg, acid soluble phosphorus from 7.3 to 10.92/100 mg, and acid insoluble phosphorus from 2.06 to 3.088/100 mg while 7-minute hydrolyzable phosphorus ranged from 1.01 to 4.36/100 mg. The amount of chloride in two venoms was reported by GRASSET et al. (1956) to be 0.19% and 0.29%, respectively. However, a range of 0.2–2.6% was observed. Recently, EL-HAWARY and HASSAN (1974a) presented data on the chloride content of two species of *Cerastes*. The values were 0.186% and 0.392% for the two species.

There appears to be little interest in the content of nonmetallic inorganic components in snake venoms. The lack of any demonstrated physiologic function for this class of compounds may well be the reason for the lack of interest. The phosphorous content of the venoms may arise from the degradation of normal tissue constituents of the venom glands. This seems reasonable in light of the observations that many venoms contain degradative enzymes that are capable of hydrolyzing nucleic acids, phospholipids, and organic phosphate esters.

C. Organic Constituents

I. Lipids

Reports that lipids are present in snake venoms are rather limited in number. GANGULY and MALKANA (1936) reported that cobra venom contained cholesterol and lecithin. The presence of lipids in venoms was proposed, based on the presence of two components that gave positive staining reactions with Fettschwarz and rouge cérol after the venom had been subjected to electrophoresis (GRASSET et al., 1956). DEVI (1968) in the review cited earlier presented unpublished results that demonstrated the presence of lipids in venoms from *N. naja*, Russell's viper, and *C. terrificus terrificus*. The results were obtained by extracting the venoms with a mixture of chloroform and methanol, then showing that the extract contained organic material that contained phosphorous. Whether the 1.0–2.5% values reported as lipid phosphorus referred to percent of total organic matter or to percent of total phosphorus is not clear. The presence of glycerophosphate among the phosphorylated compounds tentatively identified after 7-minute hydrolysis supports the suggestion that phosphoglycerides may have been present in the venoms.

II. Carbohydrates

There is very little information in the literature on carbohydrate contents of snake venoms. Whether this reflects the paucity of carbohydrates or whether it is an indication of a neglected area of research is not clear. Considering the extensive analyses that have been done on venoms from many different species of snakes, the former seems to be the more likely possibility. Again referring to the review by DEVI (1968), reference is made to extensive studies in their laboratory on organic constituents of snake venoms. Tabular data showed that galactose was present in venoms from *N. naja*, Russell's viper, and *C. terrificus terrificus* when the venoms were subjected to paper chromatography and cysteine-sulfuric acid was used for detection of carbohydrates. Use of similar techniques established that glucose was present in Russell's viper venom and that venoms from Russell's viper and *N. naja* contained both mannose and fucose. Analysis of the trichloracetic acid soluble fractions from the same three venoms showed that 7-minute acid hydrolysis released little phosphate, indicating that labile sugar phosphates were not available. More stable acid soluble organic phosphate compounds were observed including hexose phosphates and possibly glycerolphosphate. A positive test with orcinol reagent for all three venoms indicated that they contained ribose, but the possibility exists that the ribose may have been present as nucleosides (see C. IV). However, the usual orcinol procedure will not provide a positive ribose test with pyrimidine nucleosides and thus it remains to be established whether some of the ribose was present in a nonglycoside form.

Recent papers demonstrated the presence of complex polysaccharides in the poison apparatus of snakes but not in the venom itself. RHOADES et al. (1967) found a strongly acidic mucopolysaccharide that contained sulfonated uronic acid in the accessory gland of the poison apparatus from *A. piscivorus piscivorus*. ZAKAROV (1971) demonstrated that the veneniferous glands from several adders contained complex carbohydrates. Histochemical investigations showed the anterior regions contained acidic sulfomucins as well as neutral and basic mucopolysaccharides while the posterior areas had only neutral mucosaccharides and some mucoproteins. In comparison, the gland from *N. naja oxiana* had acidic mucopolysaccharides in the anterior regions, but such materials were not present in detectable quantities in the posterior portions of the gland. Whether the insoluble residue that is present when dried snake venom is dissolved in saline or buffer solutions is made up in part by complex carbohydrates has not been investigated. Considering the existence of these compounds in the glands from those species that have been examined, it seems this might be a reasonable suggestion.

III. Riboflavin

The general yellow color exhibited by most snake venoms is due to the presence of riboflavin. An extensive literature exists concerning the riboflavin content of snake venoms, particularily with respect to its role as a coenzyme for snake venom L-amino acid oxidase. This enzyme has been found in snake venoms from many different genera of snakes. A brief review of amino acid oxidases in snake venoms has appeared (SARKAR and DEVI, 1968).

ZELLER (1948) observed that there was a fairly close correspondance between the flavin content and the L-amino acid oxidase activity of snake venom. In general, the venoms that show little yellow color have relatively low riboflavin concentrations and the so-called "white venoms" do not contain riboflavin or amino acid oxidase activity. SINGER and KEARNEY (1950) found flavin adenine dinucleotide (FAD) to be the prosthetic group of L-amino acid oxidase from water moccasin venom and that all of the flavin in the crude venom (4×10^{-1} μmol/g) was in the form of FAD and was bound to amino acid oxidase. Recently, INAMASU et al. (1974) established that the prosthetic group of the L-amino acid oxidase from habu venom did not activate the L-amino acid oxidase apoenzyme derived from hog kidney, whereas FAD did activate the enzyme. Measurements of the ratio of flavin to phosphate for the habu-derived prosthetic group showed a 1:1 correspondance indicating that flavin mononucleotide (FMN) served as the prosthetic group for the enzyme. These results corroborated the earlier findings of INAMASU et al. (1973) that indicated FMN was the cofactor based on thin layer chromatography, absorption spectra, and fluorescence spectra.

A well-defined role for L-amino acid oxidase in the toxic action of snake venoms has not been established, and there is little, if any, evidence in the literature that correlates levels of L-amino acid oxidase activity with venom toxicity. It has been suggested but not conclusively demonstrated that L-amino acid oxidase might activate protease activities in snake venoms (ZELLER, 1951). It might be of some interest to examine the effects of L-amino acid oxidase on some of the small pyroglutamyl peptides that are present in snake venoms (Sect. C.V) and the effects that these compounds have on snake venom L-amino acid oxidase activity.

IV. Nucleosides and Nucleotides

The older literature on this subject has been reviewed by DEVI (1968). The presence of substances that absorb strongly in the ultraviolet region of the spectrum is indicated. The venoms of *N. naja* and *C. terrificus terrificus* had absorption peaks near 240 nm while Russell's viper venom had a substantial absorption near 260 nm. Traces of guanosine triphosphate were reported for the first two venoms while uridine triphosphate was reported to be present at relatively high levels in the latter. The results were obtained by paper chromatographic separation of the venom components, but the details of the treatment of the venoms and the composition of the solvent system used for separation were not described. A positive test for ribose is consistent with the presence of nucleotides in these venoms. LO and CH'EN (1966) reported that guanosine, adenosine, and inosine were detected in venom samples obtained from the Formosan cobra. By chromatographic separation and spectral studies, these compounds were shown to be present in the ratio of 7:2.5:1, respectively. LIN and LEE (1971) suggested that nucleoside contamination of purified toxins may be the reason for the detection of carbohydrate in these purified proteins. ETEROVIC et al. (1975) showed that the venom of *B. multicinctus* contained substantial quantities of guanosine. The guanosine accounted for 10% of the total absorbancy of the venom at 280 nm and was eluted from a CM-Sephadex column with the initial buffer. It was conclusively identified as guanosine by ultraviolet absorbance spectrophotometry. The results presented agree with the results of separations achieved by LEE et al. (1972). Guanosine was found in venoms from *B. multicinctus* and *A. acutus* and the venom of *Naja naja atra* also contains nucleosides (LO, 1972). These results substantiate the earlier work of WEI and LEE (1965) who showed that *B. multicinctus* venom contained $1.1 \pm 0.15\%$ guanosine. Earlier work by FISCHER and DORFEL (1954) demonstrated the presence of adenosine in the venoms from *Bitis arietans* and *Dendroaspis viridis* and qualitative results showed that *Bothrops* venom and several viperid venoms contained sugars. Whether the sugars were present in nucleoside form was not established. Purine compounds were present in five of eight venoms examined (DOERY, 1954). Hypoxanthine, a purine base that had not been reported previously, was observed in venom from the tiger snake (DOERY, 1957).

V. Amino Acids and Peptides

This classification of substances includes the most biologically active of the nonprotein constituents found in snake venom, namely a group of small peptides that have potent vasoactive effects on biologic systems. These substances will be discussed after reviewing the occurrence of free amino acids in snake venoms.

1. Amino Acids

SHIPOLINI et al. (1965) demonstrated that *V. ammodytes* venom contained a number of amino acids. Glycine, alanine, serine, aspartic acid, glutamic acid, and histidine were detected in this venom. In the review by DEVI (1968), results presented showed that ninhydrin-positive materials were present in the acid-soluble extracts of venoms from *N. naja*, *V. russellii*, and *C. terrificus terrificus*. Paper chromatography and paper electrophoresis were used as tools for separation and identification of glycine, leucine, glutamic acid, histidine, lysine, and tyrosine. Not all of these amino acids were found in each of the venom extracts. The largest number in one extract was five, that being from *V. russellii*. NIGAMATOV (1969) detected a number of amino acids after fractionation of venom extracts by chromatography. Included among the

14 amino acids were glycine, alanine, cysteine, cystine, serine, threonine, proline, valine, leucine, isoleucine, methionine, glutamic acid, lysine, and histidine. Venoms from *V. lebetina*, *N. n. oxiana*, *V. urisini*, *E. carinatus*, and *A. halys* were used in the studies. Recent studies of venoms from *C. cerastes* and *C. vipera* led to the conclusion that traces of four amino acids were present (EL-HAWARY and HASSAN, 1974b).

The results obtained from the studies cited suggest that most, if not all, of the amino acids that occur in proteins are present in free form in snake venoms. Whether the occurrence of free amino acids in venoms resulted from their release from proteins by venom protease action or by some other physiologic process could not be ascertained by the experiments that have been done. This would be an interesting problem to pursue by suitable methods although it seems rather unlikely that the free amino acids contribute to the toxic action of the venoms. It is possible, however, that the release of amino acids from venom proteins by venom proteases could play a role in activation of certain proteins.

2. Peptides

The most prominent physiologically active nonprotein components in snake venoms are a group of closely related low molecular weight peptides. These peptides are quite widely distributed in venoms from many species. In the literature, they are classified into two general types, namely, bradykinin-potentiating peptides and those which inhibit the conversion of angiotensin I to angiotensin II. The relationship between these two types of peptides will be discussed after the recent literature in this area of research has been briefly reviewed.

Bradykinin, a nonapeptide, is a plasma kinin that induces smooth muscle contraction and causes increased capillary permeability and vasodilation. Bradykinin is released from a precursor protein, a kininogen, by specific releasing enzymes and is inactivated by a kinin-specific protease. There is substantial evidence to suggest that the kinin system and the angiotensin system are important physiologic regulators of the vascular and circulatory system (MCGIFF and NASJLETTI, 1976). The relationship of these compounds to other important physiologic mediators is not well-understood and is an area of research that is being actively pursued. The vasoactive peptides from snake venoms may be of considerable use in such studies.

FERREIRA (1965) was the first to show that the venom from *B. jararaca* had an alcohol-soluble fraction that enhanced bradykinin activity both in vivo and in vitro. SHIPOLINI et al. (1965) isolated two peptides from the dialyzable fraction of venom from *V. ammodytes*. Both were shown to contain glutamic acid after hydrolysis but were not examined to determine whether they had any physiologic activity. KATO et al. (1966) isolated two tripeptides, A and B, from the venoms of *A. halys blomhoffi*, *C. adamanteus*, *B. jararaca*, and *T. flavoviridis*. Venom from *V. russellii* had only the B peptide while *N. naja* venom did not contain either peptide. Both peptides, A and B, were devoid of a free amino group at the amino terminal end of the peptide chain.

a) Structural Studies

The studies of KATO et al. (1966) showed that the amino terminal position of peptides A and B they had isolated was a cyclized glutamic acid residue. The presence of pyroglutamic acid at the amino terminus is characteristic of the bradykinin-poten-

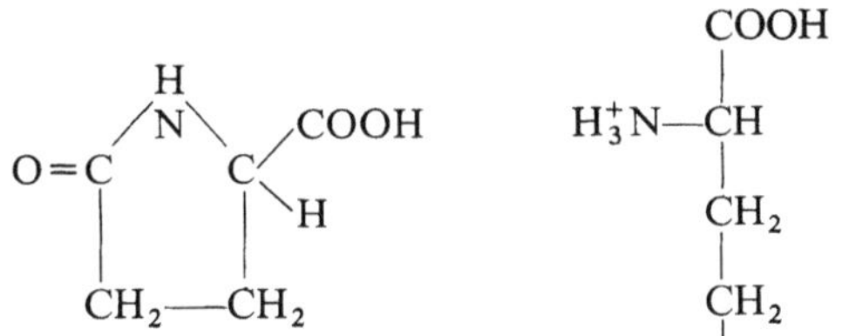

pyroglutamic acid or 2-pyrrollidone-5-carboxylic acid

glutamic acid

Fig. 1

tiating peptides and the peptides which inhibit the conversion of angiotensin I to angiotensin II. The structure of pyroglutamic acid is shown in Figure 1.

This amino terminal residue is formed by amide formation between the γ-carboxyl group of the glutamic acid side chain and the α-amino group of glutamic acid. The presence of this cyclic structure at the amino terminus accounts for the fact that amino terminal amino acids were not detectable by the usual techniques used in protein sequence studies. Another unusual feature of these peptides is the unusually high proline content found in the large ones.

KATO and SUZUKI (1969) isolated five distinct peptides from the venom of *A. halys blomhoffii*. The peptides had between eight and ten amino acid residues. Each was shown to contain one glutamic acid residue and four proline residues. The amino acid sequence of one of these peptides, B, was established and was shown to have pyroglutamic acid at the amino terminus (KATO and SUZUKI, 1970a). The sequence of peptide E was reported by KATO and SUZUKI (1970b), and its structure was confirmed by chemical synthesis (KATO and SUZUKI, 1971a). FERREIRA et al. (1970) isolated and purified nine peptides from the venom of *B. jararaca*. The number of amino acids in these peptides ranged from five in the smallest to 13 in the largest. The sequence of one of the nine was established and shown to contain pyroglutamic acid. Nine peptides were also isolated from *B. jararaca* venom by chromatographic techniques (GREENE et al., 1970). All contained glutamic acid, proline, and tryptophan but none gave positive tests with ninhydrin reagent or with Edman reagent, consistent with the presence of pyroglutamate as the N terminal amino acid. The sequences of peptides B and C were established by the work of KATO and SUZUKI (1971b). The penta-, nona-, and decapeptides from the venom of *B. jararaca* were synthesized by chemical means (BAKHLE, 1971), thus confirming the structures of these peptides. Solid state synthesis of peptides that are identic to those isolated from *B. jararaca* venom has been achieved (ONDETTI et al., 1971). The products were identic in all respects to those isolated from the venom. Peptides that contain a pyroglutamyl residue have also been isolated from *T. mucrosquamatus* and *T. gramineus* and the sequences have been established (LO, 1972). Peptides were also obtained from venoms of *B. multicinctus* and *A. acutus*, but the structures of these compounds were not determined.

The tool of mass spectrometry has been applied to the sequence determination of peptides from snake venoms. KATO et al. (1973) used mass spectral analyses to study the sequence of peptide A from *A. halys blomhoffii* and the structure was identic to that determined by dansyl Edman degradation procedures. Sequences of peptides B,

C, and E isolated from the venom of *A. halys blomhoffii* were confirmed by enzyme cleavage combined with mass spectrometry (OKADA et al., 1973). Recently, the sequence of a new pyroglutamyl peptide isolated from *A. halys blomhoffii* was elucidated (OKADA et al., 1974). Mass spectral data clearly showed the N terminal position to be pyroglutamic acid by the intense M/e 98 peak for N-methylpyrrolidone ion and the M/e 126 peak from N-methylpyrrolidone carbonyl ion. The application of instrumental methods such as mass spectrometry to the study of small peptides from snake venoms should lead to rapid progress in the area of structural studies of these compounds. Table 1 summarizes the sequences of known potentiating peptides isolated from snake venoms. Examination of the data in the table shows the consistent occurrence of pyroglutamic acid at the amino terminus and the high content of proline in the peptides that have more than five amino acids. Another interesting structural aspect is the fact that glutamine and asparagine occur quite frequently, but the acidic amino acids from which they are derived are not found to any extent except for the cyclic form of glutamic acid at the amino terminus. Some aspects of the structural activity relationships will be examined in the next section.

b) Physiologic Studies

The first demonstration of bradykinin potentiation by snake venom components both in vitro and in vivo was done with *B. jararaca* venom (FERREIRA, 1965). Peptides isolated from the venom of *A. halys blomhoffii* potentiated the action of bradykinin when tested on isolated guinea pig ileum (KATO and SUZUKI, 1969). FERREIRA et al. (1970) demonstrated that the nine purified peptides, isolated from the venom of *B. jararaca*, each enhanced the effects of bradykinin on isolated guinea pig ileum. It was reported that some of the peptides inhibited a partially purified enzyme from dog lung that converted angiotensin I to angiotensin II. With peptide IV-1-D, 50% inhibition was noted at a concentration of 2×10^{-8} M. Pulmonary conversion of angiotensin I to angiotensin II was also inhibited in vivo in the rat. The suggestion was made that these snake venom peptides function by inhibiting certain proteolytic enzymes at concentrations in the range of 10^{-6} M–10^{-8} M. Evidence has been obtained that indicates that the potentiation of bradykinin activity may be due to inhibition of enzymes that normally inactivate bradykinin (FERREIRA and VANE, 1967). Six peptides isolated from the venom of *B. jararaca* inhibited conversion of angiotensin I to angiotensin II, in vitro (ONDETTI et al., 1971). Some of the peptides examined were identic to those used by FERREIRA et al. (1970). The pentapeptide, V-3-A, caused a transient block of the pressor response produced by angiotensin while the large peptides had a more marked, longer-lasting effect. The longer peptides appear to have a higher inherent resistance to enzymic degradation by proteases.

Penta-, nona-, and decapeptides of *B. jararaca* were synthesized chemically and their biologic activities studied (BAKHLE, 1971). These compounds inhibited conversion of angiotensin I to angiotensin II but with different absolute potencies in two different test systems, namely dog lung homogenates and isolated guinea pig lung. Studies with peptides B and C from *A. halys blomhoffii* showed that they both potentiated the effect of bradykinin but neither caused smooth muscle contraction in the absence of bradykinin (KATO and SUZUKI, 1971b). Two snake venom peptides were studied to determine their effects on the centrally induced pressor activities of angiotensin I and angiotensin II (SOLOMON et al., 1974). Both attenuated the effects produced by the angiotensins, and this seemed to be a central nervous system effect. The suggestion was made that the effects may be more complex than just inhibition

Table 1. Sequences of peptides isolated from snake venoms

Pyr · Lys · Ser	OKADA et al. (1974)
Pyr · Gln · Trp	KATO et al. (1966)
Pyr · Asn · Trp	
Pyr · Trp · Lys	LO (1972)
Pyr · Glu · Trp	
Pyr · Asp · Trp	
Pyr · Lys · Trp · Ala · Pro	FERREIRA et al. (1970)
Pyr · Gly · Leu_2 · Arg · Pro · Lys · Ile · Pro_2	KATO and SUZUKI (1970a)
Pyr · Lys · Trp · Asp · Pro_3 · Val · Ser · Pro_2	KATO and SUZUKI (1970b)
Pyr · Leu · Pro_2 · Arg · Pro · Lys · Ile · Pro_2	KATO and SUZUKI (1971b)
Pyr · Gly · Leu · Pro_2 · Gly · Pro_2 · Ile · Pro_2	
Pyr · Gly · Arg · Pro_2 · Gly · Pro_2 · Ile · Pro	KATO et al. (1973)
Pyr · Trp · Pro · Arg · Pro · Gln · Ile · Pro_2	ONDETTI et al. (1971)
Pyr · Asn · Trp · Pro · Arg · Pro · Gln · Ile · Pro_2	
Pyr · Asn · Trp · Pro · His · Pro · Gln · Ile · Pro_2	
Pyr · Ser · Trp · Pro · Gly · Pro · Asn · Ile · Pro_2	
Pyr · Trp · Pro · Arg · Pro · Thr · Pro · Gln · Ile · Pro_2	
Pyr · Gly_2 · Trp · Pro · Arg · Pro · Gly · Pro · Glu · Ile · Pro_2	

of conversion of angiotensins. The possibility of blocked angiotensin receptors was suggested. Recent work with synthetic penta- and undecapeptides, identic with those isolated from snake venoms, have been studied with respect to biologic activities (PASHKINA et al., 1975). They did not inhibit the hydrolysis of artificial substrates of carboxypeptidase N, nor did they inhibit the kininase of diluted human blood. They did not inhibit the release of the C terminus of bradykinin even at a concentration of 2 mM. The C terminal peptide fragment of bradykinin did cause inhibition of the peptidase action. The snake venom peptides caused constriction of the rat uterus at very high concentrations.

A limited amount of work has been done on the structure-activity relationships with some of the venom-derived peptides. The longer peptides appear to produce a longer and more marked physiologic effect (ONDETTI et al., 1971). The longer peptides, in addition to having a common amino terminus also have a common carboxyl terminus, namely X · Pro_2 and with one exception, X is isoleucine (see Table 1). The presence of a basic amino acid residue somewhere in the middle of the peptide greatly enhances the inhibitory effect on conversion of angiotensin I to angiotensin II. These results seem to parallel the work with peptides from *A. halys blomhoffi* that showed that the presence of a basic amino acid residue was critical for inhibition of angiotensin-converting activity (BAKHLE, 1972). The relationship between chain length, amino acid composition, and activity will not be understood until much more research has been done. The validity of the latter statement is supported by the data that show the absolute potencies of a given peptide are different when tested in two distinct test systems (BAKHLE, 1971).

VI. Amines

Several biologically significant amines other than those normally found as constituents of nucleic acids and proteins occur in venoms. Serotonin, bufotenine, and N-methyltryptophan were present in some venoms examined by WELSH (1966). Twenty species were used as venom sources including *Elapidae*, *Viperidae*, and *Crotalidae*. Examination of tissues and venoms from two vipers showed that the tissues contained norepinepherine and serotonin at the expected levels but that the venoms contained little, if any, of these two compounds (ANTON and GENNARO, 1965). Acetylcholine was found in substantial quantities in venoms from three species, *D. polylepsis*, *D. jamesoni*, and *D. angusticeps*. Smaller quantities of acetylcholine-like substances were detected in venoms from *Naja*, *Crotalus*, *Sistrurus*, and *Agkistrodon* species (WELSH, 1967).

D. Summary

A variety of nonprotein consituents are found in the venoms from snakes. These compounds include some inorganic salts, including a variety of metal ions. Some of the metal ions are firmly bound to some venom proteins and may well serve as mandatory cofactors for the function of those proteins. This appears to be the case for certain proteolytic enzymes and possibly for some hemorrhagic protein fractions. No clear-cut demonstrable function for the inorganic anions has been established.

The nonprotein organic compounds include carbohydrates, lipids, nucleic acid components, amino acids, peptides, and some biologically important amines. It is difficult to assess whether these arise simply from degradation of tissue components and as such contaminate the venom solution or whether they are synthesized specifically for inclusion in the venom. Of the nonprotein constituents isolated from venoms, only the peptide fraction appears to have a major function in venom action. This group of unusual peptides all have pyroglutamic acid as the amino terminal amino acid and the larger ones all contain unusually high concentrations of proline. They appear to function by potentiating the physiologic effects caused by bradykinin. The potentiation is achieved by inhibiting specific proteases that degrade bradykinin or those that function in the conversion of angiotensin I to angiotensin II. The presence of other amines has not been considered to be very significant although if high concentrations of acetylcholine were present, a significant physiologic response might be expected.

In general, the protein components of snake venoms are the most important functional components from the physiologic standpoint. This is not too surprising when one considers that the major dry weight portion of the venom is made up of proteins, some of which are extremely toxic. The nonprotein constituents, on the other hand, make up only a minor fraction of the dry weight and only a limited number of these have potent physiologic activity.

References

Anton, A. H., Gennaro, J. F.: Norepinepherine and serotonin in the tissues and venoms of two pit vipers. Nature (Lond.) **208**, 1174—1175 (1965)

Bakhle, Y. S.: Inhibition of angiotensin I converting enzyme by venom peptides. Brit. J. Pharmacol. **43**, 252—254 (1971)

Bakhle, Y. S.: Inhibition of converting enzyme by venom peptides. In: Genest, J. (Ed.): Hypertension (Proc. Symp.), pp. 541—547. Berlin-Heidelberg-New York: Springer 1972

Devi, A.: The protein and nonprotein constituents of snake venoms. In: Bücherl, W., Buckley, E. E., Deulofeu, V. (Eds.): Venomous Animals and Their Venoms, Vol. I, pp. 119—165. New York: Academic Press 1968
Doery, H. M.: Purine compounds in snake venoms. Nature (Lond.) **177**, 381—382 (1954)
Doery, H. M.: Additional purine compounds in the venom of the tiger snake *(Notechis scutatus)*. Nature (Lond.) **180**, 799—800 (1957)
El-Hawary, M. F. S., Hassan, F.: Physiochemical properties of venoms of *Cerastes cerastes* and *Cerastes vipera*. Egypt. J. Phys. Sci. **1**, 9—18 (1974a)
El-Hawary, M. F. S., Hassan, F.: Proteins and amino acids of *Cerastes cerastes* and *Cerastes vipera* venoms. Egypt. J. Phys. Sci. **1**, 19—37 (1974b)
Eterovic, V. A., Hebert, M. S., Hanley, M. R., Bennett, E. L.: The lethality and spectroscopic properties of toxins from *Bungarus multicinctus* (Blyth) venom. Toxicon **13**, 37—48 (1975)
Ferreira, S. H.: A bradykinin-potentiating factor present in the venom of *Bothrops jararaca*. Brit. J. Pharmacol. **24**, 163—169 (1965)
Ferreira, S. H., Bartlet, D. C., Greene, L. J.: Isolation of bradykinin-potentiating peptides from *Bothrops jararaca* venom. Biochemistry **9**, 2583—2593 (1970)
Ferreira, S. H., Vane, J. R.: The detection and estimation of bradykinin in the circulating blood. Brit. J. Pharmacol. **29**, 267—377 (1967)
Fischer, F. G., Dorfel, H.: Adenosine in *Bitis arietans* and *Dendroaspis viridis*. Hoppe Seylers Z. physiol. Chem. **297**, 278—282 (1954)
Friedrich, C., Tu, A. T.: Role of metals in snake venoms for hemorrhagic, esterase, and proteolytic activities. Biochem. Pharmacol. **20**, 1549—1556 (1971)
Ganguly, S. N., Malkana, M. T.: Indian snake venoms. II. Cobra venom: its chemical composition, protein fractions and their physiological actions. Ind. J. med. Res. **24**, 281—286 (1936)
Gitter, S., Amiel, S., Gilat, G., Sonnino, T., Welwart, Y.: Neutron activation of snake venoms: copper. Nature (Lond.) **197**, 383—384 (1963)
Grasset, E., Brechbuhler, T., Schwarz, D. E., Pongranz, E.: Comparative analysis and electrophoretic fractionations of snake venoms with special reference to *Vipera russelli* and *Vipera aspis* venoms: In: Buckely, E. E., Porges, N. (Eds.): Venoms, pp. 153—169. American Association for the Advancement of Science Publication 44, Washington D.C. 1956
Greene, L. J., Stewart, J. M., Ferreira, S. H.: Bradykinin-potentiating peptides from the venom of *Bothrops jararaca*. Advanc. exp. Med. Biol. **8**, 81—87 (1970)
Hirakawa, Y.: Venom of *Trimeresurus elegans* and *Trimeresurus flavoviridis*. Kagoshima Daigaku Igaku Zasshi **26**, 611—623 (1974)
Inamasu, Y., Nakano, K., Kobayashi, M., Sameshima, Y., Obo, F.: Nature of the prosthetic group of the L-amino acid oxidase from habu snake *(Trimeresurus flavoviridis)* venom. I. Acta Med. Univ. Kagoshima **16**, 23—26 (1973)
Inamasu, Y., Nakano, K., Kobayashi, M., Sameshima, Y., Obo, F.: Nature of the prosthetic group of the L-amino acid oxidase from habu snake *(Trimeresurus flavoviridis)* venom. II. Acta Med. Univ. Kagoshima **16**, 145—154 (1974)
Kato, H., Iwanaga, S., Suzuki, T.: The isolation and amino acid sequences of new pyroglutamyl peptides from snake venoms. Experientia (Basel) **22**, 49—50 (1966)
Kato, H., Suzuki, T.: Bradykinin-potentiating peptides from the venom of *Agkistrodon halys blomhoffii* Experientia (Basel) **25**, 694—695 (1969)
Kato, H., Suzuki, T.: Amino acid sequence of a bradykinin-potentiating peptide isolated from the venom of *Agkistrodon halys blomhoffii* Proc. Jap. Acad. **46**, 176—181 (1970a)
Kato, H., Suzuki, T.: Structure of a bradykinin-potentiating peptide containing tryptophan from the venom of *Agkistrodon halys blomhoffi*. Experientia (Basel) **26**, 1205—1206 (1970b)
Kato, H., Suzuki, T.: Structure of bradykinin-potentiating peptides from the venom of *Agkistrodon halys blomhoffii*. Advanc. exp. Med. Biol. **8**, 101—105 (1970c)
Kato, H., Suzuki, T.: Bradykinin-potentiating peptides from the venom of *Agkistrodon halys blomhoffii*. Cienc. Cult. (Sao Paulo) **23**, 527—533 (1971a)
Kato, H., Suzuki, T.: Bradykinin-potentiating peptides from the venom of *Agkistrodon halys blomhoffii*. Biochemistry **10**, 972—980 (1971b)
Kato, H., Suzuki, T., Okada, K., Kimura, T., Sakakibara, S.: Structure of potentiator A, one of the five bradykinin potentiating peptides from the venom of *Agkistrodon halys blomhoffii*. Experientia (Basel) **29**, 574—575 (1973)

Lee, C. Y., Chang, S. L., Kau, S. T., Luh, S. H.: Chromatographic separation of the venom of *Bungarus multicinctus* and characterization of its components. J. Chromatog. **72**, 71—82 (1972)
Lin, S. Y., Lee, C. Y.: Are neurotoxins from elapid venoms glycoproteins? Toxicon **9**, 295—296 (1971)
Lo, T. P., Ch'en, I. H.: Chemical studies of Formosan cobra *(Naja naja atra)* venom. II. J. Chin. Chem. Soc. (Taipei) **13**, 195—202 (1966)
Lo, T. P.: Chemical studies of Formosan snake venoms. J. Chin. biochem. Soc. **1**, 39—46 (1972)
McGiff, J. C., Nasjletti, A.: Kinins, renal function and blood pressure regulation. Fed. Proc. **35**, 71—82 (1976)
Moav, B., Gilter, S., Wellwart, Y., Amiel, S.: Tracing and trace element composition of snake venom by activation analysis. Radiochem. Meth. Anal. Proc. Symp. (Salzburg) **1**, 205—215 (1964)
Nigmatov, Z.: Qualitative determination of amino acid composition of central Asian snake venoms. Ekol. Biol. Zhivotn. Uzb. 8—11 (1969)
Okada, K., Nagai, S., Kato, H.: New pyroglutamyl peptide (pyr·lys·ser) isolated from the venom of *Agkistrodon halys blomhoffi*. Experientia (Basel) **30**, 459—460 (1974)
Okada, K., Uyehara, T., Hiramoto, M., Kato, H., Suzuki, T.: Application of mass spectrometry to sequence analysis of pyroglutamyl peptides from snake venom. Chem. Pharm. Bull. (Tokyo) **21**, 2217—2223 (1973)
Ondetti, M. A., Williams, N. J., Sabo, E. F., Pluscec, J., Weaver, E. R., Kocy, O.: Angiotensin-converting enzyme inhibitors from the venom of *Bothrops jararaca*. Isolation, elucidation of structure and synthesis. Biochemistry **10**, 4033—4039 (1971)
Pashkina, T. S., Trapenznikova, S. S., Egapova, T. P., Morozova, N. A.: Effect of bradykinin-potentiating snake venom peptides and C-terminal pentapeptide fragment of bradykinin on carboxypeptidase N and kinanase activities of human blood serum. Biokhimiya **40**, 844—853 (1975)
Rhoades, R., Lorincz, A. E., Gennaro, J. F.: Polysaccharide content of the poison apparatus of the cottonmouth moccasin *Agkistrodon piscivorus piscivorus*. Toxicon **5**, 125—131 (1967)
Sarkar, N. K., Devi, A.: Enzymes in snake venoms. In: Bucherl, W., Buckley, E. E., Deulofeu, V. (Eds.): Venomous animals and their venoms, pp. 167—216. New York-London: Academic Press 1968
Shipolini, R., Ivanov, Ch. P., Dimitrov, G., Aleksiev, B. V.: Composition of the low molecular weight fraction of Bulgarian viper venom. Biochim. biophys. Acta (Amst.) **104**, 292—295 (1965)
Singer, T. P., Kearney, E. B.: L-amino acid oxidases of snake venom. I. Prosthetic group of L-amino acid oxidase of moccasin venom. Arch. Biochem. **27**, 348—363 (1950)
Solomon, T. A., Cavero, I., Buckley, J. P.: Inhibition of central pressor effects of angiotensin I and II. J. Pharm. Sci. **63**, 511—515 (1974)
Wei, A. L., Lee, C. Y.: A nucleoside isolated from the venom of *Bungarus multicinctus*. Toxicon **3**, 1—4 (1965)
Welsh, J. H.: Serotonin and related tryptamine derivatives in snake venoms. Mem. Inst. Butantan (São Paulo) **33**, 509—518 (1966)
Welsh, J. H.: Acetylcholine in Snake Venoms. In: Russell, F. E., Saunders, P. R. (Eds.): Animal Toxins, pp. 363—368. New York: Pergamon Press 1967
Zakarov, A. M.: Hisochemical investigation of polysaccharides in veneniferous gland in the adder. Arkh. Anat. Gistol. Embriol. **60**, 85—88 (1971)
Zeller, E. A.: Enzymes of snake venoms and their biological significance. Advanc. Enzymol. **8**, 459—495. Interscience Publishers 1948
Zeller, E. A.: Enzymes as essential components of bacterial and animal toxins. In: The Enzymes, Vol. I, pp. 986—1013. New York: Academic Press 1951

Part III

Pharmacology of Snake Venoms

CHAPTER 10

The Action of Snake Venoms on Nerve and Muscle

C. C. CHANG

A. Introduction

Snake venoms, especially of *Elapidae* and *Hydrophiidae*, have been known for centuries to produce symptoms relevant to nervous systems in the envenomed subject. As described in detail in Chapter 24 and 25, the most characteristic symptom is the paralysis of voluntary muscle which results in respiratory failure. Neurotoxins are believed to be the causative factor of these snake venoms dismissing voluntary muscle from nervous control and, in general, are the major principle for their lethal toxicity. Although venoms of viperid and crotalid snakes cause death by their detrimental effects on the cardiovascular system, on blood coagulation, or by hemorrhage (see Chaps. 14, 15, 18), a few of these also contain neurotoxins and kill the victims in a way similar to venoms of elapid and hydrophid snakes, causing neuromuscular paralysis. Interestingly, there are some microbial toxins and venoms from other animals which also cause respiratory paralysis on intoxication. Apparently, nature has chosen this vital system as a target for the effective toxic action during evolution.

The pharmacologic actions of many of these venoms and their purified toxins have been elucidated in recent years, and the sites of action when injected peripherally are mostly localized within the neuromuscular junction, a site most vulnerable to the action of chemical agents. In this chapter, emphasis will be placed on the actions on the neuromuscular junction of skeletal muscle. The actions of various types of neurotoxins on this site are now known to be very specific, and indeed, some purified toxins have been currently used as a powerful tool for physiologic and chemical studies of acetylcholine receptors (see Chap. 11). The pharmacologic actions of whole venoms, however, are in general very complicated since other constituents of the venoms, such as cardiotoxins, other related membrane toxins, and phospholipase A, may affect the nerve and muscular structure specifically or nonspecifically if sufficient concentrations and action time are allowed. In order to avoid confusion due to the multiplex actions of the whole venoms, the actions of purified components, if available, will be dealt with in more detail and the effects of whole venom compared with the contained toxins. Pharmacologic actions of snake venoms and the constituents on other nervous systems will be briefly described. Some constituents of snake venoms may not contribute significantly to the lethal toxicity when administered systemically but show very pronounced effects when applied directly on the brain. These constituents may in the future become a useful pharmacologic tool when the mode of action is established.

The term "neurotoxin" is frequently used in the literature on snake venoms to describe a venom or a venom fraction which produces paralysis or convulsion before death or any change of the animal behavior. However, these "neurotoxic" symptoms could be secondary effects resulting from actions on other organs rather than on the nervous structure per se. Indeed, the major group of neurotoxins isolated from elapid and hydrophid venoms acts on the acetylcholine receptor of motor endplate on the muscle membrane rather than on any structure of motor neurons. "Postsynaptic toxin" is, therefore, used for this type of neurotoxins because it is more indicative and definitive than neurotoxin.

There have been several reviews in recent years describing the effects of snake venoms and their isolated toxins on the nerve and muscle (BOQUET, 1964; MELDRUM, 1965a; JIMÉNEZ-PORRAS, 1968; HENRIQUES and HENRIQUES, 1971; VITAL BRAZIL, 1972; LEE, 1971, 1972, 1973; CHEYMOL et al., 1972b; CAMPBELL, 1975).

B. Pharmacokinetics of Snake Venoms

The difficulties for a study of absorption, distribution, fate, and excretion of whole snake venoms are obvious since snake venoms are complex mixtures of polypeptides. The results obtained from studies by using isotopically labeled whole venom are usually not definitive since the components of the venom are not equally labeled and their pharmacokinetic properties could be different from one component to another.

I. Absorption

Being the polypeptide nature of their toxic principle, snake venoms introduced by the oral route are usually nontoxic (EPSTEIN, 1930; CHOPRA and ISWARIAH, 1931), while lethal effect may result if a sufficiently large dose of cobra venom is introduced (BRUNTON and FAYRER, 1874; CHRISTENSEN, 1955). It is unknown, however, whether this effect is due to absorption from the gastrointestinal tract or to a local effect of the venom. BARNES and TRUETA (1941) studied the absorption of elapid venoms in rabbits after subcutaneous injection. By blocking the lymphatic circulation of the region into which the venom was injected, the absorption of black tiger snake (*Notechis scutatus niger*) venom was delayed as judged from the delay of death. The action of cobra venom, however, was not hindered. These authors speculated that the absorption of tiger snake venom is mainly from the lymphatic system presumably because of its high molecular weight whereas cobra venom can be absorbed through the capillaries due to the smaller molecular weight of its neurotoxin. TSENG et al. (1968) compared the absorption of I^{131}-labeled postsynaptic toxin and cardiotoxin of cobra venom in mice after subcutaneous injection. The absorption of postsynaptic toxin was about 60% within 2 h whereas that of highly basic cardiotoxin was only 30% in 4 h. Since the molecular weights of both toxins are about the same (7000), the delay of absorption of cardiotoxin is unlikely due to a difference in the route of absorption but rather to the strong affinity of cardiotoxin to tissues at the site of injection. Probably for this reason, the toxicity of cardiotoxin is much higher when injected intravenously than when injected subcutaneously. On the other hand, the toxicity of postsynaptic toxin is not so dependent on the route of injection.

For those venoms which cause local lesions, the spreading by diffusion from the site of envenomation may be more important than absorption into the blood.

McCollough and Gennaro (1963) found that, after injection of North American crotalid venoms into the lateral thigh of the dog, the underlying muscles from the knee to hip were all involved in its action within 1 h.

II. Distribution

1. Elapid Venoms and Postsynaptic Toxins

When radioiodine-labeled cobra venom, or its component cobrotoxin (a postsynaptic toxin) and cardiotoxin, was injected into mice or rabbits, the highest concentration of radioactivity was always found in the kidney (Sumyk et al., 1963; Tseng et al., 1968) with marked localization in the cortex. Cardiotoxin was more concentrated in the liver, spleen, lung, and intestine than cobrotoxin. The concentrations of cobrotoxin in the diaphragm and other skeletal muscles were even lower than in other tissues except the brain despite the fact that the pharmacologic effect of cobrotoxin originates principally from the action on the endplate of muscles. The pattern of distribution of α-bungarotoxin, labeled with either I^{131} (Lee and Tseng, 1966) or [^{3}H]-acetyl group (Huang and Chang, unpublished), is similar to that of cobrotoxin. The concentration of [^{3}H]-acetyl α-bungarotoxin in the kidney of rats was 20–30 times that in other organs 1 h after intravenous administration, but rapidly declined to one-third at 3 h and thereafter declined slowly. On the other hand, the decline of radioactivity in the spleen, liver, lung, intestine, and heart was very slow so that 30–50% of the amount found in 1 h remained even 3 days after injection. In skeletal muscles, α-bungarotoxin and cobra and sea snake postsynaptic toxins have been shown to bind specifically at the endplate where the acetylcholine receptor is localized (Lee and Tseng, 1966; Lee et al., 1967; Tseng et al., 1968; Sato et al., 1970; Miledi and Potter, 1971; Berg et al., 1972; Barnard et al., 1971; Fambrough and Hartzell, 1972; Chang et al., 1973a). The binding at the nonendplate area of sarcolemma is extremely low in the normally innervated muscle.

2. Viperid and Crotalid Venoms

Gennaro and Ramsey (1959) studied the distribution of I^{131}-labeled *Agkistrodon piscivorus* venom in mice after intravenous administration. In contrast to the distribution of elapid venoms, the greatest accumulation of venom was in the lung, followed closely by the kidney and then the heart, thymus, lymphnode, liver, and thyroid gland. The whole venom of *Vipera ammodytes* labeled with Zn^{65} and a basic protein of the venom labeled with Se^{75}-methionine were found to be highly concentrated in the liver, kidney, and spleen (Lebez et al., 1968, 1972). The distribution in the heart was slightly lower than in the above-mentioned organs, whereas the radioactivity in skeletal muscles was always much lower.

The distribution of I^{125}-labeled basic phospholipase A and acidic crotapotin, the two components of crotoxin, were compared in mice by Habermann et al. (1972). Both components left the circulation very quickly after intravenous administration. Phospholipase A was greatly concentrated in the liver (46% of the dose), but the enzyme was partially diverted to the kidney when crotapotin was simultaneously administered, and the amount of the enzyme in the liver decreased to 16%. Lung, spleen, and kidney were the next highest of tissues containing the enzyme component. Skeletal muscle and heart contained still lower amount of the enzyme. Crotapotin, when injected alone, was concentrated in the kidney and stomach. This experiment raises a possibility that the distribution of an active principle of a venom could be influenced by other constituents in the same venom.

3. Distribution in the Central Nervous System

The distribution of cobrotoxin, cardiotoxin, and α-bungarotoxin in the brain of rabbits and mice 1–2 h after administration were quite low and the ratios of concentration, as judged by the radioactivity, in the cerebrospinal fluid to that in plasma were 0.015, 0.033, and 0.029, respectively (LEE and TSENG, 1966; TSENG et al., 1968). Since some of the radioactivity might be due to the detached isotopic iodine, the value could be still lower. In contrast to other peripheral organs, the concentration of $[^3H]$α-bungarotoxin in the brain of rats increased gradually during the first 3 h after intravenous injection (HUANG and CHANG, unpublished). The phospholipase A of crotoxin distributed to the whole brain of mice was 0.1% of the amount administered (HABERMANN et al., 1972). Again this value included the detached ^{125}I. LEBEZ et al. (1968, 1972) reported that no labeled venom of *V. ammodytes* or only a trace of the basic fraction was found in the brain. It is apparent that the venom polypeptides pass the blood-brain barrier with difficulties, but it is not true to say that none of them can penetrate the blood-brain barrier. The interaction of hyaluronidase, proteolytic enzymes, and phospholipase A of the venom constituents must be considered for the distribution of venom since these enzymes have been shown to increase the permeability of the blood-brain barrier (BEILER et al., 1956). Indeed, cobra venom given into carotid artery of guinea-pigs or rabbits increased the permeability of the cerebral vessels, enabling trypan blue to enter the brain tissue (BROMAN and LINDBERG-BROMAN, 1945). Therefore, the distribution of particular toxins of snake venoms to the brain could be different whether they are in purified form or in the whole venom. The striking effect of crotalid venoms in increasing capillary permeability (Chap. 14) is in support of this view.

III. Fate and Excretion

SHÜ et al. (1968) showed that most of the radioactivity excreted in the urine within 20 min after injection of ^{131}I cobrotoxin was the intact toxin, whereas half of the radioactivity was in the detached iodine fraction if the urine was collected 4 h after injection. Whether this is due to a simple deiodination from the polypeptide molecule or to a metabolic breakdown of the peptide chain is not known. An experiment with $[^3H]$α-bungarotoxin also shows that the radioactivity excreted in the urine during 24 h is mostly in the degraded fraction (HUANG and CHANG, unpublished). Monoiodotyrosine was found as a metabolite of ^{125}I-α-bungarotoxin bound to acetylcholine receptors of skeletal muscle (BERG and HALL, 1975). The excretion of cobrotoxin, either unchanged or metabolized appears to be quite fast, about 30% being excreted within 2 h (TSENG et al., 1968) and 70% within 5 h (SHÜ et al., 1968).

These results, however, should not be taken to mean that the toxin bound to the target site is rapidly removed. The labeled α-bungarotoxin bound at the junctional acetylcholine receptors of endplate area of rat diaphragm declined very slowly. The half-time was about a week, whereas toxin bound with extrajunctional acetylcholine receptors of nonendplate zone of denervated muscle declined more rapidly with a half-time of 19 h (CHANG and HUANG, 1975; BERG and HALL, 1975).

C. Toxicity and Cause of Death

I. Cobra Venoms

Among the venoms of cobra, those of *Naja naja*, *N.n.atra*, *N. haje*, *N. nigricollis*, and *Hemachatus haemachatus* have been most extensively studied. Although the toxicity, pharmacologic properties, and chemical constituents of cobra venoms may vary quantitatively from one species to another, there appears to be no marked qualitative difference. Postsynaptic toxins have been shown to be the main lethal principle in various animals. Other constituents, such as cardiotoxins and phospholipase A, may contribute to the overall toxicity of the venoms.

1. Toxicity

Lethal doses of cobra venoms for various laboratory animals are compared in Table 1. The lethal toxicities of various venoms are rather close although those of *N. naja*, *N.n.atra*, and *N. nivea* appear to be slightly more potent. It is apparent that the lethal doses do not differ greatly among most warm-blooded animals except the cat. The difference of toxicity between subcutaneous and intravenous injections is

Table 1. The toxicity and average yield of venoms from different cobras and related elapid snakes

Snake	Venom yield (dried, mg)	Toxicity (LD_{50-100}, mg/kg)						
		Mouse		Rat s.c.	Rabbit s.c.	Cat	Pigeon	Frog s.c.
		s.c.	i.v.					
Naja naja	220[a]	0.45[b]	0.25–0.45[b]	0.66[b]	0.3–0.5[b]	2.0 i.m.[c]	0.5 i.m.[c]	10[b]
Naja naja atra	184[d]	0.67[e]	0.40[f]	0.7[g]	0.35[g]	20 s.c.[g]	0.43 s.c.[f]	70[g]
Naja nivea		0.72[b]	0.57[b]	0.75[h]	0.33[b]	3.5 s.c.[h]	1.25 s.c.[b]	4[b]
Naja nigricollis		2.8[b]	0.72[i]	1.5[b]	1.6[b]		0.33 i.v.[b]	
Naja haje	19–48[a]	0.6–1.7[a]	0.42[i]	1.5[b]			2.5 s.c.[b]	
Naja hannah	421[a]	1.7[a]	1.3–1.6[a]					
Hemachatus haemachatus	100[a]	1.8–3.7[b]	1.7[b]	1.25[b]	1.3[b]	15 s.c.[b]	1.9–3.3 s.c.[b]	1.2[b]
Dendroaspis viridis		0.7[a]	0.8[a]		0.7 i.v.[a]			
Walterinnesia aegyptia		0.4[a]			0.4 i.v.[a]			

[a] Cited in BROWN (1973).
[b] Cited in LEE (1971).
[c] CHOPRA and ISWARIAH (1931).
[d] TU (1959).
[e] LEE et al. (1962).
[f] LEE and TSENG (1969).
[g] OH (1942).
[h] EPSTEIN (1930).
[i] CHEYMOL et al. (1967a).

not marked, in contrast to the venoms of *Viperidae* and *Crotalidae*. In most of these animals, the postsynaptic toxin appears to be the main constituent responsible for the respiratory paralysis and thereby the toxicity. These purified toxins have an LD_{50} in mice ranging 50–150 µg/kg (YANG, 1974) and are about three to ten times more toxic than the whole venom, depending on the content of the toxin.

The cat, on the other hand, is rather resistant to many cobra venoms, especially when the venom is injected subcutaneously. This is due to the fact that its skeletal muscle is resistant to the neuromuscular blocking action of short-chain postsynaptic toxins (LEE and CHEN, 1976; cf. Table 3), and the absorption of cardiotoxin is delayed by this route of administration (TSENG et al., 1968). Cobra venom causes circulatory failure rather than respiratory paralysis in the cat when given intravenously (EPSTEIN, 1930; LEE and PENG, 1961). Evidently, cardiotoxin and phospholipase A contribute a great deal to the toxicity in this species. The frog is also resistant to cobra venoms, as well as to other elapid venoms (KELLAWAY and HOLDEN, 1932), because its unique cutaneous respiratory mechanism may preclude skeletal muscle paralysis as a primary cause of death. In addition, skeletal muscles of some frog species are extremely resistant to postsynaptic toxins of short peptide chain (cf. Table 3; LEE and CHEN, 1976). The lethality of the purified toxin from *N.n.atra* in a species of frog *(Rana tigrina)* is thus not greater than that of the whole venom (PENG, 1951; SU et al., 1967).

2. Symptoms

The clinical symptoms of cobra bite in human are dealt with in detail in Chapter 24. In animals, except in cats, flaccid paralysis is the main symptom after subcutaneous injection of cobra venoms (BRUNTON and FAYRER, 1873; EPSTEIN, 1930; PENG, 1952). There is usually an initial period of restlessness and excitement, presumably due to a local irritation by cardiotoxin. The animals become dull with unsteady movements and dropping head. The respiration is markedly labored and the animals die of respiratory paralysis which is often heralded by asphyxial convulsions. The heart continues to beat for hours if an adequate artificial respiration is applied.

3. Cause of Respiratory Paralysis

As early as in 1870s, FAYRER (1872, 1873) and BRUNTON and FAYRER (1873, 1874) found that artificial respiration had beneficial effect on the convulsion and cyanosis occurring in animals paralyzed by Indian cobra venoms and noted the similarity between the action of cobra venom and that of curare. The survival rate of dogs envenomed with Indian cobra venom can indeed be increased by artificial ventilation (GODE et al., 1968). The importance of respiratory failure in causing death after cobra bite was soon emphasized (WALL, 1883). Because of the predominant involvement of bulbar muscles in the course of envenomation, these pioneer workers concluded that the venom had a particular affinity for the medullary centers including the respiratory center although the experimental animals showed paralysis in skeletal muscle by a peripheral action. RAGOTZI (1890) was the first to recognize the importance of this peripheral action of cobra venom. He observed respiratory movements of the alae nasi in animals under artificial respiration after the diaphragm and costal muscles had been paralyzed by the venom, and put this forward as evidence that the central respiratory mechanism was still active. The question whether the respiratory paralysis produced by the cobra and other elapid venoms is due, at least in part, to a central effect (ROGERS, 1903, 1904; ELLIOT, 1905; FRASER and GUNN, 1909; ACTON and KNOWLES, 1921; EPSTEIN, 1930; CHOPRA and ISWARIAH, 1931; VENKATACHALAM and RATNAGIRISWARAN, 1934; BICHER, 1966) or due entirely to peripheral action (ARTHUS, 1910; CUSHNY and YAGI, 1918; KELLAWAY et al., 1932; KELLAWAY and HOLDEN, 1932; GAUTRELET et al., 1934; LEE and PENG, 1961; VICK et al., 1965) has been debated. The arguments against the theory of peripheral action came from the observations that the respiratory rate was first increased after envenomation and the stimulation of the phrenic nerve in the animal dying from cobra venom still evoked a perceptible contraction of the diaphragm though weaker than untreated, and that direct application of small doses of the venom to the floor of the fourth ventricle produced a respiratory arrest. CUSHNY and YAGI (1918), on the other hand, noted reflex movements of the diaphragm in envenomed animals under artificial respiration and regarded these Hering-Breuer reflexes as an indication of the activity of the respiratory center. More crucial evidence established later by KELLAWAY et al. (1932) clearly indicates that the respiratory failure produced by the venom stems from a peripheral action. These authors elegantly recorded the action potentials from the phrenic nerve in rabbits by an audiosystem and found that the potentials coming from the center were undeclined at a time when electromyograms of the diaphragm and intercostal muscle completely disappeared. The intensity of the action potentials even increased during asphyxia produced by interrupting artificial respiration or during administration of 5% CO_2. These observations were later confirmed by LEE and PENG (1961) and VICK et al. (1965) in dogs, but not in cats. VENKATACHALAM and RATNAGIRISWARAN (1934) concluded that the cat died of respiratory paralysis of central origin when injected with large doses of *N. tripudians* venom but of peripheral paralysis when small doses were used. EPSTEIN (1930), while confirming the curare-like nature of the respiratory paralysis by Cape cobra venom in the frog and rabbit, was also unable to confirm this in the cat. The death of cats envenomed with cobra venom was attributed to its cardiovascular effect rather than respiratory paralysis (EPSTEIN, 1930; LEE and PENG, 1961). Even in the dog, all animals subsequently die of cardiovascular failure if envenomed with a sufficient dose of cobra venom though the survival time can be increased by artificial respiration (VICK et al., 1965).

II. Krait Venoms

The clinical picture of krait envenomation (see Chap. 24) is similar to that of cobra and Australian elapid venoms (CAMPBELL, 1975), except that pain and local effects are usually absent at the site of bite. In accordance with the clinical symptoms, no cardiotoxin-like substance has been found in the venoms of the Indian *(Bungarus caeruleus)* and Formosan krait *(B. multicinctus)* (CHANG and LEE, 1963; LEE et al., 1972b, 1976c). The venom of the banded krait *(B. fasciatus)*, however, contains cardiotoxin-like substances (LIN SHIAU et al., 1972, 1975; LU and LO, 1974). The effects on the cardiovascular system of cats and dogs by the venoms of Formosan (LEE and PENG, 1961) and Indian (VICK et al., 1967) kraits are not as marked nor as persistent as with cobra venoms. All symptoms appear to be related to the respiratory paralysis, which has been shown to be peripheral in origin (KELLAWAY et al., 1932; LEE and PENG, 1961). When complete paralysis ensued after systemic administration of the venom, the discharges on the phrenic nerve persisted for a few hours if artificial respiration was maintained. Both the postsynaptic toxin, α-bungarotoxin, and the presynaptic toxin, β-bungarotoxin, contained in the Formosan krait (CHANG and LEE, 1963) or in the common krait venom (LEE et al., 1976c) are responsible for the peripheral paralysis. When injected with a dose 8–20 times that of the certainly lethal dose of the common krait venom, however, KELLAWAY et al. (1932) recorded no phrenic nerve discharges when respiratory movements failed in 23–75 min. There was also no evidence of curarization of the diaphragm at this time. The dose of *B. multicinctus* venom to kill a rabbit by injection into the cerebellomedullary cistern was only 1/40th that by intravenous injection and no curare-like effect was noticed (OUYANG, 1950). These results together suggest that the krait venoms may contain a principle which is highly toxic when directly applied to the brain and that, if a large enough dose is given intravenously, it may penetrate the blood-brain barrier in sufficient amount to kill the animal.

The common and Formosan krait venoms are more toxic in mice and other mammals than are cobra venoms, especially when administered intravenously (Table 2), whereas the average yield of these two krait venoms is much less than that of the latter. The Formosan krait venom is extremely toxic in birds and guinea pigs (TO and TIN, 1943), and there is a long latent period before the onset of toxicity in mice, characteristic of action of presynaptic toxin, β-bungarotoxin (CHANG and LEE, 1963; LEE and TSENG, 1969). On the other hand, the banded krait *(B. fasciatus)* produces about ten times the yield of venom, but its toxicity is only one-tenth that of the other two krait venoms in mice and 1/1000th in birds (computed from data in LEE and TSENG, 1969; and LIN SHIAU et al., 1972). In accordance with this species difference of toxicity, no β-bungarotoxin-like principle has been found in *B. fasciatus* venom.

III. Australian Snake Venoms

The elapid snakes of Australia present a gradual transition in morphologic characters toward the viperine type (KELLAWAY, 1933). Most of the venoms studied by KELLAWAY et al. (1932) show a similar pattern of effects as krait venoms in the delayed onset of action and flaccid muscle paralysis except *Pseudechis australis* venom which has a powerful direct action upon the heart muscle. The cause of death in rabbits was shown clearly by KELLAWAY et al. (1932) to be the peripheral blockade of respiratory muscles after subcutaneous injections of the venoms of the tiger snake *(Notechis scutatus, N. s. var. nigher)*, copperhead *(Denisonia superba)*, death adder *(Acanthophis antarcticus)*, common black snake *(Pseudechis porphyriacus)*, common brown snake *(Demansia textilis)*, and the taipan *(Oxyuranus scutellatus)*. When injected intravenously into anesthetized animals, death occurred with heart failure in the case of *D. superba* venom or with intravascular clotting by a thrombin-like effect in the case with venoms of *D. textilis*, *N. scutatus*, and *P. porphyriacus* (MARTIN, 1893; KELLAWAY et al., 1932; EAGLE, 1937). In this respect, these venoms seem to be different from those of kraits and sea snakes but resemble viperid and crotalid venoms. At larger doses, peripheral action of the venom on the blood vessel, with profound fall of blood pressure, may also lead to a fatal issue. Based on the difference of effectiveness of antisera in antagonizing the paralysis produced after envenomation, CAMPBELL (1975) has proposed that the neurotoxins of Australian venoms can be divided into at least two groups. He found that those patients bitten by taipan or Papuan black snakes *(Pseudechis papuanus)* did not respond to antivenom and the paralysis either developed after the administration of the antivenom or continued to progress in spite of it. On the other hand, patients bitten by death adders showed a quite dramatic reversal of paralysis after injection of the antivenom. In relevance with this difference are the recent findings that while taipan and tiger snake venoms contain presynaptic toxins (KARLSSON, 1972b; EAKER, 1974; MEBS et al., 1976), the copperhead and death adder venoms contain only postsynaptic toxins (MEBS et al., 1976).

IV. Other Elapid Venoms

1. Desert Cobra (Walterinnesia aegyptia) Venoms

GITTER et al. (1962) reported that a small dose (6 µg/mouse) of the venom produced increasing muscle weakness, paralysis of the hind legs and death within about 90 min in mice. At higher doses (20–30 µg) perivascular hemorrhages were noted in the liver and brain (GITTER and DE VRIES, 1968). Postsynaptic toxins were found in this venom (LEE et al., 1976a), but neither presynaptic toxin nor cardiotoxin was found. The cause of death from envenomation of this venom is likely the peripheral paralysis of respiratory muscle as most of other elapid venoms.

2. Coral Snake (Micrurus) Venoms

Envenomation in cats with the venom of a coral snake *(M. fulvius)* caused respiratory paralysis prior to cardiac failure (WEIS and MCISAAC, 1971). The clinical pictures of envenomation also involve the paralysis of eye and bulbar muscles, proceeding to a complete peripheral muscular paralysis (SHAW, 1971). It was found that depression of the response of the skeletal muscle to nerve stimulation paralleled that of respiration, indicating that the respiratory failure is due to a peripheral action of the venom. A postsynaptic toxin has been isolated by SNYDER et al. (1973).

3. Mamba (Dendroaspis) Venoms

Like most of other elapid venoms, envenomation in human produces paralysis with slurring of speach, diplopia, dysphagia, and bulbar paralysis (EIGENBERGER, 1928). Both postsynaptic and membrane-depolarizing toxins have been isolated from the venoms of *D. jamesoni* (EXCELL and PATEL, 1972; PATEL and EXCELL, 1975) and *D. polylepis polylepis* (STRYDOM, 1972).

V. Sea Snake (Hydrophiid) Venoms

The sea snake venoms appear to be more toxic than the cobra venoms on the weight basis (Table 2; ROGERS, 1903; BARME, 1968). The yield of venom, however, is much

Table 2. The toxicity and average yield of venoms of *Bungarus*, *Micrurus*, Australian, and sea snakes

Snake	Venom yield (dired, mg)	Toxicity (LD_{50-100}, mg/kg)			
		Mouse		Rabbit	Guinea pig
		i.v.	s.c.		s.c.
Bungarus caeruleus (Common krait)	10[a]	0.09[a]–0.2[c]	0.4[a]	0.05[b]–0.4 i.v.[a]	
Bungarus multicinctus (Formosan krait)	11[d]	0.07[g]	0.16[f]	0.2 i.v.[g]	0.005[g]
Bungarus fasciatus (Banded krait)	114[a]	1.2[a]	3.6[a]	4.0 i.v.[b]	
Micrurus fulvius (Coral snake)	2[e]	0.2–0.4[a]	1.3[a]		
Notechis scutatus (Tiger snake)	28[i]	0.04[j]	0.25[j]	0.045 s.c.[j] 0.002 i.v.[j]	0.02[j] 0.007 i.v.[j]
Oxyuranus scutellatus (Taipan)	120[k]		0.12[a]	<0.5 s.c.[b]	
Denisonia superba (Copper head)	25[k]		1.0[a]	<0.3 s.c.[b]	
Pseudechis porphyriacus (Black snake)	30[i]		1.8[m]	0.04 s.c.[m]	0.11[m]
Acanthophis antarcticus (Death adder)	80[k]		0.5[a]		
Enhydrina schistosa (Common sea snake)	8[a]	0.01–0.09[a]	0.05–0.2[a]	0.03 i.v.[h]	
Laticauda semifasciata (Erabu snake)	14[a]	0.2[a]	0.2–0.5[a]	0.025 s.c.[d]	

[a] Cited in BROWN (1973).
[b] KELLAWAY et al. (1932).
[c] VICK et al. (1967).
[d] TU (1959).
[e] RUSSELL (1964).
[f] LEE et al. (1962).
[g] TO and TIN (1943).
[h] BOQUET (1964).
[i] FREEMAN and KELLAWAY (1934).
[j] KELLAWAY (1929).
[k] GARNET (1970).
[m] KELLAWAY (1930) (calculated from dose/animal to dose/kg).

lower (Table 2). The cause of death by *Enhydrina schistosa* venom in rabbits was shown to be a peripheral paralysis of respiratory muscles (KELLAWAY et al., 1932), although in addition a central site of action was also postulated in the earlier literature (FRASER and ELLIOT, 1904, 1905; ROGERS, 1903, 1904). CAREY and WRIGHT (1960a, 1961) and CHEYMOL et al. (1967b, 1969a) confirmed that the venoms of *E. schistosa*, *Hydrophis cyanocinctus*, *Lapemis hardwickii*, and *Laticauda semifasciata* produce a flaccid muscular paralysis of peripheral origin in laboratory animals. The heart usually continues to beat for a long time after the respiratory failure if maintained by artificial respiration. Postsynaptic toxins with short amino acid chain have been found in all of the sea snake venoms studied (see Chap. 5 and TAMIYA, 1975). Neither presynaptic toxin nor cardiotoxin-like polypeptide have been found.

Unlike in the experiments with laboratory animals (CAREY and WRIGHT, 1960a; CHEYMOL et al., 1966a; BARME, 1968), muscle pain, myoglobinuria, and widespread but focal hyaline necrosis of skeletal muscle have been generally observed among the fishermen in Malaya bitten mostly by *E. schistosa* (REID, 1961; MARSDEN and REID, 1961). These clinical findings, however, were not encountered among the victims in Vietnam waters where *L. hardwicki* predominates (BARME, 1968). REID (1961) put forward the hypothesis that, in the human cases, death caused by *E. schistosa* envenomation results from respiratory failure or acute hyperkalemia, both due to muscle destruction or from acute renal failure. Since the animal experiments are usually carried out for short term, it is possible that the acute death is due to respiratory paralysis caused by neuromuscular blockade by the postsynaptic toxins.

On the other hand, the necrotic effect on skeletal muscle may progress slowly and become evident in human who would not die of its acute paralytic effect because of their large body weight.

VI. Viperid and Crotalid Venoms

The venoms of most crotalid and viperid snakes except those of *Crotalus scutulatus* and *C. durissus terrificus*, are less toxic than those of elapid and hydrophid if administered subcutaneously (BROWN, 1973). Nevertheless, some venoms are highly toxic when intravenously administered. Unlike in the case with elapid and sea snake venoms, the life of animals envenomed with *Echis carinatus* or *Crotalus adamanteus* cannot be maintained on artificial respiration (KELLAWAY et al., 1932), suggesting that the lethal effect is not due to respiratory paralysis of central or pheripheral origin. CHEYMOL et al. (1968) also found no paralytic action on skeletal muscle with lethal doses of the venoms of *Bothrops jararaca*, *B. atrox*, *B. lanceolatus*, or *B. carribeus*. The cause of death upon envenomation is generally due to hemorrhage, circulatory collapse, local necrotic effect, or disturbance in blood coagulation (see Chaps. 14, 15, 18, 26, 27). The most well-documented exception is the venom from the South American rattlesnake, which contains a presynaptic neurotoxin, crotoxin (SLOTTA and FRAENKEL-CONRAT, 1938; VITAL-BRAZIL and EXCELL, 1971; CHANG and LEE, 1977). This venom produces respiratory paralysis of peripheral origin (BARRIO and VITAL-BRAZIL, 1951; CHEYMOL et al., 1969b) with or without initial convulsion and spasm depending on the source of the venom. VICK (1970) studied the effects of ten crotalid and four viperid venoms on the dog. He found that whereas the tissue destruction and necrosis at the bitten site were characteristics of viperid envenomation, respiratory failure was the principal symptom for crotalid envenomation.

D. Effects on Neuromuscular Transmission

The effect on neuromuscular transmission of snake venoms has been frequently compared with that of curare. In the old literature on snake venoms, the term "curare-like" was used indiscriminately for the neuromuscular blocking effect without knowing whether the presynaptic or postsynaptic site was affected. Indeed, even the site of action of D-tubocurarine was not established until the mode of neurohumoral transmission from the motor nerve to skeletal muscle, with acetylcholine as the chemical mediator, was convincingly established. DALE et al. (1936) first proved that the release of acetylcholine from the nerve terminal is not affected by D-tubocurarine. The work by FAYRER (1872, 1873) and BRUNTON and FAYRER (1873) on the curare-like effect of Indian cobra venom almost dated back to the time of BERNARD's study on the curare in 1856.

I. Introduction to Pharmacology of Neuromuscular Transmission

To facilitate the understanding of different modes of action of snake venoms on the neuromuscular junction, the current concept on the events carrying on the signal transmittance from the nerve to muscle will be briefly summarized. Details of it can be found in the recent reviews by HUBBARD (1973), HUBBARD and QUASTEL (1973) and GAGE (1976).

The arrival of action potentials at the axon terminal initiates a series of events that effect the neurohumoral transmission. The chemical mediator acetylcholine is manufactured in the motor nerve terminal cytoplasm from acetyl coenzyme A of mitochondrial origin and choline derived from extracellular fluid by an active transport mechanism. A cytoplasmic enzyme, choline acetyltransferase catalyzes synthesis of the transmitter and the product is then stored in synaptic vesicles by an unknown mechanism. The vesicles, like the mitochondria and choline acetyltransferase, are derived from the cell body by transport along the axon. The vesicles may then come into contact and fuse with the terminal axon membrane and empty their contents into the synaptic cleft. The vesicle membrane is then incorporated into the terminal membrane and later recovered as a complex coated vesicle, which in turn sheds its coat to reveal a synaptic vesicle. The latter is refilled with acetylcholine and recycled (HEUSER and REESE, 1973). Superimposed on these mechanisms is the nerve impulse, enormously increasing the rate of release by a mechanism of which only the first two steps are known. These are the depolarization of the nerve terminals, which increases their calcium permeability, and the entry of Ca^{2+} which triggers the process called excitation—secretion coupling to cause a sudden increase of the transmitter release. Soluble acidic proteins and adenosine triphosphate, which may play some role in the binding of acetylcholine in vesicles (MUSICK and HUBBARD, 1972; SILINSKY and HUBBARD, 1973), are released together with acetylcholine.

Released acetylcholine now diffuses away from nerve terminals or is broken down by acetylcholinesterase superficially located in relation to the folded muscle membrane which formes the synaptic cleft. Following the hydrolysis, some choline molecules are taken up by nerve terminals and reincorporated into acetylcholine as described above. Before diffusing away or being hydrolyzed, however, acetylcholine molecules combine with specific macromolecules in the subsynaptic membrane of motor endplate, acetylcholine receptors. This combination results in an increase of muscle membrane conductance for Na^+ and K^+. The role of acetylcholine receptor is to recognize the molecule of chemical mediator. It is not clear at the present time whether the receptor is also the same molecule which leads to the increase of membrane conductance, or whether another molecule, an ionophore, provides such ionic channels upon combination of acetylcholine with the receptor. In any event, each receptor-acetylcholine interaction appears to effect the net passage of some 50000 cations, thus generating a 0.2 μV depolarization (KATZ and MILEDI, 1970, 1971). The result of a large number of such elementary events is a rapidly increasing membrane depolarization, the endplate potential (EPP). In the meantime, the acetylcholine molecule remaining in the synaptic cleft is rapidly hydrolyzed by acetylcholinesterase and a passive recharging of the depolarized muscle membrane follows, so that the EPP decays with the time constant of the muscle membrane. Approximately, there are about 5×10^6 molecules of acetylcholine released at each nerve terminal by a nerve impulse and about 2×10^7 receptors in one motor endplate. Spontaneous release of acetylcholine of a single vesicle may take place without nerve impulse, and the depolarization of endplate thus elicited is the so-called miniature endplate potential (MEPP).

In the focally innervated skeletal muscle where only one or two synaptic contacts exist between the nerve and muscle, the action potential of muscle is initiated when the EPP reaches a critical threshold level and the whole muscle membrane is thus excited and contraction of muscle ensues. Usually, the amplitude of EPP is well above the threshold and the safety factor for neuromuscular transmission in the rat diaphragm is three to five (CHANG et al., 1975). In the multiply innervated skeletal muscle, such as in amphibian and avian muscles, action potential may or may not be initiated, and contraction can be evoked just by the interaction of acetylcholine with the receptor.

From the current concept of neuromuscular transmission, it is obvious that the transmission can be impaired at any point, either presynaptic or postsynaptic (HUBBARD and QUASTEL, 1973). Before the establishment of the mode of neuromuscular transmission, the site of action of curare was indeed thought to be at the nerve ending (BERNARD, 1856). It is now beyond doubt that this agent blocks the transmission by competing at the acetylcholine receptor with the nerve impulse-released acetylcholine. The "curare-like" action of snake venoms in the old literature should therefore be interpreted to mean simply the "neuromuscular blocking" action.

Characteristics of neuromuscular blockade by D-tubocurarine include the following: the more rapid paralysis of those small muscles innervated by cranial nerve whereas the respiratory muscles are the last to be blocked, the effect is easily overcome by anticholinesterase agents and the parallel shift of acetylcholine dose-response curve to the right. The amplitudes of successive EPPs evoked by repetitive stimulation decline rapidly in the muscle treated with D-tubocurarine (OTSUKA et al., 1962). When treated with a high concentration of Mg^{2+}, which inhibits the release of transmitter, the amplitudes of EPPs are well-sustained (DEL CASTILLO and KATZ, 1954). D-Tubocurarine neither inhibits the release of acetylcholine nor depresses the contraction of skeletal muscle induced by direct stimulation or by K^+.

Controversies may arise in the study of neuromuscular blocking action of whole snake venoms because of involvement of different effects on nerve-muscle preparation by various constituents of venoms. Inappropriate selection of the nerve-muscle preparation may as well result in an artifact. Since the active venom components are of large molecular weight, penetration into the tissue may not be as easy as the small molecule like D-tubocurarine and acetylcholine, and consequently the effect of venom components on each of nerve-muscle unit may not be as uniform as in the case with D-tubocurarine.

II. Cobra Venoms and Cobra Neurotoxins

1. Whole Venom

It has long been established that cobra venom has a potent "curare-like" but irreversible paralytic effect on skeletal muscle (see Sect. C.I.3 for references). Since the contractile response to indirect stimulation of nerve is blocked before the depression of the response to direct stimulation of muscle, the site of primary blockade occurs obviously at the neuromuscular junction. At relatively low concentrations which induce complete neuromuscular blockade without significant effect on the muscle, the contractile response to acetylcholine of the frog rectus muscle (SU, 1960) and the chick biventer cervicis muscle (SU et al., 1967) is antagonized by Formosan cobra *(N.n.atra)* venom and that of the denervated rat diaphragm abolished by venoms of Indian cobra *(N.naja)*, black-necked spitting cobra *(N. nigricollis)*, and Egyptian cobra *(N. haje)* (CHEYMOL et al., 1967a). The depolarization of endplate of frog sartorius muscle evoked by acetylcholine or carbachol is likewise abolished (PENG, 1960; MELDRUM, 1965b). There seems to be no qualitative difference between the action of various cobra venoms, and all of the authors agree that the effect of cobra venom is primarily on the postsynaptic motor endplate. The depolarization of the muscle induced by high K^+ concentration, however, is not antagonized by the venom (PENG, 1960). The observation that saturation of the acetylcholine receptor of the frog muscle with D-tubocurarine can effectively prevent the irreversible depression by cobra venom (SU, 1960) indicates beyond doubt that similar binding sites of the acetylcholine receptor are involved in the action of D-tubocurarine and the active venom constituent. By treatment of the whole venom with various group-specific reagents, the venom loses its toxicity and neuromuscular blocking activity to a parallel extent (LEE et al., 1960), indicating that the latter activity plays an important role for the lethal toxicity. This effect of cobra venoms is due to the presence of postsynaptic toxins. Although the envenomed animal may recover generally within 2 day from the paralysis if death does not take place, a prolonged residual effect, up to 10 days, is evident as revealed by the reduced dose of D-tubocurarine in causing head drop in envenomed rabbits (SCHMIDT et al., 1964; CHEYMOL et al., 1966b).

The action of cobra venom on the nerve-muscle preparation is, however, apparently different from that of D-tubocurarine. Anticholinesterase agents are generally less effective or ineffective in antagonizing the paralytic effect of cobra venom. The dose-response curve for acetylcholine is shifted to the right with appreciable depression of the maximum height, and a sustained contraction is elicited on repetitive stimulation of the nerve (SU, 1960) instead of Wedensky inhibition as generally seen with the curare-treated muscle. These results may be accounted for partly by the relative irreversibility of the action of postsynaptic toxins, by the uneven blockage of various synapses due to the slow diffusion of the latter toxins in penetrating the nerve-muscle preparation, and partly by the action of other constituents of the venom such as phospholipase A and cardiotoxins which inhibit the muscle directly. When strong concentrations of venom are used, the response of the muscle to direct stimulation starts to decline before neuromuscular block and contracture develops (HOUSSAY et al., 1922; CUSHNY and YAGI, 1918; SU, 1960; CHEYMOL et al., 1967a; SU et al., 1967). This direct effect of cobra venom on the skeletal muscle is largely due to cardiotoxin (SARKAR and MAITRE, 1950; LEE et al., 1968; CHANG et al., 1972) and will be discussed further in Section E.

In addition to the inhibitory effect on the acetylcholine receptor of endplate and on the muscle fiber, CHEYMOL et al. (1967a) have speculated an existence of presynaptically acting component in cobra venom. Indeed, the release of acetylcholine from the rat phrenic nerve ending is reduced by Formosan cobra venom to one-half at a concentration ten times higher than that necessary for complete neuromuscular blockade (SU et al., 1967); nevertheless, it is unlikely that this effect contributes significantly to the neuromuscular blocking effect of cobra venom. So far, no neurotoxin acting on the presynaptic site has been isolated from any cobra venom. The inhibition of transmitter release by cobra venom may be due either to the action of cardiotoxin which depresses the nerve terminal potential of superficial muscle fibers (CHANG and LEE, 1966) or to the effect of basic phospholipase A since the enzyme isolated from *N. nigricollis* venom (DUMAREY et al., 1975) has a presynaptic blocking action (BOQUET, personal communication).

The blocking activity of three cobra *(N. nigricollis, N. naja, N. hannah)* venoms in the crustacean muscle is presynaptic rather than postsynaptic, since following blockade of the indirectly stimulated spikes, the crustacean muscle still responds to glutamate (RUSSELL, 1967; PARNAS and RUSSELL, 1967). This seemingly contradictory result may be accounted for by the specificity of the action of postsynaptic toxin of cobra venom which acts only on the nicotinic acetylcholine receptor but not on other types of receptors. The neuromuscular transmission in the crustacean muscle is glutaminergic rather than cholinergic (TAKEUCHI and TAKEUCHI, 1964).

2. Postsynaptic Toxins

A group of basic polypeptide toxins consisting of either 61–62 (short chain) or 71–73 (long chain) amino acid residues are universally found in all cobra venoms. Details of the chemistry of these toxins can be found in Chapter 5. This group of toxins is highly toxic and undoubtedly the principal lethal factor of cobra venoms. Although pharmacologic analysis of the mode of paralytic action on voluntary muscle has not been carried out on all of these toxins, the close similarity of their amino acid sequences enables one to classify them in a group as postsynaptic toxins on the basis of the specific action on the acetylcholine receptor of motor endplate.

Purified or partially purified toxins of cobra venoms so far studied pharmacologically are cobrotoxin from *N. n. atra* (CHANG and LEE, 1966; SU et al., 1967; CHANG et al., 1972), toxin 3 from *N. n. siamensis* (LESTER, 1970, 1972a, b; EAKER et al., 1971), toxin α from *N. nigricollis* (TAZIEFF-DEPIERRE and PIERRE, 1966; LESTER, 1970), toxins from *N. nivea* (EARL and EXCELL, 1971, 1972), and a toxin fraction from *N. naja* (MELDRUM, 1963, 1965b) and *N. n. siamensis* (SILVAMOGSTHAM and TEJASEN, 1972). In contrast to the whole venom or cardiotoxin, the axonal conduction in the rat phrenic nerve is not affected by the postsynaptic toxin at a concentration 1000 times that for blockade of neuromuscular transmission (CHANG et al., 1972). Neither the terminal nerve spike (CHANG and LEE, 1966; LESTER, 1972a) nor the release of acetylcholine (SU et al., 1967) are affected, indicating no presynaptic event of transmission is disturbed by the toxin. However, as with D-tubocurarine, the antidromic potential evoked by nerve impulse in the presence of neostigmine is abolished (CHANG and LEE, 1966). The resting membrane potential, action potential, and contractility of frog sartorius or rat diaphragm muscles are not affected (CHANG and LEE, 1966; SU et al., 1967; EAKER et al., 1971; LESTER, 1972a, EARL and EXCELL, 1972). Depolarization and direct inhibitory action on muscle by the less purified toxic fraction of cobra venom (MELDRUM, 1963, 1965b; LOOTS et al., 1973) must be due to contamination with cardiotoxin, a potent membrane depolarizing component in cobra venom (see Sect. E.II). Furthermore, the passive electric properties of muscle membrane are unchanged by the postsynaptic toxin (LESTER, 1972a). The amplitudes of EPPs, MEPPs, and acetylcholine potential are depressed by the toxin, whereas the quantal contents of EPPs are not reduced (CHANG and LEE, 1966; EAKER et al., 1971; LESTER, 1970, 1972a; EARL and EXCELL, 1972). The dose-response curve for acetylcholine is shifted to the right in parallel (SU et al., 1967). All of these results clearly indicate that the toxins block neuromuscular transmission by a specific effect on the postsynaptic acetylcholine receptor without affecting the presynaptic site or muscle fiber itself. It is further demonstrated that this blocking action of toxins can be prevented when the preparation is pretreated with D-tubocurarine (SU et al., 1967) or desensitized by carbachol (LESTER, 1972a). The specificity of the action is further substantiated by the specific binding of the labeled toxins. Binding occurs only at the endplate of muscle fiber (LEE et al., 1967; TSENG et al., 1968) as that of D-tubocurarine (WASER and LÜTHI, 1957). The difference between the effects of postsynaptic toxins and D-tubocurarine becomes less and less as purer toxins are used. Neostigmine now effectively increases the amplitude and time-course of EPPs depressed by the toxin (CHANG and LEE, 1966), shifts the acetylcholine dose-response curve back to control (SU et al., 1967), and restores the neuromuscular transmission (TAZIEFF-DEPIERRE and PIERRE, 1966; TAZIEFF-DEPIERRE et al., 1969). The amplitudes of successive EPPs on repetitive stimulation also decline as rapidly as in the D-tubocurarine-treated preparation. The differences between the actions of D-tubocurarine and those of postsynaptic toxins will be further discussed in Section D. VIII.

III. Krait (Bungarus) Venoms and Their Toxins

1. Formosan Krait (Bungarus multicinctus) Venom

The neuromuscular blocking action of *B. multicinctus* venom (CHANG, 1960a, b) is about twice as potent as cobra venom in the rat diaphragm preparation. Unlike cobra venom, no contracture is evoked. The muscle is able to respond to the direct stimulation and high concentration of K^+ as well as the untreated control even after treatment with the venom at a concentration 100 times that needed for the neuromuscular blockade. Immersion of the nerve alone in the venom solution is without effect. The dose-response curve of acetylcholine in the frog rectus abdominis can be shifted parallel to the right for more than 1 log and the shift can be subsequently counteracted by addition of physostigmine. The inhibition of acetylcholine response by the venom cannot be restored by washings but can be prevented by pretreating the preparation with dimethyltubocurarine. Unlike cobra venom, however, this krait venom also completely inhibits the release of acetylcholine from the rat phrenic nerve (CHANG, 1960a) although the action is delayed and not apparent until 60–80 min after application of the venom. A sustained tetanus occurs on repetitive stimulation of the phrenic nerve when the rat diaphragm is quickly paralyzed by incubation with a high concentration (10 µg/ml). With low concentrations (0.3–1 µg/ml), however, Wedensky inhibition and posttetanic potentiation, characteristics of β-bungarotoxin effects (Fig. 1), are evident. The inhibitory effect on the acetylcholine response can be stopped by washing out of the venom though not reversed, whereas the blocking action on neuromuscular transmission still progresses to complete paralysis even after washing out of the venom after 15 min incubation. These observations indicate that, in addition to the postsynaptic toxin, there is another type of neurotoxin which blocks neuromuscular transmission by an inhibition of the transmitter release. Antiserum of this venom can neutralize the progress of action of the bound toxin if added immediately after binding (CHANG, 1960a). CHANG and LEE

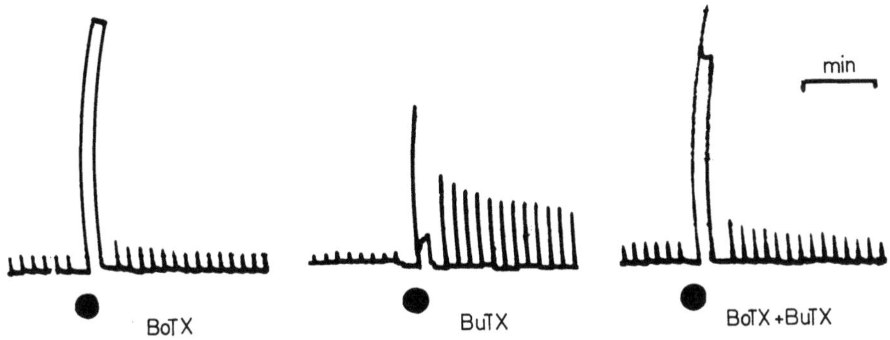

Fig. 1. Comparison of the contractile responses to repetitive stimulation of rat diaphragms treated with β-bungarotoxin (BuTX) and type A botulinum toxin (BoTX), alone or in combination. Left panel: 140 min after 0.1 μg/ml botulinum toxin; middle panel: 130 min after 1 μg/ml β-bungarotoxin; right panel: 150 min and 120 min, respectively, after botulinum toxin and β-bungarotoxin. At ●, repetitive nerve stimulation at 100 Hz for 10 s was given. Twitches were elicited by single stimulation every 10 s and were depressed by about 85–90% at the time shown. Note the typical Wedensky inhibition and posttetanic potentiation in the preparation treated with β-bungarotoxin (from CHANG and HUANG, 1974)

(1963) succeeded in isolating one postsynaptic toxin, called α-bungarotoxin, and two presynaptic toxins, β- and γ-bungarotoxins, and studied the mode of action of these two types of toxins. The blocking actions of Formosan krait venom on neuromuscular transmission can be well-explained on the basis of its toxin constituents. No cardiotoxin-like principle seems to exist in this venom. Based on the difference of the times necessary to kill mice or to cause neuromuscular block, the relative contents, and the potency of neuromuscular block for each toxin, it is likely that the Formosan krait venom kills the envenomed animal by α-bungarotoxin when the animal is small or the dose is high, but by β-bungarotoxin when the dose is small or the animal is big.

2. Indian Krait (Bungarus caeruleus) Venom

Although its potent peripheral depressant effect on respiration has been known since the study by KELLAWAY et al. in 1932, no pharmacologic analysis has been performed on the mode of its neuromuscular blocking action until recently. MEBS et al. (1974) and LEE et al. (1976c) have fractionated the venom and studied the isolated principles. Two highly toxic fractions, presumably β-bungarotoxin-like, block the transmission in the chick muscle without reducing the response to acetylcholine, and still two other toxic fractions block the transmission by abolishing the response to acetylcholine. It is obvious that the Indian krait venom, like Formosan krait venom, also contains both postsynaptic toxins and presynaptic toxins.

Recently, BON and CHANGEUX (1975) and BON (1976) reported the isolation of a highly lethal acidic neurotoxin, called ceruleotoxin, which accounts for at least 35% of the total toxicity of the venom. This toxin inhibits the depolarization and Na^+ efflux evoked by carbachol on microsac preparation prepared from *Torpedo marmorate* without inhibiting the binding of a labeled postsynaptic toxin. It is inferred that ceruleotoxin is a new type of neurotoxin acting on the postsynaptic site without binding to the acetylcholine receptor. In view of its molecular weight (14000 daltons for the single unit) and the long delay in killing mice, and since carbachol may act on the presynaptic site as in the chick biventer nerve-muscle preparations (CHANG et al., 1976), the possibility of ceruleotoxin being a presynaptic toxin, like β-bungarotoxin, or a phospholipase A cannot be ruled out. Moreover, the presence of such presynaptic toxin in this venom has been noted (MEBS et al., 1974; LEE et al., 1976c).

3. Banded Krait (Bungarus fasciatus) Venom

No report is available on the neuromuscular action of banded krait venom except that it may have curare-like as well as direct actions (HOUSSAY et al., 1922; KELLAWAY and HOLDEN, 1932) and induces contracture of skeletal muscle because of its cardiotoxin-like principles (LIN SHIAU et al., 1972, 1975a). In accordance with its relatively low toxicity (Table 2), the content of neurotoxins in this venom is found to be low (LIN SHIAU et al., 1972; LU and LO, 1974). None of the isolated fractions is as active as other elapid postsynaptic toxins or presynaptic toxins. MOORE and LOY (1972) reported an isolation of toxin similar to α-bungarotoxin in its binding capacity with electroplax, but no other pharmacologic study was performed.

4. α-Bungarotoxin

α-Bungarotoxin of *B. multicinctus* venom, consisting of 74 amino acid residues with five disulfides (MEBS et al., 1972), is one of the first postsynaptic toxins to be isolated from elapid venoms and its mode of neuromuscular blocking action analyzed (CHANG and LEE, 1963; LEE and CHANG, 1966). It blocks the transmission irreversibly by inhibiting the response of acetylcholine receptor on the motor endplate. In contrast to the whole venom, the release of acetylcholine from the motor nerve ending is not affected. No effect on the muscle itself can be demonstrated. Membrane potential and action potential of the muscle remain unchanged. The pharmacologic action is thus almost the same as other postsynaptic toxins found in cobra and sea snake venoms. The specific action of α-bungarotoxin on the acetylcholine receptor of vertebrate skeletal muscle is further substantiated by the specific binding on the endplate (LEE et al., 1967; MILEDI and POTTER, 1971; BARNARD et al., 1971; BERG et al., 1972; CHANG et al., 1973a; FAMBROUGH and HARTZELL, 1972; HARTZELL and FAMBROUGH, 1972). The density of α-bungarotoxin bound outside of the endplate is very low, being only about 1/1000th of that at the endplate in normal innervated muscle (HARTZELL and FAMBROUGH, 1972). The pharmacologic effect as well as the binding can be effectively prevented in the presence of D-tubocurarine and acetylcholine, suggesting that the same binding site is involved (LEE and CHANG, 1966; DRYDEN and HARVEY, 1974). α-Bungarotoxin, however, does not block the cholinergic transmission other than that in skeletal muscle. The muscarinic acetylcholine receptor in smooth muscles and nicotinic receptor in the autonomic ganglia are not blocked.

On the other hand, the antidromic potentials in the motor nerve evoked after orthodromic impulse is blocked as with D-tubocurarine (LEE and CHANG, 1966). Interestingly, a binding of the toxin on the nerve terminal has been also reported (LENTZ et al., 1975). These results together suggest that there may be also some receptors on the nerve terminal. This is in line with the effect of acetylcholine on nerve terminal (HUBBARD et al., 1965). Electron-microscopic study reveals that no ultrastructural change occurs at the motor endplate after complete muscular paralysis by this toxin (CHEN and LEE, 1970; TSAI, 1975).

5. β-Bungarotoxin

More than one fraction of *B. multicinctus* and *B. caeruleus* venoms show the biologic activity exemplified by β-bungarotoxin (CHANG and LEE, 1963; LEE et al., 1972b, 1976c; MEBS et al., 1974). They are more potent in blocking neuromuscular transmission and act differently from α-bungarotoxin (CHANG and LEE, 1963; LEE and CHANG, 1966; CHANG et al., 1973; CHANG and HUANG, 1974). The neuromuscular blockade proceeds slowly with a latent period lasting as long as 60 min in the rat and mouse diaphragm preparations no matter how high a concentration is used. The time to death in mice is longer than 80 min even after subcutaneous injection of $20 \times LD_{50}$ dose of β-bungarotoxin, whereas it takes only 20 min after a comparable dose of α-bungarotoxin. The chick muscle is extremely sensitive to this toxin, and the blockade in this species proceeds without such a long latency (LEE and TSENG, 1969; CHANG and HUANG, 1974). The high toxicity of the whole venom in birds (TO and TIN, 1943) is apparently due to the presence of β-bungarotoxin.

a) Electrophysiologic Study

The blockade by this toxin is usually preceded by a period of facilitation in the rat muscle (also in mouse muscle, though less marked) particularly when the neuromuscular transmission is partially impaired by decreasing the release of transmitter by lowering the Ca^{2+} concentration (CHANG et al., 1973; CHANG and HUANG, 1974). The quantal content of EPPs is first increased and the transmission improved without altering the sensitivity of endplate to acetylcholine. The frequency of MEPPs is also increased during this period. This phenomenon is even more evident in the bathing media devoid of Ca^{2+} or with high concentration of Mg^{2+}. Since the increase of MEPP frequency by depolarization of the nerve terminal is dependent on the presence of Ca^{2+} and is blocked by high Mg^{2+} concentration (LILEY, 1956), it is unlikely that the effect of β-bungarotoxin is caused by a depolarization. A similar inference is proposed for the similar effect of black widow spider venom (KAWAI et al., 1972). Thereafter, the release of transmitter declines as revealed by the decrease of acetylcholine output measured by bioassay (CHANG and LEE, 1963) or by the reduction of quantal contents of EPPs (CHANG et al., 1973; CHANG and HUANG, 1974) which eventually become as small as the MEPP before resulting in complete failure of the transmitter release. As in the case of blockade by high Mg^{2+} concentration, the amplitude of successive EPPs during repetitive stimulation does not decline one after another (Fig. 2) when the transmitter release is depressed, suggesting an inhibition of the transmitter release mechanism rather than a decrease in the available store of transmitter (CHANG et al., 1973). During the first phase of facilitatory effect, the successive decline of EPPs during repetitive stimulation is, on the contrary, more marked (CHANG and HUANG, 1974), a phenomenon similar to that evoked by increasing Ca^{2+} concentration which facilitates the release of transmitter (LUNDBERG and QUILISCH, 1953). It is thus evident that β-bungarotoxin first induces Ca^{2+}-like

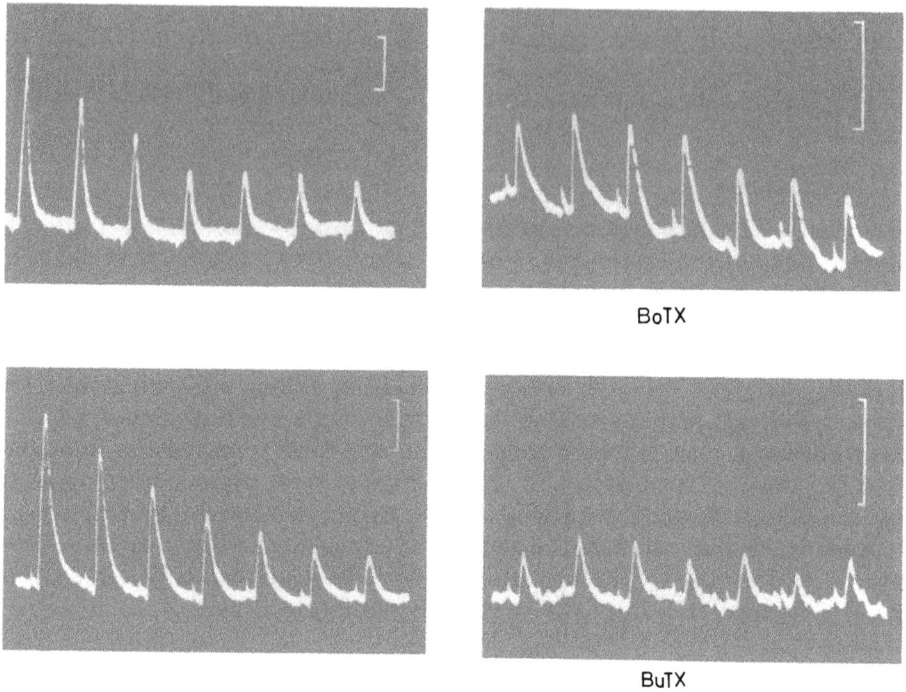

Fig. 2. Trains of EPPs of isolated rat diaphragm preparations affected either by β-bungarotoxin (BuTX, 3 μg/ml) or type A botulinum toxin (BoTX, 0.3 μg/ml). Left panels show the controls equilibrated with 0.8 μg/ml D-tubocurarine before addition of toxins. EPPs were elicited at 100 Hz. Calibrations: 1 mV (from CHANG and HUANG, 1974)

facilitation and then Mg^{2+}-like depression of transmitter release in the rat muscle. Immediately after the complete failure of transmitter release, the content of acetylcholine in the nerve terminal is within normal limits (CHANG et al., 1973). The frequency of MEPPs declines after the initial facilitatory phase and they finally disappear. ALDERICE and VOLLE (1975) have observed similar biphasic effects of β-bungarotoxin on MEPP frequency in the frog sartorius muscle and found a paradoxic effect of Ca^{2+} in the facilitatory phase of toxin effect, i.e., increasing Ca^{2+} from 0.5 to 2.0 mM depresses MEPP frequency instead of an increase as seen in normal muscle. This effect of toxin is similar to that induced by La^{3+}. The amplitude of MEPPs, however, is not reduced and occasionally giant MEPPs are observed. There are also bursts of MEPPs in some of the blocked junction. At many of the blocked junctions, high K^+ (40 mM) is still able to evoke burst of MEPPs although it does not seem to last as long as the normal junction (CHANG et al., 1973). All of these results indicate that the inhibition of the transmitter release by β-bungarotoxin is not due primarily to depletion of transmitter, inhibition of its synthesis or inhibition of recycling of the synaptic vesicles (see Sect. D.I). Since the nerve terminal spikes are not affected and the frequency of MEPPs can still be increased on repetitive nerve stimulation at the junction immediately after the failure of transmitter release (CHANG et al., 1973), it is obvious that the conduction of impulse to the nerve terminal is not impaired by the toxin. The depolarization-secretion coupling induced by high K^+ is not significantly affected at the time when that induced by nerve action potential is preferentially disturbed. In the chick biventer cervicis muscle, the release of neurotransmitter by carbachol is also depressed by β-bungarotoxin (CHANG et al., 1976). This block, however, takes place much later after the complete blockade of neuromuscular transmission. It is thus unlikely that the primary cause of neuromuscular blocking action of this toxin is depletion of the transmitter or any general destruction of the nerve terminal although these effects may eventually occur in the advanced course of its action.

b) *Ultrastructural Effects*

The ultrastructure of the motor nerve terminal in the diaphragm of mouse injected intraperitoneally with a lethal dose of β-bungarotoxin is markedly changed (CHEN and LEE, 1970). One hour after injection, the number of synaptic vesicles is decreased and increased profiles of Ω-shaped indentations similar in size to synaptic vesicles are found on the axolemma. The mitochondria are swollen and the synaptic vesicles are nearly completely depleted 2–4 h after the toxin administration. By contrast, the structures of muscle fibers, fibrocytes, endothelial cells, and myelinated axons in the diaphragm are unaffected. CHEN and LEE (1970) inferred accordingly that the inhibition of transmitter release by β-bungarotoxin is the result of the depletion of synaptic vesicles. This inference, however, is in conflict with the pharmacologic and electrophysiologic findings (LEE and CHANG, 1966; CHANG et al., 1973) which show that the transmitter is not depleted at the time when the neuromuscular transmission is blocked. In a recent study, the change of ultrastructure in the motor nerve terminal of mouse and rat diaphragms treated either in vivo or in vitro with the toxin is correlated with the inhibition of the neuromuscular transmission (TSAI, 1975). The axonal terminal appears to be quite normal until the time of complete neuromuscular blockade and the change observed by CHEN and LEE (1970) is found to occur only after the blockade of transmission. Artificial respiration increases the appearance of Ω vesicles, whereas the depletion of synaptic vesicles and swelling of mitochondria is much less marked. Since treatment with α-bungarotoxin does not induce similar change of ultrastructure, the change induced by β-bungarotoxin is unlikely due simply to asphyxia. When the phrenic nerve is cut, the structural changes are less marked, suggesting that the nerve impulse has a synergistic effect as in the case with functional blockade. Since the Ω vesicles are mostly of a coated type, these vesicles may represent the process of endocytosis rather than exocytosis according to the hypothesis of synaptic vesicle membrane recycling (HEUSER and REESE, 1973). In conclusion, it is unlikely that the depletion of synaptic vesicles is the primary cause of inhibition of transmitter release by β-bungarotoxin. The structural change, however, appears to be the result of an advanced effect of the toxin, following the functional blockade.

c) *Kinetic Study and Mode of Action*

The prolonged latent period of the blocking action of β-bungarotoxin in the rat and mouse is apparently not due to a slow binding of the toxin with its target site since washout of the toxin after incubation for only 20–30 min does not change the time-course of neuromuscular block significantly (CHANG and LEE, 1963; CHANG et al.,

1973; CHANG and HUANG, 1974). Undoubtedly, the binding during the short incubation period is enough for the subsequent blocking effect on nerve terminal to take place. It may be speculated that the macromolecule of the terminal axolemma undergoes some kind of change after the toxin is bound. The change could be due to an interaction between the toxin molecule and the axolemma per se or to an enzymic breakdown of the membrane component, such as phospholipid, since β-bungarotoxin has phospholipase A activity (WERNICKE et al., 1975; WAGNER et al., 1975; TOBIAS et al., 1976; STRONG et al., 1976a), or alternatively, to the breakdown product of the phospholipid (HOWARD, 1975; WERNICKE et al., 1975). The initial facilitatory effect of the toxin could be a transitional state of the change of the nerve terminal. It is unknown whether the toxin is acting inside or outside the axolemma. It is interesting in this respect that the horseradish peroxidase bound to β-bungarotoxin was found to be able to penetrate the axolemma (STRONG et al., 1976b). Although the inhibitory effect of β-bungarotoxin can be markedly slowed down by antivenom if added after 20 min incubation (CHANG, 1960a; TSAI, 1975), antivenom has no antagonistic effect if added after 100 min incubation (CHANG and SU, unpublished) when the inhibitory effect has emerged. This result may suggest that the toxin is first bound on the surface of the axolemma and then incorporated into or inside the nerve terminal membrane.

The process of inhibitory change which takes place after binding of β-bungarotoxin is temperature dependent and can be greatly accelerated by nerve impulses (CHANG et al., 1973; CHANG and HUANG, 1974). Reduction of Ca^{2+}, as well as increase of Mg^{2+} concentration, decreases the activity of transmitter release mechanism and also greatly slows down the process of toxin-induced inhibitory change. It seems evident that the process of transmitter release accelerates the change of the nerve terminal membrane. One may speculate that the process of transmitter release, which probably involves a conformational change of the axolemma, accelerates the toxin-induced change of the latter structure. The process of transmitter release may increase the recycling of the synaptic vesicles (HEUSER and REESE, 1973) and thus increase the incorporation of the toxin bound on the axolemma into the axon. It is also possible that the conformational change increases the accessibility of buried phospholipid to the enzymic action of the toxin. Alternatively, the increased influx of Ca^{2+} associated with the release mechanism may enhance the enzyme activity within the nerve terminal since Ca^{2+} is essential for the activity of phospholipase A (STRONG et al., 1976; TOBIAS et al., 1976). Interestingly, all of the presynaptic toxins isolated from either elapid or *Crotalus* venom, such as notexin from *Notechis scutatus* (KARLSSON et al., 1972b), taipoxin from *Oxyuranus scutellatus* (FOHLMAN et al., 1976), and crotoxin (SLOTTA and FRAENKEL-CONRAT, 1938) from *Crotalus durissus terrificus*, are known to have activity of phospholipase A. For further discussion on presynaptic toxins in general, the reader is referred to Section D. IX.

d) Specificity of Action

The twitch response of the guinea pig ileum (cholinergic) (CHANG and LEE, 1963) and of the cat nictitating membrane to sympathetic preganglionic nerve stimulation (LEE and LEE, unpublished) are not affected by β-bungarotoxin even at a concentration 100 times higher than that for neuromuscular blockade. The action is, therefore, confined only to the motor nerve terminal innervating the skeletal muscle. Sympathetic and parasympathetic neurons, whether cholinergic or adrenergic, appear not to be affected.

In contrast to its specificity in intact peripheral organs, β-bungarotoxin causes efflux of acetylcholine (SEN and COOPER, 1975; SEN et al., 1976), noradrenaline, γ-aminobutyric acid, and serotonin (WERNICKE et al., 1974, 1975) from the brain minces or synaptosomes in vitro and blocks the uptake of these putative transmitters. No change of ultrastructure of the tissue has been noted. This experiment raises the possibility that in the central nervous system, β-bungarotoxin may act on nerve terminals nonspecifically if it gains access to the brain. Indeed, β-bungarotoxin is much more toxic in rats if intraventricularly administered (CHANG, SU and TSENG, unpublished). Unlike notexin (HARRIS et al., 1975), however, no local effect on muscle can be found in rats after subcutaneous injection of β-bungarotoxin (SU and CHANG, unpublished).

e) Biochemical Study

The accumulation of Ca^{2+} by the rat brain mitochondria (WAGNER et al., 1974, 1975) and by the sarcoplasmic reticulum of rabbit skeletal muscle (LAU et al., 1974) are depressed by β-bungarotoxin. It is possible that this action may be related to the initial facilitatory effect of the toxin. Mitochondrial oxidative phosphorylation is uncoupled at low concentration of the toxin, the production of CO_2 by brain synaptosomes is increased, and the concentration of adenosin triphosphate decreased (WERNICKE et al., 1975; HOWARD, 1975). WERNICKE et al. (1975) have shown that β-bungarotoxin acts on synaptosomes to cause an efflux of newly accumulated γ-aminobutyric acid and 2-deoxyglucose. This activity of the toxin is Ca^{2+} dependent. Incubation of various subcellular membrane fractions with β-bungarotoxin produces a factor, presumably oleic acid, which uncouples oxidative phosphorylation when added to mitochondria. These authors speculate that the neuromuscular blockade by β-bungarotoxin may be caused by a depletion of energy stores, a consequence of the uncoupling activity. Since phospholipase A fraction isolated from *Vipera russellii* venom also exhibits the same biochemical effect, the above actions of β-bungarotoxin are attributed to its phospholipase activity (HOWARD, 1975). However, since the phospholipase A fractions from various venom sources do not possess the same presynaptic effect as β-bungarotoxin, it is inferred that β-bungarotoxin preferentially attack the phospholipids of the neuronal membrane (WERNICKE et al., 1975).

IV. Australian Snake Venoms and Their Toxins

1. Tiger Snake (Notechis scutatus) Venom and Notexin

Although it has been known for a long time that most of the Australian snake venoms have powerful neuromuscular blocking action, except that of *Pseudechis australis* (ARTHUS, 1911; HOUSSAY and PAVE, 1922; KELLAWAY and HOLDEN, 1932; KELLAWAY et al., 1932), the mode of action had not been elucidated until recently by DATYNER and GAGE (1973a, b). The whole venom of the tiger snake at a high concentration (50 µg/ml) rapidly blocks the response to indirect stimulation in the toad nerve-muscle preparation without affecting the action potentials in the sciatic nerve and muscle. Lower concentrations (1–10 μg/ml) of the venom reduce the amplitude of MEPPs and inhibit the depolarization of muscle fiber caused by carbachol. These effects can be attributed to the presence of postsynaptic toxin in this venom. At a still lower concentration (1 μg/ml), the frequency of MEPPs is first increased and then decreased. The quantal contents of EPPs are reduced markedly with occasional initial increase. No effect on the nerve terminal spike is observed when EPP is abolished. Twenty minutes after addition of the venom (1 μg/ml), the number of synaptic vesicles begins to decline and degenerative changes occur after 2 h incubation (LANE and GAGE, 1973). At higher concentrations (10–100 μg/ml), there are clamped or agglutinated vesicles but no complete depletion of vesicles.

This venom is, therefore, similar to Formosan krait venom in that it contains both postsynaptic and presynaptic toxins and that when the venom concentration is high, the paralytic effect results mainly by the former toxin, while at low concentrations the presynaptic toxin becomes more important. Two postsynaptic toxins with 61 and 72 amino acid residues, respectively and a basic presynaptic toxin (notexin) with 119 amino acid residues have been isolated (KARLSSON et al., 1972b). The resting membrane potential and action potential of extensor digitorum longus muscle isolated from mice intoxicated with notexin for 20 min or more are normal (HARRIS et al., 1973). The frequency of MEPPs is, however, reduced though the amplitude distribution is widened (CULL-CANDY et al., 1976). The EPP is reduced to a quantal size. High K^+ (20 mM) does not increase MEPP frequency in an intoxicated preparation. Like β-bungarotoxin, the action of notexin needs a latent period and is accelerated by nerve impulse. The binding of the toxin to mouse diaphragm is rapid and irreversible (CULL-CANDY et al., 1976). The changes of fine structure of nerve terminals of the diaphragm of notexin-treated mice at death are almost identic with those induced by β-bungarotoxin except that depletion of synaptic vesicles is not marked. It is thus evident that notexin acts primarily on the presynaptic site by an inhibition of the transmitter release. However, there appears to be some discrepancy between the results obtained by DATYNER and GAGE (1973) by using the whole venom and those by HARRIS et al. (1973) by using the purified toxin. While DATYNER and GAGE recorded no depolarization of the frog muscle in vitro with a venom concentration as high as 50 μg/ml, the purified toxin causes a slight depolarization in the mouse muscle at 1–2.5 μg/ml. The whole venom at 1 μg/ml causes initial increase then decrease of the frequency of MEPPs as well as the quantal content of EPPs, whereas the purified toxin at 1–5 μg/ml does not show such initial facilitatory effects. This discrepancy may be due to the species difference of the animals employed. In contrast to other presynaptic toxins, notexin causes a degenerative necrosis of muscle 12–24 h after subcutaneous injection (HARRIS et al., 1975) and inhibits the response of the denervated diaphragm to direct stimulation and to acetylcholine (LEE et al., 1976a).

2. Taipan (Oxyuranus scutellatus) Venom and Taipoxin

An acidic neurotoxin, called taipoxin, is contained in Taipan venom (CULL-CANDY et al., 1976; FOHLMAN et al., 1976; KAMENSKAYA and THESLEFF, 1974). This neurotoxin is a complex of an acidic glycoprotein with basic and neutral polypeptide chains, each consisting of 118–120 amino acid residues. Taipoxin is extremely toxic (Table 4) and produces flaccid paralysis and respiratory arrest after a latent period, which can be greatly reduced by an increase of nerve impulses and temperature. Immediately after neuromuscular block, depolarization of the nerve terminal by high K^+ (20 mM) still induced an increase of MEPPs in the isolated mouse diaphragm, though not as marked as in the normal muscle (CHANG et al., 1977). No such response was observed, however, in the diaphragm isolated from the mouse poisoned with the toxin (KAMENSKAYA and THESLEFF, 1974). Although KAMENSKAYA and THESLEFF (1974) and CULL-CANDY et al. (1976) observed no initial facilitatory effect by taipoxin, a recent study (CHANG et al., 1977) revealed that this toxin increased the frequency of MEPPs about twofold and improved the neuromuscular transmission in the mouse diaphragm in a low Ca^{2+} bathing medium as β-bungarotoxin does. Like in the case with β-bungarotoxin, the effect of taipoxin continues to progress even when the preparation is removed from the treated animal and placed in a toxin-free bathing medium or after incubation for only 10–15 min. The progress of blocking action is accelerated by increasing nerve activity. This toxin is bound irreversibly during the latent period and then induces inhibitory changes of the nerve terminal. Ultrastructurally, the endplates are altered in the presynaptic site but the postsynaptic parts are unchanged. The axolemma has an increased number of Ω-shaped identations and, at a later stage, the synaptic vesicles are greatly reduced in number (CULL-CANDY et al., 1976). Like in the case with β-bungarotoxin, when the phrenic nerve is cut, there is no reduction in the number of vesicles. In addition to this presynaptic neurotoxin, MEBS et al. (1976) isolated a fraction of the venom acting on the postsynaptic site.

3. Death Adder (Acanthophis antarcticus) and Copperhead (Denisonia superba) Venoms

The four toxic fractions isolated by MEBS et al. (1976) from these two venoms block the neuromuscular transmission in the chick biventer cervicis nerve-muscle preparation by acting on the postsynaptic site and inhibit the response to exogenous acetylcholine. The lethal toxicities in mice of these fractions are only one-third to one-half those of most other postsynaptic toxins. Whether these fractions have amino acid sequences similar to those of postsynaptic toxins remains to be elucidated. These two venoms probably do not contain potent presynaptic toxin as judged from the dramatic reversal of paralysis after the injection of antivenom (CAMPBELL, 1975).

V. Other Elapid Venoms

1. Mamba (Dendroaspis) Venoms

Three fractions of *D. jamensoni* venom rapidly block MEPPs of frog and rat muscles without affecting the resting membrane potential (EXCELL and PATEL, 1972; PATEL and EXCELL, 1975). As judged from the rapidity of effect in blocking MEPPs, these fractions are likely acting at the postsynaptic site. One other fraction depolarizes the muscle quickly and has local necrotic effect (DUCHEN et al., 1974) like cardiotoxin of cobra venom. The mamba venom is thus similar in its pharmacologic action to that of cobra venom. Two toxins having 72 amino acids with the sequences similar to other postsynaptic toxins have been isolated from the venom of black mamba *(D. p. polylepis)* (STRYDOM, 1972).

2. Desert Cobra (Walterinnesia aegyptia) Venoms

The venom of the desert black snake produces muscular paralysis in mice like other elapid venoms (GITTER et al., 1962). The neuromuscular block is irreversible and has been attributed to a presynaptic effect by MOHAMED and ZAKI (1958) by experimenting with the isolated toad gastrocnemius preparation. The motor endplate was reported to remain sensitive to acetylcholine when neuromuscular block occurred. LEE et al. (1971a) and LEE and TSAI (1972) have repeated the experiment with isolated and in situ nerve-muscle preparations of the frog, chick, rat, and cat. They found, however, that the response to acetylcholine was always selectively blocked, whereas neither the release of acetylcholine nor the excitability of muscle was affected. Furthermore, all of the three toxins isolated from this venom (LEE et al., 1976b) act on the postsynaptic site. It is likely, therefore, that the presynaptic effect observed by MOHAMED and ZAKI (1958) is an artifact resulting from improper selection of the test preparation. No component acting like cardiotoxin can be found in this venom (LEE et al., 1976b).

3. Coral Snake (Micrurus) Venoms

The whole venoms of *M. fulvius* (WEIS and MCISAAC, 1971) and *M. lemniscatus* (VITAL-BRAZIL, 1972) depress the twitch response of the rat diaphragm elicited by indirect stimulation. The blocking effect of *M. lemniscatus* venom is not associated with contracture and direct inhibition of muscle and is slowly reversible on washout of the venom. On the other hand, the venom of *M. fulvius* causes depolarization of muscle and hyaline degeneration in the rat soleus (WEIS and MCISAAC, 1971), an effect closely similar to that of cobra cardiotoxin. A toxic fraction isolated from *M. fulvius* venom causes flaccid paralysis and neuromuscular blockade without depolarization of the chick muscle (SNYDER et al., 1973). The blocking effect on this muscle is irreversible but can be prevented by D-tubocurarine. It is evident, therefore, that the neuromuscular blockade by this toxin is due to an effect on the motor endplate acetylcholine receptor like other postsynaptic toxins. No toxic fraction acting by inhibition of transmitter release has been isolated. The coral snake venom is thus similar to cobra venom in its pharmacologic action.

VI. Sea Snake Venoms

That the paralysis of skeletal muscle by sea snake venoms is due primarily to the blockade of neuromuscular transmission is beyond doubt from the experiments by KELLAWAY et al. (1932), CAREY and WRIGHT (1960a, b, 1961, 1962), and CHEYMOL et al. (1966a, 1967b, 1969a, 1972c). The blockade of neuromuscular transmission is of a postsynaptic type (CHEYMOL et al., 1967b, 1969a, 1972c) since the response to acetylcholine is blocked but no effect on the release of transmitter from the nerve terminal can be found. The inference that the whole venom of *Enhydrina schistosa* acts on the presynaptic site in cat muscle on the basis of its blockade of acetylcholine response

(CHAN and GEH, 1967; GEH and CHAN, 1973) is untenable based upon the current view of neuromuscular transmission. The impulse conduction in nerve and muscle is not affected. Exceptionally, with high doses of *E. schistosa* venom, permanent damage of muscle may develop after neuromuscular blockade (CAREY and WRIGHT, 1961). This venom also causes focal necrosis of skeletal muscle in human (MARSDEN and REID, 1961).

The purified toxins, erabutoxin a and b, isolated from the venom of *Laticauda semifasciata* have been also shown to act on and bind specifically with the acetylcholine receptor of motor endplate (SATO et al., 1970; CHEYMOL et al., 1972c). Some controversial observations and conclusions, however, have been reported on erabutoxin a and b. TAKAMIZAWA (1970) reported that, in contrast to the results of CHEYMOL et al. (1972c), the irritability, the tension development in response to direct stimulation, and action potentials of frog muscles were depressed by erabutoxin b. In addition, both erabutoxin a (SCHWAB and PUFFER, 1976) and erabutoxin b (TAKAMIZAWA, 1970) were reported to block the release of transmitter. Although no proper explanation can be offered for these controversial findings, they seem unlikely in view of the recent knowledge on the postsynaptic toxins. In contrast to all other postsynaptic toxins of elapid and sea snake venoms, two toxins isolated from *E. schistosa* venom are unique in that they each have one free sulfhydryl group in their molecules (TU and TOOM, 1971; KARLSSON et al., 1972a). It would not be surprising, in this regard, if these *Enhydrina* toxins have some particular pharmacologic actions not shared by others. Quite recently, GEH and TOH (1976) observed that the neurotoxins isolated from this venom caused some damage of mitochondria in the nerve terminal of guinea pig diaphragm. Since the phospholipase A fraction of the same venom is very potent in causing structural changes of mitochondria in the nerve terminal (GEH and TOH, 1976), the possibility remains that the presynaptic effect of *Enhydrina* neurotoxins may be due to a contamination from phospholipase A. The same may also apply to the presynaptic effect reported for erabutoxin a and b.

Recently, MAEDA et al. (1974) and MAEDA and TAMIYA (1974) isolated another toxin containing 66 amino acid residues from the *L. semifasciata* venom besides erabutoxin a, b, and c. This toxin acts on the postsynaptic site but is different from erabutoxins in being much less potent, and the action on neuromuscular transmission is reversible including the chick biventer cervicis muscle on which all other postsynaptic toxins act irreversibly (LEE et al., 1972a; LEE and CHEN, 1976).

VII. Viperid and Crotalid Venoms

In accordance with the cause of toxicity as mentioned previously (Sect. C.VI), most of these two groups of venoms do not have a specific blocking effect on neuromuscular transmission (ROGERS, 1905; ARTHUS, 1911; HOUSSAY and PAVE, 1922; KELLAWAY and HOLDEN, 1932; KELLAWAY et al., 1932; CHEYMOL et al., 1968, 1972a), except the venom of the South American rattlesnake which will be dealt with in detail in the next section. HOUSSAY and PAVE (1922) and KELLAWAY and HOLDEN (1932) noted a weak curarizing action in the venom of *Echis carinatus*. It was later determined that the venom from Ethiopia but not that from Pakistan has a blocking effect at the level of postsynaptic receptors in the isolated or in situ nerve-muscle preparation (CHEY-

MOL et al., 1971c, 1973a) as do the postsynaptic toxins of elapid and sea snake venoms. DETRAIT et al. (1960) and BOQUET et al. (1969) found that the neurotoxic fraction of the Ethiopian venom is related antigenically to the postsynaptic toxins of *N. naja* and *N. nigricollis* venoms. The possibility of contamination of *E. carinatus* venom obtained in Ethiopia with that of *N. nigricollis* abundant in this area, must be ruled out before one can conclude that a postsynaptic toxin is also contained in this viperid venom. A "curare-like" effect has also been reported for the venom of *Agkistrodon piscivorus* (BROWN, 1941), a toxin from the venom of *Bitis atropos* (CHRISTENSEN, 1968), and some other viperid venoms (RUSSELL and LONG, 1961). Unfortunately, no further study on the mode of neuromuscular blocking action or isolation of the active principle has been carried out. The basic toxin isolated from the venom of *Crotalus admanteus* (BONILLA et al., 1970; BONILLA and FIERO, 1971) is apparently similar to crotamine of *C. durissus terrificus* venom which has predominant action on muscle fibers (CHEYMOL et al., 1969b), except the nerve in the baby chick muscle (LEE et al., 1972c) and will be discussed in Section E.V.

1. Rattlesnake Venoms

The venom of the South American rattlesnake *(C. durissus terrificus)* is much more toxic than other viperid and crotalid venoms by causing respiratory paralysis of peripheral origin (HOUSSAY and PAVE, 1922) although the venom may also have a central effect as shown in cross-circulation experiments (HOUSSAY and HUG, 1928). A highly potent neurotoxin, crotoxin, is contained in this venom (SLOTTA and FRAENKEL-CONRAT, 1938). There are two types of venoms produced by this species, one yellowish in color, containing crotamine, and the other nearly whitish without crotamine, according to their geographic distribution in South America (VELLARD, 1939; MOUSSATCHÉ et al., 1956; SCHENBERG, 1959). When injected into rats and mice, the crotamine-positive venom produces muscular spasm and tonic convulsion before the onset of paralysis, while the crotamine-negative venom produces hypotonia and paralysis without spasm and convulsion (BARRIO and VITAL BRAZIL, 1951; CHEYMOL et al., 1969b). The paralysis in rats by the whole venom was believed to be a result of direct action on the muscle rather than a neuromuscular blockade (CHEYMOL et al., 1969b, 1971a, b). The neuromuscular transmission of the rat muscle is extremely resistant to crotoxin both in vivo and in vitro (CHANG and LEE, 1977). On the other hand, the neuromuscular block in cats by the whole venom is associated with a slight depression of acetylcholine response (CHEYMOL et al., 1969b). The mode of neuromuscular block by the whole venom has not been further studied. However, based on the mode of action of crotoxin (see Sect. D.VII.2), the primary effect is likely the presynaptic inhibition of transmitter release of respiratory muscle rather than a postsynaptic one. The toxin responsible for the muscular spasm and tonic convulsion has been isolated and identified with crotamine by MOUSSATCHÉ et al. (1956) and CHEYMOL et al. (1971a, b).

2. Crotoxin

The neuromuscular blocking action of crotoxin has been demonstrated clearly in various animals (VITAL BRAZIL, 1966; BREITHAUPT, 1976; CHANG and LEE, 1977). In the depressed preparations, the Wedensky inhibition and posttetanic potentiation are evident as observed in the preparation treated with β-bungarotoxin (CHANG and

LEE, 1963). VITAL BRAZIL (1966, 1972) inferred, however, that the neuromuscular blockade by crotoxin is postsynaptic on the basis that the acetylcholine dose-response curve of denervated rat diaphragm was shifted to the right without simultaneous inhibition of K^+ response. It is to be noted in this respect that the acetylcholine receptors on the denervated rat diaphragm are so vulnerable to repeated application of acetylcholine that VITAL BRAZIL'S result could be due to such desensitization. In the frog sartorius muscle, however, the sensitivity of endplate to acetylcholine is not changed and an inhibition of the release of acetylcholine is noted (VITAL BRAZIL and EXCELL, 1971). The frequency of MEPPs is first increased and then decreased, but their amplitudes are not reduced. Occasionally, giant spontaneous EPPs and explosive bursts of MEPPs are observed. There is no doubt that crotoxin acts on the presynaptic site, at least, in the frog muscle. After the transmission is blocked with crotoxin, high K^+ produces a fall in frequency of MEPPs instead of an increase as seen in normal muscle. This may suggest that the depolarization-secretion coupling mechanism is affected by crotoxin or that the transmitter is depleted. In view of its contradictory results concerning the action of crotoxin, the neuromuscular blocking action of crotoxin was reexamined in various species of animals (CHANG and LEE, 1977). In all of the animals tested, including the mouse, rat, cat, and chick, the response of acetylcholine receptors is not affected, whereas the quantal contents of EPPs are always depressed. These results clearly indicate that crotoxin is a presynaptic toxin just like β-bungarotoxin. Kinetic studies also revealed that the toxin is first bound to the target site in the nerve terminal and then causes change of the nerve terminal which results in the failure of the release mechanism. Although not as marked as in the case with β-bungarotoxin, an initial facilitatory effect on the release of transmitter is also noted. Increase of Mg^{2+} concentration, omission of Ca^{2+} or decrease of nerve activity all slow down the inhibitory effect of crotoxin. The mitochondria of the nerve terminal of a mouse killed by crotoxin also show marked swelling and a decrease in the number of synaptic vesicles is evident (TSAI, unpublished). The effect of crotoxin is thus very close to that of β-bungarotoxin. The rat muscle is extremely resistant to crotoxin, whereas the chick muscle is very sensitive (VITAL BRAZIL et al., 1966; CHANG and LEE, 1977).

Crotoxin is composed of two components, an acidic molecule called crotapotin and a basic phospholipase A (RÜBSAMEN et al., 1971; BREITHAUPT et al., 1974, 1975; HENDON and FRAENKEL-CONRAT, 1971). Crotactin previously isolated from crotoxin (NEUMANN and HABERMANN, 1955; HABERMANN, 1957) was once thought to be the active component of crotoxin, but is now regarded to be a mixture of crotapotin with small amount of phospholipase A (RÜBSAMEN et al., 1971). Crotapotin alone is not toxic and does not have any neuromuscular blocking activity (VITAL BRAZIL et al., 1973a). The toxicity as well as the neuromuscular blocking activity of the enzyme is greatly potentiated by crotapotin, whereas the enzyme activity is either reduced or unaffected (RÜBSAMEN et al., 1971; HENDON and FRAENKEL-CONRAT, 1971; VITAL BRAZIL et al., 1973a; BREITHAUPT, 1976; BREITHAUPT et al., 1975; CHANG and LEE, unpublished).

3. Mojave Toxin

A highly lethal acidic toxin, mojave toxin, has been isolated from the venom of the Mojave rattlesnake (*Crotalus scutulatus*) (BIEBER et al., 1975). Mojave toxin was classified as cardiotoxin because a change of EKG was observed in rabbits. However, since the respiration is eventually paralyzed and the heart continues to beat on artificial respiration, the possibility that this toxin is a neurotoxin resembling crotoxin, which is also acidic, can't be ruled out. In fact, the crude Mojave rattlesnake venom exhibits a strong presynaptic neuromuscular blocking action just like the Brazilian rattlesnake venom (HSÜ and CHANG, unpublished).

VIII. Postsynaptic Toxins, Specificity and Reversibility of Action

1. Specificity and Reversibility

Postsynaptic toxins of elapid and sea snake venoms are unique in that no similar toxin has been found in the venoms of other origins, such as scorpion, spider, bee, and frog, and no enzymic action can be found in this group of protein toxins. According to the length of their peptide chain, these toxins have been classified into two subgroups (LEE, 1972, 1973; STRYDOM, 1973; YANG, 1974). The first group is the short-chain toxins which are composed of 60–62 residues of amino acids in a single peptide chain cross-linked by four disulfides. Some cobra toxins and all of the sea snake neurotoxins belong to this group. The second group is the long-chain toxins which consist of 71–73 amino acid residues from cobra venoms or 74 residues from krait venom in a single chain cross-linked by five disulfides. These two groups of toxins have different affinity and reversibility to acetylcholine receptors of motor endplate of various species of animals (LEE et al., 1972; BURDEN et al., 1975; LEE and CHEN, 1976). As summarized in Table 3, the short-chain toxins such as cobrotoxin and erabutoxin b are less potent on kitten diaphragms than on the muscle of rats and very weak or inactive against the sartorius muscle of *Rana tigrina* though the same muscle from *R. narina* and *R. plancyi* are quite sensitive. Their neuromuscular blocking action is reversible when the toxin is removed by repetitive washing except in the case with *R. plancyi* and baby chick muscles. On the other hand, the effects of the long-chain toxins are generally less reversible, α-bungarotoxin being the most irreversible one. Although the acetylcholine receptors of skeletal muscle from some lizards (*Gekkota* and *Iguania*) are as sensitive as that of *R. pipiens* to both α-

Table 3. The neuromuscular blocking activity of postsynaptic toxins on various nerve-muscle preparation and the reversibility. Concentrations (μg/ml) of these toxins to cause complete neuromuscular blockade in 50 min are calculated from the figures in LEE et al. (1972) and LEE and CHEN (1976) by interpolation. The reversibility is shown in the bracket as the time in min to attain 50% restoration of neuromuscular transmission after complete paralysis and subsequent removal of the toxin. *i* indicates the block is irreversible

Nerve-muscle preparations	α-Bungarotoxin	Toxin A	Cobrotoxin	Erabutoxin b
Rat diaphragm	2.22 *i*	1.72 *i*	0.49 (208)	0.81 (136)
Kitten diaphragm	0.59 *i*	0.83 (143)	1.20 (77)	3.0 (23)
Frog sartorius				
Rana tigrina	4.82 *i*	8.05 (164)	11.6 (14)	100<
Rana narina	0.56 *i*	1.0 *i*	0.37 (226)	0.69 (143)
Rana plancyi	0.48 *i*	0.48 *i*	0.30 *i*	0.36 *i*
Chick biventer cervicis	0.29 *i*	0.35 *i*	0.14 *i*	0.19 *i*

bungarotoxin and cobrotoxin, some others *(Scincomorpha)* are sensitive only to α-bungarotoxin and still others *(Anguinomorpha)* are resistant to both α-bungarotoxin and cobrotoxin with at least three orders of magnitude lower affinity (BURDEN et al., 1975). The skeletal acetylcholine receptors of snakes are either sensitive only to α-bungarotoxin as *Henophidea* or to neither toxins as *Caenophidea.* These results indicate that α-bungarotoxin has more general affinity to skeletal acetylcholine receptors than the short toxins. BURDEN et al. (1975) believed that the resistance evolved phylogenetically before the appearance of postsynaptic toxins.

Since postsynaptic toxins do not have any pharmacologic effect on the smooth muscle of intestine and blood vessels and cardiac muscle, it is obvious that the muscarinic acetylcholine receptors are not affected by these toxins. The higher distribution of α-bungarotoxin or cobrotoxin in these tissues than in skeletal muscles (LEE and TSENG, 1966; TSENG et al., 1968) suggests the nonspecific binding in these tissues and cautions against the indiscriminative use of these toxins as a receptor probe.

The ganglionic transmission in cats is not blocked by purified postsynaptic toxins (CHOU and LEE, 1969; LEE and LEE, unpublished) although its acetylcholine receptors are classified as nicotinic and closer to the endplate receptors than the muscarinic one. On the other hand, the paravertebral sympathetic ganglia from chick embryo grown in a tissue culture appear to bind specifically with I^{125} α-bungarotoxin (GREEN et al., 1973). It will be of interest to see whether this is due to a species difference or to the change of the receptor structure during development. Interestingly, although the excitation of Renshaw cell in the spinal cord of frogs and mammal by acetylcholine are not blocked by cobrotoxin and α-bungarotoxin (MILEDI and SZCZEPANIAK, 1975; DUGGAN et al., 1976), both the short-chain and long-chain neurotoxins isolated from *Dendroaspis* venom are active blockers of the frog cord preparation (BANKS et al., 1976). These results suggest that the nicotinic receptors in the central nervous system have binding characteristics different from those of endplate. The binding of α-bungarotoxin with brain structures (MOORE and LOY, 1972; SALVATERRA and MOORE, 1973; SALVATERRA et al., 1975; ETEROVIC and BENNETT, 1974; POLZ-TEJERA et al., 1975), therefore, does not provide definitive evidence for the existence of nicotinic receptors in the brain until the pharmacologic actions of these toxins in the central nervous system are clarified. Indeed, the binding of α-bungarotoxin in the brain has been shown to be mostly nonspecific (SCHLEIFER and ELDEFRAWI, 1974). The specific binding of postsynaptic toxins to the acetylcholine receptors in electroplax of electric eel and torpedo is accompanied with functional blockade of transmission (CHANGEUX et al., 1970).

2. Comparison with D-Tubocurarine

In spite of the complex peptide nature, it is striking that the neuromuscular blocking action of postsynaptic toxins mimicks closely that of D-tubocurarine except that the onset of action is slower and temperature dependent (VYSKOČIL and MAGAZANIK, 1972a). After binding, the dissociation is much slower than that of D-tubocurarine though no covalent bond is formed between the toxins and the acetylcholine receptors. The snake toxins are, however, more specific in their action on the endplate since other nicotinic receptors in the autonomic ganglia and central nervous system are not affected (CHOU and LEE, 1969; MILEDI and SZCZEPANIAK, 1975; DUGGAN et al., 1976). Although the response of skeletal muscle to nerve stimulation, which involves the junctional receptor, and that to extrinsic acetylcholine, which involves the extrajunctional receptors (CHANG and TANG, 1974; CHANG and SU, 1975), are equally depressed by D-tubocurarine (DEL CASTILLO and KATZ, 1957), α-bungarotoxin blocks the response to extrinsic acetylcholine more rapidly than that to nerve stimulation in the frog and chick muscles (MAGAZANIK and VYSKOČIL, 1972a; CHANG and TANG, 1974), indicating that extrajunctional receptors may have higher affinity with the snake toxins than the junctional receptors.

VYSKOČIL and MAGAZANIK (1972b) found that the desensitization of the receptor by acetylcholine is accelerated by α-bungarotoxin applied electrophoretically on the endplate either from outside or inside of the sarcolemma but not by intracellular D-tubocurarine. It is inferred that α-bungarotoxin may have some additional action besides the binding with the acetylcholine receptors. Unlike the case with D-tubocurarine, the endplate reversal potential was found to be stabilized by the toxin and not influenced by the change of K^+ concentration (MAGAZANIK and VYSKOČIL, 1972b). These findings are so important in view of the relevance to the nature of the action of snake toxins that more evidence is needed to settle the problem. Based on the observation that the binding of labeled α-bungarotoxin with the endplate receptors can be best protected by D-tubocurarine up to 50–60% (MILEDI and POTTER, 1971; ALBUQUERQUE et al., 1973; PORTER et al., 1973) and can be further protected by histrionicotoxin (ALBUQUERQUE et al., 1973), presumably a binding agent with the ion conductance modulator, it is suggested that α-bungarotoxin binds with two sites, one which also binds with D-tubocurarine and the other with the ionophore. On the other hand, much higher protection of toxin binding by D-tubocurarine was obtained by other workers (VOGEL et al., 1972; CHANG et al., 1973a; ETEROVIČ and BENNETT, 1974; COLQUHOUN et al., 1974; DOLLY et al., 1975), indicating that the binding sites are homologous with respect to binding with α-bungarotoxin and D-tubocurarine. It is worth noting in this respect that α-bungarotoxin, like D-tubocurarine, causes no change of the spectral distribution, size, and the time-course of the elementary conductance change of the acetylcholine receptor but only a decrease of the number of the ion gate opened by acetylcholine (KATZ and MILEDI, 1973). This finding does not seem to support a pharmacologic action of postsynaptic toxins on the ionophore.

IX. Comparison of Presynaptic Toxins

1. Pharmacologic Considerations

In contrast to the universal presence of postsynaptic toxins in the venoms of elapid and sea snakes, neurotoxins acting specifically on the motor nerve terminal have been found only in the venoms of *Bungarus multicinctus* (β-bungarotoxin) (CHANG and LEE, 1963; CHANG et al., 1973b), *B. caeruleus* (LEE et al., 1976c), *Notechis scutatus* (notexin) (KARLSSON et al., 1972a; HARRIS et al., 1973), and *Oxyuranus scutellatus* (taipoxin) (KAMENSKAYA and THESLEFF, 1974; CULL-CANDY et al., 1976) of *Elapidae* and *Crotalus durissus terrificus* (crotoxin) (VITAL BRAZIL and EXCELL, 1971; CHANG and LEE, 1977) of *Crotalidae*. The presynaptic toxins are usually more toxic than the

Table 4. Toxicity of postsynaptic toxins and presynaptic toxins in the mouse and pigeon

Toxin	Snake origin	LD_{50} (mg/kg) Mouse	LD_{50} (mg/kg) Pigeon	Toxicity ratio pigeon/mouse
Postsynaptic toxins				
α-Bungarotoxin	*Bungarus multicinctus*	0.21 s.c.[a]	0.055 i.m.[b]	3.8
Cobrotoxin	*Naja naja atra*	0.091 s.c.[c]	0.057 i.m.[b]	1.6
Other toxins	*Elapidae* and *Hydrophiidae*	0.05–0.15[d]		
Presynaptic toxins				
β-Bungarotoxin	*Bungarus multicinctus*	0.040 s.c.[a]	0.00035 i.m.[b]	115
Crotoxin	*Crotalus durissus terrificus*	0.178 s.c.[e] 0.082 i.v.[e] 0.052 i.p.[f]	0.0022 i.v.[e]	81
Notexin	*Notechis scutatus scutatus*	0.017 i.v.[g]		
Taipoxin	*Oxyuranus scutellatus*	0.0021 i.v.[g]		

[a] LEE et al. (1972).
[b] LEE and TSENG (1969).
[c] SU et al. (1967).
[d] YANG (1974).
[e] VITAL BRAZIL et al. (1966).
[f] CHANG and LEE (1977).
[g] CULL-CANDY et al. (1976).

postsynaptic toxins (Table 4). Pigeons, chicks, and their isolated nerve-muscle preparations are much more sensitive than mice to β-bungarotoxin (LEE and TSENG, 1969; CHANG and HUANG, 1974) and crotoxin (VITAL BRAZIL et al., 1966; CHANG and LEE, 1977) but not to notexin and taipoxin (CHANG et al., 1977). On the other hand, the rat is more resistant than other mammal to crotoxin (VITAL BRAZIL et al., 1966; CHANG and LEE, 1977) and taipoxin (CHANG et al., 1977).

β-bungarotoxin, crotoxin, notexin, and taipoxin share many pharmacologic actions. All of them decrease the frequency of MEPPs and the quantal contents of EPPs without significant reduction of the amplitude of MEPPs and the response to the transmitter. Other common characteristics include the long latency of onset of paralysis, appearance of bursts of MEPPs, continuous progress of inhibitory action after removal of the toxin, and acceleration or enhancement of blocking action by nerve impulses. Ultrastructural changes of motor nerve terminals induced by these toxins are also identic in that the number of Ω-shaped indentations at the axolemma is increased, the number of synaptic vesicles is decreased, the electron density of axoplasma is increased, and mitochondria are swollen. The decrease of synaptic vesicles may be due to an inhibition of the recycling of membrane as suggested by CULL-CANDY et al. (1976) for notexin and taipoxin. There is reason to believe, however, that this is not the primary action of presynaptic block by this group of toxins since, when inhibition of transmitter release is just completed after treatment with β-bungarotoxin, there is still no change of ultrastructure (TSAI, 1975). As discussed in Section D.III.5.c, the depletion of synaptic vesicles may be regarded as an advanced effect of these toxins. Although studied only with β-bungarotoxin, taipoxin, and crotoxin, it also seems common that the inhibitory action is slowed down in the presence of a high concentration of Mg^{2+} which decreases the release of neurotransmitter. In mice, the diaphragm is paralyzed much earlier than other muscles probably because of the high rate of nerve impulses. The inhibitory effects of β-bungaro-

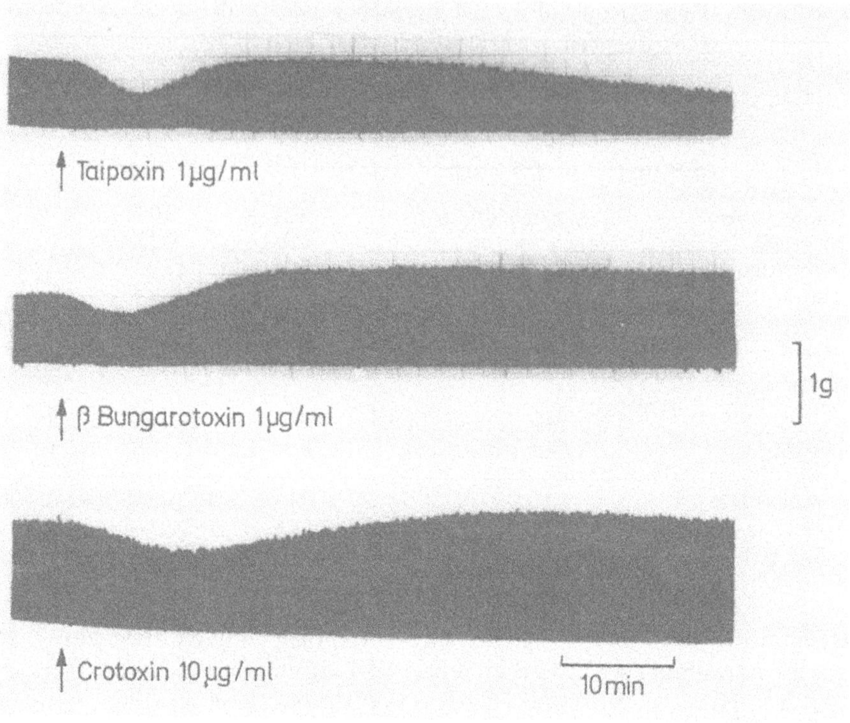

Fig. 3. Immediate effects of presynaptic toxins on the neuromuscular transmission in Sr^{2+}. The mouse phrenic nerve diaphragm preparations in Sr^{2+}-Tyrode. Indirect stimulations at 0.1 Hz

toxin, taipoxin, and crotoxin on the diaphragm of rats and mice (CHANG et al., 1973b; CHANG and HUANG, 1974; KELLY and BROWN, 1974; CHANG and LEE, 1977; CHANG et al., 1977) or on the frog sartorius (VITAL BRAZIL and EXCELL, 1971; ALDERICE and VOLLE, 1975) are all preceded by an initial facilitation of transmitter release as revealed by an increase of the frequency of MEPPs and the quantal contents of EPPs. As manifested in the frog or mammalian nerve-muscle preparations immersed in a low Ca^{2+}- or Sr^{2+}-medium (Fig. 3), the initial facilitation of these toxins is still preceded by an immediate but transient depressant effect (ABE et al., 1976; CHANG and LEE, 1977; CHANG et al., 1977). By contrast, no initial facilitation was noted with notexin in a mouse muscle (HARRIS et al., 1973; CULL-CANDY et al., 1976; CHANG and SU, unpublished). DATYNER and GAGE (1973), however, were aware of such facilitation in frogs using the whole venom of tiger snake which contains notexin. It remains to be elucidated whether the difference between the action of notexin and that of others is due to the different chemical natures of these toxins. Notexin is a basic phospholipase A, whereas the remaining three presynaptic toxins are composed of other subunits in addition to the enzyme unit (see Chap. 5). It is likely, therefore, that the initial facilitatory effect is not a prerequisite for the presynaptic inhibitory effect of presynaptic toxins and may be due directly to the binding of these complex toxins with the terminal axolemma rather than to the enzyme action. On the other hand, the presynaptic inhibitory effect of black widow spider venom seems to be causally related with its initial facilitation. There is another marked difference between notexin and other presynaptic toxins. When left in contact with the muscle for a prolonged period, notexin causes direct myotoxic effect in vivo (HARRIS et al., 1973, 1975) and in vitro (LEE et al., 1976a).

High concentration of K^+ is still able to increase the frequency of MEPPs in the diaphragm of mice or rats immediately after blockade of neuromuscular transmission treated in vitro with β-bungarotoxin (CHANG et al., 1973b), crotoxin (CHANG and LEE, 1977), or taipoxin (CHANG et al., 1977) though not as marked as in the normal diaphragm. By contrast, K^+ has no effect on the muscle treated in vivo with notexin and taipoxin (HARRIS et al., 1973; KAMENKAYA and THESLEFF, 1974). At an advanced stage of toxic effect, however, it is likely that no increase of MEPP can be induced by K^+ since all of these presynaptic toxins deplete the synaptic vesicles eventually.

2. The Relation with Phospholipase A

There have been arguments on whether the lethal effect of snake venom neurotoxins is related in any way to the phospholipase A of the venom since the first isolation of crystalline crotoxin from the tropical rattlesnake venom by SLOTTA and FRAENKEL-CONRAT (1938) who showed that the enzyme activity was not separable from the toxic effect. Subsequent success in separating the enzyme activity from the postsynaptic toxins of elapid and sea snake venoms seems to settle this argument. This question was raised again, however, when all of the four presynaptic toxins of snake venoms were shown to have some phospholipase A activity (WERNICKE et al., 1975; STRONG et al., 1976; RÜBSAMEN et al., 1971; HENDON et al., 1971; EAKER, 1974, 1976; HALPERT et al., 1976). Interestingly, the amino acid sequences of notexin (HALPERT and EAKER, 1975), taipoxin (FOHLMAN et al., 1976), and β-bungarotoxin (NARITA, personal communication) show some homology with those of phospholipase A isolated from *N. nigricollis* venom and porcine pancreatic phospholipase A (see Chap. 5). EAKER (1974, 1976) has suggested that these snake venom presynaptic toxins may be derived from the enzyme during evolution and act by the enzyme action. It will be of interest to see whether other purified phospholipase A, especially those from snake venoms, have any presynaptic inhibitory effect. There is a great difference in toxicity among various phospholipase A obtained from snake venoms (see Chap. 12). The enzyme activity of the presynaptic toxins is usually less potent in comparison with that of less toxic phospholipase A (EAKER, 1974; WERNICKE et al., 1975; STRONG et al., 1976a; HENDON et al., 1971; RÜBSAMEN et al., 1971). Moreover, the enzyme activity of phospholipase A of crotoxin is reduced when coupled with crotapotin while the toxicity increases. This result, however, cannot be taken as evidence against the hypothesis that the presynaptic toxins act by the enzyme action since the enzymic activity is dependent on the physical state of the substrate (STRONG et al., 1976a), and the toxins may have preferential enzymic activity on the phospholipid of nerve terminals. It is not even known whether the toxins act from outside or inside of the axolemma. Therefore, crotapotin in crotoxin, although it depresses the enzyme activity of the phospholipase A component when measured with isolated substrate, may, on the contrary, increase its enzyme activity on the phospholipid of the nerve terminal. It is highly possible that the subunits of complex presynaptic toxins may provide the specificity and increase affinity of the protein molecules to the nerve terminal.

So far, however, no convincing evidence has been obtained showing that the presynaptic toxins indeed act by enzyme action. Ca^{2+} is essential for the enzyme action of phospholipase A from various sources (WELLS, 1972; PIETERSON et al., 1974), including that of β-bungarotoxin (STRONG et al., 1976a), and changes the conformation of notexin (HALPERT et al., 1976), β-bungarotoxin (CHANG and SU, unpublished), and phospholipase A of *C. adamanteus* venom (WELLS, 1973). Interestingly, lower Ca^{2+} or absence of Ca^{2+} in the bathing media decreases the presynaptic action of β-bungarotoxin (CHANG et al., 1973b; CHANG and HUANG, 1974), crotoxin (CHANG and LEE, 1977), and taipoxin (CHANG et al., 1977). On the other hand, Mg^{2+}, though not an inhibitor of phospholipase A (WELLS, 1973), also antagonizes the presynaptic action of these toxins. It is thus unlikely that these cations interfere with the neuromuscular blocking action of presynaptic toxins by a direct effect on their enzyme activity. When Ca^{2+} is replaced with Sr^{2+}, the enzyme activity of β-bungarotoxin is almost completely inhibited, and the decrease of frequency of MEPPs by the toxin is also reduced. Basing on these finding, STRONG et al. (1976a) inferred that the enzymic hydrolysis of phospholipid is essential for the presynaptic action. The antagonistic effect of Sr^{2+} and Mg^{2+} and the synergistic effect of nerve activity on the inhibitory action of presynaptic toxins could be related in some way to the concentration of Ca^{2+} in the axoplasm. Mg^{2+}, by competing with the influx of Ca^{2+} and Sr^{2+}, by substituting for Ca^{2+}, may abolish the Ca^{2+} influx and thereby decrease the axoplasmic Ca^{2+} concentration. In support of this inference is the decreased effectiveness of nerve activity to enhance the action of these presynaptic toxin when Sr^{2+} is substituted for Ca^{2+} in the bathing media (CHANG and SU, in preparation). It is thus likely that the effect of presynaptic toxins is dependent on the axoplasmic Ca^{2+}. It remains to be elucidated whether the intraneuronal Ca^{2+} enhances the presynaptic effect by increasing enzyme activity or by a yet unknown mechanism not related to enzymic action. The inhibition of acetylcholine release by a Ca^{2+} ionophore (X-537A) has been attributed to an accumulation of intraneuronal Ca^{2+} (KITA and VAN DER KLOOT, 1976). It is also inferred that β-bungarotoxin might have a similar effect (ABE et al., 1976). It is worthy to note that the patients bitten by snakes which produce presynaptic toxins do not respond to antivenin and the paralysis continues to progress (CAMPBELL, 1975; ROSENFELD, 1971). This clinical situation may suggest the possibility that the toxins might act intraneuronally.

3. Presynaptic Toxins of Other Origins

Microbial toxins from *Clostridium botulinus* and *C. tetani* and the venoms of black and brown widow spiders *(Latrodectus mactaus, L. geometricus)* also affect the presynaptic site of a nerve-muscle preparation. Botulinum toxin (AMBACHE, 1949; BURGEN et al., 1949; HARRIS and MILEDI, 1971; BROOKS, 1956; HUGHES and WHALER, 1962; SIMPSON, 1971, 1973, 1974; CHANG and HUANG, 1974; BOROFF et al., 1974; KAO et al., 1976) and tetanus toxin (DUCHEN and TONGE, 1973; DUCHEN, 1973; MELLANBY, 1971; KRYZHANOVSKY, 1973) act like the presynaptic toxins of snake venoms by inhibiting the release of acetylcholine. As in the case with β-bungarotoxin, the successive EPPs on repetitive stimulation are well-maintained though at a depressed level of quantal contents (Fig. 2), suggesting that the excitation-secretion coupling is depressed rather than any inhibitory effect on the formation and storage of the transmitter. On the basis of interactions between botulinum toxin and Ca^{2+} ionophores or black widow spider venom, it was proposed that the toxin interferes with the acetylcholine release process itself but not with the Ca^{2+} entry (KAO et al., 1976). The microbial toxins, however, block the release of transmitter with neither initial facilitation (BROOKS, 1956; SPITZER, 1972; CHANG and HUANG, 1974) nor ultrastructural change of the nerve terminals (THESLEFF, 1960; ZACKS et al., 1962; DUCHEN, 1971, 1973; KRYZHANOVSKY, 1973). No Wedensky inhibition and posttetanic potentiation are observed (Fig. 1). Nevertheless, botulinum toxin and snake venom presynaptic toxins have many characteristics in common. Both toxins are bound to the nerve terminal first and then exhibit their inhibitory action progressively even after subsequent washout. The latter phase of action is accelerated by increasing nerve activity but is delayed by a decrease of temperature, decrease of Ca^{2+}, or an increase of Mg^{2+} concentration (SIMPSON, 1973; CHANG and HUANG, 1974). Botulinum and tetanus toxins, however, also affect other peripheral synaptic transmission including adrenergic neurons and ganglia (AMBACHE, 1951, 1952; KUPFER, 1958; HOLMAN and SPITZER, 1973; OSBORNE and BRADFORD, 1973; KRYZHANOVSKY, 1973) if a sufficient concentration of the toxin is used.

Unlike the snake venom presynaptic toxins, the black and brown spider venoms also act on other types of nerve terminals. The junctions in vertebrate skeletal muscle (OKAMOTO et al., 1971; LONGENECKER et al., 1970; CLARK et al., 1972; DEL CASTILLO and PAMPLIN, 1975), torpedo electric tissue (GRANATA et al., 1974), smooth muscle (FRONTALI, 1972; FRONTALI et al., 1973; EINHORN and HAMILTON, 1973), cerebral cortex slices (FRONTALI et al., 1972), and lobster neuromuscular junction (KAWAI et al., 1972) are all affected. Generally, there is an initial facilitation of the release of neurotransmitter irrespective of the chemical nature, violent but paroxysmal bursts (up to 1000 Hz) of MEPPs, and a subsequent depression of release accompanied by depletion of the synaptic vesicles (EINHORN and HAMILTON, 1973; OKAMOTO et al., 1971; CLARK et al., 1972; DEL CASTILLO and PAMPLIN, 1975). The purified toxin from a black widow spider venom was shown to have a strong affinity with an artificial lipid bilayer membrane and to increase selectively its permeability to alkali cations (FINKELSTEIN et al., 1976).

Scorpion venoms and the purified *Tityus* toxins also cause a release and depletion of acetylcholine as well as catecholamines from peripheral nerves and brain slices (MOSS et al., 1974; GOMEZ et al., 1973, 1975; TAZIEFF-DEPIERRE, 1972; TAZIEFF-DEPIERRE and ANDRILLON, 1973; DINIZ et al., 1974; LANGER et al., 1975; BLAUSTEIN, 1975; TAZIEFF-DEPIERRE and NACHON-RAUTUREAU, 1975). Apparently, there is no selectivity for the effect of scorpion venom on nerve terminals. The transmitter release may be first increased. Repetitive firing of the nerve after single stimulation and spontaneous twitchings occur in nerve-muscle preparations after treatment with scorpion venoms or *Tityus* toxins (KATZ and EDWARDS, 1972; VITAL BRAZIL et al., 1973b; LIN SHIAU et al., 1975c). Since the release of acetylcholine induced by scorpion venoms is blocked by tetrodotoxin (TAZIEFF-DEPIERRE and ANDRILLON, 1973), it is likely that the venom affects the exposed axonal membrane rather than nerve terminal per se. There are abundant observations that the axon membrane is indeed affected by the venom (NARAHASHI et al., 1972; ROMEY et al., 1975; CAHALAN, 1975;

WARNICK et al., 1976). Since the effect of scorpion venom is reduced if the Na^+ concentration is decreased, it is generally agreed that the venom modifies the Na^+ channel gating of axons. On the other hand, CHEYMOL et al. (1973b), LIN SHIAU et al. (1975c), and WARNICK et al. (1976) found that the venom of the North African scorpion and the isolated toxins also act on the muscle of rats and chickens by opening the Na^+ channel of the muscle membrane. In this regard, the scorpion venom may be better classified as a membrane toxin rather than a presynaptic toxin.

4. Mutual Antagonism Between Presynaptic Toxins

It is interesting from both the therapeutic and academic viewpoints that botulinum toxin shows mutual antagonism with β-bungarotoxin in vitro (CHANG et al., 1973c; CHANG and HUANG, 1974) and with spider venoms in vivo (STERN et al., 1974) or in vitro (KAO et al., 1976). In the isolated rat phrenic nerve-diaphragm preparation, the relative potency for neuromuscular block is reduced to less than 10% when botulinum toxin and β-bungarotoxin are added together. The antagonism occurs also when the microbial toxin is added after the preparation has been incubated with β-bungarotoxin for 30 min. This result indicates that even the venom toxin already fixed on the nerve terminal can be antagonized and that the mutual antagonism is not due to a simple chemical interaction between the two protein molecules. On the other hand, the action of botulinum toxin already bound cannot be abolished by subsequent administration of β-bungarotoxin. The binding sites for the microbial toxin and the venom toxin must be different or there would be no "mutual" antagonism. In the isolated mouse hemidiaphragm preparation pretreated with botulinum toxin and then treated with black widow spider venom, expansion and depletion of the synaptic vesicles were also present as in the preparation treated only with the venom; but in addition, clumping of vesicles at the release sites was commonly observed (KAO et al., 1976), suggesting that botulinum toxin interferes in some manner with the process of vesicle release caused by the spider venom. A further study of this antagonism may provide a clue to the presynaptic inhibitory action of these toxins.

E. Effects on Skeletal Muscle

A great variety of snake venoms have direct actions on skeletal muscle as revealed by twitching, contracture, depolarization, decrease of excitability, and necrosis. These effects have made the study of the neuromuscular blocking action of whole venom difficult and caused controversial findings in the old literature. BRUNTON and FAYRER, as early as 1873, noted that the irritability of the muscle to direct stimulation was reduced by cobra venom when curare-like action had appeared. The recognition of snake venoms as muscle poisons is largely due to the work of HOUSSAY et al. (1922), who in experiments with various snake venoms, found that the irritability of the frog muscle fell off greatly before curarization became complete. With higher concentrations of venoms, twitching and contracture were produced. They related these direct effects to the hemolytic activity of the venoms as determined by hemolysis of canine red corpuscles in the presence of homologous serum and showed that those venoms which were most active in these respects also caused the greatest imbibition of water by the frog muscle. It was suggested that phospholipase A might be responsible for the observed effects by hydrolysis of lipid constituents of the membrane. Studying a variety of Indian and Australian elapid venoms, KELLAWAY and HOLDEN (1932) confirmed the results of HOUSSAY et al. in general, except the tiger snake venom. This venom causes pronounced loss of irritability of mammalian muscle in vivo at low concentrations if sufficient time is allowed. The venom is only feebly hemolytic and causes very slight imbibition of water by isolated frog muscle. It is likely from these results that the muscle can be affected by various mechanisms. At least four constituents, such as cardiotoxins, crotamines, proteases, and phospholipase A, are now known to have an effect on the skeletal muscle.

I. Cobra, Mamba, and Coral Snake Venoms

Cobra venoms induce a sustained contracture of skeletal muscle which is not preventable by pretreatment with D-tubocurarine (SARKAR, 1951; SARKAR and MAITRE, 1950; PENG, 1951; SU, 1960; CHEYMOL et al., 1966a; SU et al., 1967). The resting membrane potential of the superficial muscle fiber of the isolated rat diaphragm and the frog sartorius is completely depolarized within 30 min by 10 μg/ml of cobra venom (MELDRUM, 1965b; CHANG and LEE, 1966; CHANG et al., 1972). The venoms of a coral snake (*Micrurus fulvius*) (WEIS and MCISAAC, 1971) and a mamba (*Dendroaspis jamesoni*) (EXCELL and PATEL, 1972) also cause marked depolarization and inhibit the excitability of skeletal muscle. These membrane-active principles are associated with the basic fractions of these venoms called cardiotoxins whereas the neurotoxins of these venoms are devoid of such membrane activity (CHANG and LEE, 1966; LEE et al., 1968; EARL and EXCELL, 1971, 1972; EXCELL and PATEL, 1972; CHANG et al., 1972; LESTER, 1970, 1972a; PATEL and EXCELL, 1975).

In addition to cardiotoxin, the phospholipase A fraction of cobra and bee venoms also depolarizes the muscle, but the action is slow and much less potent than the former (CHANG et al., 1972; ALBUQUERQUE and THESLEFF, 1968). A quantitative analysis shows that the depolarizing action of cobra venom is mostly due to the content of cardiotoxin, but phospholipase A may contribute to some extent by augmenting the action of cardiotoxin (CHANG et al., 1972). Among various cobra venoms studied, CHEYMOL et al. (1966a) found that the *N. nigricollis* venom exerted more direct effect than others.

1. Cardiotoxins—Membrane-Active Polypeptides

a) *Pharmacologic Effects*

Cardiotoxin, first isolated from the Indian cobra venom by SARKAR (1947) and so named because of its detrimental effect on the heart, has been shown, both pharmacologically and chemically, to be identic or closely related to the direct lytic factor (DLF) (CONDREA et al., 1964) which causes direct lysis of erythrocytes or cytotoxin (BRAGANCA et al., 1967) which attacks cancer cells (SLOTTA and VICK, 1969; MEL-

DRUM, 1965a; CONDREA et al., 1971; LEE et al., 1971c). All these toxins are highly basic polypeptides consisting of about 60 amino acid residues with four disulfide linkages in the molecules. Cobramine A and B of *N. naja* venom, and toxin γ of *N. nigricollis* venom also have similar chemical structures. In view of the generalized action on cell membranes of various tissues, the term "membrane-active polypeptides" was proposed by CONDREA (1974) to include all of these toxins. This term, however, is too long and not specific since there are other types of membrane-active polypeptides in snake venoms such as crotamine and phospholipase A. The term "cardiotoxin" is, therefore, retained because it was the first name proposed and represents the most important pharmacologic action when given to animals.

When a skeletal muscle is exposed to cardiotoxin (10–100 µg/ml), a slowly progressive contracture is evoked (SARKAR and MAITRE, 1950; SARKAR, 1951; LEE et al., 1968; TAZIEFF-DEPIERRE et al., 1969; LIN SHIAU et al., 1976) just like to the cobra venom. A maximum contracture is attained in several minutes to an hour and then the contracture wanes. The excitability of the muscle is abolished. The synaptic transmission is not affected until the excitability of the muscle declines (SARKAR and MAITRE, 1950; LEE et al., 1968). The nerve terminal spike of superficial fibers is also abolished after the blockade of the muscle (CHANG and LEE, 1966). The chick biventer cervicis muscle appears to be more vulnerable to cardiotoxin than the rat or frog muscle (LEE et al., 1968).

The acetylcholine receptor on the motor endplate seems not to be affected as judged from the unchanged binding of the rat diaphragm with labeled α-bungarotoxin even after treatment with a concentration as high as 100 µg/ml (CHANG and TUNG, unpublished). Acetylcholinesterase in the endplate membrane is not decreased (CHANG and SU, unpublished) though the purified enzyme in a solution of low ionic strength is inhibited by cardiotoxin (LEE et al., 1971b). The resting membrane potential of superficial muscle fibers of isolated muscle is rapidly decreased to nil at 10 µg/ml (CHANG and LEE, 1966; LEE et al., 1968; EARL and EXCELL, 1971, 1972; CHANG et al., 1972). The depolarization by cardiotoxin is, unlike that induced by cholinergic agents, not restricted to the endplate zone but is a generalized one along the whole length of muscle fiber. The propagation of action potential is retarded before the depolarization is complete. The plasma membrane of the superficial fibers appears to be rapidly disorganized. Fragmentation and vesiculation of the membrane is evident when depolarization is marked. The marked changes of composition of K^+, Na^+, and Ca^{2+} of the chick muscle treated with cardiotoxin for a prolonged time (LIN SHIAU et al., 1976) can be accounted for by the damage of membrane structure. The depolarization of deeper muscle occurs at a much slower rate, indicating that the penetration of cardiotoxin within the tissue is very much hindered.

Contracture can still be induced by cardiotoxin in a frog muscle depolarized by treating with high K^+ medium (SARKAR, 1951; LIN SHIAU et al., 1976). When the muscle membrane is removed by treating with 50% (≑7 M) glycerine, no contracture can be induced by cardiotoxin (SARKAR, 1951), but if treated with 0.8 M glycerine to disrupt only the excitation-contraction coupling, contractile response to cardiotoxin remains (LIN SHIAU et al., 1976). Actin and myosin still show precipitation on addition of adenosine triphosphate after treatment with cardiotoxin. These results together indicate that cardiotoxin induces depolarization and contracture of skeletal muscle by an effect on the membrane.

b) Antagonism by Ca^{2+} *and Other Cations*

The depolarization as well as contracture of skeletal muscle by cardiotoxin is completely prevented by increasing the Ca^{2+} concentration to 10 mM (TAZIEFF-DEPIERRE et al., 1969; EARL and EXCELL, 1971; CHANG et al., 1972; LIN SHIAU et al., 1976). After exposing the rat diaphragm to cardiotoxin (10 μg/ml) at 10 mM Ca^{2+} for 150 min, five times longer than that necessary to cause complete depolarization in normal Ca^{2+} medium (1.8 mM), no depolarization is induced when the toxin is washed out and the concentration of Ca^{2+} restored to normal (CHANG et al., 1972). It is likely that the binding of cardiotoxin to the muscle is curtailed in the presence of high Ca^{2+} concentration. By the use of ^{125}I cardiotoxin, the radioactivity retained by the chick biventer cervicis muscle is decreased by an increase of Ca^{2+} (LIN SHIAU et al., 1976). High Ca^{2+} concentration is also known to antagonize all of the pharmacologic effects of cardiotoxin, i.e., direct hemolytic action (LANKISCH et al., 1971), cytotoxic effect (PATEL et al., 1969; BOQUET, 1970; LEUNG et al., 1976), and depolarization of isolated cardiac muscle (HO et al., 1975). Administration of Ca^{2+} in vivo to rats also antagonizes the ventricular arrhythmia induced by this toxin (TAZIEFF-DEPIERRE et al., 1969; TAZIEFF-DEPIERRE and TRETHEVIE, 1975; TAZIEFF-DEPIERRE, 1975). Other cations, such as Mg^{2+}, Zn^{2+}, Mn^{2+}, and UO^{2+}, which are thought to bind with the Ca^{2+} binding site on the membrane (HAGIWARA and TAKAHASHI, 1967), are also antagonists of cardiotoxin contracture (LIN SHIAU et al., 1976). In view of this antagonism, TAZIEFF-DEPIERRE et al. (1969), EARL and EXCELL (1972), and LIN SHIAU et al. (1976) have inferred that the toxin exhibits its effect by depriving the membrane of Ca^{2+}, which has a role of stabilizing the membrane (MANERY, 1966). If deprivation of Ca^{2+} alone would result in such a marked and rapid depolarization of membrane and contracture of muscle, then one would expect that those cations except Ca^{2+} which compete at the Ca binding site with cardiotoxin should likewise result in contracture because of deprivation of membrane Ca. This, however, is not the case. The ineffectiveness of procaine to prevent the cardiotoxin contracture (TAZIEFF-DEPIERRE et al., 1969; LIN SHIAU et al., 1976) is also in conflict with the hypothesis since procaine also competes with the Ca^{2+} binding site on the membrane (BLAUSTEIN and GOLDMAN, 1966; SUAREZ-KURTZ et al., 1970).

Since at low concentrations of cardiotoxin, the membrane potential can be stabilized at a certain low level of depolarization without visible change of integrity of muscle fiber (EARL and EXCELL, 1972), an effect on ionic permeability seems to take place before the disorganization of the membrane. It is not possible to prevent either depolarization (EARL and EXCELL, 1972) or contracture (LIN SHIAU et al., 1976) induced by cardiotoxin by replacing Na^+ with choline or sucrose or by treatment with tetrodotoxin. It is thus unlikely that cardiotoxin acts by way of a specific increase of Na^+ permeability. The rapid depolarization by cardiotoxin also precludes the possibility of acting through the inhibition of the Na^+ pump. Cobramines, homologous to cardiotoxin, have been shown in many organs to inhibit the transport of various compounds against concentration gradient (LARSEN and WOLFF, 1967; WOLFF et al., 1968). It is concluded that the inhibition is due to the leakiness of the membrane. Similarly, efflux as well as influx of Ca^{2+} in skeletal muscle (TAZIEFF-

DEPIERRE et al., 1969; LIN SHIAU et al., 1976) and influx of Na^+ in erythrocytes (JACOBI et al., 1972) are all increased. The changes of ionic contents of K^+, Na^+, and Ca^{2+} of skeletal muscle (HOUSSAY and MAZZOCCO, 1926; LIN SHIAU et al., 1976) are all in the direction for leaking along the concentration gradients. It is obvious that the increased permeability induced by cardiotoxin is quite nonspecific. This leakiness may result in depolarization as well as contraction of muscle. Depolarization may not be the prerequisite for the contracture. The absence of contracture in Ca^{2+} free medium containing EDTA (LEE et al., 1968; LIN SHIAU et al., 1976) suggests that extracellular Ca^{2+} is needed for the cardiotoxin contracture.

c) *Histologic Effects*

After intramuscular injection of cobra venom in mice or rabbits, STRINGER et al. (1971) and FUKUYAMA and SAWAI (1972) found a local degeneration of the entire muscle fiber. The myofilaments coalesced to form an amorphous mass and the sarcotubular system disappeared. The mitochondria swelled into vacuoles with fragmented cristae. By injecting a supralethal dose (0.1 mg in 0.1 ml) of cardiotoxin into mice, LAI et al. (1972) noted, as early as 1 h after injection, loss of striation and hyaline degeneration of the muscle fiber and fragmentation of the sarcoplasma. After 4 h, there was diffuse hyaline degeneration and the myolysis became prominent. The effect of cardiotoxin appears to be milder than that of whole venom, and, if injected intravenously, no histologic change was noted in the heart, liver, and skeletal muscle under light microscope. When a sublethal dose of cardiotoxin from a mamba venom was injected directly into the leg muscle, the muscle fiber was selectively affected leaving the nerve terminal intact (DUCHEN et al., 1974). One early change was the loss of Z-line structure. In many places, the sarcolemmal membrane was absent so that the contents of the fiber were bound and held in place by the basement membrane. When tested in vitro on the isolated muscle, degenerative changes were evident soon after depolarization (EXCELL and PATEL, 1972).

d) *Concluding Remarks*

The membrane-disorganizing activity of cardiotoxin further suggests that its action is not simply a deprivation of sarcolemma of Ca^{2+} since other pharmacologic agents such as procaine, dibucaine, and veratrum alkaloids, which are known to compete with the negative Ca binding site on the membrane (BLAUSTEIN and GOLDMAN, 1966; SUAREZ-KURTZ et al., 1970), do not result in an effect similar to that evoked by cardiotoxin. After binding with a yet unknown component of membrane, the strong basic yet hydrophobic property of the cardiotoxin molecule may contribute to the disorganization of the membrane by interfering with the molecular interaction between phospholipids and gylcoproteins in the membrane structure. It is interesting in this respect that another strongly basic polypeptide, melittin, isolated from bee venom (HABERMANN, 1972), exhibits the same pharmacologic effects on skeletal muscle as cardiotoxin without being antagonized by a high concentration of Ca^{2+} (LIN SHIAU et al., 1975b), suggesting that the Ca binding site on the membrane is not involved in the interaction between these membrane-active polypeptides and the membrane. The most likely target for the binding of cardiotoxin in the membrane has been recently identified as the phospholipid (VINCENT et al., 1976).

2. Phospholipase A and Its Interaction with Cardiotoxin

Being the hydrolytic enzyme for the phospholipids of membrane constituents, phospholipase A had been assumed to be the main principle for the direct effect on skeletal muscle by various snake venoms (HOUSSAY et al., 1922; KELLAWAY, 1937). The purified acidic phospholipase A from cobra venom is much less potent in causing depolarization and contracture of muscles than whole venom or cardiotoxin (MELDRUM, 1965a; CHANG and LEE, 1966; CHANG et al., 1972). The enzyme, however, can enhance the biologic effect of cardiotoxin in various systems.

Phospholipase A purified from cobra venoms *(N.n.atra, N. nivea)* at 100 μg/ml causes depolarization of superficial muscle fibers of the rat diaphragm or frog sartorius slowly in 3 h and loss of excitability after incubation for more than 4 h (CHANG et al., 1972; EARL and EXCELL, 1971). A slight degree of contracture of the muscle is also observed. In contrast to the action of cardiotoxin, the depolarizing action of phospholipase A is enhanced by increasing the Ca^{2+} concentration. It is thus likely that the effect of phospholipase on the muscle membrane is due to its enzyme action, for which Ca^{2+} is essential (WELLS, 1972; PIETERSON et al., 1974). Acidic phospholipase A of cobra venoms and cardiotoxins are reported by many authors to have synergistic effect in various aspects. For example, the depolarization of muscle (CHANG and LEE, 1966; CHANG et al., 1972), axon blockade (CHANG et al., 1972), direct hemolysis (CONDREA et al., 1964), and the fibrillatory effect on the heart (SLOTTA and VICK, 1969) by cardiotoxin are all potentiated or accelerated by phospholipase A. The depolarization of the rat diaphragm by combined use of these two agents can be effectively antagonized by high Ca^{2+} concentration (CHANG et al., 1972). Since Ca^{2+} antagonizes the action of cardiotoxin but potentiates that of phospholipase A, it is evident that the enzyme is not the main active principle when combined. On the other hand, the observation by CONDREA et al. (1964) that the enhanced hemolysis induced by combined use of the DLF and phospholipase A is associated with an increased splitting of phospholipids suggests that the mutual potentiation between these two agents is highly possible. Cardiotoxin may potentiate the enzyme by binding with its target site and making the substrate within the membrane more accessible to the enzyme, whereas the action of cardiotoxin is in turn enhanced by the removal of the diffusion barrier by the enzyme. Interestingly, this mutual potentiation occurs only when both agents are present simultaneously (CHANG et al., 1972; CONDREA, 1974).

II. Krait Venoms

No cardiotoxin-like direct effect on skeletal muscle has been reported for the venoms of *Bungarus caeruleus* and *B. multicinctus*. The latter venom does not induce contracture in skeletal muscle (CHANG, 1960a, b). Neither direct myocardial effect nor local action has been noted for either venom. By contrast, the venom of *B. fasciatus* has a local action and causes contracture and swelling of frog muscles (HOUSSAY et al., 1922). LIN SHIAU et al. (1972, 1975a) and LU and LO (1974) isolated several cardiotoxin-like fractions which produce contracture of the chick muscle, local irritation on rabbit eye conjunctivae, and depression of the isolated frog heart and rat atrium. Some of these fractions are associated with phospholipase A activity. These effects are antagonized by a high concentration of Ca^{2+} as in the case with cobra cardiotoxin. The amino acid composition of krait cardiotoxin, however, is quite different from that of cobra cardiotoxin and the mode of action is probably not the same (LIN SHIAU et al., 1975a).

III. Australian Elapid Venoms

Venoms of many Australian elapid snakes, especially those of *Demansia textilis*, *Denisonia superba*, *Pseudechis porphyriacus*, and *P. australis*, have a direct depressant effect on the isolated frog skeletal muscle though less potent than cobra venoms (HOUSSAY et al., 1922; KELLAWAY and HOLDEN, 1932). The effect of tiger snake venom is less marked than that of others. However, when tiger snake venom is allowed to act upon the rabbit for a long time, the loss of irritability of the exposed muscle is greater (KELLAWAY et al., 1932). Most probably, the presynaptic toxin, notexin (HARRIS et al., 1973, 1975), is responsible for this myotoxic effect. The effect of notexin is described in Section D.IV.1. It will be of interest to see whether the potent necrotic effect of notexin is related in any way to its phospholipase A activity. Since many Australian snake venoms also appear to contain a factor which causes direct hemolysis of washed mammalian erythrocytes, a characteristic of cardiotoxin-like substances, it remains to be elucidated whether the myotoxic effect of Australian snake venoms is due to such a constituent. In line with this is the cardiotoxic effect of the venom of *P. australis* in rabbits (KELLAWAY et al., 1932). No experiment has been performed so far for the elucidation of the mode of myotoxic effect or isolation of such component.

IV. Sea Snake Venoms

The unique local muscle necrosis induced by the venom of *Enhydrina schistosa* in human (MARSDEN and REID, 1961) but not by other sea snake venoms has been described (see Sect. C.V). In animal experiments in vivo or in vitro, the venom of *E. schistosa*, *Hydrophis cyanocinctus*, *Lapemis hardwickii*, or *Laticauda semifasciata*, at a concentration sufficient for causing neuromuscular blockade, shows neither direct effect on the skeletal muscle nor an effect on the cardiovascular system (CHEYMOL et al., 1966a, 1967b, 1969a, 1972c). These experiments suggest that cardiotoxin may not be a significant constituent of the sea snake venoms, if at all. At higher concentrations of *E. schistosa* venom, a permanent damage of the rat diaphragm has been noted (CAREY and WRIGHT, 1961). Recently, GEH and TOH (1976) have shown that a phospholipase A fraction of this venom is highly myotoxic, causing marked necrosis of the diaphragm when injected intraperitoneally into a guinea pig at 100 μg/kg. They also noted that the neurotoxic fractions caused occasional breakdown of myofilament and mitochondria in isolated areas. These effects of phospholipase A and neurotoxins of *E. schistosa* venom may explain its unique clinical picture in human envenomation.

V. Viperid and Crotalid Venoms

1. Whole Venoms and Phospholipase A

HOUSSAY and PAVE (1922) and HOUSSAY et al. (1922) demonstrated in the frog gastrocnemius that venoms of these two groups depressed the irritability and caused contracture, fibrillation, and swelling. They concluded that the effect might be related to the phospholipase activity by releasing lysolecithin. CHEYMOL et al. (1971c, 1972a) observed the same musculotropic effect in the venoms of *Vipera russellii*, *Cerastes cerastes*, and *Echis carinatus*. Venoms of *V. aspis*, *V. berus*, *Bitis lachesis*, *B. gabonica*, *Bothrops jararaca*, *B. atrox*, *B. lanceolatus*, and *B. carribaeus* are either much less active or inactive in this respect (CHEYMOL et al., 1968, 1971c, 1972a). Myonecrosis is induced when the venom of *Crotalus viridis viridis* is injected into mice intramuscularly (STRINGER et al., 1972). Sarcoplasmic reticulum, myofilament, and mitochondria are all affected. A heat-stable factor of *Trimeresurus* venom, having a 20 times higher activity of phospholipase A, was reported to be very potent in causing pronounced myolysis after intramuscular injection into mice (MAENO et al., 1962). This effect is activated by Ca^{2+} but inhibited by a chelating agent.

Recently, SKET et al. (1973) have isolated a basic depressor protein fraction from the venom of *Vipera ammodytes* and shown that this toxin causes a direct depressant effect on the rat diaphragm without causing neuromuscular blockade. Whether this fraction is associated with phospholipase A has not been studied. The proteolytic enzymes which are abundant in viperid and crotalid venoms may also contribute to the direct paralysis and necrosis of skeletal muscle (HADIDIAN, 1956).

2. Crotamine and Related Basic Polypeptides

Crotamine in the venom of the South American rattlesnake is a strongly basic polypeptide (see Chap. 5) composed of 42 amino acid residues and appears to be related to the spasmodic seizure and tonic convulsion of animals envenomed with this venom (BARRIO and VITAL BRAZIL, 1951; CHEYMOL et al., 1969b, 1971a, b). Crotamine induces contracture of skeletal muscle of cats, rats, and mice, but not of chick, either in situ or isolated (MOUSSATCHÉ et al., 1956; GONCALVES, 1956; CHEYMOL et al., 1966a, 1969b, 1971a; PELLEGRINI FILHO et al., 1976). On the rat diaphragm, crotamine elicites an immediate contracture followed by spontaneous irregular contractions. This effect is inhibited by tetrodotoxin, Ca^{2+}, Mg^{2+}, and K^+, but only partly by chronic denervation or curarization. Crotamine also sensitizes the frog rectus abdominis muscle to K^+ and acetylcholine. These results indicate that the muscle fiber is the main target for the action of crotamine. The resting membrane potential was found to be reduced by about 24% with 15 μg/ml crotamine (PELLEGRINI FILHO et al., 1976). Since the depolarization was antagonized by tetrodotoxin or by reduced concentration of Na^+, it seems likely that crotamine activates the Na^+ channel. The membrane resistance of skeletal muscles was decreased and the influx of Na^+ increased (CHANG and TSENG, unpublished). Interestingly, however, the efflux of Na^+ was not increased, indicating the asymmetric nature of the action of crotamine. Crotamine will be a useful tool for the study of the resting Na^+ channel.

The small basic polypeptides isolated from the venoms of *Crotalus adamanteus*, *C.h.horridus*, and *C.v.viridis* act on skeletal muscle with close resemblance to crotamine (BONILLA and FIERO, 1971; BONILLA et al., 1970; LEE et al., 1972c). In contrast to the effect on mammalian muscles, the adult chick muscle is not affected by either crotamine or the related polypeptides. Interestingly, however, in the baby chick biventer cervicis muscle, the response to nerve stimulation is augmented, and repetitive spontaneous twitchings are elicited by these basic peptides (LEE et al., 1972c). These effects in the baby chick are completely abolished in the presence of D-tubocurarine, high (12 mM) and low (0.1 mM) Ca^{2+}, or high (10 mM) Mg^{2+}. After washing with normal Tyrode's solution, the spontaneous twitching reappears, suggesting the irreversible nature of the action. Since the effect is abolished by β-

bungarotoxin, the site of action of these peptides on the baby chick muscle is likely on the nerve fiber rather than on the muscle as in mammalian muscles. Crotamine has been referred to as neurotoxin by several authors (BONILLA et al., 1971; DOMONT et al., 1971; LEE, 1972). However, in view of its strong direct effect on mammalian skeletal muscle, it is better classified as a myotoxin though it has some effects on the nerve fiber in baby chicks (LEE, 1975).

F. Effects on Peripheral Nerve

I. Effects on Ganglionic Transmission

If administered close intra-arterially into the superior cervical ganglia of cats, cobra and mamba venoms produce contraction of the nictitating membrane (CHOU and LEE, 1969; TELANG et al., 1976). The response to preganglionic stimulation is first increased but then blocked completely within 10 min. The responses to nicotine, acetylcholine, and K^+ are abolished (CHOU and LEE, 1969) or not abolished (TELANG et al., 1976). Cardiotoxin, but not postsynaptic toxin or acidic phospholipase A of the cobra venom, has the same effect as the whole venom. The effect is presumably due to a direct depolarization of the ganglion cell as it does on skeletal muscle. It is unlikely, however, that the systemic toxicity of cobra venom entails any autonomic ganglion blockade since a lethal dose of the venom administered intravenously does not show any significant effect on the ganglionic transmission (CUSHNY and YAGI, 1918; GAUTRELET et al., 1934; CHOU and LEE, 1969; TELANG et al., 1976). A dose of *E. schistosa* venom blocks the response to acetylcholine injected into the cat ganglia without inhibiting the response elicited by preganglionic stimulation (CHAN and CHANG, 1971). With a dose very much in excess than necessary for complete neuromuscular blockade, the response to nerve stimulation could be also blocked (YEOH and WALKER, 1974). This effect, however, is not due to the neurotoxin of the venom. Postsynaptic toxins of elapid venoms and presynaptic toxin (β-bungarotoxin) are also without effect on the ganglionic transmission in the cat (F.L. LEE and C.Y. LEE, unpublished).

II. Effects on Axonal Conduction

Snake venoms do not block the conduction of mammalian nerve trunks in situ even with supralethal dose. In the frog, however, the excitability of nerve trunks could be diminished by cobra venom after systemic administration (HOUSSAY et al., 1922; GAUTRELET and HALPERN, 1933; CICARDO, 1935), probably because this species is resistant to the neuromuscular blocking action of the venom and hence high doses can be used. On the other hand, the excitability as well as conduction of impulses in isolated nerves can be depressed by cobra and crotalid venoms at a high concentration. Heated or crude cobra venom at 30–200 μg/ml abolishes the excitability or conduction in isolated nerves of frogs (NELSON, 1958; ORLOV, 1970, 1972; EVANS, 1963) and crayfish (PARNAS and RUSSELL, 1967) and giant axon of lobster and squid (TOBIAS, 1955, 1960; NARAHASHI and TOBIAS, 1964; CONDREA and ROSENBERG, 1968; CONDREA et al., 1967), and in the prenic nerve of rats (CHANG et al., 1972). While the venom of cottonmouth moccasin *(Agkistrodon piscivorus)* is more potent than cobra venom, the venoms of Russell's viper and rattlesnakes are much less potent (ROSENBERG and PODLESKI, 1962). The venoms of tiger snake *(Notechis scutatus)* and death adder *(Acanthophis antarcticus)* are also potent in this respect (ROSENBERG, 1965).

The conduction in lobster giant axons is usually blocked when the resting membrane potential is decreased to two-third of normal after treatment with cobra venom (ROSENBERG and PODLESKI, 1962; NARAHASHI and TOBIAS, 1964). The action potential, membrane resistance, and threshold potential are all decreased, indicating an increase of membrane permeability to ions. At a concentration of snake venom insufficient to cause conduction blockade, the frog sciatic nerve and the squid axon are rendered permeable to procaine, D-tubocurarine, and acetylcholine (HADIDIAN, 1956; ROSENBERG and HOSKIN, 1963; HOSKIN and ROSENBERG, 1964; ROSENBERG, 1973), and the conduction is reversibly blocked by these cholinergic ligands (ROSENBERG and EHRENPREIS, 1961; ROSENBERG and PODLESKI, 1962, 1963).

Although the effects of snake venoms on these giant axons are not exactly parallel to their phospholipase A activity, ROSENBERG and co-workers proposed that the enzyme is primarily involved based on the following evidence: the venoms retain their activity after heat treatment, the effect is associated with hydrolysis of phospholipids, lysolecithin has a similar blocking effect, and the phospholipase A-rich fraction of cobra venom is active in this respect (ROSENBERG and NG, 1963; CONDREA et al., 1967; CONDREA and ROSENBERG, 1968). On the other hand, the DLF and hyaluronidase are inactive (MARTIN and ROSENBERG, 1968). Interestingly, when the small adhering nerve fibers are removed from the giant axon, the whole venoms lose the activity of blocking the nerve conduction (CONDREA et al., 1967). Although no demonstrable change of axon was observed under the electron-microscope (NELSON, 1958), MARTIN and ROSENBERG (1968) found that the conduction blockade in squid giant axon was associated with a marked breakdown of Schwan sheath and that no change occurred if the adhering small nerve fibers were cut. There is thus a correlation between the functional blockade and the histologic changes. The DLF, although inactive by itself under experimental conditions, can potentiate the blocking action of phospholipase A (CONDREA et al., 1967; CONDREA and ROSENBERG, 1968).

In contrast to the effect on giant axons, the conduction in the phrenic nerve of rats is blocked only by cardiotoxin (CHANG et al., 1972). The postsynaptic toxin and acidic phospholipase A of the *N.n.atra* venom are all inactive up to 200 µg/ml. Phospholipase A, however, markedly accelerates the blocking action of cardiotoxin. The results with the rat phrenic nerve seem contradictory to those with giant axons at first glance. However, it may be accounted for by the difference in the ionic concentrations used since, in the experiment with giant axons, high Ca^{2+} and Mg^{2+} concentrations (9.3 and 48 mM, respectively), which inhibit the effect of cardiotoxin completely (CHANG et al., 1972; ORLOV, 1972), were used whereas, in the Ca^{2+}- or Mg^{2+}-free media, the effect of phospholipase was abolished (NARAHASHI and TOBIAS, 1964). Since the blockade of conduction of phrenic nerve by whole cobra venom is likewise blocked by high Ca^{2+} concentration, the main active principle responsible for the effect of whole venom on phrenic nerve bathed in Tyrode's solution must be cardiotoxin, whereas the blockade of giant axon bathed in artificial sea water is probably due to phospholipase A action. Phospholipase A from other sources such as mouse intestine also inhibits the conduction of the squid giant axon when applied internally but not externally. Recently, ROSENBERG (1975) has demonstrated that phospholipase A can penetrate the axolemma. The mechanism controlling the increase in membrane conductance to Na^+ is probably the site affected (ABBOTT et al., 1972).

Inability of postsynaptic toxins to block nerve conduction has been frequently reported (CHANG and LEE, 1966; CHANG et al., 1972; ROSENBERG, 1965; SU et al., 1967). The report by BICHER (1966) that the conduction in the isolated frog sciatic nerve is blocked by all three neurotoxic fractions isolated from *N. naja* venom is rather surprising. This is most probably due to coexistence of cardiotoxin in the incompletely separated neurotoxins. CHEYMOL et al. (1967b) reported that venoms of three sea snakes, *E. schistosa*, *H. cyanocinctus*, and *L. hardwickii*, did not affect the nerve fiber of cats. This may be due to the absence of cardiotoxin-like peptides in the sea snake venoms.

G. Effects on the Central Nervous System

The interest in the possible action of snake venoms on the central nervous system in the past stemmed from the central-peripheral controversy over the cause of respiratory failure in the envenomed subject (see Sect. C.I.3). From the present viewpoint, the central effects of snake venoms or their purified components are still of great interest not only because of the toxicologic effect but also the possible neurochemical as well as neurophysiologic significance resulting from the specific action of venom components. Phospholipase A, cardiotoxin, and postsynaptic and presynaptic toxins may be used as tools for elucidation of the function of the brain.

I. Central Effects After Systemic Application

1. Neuropathologic Effects

After systemic injection of various elapid and sea snake venoms into rabbits, dogs, and monkeys, it has been demonstrated that neuropathologic changes occur in the anterior horn cells, cranial nerve nuclei, and pyramidal and Purkinje cells (KILVINGTON, 1902; LAMB and HUNTER, 1907; HUNTER, 1910). The change is dependent on the type and dose of venom and the time to death. The affected cells show every stage of acute chromatolysis with ultimate cell vacuolation and nuclear degeneration. A similar change was also produced by a viperid venom (*Vipera russellii*) (HUNTER, 1910), whereas *Trimeresurus flavoviridis* venom produced severe nonspecific degenerative changes throughout the brain of the guinea pig (OKONOGI et al., 1960). Some chromatolysis in the brain and spinal cord was noted in monkeys dying 36 h after injection of *Crotalus atrox* venom (FIDLER et al., 1940). Whether these morphologic changes are due to anoxia or ischemia as suggested by KELLAWAY et al. (1932) or to a direct action of venom on the nerve cell has not been further studied. Neither has the relationship between the morphologic changes and the symptoms produced by the venom been clarified.

2. Pharmacologic Effects

The disputes on the cause of respiratory paralysis, whether of central or peripheral origin, are described in Section C. Upon envenomation in human victims, there are symptoms suggestive of central effect such as lassitude, drowsiness, clouding of consciousness, and convulsion though the possibility that these clinical symptoms are secondary to some peripheral effects is not ruled out. When a large dose of Cape cobra or death adder venom was injected into the head circulation of a semi-isolated cat head preparation, rapid loss of corneal reflex and diaphragmatic movements were observed (EPSTEIN, 1930; KELLAWAY et al., 1932). In dogs and monkeys under pentobarbital anesthesia, intravenous injection of venom of *N. naja* and *C. adamanteus* was reported to cause complete silence of electroencephalogram within 1 min (VICK et al., 1964). A similar observation was made by RUSSELL and MICKAELIS (1960) in cats with the venom of *C. adamanteus* and *C. atrox*. Although VICK et al. (1966) claimed that this loss of cortical electric activity could be elicited by toxic fractions of cobra venom independent of phospholipase A activity, BICHER (1966), CURRIE et al. (1968), SLOTTA and VICK (1969), and SLOTTA et al. (1971) all found that the cortical action was associated with the phospholipase A-rich fraction of venoms. Phospholipase of bee venom, but not of crotoxin, also shows similar cortical and hypotensive effects (SLOTTA et al., 1971). Except the bee venom phospholipase A, the effects of phospholipase A from snake venoms are reversible in about 20 min if the animal survived. Since in all of these experiments, the loss of cortical electric activity is always accompanied by a dramatic and sustained hypotension, the cerebral ischemia may contribute to a great extent (RUSSELL and MICKAELIS, 1960) and the vasoconstriction in the head circulation (KELLAWAY et al., 1932) will undoubtedly make the ischemia worse.

In contrast to the above observations in anesthetized animals, in conscious rabbits or monkeys with chronically implanted electrodes, the injection of *Naja*, *C. adamanteus* or *C. artox* venom caused initial desynchronization and activation of electroencephalogram instead of rapid depression (KRUPNICK et al., 1968; VICK and LIPP, 1970). The cortical electric activity was depressed only just before the death of the animal. It seems obvious that the rapid depression of cortical electric activity by phospholipase A in the anesthetized animal must be related in some way to the hypotension and barbiturates used for the anesthesia.

A neurotoxic fraction purified from *Vipera palestinae*, which causes a rapid and persistent fall of blood pressure with vasodilatation, abolished the action potential of the cervical sympathetic chain within 30 s (BICHER et al., 1966; BICHER, 1966). Hypotension induced by bacterial toxin, however, was accompanied with increased sympathetic firings because of vascular reflex. Since in the spinal cat, the blood pressure was increased slightly by the neurotoxin because of direct vasoconstriction, these authors concluded that the shock produced by the whole venom of *V. palestinae* could be correlated with the depression of a central autonomic vasoregulatory mechanism caused by its neurotoxic component. On the other hand, the abnormal electroencephalogram seen after injection of a basic polypeptide and the whole venom of *V. ammodytes* was attributed to anoxia of the brain due to the arterial hypotension (SKET et al., 1973).

II. Effects when Applied Directly to the Central Nervous System

ELLIOT (1905) applied dry cobra venom to the exposed medulla of rabbits and found that respiratory failure occurred before cardiac arrest in the absence of peripheral curarization. PACELLA (1923) reported that injection of the venom of *N. naja*, *C. terrificus*, or *Lachesis alternatus* into the subarachnoid space in dogs produced a rapid rise in arterial blood pressure, slowing of pulse, and later arrest of respiration. The lethal doses of Formosan cobra (PENG, 1952) and Formosan krait (OUYANG, 1950) venoms, when injected into the cerebellomedullary cistern of rabbits, were only 1/10 and 1/40, respectively, of those needed by intravenous injection. The time from injection to death was, however, unduly prolonged from 2–3 h by intravenous application to 14–32 h by cisternal application. The lethal doses that killed the animal in 2–3 h were the same for either route of administration for the cobra venom. An initial rise of blood pressure and a transient stimulation of respiration were evident instead of the fall of blood pressure after intravenous injection. GUYOT and BOQUET (1960) also found that the injection of *N. nigricollis* venom in the neighborhood of Ammon's horn in rabbits produced symptoms that were quite different from those following intravenous injection. Spasms and contractures occurred, without evidence of curarizing action. The direct application of *N. naja* venom to the exposed cerebral cortex of rats led to a long-lasting convulsion and appearance of abnormal negative waves in the somatosensory evoked potential (BHARGAVA et al., 1970), resembling those produced by strychnine and D-tubocurarine. CAREY and WRIGHT (1961) studied the effect of *E. schistosa* venom directly injected into the medulla oblongata of rabbits. The respiration was first increased in its rate, associated frequently with gasping. Some rabbits exhibited torticollis and persistent circling to the injected side. In the final stage, the respiration became very slow. Similar effects on the medulla were observed with a fraction of the venom containing phospholipase A which was nontoxic when injected intraperitoneally. On the other hand, the neurotoxin fraction, presumbly the postsynaptic toxin, which acted similarly as the whole venom when injected intraperitoneally, had virtually no effect on the medulla. LEE and CHEN (1977) found that the purified postsynaptic toxin such as cobrotoxin was no more toxic in rats when intraventricularly injected than when intravenously administered. There was strong evidence of curarization of the diaphragm, whereas the discharges in the phrenic nerve were increased when respiratory paralysis occurred, indicating that the postsynaptic toxin had no effect on the respiratory center but left the brain and acted on the motor endplate.

It is thus evident that the venoms of *Elapidae* and *Hydrophiidae* contain some constituents which act violently on the central nervous system when directly applied. Phospholipase A could be the most active of them. However, these components do not act on the central nervous system if administered systemically. Recently, LYSZ and ROSENBERG (1974) injected various components of cobra venom into rats by an intraventricular route and found that cobrotoxin (50 μg) and cardiotoxin (125 μg) caused piloerection, lacrimation, and death but no convulsion, whereas phospholipase A (25 μg) evoked tonic convulsion of the animals. In combination with cardiotoxin (5 μg), phospholipase A exhibited its effect at doses as low as 0.5 μg. A similar observation was also made by LEE and CHEN (1977). Ineffectiveness of postsynaptic toxins on cholinergic receptors in the central nervous system is further verified by microelectrode recordings of the synaptic transmission in the spinal cord for α-bungarotoxin and cobrotoxin (MILEDI and SZCZEPANIAK, 1975; DUGGAN et al., 1976) though some toxins from *Dendroaspis* venom are active (BANKS et al., 1976).

Various *Crotalus* venoms also affect the central nervous system when directly applied. The intraventricular injection in cats produced changes in behavior, motor activity, and autonomic function (RUSSELL and BOHR, 1962). The neurotoxic fraction of the South American rattlesnake venom, crotoxin, produced convulsion upon intraventricular injection instead of paralysis by systemic application in cats (VITAL BRAZIL et al., 1966).

Acknowledgements. The author is grateful to Dr. C.Y. LEE for his suggestions and criticism during the preparation of this article. This chapter would not have been completed without his encouragement. The author also wishes to thank Dr. J.H. CROSS for his reading of the manuscript.

References

Abbott, N.J., Deguchi, T., Frazier, D.T., Murayama, K., Narahashi, T., Ottolenghi, A., Wang, C.M.: The action of phospholipases on the inner and outer surface of the squid giant axon membrane. J. Physiol. (Lond.) **220**, 73—86 (1972)

Abe, T., Limbrick, A.R., Miledi, R.: Acute muscle denervation by β-bungarotoxin. Proc. roy. Soc. Lond. [Biol.] **194**, 545—553 (1976)

Acton, H.W., Knowles, R.: The nature and toxicological action of venom. In: Byam, W., Archibald, R.G. (Eds.): The Practise of Medicine in the Tropics, Vol. I, pp. 728—749. London: Henry Frowde and Hodder and Stoughton 1921

Albuquerque, E.X., Barnard, E.A., Chiu, T.H., Lapa, A.J., Dolly, J.O., Janssen, J.E., Daly, J., Witkop, B.: Acetylcholine receptor and ion conductance modulator sites at the murine neuromuscular junction: Evidence from specific toxin reactions. Proc. nat. Acad. Sci. (Wash.) **70**, 949—953 (1973)

Albuquerque, E.X., Thesleff, S.: Effects of phospholipase A and lysolecithin on some electrical properties of the muscle membrane. Acta physiol. scand. **72**, 248—252 (1968)

Alderice, M.T., Volle, R.L.: Paradoxical effects of $[Ca^{++}]_0$ on mepp frequency in muscles treated with β-bungarotoxin or La^{+++}. Neuroscience Abstract, pp. 967. New York: Society for Neuroscience 1975

Ambache, N.: The peripheral action of *Cl. botulinum* toxin. J. Physiol. (Lond.) **108**, 127—141 (1949)

Ambache, N.: A further survey of the action of *clostridium botulinum* toxin upon different types of autonomic nerve fibre. J. Physiol. (Lond.) **113**, 1—17 (1951)

Ambache, N.: Effect of botulinum toxin upon the superior cervical ganglion. J. Physiol. (Lond.) **116**, 9 (1952)

Arthus, M.: Le venin de cobra est un curare. Arch. int. Physiol. **10**, 161—191 (1910)

Arthus, M.: Physiologie comparée des intoxications par les venins de serpents. Arch. int. Physiol. **11**, 285—316 (1911)

Banks, B.E.C., Shipolini, R., Szczepaniak, A.C.: Structure-activity relations of polypeptides from a mamba venom. Bull. Inst. Pasteur. Lille **74**, 25—33 (1976)

Barme, M.: Venomous sea snakes (Hydrophiidae). In: Bücherl, W., Buckley, E., Deulofeu, V. (Eds.): Venomous Animals and Their Venoms, Vol. I, pp. 285—308. New York-London: Academic Press 1968

Barnard, E.A., Wieckowski, J., Chiu, T.H.: Cholinergic receptor molecules and cholinesterase molecules at mouse skeletal muscle junction. Nature (Lond.) **234**, 207—209 (1971)

Barnes, J.M., Trueta, J.: Absorption of bacteria toxins and snake venom from the tissues. Lancet **1941 I**, 623—626

Barrio, A., Vital Brazil, O.: Neuro-muscular action of the *Crotalus terrificus terrificus* poisons. Acta physiol. lat.-amer. **1**, 291—308 (1951)

Beiler, J. M., Brendel, R., Martin, G. J.: Enzymic modification of blood-brain barrier permeability. J. Pharmacol. exp. Ther. **118**, 415—419 (1956)

Berg, D. K., Hall, Z. W.: Loss of α-bungarotoxin from junctional and extrajunctional acetylcholine receptors in rat diaphragm muscle in vivo and in organ culture. J. Physiol. (Lond.) **252**, 771—789 (1975)

Berg, D. K., Kelly, R. B., Sargent, P. B., Williamson, P., Hall, Z. W.: Binding of α-bungarotoxin to acetylcholine receptors in mammalian muscle. Proc. nat. Acad. Sci. (Wash.) **69**, 147—151 (1972)

Bernard, C.: Analyse physiologique des propriêtés des systéms musculaire et nerveux au moyer du curare. C.R. Acad. Sci. (Paris) **43**, 825—829 (1856)

Bhargava, V. K., Horton, R. W., Meldrum, B. S.: Long-lasting convulsant effect on the cerebral cortex of *Naja naja* venom. Brit. J. Pharmacol. **39**, 455—461 (1970)

Bicher, H. I.: Specific sites of action of snake venoms in the central nervous system. Mem. Inst. Butantan **33**, 523—539 (1966)

Bicher, H. I., Klibansky, C., Shiloah, J., Gitter, S., Vries, A. de: Isolation of three different neurotoxins from Indian cobra *(Naja naja)* venom and the relation to their action to phospholipase A. Biochem. Pharmacol. **14**, 1779—1784 (1965)

Bicher, H. I., Roth, M., Gitter, S.: Neurotoxic activity of *Vipera palestinae* venom. Depression of central autonomic vasoregulatory mechanisms. Med. Pharmacol. Exp. **14**, 349—359 (1966)

Bieber, A. L., Tu, T., Tu, A. T.: Acidic cardiotoxin isolated from the venom of Mojave rattlesnake *(Crotalus scutulatus)*. Biochim. biophys. Acta (Amst.) **400**, 178—188 (1975)

Blaustein, M. P.: Effects of potassium, veratridine, and scorpion venom on calcium accumulation and transmitter release by nerve terminals in vitro. J. Physiol. (Lond.) **247**, 617—655 (1975)

Blaustein, M. P., Goldman, D. E.: Competitive action of calcium and procaine on lobster axon. J. gen. Physiol. **49**, 1043—1063 (1966)

Bon, C.: Ceruleotoxin: an acidic neurotoxin from *Bungarus caeruleus* venom which blocks postsynaptically the neuromuscular transmission without binding to the cholinergic receptor site. Bull. Inst. Pasteur Lille **74**, 41—45 (1976)

Bon, C., Changeux, J. P.: Ceruleotoxin: an acidic neurotoxin from the venom of *Bungarus caeruleus* which blocks the response to a cholinergic agonist without binding to the cholinergic receptor site. FEBS Letters **52**, 212—216 (1975)

Bonilla, C. A., Fiero, M. K.: Comparative biochemistry and pharmacology of salivary gland secretions. II. Chromatographic separation of the basic proteins from some North American rattlesnake venoms. J. Chromatog. **56**, 253—263 (1971)

Bonilla, C. A., Fiero, K., Frank, L. P.: Isolation of a basic protein neurotoxin from *Crotalus adamanteus* venom-I. Purification and biological properties. Toxicon **8**, 123 (1970)

Bonilla, C. A., Fiero, M. K., Frank, L. P.: Isolation of a basic protein neurotoxin from *Crotalus adamanteus* venom. In: Vries, A. de, Kochva, E. (Eds.): Toxins of Animal and Plant Origin, pp. 343—359. New York: Gordon and Breach 1971

Boquet, P.: Venins de serpents (1ére partie) Physiopathologie de l'envenimation et propriêtés biologiques des venins. Toxicon **2**, 5—41 (1964)

Boquet, P.: Effect of *Naja nigricollis* venom γ-toxin on KB cells cultivated in vitro. C.R. Acad. Sci. (Paris) **271**, 2422—2425 (1970)

Boquet, P., Detrait, J., Farzanpay, R.: Etude des analogues de l'antigéne alpha du venin de *N. nigricollis*. Ann. Inst. Pasteur Lille **116**, 522—542 (1969)

Boroff, D. A., Castillo, J. del, Evoy, W. H., Steinhardt, R. A.: Observation on the action of Type A botulinum toxin on frog neuromuscular junctions. J. Physiol. (Lond.) **240**, 227—253 (1974)

Braganca, B. M., Patel, N. T., Bardinath, P. G.: Isolation and properties of a cobra venom factors selectively cytotoxic to Yoshida sarcoma cells. Biochim. biophys. Acta (Amst.) **136**, 508—520 (1967)

Breithaupt, H.: Neurotoxic and myotoxic effects of *Crotalus* phospholipase A and its complex with crotapotin. Naunyn Schmiedebergs Arch. Pharmacol. **292**, 271—278 (1976)

Breithaupt, H., Omori-Satoh, T., Lang, J.: Isolation and characterization of three phospholipases A from the crotoxin complex. Biochim. biophys. Acta (Amst.) **403**, 355—369 (1975)

Breithaupt, H., Rübsamen, K., Habermann, E.: Biochemistry and pharmacology of the crotoxin complex. Biochemical analysis of crotapotin and the basic *Crotalus* phospholipase A. Europ. J. Biochem. **49**, 333—345 (1974)

Broman, T., Lindberg-Broman, A. M.: An experimental study of disorders in the permeability of the cerebral vessels (the blood-brain barrier) produced by chemical and physicochemical agents. Acta physiol. scand. **10**, 102—125 (1945)

Brooks, V. B.: An intracellular study of the action of repetitive nerve volleys and of botulinum toxin on miniature end-plate potentials. J. Physiol. (Lond.) **134**, 264—277 (1956)

Brown, J. H.: Toxicology and pharmacology of venoms from poisonous snakes, p. 184. Springfield (Illinois): C. C. Thomas 1973

Brown, R. V.: Effects of water moccasin venom on dogs. Amer. J. Physiol. **134**, 202—207 (1941)

Brunton, T. L., Fayrer, J.: On the nature and physiological action of the poison of *Naja tripudians* and other Indian venomous snakes. Part 1. Proc. roy. Soc. **21**, 358—374 (1873)

Brunton, T. L., Fayrer, J.: On the nature and physiological action of the poison of *Naja tripudians* and other Indian venomous snakes. Part 2. Proc. roy. Soc. **22**, 68—133 (1874)

Burden, S. J., Hartzell, H. C., Yoshikami, D.: Acetylcholine receptors at neuromuscular synpases. Phylogenetic differences detected by snake α-neurotoxins. Proc. nat. Acad. Sci. (Wash.) **72**, 3245—3249 (1975)

Burgen, A. S. V., Dickens, F., Zatman, L. J.: The action of botulinum toxin on the neuromuscular junction. J. Physiol. (Lond.) **109**, 10—24 (1949)

Cahalan, M. D.: Modification of sodium channel gating in frog myelinated nerve fibres by *Centruroides sculpturatus* scorpion venom. J. Physiol. (Lond.) **244**, 511—534 (1975)

Campbell, C. H.: The effects of snake venoms and their neurotoxins on the nervous system of man and animals. In: Hornabrook, R. W. (Ed.): Topics on Tropical Neurology, pp. 259—293. Philadelphia: F. A. Davis 1975

Carey, J. E., Wright, E. A.: The toxicity and immunological properties of some sea-snake venoms with particular reference to that of *Enhydrina schistosa*. Trans. roy. Soc. trop. Med. Hyg. **54**, 50—67 (1960a)

Carey, J. E., Wright, E. A.: Isolation of the neurotoxic component of the venom of the sea snake *Enhydrina schistosa*. Nature **185**, 103—104 (1960b)

Carey, J. E., Wright, E. A.: The site of action of the venom of the sea-snake *Enhydrina schistosa*. Trans. roy. Soc. trop. Med. Hyg. **55**, 153—160 (1961)

Carey, J. E., Wright, E. A.: Studies on the fractions of the venom of the seasnake *Enhydrina schistosa*. Aust. J. exp. Biol. med. Sci. **40**, 427—436 (1962)

Castillo, J. del, Katz, B.: The effect of magnesium on the activity of motor nerve endings. J. Physiol. (Lond.) **124**, 553—559 (1954)

Castillo, J. del, Katz, B.: The identity of intrinsic and extrinsic acetylcholine receptors in the motor end-plate. Proc. roy. Soc. B **146**, 357—361 (1957)

Castillo, J. del, Pumplin, D. W.: Discrete and discontinous action of brown widow spider venom on the presynaptic nerve terminals of frog muscle. J. Physiol. (Lond.) **252**, 491—508 (1975)

Chan, K. E., Chang, P.: Normal ganglionic transmission in the presence of ACh block by sea snake *(Enhydrina schistosa)* venom. Europ. J. Pharmacol. **13**, 277—279 (1971)

Chan, K. E., Geh, S. L.: Antagonism of intra-arterial acetylcholine induced contraction of skeletal muscle by sea snake venom. Nature (Lond.) **213**, 1147—1148 (1967)

Chang, C. C.: Studies on the mechanism of curare-like action of *Bungarus multicinctus* venom. I. Effect on the phrenic nerve diaphragm preparation of the rat. J. Formosan med. Ass. **59**, 315—323 (1960a)

Chang, C. C.: Studies on the mechanism of curare-like action of *Bungarus multicinctus* venom. II. Effect on response of rectus abdominis muscle of the frog to acetylcholine. J. Formosan med. Ass. **59**, 416—422 (1960b)

Chang, C. C., Chen, T. F., Chuang, S. T.: N.O-di and N.N.O-tri [^{3}H] acetyl α-bungarotoxins as specific labelling agents of cholinergic receptors. Brit. J. Pharmacol. **47**, 147—160 (1973a)

Chang, C. C., Chen, T. F., Lee, C. Y.: Studies of the presynaptic effect of β-bungarotoxin on neuromuscular transmission. J. Pharmacol. exp. Ther. **184**, 339—345 (1973b)

Chang, C. C., Chuang, S. T., Huang, M. C.: Effects of chronic treatment with various neuromuscular blocking agents on the number and distribution of acetylcholine receptors in the rat diaphragm. J. Physiol. (Lond.) **250**, 161—173 (1975)

Chang, C. C., Chuang, S. T., Lee, C. Y., Wei, J. W.: Role of cardiotoxin and phospholipase A in the blockade of nerve conduction and depolarization of skeletal muscle induced by cobra venom. Brit. J. Pharmacol. **44**, 752—764 (1972)

Chang, C. C., Huang, M. C.: Comparison of the presynaptic actions of botulinum toxin and β-bungarotoxin on neuromuscular transmission. Naunyn-Schmiedebergs Arch. Pharmacol. **282**, 129—142 (1974)
Chang, C. C., Huang, M. C.: Turnover of junctional and extrajunctional acetylcholine receptors of the rat diaphragm. Nature (Lond.) **253**, 643—644 (1975)
Chang, C. C., Huang, M. C., Lee, C. Y.: Mutual antagonism between botulinum toxin and β-bungarotoxin. Nature (Lond.) **243**, 166—167 (1973c)
Chang, C. C., Lee, C. Y.: Isolation of neurotoxins from the venom of *Bungarus multicinctus* and their modes of neuro-muscular blocking action. Arch. Int. Pharmacodyn. **144**, 241—257 (1963)
Chang, C. C., Lee, C. Y.: Electrophysiological study of neuromuscular blocking action of cobra neurotoxin. Brit. J. Pharmacol. **28**, 172—181 (1966)
Chang, C. C., Lee, J. D.: Crotoxin, the neurotoxin of South American rattlesnake venom, is a presynaptic toxin acting like β-bungarotoxin. Naunyn-Schmidebergs Arch. Pharmacol. **296**, 159—168 (1977)
Chang, C. C., Lee, J. D., Eaker, D., Fohlman, J.: The presynaptic neuromuscular blocking action of taipoxin. A comparison with β-bungarotoxin and crotoxin. Toxicon **15**, 571—576 (1977)
Chang, C. C., Su, M. J.: Further evidence that extrinsic acetylcholine acts preferentially on extra-junctional receptors in the chick biventer cervicis muscle. Europ. J. Pharmacol. **33**, 337—344 (1975)
Chang, C. C., Su, M. J., Tang, S. S.: An analysis of the mode of action of carbachol on the chick biventer cervicis nerve muscle preparation. Europ. J. Pharmacol. **36**, 199—210 (1976)
Chang, C. C., Tang, S. S.: Differentiation between intrinsic and extrinsic acetylcholine receptors of the chick biventer cervicis muscle. Naunyn-Schmiedebergs Arch. Pharmacol. **282**, 379—388 (1974)
Changeux, J.-P., Kasai, M., Lee, C. Y.: Use of a snake venom toxin to characterize the cholinergic receptor protein. Proc. nat. Acad. Sci. (Wash.) **67**, 1241—1247 (1970)
Chen, I.-L., Lee, C. Y.: Ultrastructural changes in the motor nerve terminals caused by β-bungarotoxin. Virchows Arch. Abt. B Zellpath. **6**, 318—325 (1970)
Cheymol, J., Barme, M., Bourillet, F., Roch-Arveiller, M.: Action neuromusculaire de trois venins d'Hydrophiides. Toxicon **5**, 111—119 (1967a)
Cheymol, J., Boquet, P., Bourillet, F., Detrait, J., Roch-Arveiller, M.: Compraison des principales propriétés pharmacologiques de différents venins d'*Echis carinatus* (Vipéridés). Arch. int. Pharmacodyn. **205**, 293—304 (1973a)
Cheymol, J., Bourillet, F., Roch-Arveiller, M.: Action neuromusculaire des venins de quelques *Crotalidae, Elapidae* et *Hydrophiidae*. Mem. Inst. Butantan **33**, 541—554 (1966a)
Cheymol, J., Bourillet, F., Roch-Arveiller, M.: Venin de cobra *(Naja naja)* et paralysants neuromusculaires. Med. Pharmacol. Exp. **14**, 54—64 (1966b)
Cheymol, J., Bourillet, F., Roch-Arveiller, M.: Actions neuromusculaires comparées des venins de trois *Naja (N. haje, N. nigricollis, N. naja)*. Arch. int. Pharmacodyn. **170**, 193—215 (1967b)
Cheymol, J., Bourillet, F., Roch-Arveiller, M.: Action neuromusculaire d'un venin d'*Echis carinatus* (Viperides) originaire d'Ethiopie. Thérapie **26**, 1007—1016 (1971c)
Cheymol, J., Bourillet, F., Roch-Arveiller, M.: Recherche d'une action neuromusculaire dans divers venins de Vipéridés. C.R. Soc. Biol. **166**, 1283—1287 (1972a)
Cheymol, J., Bourillet, F., Roch-Arveiller, M.: Venins et toxines de serpents effects neuromusculaires. Act. Pharmacol. (Paris) **25**, 179—240 (1972b)
Cheymol, J., Bourillet, F., Roch-Arveiller, M., Barme, B.: Action paralysante neuromusculaire de venins et de toxines de serpents marins des mers de chine et du Japon. Ann. Med. Nancy **8**, 361—364 (1969a)
Cheymol, J., Bourillet, F., Roch-Arveiller, M., Heckle, J.: Neuromuscular action of three venoms of North African scorpions and two toxin isolated from one of them. Toxicon **11**, 277—282 (1973b)
Cheymol, J., Bourillet, F., Roch-Arveiller, M., Toan, T.: Effects neuromusculaires des venins des deux varietes de *Crotalus durissus terrificus*. Arch. int. Pharmacodyn. **179**, 40—55 (1969b)
Cheymol, J., Gonçalves, J. M., Bourillet, F., Roch-Arveiller, M.: Action neuromusculaire comparée de la crotamine et du venin de *Crotalus durissus terrificus var. crotamincus* I. Sur preparations neuromusculaires in situ. Toxicon **9**, 279—286 (1971a)

Cheymol, J., Gonçalves, J.M., Bourillet, F., Roch-Arveiller, M.: Action neuromusculaire comparee de la crotamine et du venin du *Crotalus durissus terrificus var. crotaminicus* II. Sur preparations isolees. Toxicon **9**, 287—289 (1971 b)

Cheymol, J., Mille, R., Bourillet, F., Suga, T., Labourdette, E.: Sur quelques proprietés pharmacodynamiques et biologiques de venins de serpents du genre *Bothrops (B. jararaca, B. atrox, B. lanceolatus* et *B. Carribaeus)*. Bull. Soc. Pathol. Exot. **61**, 673—689 (1968)

Cheymol, J., Tamiya, N., Bourillet, F., Roch-Arveiller, M.: Neuromuscular action of venom of the sea snake "erabu" *(Laticauda semifasciata)* and erabutoxins a and b. Toxicon **10**, 125—131 (1972 c)

Chopra, R.N., Iswariah, V.: An experimental investigation into the action of the venom of the Indian cobra *(Naja naja vel tripudians)*. Indian J. med. Res. **18**, 1113—1125 (1931)

Chou, T.C., Lee, C.Y.: Effect of whole and fractionated cobra venom on sympathetic ganglionic transmission. Europ. J. Pharmacol. **8**, 326—330 (1969)

Christensen, P.A.: South African Snake Venoms and Antivenoms, pp. 1—129. Johannesburg: South African Institute for Medical Research 1955

Christensen, P.A.: The venoms of Central and South African snakes. In: Bücherl, W., Buckley, E.F., Deulofeu, V. (Eds.): Venomous Animals and their Venoms, Vol. I, pp. 437—461. New York-London: Academic Press 1968

Cicardo, V.H.: Modification de l'excitabilite nerveuse par action du venin de cobra. C.R. Soc. Biol. (Paris) **120**, 732—733 (1935)

Clark, A.W., Hurlbut, W.P., Mauro, A.: Changes in the fine structure of the neuromuscular junction of the frog caused by black widow spider venom. J. Cell Biol. **52**, 1—14 (1972)

Colquhoun, D., Rang, H.P., Ritchie, J.M.: The binding of tetrodotoxin and α-bungarotoxin to normal and denervated mammalian muscle. J. Physiol. (Lond.) **240**, 199—226 (1974)

Condrea, E.: Membrane active polypeptides from snake venom. Cardiotoxins and hemocytotoxins. Experientia (Basel) **30**, 121—129 (1974)

Condrea, E., Barzilay, M., Vries, A. de: Cobra basic polypeptides (DLF) as a mediator in the hydrolysis of membrane phospholipids by phospholipase A. In: Vries, A. de, Kochva, E. (Eds.): Toxins of Animal and Plant Origin, pp. 437—447. New York: Gordon and Breach 1971

Condrea, E., Rosenberg, P.: Demonstration of phospholipid splitting as the factor responsible for increased permeability and block of axonal conduction induced by snake venoms. II. Study on squid axons. Biochim. biophys. Acta (Amst.) **150**, 271—284 (1968)

Condrea, E., Rosenberg, P., Dettbarn, W.D.: Demonstration of phospholipid splitting as the factor responsible for increased permeability and block of axonal conduction induced by snake venom. I. Study of lobster axons. Biochim. biophys. Acta (Amst.) **135**, 669—681 (1967)

Condrea, E., Vries, A. de, Mager, J.: Hemolysis and splitting of human erythrocyte phospholipids by snake venoms. Biochim. biophys. Acta (Amst.) **84**, 60—73 (1964)

Cull-Candy, S.G., Fohlman, J., Gustavsson, D., Lüllmann-Ranch, R., Thesleff, S.: The effect of taipoxin and notexin on the function and fine structure of the murine neuromuscular junction. J. Neurosci. **1**, 175—180 (1976)

Currie, B.T., Oakley, D.E., Broomfield, C.A.: Crystalline phospholipase A associated with a cobra venom toxin. Nature (Lond.) **220**, 371 (1968)

Cushny, A.R., Yagi, S.: On the action of cobra venom. Phil. Trans. roy. Soc. **208**, 1—36 (1918)

Dale, H.H., Feldberg, W., Vogt, M.: Release of acetylcholine at voluntary motor nerve endings. J. Physiol. (Lond.) **86**, 353—380 (1936)

Datyner, M.E., Gage, P.W.: Australian tiger snake venom—an inhibitor of transmitter release. Nature (Lond.) New Biol. **241**, 246—247 (1973 a)

Datyner, M.E., Gage, P.W.: Presynaptic and post-synaptic effects of the venom of the Australian tiger snake at the neuromuscular junction. Brit. J. Pharmacol. **49**, 340—354 (1973 b)

Detrait, J., Izard, Y., Boquet, P.: Relations antigeniques entre un facteur lethal du venin d'*Echis carinata* et les neurotoxins des venins de *Naja naja* et de *Naja nigricollis*. C.R. Soc. Biol. (Paris) **154**, 1163—1165 (1960)

Diniz, C.R., Pimenta, O.F., Continho-Nett, J., Pompolo, S., Gomez, M.V., Bohm, G.M.: Effect of scorpion venom from *Tityus serrulatus* (Tityustoxin) on the acetylcholine release and fine structure of the nerve terminals. Experientia (Basel) **30**, 1304—1305 (1974)

Dolly, Y. O., Albuquerque, E. X., Sarvey, J. M., Barnard, E. A.: Interaction of α-bungarotoxin, D-tubocurarine and perhydrohistrionicotoxin with acetylcholine and ion conductance modulator sites. Proc. 6th Intern. Congress Pharmacol. Helsinki, Finland, July 20—25, 1975, pp. 562

Domont, G. B., Guimaraes, V. M., Silva, M. H., Perrone, J. C.: Analytical and preparative fractionation of snake venoms. Isolation of crotamine, a neurotoxin from *Crotalus durissus terrificus* venom. An. Acad. Bras. Cienc. **43**, 587—598 (1971)

Dryden, W. F., Harvey, A. L.: Effect of receptor desensitization on the action of α-bungarotoxin on cultured skeletal muscle. Brit. J. Pharmacol. **51**, 456—458 (1974)

Duchen, L. W.: An electron microscopic study of the changes induced by botulinum toxin in the motor endplates of slow and fast skeletal fibres of the mouse. J. Neurol. Sci. **14**, 47—60 (1971)

Duchen, L. W.: The effects of tetanus toxin on the motor endplates of the mouse: an electronmicroscopic study. J. Neurol. Sci. **19**, 153—167 (1973)

Duchen, L. W., Excell, B. J., Patel, R., Smith, B.: Changes in motor endplates resulting from muscle fibre necrosis and regeneration. A light and electron microscopic study of the effects of the depolarizing fraction (cardiotoxin) of *Dendroaspis jamesoni* venom. J. Neurol. Sci. **21**, 391—417 (1974)

Duchen, L. W., Tonge, D. A.: The effects of tetanus toxin on neuromuscular transmission and on the morphology of motor endplates in slow and fast skeletal muscle of the mouse. J. Physiol. (Lond.) **228**, 157—172 (1973)

Duggan, A. W., Hall, J. G., Lee, C. Y.: α-Bungarotoxin, cobra neurotoxin and excitation of Renshow cells by acetylcholine. Brain Res. **107**, 166—170 (1976)

Dumarey, C., Sket, D., Joseph, D., Boquet, P.: Etude d'une phospholipase basique du venin de *Naja nigricollis*. C.R. Acad. Sci. [D] (Paris) **280**, 1633—1635 (1975)

Eagle, H.: The coagulation of blood by snake venoms and its physiological significance. J. exp. Med. **65**, 613—639 (1937)

Eaker, D.: Structural nature of pre-synaptic neurotoxins from Australian elapid venoms. 4th Intern. Symp. on Animal and Microbial Toxins, Tokyo, 1974, Abstract, pp. 49—50

Eaker, D.: Snake venom toxins reacting post- and presynaptically at the neuromuscular junction. Bull. Inst. Pasteur Lille **74**, 7—9 (1976)

Eaker, D., Harris, J. B., Thesleff, S.: Action of a cobra neurotoxin on denervated rat skeletal muscle. Europ. J. Pharmacol. **15**, 254—256 (1971)

Earl, J. E., Excell, B. J.: The action of a depolarizing fraction from *Naja nivea* venom on frog skeletal muscle. J. Physiol. (Lond.) **214**, 27p—28p (1971)

Earl, J. E., Excell, B. J.: The effects of toxic components of *Naja nivea* (Cape cobra) venom on neuromuscular transmission and muscle membrane permeability. Comp. Biochem. Physiol. [A] **41**, 597—615 (1972)

Eigenberger, F.: Some clinical observations on the action of mamba venom. Bull. Antiv. Inst. Amer. **2**, 45—46 (1928)

Einhorn, V. F., Hamilton, R.: Transmitter release by red back spider venom. J. Pharm. Pharmacol. **25**, 284—286 (1973)

Elliot, R. H.: A contribution to the study of the action of Indian cobra venom. Phil. trans. roy. Soc. **197**, 361—406 (1905)

Epstein, D.: The pharmacology of the venom of the Cape cobra *(Naja flava)*. Quart. J. exp. Physiol. **20**, 7—19 (1930)

Eterović, V. A., Bennett, E. L.: Nicotinic cholinergic receptor in brain detected by binding of α[^{3}H] bungarotoxin. Biochim. biophys. Acta (Amst.) **362**, 345—365 (1974)

Evans, M. H.: Measuring small rapid changes in nerve threshold during exposure to snake venom. Nature (Lond.) **200**, 368 (1963)

Excell, B. J., Patel, R.: Characterization of toxic fractions of *Dendroaspis jamesoni* venoms. J. Physiol. (Lond.) **229**, 29p—30p (1972)

Fambrough, D. M., Hartzell, H. C.: Acetylcholine receptor: number and distribution at neuromuscular junctions in rat diaphragm. Science **176**, 189—191 (1972)

Fayrer, J.: Treatment of snake-poisoning by artificial respiration. Indian Med. Gaz. **7**, 218 (1872)

Fayrer, J.: Experiments on cobra poisoning and on a reputed antidote. Indian Med. Gaz. **8**, 6—7 (1873)

Fidler, H. K., Glasgow, R. D., Carmichael, E. B.: Pathological changes produced by the subcutaneous injection of rattlesnake *(Crotalus)* venom into *Macaca mulata* monkeys. Amer. J. Path. **16**, 355—364 (1940)

Finkelstein, A., Rubin, L. L., Tseng, M. C.: Black widow spider venom: effect of purified toxin on lipid bilayer membranes. Science **193**, 1009—1011 (1976)

Fohlman, J., Eaker, D., Karlsson, E., Thesleff, S.: Taipoxin, an extremely potent presynaptic neurotoxin from the venom of the Australian snake Taipan *(Oxyuranus s. scutellatus)*. Isolation, characterization, quaternary structure and pharmacological properties. Europ. J. Biochem. **68**, 457—469 (1976)

Fraser, T. R., Elliot, R. H.: Contributions to the study of the action of seasnake venoms. Proc. roy. Soc. **74**, 104—108 (1904)

Fraser, T. R., Elliot, R. H.: Enhydrina venom-its action on the blood circulation, motor nerves, and respiration. Phil. Trans. roy. Soc. [B] **197**, 249—279 (1905)

Fraser, T. R., Gunn, J. A.: Action of the venom of *Sepedon haemachates* of South Africa. Phil. Trans. roy. Soc. [B] **200**, 241—269 (1909)

Freeman, M., Kellaway, C. H.: The venom yields of common Australian poisonous snakes in captivity. Med. J. Aust. **21**, 373—377 (1934)

Frontali, N.: Catecholamine-depleting effect of black widow spider venom on iris nerve fibres. Brain Res. **37**, 146—148 (1972)

Frontali, N., Granata, F., Parisi, P.: Effects of black widow spider venom on ACh release from rat cerebral cortex slices in vitro. Biochem. Pharmacol. **21**, 969—974 (1972)

Frontali, N., Granata, F., Traina, M. E., Bellino, M.: Catecholamine depleting effect of black widow spider venom on fibres innervating different guinea pig tissues. Experientia (Basel) **29**, 1525—1527 (1973)

Fukuyama, T., Sawai, Y.: Local necrosis induced by cobra *(Naja naja atra)* venom. Jap. J. med. Sci. Biol. **25**, 211—214 (1972)

Gage, P. W.: Generation of end-plate potentials. Physiol. Rev. **56**, 177—247 (1976)

Garnet, J. R.: Venomous Australian Animals Dangerous to Man. Parkville (Victoria): Commonwealth Serum Lab. 1970

Gautrelet, J., Halpern, N.: Action du venin de cobra sur l'excitabilité neuromusculaire de la grenouille. C.R. Soc. Biol. (Paris) **113**, 1486—1488 (1933)

Gautrelet, J., Halpern, N., Corteggiani, E.: Du mécanisme d'action des doses physiologiques de venin de cobra sur la circulation, la respiration et l'excitabilité neuromusculaire. Arch. int. Physiol. **38**, 293—352 (1934)

Geh, S. L., Chan, K. E.: The prejunctional site of action of *Enhydrina schistosa* venom at the neuromuscular junction. Europ. J. Pharmacol. **21**, 115—120 (1973)

Geh, S. L., Toh, H. T.: The effect of sea snake neurotoxins and a phospholipase fraction on the ultrastructure of mammalian skeletal muscle. South-East Asian/Western Pacific Regional Meeting of Pharmacologists Singapore, May 1976, Abst. No. 33, 1976

Gennaro, J., Jr., Ramsey, H. W.: Distribution in the mouse of lethal and sublethal doses of cottonmouth moccasin venom labelled with iodine-131. Nature (Lond.) **184**, 1244 (1959)

Gitter, S., Moroz-Perlmutter, C., Boss, J. H., Livni, E., Rechnic, J., Goldblum, N., Vries, A. de: Studies on the snake venoms of the Near East: *Walterinnesia aegyptia* and *Pseudocerastes fieldii*. Amer. J. trop. Med. Hyg. **11**, 861—868 (1962)

Gitter, S., Vries, A. de: Symptomatology, pathology, and treatment of bites by Near Eastern, European, and North African snakes. In: Bücherl, W., Buckley, E. E., Deulofeu, V. (Eds.): Venomous Animals and Their Venoms, Vol. I, pp. 359—401. New York: Academic Press 1968

Gode, G. R., Tandan, G. C., Bhide, N. K.: Role of artificial ventilation in experimental cobra envenomation in the dog. Brit. J. Anaesth. **40**, 850—852 (1968)

Gomez, M. V., Dai, M. E. M., Diniz, C. R.: Effect of scorpion venom, tityus toxin, on the release of acetylcholine from incubated slices of rat brain. J. Neurochem. **20**, 1051—1061 (1973)

Gomez, M. V., Diniz, C. R., Barbosa, T. S.: Comparison of the effects of scorpion venom tityus toxin and ouabain on the release of acetylcholine from incubated slices of rat brain. J. Neurochem. **24**, 331—336 (1975)

Gonçalves, J. M.: Purification and properties of crotamine. In: Buckley, E. E., Porges, N. (Eds.): Venoms, No. 44, pp. 261—273. Washington: Am. Assoc. Adv. Sci. 1956

Granata, F., Traina, M. E., Frontali, N., Bertolini, B.: Effect of black widow spider venom on acetylcholine release from torpedo electric tissue slices and subcellular fractions in vitro. Comp. Biochem. Physiol. [A] **48**, 1—7 (1974)

Green, L. A., Sytokowski, A. J., Vogel, Z., Nirenberg, M. W.: α-Bungarotoxin used as a probe for acetylcholine receptors of cultured neurones. Nature (Lond.) **243**, 163—166 (1973)

Guyot, P., Boquet, P.: Envenimation experimentale du lapin par injection intracerebrale d'un venin d'Elapidae. C.R. Acad. Sci. (Paris) **251**, 1822—1824 (1960)

Habermann, E.: Zur Pharmakologie des Giftes der brasilianischen Klapperschlange. Naunyn-Schmiedebergs Arch. exp. Path. Pharmak. **232**, 244—245 (1957)

Habermann, E.: Bee and wasp venom. Science **177**, 314—322 (1972)

Habermann, E., Walsch, P., Breithaupt, H.: Biochemistry and pharmacology of the crotoxin complex. II. Possible interrelationships between toxicity and organ distribution of phospholipase A, crotapotin and their combination. Naunyn-Schmiedebergs Arch. Pharmacol. **273**, 313—330 (1972)

Hadidian, Z.: Proteolytic activity and physiologic and pharmacologic actions of *Agkistrodon piscivorous* venom. In: Buckley, E. E., Porges, N. (Eds.): Venoms, pp. 205—215. Washington: Am. Assoc. Adv. Sci. 1956

Hagiwara, S., Takahashi, K.: Surface density of calcium ions and calcium spike in the barnacle muscle fiber membrane. J. gen. Physiol. **50**, 583—601 (1967)

Halpert, J., Eaker, D.: Amino acid sequence of presynaptic neurotoxin from the venom of *Notechis scutatus scutatus* (Australian tiger snake). J. biol. Chem. **250**, 6990—6997 (1975)

Halpert, J., Eaker, D., Karlsson, E.: The role of phospholipase activity in the action of a presynaptic neurotoxin from the venom of *Notechis scutatus scutatus* (Australian tiger snake). FEBS Letters **61**, 72—76 (1976)

Harris, J. B., Johnson, M. A., Karlsson, E.: Pathological responses of rat skeletal muscle to a single subcutaneous injection of a toxin isolated from the venom of the Australian tiger snake, *Notechis scutatus*. Clin. exp. Pharmacol. Physiol. **2**, 383—404 (1975)

Harris, J. B., Karlsson, E., Thesleff, S.: Effects of an isolated toxin from Australian tiger snake *(Notechis scutatus scutatus)* venom at the mammalian neuromuscular junction. Brit. J. Pharmacol. **47**, 141—146 (1973)

Harris, A. J., Miledi, R.: The effect of type D botulinum toxin on frog neuromuscular junctions. J. Physiol. (Lond.) **217**, 497—515 (1971)

Hartzell, H. C., Fambrough, D. M.: Acetylcholine receptors, distribution, and extra-junctional density in rat diaphragm after denervation correlated with acetylcholine sensitivity. J. gen. Physiol. **60**, 248—262 (1972)

Hendon, R. A., Fraenkel-Conrat, H.: Biological roles of the two components of crotoxin. Proc. nat. Acad. Sci. (Wash.) **68**, 1560—1563 (1971)

Henriques, S. B., Henriques, O. B.: Pharmacology and toxicology of snake venoms. In: Rašková, H. (Ed.): Pharmacology and Toxicology of Naturally Occurring Toxins, International Encyclopedia of Pharmacology and Therapeutics, section 71, Vol. I, pp. 215—368. New York: Pergamon Pr. 1971

Heuser, J., Reese, T. S.: Evidence for recycling of synaptic vesicle membrane during transmitter release at the frog neuromuscular junction. J. Cell Biol. **57**, 315—344 (1973)

Ho, C. L., Lee, C. Y., Lu, H. H.: Electrophysiological effects of cobra cardiotoxin on rabbit heart cells. Toxicon **13**, 437—446 (1975)

Holman, M. E., Spitzer, N. C.: Action of botulinum toxin on transmission from sympathetic nerves to the vas deferens. Brit. J. Pharmacol. **47**, 431—433 (1973)

Hoskin, F. C. G., Rosenberg, P.: Alteration of acetylcholine penetration into and effects on venom-treated squid axons by physostigmine and related compounds. J. gen. Physiol. **47**, 1117—1127 (1964)

Houssay, B. A., Hug, E.: Action de l'apomorphine et du venin de Crotale sur les centres respiratoires et vagaux de la tête isolée. C.R. Soc. Biol. (Paris) **99**, 1509—1511 (1928)

Houssay, B. A., Mazzocco, Y. P.: Acción de las ponzoñas de serpientes sobre la difusion del potasio, fósforo y hemoglobina y formación de acido láctico de diversos órganos. Rev. Soc. Argentina Biol. **2**, 383—391 (1926)

Houssay, B. A., Negrete, J., Mazzocco, Y. P.: Actión des venins de serpents sur le nearf et le muscle strié isolé. C. R. Soc. Biol. (Paris) **87**, 823—824 (1922)

Houssay, B. A., Pave, S.: Action curarisante des venins de serpents chez la grenouille. C. R. Soc. Biol. (Paris) **87**, 821—823 (1922)
Howard, B. D.: Effects of β-bungarotoxin on mitochondrial respiration are caused by associated phospholipase A activity. Biochem. biophys. Res. Commun. **67**, 58—65 (1975)
Hubbard, J. I.: Microphysiology of vertebrate neuromuscular transmission. Physiol. Rev. **53**, 674—723 (1973)
Hubbard, J. I., Quastel, D. M. J.: Micropharmacology of vertebrate neuromuscular transmission. Ann. Rev. Pharmacol. **13**, 199—216 (1973)
Hubbard, J. I., Schmidt, R. F., Yokota, T.: The effect of acetylcholine upon mammalian motor nerve terminals. J. Physiol. (Lond.) **181**, 810—829 (1965)
Hughes, R., Whaler, B. C.: Influence of nerve ending activity and of drugs on the rate of paralysis of rat diaphragm preparations by *Cl. botulinum* type A toxin. J. Physiol. (Lond.) **160**, 221—233 (1962)
Hunter, W. K.: Acute degenerative changes in the nervous system as illustrated by snake-venom poisoning. Proc. roy. Soc. Med. **3**, 105—115 (1910)
Jacobi, C., Lankisch, P.-G., Schoner, K., Vogt, W.: Changes in Na^+ and K^+ permeability of red cells induced by the direct lytic factor of cobra venom and phospholipase A. Naunyn-Schmiedebergs Arch. Pharmacol. **274**, 81—90 (1972)
Jimènez-Porras, J. M.: Pharmacology of peptides and proteins in snake venoms. Ann. Rev. Pharmacol. **8**, 299—318 (1968)
Kamenskaya, M. A., Thesleff, S.: Neuromuscular blocking action of an isolated toxin from the elapid *(Oxyuranus scutellatus)*. Acta physiol. scand. **90**, 716—724 (1974)
Kao, I., Drachman, D. B., Price, D. L.: Botulinum toxin: Mechanism of presynaptic blockade. Science **193**, 1256—1258 (1976)
Karlsson, E., Eaker, D., Fryklund, L., Kadin, S.: Chromatographic separation of *Enhydrina schistosa* (Common sea snake) venom and the characterization of two principle neurotoxins. Biochemistry **11**, 4628—4633 (1972a)
Karlsson, E., Eaker, D., Ryden, L.: Purification of a presynaptic neurotoxin from the venom of the Australian tiger snake *Notechis scutatus scutatus*. Toxicon **10**, 405—413 (1972b)
Katz, B., Miledi, R.: Membrane noise produced by acetylcholine. Nature (Lond.) New Biol. **226**, 962—963 (1970)
Katz, B., Miledi, R.: Acetylcholine noise. Nature (Lond.) New Biol. **232**, 124—126 (1971)
Katz, B., Miledi, R.: The effect of α-bungarotoxin on acetylcholine receptor. Brit. J. Pharmacol. **49**, 138—139 (1973)
Katz, N. L., Edwards, C.: The effect of scorpion venom on the neuromuscular junction of the frog. Toxicon **10**, 133—137 (1972)
Kawai, N., Mauro, A., Grundfest, H.: Effect of black widow spider venom on lobster neuromuscular junction. J. gen. Physiol. **60**, 650—664 (1972)
Kellaway, C. H.: The venom of *Notechis scutatus*. Med. J. Aust. **1**, 348—354 (1929)
Kellaway, C. H.: Observations on the certainly lethal dose of the venom of the black snake *(Pseudechis porphyriacus)* for the common laboratory animals. Med. J. Aust. **17**, 33—41 (1930)
Kellaway, C. H.: Some peculiarities of Australian snake venoms. Trans. roy. Soc. trop. Med. Hyg. **27**, 9—34 (1933)
Kellaway, C. H.: Snake venoms. II. Their peripheral action. Johns Hopkins Med. J. **60**, 18—39 (1937)
Kellaway, C. H., Cherry, R. O., Williams, F. E.: The peripheral action of Australian snake venoms. II. The curare-like action in mammals. Aust. J. exp. Biol. med. Sci. **10**, 181—194 (1932)
Kellaway, C. H., Holden, H. F.: The peripheral action of Australian snake venoms. I. The curare-like action in frogs. Aust. J. exp. Biol. med. Sci. **10**, 167—179 (1932)
Kelly, R. B., Brown, F. R.: Biochemical and physiological properties of a purified snake venom neurotoxin which acts presynaptically. J. Neurobiol. **5**, 135—150 (1974)
Kilvington, B.: A preliminary communication on the changes in nerve cells after poisoning with the venom of the Australian tiger snake *(Hoplocephalus curtis)*. J. Physiol. (Lond.) **28**, 426—430 (1902)
Kita, H., Kloot, W. Van der: Effects of the ionophore X-537 A on acetylcholine release at the frog neuromuscular junction. J. Physiol. (Lond.) **259**, 177—198 (1976)

Krupnick, J., Bicher, H. I., Gitter, S.: Central neurotoxic effects of the venoms of *Naja naja* and *Vipera palestinae*. Toxicon **6**, 11—16 (1968)
Kryzhanovsky, G. N.: The mechanism of action of tetanus toxin: Effect on synaptic processes and some particular features of toxin binding by the nervous tissue. Naunyn-Schmiedebergs Arch. Pharmacol. **276**, 247—270 (1973)
Kupfer, C.: Selective block of synaptic transmission in ciliary ganglion by type A botulinus toxin in rabbits. Proc. Soc. exp. Biol. (N.Y.) **99**, 474—476 (1958)
Lai, M. K., Wen, C. Y., Lee, C. Y.: Local lesion caused by cardiotoxin isolated from Formosan cobra venom. J. Formosan med. Ass. **71**, 328—332 (1972)
Lamb, G., Hunter, W. K.: On the action of venoms of different species of poisonous snakes on the nervous system. VI. Venom of *Enhydrina Valakadien*. Lancet **1907 II**, 1017—1019
Lane, N. J., Gage, P. W.: Effects of tiger snake venom on the ultrastructure of motor nerve terminals. Nature [New Biol.] **244**, 94—96 (1973)
Langer, S. Z., Adler-Graschinsky, E., Almeida, A. P., Diniz, C. R.: Prejunctional effects of a purified toxin from the scorpion *Tityus serrulatus*. Release of [^{3}H] noradrenaline and enhancement of transmitter overflow elicited by nerve stimulation. Naunyn-Schmiedebergs Arch. Pharmacol. **287**, 243—259 (1975)
Lankisch, P. G., Lege, L., Oldigs, H. D., Vogt, W.: Binding of phospholipase A to the direct lytic factor revealed by the interaction of Ca^{2+} with the hemolytic effect. Biochim. biophys. Acta (Amst.) **239**, 267—272 (1971)
Larsen, P. R., Wolff, J.: Inhibition of accumulative transport by a protein from cobra venom. Biochem. Pharmacol. **16**, 2003—2009 (1967)
Lau, Y. H., Chiu, T. H., Caswell, A. H., Potter, L. T.: Effects of β-bungarotoxin on calcium uptake by sarcoplasmic reticulum from rabbit skeletal muscle. Biochem. biophys. Res. Commun. **61**, 460—466 (1974)
Lebez, D., Gubenšek, F., Maretič, Z.: Studies on labeled animal poisons. III. Possibility of labeling snake venoms in vivo with radioactive isotopes. Toxicon **5**, 263—266 (1968)
Lebez, D., Gubenšek, F., Turk, V.: Distribution of some toxic fractions of ^{75}Se labeled *Vipera ammodytes* venom in experimental animals. In: Vries, A. de, Kochva, E. (Eds.): Toxins of Animal and Plant Origin, pp. 1067—1074. New York: Gordon and Breach 1972
Lee, C. Y.: Mode of action of cobra venom and its purified toxins. In: Simpson, L. L. (Ed.): Neuropoisons, Vol. I, pp. 21—70. New York: Plenum Press 1971
Lee, C. Y.: Chemistry and pharmacology of polypeptide toxins in snake venoms. Ann. Rev. Pharmacol. **12**, 265—284 (1972)
Lee, C. Y.: Chemissry and pharmacology of purified toxins from elapid and sea snake venoms. 5th Int. Congr. Pharmacol., San Francisco, 1972, Abstract 2, pp. 210—232. Basel: Karger 1973
Lee, C. Y.: Pharmacological classification of toxic proteins from snake venoms. Jap. J. trop. Med. Hyg. **3**, 219—225 (1975)
Lee, C. Y., Chang, C. C.: Modes of actions of purified toxins from elapid venoms on neuromuscular transmission. Mem. Inst. Butantan **33**, 555—572 (1966)
Lee, C. Y., Chang, C. C., Chen, Y. M.: Reversibility of neuromuscular blockade by neurotoxins from elapid and sea snake venoms. J. Formosan med. Ass. **71**, 344—349 (1972a)
Lee, C. Y., Chang, C. C., Chiu, T. H., Chiu, P. J. S., Tseng, T. C., Lee, S. Y.: Pharmacological properties of cardiotoxin isolated from Formosan cobra venom. Naunyn-Schmiedebergs Arch. Pharmacol. **259**, 360—374 (1968)
Lee, C. Y., Chang, C. C., Su, C.: Effect of group specific reagents on toxicity and curare-like activity of elapid venoms. J. Formosan med. Ass. **59**, 1065—1072 (1960)
Lee, C. Y., Chang, C. C., Su, C., Chen, Y. W.: The toxicity and thermostability of Formosan snake venoms. J. Formosan med. Ass. **61**, 239—244 (1962)
Lee, C. Y., Chang, S. L., Kau, S. T., Luh, S. H.: Chromatographic separation of the venom of *Bungarus multicinctus* and characterization of its components. J. Chromatog. **72**, 71—82 (1972b)
Lee, C. Y., Chen, Y. M.: Species differences in reversibility of neuromuscular blockade by elapid and sea snake neurotoxins. In: Ohsaka, A., Hayashi, K., Sawai, Y. (Eds.): Animal, Plants, and Microbial Toxins, Vol. II, pp. 193—203. New York: Plenum Press 1976
Lee, C. Y., Chen, Y. M.: Central neurotoxicity of cobra neurotoxin, cardiotoxin, and phospholipase A_2. Toxicon **15**, 395—401 (1977)

Lee, C. Y., Chen, Y. M., Karlsson, E.: Postsynaptic and musculotropic effects of notexin, a presynaptic neurotoxin from the venom of *Notechis scutatus scutatus* (Australian tiger snake). Toxicon **14**, 493—494 (1976a)

Lee, C. Y., Chen, Y. M., Mebs, D.: Chromatographic separation of the venom of Egyptian black snake (*Walterinnesia aegyptia*) and pharmacological characterization of its components. Toxicon **14**, 275—281 (1976b)

Lee, C. Y., Chen, Y. M., Mebs, D.: Chromatographic separation of the venom of *Bungarus caeruleus* and pharmacological characterization of its components. Toxicon **14**, 451—457 (1976c)

Lee, C. Y., Huang, M. C., Bonilla, C. A.: Mode of action of purified basic proteins from three rattlesnake venoms on neuromuscular junction of the chick biventer cervicis muscle. In: Kaiser, E. (Ed.): Tier- und Pflanzengift, pp. 173—178. München: Wilhelm Goldmann Verlag 1972c

Lee, C. Y., Huang, P. F., Tsai, M. C.: Mode of neuromuscular blocking action of the desert black snake venom. Toxicon **9**, 429—430 (1971a)

Lee, C. Y., Liao, C., Lin, S. Y.: Identification of cholinesterase inactivating factor in cobra venom with cardiotoxin. Proc. 18th Symp. Toxin, Tokyo, 1971b

Lee, C. Y., Lin, J. S., Wei, J. W.: Identification of cardiotoxin with cobramine B, DLF, toxin γ, and cobra venom cytotoxin. In: Vries, A. de, Kochva, E. (Eds.): Toxins of Animal and Plant Origin, pp. 307—318. New York: Gordon and Breach 1971c

Lee, C. Y., Peng, M. T.: An analysis of the respiratory failure produced by the Formosan elapid venom. Arch. intern. Pharmacodyn. **133**, 180—192 (1961)

Lee, C. Y., Tsai, M. C.: Does the desert black snake venom inhibit release of acetylcholine from motor nerve endings. Toxicon **10**, 659—660 (1972)

Lee, C. Y., Tseng, L. F.: Distribution of *Bungarus multicinctus* venom following envenomation. Toxicon **3**, 281—290 (1966)

Lee, C. Y., Tseng, L. F.: Species differences in susceptibility to elapid venoms. Toxicon **7**, 89—93 (1969)

Lee, C. Y., Tseng, L. F., Chiu, T. H.: Influence of denervation on localization of neurotoxins from elapid venoms in rat diaphragm. Nature (Lond.) **215**, 1177—1178 (1967)

Lentz, T. L., Rosenthal, J., Mazurkiewicz, J. E.: Cytochemical localization of acetylcholine receptors by means of peroxidase-labelled α-bungarotoxin. Neurosci. Abstr. Soc. for Neurosci. **976** (1975)

Lester, H. A.: Postsynaptic action of cobra toxin at the myoneural junction. Nature (Lond.) **227**, 727—728 (1970)

Lester, H. A.: Blockade of acetylcholine receptors by cobra toxin: electrophysiological studies. Molec. Pharmacol. **8**, 623—631 (1972a)

Lester, H. A.: Vulnerability of desensitized or curare-treated acetylcholine receptors to irreversible blockade by cobra toxin. Molec. Pharmacol. **8**, 632—644 (1972b)

Leung, W. W., Keung, W. M., Kong, Y. C.: The cytolytic effect of cobra cardiotoxin on Ehrich ascites tumor cells and its inhibition by Ca^{2+}. Naunyn-Schmiedebergs Arch. Pharmacol. **292**, 193—198 (1976)

Liley, A. W.: The effects of presynaptic polarization on the spontaneous activity at the neuromuscular junction. J. Physiol. (Lond.) **134**, 427—443 (1956)

Lin Shiau, S. Y., Huang, M. C., Lee, C. Y.: Isolation of cardiotoxin and neurotoxic principles from the venom of *Bungarus fasciatus*. J. Formosan med. Ass. **71**, 350—357 (1972)

Lin Shiau, S. Y., Huang, M. C., Lee, C. Y.: A study of cardiotoxic principles from the venom of *Bungarus fasciatus* (Schneider). Toxicon **13**, 189—196 (1975a)

Lin Shiau, S. Y., Huang, M. C., Lee, C. Y.: Mechanism of action of cobra cardiotoxin in the skeletal muscle. J. Pharmacol. exp. Ther. **196**, 758—770 (1976)

Lin Shiau, S. Y., Huang, M. C., Tseng, W. C., Lee, C. Y.: Comparative studies on the biological activities of cardiotoxin, melittin, and prymnesin. Naunyn-Schmiedebergs Arch. Pharmacol. **287**, 349—358 (1975b)

Lin Shiau, S. Y., Tseng, W. C., Lee, C. Y.: Pharmacology of scorpion toxin II in the skeletal muscle. Naunyn-Schmiedebergs Arch. Pharmacol. **289**, 359—368 (1975c)

Longenecker, H. E., Hurlbut, W. P., Mauro, A., Clark, A. W.: Effects of black widow spider venom on the frog neuromuscular junction. Nature (Lond.) **225**, 701 (1970)

Loots, J. M., Meij, H. S., Meyer, B. J.: Effects of *Naja nivea* venom on nerve, cardiac, and skeletal muscle activity of the frog. Brit. J. Pharmacol. **47**, 576—585 (1973)

Lu, H. S., Lo, T. B.: Chromatographic separation of *Bungarus fasciatus* venom and preliminary characterization of its components. J. Chinese biochem. Soc. **3**, 57—68 (1974)

Lundberg, A., Quilisch, H.: On the effect of calcium on presynaptic potentiation and depression at the neuro-muscular junction. Acta physiol. scand. **30** [Suppl. III], 121—129 (1953)

Lysz, T. W., Rosenberg, P.: Convulsant activity of *Naja naja* venom and its phospholipase A component. Toxicon **12**, 253—265 (1974)

Maeno, H., Mitsuhashi, S., Okonogi, T., Hoshi, S., Homma, M.: Studies on snake venom. V. Myolysis caused by phospholipase A in Habu snake venom. Jap. J. exp. Med. **32**, 55—64 (1962)

Maeda, N., Takagi, K., Tamiya, N., Chen, Y. M., Lee, C. Y.: The isolation of an easily reversible post-synaptic toxin from the venom of a sea snake, *Laticauda semifasciata*. Biochem. J. **141**, 383—387 (1974)

Maeda, N., Tamiya, N.: Primary structure of the toxin Laticauda semifasciata III. a weak and reversibly acting neurotoxin from the venom of sea snake, *Laticauda semifasciata*. Biochem. J. **141**, 389—400 (1974)

Magazanik, L. G., Vyskočil, F.: The loci of α-bungarotoxin action on the muscle postjunctional membrane. Brain Res. **48**, 420—423 (1972a)

Magazanik, L. G., Vyskočil, F.: Characteristics of endplate potentials after partial blockade by α-bungarotoxin in *Rana temporaria*. Experientia (Basel) **29**, 157—158 (1972b)

Manery, J. F.: Effects of Ca ions on membranes. Fed. Proc. **25**, 1804—1810 (1966)

Marsden, A. T. H., Reid, H. A.: Pathology of sea snake poisoning. Brit. med. J. **1**, 1290—1293 (1961)

Martin, C. J.: On some effects upon the blood produced by venom of the Australian black snake. J. Physiol. (Lond.) **15**, 380 (1893)

Martin, R., Rosenberg, P.: Fine structural alterations associated with venom action on squid giant nerve fibres. J. Cell Biol. **36**, 341—353 (1968)

McCollough, N. C., Gennaro, Jr., J. F.: Evaluation of venomous snake bite in the Southern United States from parallel clinical and laboratory investigations. J. Florida med. Ass. **49**, 959—967 (1963)

Mebs, D., Chen, Y. M., Lee, C. Y.: Biochemistry and pharmacology of toxins from Australian snake venoms. 5th Int. Symp. on Animal, Plant, and Microbial Toxins. San Jose, Costa Rica, 1976

Mebs, D., Lee, C. Y., Chen, Y. M., Iwanaga, S.: Chemical and pharmacological characterization of toxic polypeptides from four Elapidae venoms. 4th Int. Symp. on Animal, Plant, and Microbial Toxins, Tokyo, 1974

Mebs, D., Narita, K., Iwanaga, S., Samejima, Y., Lee, C. Y.: Purification, properties, and amino acid sequence of α-bungarotoxin from the venom of *Bungarus multicinctus*. Hoppe Seylers Z. physiol. Chem. **353**, 243—262 (1972)

Meldrum, B. S.: Depolarization of skeletal muscle by a toxin from cobra *(Naja naja)* venom. J. Physiol. (Lond.) **168**, 49—50 (1963)

Meldrum, B. S.: The actions of snake venom on nerve and muscle. The pharmacology of phospholipase A and of polypeptide toxins. Pharmacol. Rev. **17**, 393—445 (1965a)

Meldrum, B. S.: Actions of whole and fractionated Indian cobra *(Naja naja)* venom on skeletal muscle. Brit. J. Pharmacol. **25**, 197—205 (1965b)

Mellanby, J. H.: Presynaptic effect of tetanus toxin at the neuromuscular junction. J. Physiol. (Lond.) **218**, 68—69 (1971)

Miledi, R., Potter, L. T.: Acetylcholine receptors in muscle fibres. Nature (Lond.) **233**, 599—603 (1971)

Miledi, R., Szczepaniak, A. C.: Effect of *Dendroaspis* neurotoxins on synaptic transmission in the spinal cord of the frog. Proc. roy. Soc. Lond. [Biol.] **190**, 267—274 (1975)

Mohamed, A. H., Zaki, O.: Effect of the black snake toxin on the gastrocnemius-sciatic preparation. J. exp. Biol. **35**, 20—26 (1958)

Moore, W. J., Loy, N. J.: Irreversible binding of a krait neurotoxin to membrane proteins from electroplax and hog brain. Biochem. biophys. Res. Commun. **46**, 2093—2099 (1972)

Moss, J., Thoa, N. B., Kopin, I. J.: Mechanism of scorpion toxin induced release of norepinephrine from peripheral adrenergic neurons. J. Pharmacol. Exp. Ther. **190**, 39—48 (1974)
Moussatché, H., Gonçalves, J. M., Vieira, G. D., Hasson, H.: Pharmacological actions of two proteins from Brazilian rattlesnake venom. In: Buckley, E. E., Porges, N. (Eds.): Venoms, pp. 275—279. Washington: Am. Ass. Adv. Sci. 1956
Musick, J., Hubbard, J. I.: Release of protein from mouse motor nerve terminals. Nature **237**, 279—281 (1972)
Narahashi, T., Shapiro, B. I., Deguchi, T., Senka, M., Wang, C. M.: Effects of scorpion venom on squid axon membranes. Am. J. Physiol. **222**, 850—857 (1972)
Narahashi, T., Tobias, J. M.: Properties of axon membrane as affected by cobra venom, digitonin, and proteases. Am. J. Physiol. **207**, 1441—1446 (1964)
Nelson, P. G.: Effects of certain enzymes on node of Ranvier excitability with observations on submicroscopic structure. J. Cell comp. Physiol. **52**, 127—146 (1958)
Neumann, W. P., Habermann, E.: Über Crotactin, das Haupttoxin des Giftes der brasilianischen Klapperschlange *(Crotalus d. terrificus)*. Biochem. Z. **327**, 170—185 (1955)
Oh, Y.: Über die Letaldosis des Giftes von *Naja naja atra* bei verschiedenen Tieren. J. Formosan med. Ass. **41**, 1185—1198 (1942)
Okamoto, M., Longenecker, H. E., Riker, W. F., Song, S. K.: Destruction of mammalian motor nerve terminals by black widow spider venom. Science **172**, 733—736 (1971)
Okonogi, T., Hoshi, S., Homma, M., Mitsuhashi, S., Maeno, H., Sawai, Y.: Experimental studies on Habu snake venom. III-3. Experimental histopathological studies on the central nerve system of guinea pigs. Jap. J. Microbiol. **4**, 297—302 (1960)
Orlov, B.: Effect of calcium ions on the development of the depressant action of cobra venom on nerve trunks. Uch. Zap. Gor'k Gos. Univ. **140**, 40—43 (1972)
Orlov, B. N.: Depolarization activity of animal venoms. Uch. Zap. Gor'k Gos. Univ. **101**, 197—203 (1970)
Osborne, R. H., Bradford, H. F.: Tetanus toxin inhibits amino acid release from nerve endings in vitro. Nature (Lond.) New Biol. **244**, 157 (1973)
Otsuka, M., Endo, M., Nonomura, Y.: Presynaptic nature of neuromuscular depression. Jap. J. Physiol. **12**, 573—584 (1962)
Ouyang, C.: On the cause of death due to the venom of *Bungarus multicinctus Blyth* in rabbits. Mem. Fac. Med. Nat. Taiwan Univ. **1**, 121—127 (1950)
Pacella, G.: Action des venins de serpents sur les centres bulbaires. C. R. Soc. Biol. (Paris) **88**, 366—367 (1923)
Parnas, I., Russell, F. E.: Effects of venoms on nerve, muscle, and neuromuscular junction. In: Russell, F. E., Saunders, P. R. (Eds.): Animal Toxins, pp. 401—415. Oxford: Pergamon Pr. 1967
Patel, R., Excell, B.: The effects of lethal components of *Dendroaspis jamensoni* snake venom on neuromuscular transmission and muscle membrane permeability. Toxicon **13**, 295—304 (1975)
Patel, T. N., Braganca, B. M., Bellare, R. A.: Changes produced by cobra venom cytotoxin on the morphology of Yoshida sarcoma cells. Exp. Cell Res. **57**, 289—297 (1969)
Pellegrini Filho, A., Vital Brazil, O., Laure, C. J.: The action of crotamine on skeletal muscle: an electrophysiological study. 5th International Symposium on Animal, Plant and Microbial Toxins, Costa Rica, 1976, Abstract, p. 94
Peng, M. T.: A toxicological study of the fractionated venom of *Naja naja atra*. Mem. Fac. Med. Nat. Taiwan Univ. **1**, 200—214 (1951)
Peng, M. T.: Action of the venom of *Naja naja atra* on respiration and circulation. Mem. Fac. Med. Nat. Taiwan Univ. **2**, 170—182 (1952)
Peng, M. T.: Effect of Formosan snake venoms on the depolarizing action of acetylcholine at motor end-plate. J. Formosan med. Ass. **59**, 1073—1082 (1960)
Pieterson, W. A., Volwerk, J. J., Haas, G. H. de: Interaction of phospholipase A_2 and its zymogen with divalent metal ions. Biochemistry **13**, 1439—1445 (1974)
Polz-Tejera, G., Schmidt, J., Karten, H. J.: Autoradiographic localization of α-bungarotoxin-binding sites in the central nervous system. Nature (Lond.) **258**, 349—351 (1975)
Porter, C. W., Chiu, T. H., Wieckowshi, J., Barnard, E. A.: Types and locations of cholinergic receptor-like molecules in muscle fibres. Nature (Lond.) Biol. **241**, 3—7 (1973)

Ragotzi, V.: Über die Wirkung des Giftes der *Naja tripudians*. Virchows Arch. **122**, 201—234 (1890)
Reid, H. A.: Myoglobinuria and sea snake poisoning. Br. Med. J. **1**, 1284—1289 (1961)
Rogers, L.: On the physiological action of the poison of the Hydrophidae. Proc. roy. Soc. (Lond.) [Biol.] **71**, 481—496 (1903)
Rogers, L.: On the physiological action of the poison of the Hydrophidae. II-Action on the circulatory, respiratory and nervous systems. Proc. roy. Soc. Lond. [Biol.] **72**, 305—319 (1904)
Rogers, L.: The physiological action and antidotes of colubrine and vinerine snake venoms. Phil. Trans. roy. Soc. [B] **197**, 123—191 (1905)
Romey, G., Chicheportiche, R., Lazdunski, M., Rochat, H., Miranda, F., Lissitzky, S.: Scorpion neurotoxin, presynaptic toxin which affects both sodium ion and potassium ion channels in axons. Biochem. biophys. Res. Commun. **64**, 115—121 (1975)
Rosenberg, P.: Effects of venoms on the squid giant axon. Toxicon **3**, 125—131 (1965)
Rosenberg, P.: Venoms and enzymes. Effects on permeability of isolated single electroplax. Toxicon **11**, 149—154 (1973)
Rosenberg, P.: Penetration of phospholipase A_2 and C into the squid *(Loligo peolii)* giant axon. Experientia (Basel) **31**, 1401—1403 (1975)
Rosenberg, P., Ehrenpreis, S.: Reversible block of axonal conduction by curare after treatment with cobra venom. Biochem. Pharmacol. **8**, 192—206 (1961)
Rosenberg, P., Hoskin, F. C. G.: Demonstration of increased permeability as a factor in the effect of acetylcholine on the electrical activity of venom-treated axons. J. gen. Physiol. **46**, 1065—1073 (1963)
Rosenberg, P., Ng, K. Y.: Factors in venoms leading to block of axonal conduction by curare. Biochim. biophys. Acta (Amst.) **75**, 116—128 (1963)
Rosenberg, P., Podleski, T. R.: Block of conduction by acetylcholine and D-tubocurarine after treatment of squid axon with cotton-mouth moccasin venom. J. Pharmacol. exp. Ther. **137**, 249—262 (1962)
Rosenberg, P., Podleski, T. R.: Ability of venoms to render squid axons sensitive to curare and acetylcholine. Biochim. biophys. Acta (Amst.) **75**, 104—115 (1963)
Rosenfeld, G.: Symptomatology, pathology, and treatment of snake bites in South America. In: Bücherl, W., Buckley, E. E. (Eds.): Venomous Animals and Their Venoms, Vol. II, pp. 345—384. New York: Academic Pr. 1971
Russell, F. E.: Venomous animals and their toxins. Ann. Rep. Smithsonian Inst. **1964**, 477—487 (1964)
Russell, F. E.: Comparative pharmacology of some animal toxins. Fed. Proc. **26**, 1206—1224 (1967)
Russell, F. E., Bohr, V. C.: Intraventricular injection of venom. Toxicol. Appl. Pharmacol. **4**, 165—173 (1962)
Russell, F. E., Long, T. E.: Effect of venoms on neuromuscular transmission. In: Viets, H. R. (Ed.): Myasthenia Gravis, Vol. I, pp. 101—116. Springfield: C. C. Thomas 1961
Russell, F. E., Mickaelis, B. A.: Cardiovascular effects of *Crotalus* venom. Med. Arts Sci. **14**, 119—121 (1960)
Rübsamen, K., Breithaupt, H., Habermann, E.: Biochemistry and pharmacology of the crotoxin complex. I. Subfractionation and recombination of the crotoxin complex. Naunyn-Schmiedebergs Arch. Pharmacol. **270**, 274—288 (1971)
Salvaterra, P. M., Mahler, H. R., Moore, W. J.: Subcellular and regional distribution of iodine^{125}-labelled α-bungarotoxin binding in rat brain and its relation to acetylcholinesterase and choline acetyltransferase. J. biol. Chem. **250**, 6469—6475 (1975)
Salvaterra, P. M., Moore, W. J.: Binding of iodine-125 labelled α-bungarotoxin to particulate fractions of rat and guinea pig brain. Biochem. biophys. Res. Commun. **55**, 1311—1318 (1973)
Sarkar, N. K.: Isolation of cardiotoxin from cobra venom *(Naja tripudians)* monocellate variety. J. Ind. chem. Soc. **24**, 227—232 (1947)
Sarkar, N. K.: Action mechanism of cobra venom, cardiotoxin, and allied substance on muscle contraction. Proc. Soc. exp. Biol. (N.Y.) **78**, 469—471 (1951)
Sarkar, N. K., Maitre, S. R.: Action of cobra venom and cardiotoxin on gastrocnemius-sciatic preparation of forg. Amer. J. Physiol. **163**, 209—211 (1950)

Sato, S., Abe, T., Tamiya, N.: Binding of iodinated erabutoxin b, a sea snake toxin, to the endplates of the mouse diaphragm. Toxicon **8**, 313—314 (1970)
Schenberg, S.: Geographical pattern of crotamine distribution in the same rattlesnake subspecies. Science **129**, 1361—1363 (1959)
Schleifer, L. S., Eldefrawi, M. E.: Identification of the nicotinic and muscarinic acetylcholine receptors in subcellular fractions of mouse brain. Neuropharmacology **13**, 53—64 (1974)
Schmidt, J. L., Goodsell, E. B., Brondyk, H. D., Kueter, K. E., Richards, R. K.: The prolonged effect of cobra venom on the sensitivity to D-tubocurarine. Arch. int. Pharmacodyn. **147**, 569—575 (1964)
Schwab, M. S., Puffer, H. W.: A study of the site of blockade of the vertebrate neuromuscular junction by erabutoxin a. Fed. Proc. **35**, 800 (1976)
Sen, I., Cooper, J. R.: Effect of β-bungarotoxin on the release of acetylcholine from brain synaptosomal preparations. Biochem. Pharmacol. **24**, 2107—2109 (1975)
Sen, I., Grantham, P. A., Cooper, J. R.: Mechanism of action of β-bungarotoxin on synaptosomal preparations. Proc. nat. Acad. Sci. USA **73**, 2664—2668 (1976)
Shaw, C. E.: The coral snakes, genera *Micrurus* and *Micruroides*, of the United States and Northern Mexico. In: Bücherl, W., Buckley, E. E. (Eds.): Venomous Animals and Their Venoms, Vol. II, pp. 157—172. New York: Academic Pr. 1971
Shü, I. C., Ling, K. H., Yang, C. C.: Study of iodine-131 labeled cobrotoxin. Toxicon **5**, 295—301 (1968)
Silinsky, E. M., Hubbard, J. I.: Release of ATP from rat motor nerve terminals. Nature **243**, 404—405 (1973)
Simpson, L. L.: Ionic requirements for the neuromuscular blocking action of botulinum toxin: implications with regard to synaptic transmission. Neuropharmacology **10**, 673—684 (1971)
Simpson, L. L.: The interaction between divalent cations and botulinum toxin type A in the paralysis of the rat phrenic nerve hemidiaphragm preparation. Neuropharmacology **12**, 165—176 (1973)
Simpson, L. L.: Studies on the binding of botulinum toxin type A to the rat phrenic nerve-hemidiaphragm preparation. Neuropharmacology **13**, 683—691 (1974)
Sivamogstham, P., Tejasen, P.: Isolation and pharmacological studies of the neurotoxic principle of *Naja naja siamensis* (cobra) venom from Thailand. Chian Mai Med. Bull. **11**, 135—150 (1972)
Sket, D., Gubenšek, F., Adamič, Š., Lebez, D.: Action of a partially purified basic protein fraction from *Vipera ammodytes* venom. Toxicon **11**, 47—53 (1973)
Slotta, K., Fraenkel-Conrat, H.: Schlangengifte. III. Reinigung und Krystallisation von Klapperschlangengift. Ber. Dtsch. Chem. Ges. **71**, 1076—1081 (1938)
Slotta, K. H., Vick, J. A.: Identification of the direct lytic factor from cobra venom as cardiotoxin. Toxicon **6**, 167—173 (1969)
Slotta, K. H., Vick, J. A., Ginsberg, N. J.: Enzymatic and toxic activity of phospholipase A. In: Vries, A. de, Kochva, E. (Eds.): Toxins of Animal and Plant Origin, Vol. I, pp. 401—417. New York: Gordon and Breach 1971
Snyder, G. K., Ramsey, H. W., Taylor, W. J., Chiou, C. Y.: Neuromuscular blockade of chick biventer cervicis nerve-muscle preparations by a fraction from coral snake venom. Toxicon **11**, 505—508 (1973)
Spitzer, N.: Miniature endplate potentials at mammalian neuromuscular junctions poisoned by botulinum toxin. Nature (Lond.) New Biol. **237**, 26—27 (1972)
Stern, P., Valjevac, K., Dursum, K., Dučić, V.: Mice cured definitely from Botulinus intoxication. Naunyn-Schmiedebergs Arch. Pharmacol. **282** [Suppl. R], 96 (1974)
Stringer, J. M., Kainer, R. A., Tu, A. T.: Ultrastructural studies of myonecrosis induced by cobra venom in mice. Toxicol. Appl. Pharmacol. **18**, 442—450 (1971)
Stringer, J. M., Kainer, R. A., Tu, A. T.: Myonecrosis induced by rattlesnake venom. Am. J. Pathol. **67**, 127—136 (1972)
Strong, P. N., Goerke, J., Oberg, S. G., Kelly, R. B.: β-Bungarotoxin, a presynaptic toxin with enzymatic activity. Proc. nat. Acad. Sci. (Wash.) **73**, 178—182 (1976a)
Strong, P. N., Heuser, J. E., Oberg, S. G., Kelly, R. B.: β-Bungarotoxin: Phospholipase activity is responsible for presynaptic action. 5th International Symposium on Animal, Plant, and Microbial Toxins, Costa Rica, 1976b, Abstract, p. 92

Strydom, D. J.: Snake venom toxins. The amino acid sequences of two toxins from *Dendroaspis polylepis polylepis* (black mamba) venom. J. biol. Chem. **247**, 4029—4042 (1972)
Strydom, D. J.: Snake venom toxins. Structure-function relationships and phylogenetics. Comp. Biochem. Physiol. [B] **44**, 269—281 (1973)
Su, C.: Mode of curare-like action of cobra venom. J. Formosan med. Ass. **59**, 1083—1091 (1960)
Su, C., Chang, C. C., Lee, C. Y.: Pharmacological properties of the neurotoxin of cobra venom. In: Russell, F. E., Saunders, P. R. (Eds.): Animal Toxins, pp. 259—267. Oxford: Pergamon Press 1967
Suarez-Kurtz, G., Bianchi, C. P., Krupp, P.: Effect of local anesthetics on radiocalcium binding in nerve. Europ. J. Pharmacol. **10**, 91—100 (1970)
Sumyk, G., Lal, H., Hawrylewicz, E. J.: Whole animal autoradiographic localization of radioiodine labelled cobra venom in mice. Fed. Proc. **22**, 668 (1963)
Takamizawa, T.: Effects of erabutoxin B on the membrane properties of frog sartorius muscle cells. Tohoku J. exp. Med. **101**, 339—350 (1970)
Takeuchi, A., Takeuchi, N.: The effect on crayfish muscle of iontophoretically applied glutamate. J. Physiol. (Lond.) **170**, 296—317 (1964)
Tamiya, N.: Sea snake venoms and toxins. In: Dunson, W. A. (Ed.): The Biology of Sea Snake, pp. 385—415. Baltimore: Univ. Park Pr. 1975
Tazieff-Depierre, F.: Scorpion venom, calcium, and ACh release by nerve fibers in the guinea pig ileum. C.R. Acad. Sci. [D] (Paris) **275**, 3021—3024 (1972)
Tazieff-Depierre, F.: Cardiotoxicité chez le Rat de la toxin γ purifiée, isolée du venin de *Naja nigricollis* et des toxines extraites du venin de scorpion. C.R. Acad. Sci. [D] (Paris) **280**, 1181—1184 (1975)
Tazieff-Depierre, F., Andrillon, P.: Sécrétion d'acétylcholine provoguée par le venin de Scorpion dans l'iléon de Cobaye et sa suppression par la tétrodotoxine. C.R. Acad. Sci. [D] (Paris) **276**, 1631—1633 (1973)
Tazieff-Depierre, F., Czajka, M., Lowagie, C.: Action pharmacologique de fractions pures de venin de *Naja nigricollis* et libération de calcium dans les muscles striés. C.R. Acad. Sci. [D] (Paris) **268**, 2511—2514 (1969)
Tazieff-Depierre, F., Pierre, J.: Action curarisante de la toxin alfa de *Naja nigricollis*. C.R. Acad. Sci. [D] (Paris) **263**, 1785—1788 (1966)
Tazieff-Depierre, F., Nachon-Rautureau, C.: Action du venin de scorpion *(Androctonus australis)* sur une préparation neuromusculaire de grenouille. C.R. Acad. Sci. [D] (Paris) **280**, 1745—1748 (1975)
Tazieff-Depierre, F., Trethewie, E. R.: Action du chlorure de calcium sur la cardiotoxicité chez le rat de la toxin γ, purifiée, isolatée du venin de *Naja nigricollis*. C.R. Acad. Sci. [D] (Paris) **280**, 137—140 (1975)
Telang, B. V., Galzigna, L., Maina, G., Ngángá, J. N.: Mechanism of action of Jameson's mamba venom on the superior cervical ganglion of cat. Toxicon **14**, 15—26 (1976)
Thesleff, S.: Supersensitivity of skeletal muscle produced by botulinum toxin. J. Physiol. (Lond.) **151**, 598—607 (1960)
To, S., Tin, S.: Toxikologische Untersuchungen betreffs des Giftes von *Bungarus multicinctus*. J. Formosan med. Ass. **42**, [Suppl.] 1—16 (1943)
Tobias, J. M.: Effects of phospholipases, collagenase, and chymotrypsin on impulse conduction and resting potential in the lobster axon with parallel experiments on frog muscle. J. Cell Comp. Physiol. **46**, 183—207 (1955)
Tobias, J. M.: Further studies on the nature of the excitable system in nerve. III. Effects of proteases and of phospholipases on lobster giant axon resistance and capacity. J. Gen. Physiol. **43**, 57—71 (1960)
Tobias, G. S., Donlon, M., Shain, W., Catravas, G.: β-Bungarotoxin: Relationship of phospholipase A activity to toxicity. Fed. Proc. **35**, 800 (1976)
Tsai, M. C.: Studies on the ultrastructual changes in the motor nerve terminals caused by β-bungarotoxin. Ph.D. Dissertation, National Taiwan Univ., Taipei, 1975
Tseng, L. F., Chiu, T. H., Lee, C. Y.: Absorption and distribution of ^{131}I-labelled cobra venom and its purified toxins. Toxicol. Appl. Pharmacol. **12**, 526—535 (1968)
Tu, T.: Toxicological studies on the venom of a sea snake, *Laticauda semifasciata* (Reinwardt) in Formosan waters. J. Formosan med. Ass. **58**, 182—203 (1959)

Tu, A. T., Toom, P. M.: Isolation and characterization of the toxic component of *Enhydrina schistosa* (common sea snake) venom. J. biol. Chem. **246**, 1012—1016 (1971)
Vellard, J.: Variations geographiques de venin de *Crotalus terrificus*. C.R. Soc. Biol. (Paris) **130**, 463—464 (1939)
Venkatachalam, K., Ratnagiriswaran, A. N.: Some experimental observations on the venom of the Indian cobra. Indian J. med. Res. **22**, 289—294 (1934)
Vick, J. A.: Effects of actual snake bite and venom injection on vital physiological function. Toxicon **8**, 159 (1970)
Vick, J. A.: Ciuchta, H. P., Broomfield, C., Currie, B. T.: Isolation and identification of toxic fractions of cobra venom. Toxicon **3**, 237—241 (1966)
Vick, J. A., Ciuchta, H. P., Manthei, J. H.: Pathophysiological studies of ten snake venoms. In: Russell, E. E., Sanders, P. R. (Eds.): Animal Toxins, pp. 269—282. New York: Pergamon Pr. 1967
Vick, J. A., Ciuchta, H. P., Polley, E. H.: Effect of snake venom and endotoxin on cortical electrical activity. Nature (Lond.) **203**, 1387—1388 (1964)
Vick, J. A., Ciuchta, H. P., Polley, E. H.: The effect of cobra venom on the respiratory mechanism of the dog. Arch. int. Pharmacodyn. **153**, 424—429 (1965)
Vick, J. A., Lipp, J.: Effect of cobra and rattlesnake venoms on the central nervous system of the primate. Toxicon **8**, 33—39 (1970)
Vincent, J. P., Schweitz, H., Chicheportishe, R., Fosset, M., Balerna, M., Lenoir, M. C., Lazdunski, M.: Molecular mechanism of cardiotoxin action on axonal membranes. Biochemistry **15**, 3171—3175 (1976)
Vital Brazil, O.: Pharmacology of crystalline crotoxin. II. Neuromuscular blocking action. Mem. Inst. Butantan **33**, 981—992 (1966)
Vital Brazil, O.: Venoms. Their inhibitory action on neuromuscular transmittance. Int. Encylc. Pharmacol. Ther. **14**, 145—167 (1972)
Vital Brazil, O., Excell, B. J.: Action of crotoxin and crotactin from the venom of *Crotalus durissus terrificus* (South American rattlesnake) on the frog neuromuscular junction. J. Physiol. (Lond.) **212**, 34—35 (1971)
Vital Brazil, O., Excell, B. J., Sanatana de SaS.: The importance of phospholipase A in the action of the crotoxin complex at the frog neuromuscular junction. J. Physiol. (Lond.) **234**, 63p—64p (1973a)
Vital Brazil, O., Franceschi, J. P., Waisbich, E.: Pharmacology of crystalline crotoxin. I. Toxicity. Mem. Inst. Butantan **33**, 973—980 (1966)
Vital Brazil, O., Neder, A. C., Corrado, A. P.: Effects and mechanism of action of *Tityus serrulatus* venom on skeletal muscle. Pharmacol. Res. Commun. **5**, 137—150 (1973b)
Vogel, Z., Sytkowski, A. J., Nirenberg, M. W.: Acetylcholine receptors of muscle grown in vitro. Proc. nat. Acad. Sci. (Wash.) **69**, 3180—3184 (1972)
Vyskočil, F., Magazanik, L. G.: Temperature dependence of *Naja* toxin blocking effect in *Rana temporaria*. Experientia (Basel) **29**, 158—160 (1972a)
Vyskočil, F., Magazanik, L. G.: The desensitization of post-junctional muscle membrane after intracellular application of membrane stabilizers and snake venom polypeptides. Brain Res. **48**, 417—419 (1972b)
Wagner, G. H., Mart, P. E., Kelly, R. B.: β-Bungarotoxin inhibition of calcium accumulation by rat brain mitochondria. Biochem. biophys. Res. Commun. **58**, 475—481 (1974)
Wagner, G. M., Strong, P. N., Kelly, R. B.: The mechanism of action of β-bungarotoxin. Neurosci. Abstr., pp. 968. New York: Soc. for Neurosc. 1975
Wall, A. J.: Indian Snake Poisons. Their Nature and Effects, pp. 171. London: W. H. Allen 1883
Warnick, J. E., Albuquerque, E. X., Diniz, C. R.: Electrophysiological observations on the action of the purified scorpion venom, tityus toxin, on nerve and muscle of the rat. J. Pharmacol. exp. Ther. **198**, 155—167 (1976)
Waser, P. G., Lüthi, U.: Autoradiographische Lokalisation von C^{14}-Calebassencurarin I und C^{14}-Decamethonium in der motorischen Endplatte. Arch. int. Pharmacodyn. Ther. **112**, 272—296 (1957)
Weis, R., McIsaac, R. J.: Cardiovascular and muscular effects of venom from coral snake, *Micrurus fulvius*. Toxicon **9**, 219—228 (1971)

Wells, M. A.: A kinetic study of the phospholipase A_2 *(Crotalus adamanteus)* catalysed hydrolysis of 1.2-dibutyryl-sn-glycero-3-phosphoryl choline. Biochemistry **11**, 1030—1041 (1972)
Wells, M. A.: Spectral perturbations of *Crotalus adamanteus* phospholipase A_2 induced by divalent cation binding. Biochemistry **12**, 1080—1085 (1973)
Wernicke, J. F., Oberjat, T., Howard, B. D.: β-Bungarotoxin reduces neurotransmitter storage in brain synapses. J. Neurochem. **22**, 781—788 (1974)
Wernicke, J. F., Vanker, A. D., Howard, B. D.: The mechanism of action of β-bungarotoxin. J. Neurochem. **25**, 483—496 (1975)
Wolff, J., Salabè, H., Ambrose, M., Larsen, P. R.: The basic proteins of cobra venom. II. Mechanism of action of cobramine B on thyroid tissue. J. biol. Chem. **243**, 1290—1296 (1968)
Yang, C. C.: Chemistry and evolution of toxins in snake venoms. Toxicon **12**, 1—43 (1974)
Yeoh, P. N., Walker, M. J. A.: Effect of a sea snake *(Enhydrina schistosa)* venom on the ganglionic nicotinic actions of acetylcholine. J. Pharm. Pharmacol. **26**, 441—447 (1974)
Zacks, S. L., Metzger, J. F., Smith, C. W., Blumberg, J. M.: Localization of ferritin-labeled botulinus toxin in the neuromuscular junction of the mouse. J. Neuropathol. exp. Neurol. **21**, 610—633 (1962)

CHAPTER 11

The Use of Snake Toxins for the Study of the Acetylcholine Receptor and its Ion-Conductance Modulator

E. X. ALBUQUERQUE, A. T. ELDEFRAWI, and M. E. ELDEFRAWI *

A. Introduction

Although the venoms of several snakes have been known for many years to cause muscular paralysis, their molecular and cellular sites of action have not been fully explored until recently (LEE, 1971). The venom of an elapid snake from Formosa, *Bungarus multicinctus*, was found to cause respiratory paralysis in rabbits when applied by cisternal injection, and death with much greater delay than when the venom was applied by intravenous injection (OUYANG, 1950). This led LEE and PENG (1961) to search for its sites of action. They found that the phrenic nerve discharge was intensified and prolonged after the action potentials of both the intercostal and diaphragm muscles had disappeared, which led them to suggest that respiratory failure was peripheral in origin. Subsequently, several components were isolated from the venom, which were found to inhibit neuromuscular transmission by attacking different targets. The major active component of this venom, i.e., α-bungarotoxin (α-BGT), was isolated in 1963 by CHANG and LEE by means of zone electrophoresis on starch. It was found to block skeletal neuromuscular transmission, as was another neurotoxin isolated from the venom of the cobra, *Naja naja atra* (CHANG and LEE, 1966). This block was by an antidepolarizing action similar to that of D-tubocurarine, a well-known neuromuscular nicotinic receptor antagonist. Radiolabeling of α-BGT with ^{131}I, accomplished by LEE and TSENG in 1966, permitted studies on distribution of this toxin. It was found localized at the motor endplate zone of the mouse diaphragm (LEE et al., 1967).

At that time, there were very few attempts to isolate acetylcholine (ACh) receptors, and all of them had failed because of the use of relatively nonspecific radiolabeled drugs (e.g., D-tubocurarine or gallamine) for identification of ACh receptors. Subsequent attempts with more specific reversibly binding drugs were successful (O'BRIEN et al., 1970). These two lines of research, i.e., toxin research and ACh receptor identification, crossed at this point when α-BGT was utilized to identify ACh receptors in vitro (CHANGEUX et al., 1970).

α-BGT proved to be a very specific label of the nicotinic neuromuscular type ACh receptor in situ. In fact, it was so good that any α-BGT binding protein was accepted by some to be synonymous with nicotinic ACh receptor. Its success is due mainly to two of its properties. One is the high affinity and irreversible pharmacological action, though very slowly reversible binding, of α-BGT to this receptor. Appar-

* Our research described in this chapter was financed in part by National Science Foundation grant BNS76-21683, National Institutes of Health grants NS-12063, NS-13231, and AI-13640, Muscular Dystrophy Association of America and Paralyzed Veterans of America.

ently this binding is not due to formation of covalent bonds, since treatment with SDS dissociates α-BGT from the receptor, but to multiple bond formation adding to a very high affinity. Second is the high specificity of this toxin for the nicotinic neuromuscular-type ACh receptor. These properties made α-BGT extremely useful for identifying ACh receptors in vitro, for determining numbers of ACh receptors in, and within, different tissues and during their development, and also as a specific label for quick identification of the receptor in fractions separated during purification.

The present review will describe the application of highly specific snake venom toxins to the investigation of ACh receptors located at the muscle endplates, sympathetic ganglia and central nervous system tissue, as well as the relationship between these receptor macromolecules and the macromolecules involved in ion transduction, defined as the ion-conductance modulator, ionic channel or ionophore.

B. Isolation and Radiolabeling of Neurotoxins

Neurotoxins that produce antidepolarizing neuromuscular block of skeletal neuromuscular transmission are named according to their zoological origin (e.g., cobrotoxin, bungarotoxin), and/or the order of their elution during chromatographic purification (e.g., α, β, γ or I, II, III). They are basic polypeptides found in venoms of sea snakes, cobras, kraits *(Bungarus)*, black snake, and most other elapid venoms (LEE, 1972). They are made up either of 71 to 74 amino acid residues in a single chain cross-linked by five disulfide bridges (examples of these are α-BGT, toxin III from *N. haje* (MIRANDA et al., 1970) and the principal neurotoxins from venoms of the cobras, *Naja naja siamensis, N.n. naja* [KARLSSON et al., 1971]), or of 60 to 62 amino acid residues in a single chain cross-linked by four disulfide bridges (examples are the sea snake neurotoxins [SATO and TAMIYA, 1971; TU et al., 1971], minor neurotoxins in the venom of *N. naja siamensis* [KARLSSON et al., 1971], cobrotoxin of *N.n. atra* [YANG et al., 1969], and the principal neurotoxins of the venoms of most cobra species [see LEE, 1972; YANG, 1974], including toxin α of the venom of *N. haje haje* and *N. nigricollis* [BOTES and STRYDOM, 1969]).

The neurotoxins of cobra and krait venoms have been purified by several techniques that take advantage of the basic nature of these toxins. Thus, electrophoresis (CHANG and LEE, 1963; CLARK et al., 1972a), electrofocusing (ELDEFRAWI and FERTUCK, 1974) and cation exchange chromatography (KARLSSON et al., 1971; KLETT et al., 1973) have been successfully utilized. The most widely used method is chromatography on carboxymethylcellulose (VOGEL et al., 1972; MOLINOFF and POTTER, 1972) and phosphocellulose (COOPER and REICH, 1972) or polycarboxylic resin (KARLSSON et al., 1971; POTTER, 1974) coupled with chromatography on Sephadex gels.

Purification of neurotoxins of the venom of the cobra *Naja naja siamensis* by chromatography on carboxymethylcellulose using ammonium acetate gradient yielded 15 protein peaks (Fig. 1). Four of these peaks inhibited 75–100% of the binding of [^{3}H]ACh to its membrane-bound receptor of the electric organ of *Torpedo ocellata.* MILEDI et al. (1971) had also reported that, of the 12 proteins isolated from the dried venom of *B. multicinctus*, four blocked the action of ACh on frog

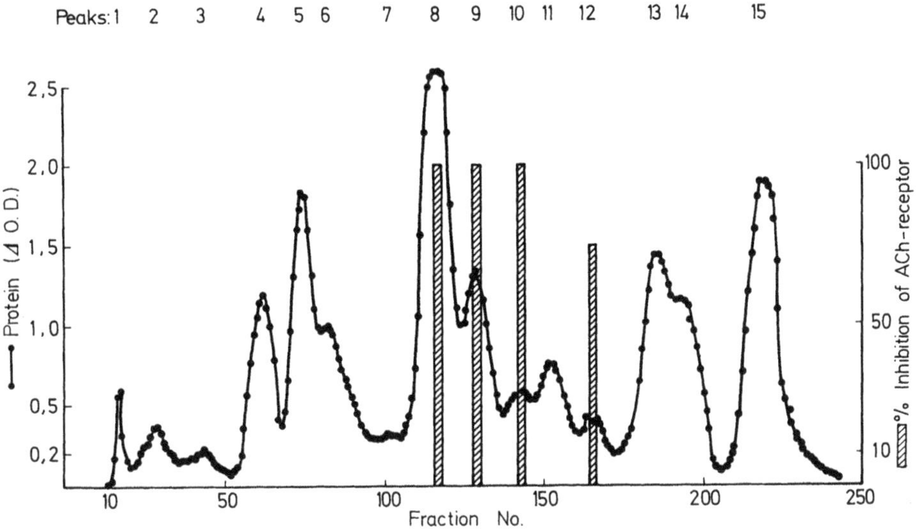

Fig. 1. Fractionation of venom of *Naja naja siamensis* by ion exchange chromatography on Sephadex CM-50 with gradient of 0.05-1 M ammonium acetate (pH 6.7). Each fraction was 5 ml. Percent inhibition of ACh receptor was obtained by measuring binding of [^{3}H]ACh to *Torpedo* electric organ membranes (pretreated with 0.1 mM diisopropylfluorophosphate). To determine inhibiting effect of each protein peak obtained, samples of electric organ membrane preparations (1 ml obtained from 1 g) were incubated for 1 h with 10 μg of protein from each venom fraction, then binding of [^{3}H]ACh (10^{-6} M) to membranes determined and compared with untreated membranes

sartorius neuromuscular junctions. Thus apparently not only the first neurotoxin peak (α), but others as well, may bind specifically to nicotinic ACh receptors.

The cobra venom neurotoxins and α-BGT have been radiolabeled by iodination with [^{131}I] (LEE and TSENG, 1966; LEE et al., 1967; MILEDI et al., 1971) or [^{125}I] (BERG et al., 1972; ELDEFRAWI and FERTUCK, 1974) with chloramine-T, or by lactoperoxidase. Iodination occurs at the 54th residue, which is tyrosine. The toxins have also been tritiated by acetylation with [^{3}H]acetic anhydride (BARNARD et al., 1971; ALBUQUERQUE et al., 1974) or by exposure of the [^{125}I]-labeled *Naja nigrocollis* α-neurotoxin to tritium gas (MENEZ et al., 1971). The mono-[^{3}H]-acetylated toxin preserves an equivalent action and potency to that of the nonradioactive material (CHIU et al., 1974; DOLLY et al., 1977). Another radiolabeling method used was reaction with pyridoxal phosphate followed by reduction of the Schiff's base with [^{3}H]sodium borohydride (COOPER and REICH, 1972). In the process, more than one product is often obtained, e.g., mono- and di-iodinated α-BGT (VOGEL et al., 1972) or multiply acetylated α-BGT (CHANG et al., 1973). Usually these products have been separated prior to utilization for ACh receptor identification or localization. High specific activities have been obtained; an example is the diiodo-α-BGT, having a specific activity of 500 Ci/mmol (KOUVELAS and GREENE, 1976).

Nearly always, the procedure used in radiolabeling causes decreased activity of the toxin and in some cases reduced specificity as well. COOPER and REICH (1972) found that the pyridoxal phosphate coupled toxin retained only 50% of its original potency. CHANG et al. (1973) reported that acetylation of α-BGT with [^{3}H]acetic anhydride produced tri-*N*-acetyl derivatives, while acetylation with *N*-[^{3}H]acetyl imidazole produced *N*,*O*-di,*N*,*N*,*O*-tri and *N*,*N*,*N*,*O*-tetraacetyl derivatives. All the derivatives exhibited decreased neuromuscular blocking action in rat diaphragm and frog rectus abdominis. Although the *N*,*O*-di and *N*,*N*,*O*-triacetyl toxins were localized mostly in the endplate region, the *N*,*N*,*N*,*O*-tetraacetyl and tri-*N*-acetyl toxins bound to endplates and slightly along the muscle fiber, whereas the hexa-*N*-acetyl toxin bound totally nonspecifically. Thus, it is very important to separate the products, and assay each for its effect on neuromuscular transmission and specificity. Equally important is to monitor activity and specificity of the radiolabeled toxin periodically. In addition to the half-life of the radioisotope, 60 days for ^{125}I vs. 12.3 years for tritium, the toxin itself loses its binding activity, a loss estimated to be less than 10% per month for [^{125}I]α-BGT (POTTER, 1974) or 50% after 3 months at 4° C for [^{3}H]α-neurotoxin from *Naja nigricollis* venom (MEUNIER et al., 1972).

In addition to the basic polypeptides discussed above, an acidic one was isolated from the venom of *Bungarus caeruleus* by gel filtration on QAE Sephadex A-50 equilibrated with 0.05 M Tris-HCl, pH 8.5 (BON and CHANGEUX, 1975). The basic or neutral proteins were not absorbed, and the acidic protein (ceruleotoxin) was eluted at 0.125 M NaCl by a linear salt gradient in buffer. This was further purified on Sephadex G-50 and Bio-gel P30 and its molecular weight determined at ≃ 39000. Although the molecular target of ceruleotoxin is not yet known, it has been suggested to be the ion conductance modulator of the ACh receptor (see below).

C. Neurotoxins as Specific Labels for Nicotinic ACh Receptors

I. Techniques Used for Detection of Binding

Many techniques have been utilized to determine the amount of radiolabeled α-BGT (and sometimes cobra neurotoxin) bound to the nicotinic ACh receptors, and these techniques generally depend upon the quasi-irreversible nature of this binding. The membrane-bound receptor-α-BGT complex is separated from free toxin by centrifugation (MILEDI et al., 1971; HESS et al., 1975) or by filtration on Millipore HAWP filters (FRANKLIN and POTTER, 1972). In either case, the precipitate and/or filter is rinsed several times with buffer and the filter presoaked with albumin solution to reduce nonspecific binding. We have recently used glass filters (Whatman GF/C) after presoaking in α-BGT solution and had low background (COPIO and M. ELDEFRAWI, unpublished). FRANKLIN and POTTER (1972) have utilized the filter assay method for studies of binding of α-BGT to solubilized receptor by precipitating the latter (bound and free) with 33% ammonium sulfate and retaining free α-BGT in solution. The use of DEAE cellulose filters (KLETT et al., 1973; SCHMIDT and RAFTERY, 1973) reduces the nonspecific binding of α-BGT or cobra toxin since toxin and filter are positively charged.

The large difference in molecular weight between α-BGT (≃ 8000) and toxin-receptor complex (≃ 330000) has also been utilized to separate them either by sucrose density gradient centrifugation (MILEDI et al., 1971; LINDSTROM and PATRICK, 1974) or by gel filtration on Sephadex G-75 (CLARK et al., 1972b) or G-200 (ALMON et al., 1974a). Cation exchange chromatography (on carboxymethylcellulose CM-52) in

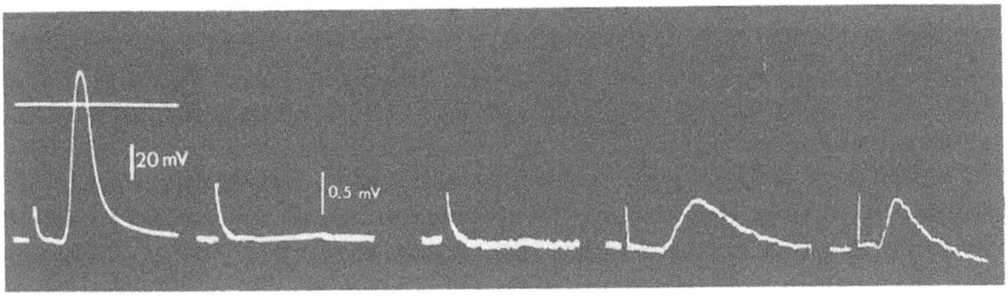

Fig. 2. Partial recovery of phrenic nerve diaphragm muscle of rat after exposure to α-BGT (5 μg/ml). At zero time, the first trace shows a control record of indirectly elicited action potential. The second trace shows a record after 30 min incubation with α-BGT. Reaction of α-BGT with acetylcholine receptor was terminated by washing of muscle with 140×10^{-6} M dTC for 30–60 min followed by washing with Ringer's solution without dTC. Third to fifth traces show records obtained 1 to 4 h from beginning of wash without drugs. (From SARVEY et al., 1978)

minicolumns of disposable Pasteur pipets proved to be a simple and rapid method. It allowed the study of binding of α-BGT to either membrane bound or soluble ACh receptors and gave consistent low blank and accomplished complete recovery of reacted and unreacted species (KOHANSKI et al., 1977).

It is not appropriate to use equilibrium dialysis for the determination of the amount of neurotoxin bound to the ACh receptor since the large size of the toxin and its aggregation would slow the penetration even if the tubing allows molecules with molecular weights up to 10000 to pass through.

Although binding of α-BGT is very specific for nicotinic neuromuscular ACh receptors, the toxin binds to other components, even foreign ones such as glass (VOGEL et al., 1972; POTTER, 1974), Diaflo membranes, polyethylene, and Sephadex gel (COPIO and ELDEFRAWI, unpublished). Thus, one has to be very careful in making sure that the binding observed is delayed or blocked by nicotinic cholinergic drugs and essentially not by muscarinic or other drugs, before concluding tentatively that the binding observed may be to the nicotinic ACh receptor. α-BGT has been reported to bind at micromolar concentrations to axons of lobster walking leg (DENBURG et al., 1972), to mammalian muscle cytoplasm (PORTER et al., 1973), and to serum proteins containing polyanions which bind *Naja* neurotoxin with low affinity and adsorb onto DEAE filters (KLETT et al., 1973). The binding of α-BGT to cellular components other than ACh receptors is evident from the large percentage of its binding that is not inhibited by curare; an amount that varies between tissues.

The actions of neurotoxins are studied by electrophysiological techniques. Their effects are determined on twitch tension, endplate potential, endplate current, miniature endplate potential, and ACh sensitivity (LAPA et al., 1974; BARNARD et al., 1975). Although α-BGT reaction with the ACh receptor is virtually irreversible, a fraction of the toxin reacts reversibly. Indeed, α-BGT at a concentration of 5 μg/ml completely blocked the endplate potential and extrajunctional ACh sensitivity of surface fibers in normal and chronically denervated mammalian muscles, respectively, in about 35 min (SARVEY et al., 1978). However, a 0.72 ± 0.033 mV amplitude endplate potential returned in normal muscle fibers after 6.5 h of washout of α-BGT (Fig. 2), while an ACh sensitivity of 41.02 ± 3.95 mV/nC was recorded in denervated muscle after 8 h of washout (control being 1246±117 mV/nC). We have found in many experiments that this reversibility of about 1% of the α-BGT binding to mammalian skeletal muscle is a very sensitive index of the potency of α-BGT. Aging of the toxin usually results in an increase in the portion of reversible binding (ALBUQUERQUE and OLIVEIRA, unpublished).

Combination of histological techniques with autoradiography or immunofluorescence proved to be very useful in identifying the subcellular localization of nicotinic ACh receptors. Frozen sections (BOURGEOIS et al., 1971, 1972) or the whole tissue, in vivo or in vitro (BARNARD et al., 1971; FERTUCK and SALPETER, 1976), are exposed to the toxin, and then sections are exposed to the film emulsion. Because of the semi-irreversible binding nature of many of the neurotoxins (BARNARD et al., 1975; SARVEY et al., 1978; LAPA et al., 1974), excessive washing of the tissue after its exposure to radiolabeled toxin removes nonspecific binding, while the toxins that are bound specifically to the ACh receptors remain. A higher sensitivity is obtained in electron-microscope autoradiography with ^{125}I than with tritium, because of the higher ratio of low-energy electrons to nuclear decays and the more favorable range of the low-energy electrons (FERTUCK and SALPETER, 1974). This method has been extremely useful and widely used in studies of development of ACh receptors and studies of effects of denervation and trophic factors.

II. Use in Identification and Localization of ACh Receptors

One of the most significant uses of snake venom neurotoxins has been in determining the densities of nicotinic ACh receptors in various tissues and in following the changes in their concentrations during development, denervation, and other treatments. Their densities vary greatly, ranging from about 1 pmol/g tissue in muscle or mammalian brain to 1000 or more pmol/g tissue in the electric organs of *Torpedo* or *Narcine* (Table 1).

α-BGT was first used for the in vitro identification of ACh receptors in membranes of *Electrophorus* electroplax by virtue of its blockade of the specific [^{3}H]decamethonium binding (CHANGEUX et al., 1970). When direct binding of [^{131}I]-α-BGT was studied, MILEDI et al. (1971) found that it bound to *Torpedo marmorata* electroplax membranes with characteristics identifiable with ACh receptors. The binding was saturable and slowed by the presence of the cholinergic drug D-tubocurarine or carbamylcholine. The concentration obtained for α-BGT binding sites of about 1 nmol per g tissue was the same as that obtained for the sites in this tissue that bound reversibly ACh receptor agonists such as [^{3}H]muscarone (O'BRIEN et al., 1970) and [^{3}H]-ACh (ELDEFRAWI et al., 1971 a). Again, the density of the sites that bound the α-neurotoxin of *Naja nigricollis* in *Electrophorus* electroplax (i.e., 17–23 pmol/g tissue) (Table 1), was similar to that of the sites that bound reversible cholinergic drugs (i.e., 21–33 pmol/g tissue) (RAFTERY et al., 1971; ELDEFRAWI et al., 1971 b). The binding of these α-neurotoxins was localized to synapses (BOURGEOIS et al., 1972) and was also specific and blocked by cholinergic drugs.

The use of autoradiography of radiolabeled α-BGT allowed the determination of the mean density of ACh receptors in postsynaptic membranes of endplates. It averaged 8700/μm^2 (ALBUQUERQUE et al., 1974) in the various skeletal muscle endplates, whose overall sizes varied from 400 to 1300 μm^2. However, since the developed

Table 1. The concentration of α-neurotoxin (*Bungarus* or *Naja*) binding sites in different tissues

Tissue	Concentration of neurotoxin binding sites pmol bound/g tissue	Reference
Electric Organs:		
Torpedo	1100; 500–1000	MILEDI et al. (1971); RAFTERY et al. (1972)
Narcine	1300	POTTER (1974)
Electrophorus	17–23[a]; 35	BOURGEOIS et al. (1972); RAFTERY et al. (1971)
Muscles:		
Rat diaphragm	3[b]	BERG et al. (1972); MILEDI and POTTER (1971)
Denervated rat diaphragm	60[c]	HARTZELL and FAMBROUGH (1972); MILEDI and POTTER (1971)
Frog sartorius	1[d]	MILEDI and POTTER (1971)
Brain:		
Rat brain	1.6; 2	POLZ-TEJERA et al. (1975); MOORE and BRADY (1976)
Rat cortex	1–1.5[e]; 2–4	ETOROVIĆ and BENNETT (1974); SALVATERRA et al. (1975)
Chick brain	7.5	POLZ-TEJERA et al. (1975)
Chick optic tectum and retina	60–70[f]	WANG and SCHMIDT (1976)

[a] Calculated from the number of *Naja nigricollis* α-neurotoxin molecules bound per mg tissue of $1.62\text{–}2.64 \times 10^{11}$ (BOURGEOIS et al., 1972).

[b] Calculated from the reported values of 0.2–0.4 pmol (BERG et al., 1972) and 1.6 pmol (MILEDI and POTTER, 1971) α-BGT binding sites per rat diaphragm.

[c] The highest density of extrajunctional α-BGT binding sites in denervated rat diaphragm was 653 sites/μm^2 (Fambrough, 1974) compared to a density of 20000–40000 sites per μm^2 at the crest of the junctional folds in innervated rat diaphragm (BARNARD et al., 1975; FERTUCK and SALPETER, 1976). But since the postjunctional membrane is much larger than the endplate area, the total number of α-BGT binding sites is calculated to be 60 pmol/g tissue.

[d] Calculated from the reported value of 1.2×10^{12} α-BGT binding sites per sartorius muscle.

[e] Calculated from values of 40–60 fmol α-BGT bound per mg protein and 4.3 mg protein per ml.

[f] These are the maximal concentrations which are reached on hatching day, and are decreased later to about 10 pmol of α-BGT binding sites/g tissue in the adult.

silver grains in emulsion films were found to coincide with the thickened portion of the postsynaptic membrane situated at the top of the junctional folds, the local concentration of ACh receptors in this dense membrane was recalculated to be 20000–40000 sites/μm^2 (ALBUQUERQUE et al., 1974; BARNARD et al., 1975; FERTUCK and SALPETER, 1976). The relative area occupied by the thickened membrane differs amongst the various endplates, ranging from 25–30% in sternomastoid and diaphragm to 50–60% in extraocular muscle. The local density of ACh receptors at the tops of the folds may differ in the various endplates.

Not only were the neurotoxins successful in identifying ACh receptors in vitro, in determining their concentrations and localization, but the data made it possible to relate the numbers of receptors in an endplate to the ACh molecules released per impulse and the amount of cation flux resulting from the interaction of a single receptor molecule.

They were also instrumental in demonstrating that ACh receptors were synthesized by muscle cells in the absence of any neuronal influence (VOGEL et al., 1972). In cultured embryonic chick and rat skeletal muscle cells no binding of α-BGT was detected to the membranes of the mononucleated dividing cells, the myoblasts. However, in the fused and multinucleated nondividing cells, the myotubes, [^{125}I]α-BGT bound to 150–1000 and 14–52 fmol of sites per mg protein in chick embryo and rat muscles, respectively. This binding showed the characteristics of binding to a nicotinic receptor, being blocked by nicotine, carbamylcholine, decamethonium, D-tubocurarine and ACh but not by equal concentrations of atropine or pilocarpine (VOGEL et al., 1972). Although the binding sites were at first evenly distributed, clusters of high-density sites developed, similar to the areas of elevated ACh sensitivity that had been detected electrophysiologically in these cells (FISCHBACH et al., 1973). These clusters represented increased α-BGT binding sites per unit area of membrane, and not increased membrane area of unchanged α-BGT binding sites (VOGEL and DANIELS, 1976). Using the fluorescent tetramethylrhodamine-labeled α-BGT, AXELROD et al. (1976) found that whereas the uniformly distributed ACh receptors on rat myotubes were labile, the dense, highly granular ACh receptors in patches measuring 10–60 μm that appeared shortly after fusion were immobile and disappeared after myotubes became extensively interconnected. ACh receptors were also shown to be synthesized in chick embryo retina before synapses appeared (VOGEL and NIRENBERG, 1976).

When the distribution of α-BGT binding sites on mammalian skeletal muscle developing in vivo in embryonic and neonatal rats was studied, there was uniform distribution at first, then by day 16 additional α-BGT binding sites accumulated in the mid-region of muscle fibers (BEVAN and STEINBACH, 1977). This accumulation became more pronounced and circumscribed with embryonic development with extrajunctional α-BGT binding sites disappearing by one week after birth. The results suggested that the high junctional receptor density found on adult innervated skeletal muscle fibers developed after the formation of the neuromuscular junction.

Attempts to block nicotinic ACh receptors in spinal cords of frog (MILEDI and SZCZEPANIAK, 1975) and cat (DUGGAN et al., 1976) by administration of α-BGT or cobra neurotoxin failed, and death from cisternal injection of cobra neurotoxin was due to peripheral effects (LEE and CHEN, 1977). It is unlikely that these observations are due to barriers in the central nervous tissue against penetration of neurotoxin to its target receptors, since labeled α-BGT readily penetrated the isolated frog spinal cord (MILEDI and SZCZEPANIAK, 1975). Thus, identification of α-BGT binding proteins in brain, spinal cord, or ganglia as nicotinic ACh receptors is premature in the absence of demonstrable electrophysiological effect.[1]

[1] *Note added in proof:* Two recent papers have added to the doubt in using α-BGT binding as an index for ACh receptors in neurons. α-BGT bound to, but did not affect the agonist-stimulated Na^+ uptake, by cultured rat sympathetic neurons, while antibodies against eel ACh receptor inhibited the Na^+ influx but not [^{125}I]α-BGT binding (PATRICK, J., STALLCUP, W. B.: Proc. nat. Acad. Sci. (Wash.) **74**, 4689, 1977). Also, α-BGT bound to cultured chick sympathetic neurons but did not affect their response to ACh (CARBONETTO, S. T., FAMBROUGH, D. M., MULLER, K. J.: Proc. nat. Acad. Sci. (Wash.) **75**, 1016, 1978).

In recent years, α-BGT has been utilized as an in vitro label for the nicotinic ACh receptors in central nervous system tissue and ganglia after proof that this binding was strongly inhibited by nicotinic drugs but poorly so by muscarinic ones (GREENE et al., 1973; LOWY et al., 1976; SCHMIDT, 1977). The α-BGT binding proteins had an isoelectric point similar to that of peripheral nicotinic ACh receptor (LOWY et al., 1976). α-BGT was found to bind to synaptosomes of rat brain (MOORE and BRADY, 1976), cerebral cortex (ETOROVIĆ and BENNETT, 1974; SALVATERRA et al., 1975) and other parts of the brain with a regional distribution corresponding to that of the nicotinic ACh receptors in brain determined electrophysiologically (CURTIS and CRAWFORD, 1969; PHILLIS, 1970; WANG and SCHMIDT, 1976). α-BGT binding was also detected in chick sympathetic ganglia (GREENE, 1976) and in cultures of chick embryo ganglion neurons (GREENE et al., 1973). They were evenly distributed in the latter, as shown by autoradiography, and their concentration was 100–300 per μm^2.

Binding of α-BGT was also utilized to study the ontogeny of the putative brain and ganglionic nicotinic receptors in chicks. They reached maximal levels in ovo in all brain regions except in cerebellum and hemispheres, where they continued to increase after hatching to maturity (KOUVELAS and GREENE, 1976). Major increases occurred between days 12 and 15, 19, or 20 in optic lobes, brain stem and sympathetic ganglia (GREENE, 1976), respectively. The concentration in optic tectum and retina dropped sharply after hatching (WANG and SCHMIDT, 1976).

To reconcile the nicotinic pharmacology of the α-BGT binding proteins of central nervous tissue and ganglia with the lack of in situ effect of α-BGT and cobra neurotoxin, SCHMIDT (1977) has recently suggested that there might be two kinds of central nicotinic receptors, only one of which might be sensitive to α-BGT. To resolve this controversy, it may be advantageous to use other neurotoxins which have already been shown to block central nicotinic receptors; examples are four neurotoxins from the venom of the elapid snake *Dendroaspis viridis* (MILEDI and SZCZEPANIAK, 1975). These dendrotoxins may be useful in identifying and isolating ACh receptors from central nervous tissue.

Not all ACh receptors are inhibited by α-BGT. In *Aplysia* central neurons three types of cholinergic responses are the result of distinct changes in ionic permeability, selective increases in permeability to Na^+, Cl^-, and K^+. α-BGT completely and reversibly blocks the response resulting from increased Cl^- permeability, but does not affect either of the other two responses (KEHOE et al., 1976). Other putative ACh receptors, whose binding of cholinergic drugs is not inhibited by α-BGT, are the ones isolated from housefly brain (ELDEFRAWI and O'BRIEN, 1970; MANSOUR et al., 1977). These ACh receptor molecules are nicotinic as well as muscarinic in their pharmacology (ELDEFRAWI et al., 1971a). SANES et al. (1977) detected α-BGT binding in *Manduca* moth antennal lobes, which was inhibited by nicotinic as well as muscarinic drugs. The relationship of this α-BGT binding to the non-α-BGT binding, but ACh, nicotine, curare, and atropine binding protein of housefly brain remains to be seen.

III. Use in Purification and Characterization of Nicotinic ACh Receptors

At a time when it was uncertain whether receptors could ever be taken out of their membrane environment and still retain their stereo-specificity, α-BGT played an important role in the solubilization of ACh receptors. MILEDI et al. (1971) demonstrated that Triton X-100 could solubilize all of the α-BGT binding proteins (i.e., ACh receptors) in electric organ membranes. Triton X-100 (LOWY et al., 1976) or emulphogene (MOORE and BRADY, 1976) also solubilized the α-BGT binding proteins of mammalian brain.

When it proved impossible to obtain a pure ACh receptor with column chromatography, electrophoresis, or isoelectrofocusing, affinity chromatography was adopted successfully. One of the most efficient affinity gels used was the one containing α-neurotoxin from *Naja* venom covalently bound to the Sepharose gel (ELDEFRAWI and ELDEFRAWI, 1973; KLETT et al., 1973). It is stable for up to 6 months at 4° C in presence of 0.02% NaN_3 and gives good recoveries of the receptor. α-BGT has been used to desorb the ACh receptor (RAFTERY, 1973); however, more reversible cholinergic drugs (e.g., carbamylcholine) are commonly used, so as to obtain functional ACh receptors. ACh receptors obtained by use of this affinity gel have specific binding of 1.8 (HEILBRONN and MATTSON, 1974), 4.1 (LINDSTROM and PATRICK, 1974), 6.6 (KLETT et al., 1973), 10–12 (ELDEFRAWI and ELDEFRAWI, 1973; RÜBSAMEN et al., 1976b) and 12.2 (ONG and BRADY, 1974) nmol per mg protein.

The specific binding of radiolabeled α-BGT has been used as a label for the ACh receptor in studies on its molecular weight based on sodium dodecyl sulfate disc gel electrophoresis. Because sodium dodecyl sulfate dissociates α-BGT or *Naja* toxin from the ACh receptor, glutaraldehyde (BIESECKER, 1973) or suberimidate (HUCHO and CHANGEUX, 1973) had to be used to attach the neurotoxin covalently to the receptor as well as to retain the receptor subunits together. Estimates obtained for the molecular weight of the ACh receptor were 260000 and 275000, respectively. This compares with the value of 330000 obtained by sedimentation equilibrium (EDELSTEIN et al., 1975).

Radiolabeled α-BGT was used to identify the ACh receptor in detergent extracts of membranes and to determine its molecular weight, by using sucrose density gradient centrifugation (GIBSON et al., 1976) and gel filtration (MILEDI et al., 1971; MEUNIER et al., 1972), as well its isoelectric point (RAFTERY et al., 1971).

D. Utilization of Neurotoxins to Compare Junctional and Extrajunctional ACh Receptors

When binding of α-BGT to mammalian and frog skeletal muscles was studied before and after denervation, it was noted that the numbers of toxin-binding sites increased, and the increase was in extrajunctional areas (LEE et al., 1967; HARTZELL and FAMBROUGH, 1972; FAMBROUGH, 1974; MILEDI and POTTER, 1971; WARNICK et al., 1977). This agreed with the increase in extrajunctional ACh sensitivity which occurred in denervated mammalian muscles and was detected by electrophysiological techniques (ALBUQUERQUE and MCISAAC, 1969, 1970; WARNICK et al., 1977). The increase was progressive and reached a maximum at about 15 days after denervation. The extrajunctional ACh receptors were distributed in patches of high and low density, such that it was possible to detect high-density areas corresponding to about 1500 mV/nC and low-density areas with ACh sensitivities as low as 100–200 mV/nC. It should be noted that these new high levels of ACh sensitivity were obtained with high-resistance ACh pipettes, in contrast to earlier observations where the high levels were obtained with low-resistance ACh pipettes. Needless to say, the phenomenon is observed in either circumstance. When degeneration progressed, the ACh sensitivity along the extrajunctional membrane decreased, and this decrease was mostly due to absence of ACh receptors (ALBUQUERQUE and MCISAAC, 1969, 1970; MILEDI and POTTER, 1971).

The patches of high- and low-density ACh-sensitivity in denervated muscle observed by ALBUQUERQUE and MCISAAC (1969, 1970) by electrophysiological means were very recently confirmed by KO et al. (1977) by means of an autoradiographic technique using $[^{125}I]\alpha$-BGT. They also found that the patches varied in size from less than 1–30 μm, depending on the muscle and the period of denervation. Within the patches the ACh receptor density was 20 times greater than elsewhere along the muscle fiber, and probably approached that in the postsynaptic membrane. They further suggested that ACh receptors could move within the sarcolemma and that at sites of high packing density their mobility was significantly restricted. A similar conclusion was reached for the patches of high receptor density found in myotubes when AXELROD et al. (1976) used tetramethylrhodamine-labeled α-BGT.

The extrajunctional increase in density of ACh receptors is apparently due to de novo synthesis as evidenced by incorporation of L-$[^{35}S]$methionine into ACh receptors of embryonic myogenic cells (MERLIE et al., 1975), and reappearance of extrajunctional ACh sensitivity in denervated rat muscle after blockade with α-BGT (SAKMANN, 1975). However, the fact that the increase in toxin binding sites is only about 20-fold (Table 1), whereas the increase in ACh sensitivity is probably at least 1000-fold (ALBUQUERQUE and MCISAAC, 1969, 1970; WARNICK et al., 1977), has not yet been explained. Chronic administration of α-BGT or curare produces effects similar to denervation in skeletal muscles, i.e. increased numbers and spread of ACh receptors (BERG and HALL, 1975; CHANG et al., 1975).

Contrary to the effects observed in muscles, denervation of *Electrophorus* electric organ by destruction of the caudal part of the spinal cord did not increase the binding sites for $[^{3}H]\alpha$-neurotoxin of *Naja nigricollis* for up to 142 days. Nor was there any morphological modification of the electroplax or any change in denervation supersensitivity, though membrane resistance increased (BOURGEOIS et al., 1973). This is despite the fact that this electric organ is embryonically derived from skeletal muscle.

Junctional and extrajunctional muscle ACh receptors bind ACh and respond by depolarizing the membrane, they have similar molecular weights, and they bind concanavalin A, which is indicative of the presence of sugars (BROCKES and HALL, 1975). However, many differences have been found between junctional and extrajunctional ACh receptors. The extrajunctional receptor has an isoelectric point that is 0.15 units higher (BROCKES and HALL, 1975), and has a faster turnover rate, a half-life of 19–24 h compared to at least 6 days (CHANG and HUANG, 1975; BERG and HALL, 1974, 1975; DEVREOTES and FAMBROUGH, 1975; MERLIE et al., 1976). In addition, the open time for extrajunctional channels was found to be 3–5-fold that for junctional channels (NEHER and SAKMANN, 1976). Antibodies from rats injected with pure *Torpedo* receptor bound selectively to rat and human junctional receptors and not to extrajunctional ones (TROTTER et al., 1977), while antibodies from myasthenic patients bound more selectively to rat extrajunctional solubilized ACh receptors

(ALMON and APPEL, 1975; ALBUQUERQUE et al., 1976). In addition to differences between the proteins, it is possible that there may be differences between the lipids in junctional and extrajunctional areas, which may contribute of some of the observed differences between the two receptors and their ionic conductance modulators.

The rate of binding of [^{125}I]α-BGT to homogenates or Triton extracts of skeletal muscles was the same in innervated as in denervated muscles ($2–5 \times 10^6$ M^{-1} min^{-1}), and so was the ability of carbamylcholine, decamethonium, or D-tubocurarine to slow this binding (ALPER et al., 1974; COLQUHOUN and RANG, 1976; SARVEY et al., 1978). However, the two could be distinguished in electrophysiological studies by means of the reduced potency of cholinergic drugs in protecting the extrajunctional receptors against α-BGT (LAPA et al., 1974; BERÁNEK and VYSKOCIL, 1967; SARVEY et al., 1978). Measurements of acetylcholine sensitivity of chronically denervated rat soleus muscle demonstrated that carbamylcholine, decamethonium, hexamethonium, and D-tubocurarine were much less potent in protecting against blockade by α-BGT than they were in the case of innervated muscles (SARVEY et al., 1978).

E. Neurotoxins as a Tool for Studies of Drug-Receptor Interactions

The number of binding sites that the membrane-bound or purified ACh receptor of electric organs has for its transmitter ACh is equal to those it carries for venom neurotoxins (ELDEFRAWI et al., 1975; SUGIYAMA and CHANGEUX, 1975).

Some believe that the ratio of ACh to α-BGT binding sites is 0.5 (MOODY et al., 1973), but this may be due to the ease of loss of ACh binding by many denaturing conditions that do not affect α-BGT binding. For example, methylmercury (at 100 μM) (ELDEFRAWI et al., 1977), benzoquinonium (at 10 mM) (ELDEFRAWI and ELDEFRAWI, 1973), Zn^{2+} (at 0.4 mM) or ethylenediamino-tetra-acetate (at 10 mM) (O'BRIEN et al., 1974) inhibited ACh binding totally without affecting α-BGT binding. Apparently small alterations in the receptor molecule greatly affect its ACh binding but not its α-BGT binding.

The characteristics of the in vitro binding of radiolabeled neurotoxins to the ACh receptor have been studied under equilibrium and kinetic conditions. One proposal is that the reaction is a simple bimolecular one and that the ACh receptor carries one kind of binding site for both activators and inhibitors (KLETT et al., 1973; WEBER and CHANGEUX, 1974a). This was made for binding of [^{3}H]α-neurotoxin of *Naja nigricollis* to *Electrophorus* and *Torpedo* electric organ membranes (WEBER and CHANGEUX, 1974b) and [^{125}I]α-BGT binding to homogenates and detergent extracts of ACh receptors from normal and denervated rat diaphragms (COLQUHOUN and RANG, 1976).

On the other hand, several findings point to sites for binding receptor activators such as carbamylcholine being different from the ones that bind inhibitors, such as the neurotoxins and D-tubocurarine. The fact that a drug inhibits the effect of another in vivo is no proof that these pharmacologically competitive drugs bind to the same site on one molecule. It was found that ACh receptor activators inhibited binding of [^{3}H]ACh to *Torpedo* ACh receptors competitively (ELDEFRAWI, 1974) and [^{125}I]α-BGT to *Electrophorus* noncompetitively (BULGER and HESS, 1973). On the

Table 2. Kinetics and equilibrium parameters calculated from binding of α-neurotoxins to various tissues

Toxin	K_1 ($M^{-1}\,min^{-1}$ $\times 10^6$)	$t_{1/2}$ (h)	K_D (nM)	Reference
α-BGT, *Torpedo*	20	20	—	FRANKLIN and POTTER (1972)
	1–90[a]	—	—	SCHMIDT and RAFTERY (1974)
α-BGT, rat diaphragm[b]	2–5	—	—	COLQUHOUN and RANG (1976)
α-BGT, chick brain	2.1	5.1	1.1	KOUVELAS and GREENE (1976)
α-BGT, chick sympathetic neurons[c]	6	—	—	GREENE et al. (1973)
α-BGT, chick sympathetic ganglia	2.6	4.2	1.1	GREENE (1976)
α-BGT, rat brain	41	5.1	0.056	LOWY et al. (1976)
N. nigricollis, Torpedo	25	60[d]	0.02	WEBER and CHANGEUX (1974a)
N. n. siamensis, Electrophorus	10	2.3[e]	0.43–1	KLETT et al. (1973)
N. n. siamensis, Electrophorus	3.1	—	1.3	LINDSTROM and PATRICK (1974)

K_1, association constant (at 20–25° C); $t_{1/2}$, time for dissociation of half the bound toxin; K_D, dissociation constant.

[a] Values are dependent on concentration of NaCl.
[b] Innervated or denervated.
[c] In culture, at 37° C.
[d] In presence of excess unlabeled toxin.
[e] A second slow dissociation has $t_{1/2}$ of over 66 h.

other hand, D-tubocurarine inhibited the toxin binding competitively and [^{3}H)ACh noncompetitively and α-BGT inhibited [^{3}H]decamethonium noncompetitively (FU et al., 1974, 1977). This is in harmony with studies of RÜBSAMEN et al. (1976a and b) on the binding of the fluorescent lanthanide, terbium (Tb^{3+}) to ACh receptor purified from *T. ocellata*. Activators displaced Tb^{3+} from the Ca^{2+}-binding sites while the inhibitors D-tubocurarine or α-BGT did not. In another study utilizing the Ca^{2+} indicator murexide, the same observations were made, and in addition α-BGT caused reuptake of Ca^{2+} (CHANG and NEUMANN, 1976).

Table 2 summarizes kinetic parameters of the binding of neurotoxins with various ACh receptors. Binding of toxin 3 of *N. n. siamensis* to partially purified *Electrophorus* ACh receptors was found to be relatively reversible (KLETT et al., 1973) (as opposed to binding of α-BGT, which is almost irreversible). The affinity of receptor for neurotoxins was observed to increase during long incubations, leading to the proposal that the toxin-receptor complex transformed into a second toxin-receptor complex that dissociated more slowly than the first, and both reactions were reversible.

It is also suggested that the interaction of α-BGT with the membrane-bound or Triton-solubilized ACh receptors of electric organs proceeds in two phases; an initial fast step followed by a slower one. The ratio of the fraction of the reaction occurring in each step differed at different initial α-BGT concentrations (BULGER et al., 1977). The slow reaction phase, characterized by a high affinity for α-BGT decreased with increasing toxin concentration, while the fast phase, characterized by low affinity for the toxin increased correspondingly. This interconversion suggested that the binding was not to two different receptor molecules or to nonequivalent noninteracting sites. On the basis of equilibrium and kinetic studies, HESS and co-workers (FU et al., 1977; BULGER et al., 1977) suggested that the reaction was quite complex and not simply a bimolecular process. They proposed a simple model consisting of a minimum of two types of receptor sites and the binding of at least two α-BGT molecules per receptor molecule. Activators and inhibitors would bind to different sites and compete for only one half of the receptor sites available to them, not by overlapping of the sites, but by ligand-induced conformational changes of the receptor molecule.

Similar observations of noncompetitive inhibition of activators and inhibitors of each other's binding to the ACh receptor were made in equilibrium studies with ACh and reversible drugs (GIBSON, 1976). It was suggested that D-tubocurarine bound to a separate binding site on the receptor that allosterically altered half of the ACh-binding sites to a lower affinity. This was not explained by the induced-fit model (KOSHLAND et al., 1966) utilized by HESS and co-workers, but by an extension of the allosteric model (MONOD et al., 1965).

Another area where the study of the kinetics of *Naja* neurotoxin binding to ACh receptors is proving to be of great interest and importance is in the understanding of receptor conformational changes and possibly receptor desensitization. This is the condition where the amplitude of the receptor response to an agonist (i.e., depolarization or muscle contraction) decreases during exposure to this agonist in a high concentration or for a prolonged period. It was observed in vertebrate neuromuscular junctions (KATZ and THESLEFF, 1957), *Electrophorus* (LESTER et al., 1975) and *Torpedo* electric organs (BENNETT et al., 1961; MOREAU and CHANGEUX, 1976). CHANGEUX and co-workers (WEBER et al., 1975; SUGIYAMA et al., 1976) found that pre-exposure of *Torpedo marmorata* membranes to carbamylcholine or ACh before measurement of their binding of *Naja nigricollis* [^{3}H]α-toxin in the presence of the same agonist decreased the initial rate of toxin binding. The antagonists D-tubocurarine and flaxedil did not cause such a change. They suggested that this decrease was due not to a reduction in receptor affinity for toxin, but to an increase in the receptor's affinity for agonists. Equivalent changes in affinity were also detected in studies of $^{22}Na^+$ efflux from excitable microsacs (SUGIYAMA et al., 1976). Thus, CHANGEUX and co-workers proposed that in the membrane at rest, the ACh receptor was present in a state with low affinity for agonists, and the induced increase in affinity for agonists corresponded to pharmacologic desensitization.

A basic assumption in this hypothesis is that the ACh receptor carries one kind of binding site, which binds either an agonist or an antagonist. This may not be true, and the characteristics of binding of an inhibitor (e.g., toxin) may be affected by binding of an activator to the same ACh receptor molecule. SARVEY et al. (1978) studied endplate potential of mammalian muscles and the effect of α-BGT in the presence and absence of drugs. The presence of potentiating or desensitizing concentrations of carbamylcholine or decamethonium or inhibiting concentrations of hexamethonium converted the effect of α-BGT on neuromuscular transmission from being 99% irreversible to being reversible (Fig. 3). Wash out of the drugs

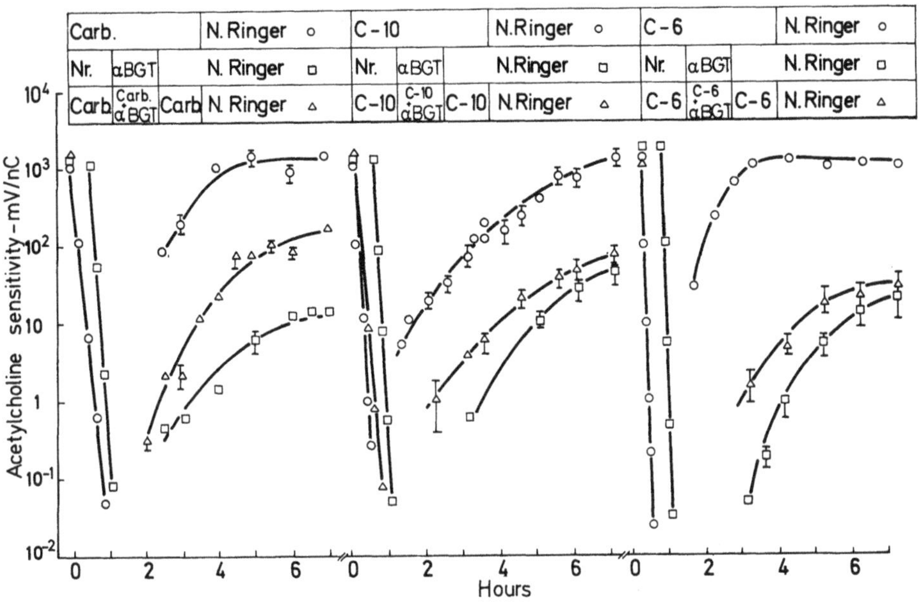

Fig. 3. Effects of carbamylcholine (Carb) decamethonium (C-10), hexamethonium (C-6) and α-bungarotoxin on extrajunctional acetylcholine sensitivity of chronically denervated (10–15 days) rat soleus muscles. Common logarithm of acetylcholine sensitivity, exposed in mV/nC, is plotted as a function of time in hours. Symbols on mean ± S.E.M. Circles (○) show effect of 90-min exposure to either carb (50 μM), C-10 (50 μM) or C-6 (50 μM) alone followed by washout with normal Ringer solution (NR). Squares (□) show effect of α-BGT (5 μg/ml) alone followed by washout. These are compared with the effect of either Carb, C-10 or C 6 used as a protective agent against α-BGT, shown by triangles (△). Temperature was 23° C. (From SARVEY et al., 1978)

restored twitch to control levels within 2 h. One explanation of these findings is that the desensitized ACh receptors exist in a different conformation which could bind α-BGT only reversibly. Accordingly, it may be that a desensitized receptor has a lower affinity for α-BGT. Furthermore, the conversion of α-BGT binding from irreversible to reversible may be regarded as a direct index for the conformational change in the desensitized receptor. Elucidation of the molecular mechanism of desensitization of the ACh receptor should be most interesting, and it is anticipated that neurotoxins will be found to play an important role.

F. Use in Studies of the Ion Conductance Modulator of the ACh Receptor

Histrionicotoxins, spiropiperidines isolated from the skin of Colombian frogs, were found to block neuromuscular transmission by inhibiting the ion conductance modulator of the ACh receptor (ALBUQUERQUE et al., 1973; LAPA et al., 1975). This modulator the molecule(s) that control(s) ACh receptor-induced ion flux across the postsynaptic membrane. These toxins were found by KATO and CHANGEUX (1976) to inhibit depolarization of the electroplax at concentrations that did not block [^{3}H]ACh or *Naja nigricollis* [^{3}H]α-toxin binding to the ACh receptor, though at very high concentrations they would block α-BGT binding (DOLLY et al., 1977). Local anesthetics (WEBER and CHANGEUX, 1974c; COHEN et al., 1974) also inhibited binding of *Naja* toxin to electric organ membranes noncompetitively, leading to the suggestion that local anesthetics and histrionicotoxins were binding to sites at the postsynaptic membrane that were different from the ACh or α-BGT binding sites. An acidic polypeptide (ceruleotoxin), isolated by BON and CHANGEUX (1975, 1977) from the venom of *Bungarus caeruleus*, was found to be quite toxic to mice and to block agonist-induced depolarization of *Electrophorus* electroplax and $^{22}Na^+$ efflux from receptor rich microsacs, without binding to the ACh or α-BGT binding sites. All these data suggested that histrionicotoxins, local anesthetics, and possibly ceruleotoxin might be binding to the ion-conductance modulator of the ACh receptor. We have found that ceruleotoxin, which we isolated from *Bungarus caeruleus* venom (obtained from the Miami Serpentarium), was nontoxic to mice, and in high concentrations (10^{-5} M) caused a slight decrease in endplate current amplitude and affected its half-decay time. However, at the concentration used, the toxin produced direct effects on the sarcolemmal and presynaptic membrane of muscle and nerve, respectively. These effects on muscles, nerves, and ACh receptors-ion-conductance modulator complex were similar to the action of phospholipase A and lysolecithin (ALBUQUERQUE et al., unpublished). Further electrophysiological testing is required to elucidate the molecular target of ceruleotoxin.

The ion-conductance modulator appears to be a molecule(s) that is separable from the ACh receptor, though closely associated with it in the membrane. The molecule has its own drug specificity, as judged by its specific binding of [^{3}H]-perhydrohistrionicotoxin, the completely reduced analog of histrionicotoxin. Binding of [^{3}H]perhydrohistrionicotoxin to *Torpedo* electric organ membranes is inhibited by drugs that modulate the endplate current e.g. local anesthetics, tetraethylammonium, amantadine, atropine, and scopolamine, but not by α-BGT or curare at the low concentrations which inhibit the ACh receptor (ELDEFRAWI et al., 1977).

A working model (ADLER et al., 1976, 1978) for the sequence of events occurring at the neuromuscular junction during the action of some of these agents (in particular atropine and scopolamine) is as follows:

$$\text{release} \rightarrow [\text{nACh}] + [\text{R}] \underset{k_{-1}}{\overset{k_1}{\rightleftharpoons}} \text{ACh}_n\text{R} \underset{k_{-2}}{\overset{k_2}{\rightleftharpoons}} \text{ACh}_n\text{R}^* \underset{\text{D}\;\;k_{-3}}{\overset{\text{D}\;\;k_3}{\rightleftharpoons}} \text{AChR}^*\text{D}$$

$[\text{nACh}] \xrightarrow{k_h}$ diffusion & hydrolysis

α-BGT $\rightarrow [\text{R}]$

where R is receptor; R* is activated receptor; D is drug; R*D is assumed to be inactive irrespective of the drug used. The dissociation of this species is assumed to be by removal of D and restoration of ACh_nR^*, instead of dissociation to nACh, R, and D (ADLER et al., 1978). Thus, released ACh causes a rather brief increase in the synaptic cleft concentration of ACh, which binds to its receptor, allowing the ion conductance modulator to go from closed to open conformation (with possible intermediate conformational changes). ACh is removed from the cleft by diffusion and esterase action, and the modulator reverts to its closed conformation. Drugs inhibiting the modulator appear to bind to the activated transmitter-receptor complex in a voltage-dependent manner to produce an inactive ternary complex (ALBUQUERQUE et al., 1974; MASUKAWA and ALBUQUERQUE, 1978). Histrionicotoxin also appears to bind to the closed form of ionconductance modulator. If elimination of drug from this complex is slow relative to the normal closing rate of channels, the resulting endplate current (EPC) will show the abbreviated exponential decay characteristic of the responses of EPC to HTX and to atropine (ADLER and ALBUQUERQUE, 1976). A more rapid elimination will lead to a secondary accumulation of AChR*, and hence to a terminal component characteristic of drugs such as DFP (KUBA et al., 1973, 1974), scopolamine (ADLER and ALBUQUERQUE, 1976) and certain local anesthetics (RUFF, 1977; KATZ and MILEDI, 1975). Thus, although the EPCs appear different in the presence of drugs, their underlying mechanism may be similarly affecting the ion-conductance modulator.

G. Use of Neurotoxins in Myasthenia Gravis Research

Neurotoxins were utilized in immunological studies to detect nicotinic ACh receptors and/or their antibodies in research related to myasthenia gravis. This is a human disease characterized by easy fatigability of skeletal muscles, improvement with anticholinesterases, reduced amplitude of miniature endplate potentials, increased curare sensitivity, and progressive reduction of muscle action potential response to repetitive nerve stimulation. The same symptoms occur in animals (rabbits, rats, guinea-pigs, goats, and sheep) (LINDSTROM, 1976; SANDERS et al., 1976) that are inoculated with ACh receptors purified from electric organs. It is now believed that myasthenia gravis is an autoimmune disease where there are fewer ACh receptors and the postsynaptic membranes of skeletal neuromuscular junctions are partially destroyed (ALBUQUERQUE et al., 1976; RASH et al., 1976).

Neurotoxins have been used to detect ACh receptors in thin sections of muscles and in solutions, and to study antibodies against these receptors and their effects. In thin sections, either autoradiography of radiolabeled toxin or a histologic technique is used. In the latter, muscle sections are incubated successively in α-BGT, rabbit antibody to α-BGT, and peroxidase-conjugated goat antibody to rabbit immunoglobulin, an enzyme whose reaction, produced with 3,3′-diamino-benzidine, is golden-brown, revealed by light microscopy (BENDER et al., 1975). Alternatively, the method can be simplified by substituting the first two incubations with one of rabbit antibody to ACh receptors (TROTTER et al., 1977). In solution, small amounts of ACh receptors could be detected directly by their binding of radiolabeled α-BGT (ALMON et al., 1974b) or better still by radioimmunoassay. The radiolabeled toxin is allowed to bind to the receptor, then the complex reacted with rabbit antireceptor antisera and then precipitated with goat anti-rabbit immunoglobulin G antiserum (PATRICK et al., 1973). Conversely, the titer of receptor antibodies can be determined by the same immunoprecipitin test.

With such methods it was discovered that skeletal neuromuscular junctions of myasthenics constained 11–30% as many ACh receptors as in normal muscles (FAMBROUGH et al., 1973). Simultaneously, electrophysiological studies disclosed that at the junctional region of intercostal muscles of patients with myasthenia gravis a significant decrease in ACh sensitivity was observed (ALBUQUERQUE et al., 1976). This decrease in ACh sensitivity was attributed to a reaction of immunoglobulin with the ACh receptor-modulator complex and morphological destruction of the synaptic folds (ALBUQUERQUE et al., 1976; RASH et al., 1976). In addition myasthenic sera, as well as those from animals inoculated with ACh receptors, contained anti-receptor antibodies (BENDER et al., 1975; APPEL et al., 1975; LINDSTROM et al., 1976). Interestingly, the half-life of ACh receptors was 18.5 h in cultured rat myotubes in the presence or absence of control sera, but was only 6 h in the presence of myasthenic sera. This, plus data on the effects of puromycin and temperature led to the suggestion that myasthenic sera accelerated the rate of degradation of ACh receptors (APPEL et al., 1977).

Not only are such tests useful in studies of myasthenia gravis and its animal model, but they are also beneficial in study of the ACh receptor molecule itself. Antibodies against eel ACh receptors cross-reacted with those from elasmobranch, bony fish and birds (SUGIYAMA et al., 1973). Also sera from animals immunized with *Electrophorus* electric organ ACh receptors had a titer of antibodies against the same receptor 1000 times the titer of antibodies against rat muscle ACh receptors (LINDSTROM, 1976). Thus it was concluded by LINDSTROM that there was sufficient homology between the two nicotinic receptors to induce an autoimmune response, but the degree of homology demonstrable serologically was quite small. He also found that the majority of antibodies in receptor immunized animals or myasthenic sera were found to be directed predominantly at sites on the ACh receptor other than the α-BGT binding sites.

H. Conclusion

One may imagine how far behind our knowledge of the structure and function of nicotinic ACh receptors would be at this time were it not for the discovery and utilization of the snake venom neurotoxins that specifically bind to these receptors. α-BGT and/or cobra neurotoxins were used to identify nicotinic ACh receptors in vitro, to make affinity gel for their purification, and to study their conformational changes and kinetics of interactions, their molecular weights, synthesis and metabolism, and their roles in diseases. It was even assumed at times that any protein that bound the toxin specifically must be an ACh receptor, and that binding of α-BGT was a better index of an ACh receptor in vitro than binding of ACh, its natural transmitter. However, the pitfalls involved in using these toxins are now better understood.

Other elapid snake venom toxins have recently been discovered, such as ceruleotoxin and those of *Dendroaspis*, which may be specific labels for the ion conductance modulator and central nicotinic ACh receptors, respectively. Definitely, snake venoms are a valuable source of toxins, some yet to be discovered, that will aid our search for knowledge on various ACh receptors and their ion conductance modulators.

References

Adler, M., Albuquerque, E. X.: An analysis of the action of atropine and scopolamine on the endplate current of frog sartorius muscle. J. Pharmacol. exp. Ther. **196**, 360—372 (1976)

Adler, M., Albuquerque, E. X., Lebeda, F. J.: A kinetic description of endplate currents. An evaluation of three models for the action of atropine and scopolamine. Neurosci. Abs. **2** (1976)

Adler, M., Albuquerque, E. X., Lebeda, F. J.: Kinetic analysis of endplate currents altered by atropine and scopolamine. Molec. Pharmacol. **14**, 514—529 (1978)

Albuquerque, E. X., Barnard, E. A., Chiu, T. H., Lapa, A. J., Dolly, J. O., Jansson, S.-E., Daly, J., Witkop, B.: Acetylcholine receptor and ion conductance modulator sites at the murine neuromuscular junction: Evidence from specific toxin reactions. Proc. nat. Acad. Sci. (Wash.) **70**, 949—953 (1973)

Albuquerque, E. X., Barnard, E. A., Porter, C. W., Warnick, J. E.: The density of acetylcholine receptors and their sensitivity in the postsynaptic membrane of muscle endplates. Proc. nat. Acad. Sci. (Wash.) **71**, 2818—2822 (1974)

Albuquerque, E. X., McIsaac, R. J.: Early development of acetylcholine receptors on fast and slow mammalian skeletal muscle. Life Sci. **8**, 409—416 (1969)

Albuquerque, E. X., McIsaac, R. J.: Fast and slow mammalian muscles after denervation. Exp. Neurol. **26**, 183—202 (1970)

Albuquerque, E. X., Rash, J. E., Mayer, R. F., Satterfield, J. R.: An electrophysiological and morphological study of the neuromuscular junction in patients with myasthenia gravis. Exp. Neurol. **51**, 536—563 (1976)

Almon, R. R., Andrew, C. G., Appel, S. H.: Acetylcholine receptor in normal and denervated slow and fast muscle. Biochemistry **13**, 5522—5528 (1974a)

Almon, R. R., Andrew, C. G., Appel, S. H.: Serum globulin in myasthenia gravis: Inhibition of α-bungarotoxin binding to acetylcholine receptors. Science **186**, 55—57 (1974b)

Almon, R. R., Appel, S. H.: Interaction of myasthenic serum globulin with the acetylcholine receptor. Biochem. biophys. Res. Commun. **393**, 66—77 (1975)

Alper, R., Lowy, J., Schmidt, J.: Binding properties of acetylcholine receptors extracted from normal and from denervated rat diaphragm. FEBS Letters **48**, 130—132 (1974)

Appel, S., Almon, R., Levy, N.: Acetylcholine receptor antibodies in myasthenia gravis. New Engl. J. Med. **293**, 760—761 (1975)

Appel, S. H., Anwyl, R., McAdams, M. W., Elias, S.: Accelerated degradation of acetylcholine receptor from cultured rat myotubes with myasthenia gravis sera and globulins. Proc. nat. Acad. Sci. (Wash.) **74**, 2130—2134 (1977)

Axelrod, D., Ravdin, P., Koppel, D. E., Schlessinger, J., Webb, W. W., Elson, E. L., Podleski, T. R.: Lateral motion of fluorescently labeled acetylcholine receptors in membranes of developing muscle fibers. Proc. nat. Acad. Sci. (Wash.) **73**, 4594—4598 (1976)

Barnard, E. A., Dolly, J. O., Porter, C. W., Albuquerque, E. X.: The acetylcholine receptor and the ionic conductance modulation system of skeletal muscle. Exp. Neurol. **48**, 1—28 (1975)

Barnard, E. A., Wieckowski, J., Chiu, T. H.: Cholinergic receptor molecules and cholinesterase molecules at mouse skeletal muscle junctions. Nature (Lond.) **234**, 207—209 (1971)

Bender, A. N., Ringel, S. P., Engel, W. K., Daniels, M. P., Vogel, Z.: Myasthenia gravis: A serum factor blocking acetylcholine receptors of the human neuromuscular junction. Lancet **1975I**, 607—608

Bennett, M. V. L., Wurzel, M., Grundfest, H.: The electrophysiology of electric organs of marine electric fishes. I. Properties of electroplaques of *Torpedo nobiliana*. J. gen. Physiol. **44**, 757—804 (1961)

Beranek, R., Vyskocil, F.: The action of tubocurarine and atropine on the normal and denervated rat diaphragm. J. Physiol. (Lond.) **188**, 53—66 (1967)

Berg, D. K., Hall, Z. W.: Fate of α-bungarotoxin bound to acetylcholine receptors of normal and denervated muscle. Science **184**, 473—475 (1974)

Berg, D. K., Hall, Z.: Increased extrajunctional acetylcholine sensitivity produced by chronic post-synaptic neuromuscular blockade. J. Physiol. (Lond.) **244**, 659—676 (1975)

Berg, D. K., Kelly, R. B., Sargent, P. B., Williamson, P., Hall, Z. W.: Binding of α-bungarotoxin to acetylcholine receptors in mammalian muscle. Proc. nat. Acad. Sci. (Wash.) **69**, 147—151 (1972)

Bevan, S., Steinbach, J. H.: The distribution of α-bungarotoxin binding sites on mammalian skeletal muscle developing in vivo. J. Physiol. (Lond.) **267**, 195—213 (1977)

Biesecker, G.: Molecular properties of the cholinergic receptor purified from *Electrophorus electricus*. Biochemistry **12**, 4403—4409 (1973)

Bon, C., Changeux, J.-P.: Ceruleotoxin: An acidic neurotoxin from the venom of *Bungarus caeruleus* which blocks the response to a cholinergic agonist without binding to the cholinergic receptor site. FEBS Letters **59**, 212—216 (1975)

Bon, C., Changeux, J.-P.: Ceruleotoxin: A possible marker of the cholinergic ionophore. Europ. J. Biochem. **74**, 43—51 (1977)

Botes, D. P., Strydom, D. J.: A neurotoxin, toxin α- from Egyptian cobra *(Naja naja haje)* venom. I. Purification, properties, and complete amino acid sequence. J. biol. Chem. **244**, 4147—4157 (1969)

Bourgeois, J. P., Popot, J. L., Ryter, A., Changeux, J.-P.: Consequences of denervation on the distribution of the cholinergic (nicotinic) receptor sites from *Electrophorus electricus* revealed by high resolution autoradiography. Brain Res. **62**, 557—563 (1973)

Bourgeois, J.-P., Ryter, A., Menez, A., Fromageot, P., Boquet, P., Changeux, J.-P.: Localization of the cholinergic receptor protein in *Electrophorus* electroplax by high resolution autoradiography. FEBS Letters **25**, 127—133 (1972)

Bourgeois, J.-P., Tsuji, S., Boquet, P., Pillot, J., Ryter, A., Changeux, J.-P.: Localization of the cholinergic receptor protein by immunofluorescence in eel electroplax. FEBS Letters **16**, 92—94 (1971)

Brockes, J. P., Hall, Z. W.: Acetylcholine receptors in normal and denervated rat diaphragm II. Comparison of junctional and extrajunctional receptors. Biochemistry **14**, 2100—2106 (1975)

Bulger, J. E., Fu, J.-J. L., Hindy, E. F., Silberstein, R. L., Hess, G. P.: Allosteric interactions between the membrane-bound acetylcholine receptor and chemical mediators. Kinetic studies. Biochemistry **16**, 684—692 (1977)

Bulger, J. E., Hess, G. P.: Evidence for separate initiation and inhibitory sites in the regulation of membrane potential of electroplax. I. Kinetic studies with α-bungarotoxin. Biochem. biophys. Res. Commun. **54**, 677—684 (1973)

Chang, C. C., Chen, T. F., Chuang, S.-T.: *N,O*-di and *N,N,O*-tri[^{3}H]acetyl α-bungarotoxins as specific labelling agents of cholinergic receptors. Brit. J. Pharmacol. **47**, 147—160 (1973)

Chang, C. C., Chuang, S. T., Huang, M. C.: Effects of chronic treatment with various neuromuscular blocking agents on the number and distribution of acetylcholine receptors in the rat diaphragm. J. Physiol. (Lond.) **250**, 161—173 (1975)

Chang, C. C., Huang, M. C.: Turnover of junctional and extrajunctional acetylcholine receptors of the rat diaphragm. Nature (Lond.) **253**, 643—644 (1975)

Chang, C. C., Lee, C. Y.: Isolation of neurotoxins from the venom of *Bungarus multicinctus* and their modes of neuromuscular blocking action. Arch. Int. Pharmacodyn. Ther. **144**, 241—257 (1963)

Chang, C. C., Lee, C. Y.: Electrophysiological study of neuromuscular blocking action of cobra neurotoxin. Brit. J. Pharmacol. **28**, 172—181 (1966)

Chang, H. W., Neumann, E.: Dynamic properties of isolated acetylcholine receptor proteins: Release of calcium ions caused by acetylcholine binding. Proc. nat. Acad. Sci. (Wash.) **73**, 3364—3368 (1976)

Changeux, J.-P., Kasai, M., Lee, C. Y.: Use of a snake venom toxin to characterize the cholinergic receptor protein. Proc. nat. Acad. Sci. (Wash.) **67**, 1241—1247 (1970)

Chiu, T. H., Lapa, A. J., Barnard, E. A., Albuquerque, E. X.: Binding of D-tubocurarine and α-bungarotoxin in normal and denervated mouse muscle. Exp. Neurol. **43**, 399—413 (1974)

Clark, D. G., MacMurchie, D. D., Elliott, E., Wolcott, R. G., Landel, A. M., Raftery, M. A.: Elapid neurotoxin. Purification, characterization, and immunochemical studies of α-bungarotoxin Biochemistry **11**, 1663—1668 (1972a)

Clark, D. G., Wolcott, R. G., Raftery, M. A.: Partial characterization of an α-bungarotoxin-binding component of electroplax membranes. Biochem. biophys. Res. Commun. **48**, 1061—1067 (1972b)

Cohen, J. B., Weber, M., Changeux, J.-P.: Effects of local anesthetics and calcium on the interaction of cholinergic ligands with the nicotinic receptor protein from *Torpedo marmorata*. Molec. Pharmacol. **10**, 904—932 (1974)

Colquhoun, D., Rang, H.P.: Effects of inhibitors on the binding of iodinated α-bungarotoxin to acetylcholine receptors in rat muscle. Molec. Pharmacol. **12**, 519—535 (1976)

Cooper, D., Reich, E.: Neurotoxin from venom of the cobra, *Naja naja siamensis*. Purification and radioactive labeling. J. biol. Chem. **247**, 3008—3013 (1972)

Curtis, D.R., Crawford, J.M.: Central synaptic transmission—Microelectrophoretic studies. Ann. Rev. Pharmacol. **9**, 209—240 (1969)

Denburg, J.L., Eldefrawi, M.E., O'Brien, R.D.: Macromolecules from lobster axon membranes that bind cholinergic ligands and local anesthetics. Proc. nat. Acad. Sci. (Wash.) **69**, 177—181 (1972)

Devreotes, P.N., Fambrough, D.M.: Acetylcholine receptor turnover in membranes of developing muscle fibers. J. Cell Biol. **65**, 335—358 (1975)

Dolly, J.O., Albuquerque, E.X., Sarvey, J.M., Mallick, B., Barnard, E.A.: Binding of perhydrohistrionicotoxin to the postsynaptic membrane of skeletal muscle in relation to its blockade of acetylcholine-induced depolarization. Molec. Pharmacol. **13**, 1—14 (1977)

Duggan, A.W., Hall, J.G., Lee, C.Y.: Alpha-bungarotoxin, cobra neurotoxin, and excitation of Renshaw cells by acetylcholine. Brain Res. **107**, 166—170 (1976)

Edelstein, S.J., Beyer, W.B., Eldefrawi, A.T., Eldefrawi, M.E.: Molecular weight of the acetylcholine receptors of electric organs and the effect of Triton X-100. J. biol. Chem. **250**, 6101—6106 (1975)

Eldefrawi, A.T., Eldefrawi, M.E., Albuquerque, E.X., Oliveira, A.C., Mansour, N., Adler, M., Daly, J.W., Brown, G.B., Burgermeister, W., Witkop, B.: Perhydrohistrionicotoxin: A potential ligand for the ion conductance modulator of the acetylcholine receptor. Proc. nat. Acad. Sci. (Wash.) **74**, 2172—2176 (1977)

Eldefrawi, A.T., O'Brien, R.D.: Binding of muscarone by extracts of housefly brain: Relationship to receptors for acetylcholine. J. Neurochem. **17**, 1287—1293 (1970)

Eldefrawi, M.: Neuromuscular transmission—The transmitter-receptor combination. In: Hubbard, J.L. (Ed.): The Peripheral Nervous System, pp. 181—200. New York: Plenum 1974

Eldefrawi, M.E., Britten, A.G., Eldefrawi, A.T.: Acetylcholine binding to *Torpedo* electroplax: Relationship to acetylcholine receptors. Science **73**, 338—340 (1971a)

Eldefrawi, M.E., Eldefrawi, A.T.: Purification and molecular properties of the acetylcholine receptor from *Torpedo* electroplax. Arch. Biochem. Biophys. **159**, 362—373 (1973)

Eldefrawi, M.E., Eldefrawi, A.T.: Acetylcholine receptors. In: Cuatrecasas, P., Greaves, M.F. (Eds.): Receptors and Recognition, pp. 197—258. London: Chapmann and Hall 1977

Eldefrawi, M.E., Eldefrawi, A.T., Gilmour, L.P., O'Brien, R.D.: Multiple affinities for binding of cholinergic ligands to a particulate fraction of *Torpedo* electroplax. Molec. Pharmacol. **7**, 420—428 (1971c)

Eldefrawi, M.E., Eldefrawi, A.T., O'Brien, R.D.: Binding sites for cholinergic ligands in a particulate fraction of *Electrophorus* electroplax. Proc. nat. Acad. Sci. (Wash.) **68**, 1047—1050 (1971b)

Eldefrawi, M.E., Eldefrawi, A.T., Wilson, D.B.: Tryptophan and cysteine residues of the acetylcholine receptors of *Torpedo* species. Relationship to binding of cholinergic ligands. Biochemistry **14**, 4304—4310 (1975)

Eldefrawi, M.E., Fertuck, H.C.: A rapid method for the preparation of $[^{125}I]$α-bungarotoxin. Analyt. Biochem. **58**, 63—70 (1974)

Eldefrawi, M.E., Mansour, N.A., Eldefrawi, A.T.: Interactions of acetylcholine receptors with organic mercury compounds. In: Miller, M.W., Shamoo, A.E. (Eds.): Membrane Toxicity, pp. 449—462. New York: Plenum Press 1977

Etorovic, V.A., Bennett, E.L.: Nicotinic cholinergic receptor in brain detected by binding of α-$[^{3}H]$bungarotoxin. Biochim. biophys. Acta (Amst.) **362**, 346—355 (1974)

Fambrough, D.M.: Revised estimates of extrajunctional receptor density in denervated rat diaphragm. J. gen. Physiol. **64**, 468—472 (1974)

Fambrough, D.M., Drachman, D.B., Satymurti, S.: Neuromuscular junction in myasthenia gravis: Decreased acetylcholine receptors. Science **182**, 293—295 (1973)

Fertuck, H.C., Salpeter, M.M.: Sensitivity in electron microscope autoradiography for ^{125}I. J. Histochem. Cytochem. **22**, 80—87 (1974)

Fertuck, H. C., Salpeter, M. M.: Quantitation of junctional and extrajunctional acetylcholine receptors by electron microscope autoradiography after ^{125}I-α-bungarotoxin binding at mouse neuromuscular junctions. J. Cell Biol. **69**, 144—158 (1976)

Fischbach, G. D., Fambrough, D., Nelson, P. G.: A discussion of neuron and muscle cell cultures. Fed. Proc. **32**, 1636—1642 (1973)

Franklin, G. I., Potter, L. T.: Studies of the binding of α-bungarotoxin to membrane-bound and detergent-dispersed acetylcholine receptors from *Torpedo* electric tissue. FEBS Letters **28**, 101—106 (1972)

Fu, J.-J. L., Donner, D. B., Hess, G. P.: Half-of-the-sites reactivity of the membrane-bound *Electrophorus electricus* acetylcholine receptor. Biochem. biophys. Res. Commun. **60**, 1072—1080 (1974)

Fu, J.-J. L., Donner, D. B., Moore, D. E., Hess, G. P.: Allosteric interactions between the membrane-bound acetylcholine receptor and chemical mediators: Equilibrium measurements. Biochemistry **16**, 678—684 (1977)

Gibson, R. E.: Ligand interactions with the acetylcholine receptor from *Torpedo californica*. Extensions of the allosteric model for cooperativity to half-of-site activity. Biochemistry **15**, 3890—3901 (1976)

Gibson, R. E., O'Brien, R. D., Edelstein, S. J., Thompson, W. R.: Acetylcholine receptor oligomers from electroplax of *Torpedo* species. Biochemistry **15**, 2377—2383 (1976)

Greene, L., Sytkowski, A. J., Vogel, Z., Nirenberg, M. W.: α-Bungarotoxin used as a probe for acetylcholine receptors of cultured neurones. Nature (Lond.) **243**, 163—166 (1973)

Greene, L. A.: Binding of α-bungarotoxin to chick sympathetic ganglia: Properties of the receptor and its rate of appearance during development. Brain Res. **111**, 135—145 (1976)

Hartzell, H. C., Fambrough, D. M.: Acetylcholine receptors. Distribution and extrajunctional density in rat diaphragm after denervation correlated with acetylcholine sensitivity. J. gen. Physiol. **60**, 248—262 (1972)

Hess, G. P., Bulger, J. E., Fu, J.-J. L., Hindy, E. F., Silberstein, R. J.: Allosteric interactions of the membrane-bound acetylcholine receptor; kinetic studies with α-bungarotoxin. Biochem. biophys. Res. Commun. **64**, 1018—1027 (1975)

Heilbronn, E., Mattson, C.: The nicotinic cholinergic receptor protein: improved purification method, preliminary amino acid composition and observed auto-immune response. J. Neurochem. **22**, 315—317 (1974)

Hucho, F., Changeux, J.-P.: Molecular weight and quaternary structure of the cholinergic receptor protein extracted by detergents from *Electrophorus electricus* electric tissue. FEBS Letters **38**, 11—15 (1973)

Karlsson, E., Arnberg, H., Eaker, D.: Isolation of the principal neurotroxins of two *Naja naja* subspecies. Europ. J. Biochem. **21**, 1—16 (1971)

Kato, G., Changeux, J.-P.: Studies on the effect of histrionicotoxin on the monocellular electroplax from *Electrophorus electricus* and on the binding of [^{3}H]acetylcholine to membrane fragments from *Torpedo marmorata*. Molec. Pharmacol. **12**, 92—100 (1976)

Katz, B., Miledi, R.: The effect of procaine on the action of acetylcholine at the neuromuscular junction. J. Physiol. (Lond.) **249**, 269—284 (1975)

Katz, B., Thesleff, S.: A study of the "desensitization" produced by acetylcholine at the motor end-plate. J. Physiol. (Lond.) **138**, 63—80 (1957)

Kehoe, J., Sealock, R., Bon, C.: Effects of α-toxins from *Bungaris multicinctus* and *Bungarus caeruleus* on cholinergic responses in Aplysia neurones. Brain Res. **107**, 527—540 (1976)

Klett, R. P., Fulpius, B. W., Cooper, D., Smith, M., Reich, E., Possani, L. D.: The acetylcholine receptor. I. Purification and characterization of a macromolecule isolated from *Electrophorus electricus*. J. biol. Chem. **248**, 6841—6853 (1973)

Ko, P. K., Anderson, M. J., Cohen, M. W.: Denervated skeletal muscle fibers develop discrete patches of high acetylcholine density. Science **196**, 540—542 (1977)

Kohanski, R. A., Andrews, J. P., Wins, P., Eldefrawi, M. E., Hess, G. P.: A simple quantitative assay of ^{125}I-labeled α-bungarotoxin binding to soluble and membrane-bound acetylcholine receptor protein. Analyt. Biochem. **80**, 531—539 (1977)

Koshland, D. E., Nemethy, G., Filmer, D.: Comparison of experimental binding data and theoretical models in proteins containing subunits. Biochemistry **5**, 365—385 (1966)

Kouvelas, E. D., Greene, L. A.: The binding properties and regional ontogeny of receptors for α-bungarotoxin in chick brain. Brain Res. **113**, 111—126 (1976)

Kuba, K., Albuquerque, E. X., Barnard, E. A.: Diisopropylfluorophosphate: Suppression of ionic conductance of the cholingeric receptor. Science **181**, 853—856 (1973)

Kuba, K., Albuquerque, E. X., Daly, J., Barnard, E. A.: A study of the irreversible cholinesterase inhibitor, diisopropylfluorophosphate, on time course of end-plate currents in frog sartorius muscle. J. Pharmacol. exp. Ther. **189**, 499—512 (1974)

Lapa, A. J., Albuquerque, E. X., Daly, J.: An electrophysiological study of the effects of D-tubocurarine, atropine, and α-bungarotoxin on the cholinergic receptor in innervated and chronically denervated mammalian skeletal muscles. Exp. Neurol. **43**, 375—398 (1974)

Lapa, A. J., Albuquerque, E. X., Sarvey, J. M., Daly, J., Witkop, B.: Effects of histrionicotoxin on the chemosensitive and electrical properties of skeletal muscle. Exp. Neurol. **47**, 558—580 (1975)

Lee, C. Y.: Mode of action of cobra venom and its purified toxins. In: Simpson, L. L. (Ed.): Neuropoisons: Their Pathophysiological Actions, pp. 21—70. New York: Plenum 1971

Lee, C. Y.: Chemistry and pharmacology of polypeptide toxins in snake venoms. Ann. Rev. Pharmacol. **12**, 265—286 (1972)

Lee, C. Y., Chen, Y. M.: Central neurotoxicity of cobra neurotoxin, cardiotoxin, and phospholipase A_2. Toxicon **15**, 395—401 (1977)

Lee, C. Y., Peng, M. T.: An analysis of the respiratory failure produced by the Formosan elapid venoms. Arch. int. Pharmacodyn. Ther. **133**, 182—192 (1961)

Lee, C. Y., Tseng, L. F.: Distribution of *Bungarus multicinctus* venom following envenomation. Toxicon **3**, 281—290 (1966)

Lee, C. Y., Tseng, L. F., Chiu, T. H.: Influence of denervation on localization of neurotoxins from elapid venoms in rat diaphragm. Nature (Lond.) **215**, 1177—1178 (1967)

Lester, H. A., Changeux, J.-P., Sheridan, R. E.: Conductance increases produced by bath application of cholinergic agonists to *Electrophorus* electroplaques. J. gen. Physiol. **65**, 797—816 (1975)

Lindstrom, J.: Immunological studies of acetylcholine receptors. J. supramolec. Struct. **4**, 389—403 (1976)

Lindstrom, J., Patrick, J.: Purification of the acetylcholine receptor by affinity chromatography. In: Bennett, M. V. L. (Ed.): Synaptic Transmission and Neuronal Interaction, pp. 191—216. New York: Raven 1974

Lindstrom, J. M., Seybold, M. E., Lennon, V. A., Whittingham, S., Duane, D. D.: Antibody to acetylcholine receptor in myasthenia gravis. Neurology **26**, 1054—1059 (1976)

Lowy, J., McGregor, J., Rosenstone, J., Schmidt, J.: Solubilization of an α-bungarotoxin-binding component from rat brain. Biochemistry **15**, 1522—1527 (1976)

Mansour, N. A., Eldefrawi, M. E., Eldefrawi, A. T.: Isolation of putative acetylcholine receptor proteins from housefly brain. Biochemistry **16**, 4126—4132 (1977)

Masukawa, L., Albuquerque, E. X.: Voltage and time-dependent action of histrionicotoxin on the endplate current of the frog muscle. J. gen. Physiol. **72**, 351—367 (1978)

Menez, A., Morgat, J.-L., Fromageot, P., Ronsseray, A.-M., Boquet, P., Changeux, J.-P.: Tritium labelling of the α-neurotoxin of *Naja nigricollis*. FEBS Letters **17**, 333—335 (1971)

Merlie, J. P., Changeux, J.-P., Gros, F.: Acetylcholine receptor degradation measured by pulse chase labelling. Science **264**, 74—76 (1976)

Merlie, J. P., Sobel, A., Changeux, J.-P., Gros, F.: Synthesis of acetylcholine receptor during differentiation of cultured embryonic muscle cells. Proc. nat. Acad. Sci. (Wash.) **72**, 4028—4032 (1975)

Meunier, J.-C., Olsen, R. W., Menez, A., Fromageot, P., Boquet, P., Changeux, J.-P.: Some physical properties of the cholinergic receptor protein from *Electrophorus electricus* revealed by a titrated α-toxin from *Naja nigricollis* venom. Biochemistry **11**, 1200—1209 (1972)

Miledi, R., Molinoff, P., Potter, L. T.: Isolation of the cholinergic receptor protein of *Torpedo* electric tissue. Nature (Lond.) **229**, 554—557 (1971)

Miledi, R., Potter, L. T.: Acetylcholine receptors in muscle fibers. Nature (Lond.) **233**, 599—603 (1971)

Miledi, R., Szczepaniak, A.C.: Effect of *Dendroaspis* neurotoxins on synaptic transmission in the spinal cord on the frog. Proc. roy. Soc. B **190**, 267—274 (1975)

Miranda, F., Kupeyan, C., Rochat, H., Rochat, C., Lissitzky, S.: Purification of animal neurotoxins. Isolation and characterization of four neurotoxins from two different sources of *Naja haje* venom. Europ. J. Biochem. **17**, 477—484 (1970)

Molinoff, P., Potter, L.T.: Isolation of the cholinergic receptor protein of *Torpedo* electric tissue. In: Advances in Biochemical Psychopharmacology, Vol. 6, pp. 111—134. New York: Raven 1972

Monod, J., Wyman, J., Changeux, J.-P.: On the nature of allosteric transitions. A plausible model. J. molec. Biol. **12**, 88—118 (1965)

Moody, T., Schmidt, J., Raftery, M.A.: Binding of acetylcholine and related compounds to purified acetylcholine receptor from *Torpedo californica* electroplax. Biochem. biophys. Res. Commun. **53**, 761—772 (1973)

Moore, W.M., Brady, R.N.: Studies of nicotinic acetylcholine receptor protein from rat brain. Biochim. biophys. Acta (Amst.) **444**, 252—260 (1976)

Moreau, M., Changeux, J.-P.: Studies on the electrogenic action of acetylcholine with *Torpedo marmorata* electric organ. I. Pharmacological properties of the electroplaque. J. molec. Biol. **106**, 457—467 (1976)

Neher, E., Sakmann, B.: Noise analysis of drug induced voltage clamp currents in denervated frog muscle fibers. J. Physiol. (Lond.) **258**, 705—729 (1976)

O'Brien, R.D., Gilmour, L.P., Eldefrawi, M.E.: A muscarone-binding material in electroplax and its relation to the acetylcholine receptor. II. Dialysis assay. Proc. nat. Acad. Sci. (Wash.) **65**, 438—445 (1970)

O'Brien, R.D., Thompson, W.R., Gibson, R.E.: A comparison of acetylcholine and α-bungarotoxin binding to soluble *Torpedo* receptor. In: Robertis, E. de, Schacht, J. (Eds.): Neurochemistry of Cholinergic Receptors, pp. 49—62. New York: Raven 1974

Ong, D.E., Brady, R.N.: Isolation of cholinergic receptor protein(s) from *Torpedo nobiliana* by affinity chromatography. Biochemistry **13**, 2822—2827 (1974)

Ouyang, C.: On cause of death due to the venom of *Bungarus multicinctus* Blyth in rabbits. Mem. Fac. Med. Nat. Taiwan Univ. **1**, 121 (1950)

Patrick, J., Lindstrom, J., Culp, B., Mc Millan, J.: Studies on purified eel acetylcholine receptor and anti-acetylcholine receptor antibody. Proc. nat. Acad. Sci. (Wash.) **70**, 3334—3338 (1973)

Phillis, J.W.: The Pharmacology of Synapses. New York: Pergamon 1970

Polz-Tejera, G., Schmidt, J., Karten, H.J.: Autoradiographic localisation of α-bungarotoxin binding sites in the central nervous system. Nature **258**, 349—351 (1975)

Porter, C.W., Chiu, T.H., Wieckowski, J., Barnard, E.A.: Types and locations of cholinergic receptor-like molecules in muscle fibers. Nature (Lond.) New Biol. **241**, 3—7 (1973)

Potter, L.T.: α-Bungarotoxin (and similar α-neurotoxins) and nicotinic acetylcholine receptors. Methods in Enzymology **32**, 309—323 (1974)

Raftery, M.A.: Isolation of acetylcholine receptor-α-bungarotoxin complexes from *Torpedo californica* electroplax. Arch. Biochem. Biophys. **154**, 270—276 (1973)

Raftery, M.A., Schmidt, J., Clark, D.G., Wolcott, R.G.: Demonstration of a specific α-bungarotoxin binding component in *Electrophorus electricus* electroplax membranes. Biochem. biophys. Res. Commun. **45**, 1622—1629 (1971)

Raftery, M.A., Schmidt, J., Clark, D.G.: Specificity of α-bungarotoxin binding to *Torpedo californica* electroplax. Arch. Biochem. Biophys. **152**, 882—886 (1972)

Rash, J.E., Albuquerque, E.X., Hudson, C.S., Mayer, R.F., Satterfield, J.R.: Studies of human myasthenia gravis: Electrophysiological and ultrastructural evidence compatible with antibody attachment to the acetylcholine receptor complex. Proc. nat. Acad. Sci. (Wash.) **73**, 4584—4588 (1976)

Rübsamen, H., Hess, G.P., Eldefrawi, A.T., Eldefrawi, M.E.: Interaction between calcium and ligand-binding sites of the purified acetylcholine receptor studied by use of a fluorescent lanthanide. Biochem. biophys. Res. Commun. **68**, 56—63 (1976a)

Rübsamen, H., Montgomery, M., Hess, G.P., Eldefrawi, A.T., Eldefrawi, M.E.: Identification of a calcium-binding subunit of the acetylcholine receptor. Biochem. biophys. Res. Commun. **70**, 1020—1027 (1976b)

Ruff, R. L.: A quantitative analysis of local anaesthetic alteration of miniature end-plate currents and endplate current fluctuations. J. Physiol. (Lond.) **264**, 89—124 (1977)

Sakmann, B.: Reappearance of extrajunctional acetylcholine sensitivity in denervated rat muscle after blockage with α-bungarotoxin. Nature (Lond.) **255**, 415—416 (1975)

Salvaterra, P. M., Maher, H. R., Moore, W. J.: Subcellular and regional distribution of ^{125}I-labeled α-bungarotoxin binding in rat brain and its relationship to acetylcholinesterase and choline acetyltransferase. J. biol. Chem. **250**, 6469—6475 (1975)

Sanders, D. B., Schleifer, L. S., Eldefrawi, M. E., Norcross, N. L., Cobb, E. E.: An immunologically induced defect of neuromuscular transmission in rats and rabbits. Ann. N.Y. Acad. Sci. **274**, 319—336 (1976)

Sanes, J. R., Prescott, D. J., Hildebrand, J. G.: Cholinergic neurochemical development of normal and deafferented antennal lobes during metamorphosis of the moth, Manduca sexta. Brain Res. **119**, 389—402 (1977)

Sarvey, J. M., Albuquerque, E. X., Eldefrawi, A. T., Eldefrawi, M. E.: Effects of α-bungarotoxin and reversible cholinergic ligands on normal and denervated mammalian skeletal muscle. Membrane Biochem. **1**, 131—157 (1978)

Sato, S., Tamiya, N.: The amino acid sequences of erabutoxins, neurotoxic proteins of sea-snake *(Laticauda semifasciata)* venom. Biochem. J. **122**, 453—461 (1971)

Schmidt, J.: Drug binding properties of an α-bungarotoxin-binding component from rat brain. Molec. Pharmacol. **13**, 283—290 (1977)

Schmidt, J., Raftery, M. A.: A simple assay for the study of solubilized acetylcholine receptors. Analyt. Biochem. **52**, 349—354 (1973)

Schmidt, J., Raftery, M. A.: The cation sensitivity of the acetylcholine receptor from *Torpedo californica*. J. Neurochem. **23**, 617—623 (1974)

Sugiyama, H., Benda, P., Meunier, J.-C., Changeux, J.-P.: Immunological characterisation of the cholinergic receptor protein from *Electrophorus electricus*. FEBS Letters **35**, 124—128 (1973)

Sugiyama, H., Changeux, J.-P.: Interconversion between different states of affinity for acetylcholine of the cholinergic receptor protein from *Torpedo marmorata*. Europ. J. Biochem. **55**, 505—515 (1975)

Sugiyama, H., Popot, J.-L., Changeux, J.-P.: Studies on the electrogenic action of acetylcholine with *Torpedo marmorata* electric organ III. Pharmacologic desensitization in vitro of the receptor-rich membrane fragments by cholinergic agonists. J. molec. Biol. **106**, 485—496 (1976)

Trotter, J. L., Ringel, S. P., Cook, J. D., Engel, W. K., Eldefrawi, M. E., McFarlin, D. E.: Morphologic and immunologic studies in experimental autoimmune myasthenia gravis and myasthenia gravis. Neurology **27**, 1120—1124 (1977)

Tu, A. T., Hong, B.-S., Solie, T. N.: Characterization and chemical modifications of toxins isolated from the venoms of the sea snake, *Laticauda semifasciata*. Biochemistry **10**, 1295—1304 (1971)

Vogel, Z., Daniels, M. P.: Ultrastructure of acetylcholine receptor clusters on cultured muscle fibers. J. Cell Biol. **69**, 501—507 (1976)

Vogel, Z., Nirenberg, M.: Localization of acetylcholine receptors during synaptogenesis in retina. Proc. nat. Acad. Sci. (Wash.) **73**, 1806—1810 (1976)

Vogel, Z., Sytkowski, A. J., Nirenberg, M. W.: Acetylcholine receptors of muscle grown in vitro. Proc. nat. Acad. Sci. (Wash.) **69**, 3180—3184 (1972)

Wang, G.-K., Schmidt, J.: Receptors of α-bungarotoxin in the developing visual system of the chick. Brain Res. **114**, 524—529 (1976)

Warnick, J. E., Albuquerque, E. X., Guth, L.: The demonstration of neurotrophic function by application of colchicine or vinblastine to the peripheral muscle. Exp. Neurol. **57**, 622—636 (1977)

Weber, M., Changeux, J.-P.: Binding of *Naja nigricollis* [^{3}H]α-toxin to membrane fragments from *Electrophorus* and *Torpedo* electric organs. I. Binding of the tritiated α-neurotoxin in the absence of effector. Molec. Pharmacol. **10**, 1—14 (1974a)

Weber, M., Changeux, J.-P.: Binding of *Naja nigricollis* [^{3}H]α-toxin to membrane fragments from *Electrophorus* and *Torpedo* electric organs. II. Effect of cholinergic agonists and antagonists on the binding of the tritiated α-neurotoxin. Molec. Pharmacol. **10**, 15—34 (1974b)

Weber, M., Changeux, J.-P.: Binding of *Naja nigricollis* [^{3}]α-toxin to membrane fragments from *Electrophorus* and *Torpedo* electric organs. III. Effects of local anaesthetics on the binding of the tritiated α-neurotoxin. Molec. Pharmacol. **10**, 35—40 (1974c)
Weber, M., David-Pfeuty, T., Changeux, J.-P.: Regulation of binding properties of the nicotinic receptor protein by cholinergic ligands in membrane fragments from *Torpedo marmorata*. Proc. nat. Acad. Sci. (Wash.) **72**, 3443—3447 (1975)
Yang, C. C.: Chemistry and evolution of toxins in snake venoms. Toxicon **12**, 1—43 (1974)
Yang, C. C., Chang, C. C., Hayashi, K., Suzuki, T.: Amino acid composition and end group analysis of cobrotoxin. Toxicon **7**, 43—47 (1969)

CHAPTER 12

Pharmacology of Phospholipase A_2 from Snake Venoms

P. ROSENBERG

A. Introduction

I. Scope of Chapter and Prior Reviews

The effects of snake venom Ph on biologic systems have been studied with one of two major goals. In some cases there was the desire to see what the Ph of the venom contributed to the overall venom action, be that action hemolysis of red blood cells, blockade of the neuromuscular junction, inhibition of cytochrome oxidase, or any one of hundreds of other venom actions. In other experiments, snake venom Ph was used as a tool to help understand the phospholipid contribution to the structure or function of a particular membrane, tissue, or organ. In this Chapter, I shall draw upon the results obtained in both of these types of studies. It is not my purpose, however, to present an uncritical encyclopedic listing of all studies in which pharmacologic effects of snake venoms have been attributed to Ph. This would only add a "stamp of approval" to much data which is impossible to interpret or has been incorrectly interpreted by the authors. Rather, I shall place greater emphasis on the more recent studies using pure or at least purified preparations of Ph derived from snake venoms. The state of purity of the preparations used shall be commented upon since the significance of the data to this present Chapter can be evaluated only if the effects can unambiguously be related to Ph. Selected interesting older data shall, however, be mentioned, even if carried out with impure preparations of Ph, or crude

---

Abbreviations

Ph = phospholipase
PC = phosphatidylcholine
LPC = lysophosphatidylcholine; lysolecithin
PE = phosphatidylethanolamine
PI = phosphatidylinositol
PS = phosphatidylserine
ATPase = adenosinetriphosphatase
CTX = cardiotoxin; direct lytic factor
SRS = slow-reacting substance
A. = *Agkistrodon*
B. = *Bitis*
C. = *Crotalus*
E. = *Enhydrina*
H. = *Hemachatus*
L. = *Laticauda*
N. = *Naja*
O. = *Oxyuranus*
P. = *Pseudechis*
T. = *Trimeresurus*
V. = *Vipera*
A. piscivorus = cottonmouth moccasin
C. adamanteus = eastern diamondback rattlesnake
C. durissus terrificus = Brazilian rattlesnake
H. haemachatus = Ringhals cobra
N. naja = Indian cobra
N. naja atra = Formosan cobra
N. nigricollis = spitting cobra
Notechis scutatus scutatus = Australian tiger snake
P. porphyriacus = Australian black snake
V. russellii = Russell's viper

venom, as long as there is reason to believe that the effects may be due to the Ph component of the venom. This is done in an effort to stimulate the repetition of these experiments with pure Ph; however, I shall be careful to indicate the uncertainty of conclusions based upon studies with crude venom or impure preparations of Ph. I shall not discuss the pharmacology of snake venoms per se since this is considered in other Chapters. The effects of Ph from other sources (bee, bacterial, mammalian) shall not be considered, except if necessary to our understanding of an action of snake venom Ph.

Only the pharmacology of PhA_2 (phosphatide acyl hydrolase, EC 3.1.1.4) shall be considered in this Chapter. The richest sources of this enzyme are in snake venoms where it is widely distributed in all of the venomous species. Although other Phs have been reported to be present in snake venoms, their pharmacology has not been studied. PhA_1 activity has not been detected in snake venoms; this enzyme is present in other preparations including mammalian tissues (ANSELL et al., 1973). PhB (lysophospholipase; lysolecithin acyl hydrolase, EC 3.1.1.5) has been reported to be present in a number of venoms, especially Australian and Egyptian snake venoms (DOERY and PEARSON, 1964; MOHAMED et al., 1969). More definitive studies were carried out by SHILOAH et al. (1973b, c) who found PhB and PhA_2 activities in purified enzymes isolated from *V. palestinae* and *N. naja* venoms. PhA_2 and the much weaker PhB activities were clearly shown to be dual activities of a single enzyme and not activities of separate enzymes. PhC (phosphatidylcholine cholinephosphohydrolase, EC 3.1.4.3) activity was reported as being present in *Bothrops alternatus* venom (VIDAL BREARD and ELIAS, 1950); however, later studies did not confirm its presence in this venom but did report PhC activity in a fraction isolated from *N. naja* venom (BRAGANCA and KHANDEPARKAR, 1966; BRAGANCA et al., 1967). This fraction lysed Yoshida sarcoma cells and degraded purified phospholipids, liberating phosphorylated bases, as would be expected of a PhC preparation. LEE (1971), however, notes the inability of HSIEH and himself to detect PhC activity in *N. naja atra* venom. It would be of interest to systematically survey snake venoms for PhB, PhC, and PhD (phosphatidylcholine phosphatidohydrolase, EC 3.1.4.4) activities. The latter enzyme has so far only been detected in plants (ANSELL et al., 1973).

It is not possible in this Chapter to make accurate quantitative comparisons of the pharmacologic potencies of the various PhA_2 preparations used by different investigators. Since the purity of the PhA_2 used in the studies differs greatly, little is to be gained by comparing potencies in terms of concentration or weight of enzyme required for a particular pharmacologic effect. This would only be valid if pure PhA_2 were used, and even then only if it were known that no degradation or inactivation of the enzyme occurred during isolation. Theoretically at least, it would seem more desirable to relate pharmacologic potency to enzymic activity rather than to weight. Unfortunately, it is not possible to do this because in most studies the enzymic activities were not recorded. Even where such data are presented, the enzymic activities reported by different investigators cannot be compared, because there is no standardized PhA_2 assay, but rather there are a bewildering variety of methods for measuring enzymic activity. The same preparation of PhA_2 will show markedly different enzymic activities dependent upon conditions of assay (temperature, pH, ions present, aqueous or nonaqueous system, sonication, addition of ether, physical state of phospholipid substrate, i.e., membrane-associated, protein bound, or pure phospholipid free of protein). For these reasons, it is only possible to compare pharmacologic potencies within a study, where the author uses the same preparation of PhA_2 for all of the studies. In most cases, therefore, we shall have to discuss the pharmacology of snake venom PhA_2 in qualitative terms, and even where we do make quantitative comparisons, the above-described reservations as to the significance of such comparisons must be born in mind. Direct comparisons of the extent of phospholipid hydrolysis in the biologic preparation could provide the most valid basis for relating pharmacologic potency to enzymic activity. Using the same biologic preparation, one could then compare the amounts of enzyme from different sources required for equivalent phospholipid hydrolysis. At the same time, the essentiality of particular phospholipids for particular biologic functions could be evaluated. Unfortunately, most investigators studying the pharmacology of PhA_2 do not measure the hydrolysis of tissue phospholipids.

The term pharmacology shall be interpreted rather broadly, so that I shall not only consider the toxicity of PhA_2 and its effects on muscle and nerve but shall also consider its metabolic actions, effects on structure and permeability of cellular membranes, and ability to release physiologically active compounds. The effects of PhA_2 on blood (hemolytic, hemorrhagic, etc.) shall not be considered in this chapter but are covered in other chapters in this text (Chaps. 13, 14, 18) as well as in a recent review (CONDREA, 1974).

There have been several earlier reviews on venom Ph; however, it is most appropriate at this time to critically survey the field because of the recent most interesting and in many cases unexpected pharmacologic results obtained using pure preparations of PhA_2 which have relatively high toxicity. The earlier literature dealing with the presence of Ph and other enzymes in bacterial and animal venoms was well reviewed by ZELLER (1951). Later reviews also emphasized the source, isolation, chemistry, and biochemistry of Ph as well as the enzyme's effects on metabolism (VAN DEENEN and DE HAAS, 1966; DEVI, 1968; SARKAR and DEVI, 1968; JIMÉNEZ-PORRAS, 1970; HANAHAN, 1971). Some neurochemical effects of snake venoms and the possible involvement of PhA_2 in these effects was reviewed by BRAGANCA and ARAVINDAKSHAN (1962). The chemical constituents, pathophysiologic effects, and immunologic properties of venoms and their enzymes were reviewed by BOQUET (1964, 1966). The most complete and definitive information on the pharmacology of PhA_2 from snake venoms is contained in several articles and reviews dealing with the pharmacology of snake venoms and neurotoxins or the properties of venom PhA_2 (MELDRUM, 1965b; CONDREA and DE VRIES, 1965; RUSSELL, 1967; JIMÉNEZ-PORRAS, 1968; RUSSELL and PUFFER, 1970; LEE, 1971, 1972; SLOTTA et al., 1971; TU, 1971, 1973; TU and PASSAY, 1971). Proceedings of meetings devoted to venoms are also sources of information concerning snake venom PhA_2 (BUCKLEY and PORGES, 1956; RUSSELL and SAUNDERS, 1967; DE VRIES and KOCHVA, 1971). There are also excellent multiauthored texts dealing with venoms and their constituents (BUCHERL et al., 1968; SIMPSON, 1971). Recent reviews have been devoted to the chemistry of potent animal toxins (KARLSSON, 1973), animal venoms (ZLOTKIN, 1973), and membrane active polypeptides from snake venoms (CONDREA, 1974).

The use of snake venom PhA_2 as an enzymic probe in the study of the essentiality of phospholipids to the structure and function of bioelectrically excitable tissues has been reviewed (ROSENBERG, 1966, 1971, 1972, 1976b; NARAHASHI, 1974).

II. Purification, Properties, Assays, and Inhibitors of PhA_2

Any critical discussion of the pharmacology of PhA_2 must consider the sources of error in interpreting the literature data. To do this, however, we must first briefly review the purification, properties, assays, and inhibitors of PhA_2 activity even though these topics are not of primary concern in this Chapter. No attempt will be made to be inclusive; rather enough data will be presented to hopefully justify the opinion of the author as to possible sources of error.

Using primarily chromatographic, electrophoretic, and gel filtration techniques, PhA_2 has been purified to varying extents. Within the last few years, the complete amino acid sequences of a number of snake venom Phs have been determined. Partial or complete purifications of PhA_2 have been obtained from the following venoms: *A. halys blomhoffii* (KAWAUCHI et al., 1971a, 1971b; SAMEJIMA et al., 1974), *A. piscivorus* (AUGUSTYN and ELLIOTT, 1970), *B. arietans* (HOWARD, 1974), *B. gabonica* (BOTES and VILJOEN, 1974a, 1974b), *Bothrops neuwiedi* (VIDAL and STOPPANI, 1971b; VIDAL et al., 1972), *C. adamanteus* (SAITO and HANAHAN, 1962; WELLS and HANAHAN, 1969; WELLS, 1971, 1975; TSAO et al., 1975; ROCK and SNYDER, 1975), *C. atrox* (WU and TINKER, 1969; HACHIMORI et al., 1971), *H. haemachatus* (BJÖRK, 1961; JOUBERT, 1975c), *L. semifasciata* (TU et al., 1970; TU and PASSEY, 1971), *N. melanoleuca* (JOUBERT and VAN DER WALT, 1975; JOUBERT, 1975a, 1975b), *N. naja* (SUZUKI et al., 1958; BRAGANCA and SAMBRAY, 1967; BRAGANCA et al., 1969; SALACH et al., 1971a; SHILOAH et al., 1973a; DEEMS and DENNIS, 1975), *N. naja atra* (LO et al., 1972), *N. nigricollis* (WAHLSTRÖM, 1971; DUMAREY et al., 1975), *P. porphyriacus* (DOERY and PEARSON, 1961), *V. ammodytes* (SKET et al., 1973a, 1973b; GUBENŠEK et al., 1974; GUBENŠEK and LAPANJE, 1974), *V. berus* (DELORI, 1971, 1973), and *V. russellii* (SALACH et al., 1971a). The methods described in the above articles can conveniently be used when one wishes to obtain purified PhA_2 preparation to study its pharmacologic properties. I have not found commercially available preparations of PhA_2 to be of high purity or specific activity; in many cases they were no better than crude venom.

The above-referenced reports have definitely established the inadequacy of referring to all snake venom Phs as if they were identic; one must specify the venom from which the Ph is derived. Pure Phs have isoelectric points varying from 4–10, molecular weights between 8500 and 24000, and in some cases a dimer is the active form. Even within a single venom, many isoenzymes may be present; for example, nine to 14 PhA_2 isoenzymes have been found in *N. naja* venom (SALACH et al., 1971a; SHILOAH et al., 1973a). Differences in physicochemical properties of the enzyme may also be reflected by different pharmacologic properties. The complete amino acid sequences of PhA_2 from *A. halys blomhoffii* (SAMEJIMA et al., 1974), *B. gabonica* (BOTES and VILJOEN, 1974a, 1974b), *H. haemachatus* (JOUBERT, 1975c), and three PhA_2 isoenzymes from *N. melanoleuca* (JOUBERT, 1975a, 1975b) have been determined. There is a great deal of homology between their amino acid sequences; however, there are also differences, whose significance, as far as differences in pharmacologic actions, has yet to be determined. The purified venom Phs usually have 12–14 half-cystine residues, high contents of aspartic acid, glycine, and tyrosine, and tend to be deficient in histidine, methionine, and tryptophan. Recently, crystals of PhA_2 from *C. adamanteus* and *C. atrox* venoms were obtained in a size suitable for X-ray diffraction analysis (PASEK et al., 1975). Further information on the three-dimensional structure of this enzyme may, therefore, be forthcoming.

PhA_2 activities of various snake venoms show marked differences in their stabilities, phospholipid substrate preferences, and stimulation, or inhibition produced by various ions. These types of differences could possibly explain some of the pharmacologic differences we will be discussing in this Chapter. Because of these differences, it is essential to measure the actual phospholipid hydrolysis produced in the tissue or organ being studied when the pharmacologic effects of PhA_2 are being measured. There is no way to extrapolate from in vitro assay systems to the in vivo biologic situation where ionic conditions, availability of substrate, etc., cannot be controlled. Pharmacologic differences may be due to differing rates of in vivo phospholipid hydrolysis or to selective differences in ability to attack particular phospholipids. However, this can only be evaluated if phospholipids of the tissue are measured prior to and following PhA_2 application. It has been reported that PC plasmalogen is hydrolyzed by *C. atrox* PhA_2 at a much lower rate than PC, whereas no large difference in sensitivity is observed with *N. naja* PhA_2 (COLACICCO and RAPPORT, 1966). The Km values of PhA_2 from *C. atrox* for PC, PE, and PC plasmalogen were 7, 27, and 96×10^{-3} M, respectively (WOELK and DEBUCH, 1971). PhA_2 activity from *C. adamanteus* venom is greatest against PC and PE, less toward PS, and least hydrolysis is observed with PI. Ca^{2+}, Mg^{2+}, and deoxycholate enhance activity while EDTA has a direct inhibitory action (UTHE and MAGEE, 1971a, 1971b). PhA_2 activity of most venoms is inhibited amongst other agents by Cu^{2+}, Fe^{3+}, Zn^{2+}, Hg^{2+}, Ba^{2+}, EDTA, N-ethyl maleimide, diisopropylfluorophosphate, iodoacetate, and formaldehyde while Ca^{2+}, Ni^{2+}, Co^{2+}, Mg^{2+}, Cd^{2+}, trypsin, ether, and deoxycholate tend to increase activity (MARINETTI, 1965; BROWN and BOWLES, 1966; WU and TINKER, 1969; MOHAMED et al., 1969). Two PhA_2 preparations from *Bothrops neuwiedi* venom hydrolyzed PE $\geq$ PC $>$ PI $>$ PS $\gg$ cardiolipin and hydrolyzed egg yolk lipoprotein phospholipids at a faster rate than pure phospholipids (VIDAL et al., 1972). PhA_2 purified from *L. semifasciata* venom was reported able to only hydrolyze PC (TU et al., 1970; TU and PASSEY, 1971). The optimal temperature for PhA_2 activity varies between 45 and 65° C for different venoms using identic assay conditions (WU and TINKER, 1969; NAIR et al., 1976a, 1976b), while additional variations in activity are produced by altering the substrate. Variations in pH optima for PhA_2 activity should also be considered when testing the pharmacologic activity of PhA_2. Most venom Phs have a pH optimum between 6 and 8.

As discussed previously, it is not possible to relate the enzymic activities of different PhA_2 preparations to their pharmacologic potencies even if pure preparations of PhA_2 are used, unless a single standardized Ph assay system is used. Unfortunately, a variety of assay systems are used including, for example: 1. isolation and titration of free fatty acids liberated from tissue phospholipids (FAIRBAIRN, 1945) or from egg yolk (KOCHOLATY, 1966), 2. determining decrease in acyl ester bonds in a collidine-ether buffer system (MAGEE and THOMPSON, 1960) or modifications of this method involving alterations in substrate or conditions of incubation (BROWN and BOWLES, 1966; AUGUSTYN and ELLIOTT, 1969; BULOS and SACKTOR, 1971), 3. titration of free fatty acids produced in an aqueous incubation medium using a water-soluble synthetic phospholipid substrate (ROHOLT and SCHLAMOWITZ, 1961; SALACH et al., 1971a, 1971b), 4. clearing of a suspension of egg yolk under controlled assay conditions (MARINETTI, 1965), 5. hemolysis of red blood cells by lysophosphatides produced as a result of PhA_2 activity (MAENO et al., 1962; CONDREA et al., 1964), 6. and conductometric assay which appears to be rapid and sensitive (MOORES and LAWRENCE, 1972). It would greatly simplify the comparisons of data obtained by different investigators if a single standardized "official" assay could be developed.

It is of interest that natural inhibitors of PhA_2 activity are present in certain venoms, which would further complicate any attempt to derive information on the pharmacology of PhA_2 by the use of crude venom. A basic polypeptide inhibitor of PhA_2, having a mol wt of about 5000 and forming a 1:1 inactive complex with the enzyme, was isolated from *N. naja* venom (BRAGANCA et al., 1970). The relatively low activity and lag period associated with the PhA_2 of several *Bothrops* species *(atrox, jararaca, neuwiedi)* has also been related to a polypeptide inhibitor of PhA_2 which was isolated, purified, and its properties determined (VIDAL and STOPPANI, 1970, 1971 a). Synthetic inhibitors of PhA_2 have also been prepared (ROSENTHAL and GEYER, 1960; ROSENTHAL and HAN, 1970).

The best known natural inhibitor of PhA_2 is the protein crotapotin, which is a component of crotoxin. Crotoxin is a toxic crystallizable protein from *C. durissus terrificus* venom and was first described in 1938 by SLOTTA and FRAENKEL-CONRAT. Crotoxin has PhA_2 activity and could be resolved into an acidic protein which has neither neurotoxic nor hemolytic activity and a basic protein which shows high indirect hemolytic activity (HENDON and FRAENKEL-CONRAT, 1971; HORST et al., 1972). A mixture of the basic and the acidic protein restores the high toxicity of crotoxin. The complex can be reconstituted even in dilute solution, although the biologic synergism of the two components does not appear to depend upon physical complex formation (HENDON and FRAENKEL-CONRAT, 1976). Other workers (RÜBSAMEN et al., 1971) resolved crotoxin into a basic PhA_2 with lower lethality than crotoxin but with a fourfold higher specific PhA_2 activity. A second substance, crotapotin, was acidic and devoid of lethality and PhA_2 activity. Addition of crotapotin to the basic PhA_2 restored the lethality and decreased the PhA_2 activity to that observed in crotoxin (BREITHAUPT and HABERMANN, 1972). Crotapotin and the basic PhA_2 were purified to homogeneity and had isoelectric points of 3.4 and 9.7 and mol wt of about 7000 (6700–8900) and 15000 (14500–15800), respectively (BREITHAUPT et al., 1974). The physical, chemical, and enzymic properties of crotoxin, crotapotin, and PhA_2 have been studied (PARADIES and BREITHAUPT, 1975; BREITHAUPT, 1976a), and a partial amino acid sequence of the *Crotalus* PhA_2 has been presented (OMORI-SATOH et al., 1975). Three isoenzymes with PhA_2 activity, two basic and one acidic, have recently been isolated from the crotoxin complex (BREITHAUPT et al., 1975). Crotapotin inhibited the PhA_2 activity and potentiated the lethality of the two basic, but not the acidic PhA_2. The acidic PhA_2 was nontoxic and antigenically different from the basic enzymes.

III. Sources of Error in Interpreting PhA_2 Data

The previous discussion makes it clear that certain experimental protocols should be adhered to if maximum information is to be obtained from studies on the pharmacology of PhA_2. Unfortunately much of the data in the literature using snake venom

PhA_2 is either difficult to completely interpret or may have been interpreted incorrectly by the authors themselves. In the design of experiments, the following sources of error should be avoided.

1. Use of Impure Preparations of PhA_2

In many studies, impure preparations of PhA_2 were used; for example, crude venom or acid-boiled venom. The use of crude venom makes it difficult or impossible to conclusively relate pharmacologic effects to PhA_2 action since snake venoms contain many other enzymes as well as nonenzymic but pharmacologically active proteins (neurotoxin, CTX, etc.). Even if effects could be related to the action of PhA_2, no reliable index of potency could be obtained since the amount of PhA_2 in different venoms varies, and in addition, as noted previously, certain venoms contain natural inhibitors of the enzyme. If the primary interest is in studying the pharmacology of PhA_2, one must isolate and test the effects of the pure enzyme. While PhA_2 is the only known enzymic component of venom resistant to boiling at an acid pH (HUGHES, 1935; BRAGANCA and QUASTEL, 1953; MAGEE and THOMPSON, 1960; ROSENBERG and NG, 1963), other nonenzymic proteins such as CTX and toxins with specific actions at the neuromuscular junction (neurotoxins such as cobrotoxin, α-bungarotoxin, erabutoxin, etc.) are also resistant to acid boiling. As noted previously, there are now many reliable and rapid methods available for the purification of PhA_2 from venoms. There is no justification for the continued use of acid-boiled venom preparations as the PhA_2 source.

2. Neglecting Effects of Hydrolytic Products

In most studies, the pharmacologic effects of the hydrolytic products (lysophosphatides, free fatty acids) produced as a result of the action of PhA_2 on phospholipids have not been evaluated. Incorrect conclusions may, therefore, be drawn about phospholipid function since it may be supposed that pharmacologic effects are directly due to hydrolysis of phospholipids by PhA_2, whereas they are actually due to the toxic actions of the hydrolytic products. For example, lysophosphatides such as LPC have detergent properties and affect many tissues including nerve (ZELLER, 1951; TOBIAS, 1955; MORRISON and ZAMECNIK, 1950; MCARDLE et al., 1960; ROSENBERG and CONDREA, 1968). In all studies using PhA_2, the effects of lysophosphatides and free fatty acids should also be determined.

3. Failure to Quantitate Extent of Phospholipid Hydrolysis

If one wishes to quantitate and compare the pharmacologic potencies for various preparations of PhA_2 and relate them to enzymic activities, it is best to quantitate the actual extent of phospholipid hydrolysis in the biologic preparation to which PhA_2 is added. It is then possible to express enzymic potency in terms of weights of the PhA_2 preparations which give comparable extents of phospholipid hydrolysis. If pharmacologic potency is due to phospholipid hydrolysis, one might expect to find the same pharmacologic and enzymic ratios of potency for the different preparations of PhA_2.

Pharmacologic potencies may differ, however, because the PhA_2 preparations have different ratios of selectivity for the various membranal phospholipids. This can only be detected if at the same time when the pharmacologic observations are made the extent of hydrolysis of each of the phospholipids is measured. There are convenient methods available for the extraction, separation, and quantitation of phospholipids (FOLCH et al., 1957; BARTLETT, 1959; CONDREA et al., 1967; LYSZ and ROSENBERG, 1974). It is a priori impossible to use PhA_2 to evaluate the essentiality of phospholipids for a biologic process without determining the extent of phospholipid splitting associated with a particular pharmacologic action. Nevertheless, many investigators reach conclusions concerning phospholipid function or PhA_2 action without ever measuring the extent of phospholipid hydrolysis in the tissue of interest. In vitro assays of PhA_2 activity are not adequate, since enzymic activity under the conditions where pharmacologic effects are observed may be quite different from that observed in controlled in vitro assay conditions. As previously discussed, different in vitro assay systems will show varying PhA_2 activities.

4. Assumption that all Snake Venom Preparations of PhA_2 are Similar

Faulty generalizations may be made by extending data obtained using a PhA_2 from one venom, assuming that preparations of PhA_2 from other venoms will act similarly. As noted previously, the isoelectric points, molecular weights, temperature optima, and substrate specificities for PhA_2 from different venoms may vary. These physicochemical and enzymic differences could be responsible for differences in pharmacologic actions. I have heard at scientific meetings the argument made that the effects of a "toxic" or pharmacologically active PhA_2 cannot be associated with its enzymic activity because PhA_2 preparations from other venoms do not show the same activity. This conclusion neglects the great variation in properties of the different Phs.

5. Conclusions

It is because of errors such as those that I have described above that our conclusions concerning the pharmacology of snake venom PhA_2 have dramatically changed over the years. In the literature up to the 1950s it was often claimed that Ph was the component responsible for most of the venom actions. Most of these studies were, however, carried out with impure preparations, and the extent of phospholipid hydrolysis was not measured. Opinions in the 1950s and 1960s changed dramatically so that few of the venom's pharmacologic actions (other than certain effects on red blood cells) were thought to be due to PhA_2. A few pure preparations of PhA_2 were found to be pharmacologically weak, and generalizations were then made that all venom PhA_2 preparations are inactive. In contrast, as we shall discuss, recent exciting data seem to indicate that certain venoms do contain toxic PhA_2 enzymes, and some PhA_2 enzymes may have potent effects at the neuromuscular junction. We finally may be able to draw more balanced and reliable conclusions concerning the pharmacology of PhA_2 as a result of the realization that Ph preparations from different venoms may have different pharmacologic and enzymic properties.

B. Lethality of PhA_2

Most of the studies, at least up until the 1950s, which showed that PhA_2 was lethal at low doses were in error because boiled venom-preparations were used and contaminated with CTX and neurotoxins. For example, BRAGANCA and QUASTEL (1952, 1953) claimed that PhA_2 was responsible for the neurotoxic activity of cobra venom, because boiled cobra venom maintained both activities, while other enzymes were inactivated by boiling.

In later studies, however, using at least partially purified preparations of PhA_2, several investigators found that PhA activity and lethality were clearly separable. Studies on Formosan cobra venom by SASAKI (1957, 1958) indicated that the distribution of PhA_2 did not parallel the distribution of lethal potencies. A toxic component with little PhA_2 activity had a "minimum lethal dose" in mice of about 0.1 mg/kg, whereas a fraction rich in PhA_2 activity had a minimum lethal dose of 12 mg/kg. Two fractions were separated from *N. naja atra* venom, one rich in enzymes including PhA_2 but low in toxicity, while the other fraction was low in enzymic activity but more toxic. It was concluded that enzymes are not responsible for the toxic actions of the venoms. Similar conclusions were reached using *Notechis scutatus scutatus* venom (DOERY, 1958). YANG and co-workers carried out extensive studies on Formosan snake venoms using zone electrophoretic techniques to elucidate the relationship between enzyme activity and lethality as judged by intraperitoneal injections into mice. PhA_2 did not appear to be responsible for the toxicity of Formosan venoms including *N. naja atra* (YANG et al., 1959a), *A. acutus* (YANG et al., 1959b), *Bungarus multicinctus* (YANG et al., 1960), and other venoms. A partially purified preparation of PhA_2 from *N. naja* venom was nonlethal following intraperitoneal injection into mice, even at doses of 5 mg/kg, whereas in cats the i.v. LD_{100} dose was 1 mg/kg (BICHER et al., 1965). The enzyme preparation was, however, probably not completely pure which may explain the moderate degree of lethality shown in cats. MELDRUM (1965a) and KOCHWA et al. (1960) also noted that PhA_2 preparations separated by electrophoresis or chromatography were neither toxic nor lethal. Toxic fractions from cobra and rattlesnake venoms had low PhA_2 activity (RADOMSKI and DEICHMANN, 1958).

MASTER and RAO (1961) studied the possible relationship between intravenous lethality in mice and enzymic activity of fractions separated by starch gel electrophoresis from *N. naja* and *V. russellii* venom. The lethal components giving rise to neurotoxic symptoms were not associated with PhA_2 activity nor with any other single enzymic activity. These findings support the data of other workers who were also able to separate PhA_2 from the toxic components in snake venoms (BUSSARD and COTE, 1954; NEUMANN and HABERMANN, 1955) and contradict the report of BRAGANCA and ARAVINDAKSHAN (1962) that crystalline PhA_2 from *N. naja* venom has six times the PhA_2 activity and five times the toxicity of the crude venom. The LD_{50} values (mg/kg) following intraperitoneal injection into mice of crude *N. naja* venom, pure cobrotoxin, CTX and PhA_2 isolated from the venom were 0.35, 0.065, 2.1, and 3.1 (LYSZ and ROSENBERG, 1974)—are in good agreement with those (0.44, 0.074, 1.5, >5) reported by LEE (1971). These results clearly show that the major PhA_2 from *N. naja* venom only has a low degree of lethality and is not the component responsible for lethality of the crude venom. GITTER et al. (1957) also reported a separation between PhA_2 activity and the component of *V. xanthina* venom responsible for neurotoxicity. A purified PhA_2 isolated from the sea snake *L. semifasciata* was nontoxic and nonhemorrhagic. In *E. schistosa* venom, it was found that more than 90% of the PhA_2 activity was retained within the dialysis bag, whereas more than 90% of the toxicity of the venom was lost (CAREY and WRIGHT, 1960). BREWSTER and GENNARO (1963) reported the lethal potencies following intravenous injection into mice of PhA_2 and of LPC. Unfortunately, boiling was used as the method of purifying the PhA_2 from *N. naja* venom. They reported LD_{50} of 0.39 mg/kg for PhA_2 and 100–200 mg/kg for LPC, depending on source. Because of the impurity of the PhA_2, this data cannot be used in support of the suggestion that PhA_2 is toxic through its direct action and not via the production of toxic hydrolytic products.

In contrast to the above results, which provide little or no support for the proposal that at least some PhA_2 preparations may be toxic and responsible for the lethal effects of the whole venom, the following results may be mentioned which have been obtained since 1970. As previously discussed, the toxin from certain snake venoms of the family *Crotalidae*, named crotoxin, is composed of an acidic, nontoxic component called crotapotin and a basic PhA_2. The combination of the two components is required for maximum toxicity, and the acidic component partially inhibits the PhA_2 activity of the basic component. The i.v. LD_{50} in mice of the basic PhA_2 is 0.54 mg/kg as compared to values of 0.11 and 750 mg/kg for crotoxin and crotapotin, respectively (RÜBSAMEN et al., 1971). Recombination of the pure crotapotin and the PhA_2 gave a product with an LD_{50} of 0.042 mg/kg. While this basic PhA_2 was considered relatively nontoxic as compared to crotoxin, it is more toxic than acidic PhA_2 preparations found in other venoms and discussed above. The order of sensitivity to the intravenous lethal action of the basic PhA_2 from crotoxin is chick > mouse > rabbit > rat. The toxicity was potentiated by crotapotin (BREITHAUPT, 1976b).

Three proteins with PhA_2 activity, one basic and two acidic, were purified from *V. berus* venom using ion-exchange chromatography and gel filtration (DELORI, 1971, 1973). The basic Ph was toxic having an i.v. LD_{50} in mice and guinea pigs of 0.4 and 0.025 mg/kg, respectively. It is of interest that the toxic Ph hydrolyzes PE, whereas the other two do not. This alone is not likely to account for the differences in toxicity, since other nontoxic Phs will hydrolyze PE (CONDREA et al., 1967; CONDREA and ROSENBERG, 1968; LYSZ and ROSENBERG, 1974). This finding, however, does support the suggestion made previously that differences in enzymic characteristics may exist between pharmacologically active and inactive Ph preparations.

Two toxic proteins with PhA_2 activity were isolated from *V. ammodytes* venom in addition to nontoxic Phs (SKET et al., 1973a, 1973b; GUBENŠEK and LAPANJE, 1974; GUBENŠEK et al., 1974). The i.p. LD_{50} values in mice for the two enzymes were 0.19 and 0.64 mg/kg. The spectra as determined by circular dichroism for one of the toxic and the nontoxic Ph preparations were different, indicating that structural differences could be responsible for differences in biologic activity (GUBENŠEK and LAPANJE, 1974). A Sepharose-bound form of the more toxic PhA_2 was also prepared and had about 10% of the toxicity of the free enzyme (GUBENŠEK, 1976).

Two enzymes with PhA_2 activity purified from *N. nigricollis* venom had isoelectric points of 7.8 and 5.5. The i.v. LD_{100} in mice of the acidic PhA_2 was about 0.8 mg/kg which was considered relatively nonlethal as compared to the neurotoxin from the same venom (LD_{100} = 0.09 mg/kg) (KARLSSON et al., 1966; BOQUET et al., 1967; WAHLSTRÖM, 1971). The lethality is, however, greater than that observed with other acidic PhA_2 enzymes. The isolation, Ph activity, amino acid composition, and toxicity of the basic Ph has also been described (WAHLSTRÖM, 1971; EAKER, 1975; DUMAREY et al., 1975), and its amino acid sequence recently determined (EAKER, personal communication). The i.v. LD_{50} in mice of the basic PhA_2 was reported as 0.25 mg/kg while 0.175 mg/kg in a rabbit caused death. In vitro assays showed that the basic and acidic PhA_2 preparations liberated 4.5 and 10.8 μequivalents, respectively, of free fatty acids per μg protein from an egg yolk reaction mixture.

The results obtained since 1970 suggest that basic PhA_2 enzymes are more toxic than are acidic Ph preparations; however, even among the acidic Ph enzymes, there are large variations in lethality. The pharmacologic reasons for the differences in lethality are not clear, although as noted elsewhere in this Chapter, there may be a relationship between the ability of toxins to act at the presynaptic nerve endings and their PhA_2 activity. It would be of great interest to test all toxic basic PhA_2 preparations to see if they have an action on presynaptic nerve endings altering the release of acetylcholine.

C. Actions of PhA_2 on Bioelectrically Excitable Tissues

The actions of PhA_2 on bioelectrically excitable tissues are of special interest because of the suggestions that phospholipids (GOLDMAN, 1964) or the dephosphorylation of phospholipids (HAWTHORNE and KAI, 1970) are essential for the genesis of bioelectricity. It has also been proposed that hydrolysis of phospholipids (DURRELL et al., 1969) or displacement of phospholipids from the membrane (WATKINS, 1965) may be responsible for the action of neurotransmitters such as acetylcholine. A possible phospholipid component to the acetylcholine (DE ROBERTIS, 1971) and the local anesthetic receptor sites (FEINSTEIN, 1964) have also been suggested.

I. Axons

TOBIAS (1955) first claimed to show that snake venom PhA_2 and lysophosphatides depolarize and block conduction of an axonal preparation, the lobster giant axon. It was pointed out that the effects of PhA_2 could either be due to the direct disruption of phospholipids or through the action of liberated lysophosphatides. Similar effects were found when PhA_2 was applied to the nodal region of myelinated frog sciatic axons (NELSON, 1958). In these studies, however, only crude *N. naja* venom or acid-boiled venom were used as the sources of PhA_2. These crude preparations produced no marked changes in the structural appearance of the lobster axon (TOBIAS, 1958). In later studies, using similar preparations of PhA_2, it was claimed that the decreases in resting and action potential, threshold potential, and membrane resistance, as well as the temporary increase in membrane capacitance, of lobster axons produced by PhA_2 provide evidence that phospholipid integrity is essential for membrane potential and excitability (NARAHASHI and TOBIAS, 1964). The enzyme preparations used by TOBIAS and his group probably contained a cardiotoxin and cobrotoxin in addition to PhA_2; it is, therefore, not possible to conclude that the pharmacologic actions they observed were due to PhA_2. BICHER (1966), however, also mentioned that a PhA_2 fraction obtained by paper electrophoresis from *N. naja* venom blocked conduction of the isolated frog sciatic axon.

More recently, LEE and co-workers tested the effects of purified PhA_2, CTX, cobrotoxin (all isolated from *N. naja atra* venom), and LPC on conduction of the rat phrenic nerve (CHANG et al., 1972a, 1972b). CTX (0.2 mg/ml) was the only one which blocked the axonal action potential although it was less potent than the crude venom. The other compounds were tested at concentrations of 0.5–1.0 mg/ml. The blocking action of CTX was accelerated by the simultaneous administration of PhA_2. This synergism appears analogous to that observed when the hemolytic effects of PhA_2 and CTX are tested alone and in combination (see Chap. 13). It was concluded, therefore, that the active agent mediating the effects of cobra venom on axonal conduction is CTX not PhA_2. Conduction of action potentials in the rabbit phrenic nerve was not affected by the basic *Crotalus* PhA_2 or its complex with crotapotin (BREITHAUPT, 1976).

The results referred to above appear to contradict some of the results which my co-workers and I have obtained (ROSENBERG and EHRENPREIS, 1961; ROSENBERG and PODLESKI, 1962, 1963; ROSENBERG and HOSKIN, 1963; ROSENBERG and NG, 1964; ROSENBERG, 1965; HOSKIN and ROSENBERG, 1965; ROSENBERG and MAUTNER, 1967; CONDREA et al., 1967; CONDREA and ROSENBERG, 1968; ROSENBERG and CONDREA, 1968; MARTIN and ROSENBERG, 1968). We found that various venoms in relatively low concentrations rendered squid and lobster axons sensitive to curare, acetylcholine, and other cholinergic compounds while higher concentrations irreversibly blocked conduction. In the squid axon, the venoms increased permeability to poorly penetrating compounds such as curare, acetylcholine, γ-amino-butyric acid, dopamine, sucrose, etc. (ROSENBERG and HOSKIN, 1963; HOSKIN and ROSENBERG, 1965; CONDREA et al., 1967; CONDREA and ROSENBERG, 1968; ROSENBERG, 1971, 1976; ROSENBERG, unpublished observations). The increase in permeability is associated with a swelling and fragmentation of the Schwann cell (MARTIN and ROSENBERG, 1968). All of these effects could be mimicked by a purified PhA_2 fraction isolated from *H. haemachatus* venom by paper electrophoresis. Other venom fractions including the CTX and neurotoxin containing fractions were inactive. These effects were, however, not directly due to splitting of phospholipids since the percentage of the squid giant axon phospholipid hydrolyzed was identic in finely dissected squid giant axons where the venoms and the purified PhA_2 were inactive and in the crudely dissected axons where PhA_2 and the venoms induced all of the effects described above. In the finely dissected axons, however, there is much less phospholipid substrate and, therefore, less lysophosphatides produced. Indeed, a mixture of lysophosphatides or synthetic LPC mimicked the action of PhA_2 (ROSENBERG and CONDREA, 1968). Therefore, our results indicate that in the nonmyelinated lobster axon and squid giant axon, the effects of venoms are due to their PhA_2 component hydrolyzing the axonal phospholipids and liberating lysophosphatides which exert marked effects on axonal functioning. That the effects were not due to phospholipid splitting per se was also supported in later studies where it was shown that even a much greater percent phospholipid hydrolysis by PhC than by PhA_2 did not give rise to blocking of conduction or the other effects produced by PhA_2 (ROSENBERG and CONDREA, 1968; ROSENBERG, 1970). TAKASHIMA et al. (1975) perfused squid axons with PhA_2, noting block of sodium activation and an increase in frequency-dependent and independent capacitances. They suggest that the enzyme perturbs the lipid structure and decreases its thickness. The purity of the commercially obtained PhA_2 is, however, not clear from the report, and it is unfortunate that the effects of LPC were not studied, since the effects may have been due to the detergent action of liberated lysophosphatides.

As commented upon by LEE and his group (CHANG et al., 1972a), their results on the rat phrenic nerve would appear to be at diametric variance with those which we obtained on the squid and lobster axons where PhA_2 was the active agent, whereas CTX was much weaker and did not potentiate the actions of PhA_2 (CONDREA et al., 1967; CONDREA and ROSENBERG, 1968). CHANG et al. (1972a) also proposed what I think is a quite reasonable explanation for the differences in results. In the rat studies, a Ringer's solution low in Ca^{2+} is used, whereas in the squid and lobster studies, sea water which is relatively high in Ca^{2+} was used. High Ca^{2+} would be expected to potentiate the action of PhA_2 and block the effects of CTX on axonal conduction.

We found, as discussed above, that PhA_2 rendered lobster and squid axons sensitive to curare and acetylcholine by increasing permeability, effects which could not have been observed, had the curare and acetylcholine axonal "receptors" been destroyed. In contrast, DENBURG et al. (1972) studied the effects of various enzymes on the binding of nicotine to an acetylcholine receptor-like material isolated from the lobster axon. They claimed that this material was a phospholipoprotein because both PhA_2 and protease decreased binding. Unfortunately, it appears that they used commercial crude *C. adamanteus* and bee venoms as their sources of PhA_2 which obviously contain many other components which may have interfered with binding. In the Torpedo electroplax, however, the same venom did not decrease muscarone binding (O'BRIEN et al., 1970). Commercial PhA_2 of unrecorded source or purity markedly decreased tetrodotoxin binding to a component isolated from the garfish olfactory nerve membrane (BENZER and RAFTERY, 1972). Since tetrodotoxin specifically blocks activation of the sodium channel, this result may suggest that the sodium channel has an essential phospholipid requirement.

In our studies on the squid giant axon, Phs have been extremely useful tools for studying the possible essentiality of phospholipids in axonal conduction (ROSENBERG, 1966, 1971, 1976b). It was possible to conclude that phospholipids or at least the great majority of membranal phospholipids are not essential for axonal conduction. Apparently, normal function should be maintained even though most of the phospholipids were hydrolyzed and their polar groups left the membrane.

Venom PhA_2 caused a much greater reduction in the free amino acid content of the axoplasm and envelope of the squid axon than PhC (from *Cl. perfringens*); and a concomitant greater increase in amino acids released into the incubation solutions even when PhA was used in a concentration which caused less phospholipid splitting than PhC. LPC had a much weaker effect than PhA_2 (ROSENBERG and KHAIRALLAH, 1974). It was concluded that disruption of hydrophobic binding by PhA_2 has a much greater effect on the nonlipid portion of the axonal membrane than does disruption of hydrophilic (electrostatic) forces of interaction by PhC. Purified PhA_2 also caused a marked vesiculation, swelling, and fragmentation of the Schwann cell of the squid giant axon indicative of gross membrane disruption while CTX had no significant effect (MARTIN and ROSENBERG, 1968). These results provide evidence in support of the protein crystal or fluid mosaic model of membrane structure (VANDERKOOI and GREEN, 1970; SINGER and NICOLSON, 1972), whereas they do not support the unit membrane hypothesis (ROBERTSON, 1960).

As discussed in this section, venom PhA_2 may be used as an enzymic probe to study the structural organization of axonal membranes and to search for specific functions of phospholipids. In studies on axons, however, connective tissue, Schwann cell, and myelin may interfere with the access of the externally applied enzyme to the axolemma. It has, for example, been stated that "It may be assumed that the phospholipid of axonal membrane is not accessible to phospholipase A because of the outermost layer of protein of the membrane" (CHANG et al., 1972a). However, according to the newer theories of membrane structure (SINGER and NICOLSON, 1972; VANDERKOOI and GREEN, 1970), the phospholipids are not covered by protein, which also finds support in my findings that venom PhA_2 readily penetrates in its active form from the external bathing solution into the axoplasm of the squid giant axon (ROSENBERG, 1975). Even myelin phospholipids are hydrolyzed by pure PhA_2 from *C. atrox* venom, although at a slower rate than for pure phosphoglycerides in an aqueous medium (COLES et al., 1974). The lysophosphatides and free fatty acids which are the products of PhA_2 action appeared to remain in the membrane and may have altered the subsequent activity of PhA_2. Nevertheless, all axonal phospholipids may not be maximally accessible to externally applied PhA_2; for example, tri-o-cresylphosphate induces paralysis and neuronal degeneration in the hen, effects which are preceded by the major sciatic nerve phospholipids becoming more readily hydrolyzable by the PhA_2 of *A. piscivorus* venom, indicating a change in membrane ultrastructure (MORAZAIN and ROSENBERG, 1970).

That externally applied PhA_2 can reach the axolemmal membrane was also shown on the walking leg nerves of lobsters where purified PhA_2 from *N. naja* venom markedly decreased tetrodotoxin binding in contrast to proteolytic enzymes, PhC and PhD which had minimal or no effect on tetrodotoxin binding (VILLEGAS et al., 1973). PhA_2 also decreased tetrodotoxin binding in membranes from the garfish olfactory nerve (BENZER and RAFTERY, 1972, 1973). Although PhA_2 effects were observed in the above studies, it was also clear that there can be considerable degradation of phospholipids (and proteins) of the axolemma without tetrodotoxin binding being markedly affected. This would agree with the findings on the squid giant axon that the great majority of the phospholipids are not essential for axonal conduction.

SIMPKINS et al. (1971) studied the changes in the molecular structure of the axonal membrane of the lobster as a result of treatment with an acid-boiled solution of *N. naja* venom, free of proteolytic activity, which was used as a source of PhA_2 activity. Spin labeling studies showed that the lipid region became more ordered and immobile possibly due to a more closely packed lipid array. Changes were also observed in the conformation of some of the membrane proteins. The effects of the acid-boiled venom were clearly different from those of a detergent.

PhA_2 may also affect membrane structure in nonbioelectrically excitable tissues. For example, LPC and acid-heated *Naja naja* venom alter the circular dichroism and optical rotatory dispersion spectra of the plasma membrane of Ehrlich ascites carcinoma cells and of human erythrocytes (GORDON et al., 1969). These results indicated that the protein architecture of the membrane depends upon lipid-protein interactions. A high angle x-ray diffraction study of red cell membranes after PhA_2 pretreatment indicated an alteration in the protein region of the membrane, whereas PhC primarily caused an alteration in the lipid region (BERNENGO and SIMPKINS, 1972). In contrast, on membrane vesicles from *Mycobacterium phlei* it was suggested that purified PhA_2 from *C. terrificus terrificus* altered primarily the lipid regions of the membrane with little effect on the protein regions (PRASAD et al., 1975). A change in the membrane phospholipids was also thought to be responsible for the decreased ability of hepatic plasma membranes to bind desialylated glycoproteins after exposure to a crude PhA_2 preparation from *V. russellii* venom (LUNNEY and ASHWELL, 1974). This was not an effect on the specific-binding protein since when it was solubilized the sensitivity to PhA_2 was lost.

The apparent cholinesterase activity observed in intact squid and lobster axons and in eel electroplax was increased by crude and acid-boiled cottonmouth moccasin venom and by purified PhA_2 from *H. haemachatus* venom, up to the level of activity observed in homogenates of the tissues (ROSENBERG and DETTBARN, 1964; ROSENBERG, unpublished observations). The venom and the PhA_2 which have no cholinesterase activity themselves act by decreasing permeability barriers, thereby allowing the substrate (acetylcholine) greater accessability to the enzyme. With most homogenates of tissues, venom and PhA_2 application had no effect on cholinesterase activity since there were no significant permeability barriers. The ability of PhA_2 pretreatment to allow the measurement of total cholinesterase activity in intact axons, after exposure to cholinesterase inhibitors, has been extremely useful in those studies attempting to determine whether cholinesterase is essential for axonal conduction (DETTBARN and ROSENBERG, 1962; HOSKIN et al., 1969; KREMZNER and ROSENBERG, 1971). There did not appear to be a simple and direct relationship between cholinesterase activity and electric activity. By allowing greater penetration, the potency of cholinesterase inhibitors on electric activity of the squid giant axon was also increased (HOSKIN et al., 1969). A commercial preparation of PhA_2 (unspecified source or purity) decreased the apparent molecular weight of triton solubilized erythrocyte cholinesterase suggesting a phospholipid-dependent aggregation (WHITTAKER and CHARLIER, 1972). PhA_2 has also been reported to release cholinesterase from erythrocytes (GREIG and GIBBONS, 1955).

II. Synapses

PhA_2, partially purified from *N. naja atra* venom, when injected intra-arterially had no significant effect on the contractions of the nictitating membrane evoked by preganglionic nerve stimulation of the cat superior cervical ganglion (CHOU and LEE, 1969). On the hypogastric nerve-vas deferens in vitro preparation, PhA_2 first enhanced and then depressed the response to hypogastric nerve or transmural (postganglionic) stimulation (CHOU and LEE, 1969). The effects of crude cobra venom on the above preparations appeared to be due to its CTX component, not to its neurotoxic or PhA_2 components. On the rat phrenic nerve diaphragm preparation, no neuromuscular blocking actions of PhA_2 were observed (CHANG et al., 1972a, 1972b).

On the isolated single electroplax of the electric eel *(Electrophorus electricus)*, acid-boiled *A. piscivorus* venom, a purified preparation of PhA_2 from this venom and LPC caused depolarization and block of both direct and indirect stimulation in concentrations of 0.1–0.5 mg/ml (BARTELS and ROSENBERG, 1972; ROSENBERG, unpublished observations). The endplate potential was depressed prior to failure of junctional transmission. Block of electric activity by PhA_2 was associated with 80–100% hydrolysis of PC, PE, and PS, the three major phospholipids of the cell. This may have either been directly responsible for the pharmacologic effects, or the lysophosphatides produced as a result of PhA_2 action may have mediated the pharmacologic effects. Lower concentrations of PhA_2 which did not block electric activity hydrolyzed approximately the same percent of PE and PS, but only about one-third of the PC. Block of excitability and extensive phospholipid hydrolysis was also associated with a two to threefold increase in permeability to ^{14}C choline (ROSENBERG, 1973). An acid-boiled preparation of cottonmouth moccasin venom free of protease activity and a purified PhA_2 preparation (0.2 and 2.0 mg/ml) caused mitochondrial swelling and a pinching off of the membrane inpocketings of the electroplax to form clusters of small, rounded vesicles external to the membrane. LPC had much less of an effect on the membrane ultrastructure (ROSENBERG, 1976a). These results provide evidence that phospholipids are essential for the functioning of this synaptic-containing preparation, a conclusion also reinforced by the findings that both the application of acetylcholine and electric stimulation increase the incorporation of ^{14}C glucose and ^{32}P inorganic phosphate into the phospholipids of the electroplax (ROSENBERG, 1973a). The observations on the membrane ultrastructure suggest that the binding between phospholipids and proteins is primarily hydrophobic in nature and is disrupted by PhA_2-induced hydrolysis of the β fatty acid ester of the phospholipid.

A most exciting recent development has been the studies on the relationship between the action of presynaptically acting neurotoxins and PhA_2 activity. β-bungarotoxin has been purified from *Bungarus multicinctus* venom and causes neuromuscular block by a presynaptic mode of action, first increasing the release of acetylcholine and then inhibiting release (LEE and CHANG, 1966; NARAHASHI, 1974). Analysis of phospholipids extracted from human erythrocytes after treatment with highly purified β-bungarotoxin (10 μg/ml) demonstrated that the toxin has PhA_2 activity (WERNICKE et al., 1974, 1975). Fairly strong evidence is presented that the effects are not due to contamination of the β-bungarotoxin with venom PhA_2 activity. It thus appears that the neurotoxic and Ph activities reside on the same protein. β-bungarotoxin also liberated fatty acids from synaptosomal preparations of the rat cerebral cortex thereby inhibiting oxidative phosphorylation in the mitochondria of the nerve terminals and causing an efflux from the synaptosomes of previously accumulated γ-aminobutyric acid and 2-deoxy-D-glucose (WERNICKE et al., 1975). The effects on efflux required the presence of Ca^{2+} and was inhibited by Mg^{2+} and Mn^{2+}, while the uncoupling of oxidative phosphorylation by the toxin was prevented by bovine serum albumin which binds free fatty acids. These observations support the suggestion that the pharmacologic effects of the toxin may be due either to the direct hydrolysis of phospholipids or to the fatty acids and lysophosphatides liberated as a result of PhA_2 activity. A Ca^{2+} requirement is a common characteristic of PhA_2 enzymes from various sources (GATT and BARENHOLZ, 1973), and it is, therefore, of interest that low Ca^{2+} in the media markedly increases the time required for neuromuscular block with β-bungarotoxin (LEE and CHANG, 1966). It was suggested by WERNICKE and co-workers that the initial phase of increased rate of spontaneous acetylcholine release followed by neuromuscular block after exposure to β-bungarotoxin could be due to a PhA_2-induced inhibition of oxidative phosphorylation. In studies such as these, it is of course critical to prove that the observed effects are not due to contamination of the toxin with the PhA_2 which is present in the *Bungarus multicinctus* venom. WERNICKE et al. (1975) appear to have proven this for several of the pharmacologic effects of the toxin; for example, the toxin has the same specific activity as the venom PhA_2 in reducing GABA storage in the synaptosomes, thus the activity of β-bungarotoxin on synaptosomes cannot be due to PhA_2 contamination. They also showed that the relative potencies of the uncoupling activity in erythrocyte and synaptosomal membranes differ for the toxin and for the venom PhA_2; β-bungarotoxin has greater activity on the synaptosome and PhA_2 on the erythrocyte membrane. HOWARD (1975) found that low concentrations of crude *V. russellii* venom, purified PhA_2 from the same venom, and β-bungarotoxin all caused uncoupling of mitochondrial respiration while higher concentrations had reverse acceptor control (prevented the increased respiration normally observed when ADP is added to rat cerebral cortex or liver slices). β-bungarotoxin inhibited calcium accumulation into subcellular fractions of rat brain, an effect apparently due to an action on the mitochondria (WAGNER et al., 1974).

The relationship of PhA_2 activity to toxicity of β-bungarotoxin has been noted by TOBIAS et al. (1976). Both the major bungarotoxin peak and another minor peak showed a Ca^{2+}-dependent PhA_2 activity which was destroyed by boiling at pH 8.6. Material from both peaks inhibited ADP-dependent oxygen consumption in mitochondria; however, the minor peak did not require Ca^{2+} for this effect. The binding data to mitochondrial and synaptosomal fractions suggest that toxicity is related to PhA_2 activity. STRONG et al. (1976) also demonstrated that β-bungarotoxin from *Bungarus multicinctus* venom has a potent PhA_2 activity and that it modifies the release of neurotransmitter at the neuromuscular junction. Strontium inhibited both the PhA_2 activity and the effects of β-bungarotoxin on neuromuscular transmission. In comparing the PhA_2 activity and the minimum lethal dose of β-bungarotoxin with those of *N. naja* and *V. russellii* the following PhA_2 results were obtained: μ equivalents free fatty acids liberated per min per mg protein were 133, 76, and 424 for β-bungarotoxin, *N. naja* and *V. russellii* PhA_2. The minimal lethal doses in mice were 0.01, 4, and 0.48 mg/kg, respectively, showing the much greater lethal potency of β-bungarotoxin than of the usual acidic PhA_2 preparations. Certainly, ability to liberate free fatty acids in artificial in vitro assay systems cannot be correlated with in vivo biologic potency.

The findings with β-bungarotoxin were not the first indication that some snake venom PhA_2 preparations may be associated with a presynaptic site of action. The basic *Crotalus* PhA_2 was reported to have a presynaptic action on the frog sartorius nerve-muscle preparation, causing an increase in the frequency of miniature end plate potentials (BRAZIL et al., 1973). A neuromuscular blockade and a myotoxic effect has also been noted in mammalian systems (BREITHAUPT and HABERMANN, 1973). PhA_2-crotapotin complexes decreased the contractions of isolated phrenic hemidiaphragms of rats to direct and indirect stimulation. A similar block of neuromuscular transmission was also observed in vivo (BREITHAUPT, 1976).

EAKER and his collaborators have recently carried out elegant studies clarifying the relationship between the presynaptic neurotoxic activity of notexin, the neurotoxin from the venom of the Australian tiger snake *Notechis scutatus scutatus*, and its PhA_2 activity. The complete amino acid sequence of notexin, which exhibits weak PhA_2 activity, has been elucidated and is homologous to both porcine pancreatic PhA_2 and a PhA_2 from *N. melanoleuca* venom (HALPERT and EAKER, 1975). The PhA_2 activity of pure notexin, i.e., its ability to liberate free fatty acids from egg yolk in solution has been clearly demonstrated. Homology has also been shown between notexin and two of the three subunits of taipoxin (from O. *scutellatus* venom), one of the subunits of β-bungarotoxin and one of the subunits of crotoxin (EAKER, 1976, personal communication). Some evidence has been obtained that the neurotoxic activity of notexin may be associated with its PhA_2 activity. The modification of one histidine residue in notexin by the use of p-bromophenacyl bromide caused a 99.8% loss of both PhA_2 activity and lethal neurotoxicity (HALPERT et al., 1976). The PhA_2 activity decreased from 850 to 1.8 μequivalents alkali per min per mg protein while the LD_{100} increased from 0.025 to 10 mg per kg mouse.

The above results on the relationship between presynaptic neurotoxins and PhA_2 activity suggest that all toxins with presynaptic neurotoxic activity may also have PhA_2 activity, and that in some manner this PhA_2 activity may be implicated in their neurotoxic action. EAKER has pointed out, however (HALPERT et al., 1976; EAKER, personal communication), that even if we accept the suggestion that PhA_2 activity is essential for presynaptic blockade, several questions remain to be answered. What are the structural features which make the PhA_2 of the presynaptic neurotoxins highly toxic, whereas the vast majority of the PhA_2 preparations are of no or of weak toxicity? As previously mentioned, this may be related to differences in phospholipid substrate specificity. If WERNICKE is correct and presynaptic neurotoxicity is due to PhA_2-induced inhibition of oxidative phosphorylation in the mitochondria, how do these presynaptically active proteins get into the cell, and how is their PhA_2 active at the very low concentrations of free Ca^{2+} thought to exist within the nerve terminal? Until additional and firmer evidence in support of the relationship between presynaptic activity and PhA_2 activity is obtained, we must also consider an alternative explanation for the presence of PhA_2 activity in presynaptic active neurotoxins, as hypothesized by EAKER (1975). He offers the possibility that the junctional effects of the presynaptic active toxins (notexin, taipoxin, β-bungarotoxin, etc.) are in no way related to their PhA_2 activity, but that the toxins have evolved from a more primitive PhA_2 structure, which is still present in the venoms of reptilians and the digestive glands of vertebrates, and that a residue of PhA_2 activity remains associated with the toxins. BREITHAUPT et al. (1975) support this interpretation since two toxic *Crotalus* PhA_2 preparations show significant sequence homologies with other phospholipases and neurotoxins (BREITHAUPT et al., 1975).

III. Muscles

It was suggested many years ago that the ability of snake venoms to produce contracture, loss of excitability, swelling, and release of ions from frog skeletal muscle was due to its PhA_2 component, probably through the action of LPC (HOUSSAY et al., 1922; HOUSSAY and MAZZOCCO, 1925, 1926). TOBIAS (1955) reported that acid-boiled solutions of *N. naja* venom depolarized and caused contracture of the frog sartorius muscle. Reports obtained by others, however, suggest that these results of

TOBIAS were probably due to contamination of the preparation with CTX. Employing electrophoretic techniques, HABERMANN and NEUMANN (1954) showed that the venom components acting on the frog sartorius and rat diaphragm muscle move more rapidly toward the cathode than does PhA_2, which would be in agreement with the active material being CTX. In addition, a purified PhA_2 isolated from cobra venom was either much weaker than the crude venom or completely ineffective in inducing membrane depolarization of the rat diaphragm muscle (CHANG and LEE, 1966; CHANG et al., 1972a, 1972b; MELDRUM, 1965a). In contrast, it was also shown in these studies that CTX was quite potent, and its effects were accelerated by PhA_2. It might be noted, however, that pure PhA_2 from bee venom does depolarize and decrease the resistance of the extensor digitorum longus and soleus muscles of the rat, effects which were mimicked by LPC (ALBUQUERQUE and THESLEFF, 1968). There was, however, little effect on membrane excitability or on sensitivity of denervated fibers to acetylcholine.

The reported inability of snake venom PhA_2 to depolarize the muscle membrane is probably not due to an inability to hydrolyze membranal phospholipids. Studies on axons where the permeability barriers are much greater than in muscle show that PhA_2 readily penetrates through connective tissue, Schwann cell, and the plasma membrane appearing in its active form in the axoplasm (ROSENBERG, 1975). Heated sea snake *(E. schistosa)* venom, in fact, hydrolyzed the phospholipids of intact rat diaphragm muscle (IBRAHIM, 1970). Hydrolysis of PC, PE, and PS was accompanied by the release of glutamic oxaloacetic transaminase and of intracellular protein. In these studies, however, the presence in the heated venom of a cardiotoxin-like material may have potentiated the action of PhA_2 or allowed it to penetrate better. IBRAHIM suggested, however, that the myotoxic action of sea snake venom is due to its PhA_2 component hydrolyzing muscle phospholipids. In support of this suggestion is the earlier finding by MCARDLE et al. (1960) that LPC also releases glutamic-oxaloacetic transaminase from rat diaphragm and other tissues.

Recently, some evidence has been obtained that there are PhA_2 preparations which affect muscle. *Crotalus* PhA_2 alone or in combination with crotapotin decreased contractions of the isolated chick biventer cervicis muscle, but did not cause a contracture (BREITHAUPT, 1976b), indicating that they are not depolarizing blockers. No cardiotoxic effect was observed in the Langendorff preparation of rat hearts perfused with PhA_2. SKET and GUBENŠEK (1976) found that two PhA_2 fractions, isolated from *V. ammodytes* venom, caused in very low concentrations (6.6×10^{-9} M) a contracture of the guinea pig ileum. A possible mechanism of action involving the formation of prostaglandins was suggested in this smooth muscle preparation but not proven, although indomethacin, an inhibitor of prostaglandin synthesis, blocked the contracture induced by PhA_2.

IV. Central Nervous System

It has been claimed that PhA_2 from cobra venom, and to a much lesser extent from Russell's viper venom causes a release of bound acetylcholine into the free form upon in vitro incubation with rat brain tissue (GAUTRELET and CORTEGGIANI, 1939; BRAGANCA and QUASTEL, 1952). An initial increase in acetylcholine synthesis, followed by a decrease in synthesis, probably due to depletion of ATP, was also observed

(BRAGANCA and QUASTEL, 1952). In these studies, however, only crude acid-boiled solutions of venom were used as sources of PhA_2, and it is possible that the membrane disruptive action of cardiotoxin could have contributed to the effects observed. A purified preparation of PhA_2 from *N. nigricollis* venom did, however, decrease the uptake of acetylcholine and increase the release of radioactive acetylcholine from preloaded slices of mouse cerebral cortex (HEILBRONN, 1969). The PhA_2 also caused vacuolization and the formation of electron-dense particles in the cortex slices. Histidine uptake into mouse brain slices was also decreased by a purified PhA_2 isolated from *Hemachatus haemachatus* venom (KIRSCHMANN et al., 1971), an effect which was associated with about 10–30% hydrolysis of the brain phospholipids. A partially purified PhA_2 from *V. russellii* venom markedly inhibited the uptake of norepinephrine into synaptosomes from the guinea-pig cerebral cortex and inhibited (Na+K)-ATPase activity (SUN, 1974). LPC had similar effects; however, the synaptosomal particles were not disrupted after PhA_2 treatment, so that whether these are direct effects or due to a detergent action of liberated lysophosphatides is not certain. LPC does cause a marked release of glutamic-oxaloacetic transaminase and cholinesterase from rat brain slices (MCARDLE et al., 1960). The retention of the soluble protein within a cell seems to depend on the integrity of the phospholipids of the cell membrane. Acid-heated solutions of *N. naja*, *E. schistosa*, and *A. piscivorus* venoms promote glutamic-oxaloacetic transaminase efflux from the rat cerebral cortex slices and diaphragm muscle (MELDRUM and THOMPSON, 1962).

There have been a few studies concerned with the ability of PhA_2 to alter receptor binding in the central nervous system. PASTERNAK and SNYDER (1974) studied the effects of various enzymes including PhA_2 on the stereospecific binding of [^{3}H]-naloxone to rat brain homogenates. Relatively low concentrations of PhA_2 markedly decreased binding while high concentrations of LPC were required for the observation of a similar effect. It is, however, impossible to relate in any meaningful manner the concentration of an enzyme, especially if impure, to the concentration of one of the products of its hydrolytic action. LPC might be much more potent when formed in situ than when added exogenously. PASTERNAK and SNYDER suggested that intact phospholipids may be essential for opiate binding to its receptor. These results must be interpreted with caution, however, since the source of PhA_2 used was an acid-boiled solution of *V. russellii* venom which, therefore, may have also contained heat-stable toxins. Purified PhA_2 isolated from bee venom does markedly decrease the binding of γ-aminobutyric acid to junctional complexes isolated from the rat cerebellum (GIAMBALVO and ROSENBERG, 1976). Inhibition of binding was correlated with the extent of splitting of phospholipids, and LPC had effects identical to those of PhA_2.

There have been several reports of structural changes in brain tissue induced by PhA_2. Using an uncharacterized, probably crude preparation of PhA_2, MORRISON and ZAMECNIK (1950) found in vitro demyelination when sections or blocks of rabbit spinal cord and medulla were exposed to the enzyme. These results are similar to earlier findings by WEIL (1930). Of related interest are the findings that PhA_2 (unspecified source or purity) increases the permeability of the blood-brain barrier, thereby decreasing the latent period for hexobarbital-induced loss of the righting reflex in mice (BEILER et al., 1956), and increasing the brain to plasma ratio of ^{14}C-inulin (CROUCH and WOODBURY, 1975). Similar effects were found with cobra venom and with two fractions having low and high hemolytic activities (LAL et al., 1966). The above studies should be repeated with pure PhA_2.

Ultrastructural changes in brain slices by purified snake venom PhA_2 have been noted. Synaptosomal membranes are ruptured by PhA_2 (HEILBRONN, 1969; CEDERGREN et al., 1970) as are synaptic vesicles (HEILBRONN and NILSSON, 1971), which leads to the release of acetylcholine. Synaptic areas in the motor cortex of the rat brain showed a relative resistance to a purified PhA_2 from *N. nigricollis* venom, although an increased presynaptic density, a widening of the extracellular space, a distension of the nerve terminals and mitochondria, decreased numbers of synaptic vesicles, and ruptures of the plasma membrane were observed (CEDERGREN et al., 1973). PhA_2 purified from *N. naja siamensis* venom was used for the obtaining of synaptic membrane fragments which showed a 15-fold enrichment of postsynaptic marker proteins and muscarinic and nicotinic receptors over that in an ordinary synaptic plasma membrane fraction (BARTFAI et al., 1976). The method is based on the observation that junctional membranes are more resistant to PhA_2 than are mitochondrial or plasma membranes.

It is of interest to compare the reported effects of PhA_2 on the central nervous system following peripheral and central administration. BICHER et al. (1965) claimed to have observed a diphasic circulatory shock and central nervous system effects, as manifested by electrocardiogram depression, following the intravenous administration of PhA_2 purified by paper electrophoresis from *N. naja* venom. Others have also reported decreases in cortical electric activity after the intravenous administration of PhA_2 purified from *N. naja* venom (VICK et al., 1966; SLOTTA et al., 1971). It is possible, however, that these effects on the central nervous system were indirect and secondary to peripheral changes such as cardiovascular collapse. A direct action of *N. naja* venom PhA_2 on the central nervous system would be difficult to understand in light of other studies which indicate that venom proteins can neither penetrate into nor out of the central nervous system (RUSSELL and BOHR, 1962; SUMYK et al., 1963; LEE and TSENG, 1966; TSENG et al., 1968). As noted previously, however, it has been claimed that PhA_2 can decrease the blood-brain barrier (BEILER et al., 1956), penetrate, and hydrolyze brain phospholipids (ARAVINDAKSHAN and BRAGANCA, 1961). However, it is known that purified PhA_2 from cobra venom has low lethality in mice following its peripheral administration (LEE, 1971). In rats, i.p. administration of about 1 mg (3 mg/kg) of purified PhA_2 from *N. naja* venom had no grossly observable effect, whereas the intraventricular injection of 2.5–5 μg caused convulsions and death (LYSZ and ROSENBERG, 1974). The intrathecal administration to rats of boiled cobra venom (4 mg/kg) was lethal with lower amounts producing a severe paralysis (HUDSON et al., 1960). There has been the claim that a very potent central nervous system toxin with high PhA_2 activity was isolated from *N. naja* venom (CURRIE et al., 1968). Although amino acid composition and crystal appearance are shown, pharmacologic details are lacking as are any subsequent confirmatory studies. *Crotalus* PhA_2 injected intravenously either alone or in complex with crotapotin had no effect on the rabbit respiratory center (BREITHAUPT, 1976). A detailed study on the convulsant action of PhA_2 was carried out by LYSZ and ROSENBERG (1974). It was shown that crude and acid-boiled *N. naja* venom, and a purified PhA_2 preparation from this venom, caused convulsions and death when injected intraventricularly into rats. In contrast, pure cobrotoxin and CTX caused death but no convulsions.

LPC and stearic acid did not cause convulsions. While the isolated and purified PhA_2 was less potent as a convulsant than the crude venom, the addition of CTX markedly potentiated the convulsant action of PhA_2. Phospholipid hydrolysis was noted in several brain areas of the rat after convulsive doses of PhA_2.

In relationship to the various central effects of PhA_2 discussed above, it would seem difficult to understand the results of KLIBANSKY et al. (1964). They reported that *N. naja* and *V. palestinae* venoms induce little or no phospholipid splitting when applied to cat brain slices. In contrast, *N. naja* venom and its purified PhA_2 were able to hydrolyze phospholipids in cat brain homogenates and mitochondria. The difficulty in relating central effects of venom or purified PhA_2 to phospholipid splitting may, however, be more apparent than real because of the following considerations. In their studies (KLIBANSKY et al., 1964), a small degree (10%) of phospholipid splitting may have been observed in the brain slices, which might be sufficient to induce some of the results reported above. Later studies from the same laboratory (KIRSCHMANN et al., 1971) did indeed show that a purified PhA_2 from *H. haemachatus* venom induced, depending on concentration and duration of incubation, about 10–30% hydrolysis of phospholipids from mouse brain slices. IBRAHIM et al. (1964) also reported, on the basis of increased free fatty acids, that PhA_2 hydrolyzes the phospholipids of rat brain slices. We also found, following the intraventricular administration of purified PhA_2 (LYSZ and ROSENBERG, 1974), up to 35% hydrolysis of rat brain phospholipids. The intraventricular or intrathecal administration of PhA_2 may be a more efficient method of application than is the bathing of brain slices in dilutions of PhA_2.

D. Release of Physiologically Active Compounds by PhA_2

The release of physiologically active compounds by PhA_2 is probably dependent on its ability to disrupt membranes. Various snake venoms possess histamine-liberating properties, an effect suggested as being due to the action of PhA_2 on the phospholipids of the mast cell membrane, liberating LPC, which itself can release histamine (UVNÄS, 1958). It was also suggested that PhA_2 disrupts the mast cells not by any lytic action but by triggering an energy-requiring release mechanism (UVNÄS et al., 1962; UVNÄS and ANTONSSON, 1963). The histamine-liberating properties of various snake venoms have been demonstrated in the perfused liver and lungs (FELDBERG and KELLAWAY, 1937a, 1938) and in the isolated diaphragm (DUTTA and NARAYANAN, 1952, 1954). The production of LPC suggested that PhA_2 was the active component (FELDBERG and KELLAWAY, 1938). The histamine-liberating, proteolytic, and hemolytic activities of five venoms, heated venoms, and a toxin from *N. naja atra* venom were compared (CHIANG et al., 1964). It was concluded that histamine release from the rat diaphragm preparation is due to PhA_2, in agreement with previous conclusions that bee or snake venom PhA_2 can release histamine from rat diaphragm or mast cells (HABERMANN, 1957). The capillary permeability increasing activity of *V. russellii* and *Echis carinatus* venoms has been reported as being due to their histamine and serotonin-releasing activities (FEARN et al., 1964; SOMANI and ARORA, 1964). Three fractions of *T. gramineus* venom have strong PhA_2 activity which appeared responsible for the release of histamine from the rat diaphragm preparation, which in turn increased capillary permeability (OUYANG and SHIAU, 1970). An antihistaminic markedly decreased the increase of capillary permeability. It was also pointed out, however, that a bradykinin-releasing activity of the venom may also be involved.

In contrast to the above reports, however, is the finding of ROTHSCHILD (1967) that the histamine-liberating fraction from *C. durissus terrificus* venom is chromatographically distinctly separated from the PhA_2-containing fraction. In a study of the in vivo and in vitro histamine-releasing activity of the dialyzable and nondialyzable fractions of cobra venom, it was concluded that the histamine-liberating action is not only mediated by the formation of LPC but also by a small molecular weight, highly basic molecule (MAY et al., 1967). Purified PhA from other sources (bee, pancreatic) was unable to release histamine from mast cells (FREDHOLM, 1966; HAGEN et al., 1969); however, the combination of the enzyme kallikrein and PhA_2 had a synergistic action on histamine release (AMUNDSEN et al., 1969). In other studies, it was shown that purified PhA_2 from *C. terrificus terrificus* venom did not release histamine from isolated rat peritoneal mast cells, although a synergistic release was observed when PhA_2 was combined with chymotrypsin (HINES et al., 1972). Disodium cromoglycate, which inhibits the release of spasmogens following challenge of allergic individuals, does not inhibit PhA_2 activity but probably stabilizes the mast cell membrane against the triggering action of prostaglandins released by PhA_2.

Cobra venom and LPC release adrenaline from the cat adrenal gland (FELDBERG, 1940) and releases "bound" acetylcholine from homogenates of the guinea-pig brain (GAUTRELET and CORTEGGIANI, 1939).

SRS, as well as histamine, is released from the lungs of nonsensitized guinea-pigs by various preparations prepared from *N. naja* venom; effects which were suggested as being due to PhA_2 (PHILLIPS and MIDDLETON, 1965). They reported, however, that hemolytic, histamine-liberating, and SRS-releasing activities were greater for venoms heated at pH 7 than for venoms heated at pH 5.6. The conclusion that PhA_2 is responsible for these effects might thus appear somewhat surprising considering the known heat stability of PhA_2 at acid pH. On the basis of studies using heparin to remove CTX, they concluded that this factor is not necessary for the releasing action of the venoms. LPC had similar effects as the venom, although somewhat weaker (PHILLIPS and MIDDLETON, 1965). The release of histamine and SRS did not appear to be correlated and probably originates from different cells (MIDDLETON and PHILLIPS, 1964). SRS is a mixture of unsaturated fatty acids which are formed when venoms are incubated with an egg yolk emulsion or when purified PhA_2 is incubated with PC or other phospholipids (VOGT, 1957; VARGAFTIG and DAO, 1971b). SRS causes hypotension in dogs, rabbits, cats, and guinea-pigs and an increased pulmonary resistance in the guinea-pig. They also found that antipyretic anti-inflammatory agents blocked the hypotension and duodenal contractions caused by SRS. The effects of SRS are thus similar to those caused by prostaglandins, suggesting that SRS either releases or is metabolized to prostaglandins. Studies by VOGT and his colleagues first suggested that the smooth muscle-stimulating activity of SRS is due to specific fatty acids or metabolic products, at that time thought to be hydroxy fatty acids or hydroperoxides (VOGT, 1964). SRS of two types, SRS-C and SRS-A, the latter being released during anaphylaxis and differing somewhat in its chemistry and physical properties from SRS-C (ORANGE et al., 1973, 1974), are both thought to be physiologically produced, or released, by PhA.

SRS liberates rabbit aorta contracting substance (RCS) whose short half-life and biologic properties suggested that it may be a prostaglandin, although perhaps different than the common prostaglandins E_2 and $F_{2\alpha}$ (VOGT et al., 1969; VARGAFTIG and DAO, 1971a; VANE, 1971). RCS has recently been shown to consist mainly of thromboxane A_2 and to some extent of endoperoxides. These are unstable, highly active precursors of the prostaglandins (SAMUELSSON, 1976).

Recently, an excellent study was carried out by DAMERAU et al. (1975) who compared the ability of *N. naja* venom and its purified PhA_2 and CTX components to cause mast cell degranulation, histamine release, and SRS formation. Cobra venom caused all three effects in mast cell containing rat peritoneal cell suspensions and in higher doses in the perfused guinea-pig lung. CTX was almost as active as crude cobra venom in inducing all three effects in peritoneal cell suspensions, although it was less active in guinea-pig lungs. PhA_2 caused little degranulation and no histamine release in guinea-pig lungs and only had little action on peritoneal cell suspensions. However, PhA_2 caused considerable SRS formation in both systems. In the peritoneal cell suspensions, the effects of CTX and PhA_2 appeared additive, whereas in the guinea-pig lung there appeared to be potentiation. It was concluded that CTX, not PhA_2, is the main cytotoxic principle in cobra venom. Thin layer chromatographic studies suggested that SRS activity is primarily due to a species of prostaglandin E. The authors note that PhA_2 is apparently able to cleave the fatty acids from membrane phospholipids without damaging the cells, thereby increasing the concentration of substrate available for the enzyme prostaglandin synthetase. Since CTX does not hydrolyze fatty acids from phospholipids, and since there is little stored prostaglandin in the tissues, the authors suggest that CTX increases the formation of SRS by activation of the endogenous PhA_2.

If, under certain conditions, PhA_2 does release physiologically active compounds, this may have marked effects on the circulatory system and the in vivo blood pressure. FELDBERG and KELLAWAY (1937a, 1937b) had attributed the steep fall in blood pressure after the intravenous injection of cobra venom to its PhA_2 component which was thought to act by liberating histamine from the tissues. The intravenous injection of PhA_2, partially purified from *N. naja* venom, caused a diphasic circulatory shock characterized by an initial rapid fall in arterial pressure followed after partial recovery by a delayed gradual fall together with a depression of cerebral electrocorticogram activity (BICHER et al., 1965). Unfortunately, in the above studies there is a probability that the PhA_2 preparations were contaminated with other components which may have been responsible for the effects observed. Other experiments have, however, also suggested that PhA_2 can decrease blood pressure which may be associated with increased pulmonary pressure (CHIU et al., 1968). Two purified PhA_2 fractions from *V. ammodytes* venom caused a decrease in the rat arterial blood pressure (SKET and GUBENŠEK, 1976). A PhA_2 purified from *N. naja* venom following intravenous injection in dogs caused a decrease in blood pressure, narrowing of the pulse pressure, and a marked increase in central venous pressure (SLOTTA et al., 1971). Whether these effects are due to the release of physiologically active compounds must still be clarified. *Crotalus* PhA_2 alone or in combination with crotapotin had no marked effect on blood pressure, heart rate, or electrocardiogram after slow i.v. injection into rabbits or rats, while rapid injection produced hypotension (BREITHAUPT, 1976).

E. Antimicrobial Properties of PhA_2

Microorganisms contain phospholipids which have a functional importance in the membrane (AMBRON and PIERINGER, 1973). It is, therefore, not surprising that PhA_2 has been reported to have antibacterial and antiviral activity. PhA_2 (100 μg/ml), purified from *P. porphyriacus* venom, rapidly decreased the titer of infectivity in the Murray encephalitis virus (ANDERSON and ADA, 1960) and the Rous sarcoma and MH_2 tumor viruses (DRAYTON, 1961). The ability of fractions from *Notechis scutatus* venom to antagonize the toxicity of staphylococcal toxin in vivo seemed to be in proportion to their PhA_2 activity (NORTH and DOERY, 1960). Antagonism of the lethal effects of *Cl. welchii* toxin by PhA_2 were also observed (NORTH et al., 1961). A PhA_2 from *N. nigricollis* venom partially disrupted the envelope of the influenza A_2 virus (WAHLSTRÖM, 1971). It is unfortunate that the extent of phospholipid breakdown in the above studies was not measured in order to confirm that the effects were in fact due to phospholipid hydrolysis. DOERY and NORTH (1960) reported that fractions of *P. porphyriocus* venom rich in PhA_2 activity protected mice against a lethal dose of staphylococcal toxin. The phospholipid hydrolytic products, LPC and unsaturated fatty acids, also protected mice.

Newcastle disease virus has a "fusion-inducing factor" which causes animal cells to fuse. This action was blocked by PhA_2 purified from *H. haemachatus* and *V. palestinae* venoms although the hemagglutinin, hemolysin, and neuraminidase properties of the virus were not affected (KOHN, 1965). This action was proportional to the log concentration of PhA_2 purified from *H. haemachatus* venom while PhA_2 from *N. naja* venom was as effective, and PhA_2 from *V. palestinae* venom was half as active (KOHN and KLIBANSKY, 1967). The latter PhA_2 was also less effective in hydrolyzing PC, PE, and PS of the virus. LPC mimicked the action of PhA_2, indicating that the action of PhA_2 on fusion may be indirect and mediated by the formation of lysocompounds (KOHN and KLIBANSKY, 1967). Other lipolytic agents which also destroy the integrity of the viral envelope, such as sodium dodecyl sulfate, sodium deoxycholate, and ether also destroy the fusing activity of Newcastle disease virus (KOHN, 1965; KOHN and KLIBANSKY, 1967).

Escherichia coli was completely resistant to the action of porcine pancreatic PhA or bacterial PhC unless the phospholipids of the cell are modified, for example, by pretreatment with ethylene diamine tetraacetic acid (SLEIN and LOGAN, 1967; DUCKWORTH et al., 1974). Likewise, phospholipids in the membrane of *Bacillus subtilis* were degraded by pancreatic PhA only after removal of the cell wall (OP DEN KAMP et al., 1972). These experiments should be repeated with snake venom PhA_2.

Additional experiments are required in order to further evaluate the significance of the antimicrobial activities of venom PhA_2.

F. Effects of PhA_2 on Metabolism

In our previous discussion of the mechanism of action of toxins which have both a presynaptic site of action and PhA_2 activity, we noted the suggestion of WERNICKE et al. (1975) that the presynaptic action is due to inhibition of oxidative phosphorylation by their PhA_2 activity. Many of the "nontoxic" snake venom PhA_2 preparations, however, also have effects on metabolism.

BRAGANCA and QUASTEL (1953) studied the effects of *N. naja* and other venoms heated at 100° C for 15 min on a variety of enzymes. Enzymes which were markedly inhibited included those enzymes in brain concerned with the oxidation of glucose, pyruvate, L-glutamate, succinate, α-ketoglutarate, and fructose. Pyruvic and succinic dehydrogenases of brain and heart, and cytochrome and choline oxidases of liver were all inhibited. Enzymes not inhibited included those concerned with anaerobic glycolysis in brain, glucose fermentation, pyruvic acid dismutation, hexokinase, glucose oxidase, lactic and malic dehydrogenases, urease, and cytochrome-c. The enzyme systems which are not attacked tend to be active in aqueous cell-free tissue extracts, and are not essentially dependent upon membrane structure. The inhibitory effects of the venoms were potentiated by Ca^{2+} and destroyed by boiling at an alkaline pH which is consistent with but not conclusive of PhA_2 being the active venom component. It was suggested by the authors that inhibition of enzymic activities is due to disruption of mitochondrial structure. PhA_2 (unspecified purity) from *N. naja* venom, although hydrolyzing almost all of the phospholipids of fragmented beef heart mitochondria, did not affect the activity of succinate dehydrogenase in contrast to the inhibition observed with PhC and PhD (CERLETTI et al., 1969). The reasons for the inactivity of PhA_2 in this study as contrasted to the above and several other studies noted in this section are not clear. YANG and co-workers suggested that the inhibition of the succinate cytochrome-c reductase activity of heart muscle by fractions of cobra venom and by crotoxin were not due to their PhA_2 activity because heat treatment and glutathione did not equally affect inhibitory potency and PhA_2 activity (YANG, 1954; YANG and TUNG, 1954; YANG et al., 1954).

A purified PhA_2 from *C. terrificus terrificus* venom inactivated succinoxidase of rat liver mitochondria and homogenates when only about 10% of the mitochondrial PC was hydrolyzed (NYGAARD and SUMNER, 1953; NYGAARD et al., 1954). The effect did not appear due to the formation of LPC since disruptions of the mitochondrial membrane by lysophosphatides seemed different from those caused by PhA_2. Succinic dehydrogenase, cytochrome oxidase, choline oxidase, and malic oxidase were also slowly inactivated. EDWARDS and BALL (1954) confirmed the results with cytochrome oxidase using acid-heated venom as the source of PhA_2. The addition of lipid extracts restored succinoxidase activity previously lost as a result of venom treatment (CASU and MODENA, 1964). It was later shown that the ability of crude and boiled venoms to inhibit enzymes of the mitochondrial respiratory chain exactly correlated with their PhA_2 activity (BADANO and STOPPANYI, 1971).

Purified PhA_2 from *Bothrops neuwiedi* venom markedly inhibited NADH—oxidase, succinate, and NADH—cytochrome-c reductase activities of submitochondrial heart muscle particles. Less marked inhibition of menadiol oxidase, NADH-Q reductase, and cytochrome oxidase was observed while NADH- and succinate dehydrogenase activities were not affected (VIDAL et al., 1966). In later studies, the same workers (BADANO et al., 1973) showed that this purified PhA_2 hydrolyzed PC, PC plasmalogen, PE, and PE plasmalogen (with associated increase of lysophosphatides) of heart muscle mitochondrial fragments (Keilin-Hartree preparation) while cardiolipin was not attacked. Primary enzymic inhibition occurred at the NADH-ubiquinone segment and the cytochrome-b to c segment of the respiratory chain with a third less sensitive site near cytochrome oxidase. In contrast, the activities of succinate dehydrogenase and NADH-ferricyanide reductase were increased. All effects were thought to be due to the products of phospholipid hydrolysis since lipid extracts of the digested particles, unsaturated fatty acids, and lysophospholipids mimicked the action of PhA_2, whereas human serum albumin, presumably by binding released free fatty acids, reversed some of the effects of PhA_2. The effects of *Bothrops neuwiedi* and *C. adamanteus* PhA_2 were similar, whereas in striking contrast are some of the results obtained by others with *N. naja* PhA_2.

Purified PhA_2 from *N. naja* venom markedly inhibited NADH-dehydrogenase probably due to the fatty acids released which are potent inhibitors of the enzyme while lysophosphatides were not as potent inhibitors (AWASTHI et al., 1970). In this same study, it was reported that both free and membrane-bound phospholipids were hydrolyzed in the order PE, PC, and cardiolipin. Release (solubilization) of NADH-dehydrogenase from beef heart mitochondria by *N. naja* PhA_2 correlated with hydrolysis of cardiolipin. *C. adamanteus* venom did not release the enzyme and did not hydrolyze cardiolipin. Lysophosphatides and fatty acids were also unable to release the enzyme. In other studies on enzyme leakage, it was found that PhA_2 from *N. naja* venom did not induce a significant leakage of glutamic oxaloacetic transaminase from isolated liver cells until at least 25% of the PE had been hydrolyzed; at this time little PC was hydrolyzed (GALLAI-HATSHARD and GRAY, 1968). The gross morphology of the cells appeared unaltered by hydrolysis of up to 60% of the cell's PE. PE appeared to be relatively more important than PC in maintaining the structural integrity of the cell's plasma membrane. The complex nature of the action of venom PhA_2 on mitochondrial enzymes was noted in a report where the isoenzymes of PhA_2 from *N. naja* and *V. russellii* venom were compared in their ability to affect the release and activity of mitochondrial enzymes (SALACH et al., 1971b). Marked differences were noted in regard to specificity toward membrane phospholipids. It is known of course that certain enzymes, for example β-hydroxybutyrate apodehydrogenase from beef heart mitochondria, have an absolute requirement for phospholipids, in this particular case PC, and this enzyme is released from mitochondria by acid-boiled *N. naja* venom in an inactive but lecithin activatable form (FLEISCHER et al., 1966).

Heated cottonmouth moccasin, Russell's viper and cobra venoms first stimulated and then depressed respiration of crude preparations of rat liver, kidney, or brain mitochondria and rat brain cortex slices (PETRUSHKA et al., 1959). This action was correlated with a breakdown of mitochondrial PC and PC protected against the inhibition of respiration. It was suggested that the LPC formed as a result of PhA_2 action may at least partly account for the effects observed with heated venom, which is in agreement with the observation that both LPC and cottonmouth moccasin venom inhibit oxygen uptake of rat brain slices to a greater extent than they inhibit muscle or liver uptake (MCARDLE et al., 1960). A release of the enzyme glutamic oxaloacetic transaminase from rat brain, liver, and diaphragm slices by LPC and venom and of true cholinesterase from brain slices by LPC was also observed.

Several studies have shown that PhA_2 and LPC can swell mitochondria and uncouple oxidative phosphorylation (WITTER and COTTONE, 1956; WITTER et al., 1957; PETRUSHKA et al., 1959). HABERMANN (1954) showed that oxidative phosphorylation in liver homogenates is uncoupled by heated *N. nigricollis*, *N. haje*, and *V. ammodytes* venoms. Heated *N. naja* venom decreased respiratory activity, ^{32}P incorporation and P:O ratios in spinal cord slices (HUDSON et al., 1960) but did not uncouple oxidative phosphorylation in submitochondrial fragments prepared by digitonin extraction (ARAVINDAKSHAN and BRAGANCA, 1961), indicating that the venom did not directly inhibit the phosphorylating enzyme. Both heated *N. naja* venom and crystalline PhA_2 from this venom enhanced swelling of mitochondria, both in vivo and in vitro; in the latter case, the effect was reversed by PC (ARAVINDAKSHAN and BRAGANCA, 1961). Changes in enzymic activity, P:O ratios, etc., were thought to be secondary to and caused by phospholipid hydrolysis in mitochondria leading to changes in the structure and permeability of the mitochondria. Evidence was presented that LPC, although having similar effects as PhA_2, was not produced in sufficient quantitites to account for the effects of *N. naja* venom. Various other venoms also cause swelling of rat liver mitochondria and inhibit succinate oxidation (TAUB and ELLIOTT, 1964). It is most intriguing that swelling of rat liver mitochondria induced by a purified PhA_2 from *V. russellii* venom or by *C. adamanteus* venom was inhibited by local anesthetics and other compounds (SEPPALA et al., 1971). Although not directly inhibiting PhA_2 activity, they stabilized the mitochondrial membrane, inhibiting the formation of LPC and free fatty acids when mitochondria were incubated with PhA_2. The ability of local anesthetics to stabilize the membrane and inhibit phospholipid hydrolysis is especially interesting in view of the suggestions that phospholipids or the splitting of phospholipids may be essential for the genesis of bioelectricity (HAWTHORNE and KAI, 1970; DURRELL et al., 1969; GOLDMAN, 1964; WATKINS, 1965) or that phospholipids may serve as receptor sites for local anesthetics (FEINSTEIN, 1964).

Exposure of bovine heart mitochondria to purified PhA_2 from *N. naja* venom resulted in losses of phosphorylation capacity (decreased P:O ratio), whereas respiration was not impaired as judged by the rate of oxidation of NADH or succinate (BURSTEIN et al., 1971 a). Bovine serum albumin which binds fatty acids prevented or reversed the inhibitory effects on phosphorylation of low concentrations of PhA_2, whereas neither PC nor albumin could restore phosphorylation after higher concentrations of PhA_2. Results with submitochondrial particles were quite different since the same preparation of PhA_2 impaired both the rate of phosphorylation and oxidation with NADH oxidation being more inhibited than succinate oxidation (BURSTEIN et al., 1971 b). The effects of bovine serum albumin were similar as described above.

Bungarus fasciatus venom induces in rat liver mitochondria both uncoupling of energy transfer and inhibition of respiration by ADP (reverse acceptor control) (ZIEGLER et al., 1965; ELLIOTT et al., 1966). Some evidence was presented that the former effect may be due to PhA_2, since for example acid-boiled venom caused only uncoupling. The venoms of other elapids and some viperids had a similar effect (ELLIOTT and GANS, 1967). Purified PhA_2 from *A. piscivorus* venom altered mitochondrial respiration and phosphorylation in a manner identic to that of the crude venom (AUGUSTYN et al., 1970). The early uncoupling and swelling effects of PhA_2 are attributed to the release of free fatty acids which are uncouplers, while the inhibition of respiration, membrane disruption, and loss of structural integrity at higher concentrations are attributed to the extensive hydrolysis of membrane phospholipids and release of lysophosphatides (AUGUSTYN et al., 1970). Albumin reversed the uncoupling effects by binding the free fatty acids. Electron-microscopic studies showed that alterations in mitochondrial structure paralleled the respiratory decline.

Initial swelling progressed to minor membrane disruption, extrusion of cristae, and total loss of structural integrity.

Acid-boiled *N. naja* venom in low concentrations (up to 6 μg/ml) stimulated and in higher concentrations inhibited the facilitated transport into and the metabolism of glucose in rat adipose tissue. An alteration of membrane lipoproteins was suggested although production of lysophosphatides could not be demonstrated (BLECHER, 1966). On the other hand, lysophospholipids had similar effects as the venom. Ca^{2+} were required for the venom action, and a partially purified PhA_2 had a similar action as acid-boiled venom (BLECHER, 1967). The effects of insulin were very similar to those of PhA_2, although insulin has no PhA_2 activity. Boiled *N. naja* venom antagonized the epinephrine and theophylline-stimulated hydrolysis of endogenous triglycerides; an effect similar to that caused by insulin (BLECHER, 1969). PhA_2 also inactivated the stereospecific uptake system for D-glucose by isolated human erythrocyte membranes (BANJO et al., 1974). Associated with this action was about a 25% hydrolysis of membrane phospholipids, a twofold increase in the dissociation constant of the D-glucose-membrane complex and a 34% decrease in the maximum capacity for glucose uptake. Evidence was provided that the above changes occur by two different mechanisms. When there is limited phospholipid hydrolysis, the resulting fatty acids and lysophosphatides decrease the affinity of the membrane for D-glucose and mask some of the binding sites. On the other hand, extensive cleavage of the phospholipids causes an irreversible disorganization of the membrane binding component. A commercial preparation of PhA_2 from *C. terrificus terrificus* had no effect on the uptake by rat uterus of a nonmetabolizable sugar and amino acid, whereas PhC and PhD decreased uptake in estrogen-treated animals (KOGO and AIZAWA, 1972).

Acid-heated *N. naja* venom caused in normal animals an activation of rat liver ribonuclease leading to a disaggregation of the liver polyribosomes; these effects were not observed in partially hepatectomized animals (TSUKADA et al., 1966). Purified PhA_2 from *C. atrox* venom increased RNA polymerase activity of aggregate enzyme preparations from rat brain if Mg^{2+} or Mn^{2+} was present (but not in the presence of ammonium sulfate, KCl, or NaCl), probably due to changes in the physicochemical state of the enzyme (MENON, 1971). PhA_2 also solubilized about 50% of the RNA polymerase. Prior freezing and thawing or sonication decreased the effect of PhA_2, probably because these treatments induce similar changes in the RNA polymerase complex as PhA_2. The authors note, but cannot explain, that in rat liver RNA polymerase activity is decreased by PhA_2.

C. atrox venom activated the glycosyl transferase enzyme, UDP-galactose: glycoprotein galactosyltransferase in rat liver microsomes, and in Golgi-rich membranes (MOOKERJEA and YUNG, 1974). The effects were shown to be specifically due to the production of LPC which mimicked the action of the venom while other phospholipids and lysophospholipids were inactive. LPC probably acts by solubilization of the membrane and consequently enhanced interaction of the enzyme with its substrate. LPC may be a natural regulator of glycosylation reactions in mammalian systems.

Russell's viper venom, used as a source of PhA_2, did not inhibit the Na^+-stimulated ATPase of guinea pig cerebral microsomes (SWANSON et al., 1964). A commercial PhA of unrecorded source or purity cleaved phospholipids and increased the permeability of muscle sarcoplasmic reticulum membranes for calcium, without affecting the activity of the calcium-dependent ATPase (Fiehn and Hasselbach, 1970). The split products of the PhA_2 action remained attached to the membrane, unless removed with bovine serum albumin in which case the ATPase activity was abolished but could be restored by fatty acids and LPC.

Commercial PhA (unspecified source and purity) prevented lactate and pyruvate-induced stimulation of a soluble adenylate cyclase from *Brevibacterium liquefaciens* (Chiang and Cheung, 1973). The effect was thought to be direct and not due to released products. Electron transport particles from *Mycobacterium phlei*, when treated with purified PhA_2 from *C. terrificus terrificus* venom, showed impaired rates of oxidation and phosphorylation together with 50% hydrolysis of PE and 5% hydrolysis of cardiolipin (Prasad et al., 1975). However, if the membrane was altered, by removal of the membrane-bound coupling factor-latent ATPase, then cardiolipin became much more accessible. The inhibition of phosphorylation was reversed by washing with bovine serum albumin, suggesting an action of released fatty acids.

Commercial crude PhA_2 from *V. russellii* venom in high concentrations reduced overall incorporation of 2-^{14}C mevalonic acid into a $3000 \times g$ adult rat brain supernatant, although incorporation into the steryl ester fraction was increased. In contrast, lower amounts of PhA caused a 25% increase in incorporation into the total neutral isoprenoid and free sterol fractions (Ramsey et al., 1974). Incubation of rat brain homogenates in the presence of this preparation of PhA_2 led to a tenfold increase in the percentage of cholesterol esterified. It was suggested that in demyelinating diseases, the release of lysosomal PhA may play a role in cholesteryl ester deposition (Ramsey and Davison, 1974).

Recently, the most interesting observation has been made that the effects of purified β-bungarotoxin on mitochondrial respiration are due to the PhA_2 activity associated with this neurotoxic protein (Howard, 1975). Crude *V. russellii* PhA_2, oleate, and β-bungarotoxin prevented the increased respiration normally observed when ADP is added to rat cerebral cortex or liver mitochondria. Lower amounts of these agents caused the mitochondria to become uncoupled. Bovine serum albumin protects the mitochondria against these effects.

G. Summary and Conclusions

There has developed a very extensive literature on the pharmacology of snake venom PhA_2 because of the interest in determining which of the venom effects are due to the PhA_2 component and because of the usefulness of PhA_2 as a tool to study the function of phospholipids in biologic tissues. Unfortunately, the reliability and interpretation of many of the studies with PhA_2 are subject to doubt because impure preparations of PhA_2 were used, the possible effects of the hydrolytic products of PhA_2 action were neglected, the extent of phospholipid hydrolysis by PhA_2 was not quantitated, and the assumption has often been made that all snake venom preparations of PhA_2 are similar.

Purified preparations of PhA_2 from Formosan cobra, Indian cobra, cottonmouth moccasin, Russell's viper, Ringhals, and other venoms are of relatively low toxicity and lethality ($LD_{50} > 1$ mg/kg). In contrast, there are purified preparations of PhA_2

from *C. durissus terrificus*, *V. berus*, *V. ammodytes*, and *N. nigricollis* which are of relatively high lethality ($LD_{50} < 1$ mg/kg). In general, the nontoxic PhA_2 preparations are acidic while the toxic PhA_2 enzymes are basic in nature (isoelectric points above 7).

The effects of PhA_2 on axons seem to depend on experimental conditions. In media containing a low concentration of calcium, PhA_2 may have little direct effects, although it may potentiate the action of cardiotoxin. In contrast, in media rich in calcium, such as sea water, PhA_2 causes an increased permeability, membranal disruption and blockade of the action potential; effects which are due to the detergent action of lysophospholipids. The majority of axonal phospholipids do not appear to be essential for conduction. Experiments with PhA_2 have provided evidence in support of the newer theories of membrane structure which emphasize the importance of hydrophobic rather than electrostatic binding between phospholipids and proteins.

The synaptic actions of PhA_2 have recently assumed an especial importance. PhA_2 from the Formosan cobra venom has little or no effect on sympathetic ganglia, the hypogastric-vas deferens preparation, and the rat phrenic nerve diaphragm preparation. PhA_2 from cottonmouth moccasin venom blocks conduction, increases permeability, and causes structural modifications of the isolated single electroplax. Phospholipids may be essential for the functioning of this synaptic-containing preparation. An exciting recent development is the finding that purified toxins such as β-bungarotoxin and notexin which have primarily a presynaptic site of action also have PhA_2 activity. It must now be determined whether the PhA_2 activity is responsible for the presynaptic and lethal activity of these toxins, whether other presynaptic toxins also have PhA_2 activity, and whether the basic highly toxic PhA_2 preparations have presynaptic actions.

The effects on muscle of snake venoms which contain acidic Phs are probably primarily due to their cardiotoxin rather than their PhA_2 component. In contrast, basic Phs may cause depolarization and contracture of muscle.

In slices and synaptosomes prepared from brain tissue, some preparations of PhA_2 cause decreased uptake and/or increased release of acetylcholine, norepinephrine, cholinesterase, glutamic oxaloacetic transaminase, etc. Various ultrastructural changes have also been observed. PhA_2 from cobra venom when injected intraventricularly into rats caused convulsions and death (5 μg), whereas much higher amounts injected peripherally had no effect. The central effects appear related to phospholipid hydrolysis.

The release of physiologically active compounds and solubilization of enzymes by PhA_2 is probably related to its ability to disrupt membranes. While some studies indicate that PhA_2 has histamine-liberating properties, there are several carefully controlled investigations which show that the histamine-liberating activity of certain snake venoms is not due to its PhA_2 component. SRS is formed by the action of PhA_2 upon phospholipids and is a mixture of unsaturated fatty acids which cause hypotension and increased pulmonary resistance either by a direct action or via the release of, or metabolism to prostaglandins. SRS liberates rabbit aorta contracting substance which consists primarily of highly potent prostaglandin precursors. A decrease of blood pressure has been noted with PhA_2; however, whether this effect is secondary to the release of physiologically active compounds is not known.

PhA_2 has been reported to decrease infectivity, lethal or other effects of the Murray encephalitis, influenza A_2, Newcastle disease, Rous sarcoma, and MH_2 tumor viruses, and of staphylococcal and *Cl. welchii* toxin.

PhA_2 has marked effects on metabolism, uncoupling oxidative phosphorylation, inhibiting respiration, and seeming to especially inhibit the activity of those enzymes which are membrane associated. The mechanism of action of PhA_2 is directly due to phospholipid hydrolysis in those enzymes which have an essential phospholipid requirement, whereas other metabolic actions of PhA_2 are due to the toxic effects of lysophosphatides and/or fatty acids liberated as a result of PhA_2 action. In other cases, the effects of PhA_2 on metabolism and enzymes seems to be due to its nonspecific disruption or swelling of membranes, especially mitochondrial membranes. The effects of PhA_2 on transport and metabolism of glucose in adipose tissue and on epinephrine-induced lipolysis are similar to those induced by insulin. Effects on brain and liver RNA polymerase and ribonuclease activities and on cholesterol esterification and mevalonic acid incorporation in brain have also been reported. It has recently been suggested that the presynaptic action of snake toxins may be due to inhibition of oxidative phosphorylation by their PhA_2 activity.

At one time, it was thought that PhA_2 was the component responsible for most of snake venom actions. As purer preparations of PhA_2 became available, it was clear that many of these enzymic preparations were pharmacologically weak and not able to explain many of the venom actions. Unsupported generalizations were then made that all venom PhA_2 preparations are pharmacologically inactive. It has only recently become clear that there are basic highly potent and toxic PhA_2 enzymes in several venoms. While we can make less generalizations concerning the pharmacologic actions of PhA_2 than ever before, and while our conclusions may be more complex than before, our data are more reliable and will eventually lead to a much clearer understanding of PhA_2 and venom action. We are still in the stage of data gathering; however, perhaps in the not too distant future, we will be able to categorize, systematize, and relate the pharmacologic actions of PhA_2 to its physicochemical properties and to the chemical evolution of the venom from which it is derived.

References

Albuquerque, E. X., Thesleff, S.: Effects of phospholipase A and lysolecithin on some electrical properties of the muscle membrane. Acta physiol. Scand. **72**, 248—252 (1968)

Ambron, R. T., Pieringer, R. A.: Phospholipids in microorganisms. In: Ansell, G. B., Hawthorne, J. N., Dawson, R. M. C. (Eds.): Form and Function of Phospholipids, 2nd Ed. Amsterdam: Elsevier 1973

Amundsen, E., Ofstad, E., Hagen, P. O.: Histamine release induced by synergistic action of kallikrein and PhA. Arch. int. Pharmacodyn. **178**, 104—114 (1969)

Anderson, S. G., Ada, G. L.: A lipid component of Murray Valley encephalitis virus. Nature (Lond.) **188**, 876 (1960)

Ansell, G. B., Hawthorne, J. N., Dawson, R. M. C. (Eds.): Form and Function of Phospholipids, 2nd Ed. Amsterdam: Elsevier 1973

Aravindakshan, I., Braganca, B. M.: Studies on phospholipid structures in mitochondria of animals injected with cobra venom or phospholipase A. Biochem. J. **79**, 84—90 (1961)

Augustyn, J. M., Elliott, W. B.: A modified hydroxamate assay of phospholipase A activity. Analyt. Biochem. **31**, 246—250 (1969)

Augustyn, J. M., Elliott, W. B.: Isolation of a phospholipase A from *Agkistrodon piscivorus* venom. Biochim. biophys. Acta (Amst.) **206**, 98—108 (1970)

Augustyn, J. M., Parsa, B., Elliott, W. B.: Structural and respiratory effects of *Agkistrodon piscivorus* phospholipase A on rat liver mitochondria. Biochim. biophys. Acta (Amst.) **197**, 185—196 (1970)

Awasthi, Y. C., Ruzicka, F. J., Crane, F. L.: The relation between phospholipase action and release of NADH dehydrogenase from mitochondrial membrane. Biochim. biophys. Acta (Amst.) **203**, 233—248 (1970)

Badano, B. N., Boveris, A., Stoppanyi, A. O. M., Vidal, J. C.: The action of *Bothrops neuwiedii* phospholipase A_2 on mitochondrial phospholipids and electron transfer. Molec. Cell Biochem. **2**, 157—167 (1973)

Badano, B. N., Stoppanyi, A. O. M.: Actividad de fosfolipasa a y proteases en venenos de *Bothrops* y *Crotalus*. Accion sobre la cadena respiratoria mitocondrial. Rev. Soc. Argent. Biol. **47**, 173—186 (1971)

Banjo, B., Walker, C., Rohrlick, R., Kahlenberg, A.: Studies on the mechanism and reversal of the phospholipase A_2 inactivation of D-glucose uptake by isolated human erythrocyte membranes. Canad. J. Biochem. **52**, 1097—1109 (1974)

Bartels, E., Rosenberg, P.: Correlation between electrical activity and splitting of phospholipids by snake venoms in the single electroplax. J. Neurochem. **19**, 1251—1265 (1972)

Bartfai, T., Berg, P., Schultzberg, M., Heilbronn, E.: Isolation of a synaptic membrane fraction enriched in cholinergic receptors by controlled phospholipase A_2 hydrolysis of synaptic membranes. Biochim. biophys. Acta (Amst.) **426**, 186—197 (1976)

Bartlett, G. R.: Phosphorus assay in column chromatography. J. biol. Chem. **234**, 466—468 (1959)

Beiler, J. M., Brendel, R., Martin, G. J.: Enzymic modification of blood-brain barrier permeability. J. Pharmacol. exp. Ther. **118**, 415—419 (1956)

Benzer, T. I., Raftery, M. A.: Partial characterization of a tetrodotoxin-binding component from nerve membrane. Proc. nat. Acad. Sci. (Wash.) **69**, 3634—3637 (1972)

Benzer, T. I., Raftery, M. A.: Solubilization and partial characterization of the tetrodotoxin binding component from nerve axons. Biochem. biophys. Res. Commun. **51**, 939—944 (1973)

Bernengo, J. C., Simpkins, H.: A high angle X-ray diffraction study of red cell membranes after treatment with phospholipase A_2 and C. Canad. J. Biochem. **50**, 1260—1266 (1972)

Bicher, H. I.: Specific sites of action of snake venoms in the central nervous system. Mem. Inst. Butantan **33**, 523—540 (1966)

Bicher, H. I., Klibansky, C., Shiloah, J., Gitter, S., DeVries, A.: Isolation of three different neurotoxins from Indian cobra *(Naja naja)* venom and the relation of their action to phospholipase A. Biochem. Pharmacol. **14**, 1779—1784 (1965)

Björk, W.: Partial purification of phosphodiesterase, 5'-nucleotidase, lecithinase A, and acetylcholine esterase from Ringhals-cobra venom. Biochim. biophys. Acta (Amst.) **49**, 195—204 (1961)

Blecher, M.: On the mechanism of action of phospholipase A and insulin on glucose entry into free adipose cells. Biochem. biophys. Res. Commun. **23**, 68—74 (1966)

Blecher, M.: Effects of insulin and phospholipase A on glucose transport across the plasma membrane of free adipose cells. Biochim. biophys. Acta (Amst.) **137**, 557—571 (1967)

Blecher, M.: Insulin-like, antilipolytic actions of phospholipase A in isolated rat adipose cells. Biochim. biophys. Acta (Amst.) **187**, 380—384 (1969)

Boquet, P.: Venins de serpents. Physio-pathologie de l'envenimation et properties biologigues des venins. Toxicon **2**, 5—41 (1964)

Boquet, P.: Venins de serpents. II. Constitution chimique des venins de serpents et immunite antivenimeuse. Toxicon **3**, 243—279 (1966)

Boquet, P., Izard, Y., Jouannet, M., Meaume, J.: Biochemical and immunological studies on *Naja nigricollis* venom. Ann. Inst. Pasteur (Paris) **112**, 213 (1967)

Botes, D. P., Viljoen, C. C.: Purification of phospholipase A from *Bitis gabonica* venom. Toxicon **12**, 611—619 (1974a)

Botes, D. P., Viljoen, C. C.: *Bitis gabonica* venom. The amino acid sequence of phospholipase A. J. biol. Chem. **249**, 3827—3835 (1974b)

Braganca, B. M., Aravindakshan, I.: Neurochemical effects of snake venoms. In: Elliott, K. A. C., Page, I. H., Quastel, J. H. (Eds.): Neurochemistry, pp. 840—850. Springfield (Illinois): C. C. Thomas 1962

Braganca, B. M., Khandeparkar, V. G.: Phospholipase C activity of cobra venom and lysis of Yoshida sarcoma cells. Life Sci. **5**, 1911—1920 (1966)
Braganca, B. M., Patel, N. T., Badrinath, P. G.: Isolation and properties of a cobra venom factor selectively cytotoxic to Yoshida sarcoma cells. Biochim. biophys. Acta (Amst.) **136**, 508—520 (1967)
Braganca, B. M., Quastel, J. H.: The action of snake venom on acetylcholine synthesis in brain. Nature (Lond.) **169**, 695—697 (1952)
Braganca, B. M., Quastel, J. H.: Enzyme inhibitions by snake venoms. Biochem. J. **53**, 88—101 (1953)
Braganca, B. M., Sambray, Y. M.: Multiple forms of cobra venom phospholipase A. Nature (Lond.) **216**, 1210—1211 (1967)
Braganca, B. M., Sambray, Y. M., Ghadially, R. C.: Simple method for purification of phospholipase A from cobra venom. Toxicon **7**, 151—157 (1969)
Braganca, B. M., Sambray, Y. M., Sambray, R. Y.: Isolation of polypeptide inhibitor of phospholipase A from cobra venom. Europ. J. Biochem. **13**, 410—415 (1970)
Brazil, O. V., Excell, B. J., De Sa, S. S.: The importance of phospholipase A in the action of the crotoxin complex at the frog neuromuscular junction. J. Physiol. (Lond.) **234**, 63P—64P (1973)
Breithaupt, H.: Enzymatic characteristics of *Crotalus* phospholipase A_2 and the crotoxin complex. Toxicon **14**, 221—223 (1976a)
Breithaupt, H.: Neurotoxic and myotoxic effects of *Crotalus* phospholipase A and its complex with crotapotin. Naunyn Schmiedebergs Arch. Pharmacol. **292**, 271—278 (1976b)
Breithaupt, H., Habermann, E.: Biochemistry and pharmacology of phospholipase A from *Crotalus terrificus* venom as influenced by crotapotin. Toxicon **10**, 525—526 (1972)
Breithaupt, H., Habermann, E.: Biochemistry and Pharmacology of phospholipase A from *Crotalus terrificus* venom as influenced by crotopotin. In: Kaiser, E. (Ed.): Animal and Plant Toxins, pp. 83—88. München: Goldmann 1973
Breithaupt, H., Omori-Satoh, T., Lang, J.: Isolation and characterization of three phospholipase A from the crotoxin complex. Biochim. biophys. Acta (Amst.) **403**, 355—369 (1975)
Breithaupt, H., Rübsamen, K., Habermann, E.: Biochemistry and pharmacology of the crotoxin complex. Biochemical analysis of crotapotin and the basic *Crotalus* phospholipase A. Europ. J. Biochim. **49**, 333—345 (1974)
Brewster, H. B., Gennaro, J. F., Jr.: A comparison of the toxicity of snake venom phospholipase and lysolecithin. Toxicon **1**, 123—125 (1963)
Brown, J. H., Bowles, M. E.: Studies on the phospholipase A activity of *Crotalus atrox* venom. Toxicon **3**, 205—212 (1966)
Buckley, E. E., Porges, N. (Eds.): Venoms. Washington D.C.: Amer. Ass. Advanc. Sci. 1956
Bücherl, W., Buckley, E. E., Deulofeu, V. (Eds.): Venomous Animals and Their Venoms, Vol. I, II, Venomous Vertebrates. New York: Academic Press 1968
Bulos, B. A., Sacktor, B.: Assay for phospholipase A activity of snake venom with asolectin as substrate. Analyt. Biochem. **42**, 530—534 (1971)
Burstein, C., Kandrach, A., Racker, E.: Effect of phospholipases and lipase on submitochondrial particles. J. biol. Chem. **246**, 4083—4089 (1971b)
Burstein, C., Loyter, A., Racker, E.: Effect of phospholipases on the structure and function of mitochondria. J. biol. Chem. **246**, 4075—4082 (1971a)
Bussard, A., Cote, R.: Etude de la constitution du venin de cobra *(Naja naja)*. C. R. Acad. Sci. (Paris) **239**, 915—917 (1954)
Carey, J. E., Wright, E. A.: Isolation of the neurotoxic component of the venom of the sea snake *Enhydrina schistosa*. Nature (Lond.) **185**, 103—104 (1960)
Casu, A., Modena, B.: Reactivation of succinoxidase activity in rat liver mitochondria treated with lecithinase A by lipid extracts of rat liver. Ital. J. Biochem. **13**, 197—207 (1964)
Cedergren, E., Heilbronn, E., Johansson, B., Widlund, L.: Ultrastructural stability of contact regions of phospholipase-treated synapses from rat motor cortex. Brain Res. **24**, 139—142 (1970)
Cedergren, E., Johansson, B., Heilbronn, E., Widlund, L.: Ultrastructural analysis of phospholipase A induced changes in membranes of synaptic regions in rat motor cortex. Exp. Brain Res. **16**, 400—409 (1973)

Cerletti, P., Caiafa, P., Giordano, M. G., Giovenco, M. A.: Succinate dehydrogenase. II. The effect of phospholipases on particulate and soluble succinate dehydrogenase. Biochim. biophys. Acta (Amst.) **191**, 502—508 (1969)

Chang, C. C., Chuang, S.-T., Lee, C. Y., Wei, J. W.: Role of cardiotoxin and phospholipase A in the blockade of nerve conduction and depolarization of skeletal muscle induced by cobra venom. Brit. J. Pharmacol. **44**, 752—764 (1972a)

Chang, C. C., Lee, C. Y.: Electrophysiological study of neuromuscular blocking action of cobra neurotoxin. Brit. J. Pharmacol. **28**, 172—181 (1966)

Chang, C. C., Wei, J. W., Chuang, S.-T., Lee, C. Y.: Are the blockade of nerve conduction and depolarization of skeletal muscle induced by cobra venom due to phospholipase A, neurotoxin or cardiotoxin? J. Formosan med. Ass. **71**, 323—327 (1972b)

Chiang, M. H., Cheung, W. Y.: Adenylate cyclase of *Brevibacterium liquefaciens*. Inactivation by neuraminidase, phospholipase A and phospholipase C. Biochem. biophys. Res. Commun. **55**, 187—192 (1973)

Chiang, T. S., Ho, K. J., Lee, C. Y.: Release of histamine from the rat diaphragm preparation by Formosan snake venoms. J. Formosan med. Ass. **63**, 127—132 (1964)

Chiu, T. H., Lee, C. Y., Lee, S. Y.: Hemodynamic effects of cardiotoxin isolated from Formosan cobra venom. J. Formosan med. Ass. **67**, 557 (1968)

Chou, T. C., Lee, C. Y.: Effect of whole and fractionated cobra venom on sympathetic ganglionic transmission. Europ. J. Pharmacol. **8**, 326—330 (1969)

Colacicco, G., Rapport, M. M.: Lipid mono-layers: action of phospholipase A of *Crotalus atrox* and *Naja naja* venoms on phosphatidyl choline and phosphatidal choline. J. Lipid Res. **7**, 258—263 (1966)

Coles, E., Mc Ilwain, D. L., Rapport, M. M.: The activity of pure phospholipase A_2 from *Crotalus atrox* venom on myelin and on pure phospholipids. Biochim. biophys. Acta (Amst.) **337**, 68—78 (1974)

Condrea, E.: Membrane-active polypeptides from snake venom: cardiotoxins and haemocytotoxins. Experientia (Basel) **30**, 121—129 (1974)

Condrea, E., De Vries, A.: Venom phospholipase A: a review. Toxicon **2**, 261—273 (1965)

Condrea, E., De Vries, A., Mager, J.: Hemolysis and splitting of human erythrocyte phospholipids by snake venom. Biochim. biophys. Acta (Amst.) **84**, 60—73 (1964)

Condrea, E., Rosenberg, P.: Demonstration of phospholipid splitting as the factor responsible for increased permeability and block of axonal conduction induced by snake venom. II. Study on squid axons. Biochim. biophys. Acta (Amst.) **150**, 271—284 (1968)

Condrea, E., Rosenberg, P., Dettbarn, W.-D.: Demonstration of phospholipid splitting as the factor responsible for increased permeability and block of axonal conduction induced by snake venom I. Study on lobster axons. Biochim. biophys. Acta (Amst.) **135**, 669—681 (1967)

Crouch, R., Woodbury, D.: Effects of phospholipase A on blood-brain barrier. Fed. Proc. **34**, 284 (1975)

Currie, B. T., Oakley, D. E., Broomfield, C. A.: Crystalline phospholipase A associated with a cobra venom toxin. Nature (Lond.) **220**, 371 (1968)

Damerau, B., Lege, L., Oldigs, H.-D., Vogt, W.: Histamine release, formation of prostaglandin-like activity (SRS-C) and mast cell degranulation by the direct lytic factor (DLF) and phospholipase A of cobra venom. Naunyn Schmiedebergs Arch. Pharmacol. **287**, 141—156 (1975)

Deems, R. A., Dennis, E. A.: Characterization and physical properties of the major form of phospholipase A_2 from cobra venom *(Naja naja naja)* that has a molecular weight of 11000. J. biol. Chem. **250**, 9008—9012 (1975)

Delori, P. J.: Isolement purification et étude d'une phospholipase A_2 toxique du venin de *Vipera berus*. Biochemie **53**, 941—942 (1971)

Delori, P. J.: Purification et propriétés physico-chimiques, chimiques et biologiques d'une phospholipase A_2 toxique isolée d'un venin de serpent *Viperidae Vipera berus*. Biochimie **55**, 1031—1045 (1973)

Denburg, J. L., Eldefrawi, M. E., O'Brien, R. D.: Macromolecules from lobster axon membranes that bind cholinergic ligands and local anesthetics. Proc. nat. Acad. Sci. (Wash.) **69**, 177—181 (1972)

De Robertis, E.: Molecular biology of synaptic receptors. Science **171**, 963—971 (1971)

Dettbarn, W. D., Rosenberg, P.: Sources of error in relating electrical and acetylcholinesterase activity. Biochem. Pharmacol. **11**, 1025—1030 (1962)

Devi, A.: The protein and nonprotein constituents of snake venoms. In: Bücherl, W., Buckley, E. E., Deulofeu, V. (Eds.): Venomous Animals and Their Venoms, Vol. 1, Venomous Vertebrates, Vol. 1, pp. 119—165. New York: Academic Press 1968

De Vries, A., Kochva, E. (Eds.): Toxins of Animal and Plant Origin, Vol. 1. New York: Gordon and Breach 1971

Doery, H. M.: The separation and properties of the neurotoxins from the venom of the tiger snake *Notechis scutatus scutatus*. Biochem. J. **70**, 535—543 (1958)

Doery, H. M., North, E. A.: Factors involved in the action of venoms against bacterial toxins in experimental animals. Brit. J. exp. Path. **41**, 243—250 (1960)

Doery, H. M., Pearson, J. E.: Haemolysins in venoms of Australian snakes. Observations on the haemolysins of the venoms of some Australian snakes and the separation of phospholipase A from the venom of *Pseudechis porphyriacus*. Biochem. J. **78**, 820—827 (1961)

Doery, H. M., Pearson, J. E.: Phospholipase B in snake venom and bee venom. Biochem. J. **92**, 599—602 (1964)

Drayton, H.: Inactivation of Rous virus by phospholipase A. Nature (Lond.) **192**, 896 (1961)

Duckworth, D. H., Bevers, E. M., Verkleij, A. J., Op den Kamp, J. A. F., Van Deenen, L. L. M: Action of phospholipase A_2 and phospholipase C on *Escherichia coli*. Arch. Biochem. Biophys. **165**, 379—387 (1974)

Dumarey, C., Sket, D., Joseph, D., Boquet, P.: Etude d'une phospholipase basique du venin de *Naja nigricollis*. C. R. Acad. Sci. (Paris) **280**, 1633 (1975)

Durrell, J., Garland, J. T., Friedel, R. O.: Acetylcholine action: biochemical aspects. Science **165**, 862—866 (1969)

Dutta, N. K., Narayanan, K. G. A.: Release of histamine from rat diaphragm by cobra venom. Nature (Lond.) **169**, 1064—1065 (1952)

Dutta, N. K., Narayanan, K. G. A.: Release of histamine from skeletal muscle by snake venoms. Brit. J. Pharmacol. **9**, 408—412 (1954)

Eaker, D.: Structural nature of presynaptic neurotoxins from Australia elapid venoms. Toxicon **13**, 90—91 (1975)

Eaker, D.: Snake venom toxins reacting post- and pre-synaptically at the neuromuscular junction. Bull. Inst. Pasteur Lille **74**, 9 (1976)

Edwards, S. W., Ball, E. G.: The action of phospholipases on succinate oxidase and cytochrome oxidase. J. biol. Chem. **209**, 619—633 (1954)

Elliott, W. B., Augustyn, J. M., Gans, C.: Some actions of snake venom on mitochondria. Mem. Inst. Butantan **33**, 411—424 (1966)

Elliott, W. B., Gans, C.: Production by snake venoms of uncoupling activity and reverse acceptor control in rat liver mitochondrial preparations. In: Russell, F., Saunders, P. (Eds.): Animal Toxins. New York: Pergamon Press 1967

Fairbairn, D.: The phospholipase of the venom of the cottonmouth moccasin (*Agkistrodon piscivorus L.*). J. biol. Chem. **157**, 633—644 (1945)

Fearn, H. J., Smith, C., West, G. B.: Capillary permeability responses to snake venom. J. Pharm. Pharmacol. **16**, 79—84 (1964)

Feinstein, M. B.: Reaction of local anesthetics with phospholipids: A possible chemical basis for anesthesia. J. gen. Physiol. **48**, 357—374 (1964)

Feldberg, W.: The action of bee venom, cobra venom, and lysolecithin in the adrenal medulla. J. Physiol. (Lond.) **99**, 104—118 (1940)

Feldberg, W., Kellaway, C. H.: Liberation of histamine from the perfused lung by snake venoms. J. Physiol. (Lond.) **90**, 257—279 (1937a)

Feldberg, W., Kellaway, C. H.: Circulatory effects of the venom of the Indian cobra (*Naja naja*) in cats. Aust. J. exp. Biol. med. Sci. **15**, 159—172 (1937b)

Feldberg, W., Kellaway, C. H.: Liberation of histamine and formation of lysolecithin-like substances by cobra venom. J. Physiol. (Lond.) **94**, 187—226 (1938)

Fiehn, W., Hasselbach, W.: The effect of phospholipase A on the calcium transport and the role of unsaturated fatty acids in ATPase activity of sarcoplasmic vesicles. Europ. J. Biochem. **13**, 510—518 (1970)

Fleischer, B., Casu, A., Fleischer, S.: Release of β-hydroxybutyric apodehydrogenase from beef heart mitochondria by the action of phospholipase A. Biochem. Biophys. Res. Commun. **24**, 189—194 (1966)
Folch, J., Lees, M., Sloan Stanley, G. H.: A simple method for the isolation and purification of total lipids from animal tissue. J. biol. Chem. **226**, 497—509 (1957)
Fredholm, B.: Studies on a mast cell degranulating factor in bee venom. Biochem. Pharmacol. **15**, 2037—2043 (1966)
Gallai-Hatchard, J., Gray, G. M.: The action of phospholipase A on the plasma membranes of rat liver cells. Eur. J. Biochem. **4**, 35—40 (1968)
Gatt, S., Barenholz, Y.: Enzymes of complex lipid metabolism. Ann. Rev. Biochem. **42**, 61—90 (1973)
Gautrelet, G., Corteggiani, E.: Liberation de la acetyl choline du tissu cerebrals in vitro par les venins de Cobra ou de Visperis Aspis, la lysolecithin et la saponin. C. R. Soc. Biol. (Paris) **131**, 951—954 (1939)
Giambalvo, C., Rosenberg, P.: The effect of phospholipases and proteases on the binding of γ-aminobutyric acid to junctional complexes of rat cerebellum. Biochim. biophys. Acta (Amst.) **436**, 741—756 (1976)
Gitter, S., Kochva, S., De Vries, A., Leffkowitz, M.: Studies on electrophoretic fractions of *Vipera xanthina palestinae venom*. Amer. J. trop. Med. Hyg. **6**, 180—189 (1957)
Goldman, D. E.: A molecular structural basis for the excitation properties of axons. Biophys. J. **4**, 167—188 (1964)
Gordon, A. S., Wallach, D. F. H., Straus, J. H.: The optical activity of plasma membranes and its modification by lysolecithin, phospholipase A and phospholipase C. Biochim. biophys. Acta (Amst.) **183**, 405—416 (1969)
Greig, M. E., Gibbons, A. J.: Possible mechanisms whereby phenothiazine derivatives preserve stored blood. Amer. J. Physiol. **181**, 313—318 (1955)
Gubenšek, F.: Sepharose bound toxic phospholipase A. Bull. Inst. Pasteur Lille **74**, 47—49 (1976)
Gubenšek, F., Lapanje, S.: Circular Dichroism of two phospholipases A from *Vipera ammodytes* venom. FEBS Letters **44**, 182—184 (1974)
Gubenšek, F., Sket, D., Turk, V., Lebez, D.: Fractionation of *Vipera ammodytes* venom and seasonal variation of its composition. Toxicon **12**, 167—171 (1974)
Habermann, E.: Hemmung der oxydativen Phosphorylierung durch tierische Gifte. Naturwissenschaften **41**, 429—430 (1954)
Habermann, E.: Beiträge zur Pharmakologie von Phospholipase A. Naunyn Schmiedebergs Arch. Pharmakol. **230**, 538—546 (1957)
Habermann, E., Neumann, W.: Beiträge zur Characterisierung der wirksamen Komponenten von Schlangengiften. Naunyn Schmiedebergs Arch. Pharmacol. **223**, 388—398 (1954)
Hachimori, Y., Wells, M. A., Hanahan, D. J.: Observations on the phospholipase A_2 of *Crotalus atrox*. Molecular weight and other properties. Biochemistry **10**, 4084—4089 (1971)
Hagen, P.-O., Ofstad, E., Amundsen, E.: Experimental acute pancreatitis in dogs. IV. The relationship between phospholipase A and the histamine releasing and hypotensive effects of pancreatic exudate. Scand. J. Gastroenterol. **4**, 89—96 (1969)
Halpert, J., Eaker, D.: Amino acid sequence of a presynaptic neurotoxin from the venom of *Notechis scutatus scutatus* (Australian tiger snake). J. biol. Chem. **250**, 6990—6997 (1975)
Halpert, J., Eaker, D., Karlsson, E.: The role of phospholipase activity in the action of a presynaptic neurotoxin from the venom of *Notechis scutatus scutatus* (Australian tiger snake). FEBS Letters **61**, 72—76 (1976)
Hanahan, D. J.: Phospholipases. In: Boyer, P. D. (Ed.): The Enzymes, 3rd Ed., Vol. V. New York: Academic Press 1971
Hawthorne, J. N., Kai, M.: Metabolism of phosphoinositides. In: Lajtha, A. (Ed.): Handbook of Neurochemistry, Vol. III, pp. 491—508. New York: Plenum Press 1970
Heilbronn, E.: The effect of phospholipases on the uptake of atropine and acetylcholine by slices of mouse brain cortex. J. Neurochem. **16**, 627—635 (1969)
Heilbronn, E., Nilsson, M. G.: Possible involvement of an enzyme reaction in ACh-release. Abstr. 3rd Int. Meeting of the Internat. Soc. for Neurochem., p. 392, Budapest, 1971
Hendon, R. A., Fraenkel-Conrat, H.: Biological roles of the two components of crotoxin. Proc. nat. Acad. Sci. (Wash.) **68**, 1560—1563 (1971)

Hendon, R. A., Fraenkel-Conrat, H.: The role of complex formation in the neurotoxicity of crotoxin components A and B. Toxicon **14**, 283—289 (1976)
Hines, G. C., Moss, G. F., Cox, J. S. G.: Effect of disodium cromoglycate on phospholipase A activity. Studies with egg yolk and isolated mast cell systems. Biochem. Pharmacol. **21**, 171—179 (1972)
Horst, J., Hendon, R. A., Fraenkel-Conrat, H.: The active components of crotoxin. Biochem. Biophys. Res. Commun. **46**, 1042—1047 (1972)
Hoskin, F. C. G., Kremzner, L. T., Rosenberg, P.: Effects of some cholinesterase inhibitors on the squid giant axon—Their permeability, detoxication and effects on conduction and acetylcholinesterase activity. Biochem. Pharmacol. **18**, 1727—1737 (1969)
Hoskin, F. C. G., Rosenberg, P.: Pentration of sugars, steroids, amino acids and other compounds into the interior of the squid giant axon. J. gen. Physiol. **49**, 47—56 (1965)
Houssay, B. A., Mazzoco, P.: Mecanisme de l'action des venins de serpents et de scorpions sur le muscle strie. C.R. Soc. Biol. (Paris) **93**, 1120—1122 (1925)
Houssay, B. A., Mazzocco, P.: Action of snake venoms on the diffusion of potassium, phosphates, and hemoglobin, also on the formation of lactic acid in various organs. Rev. Soc. argent. Biol. **2**, 383 (1926)
Houssay, B. A., Negrete, J., Mazzocco, P.: Action des venins de serpents sur le nerf et le muscle isoles. C.R. Soc. Biol. (Paris) **87**, 823—824 (1922)
Howard, B. D.: Effects of β-bungarotoxin on mitochondrial respiration are caused by associated phospholipase A activity. Biochem. Biophys. Res. Commun. **67**, 58—65 (1975)
Howard, N. L.: Phospholipase A_2 from puff adder *(Bitis arietans)* venom. Toxicon **13**, 21—30 (1974)
Hudson, A. J., Quastel, J. H., Scholefield, P. G.: The effects of heated snake venom on the phosphate metabolism of the rat spinal cord. J. Neurochem. **5**, 177—184 (1960)
Hughes, A.: The action of snake venoms on surface films. Biochem. J. **29**, 437—444 (1935)
Ibrahim, S. A.: A study on sea snake venom phospholipase A. Toxicon **8**, 221—224 (1970)
Ibrahim, S. A., Sanders, H., Thompson, R. H. S.: The action of phospholipase A on purified phospholipids, plasma, and tissue preparations. Biochem. J. **93**, 588—594 (1964)
Jiménez-Porras, J. M.: Pharmacology of peptides and proteins in snake venoms. Ann. Rev. Pharmacol. **8**, 299—318 (1968)
Jiménez-Porras, J. M.: Biochemistry of snake venoms. Clin. Toxicol. **3**, 389—431 (1970)
Joubert, F. J.: *Naja melanoleuca* (Forest cobra) venom. The amino acid sequence of phospholipase A, Fraction DE-III. Biochim. biophys. Acta (Amst.) **379**, 329—344 (1975a)
Joubert, F. J.: *Naja melanoleuca* (Forest cobra) venom. The amino acid sequence of phospholipase A, fractions DE-I and DE-II. Biochim. biophys. Acta (Amst.) **379**, 345—359 (1975b)
Joubert, F. J.: *Hemachatus haemachatus* (Ringhals) venom. Purification, some properties and amino-acid sequence of phospholipase A (Fraction DE-I). Europ. J. Biochem. **52**, 539—554 (1975c)
Joubert, F. J., Van der Walt, S. J.: *Naja melanoleuca* (Forest cobra) Venom. Purification and some properties of phospholipases A. Biochim. biophys. Acta (Amst.) **379**, 317—328 (1975)
Karlsson, E.: Chemistry of some potent animal toxins. Experientia (Basel) **29**, 1319—1327 (1973)
Karlsson, E., Eaker, D. L., Porath, J.: Purification of a neurotoxin from the venom of *Naja nigricollis*. Biochim. biophys. Acta (Amst.) **127**, 505—520 (1966)
Kawauchi, S., Iwanaga, S., Samejima, Y., Suzuki, T.: Isolation and characterization of two phospholipase A's from the venom of *Agkistrodon halys blomhoffii*. Biochim. biophys. Acta (Basel) **236**, 142—160 (1971a)
Kawauchi, S., Samejima, Y., Iwanaga, S.: Amino acid compositions of snake venom phospholipase A's. J. Biochem. **69**, 433—437 (1971b)
Kirschmann, C., Ten-Ami, I., Smorodinski, I., De Vries, A.: Effect of phospholipase and trypsin on histidine uptake by mouse brain slices. Biochim. biophys. Acta (Amst.) **233**, 644—651 (1971)
Klibansky, C., Shiloah, J., De Vries, A.: Action of *Naja naja* and *Vipera palestinae* venoms on cat brain phospholipids in vitro. Biochem. Pharmacol. **13**, 1107—1112 (1964)
Kocholaty, W. F.: A rapid and simple phospholipase A assay. Toxicon **4**, 1—5 (1966)
Kochwa, S., Perlmutter, C., Gitter, S., Rechnic, J., De Vries, A.: Studies on *Vipera palestinae* venom. Fractionation by ion exchange chromatography. Amer. J. trop. Med. Hyg. **9**, 374—380 (1960)

Kogo, H., Aizawa, Y.: Effect of phospholipase A, C, and D on sugar and amino acid transport in rat uterus. Jap. J. Pharmacol. **22**, 411—415 (1972)

Kohn, A.: Polykaryocytosis induced by Newcastle disease virus in monolayers of animal cells. Virology **26**, 228—245 (1965)

Kohn, A., Klibansky, C.: Studies on the inactivation of cell-fusing property of Newcastle disease virus by phospholipase A. Virology **31**, 385—388 (1967)

Kremzner, L.T., Rosenberg, P.: Relationship of acetylcholinesterase activity to axonal conduction. Biochem. Pharmacol. **20**, 2953—2958 (1971)

Lal, H., Sumyk, G., Shefner, A.: Effect of cobra venom and venom fractions on barbital-induced hypnosis in mice. Arch. int. Pharmacodyn. **159**, 452—460 (1966)

Lee, C.Y.: Mode of action of cobra venom and its purified toxins. In: Simpson, L.L. (Ed.): Neuropoisons: Their Pathophysiological Actions, Vol. I, pp. 21—70. New York: Plenum Press 1971

Lee, C.Y.: Chemistry and pharmacology of polypeptide toxins in snake venoms. Ann. Rev. Pharmacol. **12**, 265—286 (1972)

Lee, C.Y., Chang, C.C.: Modes of action of purified toxins from Elapid venoms on neuromuscular transmission. Mem. Inst. Butantan **33**, 555—572 (1966)

Lee, C.Y., Tseng, L.F.: Distribution of *Bungarus multicinctus* venom following envenomation. Toxicon **3**, 281—290 (1966)

Lo, T.B., Chang, W.C., Chang, C.S.: Chemical studies on phospholipase A from Formosan cobra *(Naja naja atra)* venom. J. Formosan med. Ass. **71**, 318—402 (1972)

Lunney, J., Ashwell, G.: The effect of phospholipase on the binding of asialoglycoproteins by rat liver plasma membranes. Biochim. biophys. Acta (Amst.) **367**, 304—315 (1974)

Lysz, T.W., Rosenberg, P.: Convulsant activity of *Naja naja* venom and its phospholipase A component. Toxicon **12**, 253—265 (1974)

McArdle, B., Thompson, R.H.S., Webster, G.R.: The action of lysolecithin and of snake venom on whole-cell preparations of brain, muscle, and liver. J. Neurochem. **5**, 135—144 (1960)

Maeno, H., Mitsuhashi, S., Okonogi, T., Hoshi, S., Homma, M.: Studies on Habu snake venom. V. Myolysis caused by phospholipase A in Habu snake venom. Jap. J. exp. Med. **32**, 55—64 (1962)

Magee, W.L., Thompson, R.H.S.: The estimation of phospholipase A activity in aqueous systems. Biochem. J. **77**, 526—534 (1960)

Marinetti, G.V.: The action of phospholipase A on lipoproteins. Biochim. biophys. Acta (Amst.) **98**, 554—565 (1965)

Martin, R., Rosenberg, P.: Fine structural alterations associated with venom action on squid giant nerve fibers. J. Cell Biol. **36**, 341—353 (1968)

Master, R.W.P., Rao, S.S.: Identification of enzymes and toxins in venoms of Indian cobra and Russell's viper after starch gel electrophoresis. J. biol. Chem. **236**, 1986—1990 (1961)

May, B., Holler, C., Westermann, E.: Über die Bedeutung der Phospholipase A für die histaminfreisetzende Wirkung des Cobragiftes. Naunyn Schmiedebergs Arch. Pharmak. exp. Path. **256**, 237—256 (1967)

Meldrum, B.S.: Actions of whole and fractionated Indian cobra *(Naja naja)* venom of skeletal muscle. Brit. J. Pharmacol. **25**, 197—205 (1965a)

Meldrum, B.S.: The actions of snake venoms on nerve and muscle. The pharmacology of phospholipase A and of polypeptide toxins. Pharmacol. Rev. **17**, 393—446 (1965b)

Meldrum, B.S., Thompson, R.H.S.: The action of snake venoms on the membrane permeability of brain, muscle, and red blood cells. Guy's Hosp. Rep. **111**, 87—97 (1962)

Menon, I.A.: Effects of phospholipases on RNA polymerase activity in preparation from rat brain. Canad. J. Biochem. **49**, 1318—1325 (1971)

Middleton, E.J.R., Phillips, G.B.: Distribution and properties of anaphylactic and venom-induced slow-reacting-substance and histamine in guinea-pigs. J. Immunol. **93**, 220—227 (1964)

Mohamed, A.H., Kamel, A., Ayobe, M.H.: Studies of phospholipase A and B activities of Egyptian snake venoms and a scorpion toxin. Toxicon **6**, 293—298 (1969)

Mookerjea, S., Yung, J.W.M.: A study of the effect of lysolecithin and phospholipase A on membrane-bound galactosyltransferase. Canad. J. Biochem. **52**, 1053—1066 (1974)

Moores, G.R., Lawrence, A.J.: Conductimetric assay of phospholipids and phospholipase A. FEBS Letters **28**, 201—204 (1972)

Morazain, R., Rosenberg, P.: Lipid changes in tri-o-cresylphosphate-induced neuropathy. Toxicol. appl. Pharmacol. **16**, 461—474 (1970)

Morrison, L. R., Zamecnik, P. C.: Experimental demyelination by means of enzymes, especially the alpha toxin of *Clostridium welchii*. Arch. Neurol. Psychiatr. **63**, 367—381 (1950)

Nair, B. C., Nair, C., Elliott, W. B.: Temperature stability of phospholipase A activity. II. Variations in optimum temperature of phospholipases A_2 from various snake venoms. Toxicon **14**, 43—47 (1976 b)

Nair, C., Hermans, J., Munjal, D., Elliott, W. B.: Temperature stability of phospholipase A activity I Bee *(Apis mellifera)* venom phospholipase A. Toxicon **14**, 35—42 (1976 a)

Narahashi, T.: Chemicals as tools in the study of excitable membranes. Physiol. Rev. **54**, 813—889 (1974)

Narahashi, T., Tobias, J. M.: Properties of axon membrane as affected by cobra venom, digitonin, and proteases. Amer. J. Physiol. **207**, 1441—1446 (1964)

Nelson, P. G.: Effects of certain enzymes on node of Ranvier excitability with observations on submicroscopic structure. J. cell. comp. Physiol. **52**, 127—145 (1958)

Neumann, W. P., Habermann, E.: Über Crotactin, das Haupttoxin des Giftes der brasilianischen Klapperschlange *(Crotalus terrificus terrificus)* Biochem. Z. **327**, 170—185 (1955)

North, E. A., Doery, H. M.: Antagonism between the action of staphylococcal toxin and the venom of certain snakes and insects in mice. Brit. J. exp. Path. **46**, 234—242 (1960)

North, E. A., Paulyszyn, G., Doery, H. M.: The action of phosphatidase A, sodium oleate and ganglioside on the exotoxins of *Cl. welchii* (Phospholipase C) and on the neurotoxin of *Shigella shigae*. Aust. J. exp. Biol. med. Sci. **39**, 259—266 (1961)

Nygaard, A. P., Dianzani, V., Bohr, G. F.: The effect of lecithinase A on the morphology of isolated mitochondria. Exp. Cell Res. **6**, 453—458 (1954)

Nygaard, A. P., Summer, J. B.: The effect of lecithinase A on the succinoxidase system. J. biol. Chem. **200**, 723—729 (1953)

O'Brien, R. D., Gilmour, L. P., Eldefrowi, M. E.: A muscarone binding material in electroplax and its relation to the acetylcholine receptor. II. Dialysis assay. Proc. nat. Acad. Sci. (Wash.) **65**, 438—445 (1970)

Omori-Satoh, T., Lang, J., Breithaupt, H., Habermann, E.: Partial amino acid sequence of the basic *Crotalus* phospholipase A. Toxicon **13**, 69—71 (1975)

Op den Kamp, J. A. F., Kauerz, M. T., Van Deenen, L. L. M.: Action of phospholipase A_2 and phospholipase C on *Bacillus subtilis* protoplasts. J. Bacteriol. **112**, 1090—1098 (1972)

Orange, R. P., Murphy, R. C., Austen, K. F.: Inactivation of slow reacting substance of anaphylaxis (SRS-A) by arylsulfatases. J. Immunol. **113**, 316—322 (1974)

Orange, R. P., Murphy, R. C., Karnovsky, M. L., Austen, K. F.: The physicochemical characteristics and purification of slow-reacting substance of anaphylaxis. J. Immunol. **110**, 760—770 (1973)

Ouyang, C., Shiau, S.-Y.: Relationship between pharmacological actions and enzymatic activities of the venom of *Trimeresurus gramineus*. Toxicon **8**, 183—191 (1970)

Paradies, H. H., Breithaupt, H.: On the subunit structure of crotoxin: Hydrodynamic and shape properties of crotoxin, phospholipase A and crotapotin. Biochem. Biophys. Res. Commun. **66**, 496—504 (1975)

Pasek, M., Keith, C., Feldman, D., Sigler, P. B.: Characterization of crystals of two venom phospholipases A_2. J. molec. Biol. **97**, 395—397 (1975)

Pasternak, G. W., Snyder, S. H.: Opiate receptor binding: effects of enzymatic treatments. Molec. Pharmacol. **10**, 183—193 (1974)

Petrushka, E., Quastel, J. H., Scholefield, P. G.: Role of phospholipids in mitochondrial respiration. Canad. J. Biochem. Physiol. **37**, 975—987 (1959)

Phillips, G. B., Middleton, E., Jr.: Release of histamine and slow-reacting substance activities from guinea pig lung. Proc. Soc. exp. Biol. (N.Y.) **119**, 465—470 (1965)

Prasad, R., Kabra, V. K., Brodie, A. F.: Effect of phospholipase A on the structure and functions of membrane vesicles from *Mycobacterium phlei*. J. biol. Chem. **250**, 3690—3698 (1975)

Radomski, J. L., Deichmann, W. B.: The relationship of certain enzymes in cobra and rattlesnake venoms to the mechanism of action of these venoms. Biochem. J. **70**, 293—297 (1958)

Ramsey, R. B., Atallah, A., Fredericks, M., Nicholas, H. J.: The effect of non-ionic detergents and phospholipase A on enzymes involved in adult rat brain sterol biosynthesis from (2-^{14}C)-mevalonic acid in vitro. Biochem. Biophys. Res. Commun. **61**, 170—177 (1974)
Ramsey, R. B., Davison, A. N.: Effect of phospholipase A upon brain cholesterol ester formation. Lipids **9**, 440—442 (1974)
Robertson, J. D.: The molecular structure and contact relationships of cell membranes. Prog. Biophys. Mol. Biol. **10**, 343—418 (1960)
Rock, C. O., Snyder, F.: Rapid purification of phospholipase A_2 from *Crotalus adamanteus* venom by affinity chromatography. J. biol. Chem. **250**, 6564—6566 (1975)
Roholt, O. A., Schlamowitz, M.: Studies of the use of dihexanoyllecithin and other lecithins as substrates for phospholipase A with addendum on aspects of micelle properties of dihexanoyllecithin. Arch. Biochem. Biophys. **94**, 364—379 (1961)
Rosenberg, P.: Effects of venoms on the squid giant axon. Toxicon **3**, 125—131 (1965)
Rosenberg, P.: Use of venoms in studies on nerve excitation. Mem. Inst. Butantan **33**, 477—508 (1966)
Rosenberg, P.: Function of phospholipids in axons: Depletion of membrane phosphorus by treatment with phospholipase C. Toxicon **8**, 235—243 (1970)
Rosenberg, P.: The use of snake venoms as pharmacological tools in studying nerve activity. In: Simpson, L. L. (Ed.): Neuropoisons: Their Pathophysiological Actions, Vol. 1, Chap. 5, pp. 111—137. New York: Plenum 1971
Rosenberg, P.: Use of phospholipases in studying nerve structure and function. In: De Vries, A., Kochva, E. (Eds.): Toxins of Animal and Plant Origin, pp. 449—461. London: Gordon and Breach 1972
Rosenberg, P.: Effect of stimulation and acetylcholine on ^{32}P and ^{14}C incorporation into phospholipids of the eel electroplax. J. Pharm. Sci. **62**, 1552—1554 (1973a)
Rosenberg, P.: Venoms and enzymes: effects on permeability of isolated single electroplax. Toxicon **11**, 149—154 (1973b)
Rosenberg, P.: Penetration of phospholipase A_2 and C into the squid *(Loligo pealii)* giant axon. Experientia (Basel) **31**, 1401—1402 (1975)
Rosenberg, P.: Effect of phospholipases A_2 and C on structure and phospholipids of the electroplax. Toxicon **14**, 319—328 (1976a)
Rosenberg, P.: Bacterial and snake venom phospholipases: enzymatic probes in the study of structure and function in bioelectrically excitable tissues. In: Ohsaka, A., Hayashi, K., Sawai, Y. (Eds.): Animal, Plant, and Microbial Toxins, Vol. II, pp. 229—261. New York: Plenum Press 1976b
Rosenberg, P., Condrea, E.: Maintenance of axonal conduction and membrane permeability in presence of extensive phospholipid splitting. Biochem. Pharmacol. **17**, 2033—2044 (1968)
Rosenberg, P., Dettbarn, W.-D.: Increased cholinesterase activity of intact cells caused by snake venoms. Biochem. Pharmacol. **13**, 1157—1165 (1964)
Rosenberg, P., Ehrenpreis, S.: Reversible block of axonal conduction by curare after treatment with cobra venom. Biochem. Pharmacol. **8**, 192—206 (1961)
Rosenberg, P., Hoskin, F. C. G.: Demonstration of increased permeability as a factor responsible for the effect of acetylcholine on the electrical activity of venom treated axons. J. gen. Physiol. **46**, 1065—1073 (1963)
Rosenberg, P., Khairallah, E. A.: Effect of phospholipases A and C on free amino acid content of the squid axon. J. Neurochem. **23**, 55—64 (1974)
Rosenberg, P., Mautner, H. G.: Acetylcholine receptor: Similarity in axons and junctions. Science **155**, 1569—1571 (1967)
Rosenberg, P., Ng, K. Y.: Factors in venoms leading to block of axonal conduction by curare. Biochim. biophys. Acta (Amst.) **75**, 116—128 (1963)
Rosenberg, P., Podleski, T. R.: Block of conduction by acetylcholine and D-tubocurarine after treatment of squid axon with cottonmouth moccasin venom. J. Pharmacol. exp. Ther. **137**, 249—262 (1962)
Rosenberg, P., Podleski, T. R.: Ability of venoms to render squid axons sensitive to curare and acetylcholine. Biochim. biophys. Acta (Amst.) **75**, 104—115 (1963)
Rosenthal, A. F., Geyer, R. P.: A synthetic inhibitor of venom lecithinase A. J. biol. Chem. **235**, 2202—2206 (1960)

Rosenthal, A. F., Han, S. C. H.: A study of phospholipase A inhibition by glycerophosphatide analogs in various systems. Biochim. biophys. Acta (Amst.) **218**, 213—220 (1970)
Rothschild, A. M.: Chromatographic separation of phospholipase A from a histamine releasing component of Brazilian rattlesnake venom *(Crotalus durissus terrificus)*. Experientia (Basel) **23**, 741—742 (1967)
Rübsamen, K., Breithaupt, H., Habermann, E.: Biochemistry and pharmacology of crotoxin complex I. Subfractionation and recombination of the crotoxin. Naunyn Schmiedebergs Arch. Pharmacol. **270**, 274—288 (1971)
Russell, F. E.: Pharmacology of animal venoms. Clin. Pharmacol. Ther. **8**, 849—873 (1967)
Russell, F. E., Bohr, V. C.: Intraventricular injection of venom. Toxicol. appl. Pharmacol. **4**, 165—173 (1962)
Russell, F. E., Puffer, H. W.: Pharmacology of snake venoms. Clin. Toxicol. **3**, 433—444 (1970)
Russell, F. E., Saunders, P. R. (Eds.): Animal Toxins. Oxford: Pergamon Press 1967
Saito, K., Hanahan, D. J.: A study of the purification and properties of the phospholipase A of *Crotalus adamanteus* venom. Biochemistry **1**, 521—532 (1962)
Salach, J. I., Seng, R., Tisdale, H., Singer, T. P.: Phospholipase A of snake venoms. II. Catalytic properties of the enzyme from *Naja naja*. J. biol. Chem. **246**, 340—347 (1971 b)
Salach, J. I., Turini, P., Seng, R., Hauber, J., Singer, T. P.: Phospholipase A of snake venoms. Isolation and molecular properties of isoenzymes from *Naja naja* and *Vipera russellii* venoms. J. biol. Chem. **246**, 331—339 (1971 a)
Samejima, Y., Iwanaga, S., Suzuki, T.: Complete amino acid sequence of phospholipase A_2—II. Isolated from *Agkistrodon halys blomhoffii* venom. FEBS Letters **47**, 348—351 (1974)
Samuelsson, B.: Prostaglandin endoperoxides and thromboxanes: short lived bio-regulators. Abstracts. 38. Am. Chem. Soc. Biol. Chem. Meeting, April, 1976
Sarker, N. K., Devi, A.: Enzymes in snake venoms. In: Bücherl, W., Buckley, E. E., Deulofeu, V. (Eds.): Venomous Animals and Their Venoms: Venomous Vertebrates, Vol. I, pp. 167—216. New York: Academic Press 1968
Sasaki, T.: Chemical studies on the poison of Formosan cobra. II. The terminal amino acid residues of purified poison (Neurotoxin). J. Pharm. Soc. Jpn. **77**, 845—847 (1957)
Sasaki, T.: Chemical studies on the poison of Formosan cobra. IV. Terminal amino acid residues, molecular weight and amino acid composition of purified lecithinase. J. Pharm. Soc. Jpn. **78**, 516—520 (1958)
Seppala, A. J., Saris, N.-E. L., Gauffin, M. L.: Inhibition of phospholipase A—induced swelling of mitochondria by local anesthetics and related agents. Biochem. Pharmacol. **20**, 305—313 (1971)
Shiloah, J., Klibansky, C., De Vries, A.: Phospholipase isoenzymes from *Naja naja* venom. I. Purification and partial characterization. Toxicon **11**, 481—490 (1973 a)
Shiloah, J., Klibansky, C., De Vries, A.: Phospholipase isoenzymes from *Naja naja* venom. II. Phospholipase A and B activities. Toxicon **11**, 491—497 (1973 b)
Shilaoh, J., Klibansky, C., De Vries, A., Berger, A.: Phospholipase B activity of a purified phospholipase A from *Vipera palestinae* venom. J. Lipid Res. **14**, 267—278 (1973 c)
Simpkins, H., Tay, S., Panko, E.: Changes in the molecular structure of axonal and red blood cell membranes following treatment with phospholipase A_2. Biochemistry **10**, 3579—3585 (1971)
Simpson, L. (Ed.): Neuropoisons, Their Pathological Actions, Vol. 1—Poisons of Animal Origin. New York: Plenum Press 1971
Singer, S. J., Nicolson, G. L.: The fluid mosaic model of the structure of cell membranes. Science **175**, 720—731 (1972)
Sket, D., Gubenšek, F.: Pharmacological study of phospholipase A from *Vipera ammodytes* venom. Toxicon **14**, 393—396 (1976)
Sket, D., Gubenšek, F., Adamič, S., Lebez, D.: Action of a partially purified basic protein fraction from *Vipera ammodytes* venom. Toxicon **11**, 47—53 (1973 b)
Sket, D., Gubenšek, F., Pavlin, R., Lebez, D.: Oxygen consumption of rat brain homogenates after in vitro and in vivo addition of the basic protein from *Vipera ammodytes* venom. Toxicon **11**, 193—196 (1973 a)
Slein, M. W., Logan, G. F.: Lysis of *Escherichia coli* by ethylenediamine tetroacetate and phospholipase as measured by β-galactosidase activity. J. Bacteriol. **94**, 934—941 (1967)

Slotta, K. H., Fraenkel-Conrat, H. L.: Schlangengifte, III. Mitteilung: Reinigung und Krystallisation des Klapperschlangen-Giftes. Ber. dtsch. Chem. Ges. **71**, 1076—1081 (1938)

Slotta, K. H., Vick, J. A., Ginsberg, N. J.: Enzymatic and toxic activity of phospholipase A. In: De Vries, A., Kochva, E. (Eds.): Toxins of Animal and Plant Origin, Vol. I, pp. 401—417. London: Gordon and Breach 1971

Somani, P., Arora, R. B.: Mechanism of increased capillary permeability induced by saw-scaled viper venom. A possible new approach to the treatment of viperine snake poisoning. J. Pharm. Pharmacol. **14**, 394—395 (1964)

Strong, P. N., Goerke, J., Oberg, S. G., Kelly, R. B.: β-Bungarotoxin, a pre-synaptic toxin with enzymatic activity. Proc. nat. Acad. Sci. (Wash.) **73**, 178—182 (1976)

Sumyk, G., Lal, H., Hawrylewicz, E. J.: Whole-animal autoradiographic localization of radio-iodine labeled cobra venom in mice. Fed. Proc. **22**, 668 (1963)

Sun, A. Y.: The effect of phospholipases on the active uptake of norepinephrine by synaptosomes isolated from the cerebral cortex of guinea-pig. J. Neurochem. **22**, 551—556 (1974)

Suzuki, T., Iwanaga, S., Kawauchi, S.: Isolation of crystalline lecithinase A (hemolysin) from Formosan cobra venom *(Naja naja atra* Cantor). J. Pharm. Soc. Jpn. **78**, 568—569 (1958)

Swanson, P. D., Bradford, H. F., Mc Ilwain, H.: Stimulation and solubilization of the sodium ion-activated adenosine triphosphatase of cerebral microsomes by surface-active agents, especially polyoxyethylene ethers. Actions of phospholipases and a neuroaminidase. Biochem. J. **92**, 235—247 (1964)

Takashima, S., Yantorno, R., Pal, N. C.: Electrical properties of squid axon membrane II. Effect of partial degradation by phospholipase A and pronase on electrical characteristics. Biochim. biophys. Acta (Amst.) **401**, 15—27 (1975)

Taub, A. M., Elliott, W. B.: Some effects of snake venoms on mitochondria. Toxicon **2**, 87—92 (1964)

Tobias, G. S., Donlon, M., Shain, W., Catravas, G.: β-Bungarotoxin: Relationship of phospholipase activity to toxicity. Fed. Proc. **35**, 800 (1976)

Tobias, J. M.: Effects of phospholipases, collagenase and chymotrypsin on impulse conduction and resting potential in the lobster axon with parallel experiments on frog muscle. J. Cell Comp. Physiol. **46**, 183—207 (1955)

Tobias, J. M.: Experimentally altered structure related to function in the lobster axon with an extrapolation to molecular mechanisms in excitation. J. Cell Comp. Physiol. **52**, 89—125 (1958)

Tsao, F. H. C., Keim, P. S., Heinrikson, R. L.: *Crotalus adamanteus* phospholipase A_2-α: Subunit structure, NH_2—terminal sequence, and homology with other phospholipases. Arch. Biochem. Biophys. **167**, 706—717 (1975)

Tseng, L. F., Chiu, T. H., Lee, C. Y.: Absorption and distribution of ^{131}I-labelled cobra venom and its purified toxins. Toxicol. appl. Pharmacol. **12**, 526—535 (1968)

Tsukada, K., Majunsdar, C., Lieberman, I.: Liver polyribosomes and phospholipase A. Biochem. Biophys. Res. Commun. **25**, 181—186 (1966)

Tu, A. T.: Neurotoxins of animal venoms: Snakes. Ann. Rev. Biochem. **42**, 235—255 (1973)

Tu, A. T.: The mechanism of snake venom actions—rattlesnakes and other crotalids. In: Simpson, L. L. (Ed.): Neuropoisons, Their Pathophysiological Actions, Poisons of Animal Origin, Vol. I, pp. 87—109. New York: Plenum Press 1971

Tu, A. T., Passey, R. B.: Phospholipase A from sea snake venom and its biological properties. In: De Vries, A., Kochva, E. (Eds.): Toxins of Animal and Plant Origin, Vol. I, pp. 419—435. London: Gordon and Breach 1971

Tu, A. T., Passey, R. B., Toom, P. M.: Isolation and characterization of phospholipase A from sea snake, *Laticauda semifasciata* venom. Arch. Biochem. Biophys. **140**, 96—106 (1970)

Uthe, J. F., Magee, W. L.: Phospholipase A_2: action on purified phospholipids as affected by deoxycholate and divalent cations. Canad. J. Biochem. **49**, 776—784 (1971 a)

Uthe, J. F., Magee, W. L.: Phospholipase A_2: Comparative action of three different enzyme preparations on selected lipoprotein systems. Canad. J. Biochem. **49**, 785—794 (1971 b)

Uvnäs, B.: The mechanism of histamine liberation. J. Pharm. Pharmacol. **10**, 1—13 (1958)

Uvnäs, B., Antonsson, J.: Triggering action of phosphatidase A and chymotrypsins on degranulation of rat mesentery mast cells. Biochem. Pharmacol. **12**, 867—873 (1963)

Uvnäs, B., Diamant, B., Hogberg, B.: Trigger action of phospholipase A on mast cells. Arch. int. Pharmacodyn. **140**, 577—580 (1962)
Van Deenen, L. L. M., De Haas, G. H.: Phosphoglycerides and phospholipases. Ann. Rev. Biochem. **35**, 157—193 (1966)
Vanderkooi, G., Green, D. E.: Biological membrane structure. I. The protein crystal model for membranes. Proc. nat. Acad. Sci. (Wash.) **66**, 615—621 (1970)
Vane, J. R.: Inhibition of prostaglandin synthesis as a mechanism of action for aspirin-like drugs. Nature (Lond.) New Biol. **231**, 232—235 (1971)
Vargaftig, B. B., Dao, N.: Release of vasoactive substances from guinea-pig lungs by slow-reacting substance C and arachidonic acid. Pharmacology **6**, 99—108 (1971 a)
Vargaftig, B. B., Dao, N.: Mode d'action et antagonisme de la "substance a contraction differée C" liberée per lo phospholipase A, a partir du jaune d'oeuf. J. Pharmacol. **2**, 287—304 (1971 b)
Vick, J. A., Cuichta, H. P., Broomfield, C., Currie, B. T.: Isolation and identification of toxic fractions of cobra venom. Toxicon **3**, 237—241 (1966)
Vidal Breard, J. J., Elias, V. E.: Bioquimica de los venonos de serpientes 1. Actividad de Lecitinase C en veneno de *Bothrops alternatus*. Arch. Farm. Bioquim. Tucman **5**, 77—85 (1950)
Vidal, J. C., Badano, B. N., Stoppani, A. O. M., Boveris, A.: Inhibition of electron transport chain by purified phospholipase A from *Bothrops neuweidi* venom. Mem. Inst. Butantan **33**, 913—920 (1966)
Vidal, J. C., Cattaneo, P., Stoppani, A. O. M.: Some characteristic properties of phospholipases A_2 from *Bothrops neuwiedii* venom. Arch. Biochem. Biophys. **151**, 168—179 (1972)
Vidal, J. C., Stoppani, A. O. M.: Inhibition of phospholipase A by a naturally occurring peptide in *Bothrops* venoms. Experientia (Basel) **26**, 831—832 (1970)
Vidal, J. C., Stoppani, A. O. M.: Isolation and properties of an inhibitor of phospholipase A from *Bothrops neuwiedii* venom. Arch. Biochem. Biophys. **147**, 66—76 (1971 a)
Vidal, J. C., Stoppani, A. O. M.: Isolation and purification of two phospholipases A from *Bothrops* venoms. Arch. Biochem. Biophys. **145**, 543—556 (1971 b)
Villegas, R., Barnola, F. V., Camejo, G.: Action of proteases and phospholipases on tetrodotoxin binding to axolemma preparations isolated from lobster nerve fibres. Biochim. biophys. Acta (Amst.) **318**, 61—68 (1973)
Vogt, W.: Pharmacologically active lipid-soluble acids of natural occurrence. Nature (Lond.) **179**, 300—304 (1957)
Vogt, W.: Liberation of pharmacology active lipids by enzymes contained in toxins. In: Raudonat, H. W. (Ed.): Recent Advances in the Pharmacology of Toxins, pp. 43—51. Oxford: Pergamon Press 1964
Vogt, W., Meyer, V., Kunze, H., Lufft, E. E., Babilli, S.: Enstehung von SRS-C in der durchströmten Meerschweinchenlunge durch Phospholipase A. Identifizierung mit Prostaglandin. Naunyn Schmiedebergs Arch. Pharmacol. **262**, 124—134 (1969)
Wagner, G. M., Mart, P. E., Kelly, R. B.: β-bungarotoxin inhibition of calcium accumulation by rat brain mitochondria. Biochem. Biophys. Res. Commun. **58**, 475—481 (1974)
Wahlström, A.: Purification and characterization of phospholipase A from the venom of *Naja nigricollis*. Toxicon **9**, 45—56 (1971)
Watkins, J. C.: Pharmacological receptors and general permeability phenomena of cell membranes. J. theor. Biol. **9**, 37—50 (1965)
Weil, A.: The effect of hemolytic toxins on nervous tissue. Arch. Path. **9**, 828—842 (1930)
Wells, M. A.: Evidence that the phospholipases A_2 of *Crotalus adamanteus* venom are dimers. Biochemistry **10**, 4074—4077 (1971)
Wells, M. A.: A simple and high yield purification of *Crotalus adamanteus* phospholipases A_2. Biochim. biophys. Acta (Amst.) **380**, 357—505 (1975)
Wells, M. A., Hanahan, D. J.: Studies on phospholipase A. I. Isolation and characterization of two enzymes from *Crotalus adamanteus* venom. Biochemistry **8**, 414—424 (1969)
Wernicke, J. F., Oberjat, T., Howard, B. D.: β neurotoxin reduces neurotransmitter storage in brain synapses. J. Neurochem. **22**, 781—788 (1974)
Wernicke, J. F., Vanker, A. D., Howard, B. D.: The mechanism of action of β-bungarotoxin. J. Neurochem. **25**, 483—496 (1975)
Whittaker, M., Charlier, A. R.: The effect of phospholipase A on human erythrocyte acetylcholinesterase. FEBS Letters **22**, 283—286 (1972)

Witter, R. F., Cottone, M. A.: The effect of lysolecithin and related compounds on the swelling of isolated mitochondria. Biochim. biophys. Acta (Amst.) **22**, 372—377 (1956)
Witter, R. F., Morrison, A., Shepardson, G. R.: Effect of lysolecithin on oxidative phosphorylation. Biochim. biophys. Acta (Amst.) **26**, 120—129 (1957)
Woelk, H., Debuch, H.: Die Wirkung der Phospholipase A aus Schlangengift auf Phosphatidylcholin, Phosphatidyläthanolamin und auf die entsprechenden Plasmalogene. Hoppe-Seylers Z. physiol. Chem. **352**, 1275—1281 (1971)
Wu, T. W., Tinker, D. O.: Phospholipase A_2 from *Crotalus atrox* venom. I. Purification and some properties. Biochemistry **8**, 1558—1568 (1969)
Yang, C. C.: Effects of crotoxin on the succinoxidase system. J. Formosan med. Ass. **53**, 59—66 (1954)
Yang, C. C., Chen, C. J., Su, C. C.: Biochemical studies on the Formosan snake venoms. IV. The toxicity of Formosan cobra venom and enzyme activities. J. Biochem. **46**, 1201—1208 (1959a)
Yang, C. C., Huang, L. C., Tung, T. C.: The activities of lecithinase A in cobra venom and crotoxin. J. Formosan med. Ass. **53**, 1—7 (1954)
Yang, C. C., Kao, K. C., Chiu, W. C.: Biochemical studies on the snake venoms. VIII. Electrophoretic studies of banded krait *(Bungarus multicinctus)* venom and the relation of toxicity with enzyme activities. J. Biochem. **48**, 714—722 (1960)
Yang, C. C., Su, C. C., Chen, C. J.: Biochemical studies on the Formosan snake venoms. V. The toxicity of hyappoda *(Agkistrodon acutus)* venom and enzyme activities. J. Biochem. **46**, 1209—1215 (1959b)
Yang, C. C., Tung, T. C.: The toxicity of Formosan snake venom on succinatecytochrome C reductase and its lecithinase A activity. J. Formosan med. Ass. **53**, 123—127 (1954)
Zeller, E. A.: Enzymes as essential components of bacterial and animal toxins. In: Sumner, J. B., Myrback, K. (Eds.): The Enzymes, Vol. 1, pt. 2, pp. 986—1013. New York: Academic Press 1951
Ziegler, F. D., Vazquez-Colon, L., Elliott, W. B., Taub, A., Gans, C.: Alteration of mitochondrial function by *Bungarus fasciatus* venom. Biochemistry **4**, 555—560 (1965)
Zlotkin, E.: Chemistry of animal venoms. Experientia (Basel) **29**, 1453—1588 (1973)

CHAPTER 13

Hemolytic Effects of Snake Venoms

E. Condrea

A. Introduction

Snake venoms evolved as specialized secretions of high efficiency in immobilizing, killing, and initiating the digestion of the prey. The red cell lysis which may develop following snakebite does not play a predominant role in the overall venom lethality, but should rather be considered as one of the manifestations of the digestive action of the venom. Snake venoms have been shown to contain factors able to attack and disorganize cellular and subcellular membranes. Hemolysis is the expression of red cell membrane distruction by the action of these venom factors which act either directly or through a complex multistep process.

The apparently controversial aspects of venom-induced hemolysis puzzled investigators for almost a century; it is only due to recently aquired knowledge on the structure of biologic membranes in general and of the red cell membrane in particular that the mechanism of hemolysis by snake venoms has been approached from a new standpoint leading to a better understanding of the events at the molecular level.

Studies on snake venoms and their components, including those involved in hemolysis, have been frequently reviewed with special emphasis on their chemistry and pharmacology (Meldrum, 1965; Jiménez-Porras, 1968, 1970; Lee, 1971, 1972; Tu, 1973). On the other hand, reviews on red cell membrane structure deal with the action of venom factors as tools in localizing the membrane phospholipids (Zwaal et al., 1973; Singer, 1974). The purpose of the present survey on venom-induced hemolysis is to integrate clinical observations with pharmacologic and biochemical data, as well as with the recent studies on red cell membrane structure.

B. Hemolysis in Envenomation

Although snake venoms are heterogenous in composition and produce multiple simultaneous effects, venoms of snakes belonging to the *Elapidae* family are predominantly neurotoxic while *Viperidae* and *Crotalidae* venoms cause mainly hemorrhages and coagulation disturbances. It has been already pointed out by Gitter and De Vries (1968) that all criteria for intravascular hemolysis, valid in the case of nonhemorrhagic venoms, may become inconclusive in the presence of internal bleeding which by itself can induce anemia, reticulocytosis, erythroid bonemarrow hyperplasia, increased indirect plasma bilirubin, increased pigment excretion, and even decreased red cell life span. Therefore, the evidence for hemolysis following snakebite or in experimental envenomation has to be carefully evaluated according to the type of venoms.

I. Elapid Venoms

Early descriptions of the hemolytic effects of elapid venoms appear in reports made by British medical officers stationed in India at the turn of the century (ROGERS, 1904; LAMB and HUNTER, 1904; CUNNINGHAM, 1968). Observing cases of snakebite in humans and experimenting with animals, it was noticed that lethal doses of cobra venom induce a decrease in red cell counts which, however, is "very far short of what would be required to produce a lethal effect" (ROGERS, 1904). It was, therefore, already clear at that time that the hemolytic action of cobra venom is of slight importance as compared with the action of venom on the nervous system. The occurrence of hemolysis following bites by various elapids has been confirmed by numerous observations. Among the snakes of the Pacific area studied by CAMPBELL (1969), the Papuan black snake, *Pseudechis papuanus*, is reported as the most strongly hemolytic, while the taipan, *Oxyuranus scutellatus*, is but weakly hemolytic. Passing of blood-stained or black urine is common following bites by Australian elapids (CAMPBELL, 1969). Reviewing the pathology of snakebites in Australia, TRETHEWIE (1971) reports evident signs of hemolysis in a lethal case of tiger *(Notechis scutatus)* snakebite and considers that the effects of hemolysis in the bite by the black snake may be extensive. In cobra bites with severe poisoning, REID (1968) found moderate hemolysis indicated by raised serum bilirubin and urine urobilinogen, a fall in hemoglobin and increased reticulocyte counts. However, in a severe krait *(Bungarus candidus)* poisoning, there was no sign of hematologic abnormality. Additional cases of probable intravascular hemolysis with hemoglobinuria in bites by elapids have been reviewed by DE VRIES and CONDREA (1971) and by GITTER and DE VRIES (1968). The role of hemolysis in the lethal effect of *Naja naja* venom has been investigated by CONDREA et al. (1969). Since, following the administration of a lethal dose of venom in mice and guinea-pigs, no evidence of hemolysis was found, the authors concluded that the more active venom components killed the animals before the hemolytic level was reached.

II. Viperid and Crotalid Venoms

Venoms of the *Viperidae* contain hemorrhagins which produce tears in the small vessels by acting directly on the vessel wall (EFRATI, 1969). Obtaining of reliable evidence for intravascular hemolysis would, therefore, require venom fractionation and administration of fractions devoid of hemorrhagins to experimental animals. However, BALOZET (1957) reported data which suggest the occurrence of intravascular hemolysis following administration of whole *Vipera lebetina* venom. In blood samples collected from envenomated guinea-pigs, the plasma was hemoglobin-colored and the red cells showed an increased osmotic fragility. Occurrence of intravascular hemolysis in dogs following intravenous administration of *Echis coloratus* venom (KLIBANSKY et al., 1966) is supported by the rise in plasma hemoglobin and the decrease in plasma haptoglobin. In the surviving animals, the maximal levels of plasma hemoglobin were reached in about 2 h following venom administration, remained elevated for at least 6 h, and returned to normal within 1 day. There was no hemoglobinuria. The red cells had a moderately increased osmotic fragility and a greatly increased mechanic fragility. It is noteworthy that inoculation of the animals with *Echis coloratus* venom devoid of procoagulant activity did not lead to hemolysis. Thus, intravascular hemolysis induced by the whole venom of *Echis coloratus* seems to be due to sensitization of the red cells by the action of the lytic factor(s) followed by trapping of the sensitized cells within the clots of fibrin promoted by the action of the procoagulant factor(s) (KLIBANSKY et al., 1966).

Like most of the vipers, venoms of snakes belonging to the *Crotalidae* family are hemorrhagic and produce anemia which is not necessarily related to intravascular hemolysis. Indeed, in systemic poisoning induced by *Agkistrodon rhodostoma*, REID (1968) reported the occurrence of anemia following hemorrhage but no hemolysis. Likewise, in monkeys injected with lethal doses of timber rattlesnake and eastern diamondback rattlesnake venoms, there was no change in hematocrit and no hemolysis (VICK, 1971). MALETTE et al. (1963) examined blood samples obtained by venous catheter from splenectomized dogs who received lethal doses of *Crotalus atrox* venom and found normal levels of plasma hemoglobin and plasma sodium. In a review on snake venoms from North America including those of the genera *Crotalus*, *Agkistrodon*, and *Sistrurus*, DEVI (1971) emphasized the contrast between their hemolytic effect in vitro and the fact that lysis in vivo is seldom observed. In a study on South American snakes, ROSENFELD (1971) reported that while there is only slight erythrocyte damage in patients bitten by *Bothrops jararaca*, envenomation due to *Crotalus durissus terrificus* leads to intense hemolysis. However, this conclusion is questionable since intravascular hemolysis is evaluated only by the degree of hemoglobinuria.

The above data indicate that hemolysis in circulating blood is more probable to occur following bites by elapids than by viperids or crotalids. Even when hemolysis does occur, its contribution to the venom toxicity is slight as compared with the venom effects on the nervous system, on the heart, the vessel walls, or on coagulation. Venoms might be lethal due to any of these effects, single or combined, well before an important hemolytic effect becomes manifest.

C. Venom Factors Involved in the Hemolytic Process

In contrast to the difficulty of obtaining definite evidence for the occurrence of intravascular hemolysis following envenomation, the addition of venom to either whole blood or to washed red blood cells was widely used as a simple and rapid means of establishing its hemolytic power. Since early work on in vitro hemolysis by snake venoms has been reviewed in detail (MELDRUM, 1965; ROSENFELD et al., 1968), the following is a brief account of the main findings.

A fundamental observation on the effects of snake venoms on red cells in vitro was made at the turn of the century. While all snake venoms are able to hemolyze human or various animal red cells "indirectly," i.e., in presence of lecithin or a source for lecithin, only a number of venoms belonging to the *Elapidae* family are lytic to washed red cells "directly," i.e., without any addition. The recognition of an enzymic reaction between a hydrolytic enzyme in venoms, phospholipase A, and lecithin as substrate accounted satisfactorily for the indirect lytic action of venoms as a two-step process: first, hydrolysis of exogenous lecithin to lysolecithin and fatty acids, second, lysis of the red blood cells by these lecithin split products (DELEZENNE and FOUR-

NEAU, 1914; DELEZENNE and LEDEBT, 1911a, b, c, d). The tendency of explaining the direct hemolysis through a similar mechanism in which the venom phospholipase acts on the lecithin contained in the red cell membrane could not account for the observation that many viperid or crotalid venoms containing a potent phospholipase A are completely inactive on washed red cells (KYES and SACHS, 1903). The mechanism of the direct hemolysis remained obscure until electrophoretic fractionation of a number of elapid venoms yielded, in addition to the phospholipase A, a protein fraction able to hemolyze red cells directly, later designated as "direct lytic factor" (DLF) (HABERMANN, 1954; HABERMANN and NEUMANN, 1954; NEUMANN and HABERMANN, 1956; GRASMANN and HANNIG, 1954; MICHL, 1954; RAUDONAT, 1955; CONDREA et al., 1964a).

The phospholipase A and the DLF are the main venom components active in hemolysis and their effects on the red cell membrane, single and in combination, will be discussed in detail.

I. Phospholipase A

Phospholipase A_2 (EC 3.1.1.4) is an esterolytic enzyme specifically catalyzing the hydrolysis of the ester bond at the C_2 position in 1,2-diacyl-sn-glycero-3-phosphatides, forming a lysoderivative and releasing a molecule of free fatty acid (VAN DEENEN and DE HAAS, 1963) (Fig. 1). The enzyme hydrolyzes naturally occurring and synthetic phosphoglycerides independently of the nature of the fatty acids present in the molecule (LONG and PENNY, 1957). Phospholipases of the A_2 type have been found in all snake venoms tested so far with the exception of the *Crotalus horridus horridus* venom (KOCHOLATY et al., 1971). The enzyme has been successfully purified from venoms of elapids, viperids, and sea snakes (see BOTES and VILJOEN, 1974a, b). BOTES and VILJOEN (1974b) were the first to establish the complete amino acid

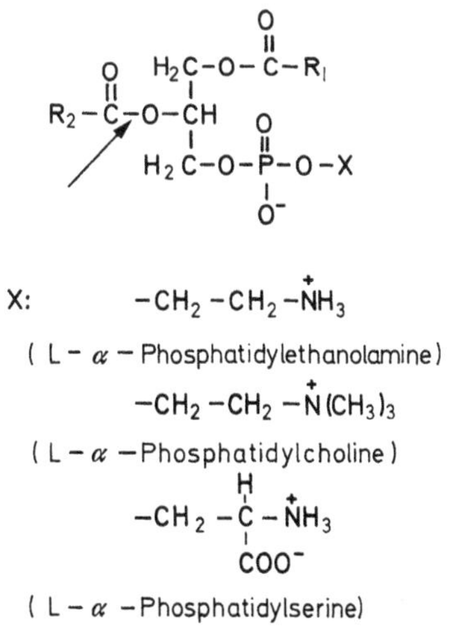

Fig. 1. Structural formula of the main phospholipid substrates for phospholipase A_2. R_1 and R_2 designate fatty acids. In naturally occurring phospholipids, R_1 is a long chain saturated fatty acid while R_2 is a long chain unsaturated one. Arrow indicates the site of enzymic hydrolysis

sequence of a snake venom phospholipase A_2, that of *Bitis gabonica*, followed by SAMEJIMA et al. (1974) who elucidated the complete amino acid sequence of the acidic phospholipase A_2-II from *Agkistrodon halys blomhoffii* venom. Molecular weight values reported for a large number of snake venom phospholipases fall within the range of 11000–14500 daltons (AUGUSTYN and ELLIOTT, 1970; TU et al., 1970; WAHLSTRÖM, 1971; SALACH et al., 1971; KAWAUCHI et al., 1971; SHILOAH et al., 1973; LO et al., 1972; HOWARD, 1975). From some venoms additional phospholipase isoenzyme with molecular weights between 20000–23000 daltons have been isolated (SALACH et al., 1971; VIDAL et al., 1972). The simultaneous presence of 15000 and 30000 dalton molecular forms in the venoms of *Crotalus atrox* (HACHIMORI et al., 1971), *Crotalus adamanteus* (WELLS, 1971, 1973), and *Bitis gabonica* (BOTES and VILJOEN, 1974a) is thought to be due to a monomer-dimer equilibrium.

While most of the phospholipases A_2 are acidic proteins, a number of basic phospholipases have been isolated from the venoms of *Crotalus durissus terrificus* (OMORI-SATOH et al., 1975), *Agkistrodon halys blomhoffii* (KAWAUCHI et al., 1971), *Naja nigricollis* (EAKER, 1975; DUMAREY et al., 1975), *Naja naja atra* (LO and CHANG, 1975), *Vipera berus* (DELORI, 1971), and *Vipera ammodytes* (GUBENSEK, 1976). Unlike the acidic phospholipases, the basic enzymes are apparently toxic (EAKER, 1975); DELORI, 1971; GUBENSEK, 1976; LO and CHANG, 1975). The data on snake venom phospholipases A_2 including methodology and enzyme characteristics, such as substrate specificity, activation by calcium and ether, inhibitors, effects of pH and buffers, heat stability, etc., have been reviewed by CONDREA and DE VRIES (1965). Recent studies on the snake venom enzyme kinetics and nature of its activation by calcium have been published by WELLS (1972) and by VILJOEN et al. (1974).

The rate of substrate hydrolysis by snake venom phospholipase A_2 is strongly dependent on the molecular packing of the phospholipid, i.e., whether present in monomeric form, aggregated in micelles or liposomes, associated with protein in soluble lipoproteins, such as in egg yolk or plasma, or in a complex structure such as in a biologic membrane.

In addition to phospholipases of the A_2 type, snake venoms also exhibit phospholipase B activity. The type B phospholipases, or lysophospholipases (EC 3.1.1.5) catalyze the hydrolysis of monoacyl phosphatides (lysophosphatides) with the release of free fatty acid and the formation of glycerophosphoryl derivatives. Phospholipase B activity in whole or boiled snake venoms has been reported by DOERY and PEARSON (1964) and by MOHAMED et al. (1969). SHILOAH et al. (1973) demonstrated phospholipase B activity in a purified phospholipase A preparation from *Vipera palestinae* venom and provided evidence for the two activities being associated with one enzyme. However, since the optimal phospholipase B activity occurs at elevated pH (over 10.5), its contribution to the degradation of membrane phospholipids at physiologic pH seems of little practical importance.

II. The Direct Lytic Factor

The DLF belongs to a group of basic polypeptides devoid of enzymic activity and of relatively low toxicity, present in the venoms of snakes belonging to the *Elapidae* family. This group of polypeptides induce a variety of pharmacologic effects which have been recognized separately in various laboratories, leading to a multiple nomenclature. Today, the basic polypeptides designated as cardiotoxin (SARKAR, 1948; LEE et al., 1968), skeletal muscle-depolarizing factor (MELDRUM, 1963), Cobramine A and B (LARSEN and WOLFF, 1968), cytotoxin (BRAGANCA et al., 1967), toxin γ (IZARD et al., 1969), DLF (CONDREA et al., 1964a), peak 12B (FRYKLUND and EAKER, 1973), and others are recognized as being closely related, if not identic (LEE et al., 1971). In a review article, CONDREA (1974) emphasized their similarity in composition and structure and, in view of their primary action being exerted at the level of the cell membrane, proposed the designation of "membrane-active polypeptides."

The membrane-active polypeptides have molecular weights ranging between 6000–7000 daltons and are, similar to phospholipase A, remarkably heat stable at acidic pH (LEE, 1972). The amino acid composition of the polypeptides from *Naja naja*, *Naja naja atra*, *Naja nigricollis*, and *Hemachatus haemachatus* venoms is similar (LEE, 1972). The amino acid sequences of cardiotoxin from *Naja naja atra* venom, of the cytotoxins I and II from *Naja naja* venom, and of the hemolytic protein 12B from *Hemachatus haemachatus* venom show remarkable homology (CONDREA, 1974). The active conformation of the molecule is stabilized by four disulfide bridges (TAKECHI and HAYASHI, 1972); reduction, carboxymethylation, or aminoethylation abolishes the direct hemolytic effect and the pharmacologic activities (HAYASHI et al., 1971; VOGT et al., 1970).

D. Nonmediated Effects of Phospholipase A and Direct Lytic Factor on the Red Cell Membrane

I. Red Cell Membrane Structure and Function

The red cell is surrounded by a membrane which forms a semipermeable boundary between the inside and the outside of the cell. One of the main functions of the red cell membrane, i.e., maintainance of an osmotic equilibrium between the hemoglobin-loaded cytoplasm and the external medium, is based on its being selectively permeable and capable of transporting solutes. Structural damage producing an alteration in the membrane's normal permeability properties and transport capacity results in entry of water, red cell swelling, stretching of the membrane, and eventually hemolysis. The total mass of the human red cell membrane consists of 49.2% protein, 43.6% lipid, and 7.6% carbohydrate (GUIDOTTI, 1972). The lipid composition and phospholipid distribution in human red cell membranes are given in Tables 1 and 2, respectively. Phosphatidylcholine (lecithin), sphingomyelin, and phosphatidylethanolamine are the major red cell phospholipids. According to a modern concept, the membrane components are organized in a fluid mosaic of lipid and protein (SINGER and NICOLSON, 1972) as illustrated in Figure 2. The membrane matrix consists of a double layer of lipid molecules whose polar ends are oriented outward while the fatty acid chain stretch inward facing each other (Fig. 2). At body temperature and in the presence of cholesterol, the membrane phospholipids are in a liquid-crystalline state presenting a remarkable degree of fluidity and lateral mobility (SINGER and NICOLSON, 1972). According to their type of association with the lipid, membrane proteins have been designated as integral and peripheral. While the integral proteins penetrate the fatty acid region of the lipid bilayer with whom they

Table 1. Lipid composition of human erythrocyte ghosts [a]

	gm × 10^{-13}/cell	μmol × 10^{-10}/cell
Total lipid	4.75	7.41
Cholesterol	1.2	3.2
Phospholipids	3.2	4.01
Glycolipids	0.18	0.2

[a] Reproduced after GUIDOTTI (1972).

Table 2. Phospholipid distribution in human erythrocyte membranes [a]

	Percent of total
Phosphatidylethanolamine	26.03
Phosphatidylcholine	28.25
Sphingomyelin	24.57
Phosphatidylserine	13.38
Phosphatidic acid	2.07
Phosphatidylinositol	1.13
Lysophosphatidylcholine	1.06
Minor components	3.52

[a] Reproduced after GUIDOTTI (1972).

interact hydrophobically, the peripheral proteins are bound by weaker, ionic bonds to the external polar region of the lipid. The structure is stabilized also by lipid-lipid and protein-protein interactions and by Ca^{++}-mediated bonds (SINGER and NICOLSON, 1972; STECK, 1974; SINGER, 1974; WALLACH, 1972). An important aspect of membrane organization is the asymmetric disposition of its components resulting in a difference in composition between the outer and inner halves of the membrane. An asymmetric arrangement of the phospholipids and cholesterol was first proposed by BRETCHER (1972a, b, 1973) and confirmed by others in studies using nonpermeant labels for the outer surface of the red cell membrane (GORDESKY and MARINETTI, 1973; WHITELEY and BERG, 1974) and by the use of phospholipases (ZWAAL et al., 1973, 1975). According to these findings, lecithin and sphingomyelin are preferentially located in the outer half of the double layer while most of phosphatidylethanolamine and all of phosphatidylserine occupy the inner, cytoplasmic half (Fig. 3). It is noteworthy that, while lecithin, phosphatidylethanolamine and phosphatidylserine are substrates for phospholipase A, sphingomyelin is not hydrolyzed by the enzyme since it does not possess the necessary structural requirements. An asymmetric arrangement has also been demonstrated for both the integral and the peripheral membrane proteins (SINGER and NICOLSON, 1972; STECK, 1974; SINGER, 1974; WALLACH, 1972).

In studies on the human red cell membrane, it was found that the integral polypeptides span the membrane exposing the N terminal, sugar-carrying end at the membrane surface, while the C terminal end extends towards the cytoplasmic side. While reaching the membrane exterior, the integral proteins do not cover the mem-

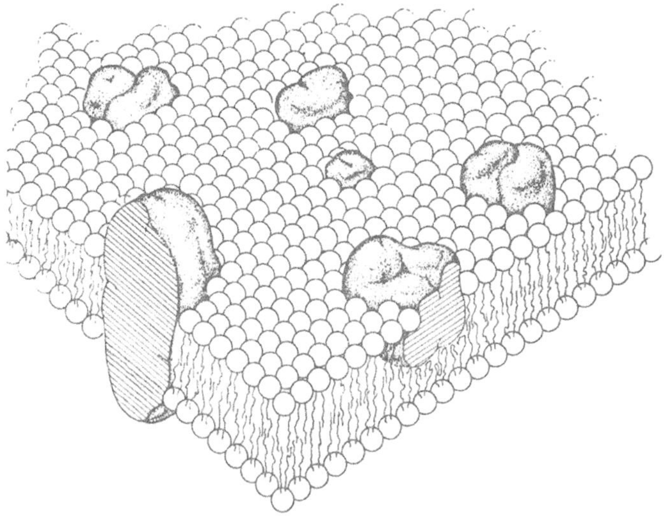

Fig. 2. The fluid mosaic model of the red cell membrane structure. The phospholipids are arranged as a discontinous bilayer, with the ionic and polar heads (open circles) in contact with water and the fatty acid chains (wavy lines) facing inward. The solid bodies, partially embedded in the lipid bilayer, represent the globular integral proteins. The peripheral proteins are not represented. After SINGER and NICOLSON (1972)

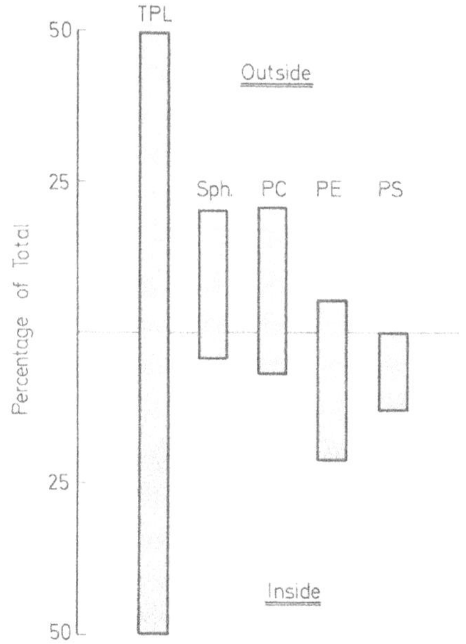

Fig. 3. Proposed distribution of phospholipids between inner and outer layer of the human erythrocyte membrane. Abbreviations: TPL, total phospholipid; Sph, sphingomyelin; PC, lecithin; PE, phosphatidylethanolamine; PS, phosphatidylserine. Reproduced after VERKLEJ et al. (1973)

brane surface (STECK, 1974). Since the peripheral proteins, mainly spectrin and actin, are localized in a network along the inner, cytoplasmic side of the membrane, it results that, at the membrane exterior, lipid is mostly exposed.

II. Action of Phospholipases on Red Cell Membrane Phospholipids

1. Nonlytic Phospholipid Degradation

Phospholipases A_2 from various snake venoms differ in their ability to hydrolyze phospholipids in washed, saline-suspended human red blood cells. Thus, *Naja naja* phospholipase hydrolyzes up to 70% of the membrane lecithin, an amount which represents about 20% of total membrane phospholipid (GUL and SMITH, 1974; ZWAAL et al., 1975). Similar results have been obtained with the bee venom phospholipase A which, in addition, hydrolyzes about 10% of the membrane phosphatidyl ethanolamine (GUL and SMITH, 1974; ZWAAL et al., 1975). From these results and from data on phospholipid labeling by nonpenetrating reagents, it was concluded that about 70% of the lecithin and 10% of the phosphatidylethanolamine are located in the outer half of the membrane and exposed to the cell exterior. In contradistinction, *Crotalus adamanteus* (ZWAAL et al., 1975) and *Vipera palestinae* (CONDREA et al., 1964a) phospholipases fail to hydrolyze any of the phospholipid substrates in intact erythrocytes. The unequal ability of phospholipases A_2 from various sources to reach and hydrolyze substrates in the membrane points to structural differences between the enzyme molecules.

It is noteworthy that degradation of phospholipids in intact human red cells by venom phospholipases is limited to the outer layer and does not result in hemolysis. Apparently, the membrane structure is preserved at a sufficient degree by the presence of an important amount of intact sphingomyelin in the outer layer, together with the fact that the phospholipid split products, lysophospholipids, and fatty acids do not leave the membrane. Indeed, removal of the lysolecithin and fatty acids from the membrane by albumin results in red cell lysis, and a good correlation between the degree of phospholipid splitting and of hemolysis is obtained (GUL and SMITH, 1974; GUL et al., 1974). It might be surprising that, while lysolecithin and fatty acids are lytic when added to red cells, their production in situ does not result in membrane lysis as long as they are retained within the membrane.

It is noteworthy that a strongly basic phospholipase A from *Naja nigricollis* venom was found able to hemolyze red cells directly (DUMAREY et al., 1975). The joined presence on the same polypeptide chain of an enzymic site, strong electropositive charge, and proper configuration might account for this unusual property.

Unlike their limited hydrolysis in the intact erythrocytes, the hydrolysis of phospholipid substrates in the membranes of osmotically prepared "leaky" ghosts by most venom phospholipases proceeds to completion (ZWAAL et al., 1975). This finding is of interest since it indicates that the membrane of osmotically prepared ghosts differs from that of the intact erythrocytes as evidenced by the increased phospholipid exposure to the enzyme action. It is not known, however, whether in leaky ghosts the enzyme penetrates the membrane and hydrolyzes the substrate from both the external and internal sides of the lipid double layer or whether the enzyme is able to "eat its way" through the thickness of the membrane starting from outside. *Vipera palestinae* (CONDREA et al., 1964a) and *Dendroaspis polylepsis* (IBRAHIM and MASR, 1975) phospholipases are so far exceptions since they do not hydrolyze phospholipids in leaky ghosts.

2. Lytic Phospholipid Degradation

We have shown above that in the membranes of intact, saline-suspended red cells, phospholipid hydrolysis is limited and hemolysis does not occur. However, if the red cell membrane is subjected to certain treatments producing little or no hemolysis per se, the phospholipase becomes able to hydrolyze extensively the phospholipid substrates and hemolysis occurs. WOODWARD and ZWAAL (1972) demonstrated that hypotonically swollen human erythrocytes expose their phospholipids to the action of pancreatic phospholipase A, with subsequent lysis of the cells. LANKISCH et al. (1972b) showed that bile salts, lysolecithin, and saponin, at sublytic concentrations, potentiate the phospholipase A-induced hemolysis probably by modifying the membrane structure and facilitating the access of the enzyme to the membrane lipid bilayer. Facilitation of phospholipid splitting in human erythrocytes ghosts by *Vipera palestinae* phospholipase in the presence of detergents had been previously described by CONDREA et al. (1964a). A special case of lytic red cell phospholipid degradation is that induced by the synergistic effect of the two venom factors, DLF and phospholipase A, which will be dealt with in more detail.

III. Action of the Direct Lytic Factor on the Red Cell Membrane

1. Direct Hemolysis

The membrane-active polypeptides isolated from snake venoms are characterized by a direct lytic effect on washed red blood cells suspended in isotonic media, thus being designated as DLFs (CONDREA et al., 1964a) or "hemolytic proteins" (FRYKLUND and EAKER, 1973). The degree of hemolysis is dependent on the type of red cells. When subjected to the action of DLF, erythrocytes from various animal species exhibit a range of sensitivities, guinea-pig and dog erythrocytes being the most susceptible, human and rabbit having a moderate susceptibility, while camel and sheep erythrocytes are entirely resistant (CONDREA et al., 1964b). The relatively low susceptibility of human erythrocytes to the lytic action of membrane-active polypeptides might explain the report on toxin γ as being nonlytic (IZARD et al., 1969). Indeed, in experiments with Ringhals *(Hemachatus haemachatus)* venom DLF, using concentrations up to 200 μg/ml, hemolysis of human erythrocytes did not exceed 10% (KLIBANSKY et al., 1968; CONDREA et al., 1970). JACOBI et al. (1972) and OLDINGS et al. (1971) showed rat erythrocytes to be completely resistant to amounts of *Naja naja* DLF which induced 26% hemolysis of guinea-pig erythrocytes; 50 times more DLF was needed to produce a similar degree of hemolysis. LEE et al. (1971) reported a range of sensitivities to the lytic action of *Naja naja atra* cardiotoxin for erythrocytes from nine species and ZAHEER et al. (1975) listed the sensitivity of erythrocytes from 15 species to the lytic action of *Naja naja* cytotoxic proteins, both being in full agreement with the previous data.

2. Attachment to Membranes

Studies with ^{131}I-DLF indicated that the polypeptide becomes bound to erythrocytes from human, guinea-pig, and sheep in amounts which correlate with their specific sensitivity towards DLF-induced hemolysis (CONDREA et al., 1965). The capacity of erythrocyte ghosts to bind DLF was found to be superior to that of the intact cells, while the amount bound per unit area bears no relationship to the type of red cell sensitivity. Studying binding of DLF to guinea-pig red cells by an immunofluorescence technique, SCHROETER et al. (1973) found that the intact cells do not bind DLF, the binding being restricted to ghosts. Thus, the small amounts bound by cell suspensions would reflect the presence of ghosts formed by lysis. The failure to find bound DLF in amounts detectable by this method does not exclude the possibility that an interaction with the intact cell does take place. The authors consider the massive binding of DLF to ghosts as probably unrelated to the actual mechanism of DLF attack on intact cells since the attachment is largely temperature-independent, while the lytic effect of DLF is completely absent at temperatures below 15° C (SCHROETER et al., 1973).

3. Effects on Membrane Permeability and Transport

The fact that membrane-active polypeptides from various snake venoms inhibit transport of various classes of compounds in a variety of tissues reflects the general nature of this phenomenon (for review see CONDREA, 1974). The question was raised as to whether membrane-active polypeptides produce this effect by interaction with specific carriers, by interference with metabolically activated pump systems, or by increasing in a nonspecific way the membrane permeability. A number of data obtained on red blood cells suggest that the DLFs induce membrane leakiness. Thus, JACOBI et al. (1972) showed that the moderate hemolysis and increased osmotic fragility of guinea-pig red cells induced by *Naja naja* DLF are accompanied by an increased passive permeability to Na^+ ions. At the same time, the activity of the pump ATPase in human and guinea pig erythrocytes is little or not affected (LANKISH et al., 1972a). Furthermore, the efflux rate of Na^+ from preloaded human erythrocytes remains normal (LARSEN and WOLFF, 1967), suggesting that inhibition of active transport is not involved in the hemolytic mechanism. These findings, however, are at variance with the data obtained on other tissues, i.e., inhibition of $(Na^+ + K^+)$-ATPase of ox brain (LANKISH et al., 1972a) and Na^+ pump of toad bladder (LARSEN and WOLFF, 1967). While an inhibition of the active Na^+ transport in intact red cells by DLF is still questioned, recent data reported by ZAHEER et al. (1975) demonstrate unequivocally that the cytotoxic protein from cobra venom is able to inactivate the $(Na^+ + K^+)$-ATPase of human and dog erythrocyte membrane preparations, the extent of the inhibition being proportional to the sensitivity of the respective red cells to the lytic action of the protein.

It can, therefore, be reasonably concluded that the DLFs initially induce a perturbation of the red cell membrane permeability which may lead, in certain cases, to an impairment of the active transport. Since cellular membranes differ in composition and organization, it is not surprising that they exhibit different sensitivities to the disrupting action of the DLFs. The membrane activity of these venom polypeptides is further exemplified by their capacity to depolarize membranes of excitable cells, to affect the activity of membrane-bound enzymes, and to produce cytotoxic effects mainly in neoplastic cells (for review, see CONDREA, 1974).

IV. Synergistic Action of Phospholipase A and the Direct Lytic Factor

We have shown above that pure venom phospholipases A produce a limited membrane phospholipid hydrolysis and are nonlytic to washed red cells, while purified DLF has no enzymic action but induces a moderate degree of hemolysis in sensitive red cells. However, human red cells treated with a mixture of phospholipase A and DLF are strongly hemolyzed (CONDREA et al., 1964a). Thus, the presence of both phospholipase A and DLF in elapid venoms explains their known ability to lyse rapidly and completely washed red blood cells from human and a number of animal species, an effect known as direct hemolysis, on whose basis the respective venoms were designated as direct lytic. The term is correct only in as far as it implies that no exogenous substance is needed for hemolysis to occur, in contrast to the indirect lytic venoms which lyse red cells only in the presence of added phospholipids. However, it should be clear that direct hemolysis by elapid venoms is the result of the synergistic action of two venom factors on the red cell membrane.

The observation by CONDREA et al. (1964a) that hemolysis induced by the combined action of DLF and phospholipase A is associated with progressive splitting of membranal phospholipids helped clarify the mechanism of the potentiated hemolysis. While in intact cells hydrolysis of the membrane phospholipid substrates by phospholipase A is limited to lecithin and phosphatidylethanolamine present in the outer half of the double layers, under the action of DLF, a membrane structural change is produced which allows access of the enzyme to the depth of the lipid matrix. When, by progressive hydrolysis, the lipid double layer is loosened and the cells start to hemolyze, the phospholipase continues its hydrolytic action on the newly formed ghosts. The capacity of DLF to modify the membrane structure as evidenced by an increased availability of its phospholipids to hydrolysis by phospholipase A has also been demonstrated on red cell osmotic ghosts. Thus, while the cobra venom phospholipase hydrolyzes freely phospholipids in osmotic ghosts, *Vipera palestinae* phospholipase does so only when supplemented with DLF (CONDREA et al., 1964a).

Synergistic actions between the membrane-active polypeptides and phospholipase A have also been demonstrated on membranes other than the red cell (CONDREA, 1974). A characteristic of the synergistic action is the necessity for the simultaneous presence of DLF and phospholipase A during the reaction (CONDREA et al., 1964a; CHANG et al., 1972).

V. Mode of Action of the Direct Lytic Factor

The membrane-active polypeptides are able to disturb the normal membrane architecture and impair membrane function. Regarding the mechanism by which this result is achieved, two different approaches have been advanced so far.

One view is concerned both with the direct lytic effect and with the phospholipid splitting-facilitating action of the polypeptide. According to this view, the electropositively charged DLF becomes first attached to the red cell membrane owing to electrostatic interactions and then penetrates the membrane structure through its lipophilic residues. It is conceivable that, in the presence of phospholipase A which initiates the hydrolysis of phospholipid substrates in the outer half of the membrane, penetration of DLF is facilitated and this, in turn, paves the way for further hydrolysis. The looseness of the initial interaction between DLF and the intact erythrocyte is suggested by its easy removal with saline washings (CONDREA et al., 1965). Removal of DLF by saline washings might also account for the failure of detecting it on the red cell membrane by immunofluorescence (SCHROETER et al., 1973). This mode of action would resemble that of the lytic protein from bee venom, melittin, which disrupts membranes by penetrating their lipid region with which it interacts hydrophobically (SESSA et al., 1969; WILLIAMS and BELL, 1972; MOLLAY and KREIL, 1973). In their studies on the cytotoxic protein P_6 from *Naja naja* venom, ZAHEER et al. (1975) expressed a similar view. Their observations are taken to indicate that the protein P_6, due to its highly basic nature and specificity of structure, is able to penetrate the membrane lipid layer and combine with the acidic phospholipids, i.e., phosphatidic acid and phosphatidylserine, thus causing a disturbance in the conformation of the $(Na^+ + K^+)$-ATPase complex. Furthermore, VINCENT et al. (1976) studied the association of *Naja mossambica* cardiotoxin with axonal membranes by direct binding measurements. The high amount of binding suggests an association of the toxin with the lipid phase of the membrane. This would occur as a two-step process: first, a rapid and reversible association, then a rearrangement of the membrane structure which induces irreversible inactivation of the $(Na^+ + K^+)$-ATPase.

More direct evidence for an interaction of the membrane-active polypeptides with the phospholipids as a prerequisite for enhanced hydrolysis by phospholipase A is derived from a study on lecithin liposomes. MOLLAY and KREIL (1974) found that hydrolysis of egg lecithin liposomes by venom phospholipase A was enhanced by the DLFs from *Naja naja* and *Hemachatus haemachatus* venoms as well as by melittin. Stimulation of the phospholipase action by the polypeptides was found closely linked with their ability of complex formation with the lecithin substrate. Both complex formation and stimulation of the phospholipase required phospholipid fluidity and were observed only at temperatures at which the substrate was in a liquid crystalline state (MOLLAY and KREIL, 1974). It might be relevant that the lytic action of DLF is also strongly temperature-dependent (SCHROETER et al., 1973). Further support for this view derives from the study of a number of synthetic basic polymers and copolymers as possible DLF substitutes in inducing direct hemolysis and promoting phospholipid splitting by phospholipase A in osmotic ghosts (KLIBANSKY et al., 1968). The common characteristic of the active copolymers is the presence of both basic and lipophilic groups such as in polyornithine-leucine, polyornithine-leucine-alanine, and polylysine-leucine. The basicity of the polypeptides is held responsible for their attachment to the membrane, whereas the lipophilic side chains are invoked in the facilitation of the approach of phospholipase to phospholipid substrates situated in the membrane. Protamine (CONDREA et al., 1964a) and the basic polymers polylysine and polyornithine (KLIBANSKY et al., 1968) failed to duplicate the synergistic action of DLF with phospholipase A on human red cell membrane but were moderately lytic and able to inhibit I^- accumulation by thyroid slices, although to a lesser extent than cobramine B (WOLFF et al., 1968). A polylysine with average molecular weight of 14000 was found optimal for the inhibitory effect.

Polyarginine was also inhibitory but the respective monomers were not. Inactive were the natural basic proteins, ribonuclease, spermine, lysosyme, and histones (WOLFF et al., 1968).

However similar, the activity of the analogues is not identic to that of the venom polypeptides, and the conclusions drawn by comparison should be cautious. Thus, the basic copolymers which promote splitting of red cell phospholipids by phospholipase A are, unlike DLF, markedly lytic. Moreover, they migrate in lipid solvents on chromatography, while DLF does not (KLIBANSKY et al., 1968).

One characteristic of the synergistic action of DLF with phospholipase A is the necessity for their simultaneous presence, which suggests that DLF participates not only as a membrane modifier but also as a mediator in binding the enzyme to the membrane substrate (CONDREA et al., 1964a, 1970). The cationic groups of the membrane-active polypeptide might perform this function in a way similar to the mechanism of enzyme activation by Ca^{++} ions through formation of an enzyme-Ca-substrate complex (DE HAAS et al., 1971). Indeed, DLF and Ca^{++} are interchangeable as activators of phospholipid splitting in erythrocyte ghosts by *Vipera palestinae* phospholipase (CONDREA et al., 1970). However, here again, the similarity is limited since DLF does not replace Ca^{++} in nonmembranal systems while Ca^{++} does not replace DLF in mediating hemolysis and phospholipid hydrolysis by phospholipase A in the intact erythrocyte (CONDREA et al., 1970; LANKISCH et al., 1971).

It has been repeatedly reported that relatively high Ca^{++} concentrations (~ 10 m*M*) antagonize a number of pharmacologic effects of the membrane-active polypeptides from snake venoms in a variety of systems (for review, see CONDREA, 1974; LIN SHIAU et al., 1973, 1975, 1976). Moreover, direct measurements with labeled cardiotoxins demonstrate that Ca^{++} in high concentrations interferes with binding of the toxins to axons (VINCENT et al., 1976) or to skeletal muscle (LIN SHIAU et al., 1976). Based on these findings, as well as on additional experimental evidence, LIN SHIAU and her group (LIN SHIAU et al., 1973, 1975, 1976) support the view that cardiotoxin acts primarily on the membrane Ca^{++} binding sites. While cardiotoxin specifically releases membrane Ca^{++}, melittin, which has similar pharmacologic actions, would induce an overall increase of the ionic permeability of the membrane (LIN SHIAU et al., 1975). This approach does not necessarily contradict the assumption of an interaction between cardiotoxin and the membrane phospholipids which are likely candidates as Ca^{++} binding sites (FORSTNER and MANERY, 1971).

A different view in interpreting the mode of action of the venom polypeptides on red cell membranes has been advanced by VOGT et al. (1970). In their view, the potentiation of phospholipase A hemolysis by DLF is due to an alteration of the red cell membrane structure caused by the interaction of DLF with SH groups in the membrane. Combination of electropositive charge with disulfide bonds is considered to be the structural feature enabling DLF and a number of peptide analogues such as an apamine fraction, vasopressin, anaphylatoxin (VOGT et al., 1970), and viscotoxin B (LANKISCH and VOGT, 1971) to promote hemolysis by phospholipase A. VOGT et al. (1970) considered the direct and the potentiated hemolysis with phospholipase A as independent of the detergent property of DLF, since, by reduction, the lytic activities are abolished while the detergent effect is not. In addition, synthetic SH reagents like p-chloromercurybenzoate and N-ethylmaleimide, which are devoid of detergent properties, mimic the action of DLF when combined with phospholipase A. However, the basic membrane-active polypeptide from bee venom, melittin, potentiates the phospholipase A while being devoid of S-S bridges. An additional argument in favor of a possible interaction between the disulfide bonds of DLF and the SH groups of membrane proteins derives from the positive correlation between glutathione reductase activity and sensitivity to DLF in erythrocytes of various animal species (SCHROETER et al., 1972). The mode by which high enzyme activity would enhance the sensitivity to DLF rather that protect the cells against it is not easily explained. SCHROETER et al. (1972) considered the possibility of a dual action; first cleavage of the S-S bonds of DLF at the membrane site, enabling binding to a membrane constituent by new S-S bridges, and second, reduction of this bond and detachment of DLF.

The interaction of the disulfide bonds in DLF with membrane SH groups is still to be directly tested. Loss of activity by reduction of DLF does not necessarily demonstrate such as interaction; an alternative interpretation might be that reduction results in unfolding of the polypeptide and loss of the proper configuration which might be instrumental for its membrane activity. As VOGT et al. (1970) pointed out, there are several possibilities of enhancing hemolysis and phospholipid cleavage by phospholipase A. The basic requisite is that the red cell membrane be modified and the access of the enzyme to its substrate in the membrane be facilitated. This has been achieved by hypotonic media which induce membrane stretching, by SH reagents which interfere with the membrane proteins, or by detergents which interact with the membrane lipid. The direct effect of venom polypeptides on protein-free liposomes (MOLLAY and KREIL, 1974) and their detergent-like properties would range them in the last category.

VI. Sensitivity of Erythrocytes from Various Animal Species to Venom-Induced Hemolysis

When washed red blood cells from various animal species are subjected to the action of a direct lytic venom, a range of sensitivities becomes evident, some red cells being easily hemolyzed, others moderately, and a number being completely resistant. Earlier reports on various red cell sensitivities were difficult to interpret for the obvious reason that the red cells were tested undiscriminately with and without addition of serum, the latter being either homologous or heterologous, fresh or following heat inactivation; furthermore, both direct and indirect lytic venoms were compared without distinction (ROSENFELD et al., 1968; KELLAWAY and WILLIAMS, 1933a, b; ROSENFELD et al., 1960–1962; KELEN et al., 1960–1962). A further source of confusion was the effect of increasing venom concentrations on the degree of hemolysis. Venoms tested in amounts as high as 20 mg/ml (ROSENFELD et al., 1960–1962) or even 40 mg/0.3 ml (KELLAWAY and WILLIAMS, 1933a) were found less hemolytic than in low concentrations. In order to account for hemolytic curves obtained with venoms ranging in concentrations up to 20 mg/ml, ROSENFELD et al. (1960–1962) had to postulate the existence of as many as seven hemolytic components and of six types of venoms.

However, regarding the red cells from various sources, a range of sensitivities emerged which is, in decreasing order: guinea pig > human > rabbit > horse > sheep, the latter being completely resistant (KELLAWAY and WILLIAMS, 1933a, b).

Table 3. Approximate ratios of leicithin: sphingomyelin in erythrocytes of various species[a]

	Lecithin: sphingomyelin ratio
Rat, dog, guinea-pig	4: 1
Horse	3: 1
Human, rabbit	3: 2
Pig, cat	1: 1
Cow, sheep, goat	1:12
Camel[b]	1: 3

[a] After ZWAAL et al. (1973).
[b] Ratio calculated from the data of LIVNE and KUIPER (1973).

The effect of *Vipera ammodytes* venom on the red cells of 73 vertebrate species, both directly and in the presence of inactivated horse serum, was reported by LIVREA (1958). The absence of direct hemolysis in most of the red cells tested is in agreement with the *Vipera* venoms being devoid of DLF and unable to induce hemolysis of washed red cells. It is noteworthy that in the red cells of only three animals—the carp, trout, and the blue-faced cercopithecus—direct hemolysis did occur, suggesting that in the membranes of these cells the phospholipid substrates are reached by the venom phospholipase directly without the mediation of DLF.

One of the first attempts to explain the range of red cell sensitivities was made by TURNER (1957), who related it to the erythrocyte lecithin content. The resistance to hemolysis by whole cobra venom of erythrocytes almost devoid of lecithin and the high susceptibility of lecithin-rich cells was taken as proof that the hemolytic venom agent is the phospholipase and that hemolysis results from the hydrolysis of the substrate in membranes. In order to account for the high resistance of lecithin-containing camel erythrocytes, TURNER et al. (1958a, b) introduced the notion of lecithin "availability" to the action of the venom enzyme. TURNER's data concerning the phospholipid composition of erythrocytes from various animal species have been confirmed and detailed by other investigators (CONDREA et al., 1974b; ZWAAL et al., 1973). Thus, in the order of decreasing sensitivities to the lytic action of cobra venom, the amount of red cell lecithin decreases, being compensated by a rise in sphingomyelin, while the other phospholipids do not change significantly. This variation is well-illustrated by the decrease in lecithin/sphingomyelin ratio which, except for the camel erythrocytes, parallels the decrease in red cell sensitivity (Table 3).

The explanation offered by TURNER (1957) and TURNER et al. (1958) was questioned when it appeared that purified cobra and sea snake venom phospholipases are unable to hemolyze washed red cells of those species which contain lecithin in high proportion (ZWAAL et al., 1973), even if most of the lecithin becomes hydrolyzed (IBRAHIM and THOMPSON, 1965; GUL and SMITH, 1972).

Recognition of the direct hemolysis as a synergistic effect due to two venom factors, phospholipase A and DLF (CONDREA et al., 1964a) prompted a different approach to the problem of red cell sensitivities. Thus, CONDREA et al. (1964b) provided evidence for the concept that red cell sensitivity to cobra venom is primarily a reflexion of their susceptibility to the action of the venom DLF. First, the sequence of sensitivities of various erythrocytes to whole cobra venom is the same as the sequence of their sensitivity to the lytic action of the DLF. The second argument is derived from the action of the DLF and *Vipera palestinae* phospholipase on osmotic ghosts. *Vipera palestinae* phospholipase is unable to attack phospholipids in ghosts derived from human (CONDREA et al., 1964a) or any of the animal erythrocytes studied (CONDREA et al., 1964b). Whereas the DLF is able to render the phospholipids in osmotic ghosts derived from sensitive erythrocytes available to the action of *Vipera palestinae* phospholipase, it is unable to do so with osmotic ghosts derived from the resistant erythrocytes (CONDREA et al., 1964b). The difference in sensitivity of the whole cells and of the osmotic ghosts to the action of the DLF is in contrast to the nonselective effect of cobra phospholipase on osmotic ghosts and of *Vipera palestinae* phospholipase on ghosts solubilized by detergents, when full phospholipid hydrolysis results irrespective of species sensitivity.

OLDINGS et al. (1971) support the view that specific sensitivities to cobra venom derive from susceptibility not only to DLF but also to the phospholipase. Comparing time/hemolysis curves of sensitive guinea-pig erythrocytes with those of more resistant rat erythrocytes, they found that similar curves can be obtained by using, with the rat cells, 50-fold more DLF and 100-fold more phospholipase.

There is little doubt that specific factors of membrane composition and organization in the red cell membranes are the basis of their different susceptibility. It is noteworthy that the sequence of red cell sensitivities to the DLF and to whole cobra venom is in good agreement with the sequence of red cell permeabilities for agents such as glycerol, ethyleneglycol, urea, and thiourea, related by the group of VAN DEENEN (KÖGL et al., 1960; DE GIER and VAN DEENEN, 1961; DE GIER et al., 1961) to variations in their lecithin and sphingomyelin content and fatty acid pattern. For the resistant camel erythrocyte, it seems that it is not the lipid distribution (LIVNE and KUIPER, 1973) but rather the unique features of protein content and organization (EITAN et al., 1976) which might account for its particular properties. Since membrane phospholipids are asymmetrically distributed with a preference of the choline-containing phospholipids, lecithin, and sphingomyelin, for the outer half, it results that, in lecithin-poor cells, there are essentially no glycerophospholipid substrates on the outside of the membrane (ZWAAL et al., 1973). It is conceivable that this particular distribution, possibly together with variations in protein composition (ZWAAL and VAN DEENEN, 1968), is responsible for their resistance to DLF per se as well as for their general low permeability. In addition, phospholipase A will not initiate hydrolysis at the cell surface and the synergistic action between the two venom factors will not proceed.

E. Mediated Effects of Venom Phospholipase A

I. The Disk-Sphere Transformation

1. In Vitro Red Cell Shape Changes

In vitro treatment of normal human blood with indirect lytic snake venoms does not produce hemolysis but initiates a marked change in the red cell morphology, the normal bidiscoids becoming spheres. As a consequence, stacking of the red cells in piles, known as rouleaux formation, is prevented and their sedimentation rate inhib-

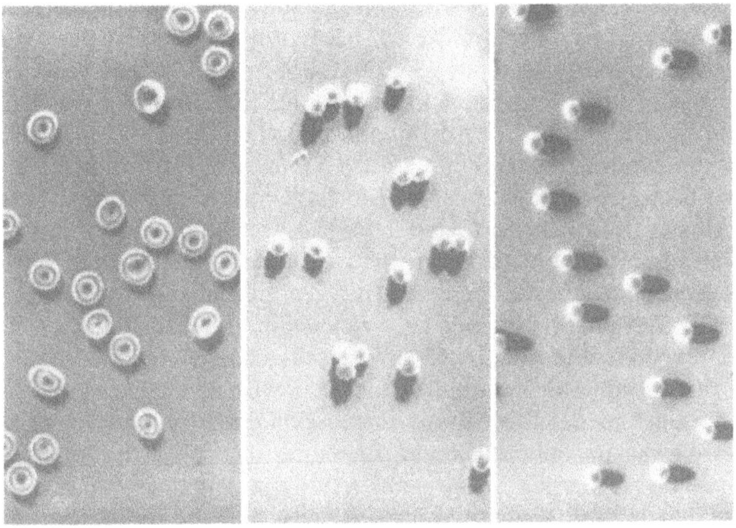

Fig. 4. Disk-sphere transformation of red cells in human blood treated with *Vipera palestinae* venom. Shadow-casted smears, all at the same magnification. Left: no venom. Normal bidiscoid red cells. Middle: 0.5 μg venom/ml blood. Crenated, spherocytic red cells. Right: 6 μg venom/ml blood. Spherocytic red cells. Reproduced after GITTER et al. (1959)

ited. This phenomenon, described in as early as 1883 by MITCHELL and REICHERT and repeatedly reported by others (for review, see BALOZET, 1962) was studied in more detail by BERGENHEM and FAHRAEUS (1936) and BERGENHEM (1939). These authors rightly attributed the red cell shape change to the production of lysolecithin by the action of a venom enzyme on plasma lecithin and considered it to be a step prior to hemolysis. More recently, investigations on the disk-sphere transformation by means of *Vipera palestinae* venom (GITTER et al., 1959) provided additional information. Thus, it was shown that as little as 5 μg of the venom added to 1 ml of whole blood causes practically instantaneous sphering of all red blood cells, prevention of rouleaux formation, and inhibition of sedimentation (Fig. 4). Washed, saline-suspended red blood cells maintain their bidiscoidal shape in the presence of venom. The sphered cells can be reversed to bidiscoids by washings with normal plasma or albumin solutions but not with saline. Sphered cells show increased osmotic and mechanical fragilities; after reversion to bidiscoids, both the osmotic and mechanical fragilities remain above normal (BERWALD, 1960; CONDREA et al., 1961). BALOZET (1962) studied a large number of snake venoms and found that, with the exception of *Dendroaspis angusticeps* venom, they were all able to induce red cell sphering, although being of variable potency. Since red cell sphering is induced by lysolecithin resulting from the action of the venom phospholipase, it follows that all venoms tested, with the exception of *Dendroaspis*, possess the enzyme.

The view of BERGENHEM and FAHRAEUS (1936) that red cell sphering is an initial stage in the process of hemolysis was at first challenged by GITTER et al. (1959) and BALOZET (1962). Their argument was that, if both the sphering factor and the hemolytic factor resulted from splitting of the plasma lecithin, the amounts of venom necessary for induction of the two phenomena should be in a constant ratio. In fact, this ratio was found to differ by several orders of magnitude between venoms from different snake families (BALOZET, 1962). Moreover, while cobra venom is strongly hemolytic, *Vipera palestinae* venom in an amount 20000 times larger than the minimal amount producing spherocytosis is still nonlytic (GITTER et al., 1959). This was taken to mean that the lysolecithin is not the common agent producing both spherocytosis and hemolysis. These apparent contradictions were clarified by subsequent studies. Using an optic method to determine the morphologic change, AVI-DOR et al. (1960) established that the sphering factor is indeed the product of an enzymic reaction between an enzyme present in the venom and the plasma phospholipids. The action of the sphering factors, i.e., lysolecithin and fatty acids, on the red cells being instantaneous, the rate at which red cells change shape reflects the rate of production of the sphering factors. The fact that, with normal human blood, red cell sphering does not proceed to hemolysis was explained by two factors: the limited amount of plasma phospholipids and, therefore, of evolved lysoproducts and the protective action of the plasma proteins (AVI-DOR et al., 1960). In a quantitative study of the interaction between human red cells and the lysolecithin produced in plasma by the action of *Vipera palestinae* venom, a correlation was established between the amount of lysolecithin attached to the cell and the cell shape (KLIBANSKY and DE VRIES, 1963). Thus, attachment of about 10^{-11} μmol lysolecithin per cell produces crenated bidiscoids and 1.3×10^{-11} μmol per cell produces crenated spheres while amounts above 2×10^{-11} μmol per cell result in smooth spheres. All these shape changes are associated with inhibition of rouleaux formation. In normal human blood, the maximal amount of lysolecithin adsorbed per cell does not exceed 2.6×10^{-11} μmol, this being below what is required for the production of hemolysis. It is noteworthy that, in human blood, only 20% of the lysolecithin produced becomes attached to the cell, the rest being associated with the plasma proteins. Reversion of the sphered red cells to bidiscoids by albumin washing is accompanied by removal of the adsorbed lysolecithin (KLIBANSKY and DE VRIES, 1963).

The other product of the enzymic hydrolysis of lecithin, the fatty acids, are also able to induce erythrocyte shape changes and inhibition of sedimentation, when present in sublytic amounts. The question has been asked whether the main sphering agent in the venom-treated blood is lysolecithin or the fatty acids. DE VRIES et al. (1960) demonstrated that in postheparin blood which contains lipoprotein lipase, red cell shape changes occur due to the attachment of fatty acids liberated from plasma triglycerides. However, while in venom-treated blood, sphering occurs at a level of 1.1 m equivalent/l of the fatty acid and correspondingly lysophospholipid, in postheparin blood in which there is no production of lysolecithin, sphering occurs only at a fatty acid level as high as 2 mequivalent/l.

A molecular mechanism for the erythrocyte shape changes induced by various agents was proposed by SHEETZ and SINGER (1974). In their concept, the membrane, whose proteins and polar lipids are distributed asymetrically in the two halves of the membrane bilayer, can act as bilayer couples, i.e., the two halves can respond differently to a perturbation. It is proposed that substances which intercalate into the lipid in the exterior half of the bilayer expand that layer relative to the cytoplasmic half, and thereby induce the cell to crenate. Fatty acids and other anionic amphipathic compounds, such as 2,4-dinitrophenol and barbiturates, together with lysolecithin

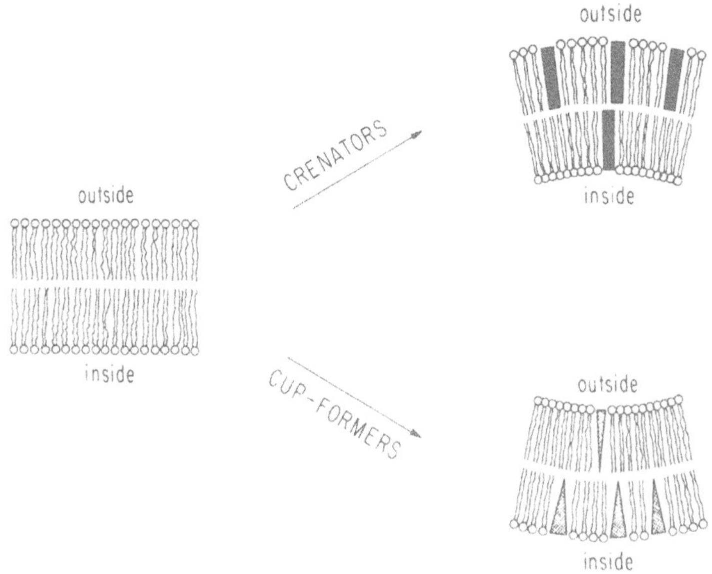

Fig. 5. Schematic representation of the proposed binding of amphipathic compounds that are crenators or cup formers to the phospholipid regions of the erythrocyte membrane. Reproduced after SHEETZ and SINGER (1974)

which is amphipathic without being anionic, belong to the class of crenators. Furthermore, it is proposed that all amphipathic compounds that bind to the membrane but cannot diffuse across it at a significant rate are crenators, since they must perforce concentrate in the lipid portion of the exterior half. Cationic amphipathic compounds, such as phenothiazine tranquilizers and local anesthetics, penetrate into the cytoplasmic half of the membrane probably interacting with phosphatidyl-serine. As a consequence, the inner layer expands and causes the cell to form cup shapes (Fig. 5). At sufficiently high concentrations, both crenators and cup formers cause the erythrocytes to become spheric and lyse (SHEETZ and SINGER, 1974).

2. In Vivo Red Cell Shape Changes

Red cell crenation, spherocytosis, and inhibition of the sedimentation rate have been observed not only in vitro but also in experimental envenomation with indirect lytic venoms. BALOZET (1962) found that intraperitoneal administration of *Vipera lebetina* venom to guinea-pigs produces such effects only at very high doses. DANON et al. (1961) showed that red cell shape changes occurred in rabbits and rats injected with both lethal and sublethal doses of *Vipera palestinae* venom. The higher the amount of venoms, the earlier the changes appeared. With sublethal doses of the venom, the deformed red cells reverted slowly to bidiscoids. In no instance were ghosts observed, indicating that the shape change was not followed by hemolysis. However, red cells sphered in vitro by the action of *Vipera* venom show increased osmotic and mechanical fragilities which remain above normal even after reversion to bidiscoids (BERWALD, 1969; CONDREA et al., 1961). The question has been asked whether in vivo hemolysis might occur as a consequence of these cells being less resistant to the trauma of circulation or being trapped by the spleen. DE VRIES et al. (1962) and KLIBANSKY et al. (1962) investigated this aspect by means of a *Vipera palestinae* phospholipase A preparation devoid of hemorrhagin which was injected into rabbits. The phospholipase A caused practically instantaneous sphering associated with attachment of lysolecithin to the red cells. Within 2 h after injection, plasma lysolecithin dropped to normal and the red cells regained bidiscoidal shape (KLIBANSKY et al., 1962). Hemolysis, however, occurred in only a minority of the animals as indicated by shortening of the red cell survival, a decrease in hemoglobin, hematocrit and red cell count, and the appearance of reticulocytosis (DE VRIES et al., 1962). Similar to the effects of *Vipera palestinae* venom in rabbits, intravenous administration of the phospholipase-containing, boiled *Echis coloratus* venom to dogs (KLIBANSKY et al., 1966) induced red cell shape changes by attachment of lysolecithin to the cells. Here again, there was none or little intravascular hemolysis. In the presence of the venom procoagulant factor, however, hemolysis did occur (see Sect. B).

One may conclude that the phospholipase-induced in vivo red cell sphering may produce but need not entail hemolysis. Several factors may determine whether hemolysis will or will not occur: first, the amount of lysolecithin attached to the red cell and the duration of the attachment which, in turn, will depend upon the initial plasma lecithin concentration and rate of plasma lysolecithin clearance; second, the level of plasma proteins known to protect sphered red cells from destruction; and third, the functional state of the spleen. The study on rabbits suggests that in the human, whose plasma phospholipid level is two to three times higher, hemolysis may occur following bite by a snake possessing indirect lytic venom (see Sect. B).

II. The Indirect Hemolysis; Lytic Effects of Lysolecithin and Fatty Acids

In the previous section, it was shown that lysolecithin and fatty acids evolved by the action of venom on whole blood distribute between the red cells and plasma proteins and that the amounts becoming attached to the red cells are at a sublytic level. In the test for indirect hemolysis, washed, saline-suspended red cells are incubated with venom in the presence of egg yolk as a rich source for lecithin and other glycerophospholipids. Hydrolysis by the phospholipase of the phospholipid substrates in naturally occurring lipoproteins such as in egg yolk proceeds at a high rate (CONDREA et al., 1962), and the amounts of lysoproducts are large enough to induce red cell lysis. Likewise, in indirect hemolysis tests performed on washed red cells and added plasma, hemolysis can be induced if the amounts of plasma are sufficiently high.

The lytic effect of lysolecithin was thought to be exerted through the membrane cholesterol, either by the formation of a cholesterol-lysolecithin complex (COLLIER, 1952; COLLIER and CHEN, 1950) or by displacement of cholesterol from the membrane (LONG and ZAKI, 1967; ZAKI and LONG, 1969). KLIBANSKY and DE VRIES (1963) found the attachment of lysolecithin to the membrane to be accompanied by a small decrease in red cell cholesterol content. LONG and ZAKI (1967) and ZAKI and LONG (1969) considered the lysolecithin-induced loss of cholesterol from the red cell membrane as the event leading to hemolysis. Experimenting with *Walterinnesia* venom which has no direct lytic action on washed red cells of the rat, the authors found that in the presence of added plasma the erythrocytes are hemolysed and membrane cholesterol decreases. However, administration of a sublethal dose of the venom in rats did not produce hemolysis, and there was no increase in plasma cholesterol, although plasma lecithin was converted to lysolecithin. Hemolysis and an increase in plasma cholesterol did occur when the same doses of the venom were injected in adrenalectomized animals, and these effects could be prevented by corticosterone administration. Thus, the authors postulated a protective effect of the adrenal cortical hormones against the lytic action of plasma lysolecithin produced by the venom phospholipase.

REMAN et al. (1969) found, however, that a lytic amount of lysolecithin does not remove amounts of cholesterol from the membrane sufficiently high to account for hemolysis. An alternative explanation for the lytic effects of lysolecithin is that proposed by LUCY (1970). According to this author, lysolecithin induces hemolysis by changing the stable bimolecular lipid layer in membranes to an unstable, micellar structure.

III. Effects of Serum Proteins on Phospholipase-Induced Hemolysis

The role of serum proteins in the occurrence of hemolysis following the action of the venom phospholipase on red blood cells has been repeatedly mentioned throughout this survey. The effects of serum proteins which are complex and vary with the type of hemolytic system under investigation can be summarized as follows:

In indirect lytic systems consisting of washed red cells, an indirect lytic venom or purified venom phospholipase and an exogenous source for phospholipids, albumin exerts a protective effect on hemolysis by binding the lytic agents produced enzymically. LUZZIO (1967) found that hemolysis of human and rabbit cells by *Crotalus* venom in the presence of egg yolk is inhibited by serum albumin but not by α-, β- or γ-globulin. These results are in agreement with the data on the erythrocyte-lysolecithin interaction in the presence of plasma or albumin solutions (GITTER et al., 1959; KLIBANSKY and DE VRIES, 1963).

In lytic systems consisting of washed red cells and venom phospholipase in the absence of exogenous substrates, albumin promotes hemolysis by removing from the membrane lysolecithin and fatty acids produced by the limited hydrolysis of phospholipids in the outer half of the membrane (GUL and SMITH, 1972; GUL and SMITH, 1974; GUL et al., 1974). GUL and SMITH (1974) showed that as much as 75% of the evolved fatty acids can be removed from the membrane by albumin without inducing hemolysis, but a further increase in the amount of fatty acids removed produces loss of hemoglobin from the cells. Since albumin, at the effective concentrations, binds both fatty acids and lysophospholipids from the membrane, it is not established whether the removal of fatty acids alone is responsible for hemolysis.

While albumin promotes hemolysis when added during or after incubation of the red cells with the phospholipase, prolonged incubation of the red cells with albumin prior to the addition of the enzyme decreases the final level of hemolysis (GUL and SMITH, 1974). This protection of the erythrocytes against hemolysis seems to be due to stabilization of the membrane by external coating, since the degradation of membrane phospholipids is not affected.

F. Hemolysis by a Cobra Venom Factor Acting Through the Complement System

In addition to the hemolytic pathways which involve the venom phospholipases and the direct lytic polypeptides, red cell lysis can be produced through an entirely different mechanism by a cobra venom factor (CVF) which is active on the complement system.

The observation that cobra venom causes hemolysis of sheep erythrocytes in the presence of guinea-pig serum, this effect being blocked by preheating of the serum at 56° C for 30 min, dates from the turn of the century (FLEXNER and NOGUCHI, 1902; KYES and SACHS, 1903; KYES, 1903). For this effect to occur, sheep erythrocytes do not have to be sensitized by incubation with antisheep erythrocyte serum. An indication for this hemolytic effect being related to the complement system came from later investigations showing that serum lacking complement factors was inefficient (VAN OSS and GÖTZE, 1963; VAN OSS and CIXOUS, 1963) and that agents which impair C3 activity abolish hemolysis (PICKERING et al., 1969). The complement-dependent hemolytic effect of cobra venom was at first attributed to the venom phospholipase A and formation of lysolecithin from substrates in serum (VAN OSS and GÖTZE, 1963) or in the red cell membrane itself. The first mechanism, however, was not consistant with the finding that preheating of the serum at 56° C prevents hemolysis. Moreover, PHILLIPS and MIDDLETON (1965) quantitated the amount of lysolecithin produced in guinea-pig serum and found it insufficient to induce hemolysis.

As to the second possibility, PHILLIPS (1970) determined the phospholipid distribution in guinea-pig red cells and found that the complement-dependent hemolysis by cobra venom is not a result of erythrocyte phospholipid breakdown.

Efforts have been made toward the identification of the CVF involved in complement-dependent hemolysis. By paper electrophoresis of cobra venom at two different pH values, PHILLIPS (1970) obtained either inactive fractions or some activity which was associated with fractions other than phospholipase A or DLF. Using DEAE cellulose and Sephadex columns, BALLOW and COCHRANE (1969) isolated from cobra venom a protein fraction, homogeneous by acrylamide gel electrophoresis and able to produce complement-dependent hemolysis of guinea-pig cells in the presence of homologous serum. This protein was shown to differ from the DLF by having a molecular weight of 140000 daltons, being nonlytic when applied to washed guinea-pig red cells in the absence of serum and having an acidic character.

The mechanism of action proposed for the CVF involves activation by cleavage of C3 and initiation of the complement sequence on the surface of the red cell leading to hemolysis (BALLOW and COCHRANE, 1969). In addition, it is suggested that, by becoming bound to the cell membrane, CVF might provide sites for complement fixation or render the membrane susceptible to the late-acting complement components (BALLOW and COCHRANE, 1969). The interaction between the CVF and component C3 requires the presence of two additional serum factors, one identified as a glycine-rich β-glycoprotein (GBG), the other a low molecular weight protein designated as factor D. LYNEN et al. (1973) and VOGT et al. (1974) produced evidence for a sequence of events leading to the cleavage of C3: the CVF binds to GBG by aid of Mg ions and induces a structural conformation of the GBG which allows its being attacked by factor D, presumably a proteolytic enzyme. The CVF remains in stable complex with the resulting fragment of the GBG cleavage and together they represent the C3 cleaving system in which the serum glycoprotein fragment is the actual enzyme.

G. Concluding Remarks

The snake venom-induced hemolysis, although being of moderate interest to the clinician, has prompted an impressive body of research which revealed some general aspects regarding the mode of action of snake venoms.

One aspect is the cooperation between venom components which, each separately being of low efficiency, may act synergistically with a high performance. Thus,

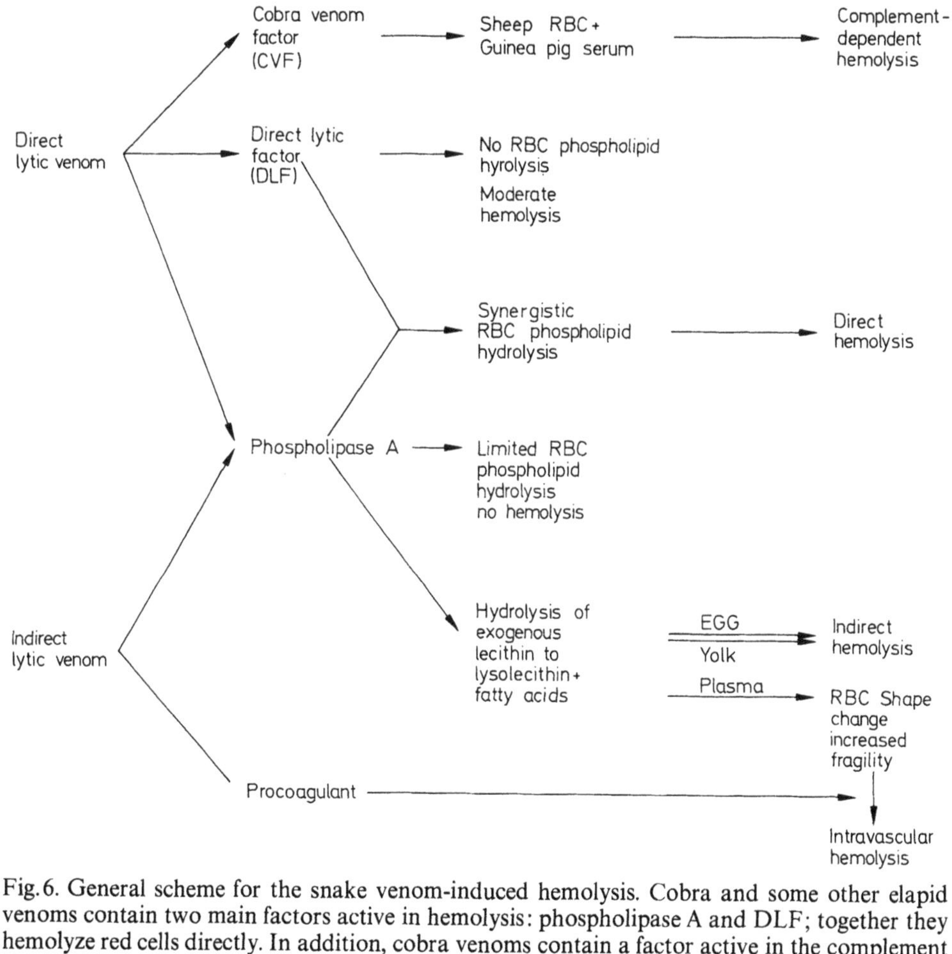

Fig. 6. General scheme for the snake venom-induced hemolysis. Cobra and some other elapid venoms contain two main factors active in hemolysis: phospholipase A and DLF; together they hemolyze red cells directly. In addition, cobra venoms contain a factor active in the complement system. Viperid and crotalid venoms contain only phospholipase A, which hemolyzes red blood cells indirectly, in the presence of egg yolk. The double arrow represents the large amounts of lysoproducts resulting from the action of the phospholipase on egg yolk. From plasma, the limited amounts of lysoproducts liberated (single arrow) induce red cell shape change. These fragile cells may hemolyze in the circulation, the process being enhanced if the venom possesses a procoagulant factor

during the evolutionary development, certain snake venoms became equipped not only with a proper enzyme, phospholipase A, but also with a detergent-like polypeptide able to render the substrates in biologic membranes amenable to the action of this enzyme.

A second aspect is the importance of the role played by environmental factors. In the case of venom-induced hemolysis, these factors are: the level of plasma phospholipids and proteins, clearance rate of lysoproducts from plasma, the flow of the red cells during circulation, and the functional state of the spleen.

Last, snake venom phospholipases have become an important tool in the study of biologic membranes. Localizing the phospholipids within the membrane by means of phospholipases helped elucidate both important aspects of membrane structure and the mode of action of venom components acting at that level.

A general scheme of the snake venom-induced hemolysis is given in Figure 6.

References

Augustyn, J. M., Elliott, W. B.: Isolation of a phospholipase A from *Agkistrodon piscivorus* venom. Biochim. biophys. Acta (Amst.) **206**, 98—108 (1970)

Avi-Dor, Y., Condrea, E., Vries, A. de: Production enzymatique dans le plasma humain d'un facteur provoquant la sphéricité des hématies par le venin de *Vipera palestinae*. Rev. Clin. Biol. **8**, 819—821 (1960)

Ballow, M., Cochrane, C. G.: Two anticomplementary factors in cobra venom: hemolysis of guinea pig erythrocytes by one of them. J. Immunol. **103**, 944—952 (1969)

Balozet, L.: La vipère lébétine et son venin. Arch. Inst. Pasteur Algér. **35**, 220—295 (1957)

Balozet, L.: Les venins, la sphérocytose des hématies et leur sédimentation. Arch. Inst. Pasteur Algér. **40**, 149—178 (1962)

Bergenhem, B.: Experimentelle Untersuchungen über die spontanen Veränderungen des Blutes in vitro hinsichtlich Suspensionsstabilität, Komplementaktivität und Antithrombinfunktion. Acta path. microbiol. scand. [Suppl.] **39**, 1—251 (1939)

Bergenhem, B., Fahraeus, R.: Über spontane Hämolysinbildung im Blut, unter besonderer Berücksichtigung der Physiologie der Milz. Z. ges. Exp. **97**, 555—587 (1936)

Berwald, J.: Effect of treatment of human blood with *Vipera palestinae* venom on the osmotic, mechanical and incubation fragilities of red blood cells. M.Sc. Thesis, Tel-Aviv Univ. 1960

Botes, D. P., Viljoen, C. C.: Purification of phospholipase A from *Bitis gabonica* venom. Toxicon **12**, 611—619 (1974 a)

Botes, D. P., Viljoen, C. C.: *Bitis gabonica* venom. The amino-acid sequence of phospholipase A. J. biol. Chem. **249**, 3827—3832 (1974 b)

Braganca, B.M., Patel, N.T., Bandrinath, P.G.: Isolation and properties of a cobra venom factor selectively cytotoxic to Yoshida sarcoma cells. Biochim. biophys. Acta (Amst.) **136**, 508—520 (1967)

Bretcher, M. S.: Asymmetrical lipid bilayer structure for biological membranes. Nature (Lond.) New Biol. **236**, 11—12 (1972 a)

Bretcher, M. S.: Phosphatidyl-ethanolamine: differential labelling in intact cells and cell ghosts of human erythrocytes by a membrane impermeable reagent. J. molec. Biol. **71**, 523—528 (1972 b)

Bretcher, M. S.: Membrane structure: some general principles. Science **181**, 622—629 (1973)

Campbell, C. H.: Clinical aspects of snake bite in the Pacific area. Toxicon **7**, 25—28 (1969)

Chang, C. C., Chuang, S.-T., Lee, C. Y., Wei, J. W.: Role of cardiotoxin and phospholipase A in the blockade of nerve conduction and depolarization of skeletal muscle induced by cobra venom. Brit. J. Pharmacol. **44**, 752—764 (1972)

Collier, H. B.: Factors affecting hemolytic action of "lysolecithin" upon rabbit erythrocytes. J. gen. Physiol. **35**, 617—628 (1952)

Collier, H. B., Chen, H. L.: On antihaemolytic value of blood of rabbits as measured by lysolecithin. Canad. J. Res. **28**, 289—297 (1950)
Condrea, E.: Membrane-active polypeptides from snake venom: cardiotoxins and haemocytotoxins. Experientia (Basel) **30**, 121—129 (1974)
Condrea, E., Barzilay, M., Mager, J.: Role of cobra venom direct lytic factor and Ca^{2+} in promoting the activity of snake venom phospholipase A. Biochim. biophys. Acta (Amst.) **210**, 65—73 (1970)
Condrea, E., Barzilay, M., de Vries, A.: Study of hemolysis in the lethal effects of *Naja naja* venom in the mouse and guinea pig. Toxicon **7**, 95—98 (1969)
Condrea, E., Kendjersky, I., de Vries, A.: Binding of ringhals venom direct hemolytic factor to erythrocytes and osmotic ghosts of various animal species. Experientia (Basel) **21**, 461—464 (1965)
Condrea, E., Livni, E., Berwald, J., de Vries, A.: Changes in red blood cell fragilities due to the action of phosphatidase and lipoprotein lipase on human blood in vitro. Arch. int. Pharmacodyn. Ther. **134**, 368—372 (1961)
Condrea, E., Mammon, Z., Aloof, S., de Vries, A.: Susceptibility of erythrocytes of various animal species to the hemolytic and phospholipid-splitting action of snake venom. Biochim. biophys. Acta (Amst.) **84**, 365—375 (1964b)
Condrea, E., de Vries, A.: Venom phospholipase A, a review. Toxicon **2**, 261—273 (1965)
Condrea, E., de Vries, A., Mager, J.: Action of snake venom phospholipase A on free and lipoprotein-bound phospholipids. Biochim. biophys. Acta (Amst.) **58**, 389—397 (1962)
Condrea, E., de Vries, A., Mager, J.: Hemolysis and splitting of human erythrocyte phospholipids by snake venoms. Biochim. biophys. Acta (Amst.) **84**, 60—73 (1964a)
Cunningham, D. D.: Snake Venoms. In: Scientific Memoirs by Medical Officers of the Army of India, No. 11, p. 1, Calcutta: Off. Govt. Print. 1968
Danon, D., Gitter, S., Rosen, M.: Deformation of red cell shape induced by *Vipera palestinae* venom in vivo. Nature (Lond.) **189**, 320—321 (1961)
De Gier, J., Van Deenen, L. L. M.: Some lipid characteristics of red cell membranes of various animal species. Biochim. biophys. Acta (Amst.) **49**, 286—296 (1961)
De Gier, J., Mulder, J., Van Deenen, L. L. M.: On the specific lipid composition of red cell membranes. Naturwissenschaften **48**, 54 (1961)
De Haas, G. H., Bonsen, P. P. M., Pieterson, W. A., Van Deenen, L. L. M.: Studies on phospholipase A and its zymogen from porcine pancreas. III. Action of the enzyme on short-chain lecithin. Biochim. biophys. Acta (Amst.) **239**, 252—266 (1971)
Delezenne, C., Fourneau, E.: Constitution du phosphatide hémolysant (lysocithine) provenant de l'action du venin de cobra sur le vitellus d'oeuf de poule. Bull. Soc. chim. Fr. **15**, 421—434 (1914)
Delezenne, C., Ledebt, S.: Les poisons libérés par les venins aux dépens du vitellus de l'oeuf. C.R. Soc. Biol. (Paris) **71**, 121—124 (1911a)
Delezenne, C., Ledebt, S.: Action du venin de cobra sur le serum de cheval. Ses rapports avec l'hémolyse. C.R. Acad. Sci. (Paris) **152**, 790—792 (1911b)
Delezenne, C., Ledebt, S.: Formation de substances hémolytiques et de substances toxiques aux dépens du vitellus de l'oeuf soumis a l'action du cobra. C.R. Acad. Sci. (Paris) **153**, 81—84 (1911c)
Delezenne, C., Ledebt, S.: Nouvelle contribution a l'étude des substances hémolytiques derivées du serum et du vitellus de l'oeuf soumis à l'action des venins. C.R. Acad. Sci. (Paris) **155**, 1101—1103 (1911d)
Delori, P. J.: Isolation, purification and study of a toxic phospholipase A_2 from *Vipera berus* venom. Biochimie **53**, 941—948 (1971)
Devi, A.: The chemistry, toxicity, biochemistry and pharmacology of North American snake venoms. In: Buckley, E. E., Bücherl, W. (Eds.): Venomous Animals and Their Venoms, Vol. II. New York-London: Academic Press 1971
De Vries, A., Condrea, E.: Clinical aspects of elapid bite. In: Simpson, L. L. (Ed.): Neuropoisons, Vol. I. New York-London: Plenum Press 1971
De Vries, A., Condrea, E., Gitter, S., Danon, D., Katachalsky, R., Kessler, J., Kochwa, S.: Crénelure des globules rouges et inhibition de la formation des rouleaux dans le sang humain en correlation avec l'activité de la lipoproteinelipase. Sang **31**, 289—302 (1960)

De Vries, A., Kirschmann, C., Klibansky, C., Condrea, E., Gitter, S.: Hemolytic action of indirect lytic snake venom in vivo. Toxicon **1**, 19—23 (1962)
Doery, H. M., Pearson, J. E.: Phospholipase B in snake venoms and bee venom. Biochem. J. **92**, 599—602 (1964)
Dumarey, C., Sket, D., Joseph, D., Boquet, P.: Etude d'une phospholipase basique du venin de *Naja nigricollis*. C.R. Acad. Sci. (Paris) **280**, 1633 (1975)
Eaker, D.: Structural nature of pre-synaptic neurotoxins from Australian elapid venoms. Abstr. of 4th Intern. Symp. on Animal, Plant, and Microbial Toxins. Toxicon **13**, 90—91 (1975)
Efrati, P.: Clinical manifestations and treatment of viper bite in Israel. Toxicon **7**, 29—31 (1969)
Eitan, A., Aloni, B., Livne, A.: Unique properties of the camel erythrocyte membrane. Organization of membrane proteins. Biochim. biophys. Acta (Amst.) **426**, 647—658 (1976)
Flexner, S., Noguchi, H.: Snake venoms in relation to haemolysis, bacteriolysis and toxicity. Univ. Padova Med. Bull. **14**, 438—441 (1902)
Forstner, J., Manery, J. F.: Calcium binding by human erythrocyte membranes. Biochem. J. **124**, 563—571 (1971)
Fryklund, L., Eaker, D.: Complete amino acid sequence of a nonneurotoxic hemolytic protein from the venom of *Hemachatus haemachatus* (African Ringhals cobra). Biochemistry **12**, 661—667 (1973)
Gitter, S., Kochwa, S., Danon, D., de Vries, A.: Disk-sphere-transformation and inhibition of rouleaux formation and of sedimentation of human red blood cells induced by *Vipera xanthina palestinae* venom. Arch. int. Pharmacodyn. Ther. **118**, 350—357 (1959)
Gitter, S., de Vries, A.: Symptomatology, pathology, and treatment of bites by Near Eastern, European, and North African snakes. In: Buckley, E. E., Bücherl, W. (Eds.): Venomous Animals and Their Venoms, Vol. I. New York-London: Academic Press 1968
Gordesky, S. E., Marinetti, G. V.: The asymmetric arrangement of phospholipids in the human erythrocyte membrane. Biochim. biophys. Res. Commun. **50**, 1027—1031 (1973)
Grassman, W., Hannig, K.: Electrophoretische Untersuchungen an Schlangen- und Insektentoxinen. Hoppe-Seylers Z. physiol. Chem. **296**, 30—44 (1954)
Gubensek, F.: Sepharose-bound toxic phospholipase A. Bull. Inst. Pasteur Lille **74**, 47—49 (1976)
Guidotti, G.: The composition of biological membrane. Arch. int. Med. **129**, 194—201 (1972)
Gul, S., Khara, J. S., Smith, A. D.: Hemolysis of washed human red cells by various snake venoms in the presence of albumin and Ca^{2+}. Toxicon **12**, 311—315 (1974)
Gul, S., Smith, A. D.: Hemolysis of washed human red cells by the combined action of phospholipase A_2 and albumin. Biochim. biophys. Acta (Amst.) **288**, 237—240 (1972)
Gul, S., Smith, A. D.: Hemolysis of intact human erythrocytes by purified cobra venom phospholipase A_2 in the presence of albumin and Ca^{2+}. Biochim. biophys. Acta (Amst.) **367**, 271—281 (1974)
Habermann, E.: Zur pharmakologischen Charakterisierung elektrophoretischer Fraktionen der Gifte von *Naja nigricollis* und *Naja naja*. Hoppe-Seylers Z. physiol. Chem. **297**, 104—107 (1954)
Habermann, E. N., Neumann, W.: Beiträge zur Charakterisierung der wirksamen Komponenten von Schlangengift. Arch. exp. Path. Pharmakol. **223**, 388—398 (1954)
Hachimori, Y., Wells, M. A., Hanahan, D. J.: Observations on the phospholipases A_2 of *Crotalus atrox*. Molecular weight and other properties. Biochemistry **10**, 4084—4089 (1971)
Hayashi, K., Takechi, M., Sasaki, T.: Amino acid sequence of cytotoxin I from the venom of the Indian cobra *(Naja naja)*. Biochim. biophys. Res. Commun. **45**, 1357—1362 (1971)
Howard, N. L.: Phospholipase A_2 from puff adder *(Bitis arietans)* venom. Toxicon **13**, 21—30 (1975)
Ibrahim, S.A., Masr, A.R.M.: Action of phospholipase A from black mamba *(Dendroaspis polylepsis)* venom on the phospholipids of human blood. Abstr. 4th Intern. Symp. on Animal, Plant and Microbial Toxins. Toxicon **13**, 99 (1975)
Ibrahim, S. A., Thomson, R. H. S.: Action of phospholipase A on human red cell ghosts and intact erythrocytes. Biochim. biophys. Acta (Amst.) **99**, 331—341 (1965)
Izard, Y., Boquet, P., Golemi, E., Goupil, D.: La toxine gamma n'est pas le facteur lytique direct du venin de *Naja nigricollis*. C.R. Acad. Sci. (Paris) **269**, 666—671 (1969a)
Izard, Y., Boquet, M., Ronsseray, A. M., Boquet, P.: Isolement d'une proteine toxique du venin de *Naja nigricollis*: la toxine γ. C.R. Acad. Sci. (Paris) **269**, 96—97 (1969b)

Jacobi, C., Lankish, P. G., Schoner, K., Vogt, W.: Changes in Na^+ and K^+ permeability of red cells induced by the direct lytic factor of cobra venom and phospholipase A. Naunyn-Schmiedebergs Arch. Pharmacol. **274**, 81—90 (1972)
Jiménez-Porras, J. M.: Pharmacology of peptides and proteins in snake venoms. Ann. Rev. Pharmacol. **8**, 299—318 (1968)
Jiménez-Porras, J. M.: Biochemistry of snake venoms. Clin. Toxicol. **3**, 389—431 (1970)
Kawauchi, S., Iwanaga, S., Samejima, Y., Suzuki, T.: Isolation and characterization of two phospholipases A from the venom of *Agkistrodon halys blomhoffii*. Biochim. biophys. Acta (Amst.) **236**, 142—160 (1971)
Kelen, E. M. A., Rosenfeld, G., Nudel, F.: Hemolytic activity of animal venoms. II. Variations in relation to erythrocyte species. Mem. Inst. Butantan. **30**, 133—140 (1960—1962)
Kellaway, C. H., Williams, F. E.: Haemolysis by Australian snake venoms. I. The comparative haemolytic power of Australian snake venoms. Aust. J. exp. Biol. med. Sci. **2**, 75—80 (1933a)
Kellaway, C. H., Williams, F. E.: Haemolysis by Australian snake venoms. II. Some peculiarities in the behaviour of the haemolysis of Australian snake venoms. Aust. J. exp. Biol. med. Sci. **2**, 81—94 (1933b)
Klibansky, C., Condrea, E., De Vries, A.: Changes in plasma phospholipids after intravenous phosphatidase A injection in the rabbit. Amer. J. Physiol. **203**, 114—118 (1962)
Klibansky, C., London, Y., Frenkel, A., De Vries, A.: Enhancing action of synthetic and natural basic plypeptides on erythrocyte-ghost phospholipid hydrolysis by phospholipase A. Biochim. biophys. Acta (Amst.) **150**, 15—23 (1968)
Klibansky, C., Ozcan, E., Joshua, H., Djaldetti, M., Bessler, H., De Vries, A.: Intravascular hemolysis in dogs induced by *Echis coloratus* venom. Toxicon **3**, 213—221 (1966)
Klibansky, C., De Vries, A.: Quantitative study of erythrocyte-lysolecithin interaction. Biochim. biophys. Acta (Amst.) **70**, 176—187 (1963)
Kocholaty, W. P., Ledford, E. B., Daly, J. G., Billings, T. A.: Toxicity and some enzymatic properties and activities in the venoms of *Crotalidae*, *Elapidae* and *Viperidae*. Toxicon **9**, 131—138 (1971)
Kögl, F., De Gier, J., Mulder, J., Van Deenen, L. L. M.: Metabolism and functions of phosphatides. Specific fatty acid composition of the red blood cell membranes. Biochim. biophys. Acta (Amst.) **43**, 95—103 (1960)
Kyes, P.: Über die Lecithide des Schlangengiftes. Berl. klin. Wschr. **40**, 956 (1903)
Kyes, P., Sachs, H.: Zur Kenntnis der Cobragift-aktivierenden Substanzen. Berl. klin. Wschr. **40**, 21—23 (1903)
Lamb, G., Hunter, W. K.: On the action of venoms of different species of poisonous snakes on the nervous system. Lancet **1904 I**, 20—22
Lankisch, P. G., Jacobi, C., Schoner, K.: Bile salts, lysolecithin and saponin-induced potentiation of phospholipase A hemolysis. FEBS Letters **23**, 61—64 (1972b)
Lankisch, P. G., Lege, L., Oldings, H. D., Vogt, W.: Binding of phospholipase A to the direct lytic factor revealed by the interaction of Ca^{2+} with the haemolytic effect. Biochim. biophys. Acta (Amst.) **239**, 267—272 (1971)
Lankisch, P. G., Schoner, K., Schoner, W., Kunze, H., Bohn, E., Vogt, W.: Inhibition of Na^+- and K^+-activated ATPase by the direct lytic factor of cobra venom *(Naja naja)*. Biochim. biophys. Acta (Amst.) **266**, 133—134 (1972a)
Lankisch, P. G., Vogt, W.: Potentiation of haemolysis by the combined action of phospholipase A and a basic peptide containing S-S-bonds (Viscotoxin B). Experientia (Basel) **27**, 122 (1971)
Larsen, P. R., Wolff, J.: Inhibition of accumulative transport by a protein from cobra venom. Biochem. Pharmacol. **16**, 2003—2009 (1967)
Larsen, P. R., Wolff, J.: The basic proteins cobra venom. I. Isolation and characterization of cobramines A and B. J. biol. Chem. **243**, 1283—1289 (1968)
Lee, C. Y.: Mode of action of cobra venom and its purified toxins. In: Simpson, L. L. (Ed.): Neuropoisons, Vol. I. New York-London: Plenum Press 1971
Lee, C. Y.: Chemistry and pharmacology of polypeptide toxins in snake venoms. Ann. Rev. Pharmacol. **12**, 265—286 (1972)
Lee, C. Y., Chang, C. C., Chiu, T. H., Chiu, P. J. S., Tseng, T. C., Lee, S. Y.: Pharmacological properties of cardiotoxin isolated from Formosan cobra venom. Naunyn-Schmiedebergs Arch. Pharmacol. **259**, 360—374 (1968)

Lee, C. Y., Lin, J. S., Wei, J. W.: Identification of cardiotoxin with cobramine B, DLF, toxin γ, and cobra venom cytotoxin. In: de Vries, A., Kochva, E. (Eds.): Toxins of animal and Plant Origin, Vol. I. New York: Gordon and Breach 1971

Lin Shiau, S. Y., Huang, M. C., Lee, C. Y.: Mechanism of action of cobra cardiotoxin in the skeletal muscle. J. Pharmacol. exp. Ther. **196**, 758—770 (1976)

Lin Shiau, S. Y., Huang, M. C., Tseng, W. C., Lee, C. Y.: Comparative studies on the biological activities of cardiotoxin, melittin, and prymnesin. Naunyn-Schmiedebergs Arch. Pharmacol. **287**, 349—358 (1975)

Lin Shiau, S. Y., Hsia, S., Lee, C. Y.: Studies on the cytotoxic action of cardiotoxin on HeLa cells. J. Chinese biochem. Soc. **2**, 38—45 (1973)

Livne, A., Kuiper, P. J. C.: Unique properties of the camel erythrocyte membrane. Biochim. biophys. Acta (Amst.) **318**, 41—49 (1973)

Livrea, G.: A comparative study of in vitro hemolysis by *Vipera ammodytes* poison conducted on 73 vertebrate species: probable implications regarding the ultrastructure of the erythrocytic membrane in the different species. Biologica Latina **11**, 141—147 (1958)

Lo, T. B., Chang, W. C.: Studies on phospholipase A from Formosan cobra *(Naja naja atra)* venom. Abstr. 4th Intern. Symp. on Animal, Plant, and Microbial Toxins. Toxicon **13**, 108 (1975)

Long, C., Penny, J. F.: The structure of the naturally occurring phosphoglycerides 3. The action of moccasin venom phospholipase A on ovolecithin and related substances. Biochem. J. **65**, 382—389 (1957)

Long, C., Zaki, O. A.: Effects of *Walterinnesia* venom on phospholipids of plasma and adrenals in rats. Amer. J. Physiol. **213**, 763—767 (1967)

Lucy, J. A.: The fusion of biological membranes. Nature (Lond.) **227**, 815—817 (1970)

Luzzio, A. J.: Inhibitory properties of serum proteins on the enzymatic sequence leading to lysis of red blood cells by snake venoms. Toxicon **5**, 97—103 (1967)

Lynen, R., Brade, V., Wolf, A., Vogt, W.: Purification and some properties of a heat-labile serum factor (VF): Identity with glycine-rich β-glycoprotein and properdin factor B. Hoppe-Seylers Z. physiol. Chem. **354**, 37—47 (1973)

Malette, W. G., Fitzgerald, J. B., Cockett, A. T. K., Glass, T. G., Glenn, W. G., Donnelly, P. V.: The pathophysiologic effects of rattlesnake venom *(Crotalus atrox)*. In: Keegan, H. L., MacFarlane, W. V. (Eds.): Venomous and Poisonous Animals and Noxious Plants of the Pacific Region. Oxford-London-New York-Paris: Pergamon Pr. 1963

Meldrum, B. S.: Depolarization of skeletal muscle by a toxin from cobra *(Naja naja)* venom. J. Physiol. (Lond.) **168**, 49—50 (1963)

Meldrum, B. S.: The actions of snake venoms on nerve and muscle. The pharmacology of phospholipase A and of polypeptide toxins. Pharmacol. Rev. **17**, 393—445 (1965)

Michl, H.: Elektrophoretische und enzymatische Untersuchungen des Jararaca-Toxins. Naturwissenschaften **41**, 403 (1954)

Mitchell, S. W., Reichert, E.: Preliminary report on the venom of serpents. Med. News **42**, 469—472 (1883)

Mohamed, A. H., Kamel, A., Ayobe, M. H.: Studies of phospholipase A and B activities of Egyptian snake venoms and a scorpion toxin. Toxicon **6**, 293—298 (1969)

Mollay, C., Kreil, G.: Fluorometric measurements on the interaction of melittin with lecithin. Biochim. biophys. Acta (Amst.) **316**, 196—203 (1973)

Mollay, C., Kreil, G.: Enhancement of bee venom phospholipase A_2 activity by melittin, direct lytic factor from cobra venom and polymyxin B. FEBS Letters **46**, 141—144 (1974)

Neumann, W., Habermann, E.: Paper electrophoresis separation of pharmacologically and biochemically active components of bee and snake venoms. In: Buckley, E. E., Porges, N. (Eds.): Venoms. Washington: Am. Assoc. Adv. Sci. 1956

Oldings, H. D., Lege, L., Lankisch, P. G.: Vergleichende Hämolyseversuche an Meerschweinchen und Rattenerythrocyten in vitro mit Phospholipase A und Direkt-Lytischen-Faktor aus Cobragift *(Naja naja)*. Naunyn-Schmiedebergs Arch. Pharmacol. **268**, 27—32 (1971)

Omori-Satoh, T., Lang, Y., Breithaupt, H., Habermann, E.: Partial amino acid sequence of the basic *Crotalus* phospholipase A. Toxicon **13**, 69—71 (1975)

Phillips, G. B.: Studies on a hemolytic factor of cobra venom requiring a heat-labile serum factor. Biochim. biophys. Acta (Amst.) **201**, 364—374 (1970)

Phillips, G. B., Middleton, E.: Studies on lysolecithin formation in immune hemolysis. J. Immunol. **94**, 40—46 (1965)
Pickering, R. J., Wolfson, M. R., Good, R. A., Gewurtz, H.: Passive hemolysis by serum and cobra venom factor: a new mechanism inducing membrane damage by complement. Proc. nat. Acad. Sci. (Wash.) **62**, 521—527 (1969)
Raudonat, H. W.: Über den dialysablen Anteil des Cobragiftes. Naturwissenschaften **42**, 648 (1955)
Reid, A. H.: Symptomatology, pathology, and treatment of land snake bite in India and Southeast Asia. In: Buckley, E. E., Bücherl, W. (Eds.): Venomous Animals and Their Venoms, Vol. I. New York-London: Academic Press 1968
Reman, F. C., Demel, R. A., de Gier, J., Van Deenen, L. L. M., Eibl, E., Westphal, O.: Studies on the lysis of red cells and bimolecular lipid leaflets by synthetic lysolecithins, lecithins, and structural analogs. Chem. Phys. Lipids **3**, 221—233 (1969)
Rogers, L.: The physiological action and antidotes of snake venoms with a practical method of treatment of snake bites. Lancet **4197**, 349—355 (1904)
Rosenfeld, G.: Symptomatology, pathology, and treatment of snake bites in South America. In: Buckley, E. E., Bücherl, W. (Eds.): Venomous Animals and Their Venoms, Vol. II. New York-London: Academic Press 1971
Rosenfeld, G., Kelen, E. M. A., Nudel, F.: Hemolytic activity of animal venoms. I. Classification in different types of activity. Mem. Inst. Butantan **30**, 103—116 (1960—1962)
Rosenfeld, G., Nahas, L., Kelen, E. M. A.: Coagulant, proteolytic, and hemolytic properties of some snake venoms. In: Buckley, E. E., Bücherl, W. (Eds.): Venomous Animals and Their Venoms, Vol. I. New York-London: Academic Press 1968
Salach, J. I., Turini, P., Seng, R., Hauber, J., Singer, T. P.: Phospholipase A of snake venoms. I. Isolation and molecular properties of isoenzymes from *Naja naja* and *Vipera russellii* venoms. J. biol. Chem. **246**, 331—339 (1971)
Samejima, Y., Iwanaga, S., Suzuki, T.: Complete amino acid sequence of the phospholipase A_2 II isolated from *Agkistrodon piscivorus* venom. FEBS Letters **47**, 348—351 (1974)
Sarkar, N. K.: Existence of cardiotoxic principle in cobra venom. Ann. Biochem. exp. Med. **8**, 11 (1948)
Schroeter, R., Damerau, B., Vogt, W.: Differences in binding of the direct lytic factor (DLF) of cobra venom *(Naja naja)* to intact red cells and ghosts. Naunyn-Schmiedebergs Arch. Pharmacol. **280**, 201—207 (1973)
Schroeter, R., Lankisch, P. G., Lege, L., Vogt, W.: Possible implication of glutathione reductase in haemolysis by the direct lytic factor of cobra venom *(Naja naja)*. Naunyn-Schmiedebergs Arch. Pharmacol. **275**, 203—211 (1972)
Sessa, G., Freer, J. H., Colacicco, G., Weissmann, G.: Interaction of a lytic polypeptide, melittin, with lipid membrane systems. J. biol. Chem. **244**, 3575—3582 (1969)
Sheetz, M. P., Singer, S. J.: Biological membranes as bilayer couples. A molecular mechanism of drug-erythrocyte interactions. Proc. nat. Acad. Sci. (Wash.) **71**, 4457—4461 (1974)
Shiloah, J., Klibansky, C., de Vries, A., Berger, A.: Phospholipase B activity of a purified phospholipase A from *Vipera palestinae* venom. J. Lipid Res. **14**, 267—278 (1973)
Singer, S. J.: The molecular organization of membranes. Ann. Rev. Biochem. **43**, 805—833 (1974)
Singer, S. J., Nicolson, G. L.: The fluid mosaic model of the structure of cell membranes. Science **175**, 720—731 (1972)
Steck, T. L.: The organization of proteins in the human red cell membrane. J. Cell Biol. **62**, 1—19 (1974)
Takechi, M., Hayashi, K.: Localization of the four disulfide bridges in cytotoxin II from the venom of the Indian cobra *(Naja naja)*. Biochim. biophys. Res. Commun. **49**, 564—590 (1972)
Trethewie, E. R.: Pathology, symptomatology, and treatment of snake bite in Australia. In: Buckley, E. E., Bücherl, W. (Eds.): Venomous Animals and Their Venoms, Vol. II. New York-London: Academic Press 1971
Tu, A. T.: The mechanism of snake venom actions; rattlesnakes and other crotalids. In: Simpson, L. L. (Ed.): Neuropoisons, Vol. 1. New York-London: Plenum Press 1971
Tu, A. T.: Neurotoxins of animal venoms: snakes. Ann. Rev. Biochem. **42**, 235—258 (1973)

Tu, A. T., Passey, R. B., Toom, P. M.: Isolation and characterization of phospholipase A from sea-snake, *Laticauda semifasciata* venom. Arch. Biochem. Biophys. **140**, 96—106 (1970)
Turner, J. C.: Absence of lecithin from the stromata of the red cells of certain animals (ruminants) and its relation to venom hemolysis. J. exp. Med. **105**, 189—195 (1957)
Turner, J. C., Anderson, H. M., Gandall, C. P.: Species differences in red blood cell phosphatides separated by column and paper chromatography. Biochim. biophys. Acta (Amst.) **30**, 130—134 (1958a)
Turner, J. C., Anderson, H. M., Gandall, C. P.: Comparative liberation of bound phosphatides from red cells of man, ox, and camel. Proc. Soc. exp. Biol. **99**, 547—550 (1958b)
Van Deenen, L. L. M., de Haas, G. H.: The substrate specificity of phospholipase A. Biochim. biophys. Acta (Amst.) **70**, 538—553 (1963)
Van Oss, C. J., Cixous, N.: Evidence for the phospholipid nature of the third component of the complement. Naturwissenschaften **50**, 500 (1963)
Van Oss, C. J., Götze, D.: Haemolytic action of cobra venom lecithinase A in the presence of whole guinea-pig serum or lecithin. Z. Immun. Forsch. **125**, 75—79 (1963)
Verkleij, A. J., Zwaal, R. F. A., Roelofsen, B., Comfurius, P., Kastelijnn, D., Van Deenen, L. L. M.: The asymmetric distribution of phospholipids in the human red cell membrane. A combined study using phospholipases and freeze-etch electron microscopy. Biochim. biophys. Acta (Amst.) **323**, 178—193 (1973)
Vick, J. A.: Symptomatology of experimental and clinical crotalid envenomation. In: Simpson, L. L. (Ed.): Neuropoisons, Vol. 1. New York-London: Plenum Press 1971
Vidal, J. C., Cattaneo, P., Stoppani, A. O. M.: Some characteristic properties of phospholipases A_2 from *Bothrops neuwiedii* venom. Arch. Biochem. Biophys. **151**, 168—179 (1972)
Viljoen, C. C., Schabort, J. C., Botes, D. P.: *Bitis gabonica* venom. A kinetic analysis of the hydrolysis by phospholipase A_2 of 1,2-dipalmitoyl-sn-glycero-3-phosphorylcholine. Biochim. biophys. Acta (Amst.) **360**, 156—165 (1974)
Vincent, J. P., Schweitz, H., Chicheportiche, R., Fosset, M., Balerna, M., Lenoir, M. C., Lazdunski, M.: Molecular mechanism of cardiotoxin action on axonal membranes. Biochemistry **15**, 3171—3175 (1976)
Vogt, W., Dieminger, L., Lynen, R., Schmidt, G.: Alternative pathway for the activation of complement in human serum. Formation and composition of the complex with cobra venom factor that cleaves the third component of complement. Hoppe-Seylers Z. physiol. Chem. **355**, 171—183 (1974)
Vogt, W., Patzer, P., Lege, L., Oldings, H. D., Wille, G.: Synergism between phospholipase A and various peptides and SH-reagents in causing haemolysis. Naunyn-Schmiedebergs Arch. Pharmacol. **265**, 442—454 (1970)
Wahlström, A.: Purification and characterization of phospholipase A from the venom of *Naja nigricollis*. Toxicon **9**, 45—56 (1971)
Wallach, D. F. H.: The disposition of proteins in the plasma membranes of animal cells: analytical approaches using controlled peptidolysis and protein labels. Biochim. biophys. Acta (Amst.) **265**, 61—83 (1972)
Wells, M. A.: Evidence that the phospholipases A_2 of *Crotalus adamanteus* venom are dimers. Biochemistry **10**, 4074—4078 (1971)
Wells, M. A.: A kinetic study of the phospholipase A_2 catalized hydrolysis of 1,2-dibutyryl-sn-glycero-3-phosphorylcholine. Biochemistry **11**, 1030—1041 (1972)
Wells, M. A.: Spectral perturbations of *Crotalus adamanteus* phospholipase A_2 induced by divalent cation binding. Biochemistry **12**, 1080—1085 (1973)
Whitely, N. M., Berg, H. C.: Amidination of the outer and inner surfaces of the human erythrocyte membrane. J. molec. Biol. **87**, 541—561 (1974)
Williams, J. C., Bell, R. M.: Membrane matrix disruption by melittin. Biochim. biophys. Acta (Amst.) **288**, 255—261 (1972)
Wolff, J., Salabe, H., Ambrose, M., Larsen, P. R.: The basic proteins of cobra venoms. II. Mechanism of action of cobramine B on thyroid slices. J. biol. Chem. **243**, 1290—1296 (1968)
Woodward, C. B., Zwaal, R. F. A.: The lytic behaviour of pure phospholipase A_2 and C towards osmotically swollen erythrocytes and released ghosts. Biochim. biophys. Acta (Amst.) **274**, 272—278 (1972)

Zaheer, A., Noronha, S. H., Hospattankar, A. V., Braganca, B. M.: Inactivation of ($Na^+ + K^+$)-stimulated ATPase by a cytotoxic protein from cobra venom in relation to its lytic effects on cells. Biochim. biophys. Acta (Amst.) **394**, 293—303 (1975)
Zaki, O. A., Long, C.: Effects of adrenalectomy on the changes in cholesterol levels in rats induced by *Walterinnesia* venom. Toxicon **6**, 255—261 (1969)
Zwaal, R. F. A., Van Deenen, L. L. M.: Protein patterns of red cell membranes from different mammalian species. Biochim. biophys. Acta (Amst.) **163**, 44—49 (1968)
Zwaal, R. F. A., Roelofsen, B., Colley, M.: Localization of red cell membrane constituents. Biochim. biophys. Acta (Amst.) **300**, 159—182 (1973)
Zwaal, R. F. A., Roelofsen, B., Confurius, P., Van Deenen, L. L. M.: Organization of phospholipids in human red cell membranes as detected by the action of various purified phospholipases. Biochim. biophys. Acta (Amst.) **406**, 83—96 (1975)

CHAPTER 14

Hemorrhagic, Necrotizing and Edema-Forming Effects of Snake Venoms

A. OHSAKA

A. Introduction

Since prehistoric times, man has suffered from envenomation from snakebite. Today, snakebite is still a medical problem of considerable magnitude. According to SWAROOP and GRAB (1954, 1956), about 30000–40000 deaths occur annually from bites of venomous snakes in those areas of the world that have national registration, covering a total population of 1122 millions.

Poisonous snakes mainly belong to four families: *Hydrophiidae*, *Elapidae*, *Viperidae* and *Crotalidae* (KLEMMER, 1963). The usual distinction between poisonous and nonpoisonous snakes depends on the ability of the snake to inject the venom into its victim (FONSECA, 1949), and so-called nonpoisonous snakes also possess extractable venom (KAISER and MICHL, 1958). To date, however, only the venoms from poisonous snakes have been studied intensively, while those from nonpoisonous snakes have received very scant attention. Accordingly, snake venoms dealt with in this article are restricted to those produced by poisonous snakes.

It is well known that snake venoms are the most complex of all known poisons. Because of the diverse biological activities of their many components, snake venoms simultaneously exert toxic and lethal effects on blood, cardiovascular, respiratory, and nervous systems. However, most snake venoms can be classified into several fundamental groups according to the main pathophysiological effect they manifest. Venoms of snakes belonging to families *Elapidae* (numerous cobra species, kraits, mambas, tiger snake, death adder, taipan, etc.) and *Hydrophiidae* (many species of sea snakes) are highly neurotoxic and produce flaccid paralysis and respiratory failure in animals (MELDRUM, 1965; JIMÉNEZ-PORRAS, 1968, 1970; LEE, 1972; also see Chap. 10). *Viperidae* (viper) and *Crotalidae* (pit viper) venoms produce, beside systemic or lethal effects, striking local effects, consisting of hemorrhage, necrosis, and edema (ROSENFELD, 1963; BOQUET, 1964, 1966; OHSAKA et al., 1966a; JIMÉNEZ-PORRAS, 1968, 1970), and often induce marked alterations of blood coagulability as well (DE VRIES and COHEN, 1969; also see Chap. 18).

Our understanding of the neurotoxic effects of *Elapidae* and *Hydrophiidae* venoms has advanced greatly in the last decade (see Chap. 10). On the other hand, the local effects of *Crotalidae* and *Viperidae* venoms are still very incompletely understood, in spite of their clinical importance in envenomation from snakebite; and only a few entities responsible for the local effects, such as those responsible for hemorrhage, have been sufficiently isolated to permit characterization. This has largely been due to the lack of specific methods for separate determination of individual principles responsible for such elementary pathophysiological changes as hemorrhage, necrosis, and edema involved in a complex local lesion (OHSAKA et al., 1966a; OHSAKA, 1973) (see Sect. B).

The present review will concentrate on the hemorrhagic, necrotizing, and edema-forming effects of snake venoms; the hemorrhagic effect of snake venoms will be described in most detail.

For a more general account of the effects of snake venoms, the reader is referred to the recent publications edited by BÜCHERL et al., 1968–1971; POLLER, 1969; RAŠKOVÁ, 1971; SUZUKI et al., 1971; DE VRIES and KOCHVA, 1971–1973; KAISER, 1973; and OHSAKA et al., 1976; and also to Memorias do Instituto Butantan **33** (1–3) (Supplemento comemorativo), 1966; Clinical Toxicology **3** (3), 1970; J. Formosan Med. Ass. **71** (6), 1972.

B. The Use of Well-Defined Lesions in Experimental Animals to Specify and Determine Local Effects of Snake Venom

The local lesion produced by the parenteral injection to animals of crotalid and viperid venoms is of a complex nature, consisting of hemorrhage, necrosis, and edema (VAN HEYNINGEN, 1954; SLOTTA, 1955). The formation of such a complex pathophysiological lesion may be due to multiple biological actions possessed by a single venom principle, or more likely, to a combined effect of two or more principles with different biological actions or the possible synergistic effect of these principles (OHSAKA, 1968, 1973).

In order to elucidate biochemically the mechanism of the diverse local effects of a snake venom, separation of the various principles that are contained in the venom and have different local actions is obviously required. For this purpose, however, it is necessary to establish experimental conditions under which the elementary changes involved in a complex lesion, e.g., hemorrhage, necrosis, and edema are reproduced separately in experimental animals. It is also necessary to develop specific methods for determining individual principles responsible for such well-defined changes (OHSAKA et al., 1966a; OHSAKA, 1968, 1973). For this purpose, one must (1) specify the experimental conditions, e.g., animal species used, amount of venom administered, route and site of administration, method of observation of the response, etc., and (2) establish a method for determining quantitatively the specific principle responsible for each specified pathophysiological change on the basis of the principle of bioassay.

For the hemorrhagic principle, these requirements were satisfied when KONDO et al. (1960) developed a method for determining hemorrhagic activity with a great improvement in precision. As described in Section E.I.1, the hemorrhagic spot observed from the inner surface is sharply demarcated (Fig. 1) (OHSAKA et al., 1971a). A definite hemorrhagic spot, visible from the inner surface, was usually produced with a small amount (0.1–0.3 μg) of *Trimeresurus flavoviridis* venom. Approximately 100 to 300 times this dose of venom was required to produce a feeble reaction which was not clearly discernible from the outer surface (KONDO et al., 1960). Histological studies performed on biopsies from the test reactions indicated that the hemorrhage was predominant in the profound layer of the corium immediately above the muscular layer. This finding clearly explains the fact that sharply demarcated hemorrhagic

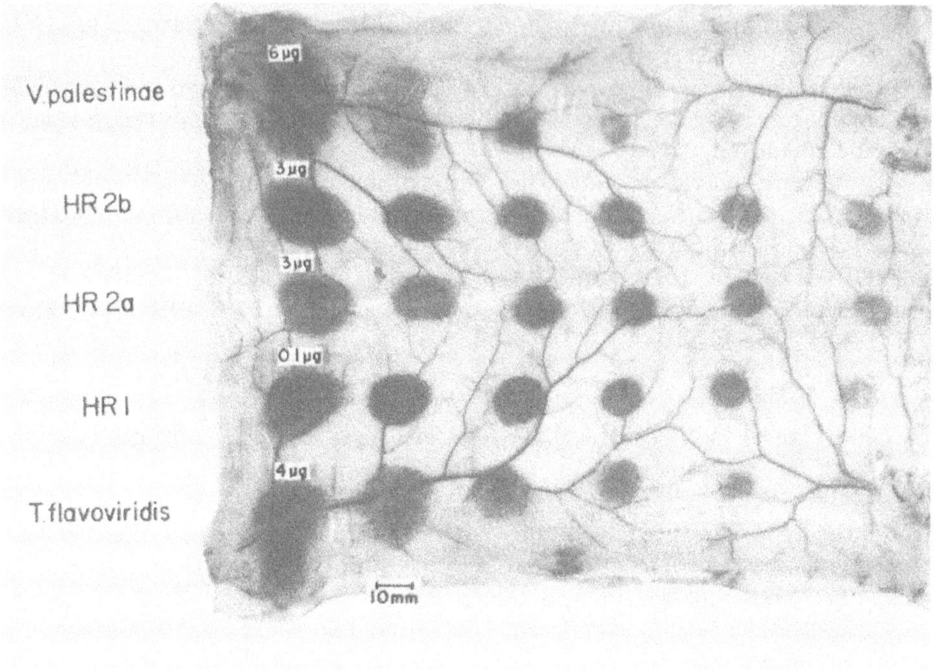

Fig. 1. Venom-produced hemorrhage observed from visceral side of rabbit skin. Aliquots (0.1 ml) from each of 3-fold dilutions of venom of *Trimeresurus flavoviridis* and purified hemorrhagic principles (HR1, HR2a and HR2b) were injected i.c. to the depilated back skin of a rabbit. The venom of *Vipera palestinae* was also injected for comparison. After 24 h, hemorrhage was observed from visceral side of removed skin (OHSAKA et al., 1971a)

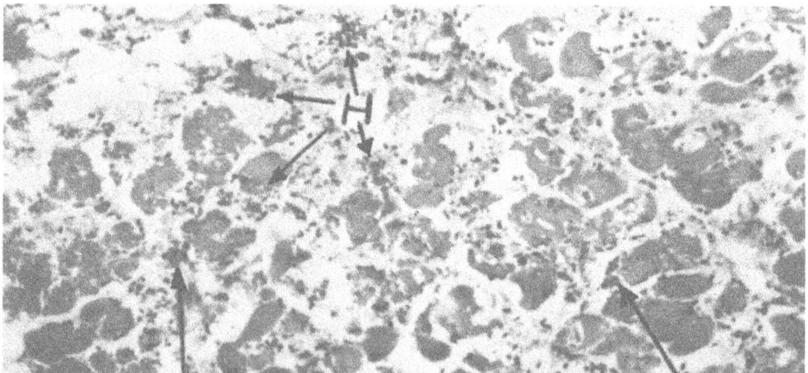

Fig. 2. Section of rabbit skin inoculated with 300 µg of *Trimeresurus flavoviridis* venom. Almost all muscle fibers show necrosis and dissolution. Diffuse infiltration of polymorphonuclear leucocytes (L) and intensive hemorrhage (H) are seen (OHSAKA et al., 1960a)

spots are visible only when observed from the inner surface of the removed skin (KONDO et al., 1960). The hemorrhage following the injection of such a large amount of venom as 300 μg spreads throughout the dermis and muscular layer, and necrosis of the muscle fibers was also observed (OHSAKA et al., 1960a) (Fig. 2). With this amount of venom, a complex local lesion, the so-called "necrosis" or "hemorrhagic necrosis" (necrosis with hemorrhage) was observable. These results indicate that the size of the hemorrhagic spot in the skin as determined from the inside, but not from the outside, is an exact measure for the intensity of the venom-induced hemorrhage under the specified conditions (KONDO et al., 1960).

Since the log dose-response curves obtained with a large number of crude venoms and their fractions proved to be linear and parallel to each other, the hemorrhagic activity of venom or venom fraction was determined relative to that of a reference venom by the parallel-line-assay method (KONDO et al., 1960).

C. Necrotizing Effect

As is usual among pathologists, the term necrosis is used here in a very restricted sense to refer to a localized process resulting in the death of a group of cells (VAN LANCKER, 1976). It is well known that venoms from *Crotalidae* and *Viperidae* exert a strong necrotizing effect. In human victims who survive snake bites, necrosis is seen at the site of the bite, with destruction of soft tissues (ROSENFELD, 1971); deep necrosis down to the bones of a foot or hand has often been reported (DEVI, 1971). Contrary to the popular belief, the main clinical feature of cobra bites in Malaya is also located necrosis (REID, 1964). The local lesion induced by cobra venom is attributable to cardiotoxin, which may be potential by phospholipase A (LAI et al., 1972).

Hemorrhage and necrosis have long been believed to be due, at least in part, to the action of proteolytic enzymes. HOUSSAY (1930) and others (KELLAWAY, 1939; ZELLER, 1948, 1951; PORGES, 1953; VAN HEYNINGEN, 1954; KAISER and MICHL, 1958) considered that proteolytic enzymes were mainly responsible for hemorrhage and necrosis at the site of bites, while SLOTTA (1955) regarded them as being attributable mainly to the joint action of proteases and phosphatases.

There are, however, clear examples of dissociation of hemorrhagic, myolytic (necrotic), and proteolytic activities in native venoms. Local necrosis, predominating over neurotoxic effects, is typical of the envenomation in man by Malayan cobras, whose venoms are neither proteolytic nor hemorrhagic (REID, 1964), whereas the venoms of *Trimeresurus okinavensis* (KURASHIGE et al., 1966), *Bitis gabonica*, *Bitis nasicornis* and *Bitis arietans* (TU et al., 1969) are all strongly hemorrhagic but only weakly myonecrotic if at all. In order to examine the relationship of necrotic activity to hemorrhagic and proteolytic activities in a snake venom, OHSAKA et al. (1960a) carefully studied histopathological changes evoked in the rabbit skin by intracutaneous injection with *Trimeresurus flavoviridis* venom and its electrophoretic fractions; they demonstrated that the muscle-degenerating effect, which leads to necrosis in its more severe forms, was related neither to hemorrhagic activity nor to proteolytic activity (on casein). Experimental induction of myolysis with venom phospholipase A (MAENO et al., 1962; SARKAR and DEVI, 1968) or lysolecithin (PHILLIPS et al.,

1965) has prompted the suggestion that the necrotic effects of snake venoms are attributable to phospholipase A (MAENO and MITSUHASHI, 1961; MAENO et al., 1962). This suggestion was later supported by the work of GEH and TOH (1976) with a phospholipase A fraction from *Enhydrina schistosa* venom, although a highly purified phospholipase A from other sea snake venom showed little, if any, myolytic or cytopathic effect (TU and PASSEY, 1971). On the other hand, heat-stable myolytic factors purified from *Trimeresurus flavoviridis* venom by KURASHIGE et al. (1966) were devoid of proteinase, phospholipase A, ribonuclease and esterase activities. In the presence of Mg^{2+} and phospholipase A, these factors caused severe myolysis.

Recently, OWNBY et al. (1976) isolated a myotoxin from *Crotalus viridis viridis* venom by gel filtration on Sephadex G-50, followed by chromatography on Sephadex G-25. The electrophoretic homogeneity of the myotoxin was demonstrated in isoelectric focusing and disc electrophoresis. White mice were injected intramuscularly with 1.5 μg/g of the purified protein. Light-microscopic examination of injected muscle revealed a series of degenerative events, including partial vacuolation of muscle cells at 6, 12, and 24 h and complete vacuolation and loss of striations at 48 and 72 h. Hemorrhage was not observed. At the electron-microscopic level the perinuclear space and sarcoplasmic reticulum were dilated in all samples. By 48 and 72 h the myofibrils lacked striations and the sarcomeres were disorganized. Plasma membranes and T tubules remained intact in all samples. These results correlated well with the myonecrosis induced by crude *Crotalus viridis viridis* venom except for several important aspects. The pure component altered skeletal muscle cells specifically, with the sarcoplasmic reticulum being the primary site of action.

From all the information we may conclude that snake venoms contain, besides hemorrhagins (see Sect. E), necrotic factors that are not necessarily proteolytic enzymes. However, in view of the findings suggesting that many proteinases such as H_2-proteinase (a venom proteinase) (TAKAHASHI and OHSAKA, unpubl.), pronase, nagarse, papain, chymotrypsin, and trypsin (TAKAHASHI and OHSAKA, 1970b) in amounts more than 50 μg induce necrosis on the back skin of the rabbit, most, if not all, proteolytic enzymes in snake venoms may also contribute, at least in part, to the necrotizing effects of the venoms. Further elucidation of the nature of venom components that induce necrosis obviously depends on the devising of a reliable method for quantitative assay of necrotic activity.

D. Edema-Forming Effect

Swelling and edema are often the paramount early features of snake venom poisoning at the affected part of the victims (REID, 1968). To date, however, extensive studies have not been made on the edema-forming principles of snake venoms (see Chaps. 16 and 17).

The local irritant action of cobra venom causing pain and swelling has been attributed to cardiotoxin of the venom; the instillation of this toxin into the rabbit's eye caused congestion of the conjunctiva, followed by edema of the palpebral and ocular conjunctiva (LEE et al., 1968). The local irritant action of cardiotoxin was also demonstrated by the rat-paw edema test; the increase in weight of the rat hind paw due to edema was found to be dose-dependent (LEE et al., 1968). The cobra venom-induced rat-paw edema was inhibited by oestriol succinate (BONTA and DE VOS, 1965; BONTA, 1969).

The edema-forming activity of some *Crotalidae* venoms has also been investigated. BHARGAVA et al. (1972) fractionated *Agkistrodon piscivorus* venom by gel filtration and separated from kininogenase a polypeptide fraction with a molecular weight of about 8000, the latter being more potent in provoking edema than the former. Time-course studies indicated that the edema induced by the venom or the polypeptide fraction is of a rapid and transient type; it reaches a maximum in as little as 30 min and thereafter starts to decline. The edema provoked by the polypeptide fraction was inhibited by Trasylol, phenylbutazone, and cyproheptadine (BHARGAVA et al., 1972). YAMAKAWA et al. (1976) investigated the edema-forming activity of the venom of *Trimeresurus elegans*. Mice in groups of 10 were injected in the right pads with 10-μl doses of 3–4 dilutions of venom graded with threefold intervals. Four h after injection, the mice were killed by chloroform inhalation. Both legs were then cut off and weighed individually. The weight of the injected leg as a percentage of the control leg was designated the "edema ratio," and was taken as a measure of the severity of the edema. When three lethal fractions, S_1, S_2, and S_3 obtained from the venom by gel filtration were injected into foot-pads of mice, swelling developed quickly and reached the maximum severity in about 30–60 min (YAMAKAWA et al., 1976). Fraction S_1 induced severe edema without causing hemorrhage, and this edema healed rapidly in 8–10 h. On the other hand, both fraction S_2 and crude venom caused intensive edema with severe hemorrhage in the foot-pads, and these changes persisted for a longer time. Fraction S_3 induced both edema and hemorrhage, but to a lesser extent. Statistical analysis demonstrated the linearity and parallelism of log dose-response curves obtained with any of the venom fractions. The common slope, $\bar{b}$, was 25.1 and the common variance, S^2, was 43.3 in 4 h of observation. The minimum edema dose (MED) was defined as the least quantity of venom causing an edema ratio of 130%.

It is worth mentioning the studies of VICK et al. (1963), who demonstrated that the pulmonary edema occurring in isolated canine lungs perfused with *Naja hannah* or *Crotalus adamanteus* venom in the presence of plasma can be prevented by heating the plasma to 56° C for 30 min or by epsilon aminocaproic acid. So far, this is the only evidence that venom-induced edema is not due to the direct action of venom on the vessel wall but occurs through activation of a plasma enzyme, which, according to the authors, is probably not identical with fibrinolysin. It would therefore be interesting to know whether the edema induced by snake venoms is due, at least in part, to direct action of venom toxin(s) or to mediation through autopharmacological action of the toxin(s), i.e., a release of histamine, serotonin, or kinins. By the early nineteen-sixties, evidence had accumulated to show that the release of 5-hydroxytryptamine (5-HT, serotonin) and histamine is the major cause of edema and increased vascular permeability occurring in rats following treatment with high-molecular-weight substances and peptides (ROWLEY and BENDITT, 1956; GÖZSY and KÁTÓ, 1957; PARRAT and WEST, 1957; SPECTOR, 1958; JORI et al., 1961; WEST, 1961). Do the same factors mediate the vascular response to snake venom?

SOMANI (1962) reported that the increased vascular permeability (blue discoloration) induced in the abdominal skin of rats by *Echis carinatus* (saw-scale viper) venom is largely mediated through the release of histamine, and to a lesser extent by the release of serotonin. This is suggested by the fact that this vascular response to the venom is blocked to a greater extent by a powerful antihistaminic drug than by an antiserotonin drug or reserpine pretreatment. Hydrocortisone pretreatment also almost completely inhibits the increased vascular permeability induced by the venom, and also that by histamine, confirming the above statement that *E. carinatus* venom acts mainly through the release of histamine (SOMANI and ARORA, 1962). The possibility that the increase in vascular permeability produced by the venom of Russell's viper *(Vipera russellii)* and *Echis carinatus* is mediated by histamine and serotonin was also suggested by FEARN et al. (1964). COHEN and his co-workers (1969) separated the hemorrhagic activity of *Echis coloratus* venom from its kinin-releasing and vascular permeability-increasing activities, the latter two being thermostable, whereas the former was thermolabile. SATO et al. (1965) isolated a substance from *Agkistrodon halys blomhoffii* venom, in a physicochemically homogeneous state, which induces an increase in vascular permeability. They concluded that this substance is identical with an arginine-ester (TAME)-hydrolase that is separable from two other hydrolases associated with bradykinin-releasing and clotting activities, respectively. However, this conclusion was not based on a quantitative comparison of the increases in specific activities of vascular-permeability-increasing and TAME-hydrolase activities during the purification. It remains to be determined whether the arginine-ester-hydrolase having the vascular permeability-increasing activity can significantly induce edema in foot pads of mice or rats.

E. Hemorrhagic Effect

The occurrence of hemorrhage is one of the most striking consequences of the parenteral injection of many snake venoms, especially crotalid and viperid venoms (EFRATI and REIF, 1953; OHSAKA and KONDO, 1960; RUSSELL, 1960; DE VRIES et al., 1962; GITTER et al., 1962; BOQUET, 1964; OHSAKA et al., 1966a; WATT and GENNARO, 1966; JIMÉNEZ-PORRAS, 1968; DE VRIES and COHEN, 1969). In less severe cases, hemorrhage is limited to the cutaneous and subcutaneous tissues at the site of injection; in severe cases, hemorrhage may even spread to cover a large portion of the involved extremity, affecting the muscle layer. Bleeding in several organs such as the brain, heart, lungs, intestines, and kidneys is often encountered (RUSSELL, 1960; MCCOLLOUGH and GENNARO, 1963).

TAUBE and ESSEX (1937) found histological evidence for swelling of the endothelial cells of capillaries, and also the disintegration of the vessel walls, in dogs injected with rattlesnake venom. In early studies on the effect of *Crotalus* venom on blood vessels, MITCHELL and REICHERT (1886) concluded that hemorrhage occurred from the capillaries only, and not from the arteries and veins, and that the escape of blood apparently occurred from filtration of the blood through the vessel wall. Using cinematography at a microscopic level FULTON et al. (1956) demonstrated that, when moccasin (cotton mouth, *Agkistrodon piscivorus piscivorus*) venom was applied to the cheek pouch of the hamster, there was an initial arteriolar constriction. Subsequently, red blood cells were seen escaping from the blood vessels one by one, as if they were escaping through holes that appeared in the intracellular cement (FULTON et al., 1956). Erythrocytic extravasation in a one-by-one fashion through pin-point holes formed in mesenteric capillaries exposed to *Trimeresurus flavoviridis* venom was also demonstrated by OHSAKA et al. (1971 b).

Crotalid and viperid venoms are known to cause disturbance in blood coagulation, and also thrombocytopenia (KLOBUSITZKY, 1961; HÄRTEL, 1963; BOQUET, 1964; INGRAM, 1964; MEAUME, 1966; DENSON, 1969; DE VRIES and COHEN, 1969). The pathogenesis of hemorrhage due to envenomation from snakebite involves, besides vessel wall damage caused by certain venom component(s) (hemorrhagins), coagulation disturbances by other venom components (anticoagulants and coagulants) and thrombocytopenia (DE VRIES and COHEN, 1969). It has been demonstrated, however, that venom-induced blood incoagulability *per se* is a relatively benign state that may exist without causing hemorrhage (RECHNIC et al., 1962; ROSENFELD, 1964; MARSTEN et al., 1966; REID, 1967), although the defect in hemostasis may aggravate hemorrhage primarily caused by the destructive action of venom on vessel walls (RECHNIC et al., 1960, 1962; DJALDETTI et al., 1964; ROSENFELD, 1964; REID, 1967; OHSAKA, 1973, 1976a, b).

The presence of snake venom components that damage the blood vessel wall has been known for about a century (MITCHELL, 1860). The term hemorrhagin (FLEXNER and NOGUCHI, 1903) or hemorrhagic principle (OHSAKA et al., 1960a) designates a venom agent causing bleeding by a direct action on the blood vessel wall, as distinct from venom agents that affect hemostasis through an action on blood coagulation (DE VRIES and COHEN, 1969).

The hemorrhagic effect of snake venoms has been attributed to the action of proteolytic enzyme(s) in the venoms (HOUSSAY, 1930; KELLAWAY, 1939; ZELLER, 1948, 1951; PORGES, 1953; VAN HEYNINGEN, 1954; SLOTTA, 1955; KAISER and MICHL, 1958). However, as pointed out by some workers (OHSAKA and KONDO, 1960; BOQUET, 1964, 1966; GITTER and DE VRIES, 1968; JIMÉNEZ-PORRAS, 1968, DE VRIES and COHEN, 1969), the only evidence in the past for ascribing hemorrhagic effects to proteolytic activities was the high protease content of many crotalid and viperid venoms endowed with potent hemorrhagic activity. The failure to isolate pure venom hemorrhagins and proteases (DE VRIES et al., 1962; GITTER et al., 1962; GOUCHER and FLOWERS, 1964; OHSAKA et al., 1966a; SUZUKI, 1966a; TU et al., 1967, 1969; OSHIMA et al., 1968) also contributed to the long-accepted notion of the identity of hemorrhagins with proteolytic enzymes.

OHSAKA et al. (1960a) measured the hemorrhagic activity of electrophoretic fractions obtained from the venom of *Trimeresurus flavoviridis*, using a quantitative assay method (skin reaction) devised by KONDO et al. (1960); they found that the venom contains two hemorrhagic principles, HR 1 and HR 2 (OHSAKA et al., 1960a), which are distinct immunologically but indistinguishable in hemorrhagic action on rabbit skin (KONDO et al., 1965b; OHSAKA et al., 1966b; OHSAKA, 1976a). As well as by electrophoresis (OHSAKA et al., 1960a, b), these hemorrhagic principles were separable from each other by ion-exchange chromatography (OHSAKA, 1960a) and gel filtration (OMORI-SATOH et al., 1967). Many authors attempted to correlate the hemorrhage induced by snake venoms with proteolytic activity in the venoms (MAENO et al., 1959a, b, 1960; KOCHWA et al., 1960; OHSAKA, 1960a; OHSAKA et al., 1960a, b, 1966a; MAENO, 1962; OMORI et al., 1964; IWANAGA et al., 1965; GROTTO et al., 1967; OMORI-SATOH et al., 1967; TU et al., 1967; TOOM et al., 1969) and some of them purified "hemorrhagic proteinases" from crotalid venoms (MAENO et al., 1959b,

1960; IWANAGA et al., 1965). On the other hand, the presence of hemorrhagic principles devoid of proteolytic activity towards conventional substrates has been reported from several laboratories (OHSAKA, 1960a; OHSAKA et al., 1960b; MAENO, 1962; OMORI et al., 1964; TOÓM et al., 1969). GROTTO et al. (1967) purified "hemorrhagin" from *Vipera palestinae* venom and distinguished between the hemorrhagic and the proteolytic activities. The lack of identity of venom proteases with hemorrhagins suggested by some workers (OHSAKA, 1960a; OHSAKA et al., 1960b, 1966a; GITTER et al., 1962; OMORI et al., 1964; SUZUKI, 1966a, b; GROTTO et al., 1967; TOOM et al., 1969; OMORI-SATOH and OHSAKA, 1970) was conclusively demonstrated by the recent isolation from *Agkistrodon halys blomhoffii* and *Trimeresurus flavoviridis* venoms of the major proteinases completely free from hemorrhagic activity (OSHIMA et al., 1968; TAKAHASHI and OHSAKA, 1970a) as well as a hemorrhagin devoid of proteolytic activity toward casein from the latter venom (TAKAHASHI and OHSAKA, 1970b). (For information on the nature and the mode of action of purified venom hemorrhagic principles, see Sect. E.III.)

Hemorrhagic principles play a minor role in the lethality of some venoms (GENNARO and RAMSEY, 1959; EMERY and RUSSELL, 1963), but they appear to be the major lethal factors in others (OMORI et al., 1964; OHSAKA et al., 1966a; OMORI-SATOH and OHSAKA, 1970), causing death in severe envenomation from bleeding in the brain, lungs, kidneys, and heart (DE VRIES et al., 1962; BICHER et al., 1966; MCCOLLOUGH and GENNARO, 1966; WATT and GENNARO, 1966; REID, 1967).

I. Methods for Determining Hemorrhagic Activity

1. Skin Reaction

KONDO et al. (1960) devised a quantitative method for determining hemorrhagic activity of snake venom. The method consists of (1) intracutaneous injection of minute amounts (0.1–30 μg) of venom into the clipped back skin of rabbits, (2) accurate measurement of the size of the hemorrhagic spots produced in 24 h from the visceral side of the removed skin, and (3) application of the parallel-line-assay method for estimating the hemorrhagic activity.

Procedure: The determination of hemorrhagic activity is made on albino rabbits of either sex weighing about 2.7–2.8 kg. One day before testing, the fur over the dorsal area is gently clipped. Three-fold dilutions of venom or venom fraction, in a volume of 0.1 ml, are injected intracutaneously into the clipped area. The injection sites are spaced at distances of about 2.5 cm in a checker-board arrangement. The large surface of the back skin of a rabbit usually permits the production of 60–70 circumscribed hemorrhagic spots. In order to control the possible variations in response due to the different sensitivities of the sites of injection and of individual rabbits, each dilution is injected to 2–3 rabbits at different sites selected at random. Twenty-four hours later, when the response has reached its maximum, the animals are killed by chloroform inhalation and the intensity of the skin response (the size of hemorrhagic spot) is estimated from the visceral side of the removed skin. The skin is spread and fixed on a glass plate so as to keep the original size. The cross-diameters of hemorrhagic spots (see Fig. 1) are measured through the glass plate and the mean of the cross-diameters of all the spots is taken as a measure for the intensity of the response.

By statistical analysis of the results obtained with a large number of venom preparations, a distinct correlation was established between log doses of venom and the size of hemorrhagic spots, and the log dose-response curves were proven to be linear and parallel with each other within a range of diameters from 10 to 18 mm (KONDO et al., 1960) (Fig. 3). The common slope $\bar{b}$

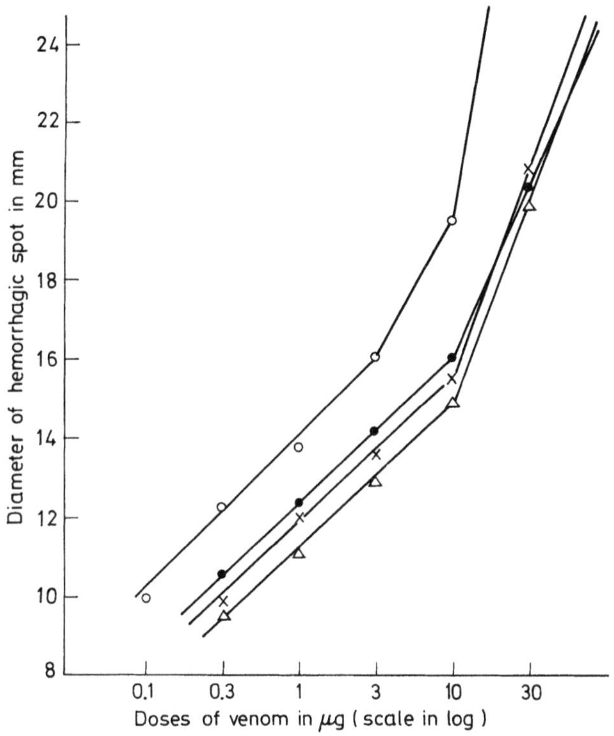

Fig. 3. Dose-response curves of hemorrhage induced by various preparations of *Trimeresurus flavoviridis* venom. ●—●, crude venom; ○—○, fraction-13; ×—×, fraction-21; △—△, fraction-26 (KONDO et al., 1960)

was 4.724 and the common variance s^2 was 0.836 with 1013 hemorrhagic spots measured (OHSAKA et al., 1966a). The curves deviate from linearity when the hemorrhagic spots are larger than 18 mm; the reactions with diameters less than 8 to 9 mm were sometimes not clearly demarcated (KONDO et al., 1960). From these results a dosage range was selected that would produce reactions of 10–18 mm in diameter.

Based on the parallel-line-assay method, the hemorrhagic activity of venom is determined in terms of relative potency to a reference venom. The fiducial limits for the relative potency are about ±50% at a 95% level of probability when three rabbits are used under the above-described conditions; in order to expect fiducial limits of less than ±30%, five rabbits should be used in one experiment (KONDO et al., 1960). The method is applicable to venoms from different species of snakes (OHSAKA et al., 1966a).

Prior to KONDO et al. (1960), MINTON (1956) and MITSUHASHI et al. (1959) also reported methods for the estimation of hemorrhagic activity. Their methods were based on the reactions on the outer surface of the skin. MINTON (1956) tried to measure the "local necrotizing effect" of various kinds of venoms by intradermal injection into the shaved belly skin of guinea-pigs, but the results thus obtained were, as he pointed out, only a rough approximation for the following reasons; (1) the areas of necrosis were irregular in shape and (2) no satisfactory way was found to compare the deep, circumscribed necrosis with the superficial, wide one. MITSUHASHI et al. (1959) tried to estimate hemorrhagic necrosis in the rabbit skin by the intracutaneous inoculation of *Trimeresurus flavoviridis* venom. The ability of venom to induce hemorrhagic necrosis was represented by the dosage of venom required to cause 100 mm^2 of hemorrhagic necrosis on the outer surface of the skin. However, in the light of the experience of KONDO et al. (1960) and MINTON (1956), this method of measurement appears to be subject to considerable variations, and therefore the accuracy of experimental results seems unsatisfactory.

More recently JUST et al. (1970) developed a new method for estimating hemorrhagic activity; a similar method was reported independently by TÁBORSKÁ (1971). The outline of the method is described here in some detail (OHSAKA et al., 1973a). Venom samples were injected intracutaneously to rabbits that had previously received ^{51}Cr-labeled erythrocytes from 16 to 18 ml blood. The animals were sacrificed 24 h after the injection, and the skin was removed; pieces of the skin around the site of injections were weighed and measured for radioactivity. The mean value for cpm/mg, calculated from 10–20 pieces, of uninjected skin was taken as background radioactivity. Net counts were calculated according to the following formula; net counts = cpm [sample]—(cpm/mg [back-ground]·mg[sample]). The average net counts calculated from five injections with each sample were taken as a measure for hemorrhagic activity. If ^{125}I-labeled albumin is previously given to the rabbits together with ^{51}Cr-labeled erythrocytes, it is possible to estimate simultaneously the extravasation not only of erythrocytes (^{51}Cr) but also of albumin (^{125}I). The method is especially useful for differentiating the local effects produced by different vasoactive agents (JUST et al., 1970).

2. Lung Surface Reaction

BONTA et al. (1970) developed a method that allowed quantitative assessment of hemorrhage induced by topical application of snake venoms to the lung surface in dog open-chest preparations.

Procedure: Filter-paper discs of 5 mm in diameter were soaked in dilute solutions of venom and applied for 3 min to the pulmonary surface. For obtaining dose-response curves, three concentrations (0.5–4 mg per ml) of venom were simultaneously applied. After removal of the filter-paper disc, the site of application was observed with unaided eye. The time between the removal of the filter paper and the appearance of distinct hemorrhage was recorded in the nearest minute. The intensity of the hemorrhage was scored according to an arbitrary scale (0 to 3) every minute, starting immediately after removal of the filter paper and ending 10 min thereafter. The large surface of the canine lung permits the production of 15–20 circumscribed hemorrhagic spots.

The method has some advantages; it gives information regarding the character and onset of the bleeding, and the rapidity of this method excludes the possibility that the hemorrhage observed was partially caused by systemic effects due to absorption of the venom. However, the onset time and the intensity of hemorrhage on the lung surface may be subject to considerable variations depending on individual dogs; this makes it difficult to quantitate the hemorrhage on the basis of the principle of bioassay. Moreover, in their method, the scoring of the hemorrhagic response was so arbitrary that the method lacked the rational basis for justifying its use in quantitative studies. Apparently, numerous fundamental problems have to be solved before the lung surface reaction can be used for quantitative assessment of hemorrhage induced by snake venoms.

Table 1. Distribution of hemorrhagic, lethal and proteolytic activities in snake venoms (OHSAKA et al., 1966a)

Snake venom	Hemorrhagic activity MHD (μg)	Lethal activity LD_{50} (μg)	Proteolytic activity (units/mg)	LD_{50}/MHD
A. contortrix contortrix	1.90	200	33.7	105
A. contortrix mokasen	1.20	125	48.1	104
A. piscivorus piscivorus	0.80	60.0	41.5	75
A. halys	0.14	16.0	35.8	114
Bothrops atrox	2.11	5.6	44.5	2.7
Bothrops jararaca	0.75	18.5	74.0	25
C. adamanteus	0.04	18.5	9.76	462
C. atrox	0.43	45.0	83.6	105
C. durissus terrificus	18.0	3.6	39.2	0.2
C. viridis viridis	0.56	21.0	39.5	38
T. flavoviridis	0.20	54.0	33.0	270
T. flavoviridis tokarensis	1.15	160	37.8	139
T. elegans	0.30	71.0	13.0	237
T. okinavensis	1.38	140	69.0	102
Vipera russellii	21.0	2.2	5.56	0.1
Vipera ammodytes	0.47	7.4	41.7	16
Vipera palestinae	0.54	7.1	4.96	13
Causus rhombeatus	0.81	>250	0.26	>309
Bitis arietans	0.15	15.0	18.7	100
Bitis gabonica	0.04	13.5	11.7	338
Ophiophagus hannah	0.84	54.0	12.0	64
Bungarus fasciatus	≫ 100[a]	18.5	0.06	≪ 0.18
Naja melanoleuca	≫ 100	6.0	7.00	≪ 0.06
Naja naja atra	≫ 100[a]	8.0	0.12	≪ 0.08
Naja naja	≫ 100	5.6	2.85	≪ 0.06

A: Agkistrodon, C: Crotalus, T: Trimeresurus

[a] A pinkish macule was observed at the site of injection.

Using such dog open-chest preparations, BONTA and his group (1970) observed that *Naja naja* and *Naja nigricollis* venoms, when applied to the lung surface, produced bleeding of a diffuse character, whereas hemorrhage caused by *Agkistrodon piscivorus* venom had the appearance of petechial bleeding. It is surprising that cobra venoms produced the pulmonary hemorrhage, since none of the cobra venoms except *Ophiophagus hannah* venom is known to contain hemorrhagic activity when tested by the skin reaction (see Table 1). According to BONTA et al. (1969), the hemorrhagic principle of *Naja naja* venom detected by the lung surface reaction is probably identical with the direct lytic factor (DLF), which renders the venom phospholipase A capable of causing diffuse bleeding on the lung surface. Fractionation of the venom of *Agkistrodon piscivorus* indicated that the venom principle responsible for pulmonary hemorrhage is a polypeptide having a molecular weight of less than 10000 (BHARGAVA et al., 1970). The results again disagree with the much higher values reported for hemorrhagic principles from some *Crotalidae* venoms detected by the skin reaction. These discrepancies may suggest that venom principles detected by the skin reaction are not necessarily the same as those detected by the lung surface reaction in respect to their action on microvessels. A full account of the work of BONTA and his group is given in Chapter 17.

II. Distribution of Hemorrhagic Activity in Venoms of Crotalidae, Viperidae and Elapidae

As shown in Table 1 (OHSAKA et al., 1966a), hemorrhagic activity as determined by the skin reaction is distributed in all venoms of both *Crotalidae* and *Viperidae*, although the ratios of LD_{50} to the minimum hemorrhagic dose (MHD), especially for the venoms of *Bothrops atrox*, *Crotalus durissus terrificus* and *Vipera russellii*, are very small; almost none of the venoms of *Elapidae* manifests hemorrhagic activity, and therefore the ratios for such venoms are much smaller. The only exception is *Ophiophagus hannah* (king cobra) venom, whose hemorrhagic activity is as high as those of *Crotalidae* and *Viperidae* venoms.

Macroscopic observation indicated similarity of hemorrhagic lesions induced by venoms from different species of snakes. The common slope ($\bar{b}$) of the log dose-response curves for the hemorrhage was 4.72 for the venom of *Trimeresurus flavoviridis*; essentially the same value was obtained with all the other venoms tested (OHSAKA et al., 1966a). These results suggest a certain similarity among hemorrhagic principles in venoms from different species of snakes. Incidentally, the results presented in Table 1 may be an indication that the hemorrhagic activity is not directly associated with the proteolytic (caseinolytic) activity or the lethal toxicity of crude venoms.

III. Purification and Characterization of Hemorrhagic Principles

In recent years, marked progress has been made in the separation and purification of hemorrhagic principles from the venoms of four species of snakes: *Agkistrodon halys blomhoffii* (Mamushi), *Bothrops jararaca*, *Trimeresurus flavoviridis* (Habu), and *Vipera palestinae*.

GROTTO et al. (1967) purified a hemorrhagin from the venom of *Vipera palestinae*. The purified preparation, which was homogeneous in immunodiffusion and in ultracentrifugal analysis, was an acidic protein with a molecular weight of 44000, calculated from the sedimentation coefficient $S_{20,\omega}$ of 3.44 and the diffusion coefficient D_{20} of 7.6×10^{-7}. Although the purified hemorrhagin had gelatinase activity, it was suggested that the hemorrhagic action of the preparation was not due to its proteolytic activity since soybean trypsin inhibitor or DFP inhibited the latter, while leaving the hemorrhagic activity intact. The authors regarded this functional difference as indicating either association of two protein molecules having distinct active sites (PARK et al., 1961), or selective blocking of a part of one active center having two distinct biological activities (COLEMAN and VALLEE, 1961).

Recently one of the hemorrhagic principles, HR 1, in the venom of *Trimeresurus flavoviridis* was highly purified (OMORI-SATOH and OHSAKA, 1970; OHSAKA et al., 1971a). The preparation possessed some proteolytic activity toward casein but this activity was ascribed to contaminant(s), as shown by inhibition studies of the preparation by EDTA (OMORI-SATOH and OHSAKA, 1970). Another hemorrhagic principle in the same venom, HR 2, which had previously been associated with the bulk of the proteolytic activity of the venom (OHSAKA et al., 1960a, b, 1966a; MAENO, 1962; OMORI-SATOH et al., 1967) was also highly purified, with concomitant resolution into two hemorrhagic principles (HR 2a and HR 2b), each being completely devoid of proteolytic activity as well as any of the enzyme activities present in the original venom (TAKAHASHI and OHSAKA, 1970b; OHSAKA et al., 1971a). Thus, substantial evidence was presented to show that hemorrhage induced by snake venom is not due to proteolytic (caseinolytic) enzyme(s) in the venom; this does not exclude, however, the possibility that a venom hemorrhagic principle might be a proteolytic enzyme having a strict substrate specificity (OHSAKA et al., 1973a, b).

Two hemorrhagic principles from the venom of *Agkistrodon halys blomhoffii* were highly purified. One of the hemorrhagic factors, HR-1, was found to be devoid of proteolytic activity as well as any of the enzyme activities known to be present in the crude venom (OSHIMA et al., 1971, 1972); whereas the other hemorrhagic factor, HR-II, was claimed to be identical with one of the proteolytic enzymes, named proteinase b, in this venom (IWANAGA et al., 1965). It was demonstrated that HR-II (proteinase b) is an acidic protein with an $S_{20,\omega}$ of 4.82 S, and differs from trypsin, chymotrypsin, and pancreatopeptidase in its action on synthetic substrates and its ability to destroy bradykinin (IWANAGA et al., 1965).

From the venom of *Bothrops jararaca*, MANDELBAUM et al. (1976) purified one of the hemorrhagic factors, HF_2; the preparation was homogeneous, as judged by several physicochemical criteria, and had an $S_{20,\omega}$ of 4.34 S and a molecular weight of 49100–50090. HF_2 was found to contain some caseinolytic activity.

It is worth describing here in greater detail the purification and characterization of hemorrhagic principles, HR 1 (OMORI-SATOH and OHSAKA, 1970) and HR 2 (HR 2a and HR 2b) (TAKAHASHI and OHSAKA, 1970b), in the venom of *Trimeresurus flavoviridis*.

1. Purification and Characterization of HR 1

a) Purification

Crude venom was dissolved to a concentration of 20% in 5 mM Tris-HCl buffer (pH 8.5) containing 0.15 M NaCl, and this was chromatographed on Sephadex G-100, as reported previously (OMORI-SATOH et al., 1967) (Fig. 4). The HR 1 fraction (crude HR 1) thus separated from HR 2 contained 63% of the hemorrhagic activity, 50% of the lethal toxicity and 7% of the proteolytic activity of the original venom. This fraction, after concentration and dialysis against 6 mM borax-HCl buffer (pH 9.0), was chromatographed on DEAE-Sephadex A-50 (Fig. 5). After a minor peak of proteolytic activity had emerged, a large protein peak containing both the hemorrhagic activity and the lethal toxicity (Tube No. 90–150) was eluted. This fraction, which contained some proteolytic activity, was chromatographed on guanidoethyl (GE)-cellulose after concentration and dialysis against 10 mM Tris-HCl buffer (pH 8.5) (Fig. 6). The first eluted peak contained not only the bulk of the hemorrhagic activity and of the lethal toxicity, but also some proteolytic activity. The same fraction was then submitted to recycling chromatography (PORATH and BENNICH, 1962) on Sephadex G-200 (Fig. 7). The preceding and trailing materials (hatched areas) were withdrawn from the recycling system in the first and second cycles. Specific hemorrhagic activity was consistently higher in the preceding mate-

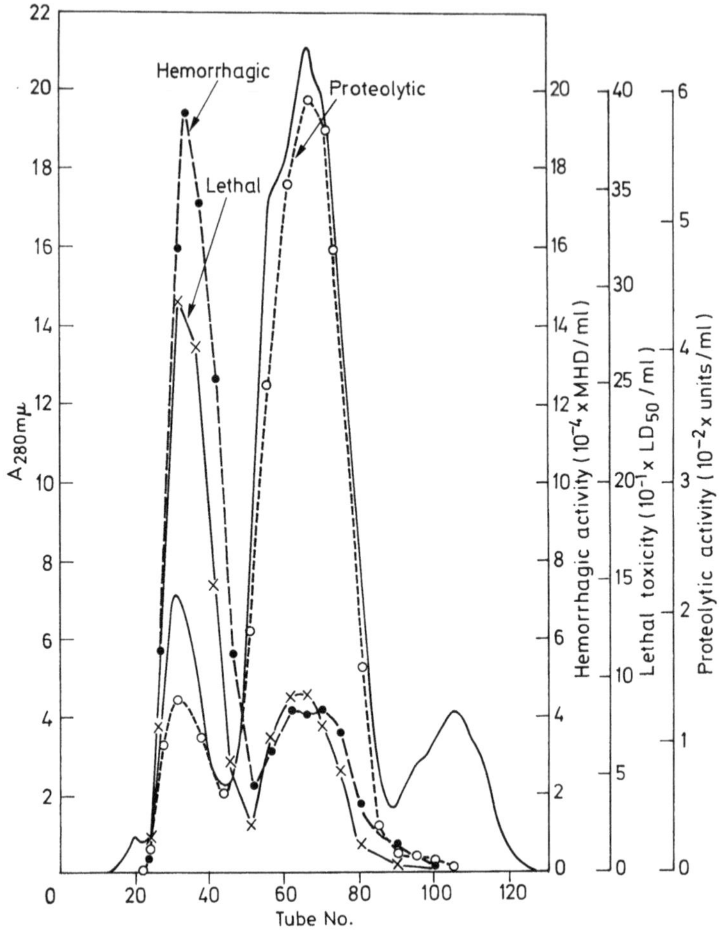

Hemorrhagic
Proteolytic
Lethal
$A_{280m\mu}$
Hemorrhagic activity (10^{-4} x MHD / ml)
Lethal toxicity (10^{-1} x LD_{50} / ml)
Proteolytic activity (10^{-2} x units / ml)
Tube No.

Fig. 4.

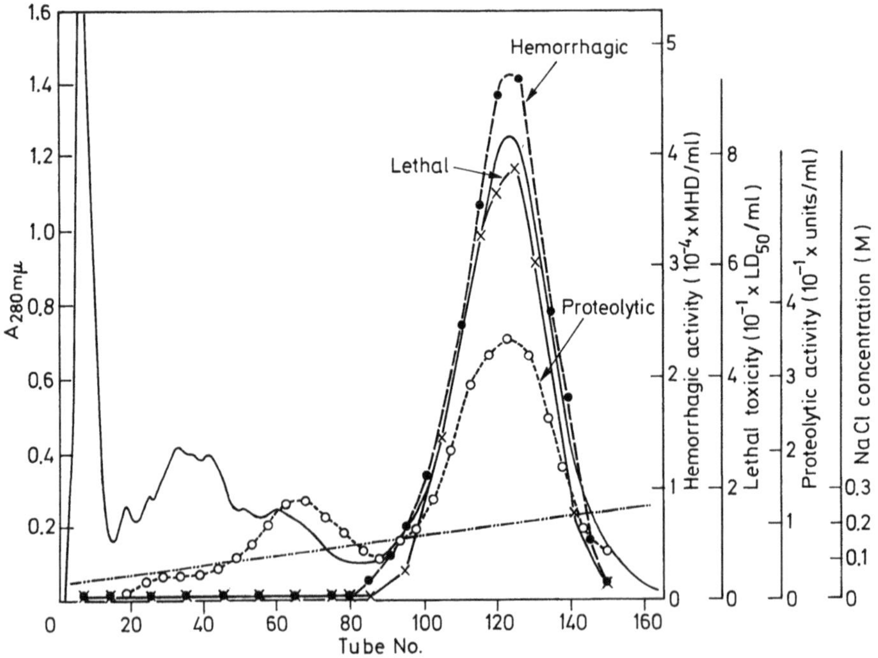

Hemorrhagic
Lethal
Proteolytic
$A_{280m\mu}$
Hemorrhagic activity (10^{-4} x MHD / ml)
Lethal toxicity (10^{-1} x LD_{50} / ml)
Proteolytic activity (10^{-1} x units / ml)
NaCl concentration (M)
Tube No.

Fig. 5.

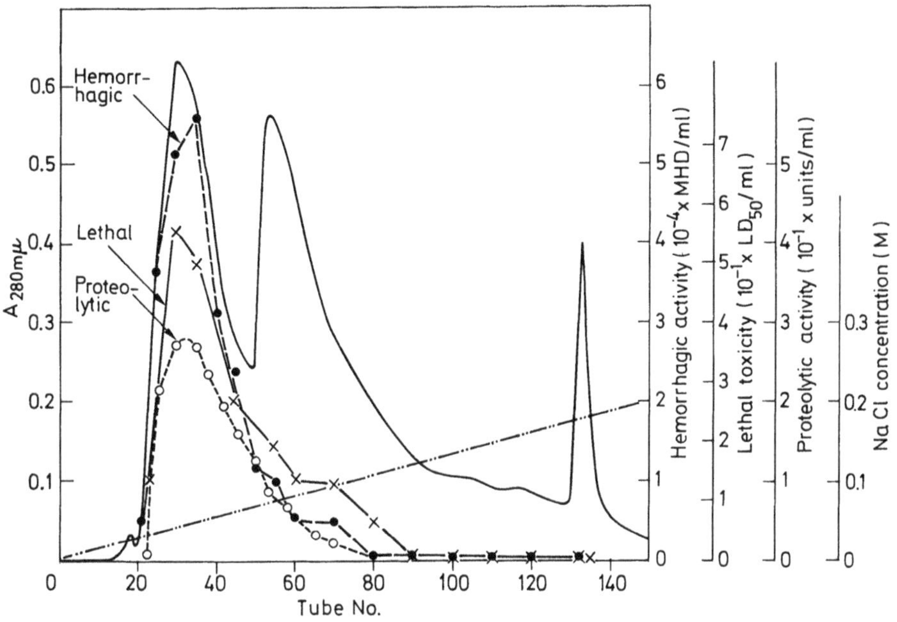

Fig. 6. Column chromatography of HR1 on GE-cellulose. Hemorrhagic fraction eluted from DEAE-Sephadex A-50 column was concentrated and dialyzed against 10 mM Tris-HCl buffer (pH 8.5). Dialysis residue (8 ml) containing 400 mg protein was applied to a column (1.5 × 52 cm) of GE-cellulose equilibrated with same buffer. Elution with linear gradient increase in NaCl concentration from 0 to 0.2 M in 1.6 liters of buffer was performed. 10-ml fractions were collected. Flow rate was 30 ml/h. ——, $A_{280\,m\mu}$; ●- - -●, hemorrhagic activity; ×—×, lethal toxicity; ○- - -○, proteolytic activity; —·-·—, NaCl concentration (OMORI-SATOH and OHSAKA, 1970)

rial than in the trailing material (see 1st and 2nd cycles); the material eluted between them, being apparently a mixture, was effectively fractionated by further recycling. In the third cycle, the protein was eluted in a symmetrical peak. The fractions 90-103, 173-183, and 260-300, with higher hemorrhagic activity, were combined. Potent lethal toxicity was also found in the combined fraction.

The extent of purification and the yield at each step are summarized in Table 2. A 43-fold purification was attained with a yield of 20% in respect to hemorrhagic

---

← Fig. 4. Separation of two hemorrhagic fractions by gel filtration. 40 ml of 20% solution of crude venom (Batch No. 65A) dissolved in 5 mM Tris-HCl buffer (pH 8.5) containing 0.15 M NaCl, after clarification by centrifugation, was placed on a column (5 × 91 cm) of Sephadex G-100. Elution was carried out with same buffer and every 15 ml of the eluate was collected. ——, $A_{280\,m\mu}$; ●- - -●, hemorrhagic activity; ×—×, lethal toxicity; ○- - -○, proteolytic activity (OHSAKA et al., 1971a)

← Fig. 5. Column chromatography of crude HR1 on DEAE-Sephadex A-50. Crude HR1 obtained by gel filtration of 8 g of crude venom on Sephadex G-100 was dialyzed against 6 mM borax-HC1 buffer (pH 9.0). After removal of precipitate by centrifugation, supernatant fluid (30 ml) containing 800 mg protein was applied to a column (2.5 × 25 cm) of DEAE-Sephadex A-50 equilibrated with same buffer. Column was eluted with linear gradient increase in NaCl concentration from 0.05 to 0.25 M in 2 liters of buffer. 12 ml fractions were collected. Flow rate was 15 ml/h. ——, $A_{280\,m\mu}$; ●- - -●, hemorrhagic activity; ×—×, lethal toxicity; ○- - -○, proteolytic activity; —·-·—, NaCl concentration (OMORI-SATOH and OHSAKA, 1970)

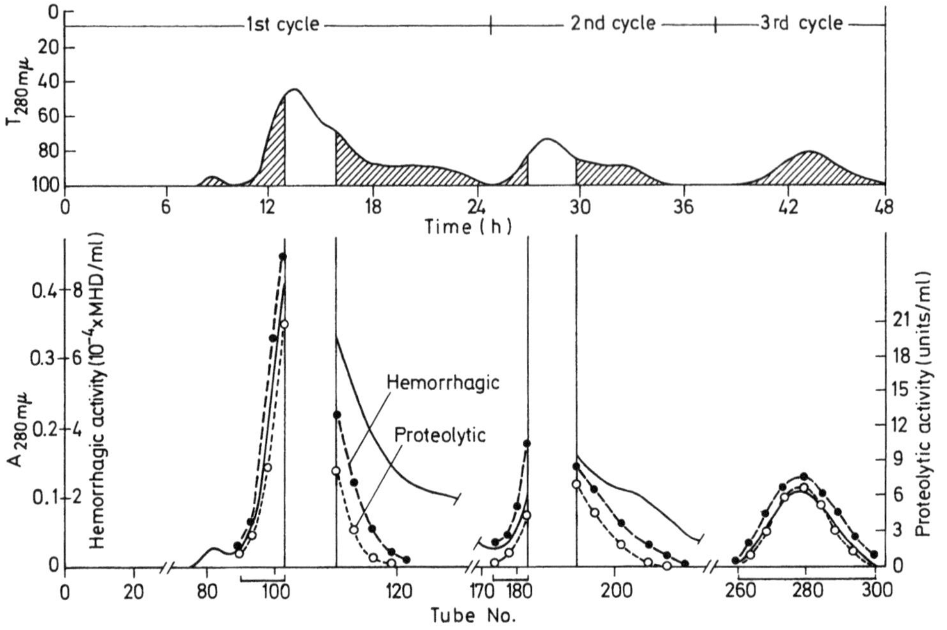

Fig. 7. Recycling chromatography of HR1 on Sephadex G-200. The hemorrhagic fraction eluted from the GE-cellulose column was concentrated. The concentrated solution (2 ml) containing 120 mg protein was applied to a column (3.2 × 90 cm) of Sephadex G-200 equilibrated with 6 mM borax-HCl buffer (pH 9.0). Recycling chromatography was carried out as described by OMORI-SATOH and OHSAKA (1970). The upper figure shows the chromatographic diagram in which protein contents are expressed in per cent transmission at 280 mμ; the lower figure shows the diagram of the hatched area in which protein contents are expressed in absorbance at 280 mμ; ——, $T_{280\,m\mu}$ or $A_{280\,m\mu}$; ●- - -●, hemorrhagic activity; ○- - -○, proteolytic activity (OMORI-SATOH and OHSAKA, 1970)

activity and 15-fold with a yield of 7% in respect to lethal toxicity. The purified preparation contained only 0.6% of the proteolytic activity. The minimum hemorrhagic dose and the 50% lethal dose were 0.0058 μg and 4.6 μg (per mouse), respectively.

The purified preparation of HR 1 was analyzed by ultracentrifugation. A single but not strictly symmetrical boundary with an $S_{20,\omega}$ of 5.8 S was observed.

The reaction of the purified preparation against antivenin by the Ouchterlony technique (OUCHTERLONY, 1948) is shown in Figure 8: a single precipitin line was observed (OHSAKA, 1976a).

Upon electrophoresis on cellulose acetate membrane at pH 8.6, the purified preparation migrated toward the anode as a single band. Isoelectric focusing (VESTERBERG and SVENSSON, 1966) of the preparation in carrier ampholytes covering a pH range of 3–6 yielded a single protein band associated with hemorrhagic activity.

b) Properties

Stability of the purified preparation was tested by exposing it to various pH values between 2.0 and 13.0 at 37° C for 1 h. The hemorrhagic activity was more stable in

Table 2. Summary of purification of HR1 (OMORI-SATOH and OHSAKA, 1970)

Step	Protein (mg)	Hemorrhagic activity				Lethal toxicity				Proteolytic activity		
		MHD (μg)	Relative activity	Total activity in MHD (10^{-6} × MHD)	Yield (%)	LD_{50} (μg)	Relative activity	Total activity (10^{-3} × LD_{50})	Yield (%)	Specific activity (units/mg protein)	Total activity (10^{-3} × units)	Yield (%)
Crude venom	8000	0.25	1.0	31.7	100	70	1.0	114	100	54.0	432	100
1. Sephadex G-100 (crude HR1)	1200	0.064	3.94	19.8	62.5	21	3.3	57	50.3	26.0	31.5	7.2
2. DEAE-Sephadex	400	0.030	8.45	13.6	42.9	13	5.4	28	24.6	27.0	10.8	2.5
3. GE-cellulose	120	0.015	16.5	7.9	25.0	9.0	7.8	13	12.0	51.2	6.2	1.4
4. Recycling chromatography	37	0.0058	43.4	6.4	20.0	4.6	15.0	8	7.0	67.5	2.6	0.6

MHD: Minimum hemorrhagic dose.

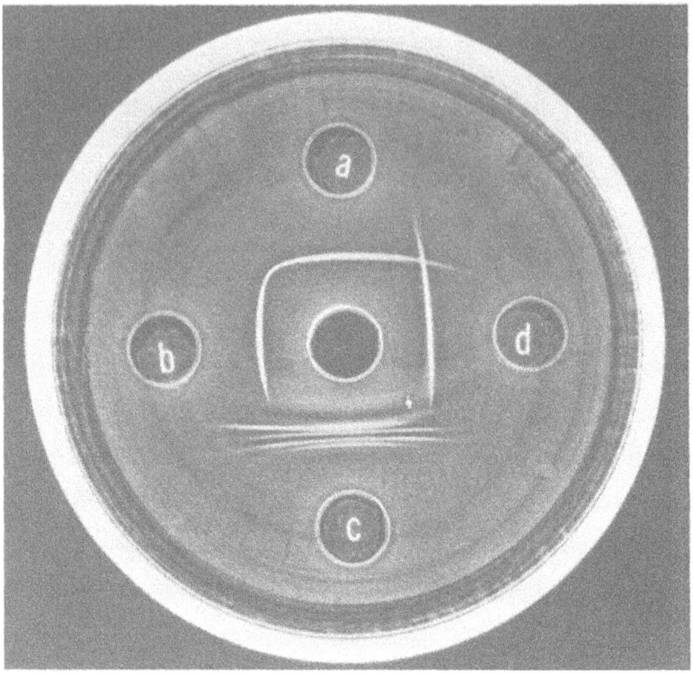

Fig. 8. Agar gel diffusion patterns demonstrating antigenic relationship among HR1, HR2a and HR2b (OHSAKA, 1976a). Center well contained 0.05 ml of antiserum to crude venom (500 units/ml). Outer wells, a, b, c, and d, contained, respectively, 0.05 ml each of HR2a (0.05%), HR2b (0.05%), crude venom (0.5%) and HR1 (0.05%)

Table 3. Effect of some reagents on hemorrhagic activity of HR1 (OMORI-SATOH and OHSAKA, 1970). The purified preparation of HR1 at 0.1 mg protein/ml was incubated at 37° C for 1 h in 10 mM Tris-HCl buffer (pH 8.5) in the presence of a given reagent at the indicated concentration. To terminate the reaction the incubation mixture was treated as follows. To the mixture containing EDTA or cysteine, $CaCl_2$ or monoiodoacetic acid, respectively, was added to give a final concentration of 5 mM. To the mixture containing formaldehyde glycine buffer (pH 8.5) was added to give a final concentration of 0.2 M. Excess DFP was removed by passing the incubation mixture through a column of Sephadex G-25. Hemorrhagic activity was expressed as a percentage of control

Reagent	Concentration	Hemorrhagic activity (%)
EDTA	0.03 mM	105
	0.1 mM	50
	1.0 mM	3
Cysteine	0.01 mM	92
	0.1 mM	45
	1.0 mM	12
Formaldehyde	10 mM	100
	30 mM	52
	100 mM	20
DFP	10 mM	105
Soybean trypsin inhibitor	0.5 mg/ml	115

DFP: Diisopropyl fluorophosphate.

the alkaline than in the acidic regions, the highest stability being at a pH of approximately 9.0.

The molecular weight was determined by the approach-to-equilibrium method (YPHANTIS, 1960). The partial specific volume of the hemorrhagic principle was assumed to be 0.75. At protein concentrations of 0.25%, 0.5%, and 1.0%, the molecular weight was estimated to be 101000, 112600, and 99500, respectively, the mean value being approximately 104000.

The isoelectric point (pI) of the purified hemorrhagic principle as determined by isoelectric focusing was about 4.3.

The purified preparation was incubated with each of the reagents shown in Table 3 at various concentrations for 1 h at 37° C. EDTA, cysteine or formaldehyde inhibited the hemorrhagic activity. The addition of an excess amount of Ca^{2+} (10 mM) did not counteract EDTA. Soybean trypsin inhibitor or DFP at concentrations that completely inhibit trypsin had no effect on the hemorrhagic activity.

Susceptibilities of the hemorrhagic activity, the lethal toxicity and the proteolytic activity of the purified preparation to heat and EDTA were compared to see whether any dissimilarity could be found among them.

The purified principle retained its full hemorrhagic activity after heating for 3 min up to 45° C but lost activity abruptly at about 55° C. The lethal toxicity and the proteolytic activity behaved similarly to the hemorrhagic activity.

The time-course of the inhibition by EDTA revealed, however, that the proteolytic activity was more susceptible than either the hemorrhagic activity or the lethal toxicity, which suggested that the entity responsible for the proteolytic activity might be different from that responsible for the hemorrhagic activity and the lethal toxicity.

2. Purification and Characterization of HR 2

a) Purification

The HR 2 fraction (crude HR 2) obtained by gel filtration of the venom on Sephadex G-100 was dialyzed against 5 mM borax-NaOH buffer (pH 9.3) containing 2 mM Ca^{2+}. The dialysis residue was chromatographed on Bio-Rex 70 with gradient elution. As shown in Figure 9, the hemorrhagic activity was separated almost completely from the proteolytic activity. The major proteinase, named H_2-proteinase (TAKAHASHI and OHSAKA, 1970a), emerged at an NaCl concentration of 0.13 M. The main part of the hemorrhagic activity was eluted at 0.17–0.20 M NaCl in two peaks, designated as HR 2a and HR 2b. HR 2a (tubes No. 162–177) and HR 2b (tubes No. 178–186) (Fig. 9) were concentrated and dialyzed against 5 mM borax-NaOH buffer (pH 9.3) containing 2 mM Ca^{2+}. HR 2b contained no proteolytic activity; HR 2a still contained a trace of the activity. Rechromatography of the HR 2a fraction on Bio-Rex 70 yielded a symmetrical protein peak containing no proteolytic activity; the specific hemorrhagic activity was constant throughout the peak. The amount of HR 2b was too small to be subjected to rechromatography. The purification procedure and the yield at each step are summarized in Table 4. A 13-fold purification was attained from crude HR 2 with a yield of 25% in HR 2a and 13-fold with a yield of 12% in HR 2b. The minimum hemorrhagic dose and the 50% lethal dose were 0.066 μg (TAKAHASHI and OHSAKA, 1970b) and 144 μg per mouse (OHSAKA et al., 1971a), respectively, with both HR 2a and HR 2b preparations.

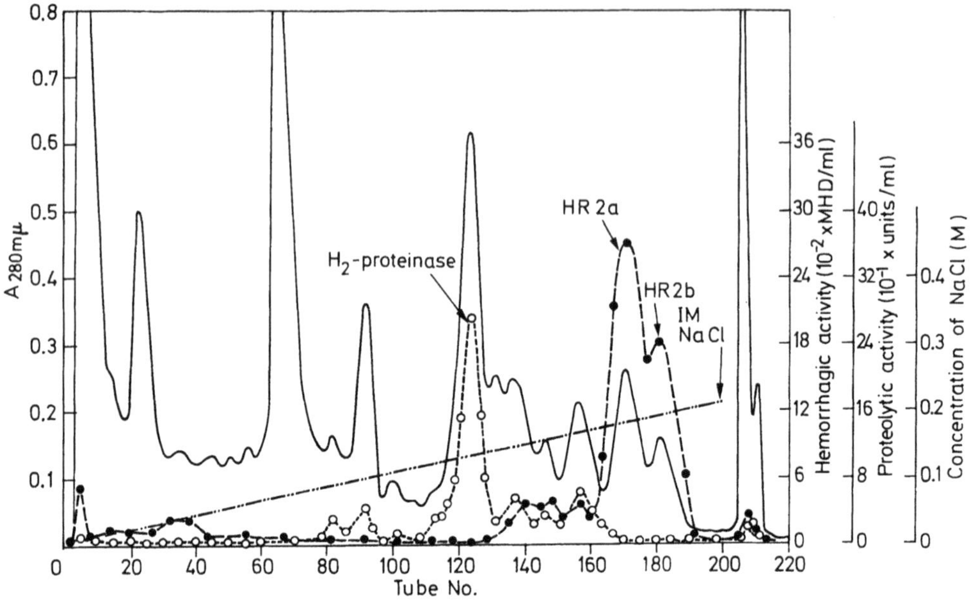

Fig. 9. Column chromatography of crude HR2 on Bio-Rex 70. Crude HR2 obtained by gel filtration of 1 g of crude venom on Sephadex G-100 was dialyzed against 5 mM borax-NaOH buffer (pH 9.3) containing 2 mM Ca^{2+}. After precipitate formed was removed by centrifugation, dialysis residue was concentrated. Concentrated solution containing 670 mg protein in 3 ml was applied to a column (1.6 × 42 cm) of Bio-Rex 70 equilibrated with same buffer. Column was eluted with linear gradient increase in NaCl concentration from 0 to 0.25 M in 2.2 liters of buffer. 10-ml fractions were collected at a flow rate of 20 ml/h. ——, $A_{280\,m\mu}$; ●- - - -●, hemorrhagic activity; ○- - - -○, proteolytic activity; —·—·—, concentration of NaCl (TAKAHASHI and OHSAKA, 1970b)

HR 2a and HR 2b were analyzed by ultracentrifugation. A single symmetrical boundary with an $S_{20,\omega}$ of 2.4 S was obtained with HR 2a, and a asymmetrical boundary with an $S_{20,\omega}$ of approximately 2.0 S appeared with HR 2b.

Each of the purified preparations of HR 2a and HR 2b formed a single coalescing precipitation band against Habu antivenin (OHSAKA, 1976a) (see Fig. 8).

Upon electrophoresis on cellulose acetate membrane at pH 9.5 and I = 0.1, the HR 2a preparation gave a single protein band migrating toward the cathode: the HR 2b preparation gave two bands, of which the major one migrated toward the cathode slightly faster than the minor one, having a mobility identical to that of HR 2a (TAKAHASHI and OHSAKA, 1970b).

Thus HR 2a behaved as a homogeneous protein but HR 2b did not, probably being contaminated with HR 2a.

b) Properties

In a mixture of HR 2a and HR 2b, none of the following enzymes contained in the original venom was detectable: proteinase, nonspecific alkaline phosphomonoesterase, phosphodiesterase, 5′-nucleotidase, L-aminoacid oxidase, hyaluronidase, and phospholipase A. Arginine ester (TAME)-hydrolyzing and tyrosine ester

Table 4. Summary of simultaneous purification of HR2a and HR2b (TAKAHASHI and OHSAKA, 1970b)

Step	Protein (mg)	Hemorrhagic activity				Proteolytic activity	
		MHD (μg)	Total activity in MHD (10^{-5} × MHD)	Specific activity (10^{-3} × MHD/mg protein)	Yield[a] (%)	Specific activity (units/mg protein)	Yield[a] (%)
Crude venom	1000	0.22	46.5	4.65	(100)	54.0	(100)
Sephadex G-100 (crude HR2)	780	0.84	9.3	1.19	100 (19.9)	58.4	100 (85.6)
Dialysis	673	0.74	9.1	1.35	98.5 (19.6)	66.5	96.0 (82.2)
Bio-Rex 70 (1st)							
HR2a	22.5	0.068	3.3	14.7	35.1 (7.0)	9.6	0.48 (0.35)
HR2b	7.2	0.066	1.1	15.3	12.0 (2.4)	None[b]	None
Bio-Rex 70 (2nd)							
HR2a	15.1	0.066	2.3	15.2	24.6 (4.9)	None[b]	None

[a] Figures are expressed as percentage of crude HR2; those in parentheses as percentage of crude venom.
[b] Activity was not detectable when tested at an amount 50 times larger than that of crude venom containing 10 units.

(BTEE)-hydrolyzing activities were also not detectable. Incidentally, the crude venom contains the former (OHSAKA et al., 1971a). Although it has been claimed that a certain bacterial collagenase causes hemorrhage (OAKLEY et al., 1948; HABERMANN, 1960; JUST et al., 1970; KAMEYAMA and AKAMA, 1971), an enzyme of this type was not detected either in the venom (OHSAKA, 1960b) or in the purified hemorrhagic principles.

The stability of HR2a and HR2b at various pH values from 2.0 to 13.0 was determined. HR2a and HR2b were similarly stable between pH 7.0 and 9.5, but completely inactivated below pH 4.0 and above pH 12.0.

Upon heating in 5 mM borax-HCl buffer (pH 8.5, I=0.1) for 5 min at various temperatures, both HR2a and HR2b retained their full activity up to 45°, but abruptly lost their activity above 50°.

The effects of some reagents on hemorrhagic activity of the principles are summarized in Table 5. The reagents tested included potent inhibitors of H_2-proteinase (TAKAHASHI and OHSAKA, 1970a) such as EDTA, cysteine, Cd^{2+}, Ni^{2+}, Cu^{2+}, and Hg^{2+}. Both HR2a and HR2b, lost their hemorrhagic activity when incubated at 37° C for 1 h in the presence of EDTA (2 mM) or cysteine (2 mM). This inhibition could not be reversed either by the addition of an excess amount of Ca^{2+} or by dialysis against 5 mM borax-HCl buffer (pH 8.5, I=0.1) containing 2 mM Ca^{2+}. The hemorrhagic activities of both HR2a and HR2b were little affected by DFP (1 mM), PCMB (2 mM) or soybean trypsin inhibitor (1 mg/ml). To examine the effects of

Table 5. Effects of some reagents on hemorrhagic activity of HR2a and HR2b (TAKAHASHI and OHSAKA, 1970b). In Experiment 1, each hemorrhagic principle at 0.3 mg/ml was incubated at 37° C for 1 h in 5 mM borax-HCl buffer (pH 8.5, I=0.1), added with a given reagent at the indicated concentration. In Experiment 2, each principle was dialyzed at 4° C for 20 h against 5 mM borax-HCl buffer (pH 8.5, I=0.1) containing a given divalent cation at the indicated concentration. The final concentration of each principle was the same as above. In both experiments hemorrhagic activity was expressed relative to that obtained with Ca^{2+}

Experiment	Reagent	Concentration	Hemorrhagic activity (%)	
			HR2a	HR2b
1	EDTA	2 mM	0	0
	DFP	1 mM	90	103
	PCMB	2 mM	110	125
	Cysteine	2 mM	0	0
	Soybean trypsin inhibitor	1 mg/ml	118	120
2	Ca^{2+}	2 mM	100	100
	Ni^{2+}	2 mM	90	88
	Cd^{2+}	2 mM	99	93
	Hg^{2+}	2 mM	92	100
	Cu^{2+}	1 mM	105	96
	Zn^{2+}	1 mM	100	96

PCMB: *p*-chloromercuribenzoate.

divalent cations, each hemorrhagic principle was dialyzed at 4° C for 20 h against 5 mM borax-HCl buffer (pH 8.5) added with each cation at the indicated concentration. None of these cations affected the activity of HR 2a or HR 2b.

Thus HR 2a is very similar to HR 2b in such properties as pH and heat stability, as well as the susceptibility to EDTA or cysteine.

IV. Dynamic Aspects of the Action of Hemorrhagic Principles on Microcirculation as Revealed by Cinematography

Using high power microscopy and motion-picture recording, FULTON and his co-workers (1956) investigated the mechanism of petechial formation in the cheek pouch of hamsters injected with moccasin *(Agkistrodon piscivorus)* venom. They demonstrated arteriolar constriction with sluggish circulation and subsequent escape of erythrocytes through the vessel wall one by one, without apparent rupture of the endothelium. No openings were visible. According to these authors, erythrocytes emerge through spaces that develop between the endothelial cells in the region of the interendothelial cement substance. Microscopic examination of the lungs after intravenous injection of *Echis colorata* venom disclosed perivascular hemorrhages with a still morphologically intact vessel wall (GITTER et al., 1960). Transitions to various stages of deterioration of the vessel wall were found. It was thought that the initial process affected the intercellular spaces, causing *per-diapedesin* hemorrhage.

By means of cinematography at a microscopic level, OHSAKA et al. (1971 b) studied in detail the effects of *Trimeresurus flavoviridis* venom on the microcirculation. Three min after application of 0.25% crude venom to the omentum or the mesentery of the rat, severe vasoconstriction of larger vessels (e.g., 200–300 μm in diameter), and especially of arterioles, occurred, as revealed by microscopy at low magnification (40×) (Fig. 10A, B). Shortly after, this was followed by vasodilatation. These vasomotor changes were usually repeated. In 7 min, hemorrhage occurred from the capillary bed (Fig. 10C). Similar vasoconstriction was described by SAGARA (1960) with the same venom. To visualize the whole process of the escape of erythrocytes from the microcirculatory system, observation was made at higher magnifications (200–500×) with both low- and high-speed movie cameras. It was demonstrated that at an early stage in the events, the erythrocytes escaped not along the capillaries, but one by one through the pin-point holes formed in true capillaries including thoroughfare ways (preferential channels), without apparent rupture of the endothelium (OHSAKA et al., 1971b). These observations agree with the earlier findings of FULTON et al. (1956) that erythrocytes escape one by one through the vessel wall without detectable openings in the vessel wall, but are apparently in disagreement with their statement that venom-induced hemorrhage occurred consistently in the venous portion of the circulation especially at venous junctions, and that the capillaries were not vulnerable. Electron-microscopic examinations of the vascular endothelial cells treated with *Trimeresurus flavoviridis* venom or venom hemorrhagic principle (HR1) revealed that the erythrocytes came out through the junctions of the endothelial cell lining, the adjacent basement membrane being disrupted to permit eventual extravasation of the erythrocytes (TSUCHIYA et al., 1974; OHSAKA et al., 1975). The extravasation of erythrocytes ceased temporarily within seconds of initiation, but with rare formation of a white thrombus (platelet plug) (OHSAKA et al., 1971b), which is known to be one of the major factors in hemostasis resulting from experimental damage to the vessel wall. Some other factor(s) must be concerned, therefore, with cessation of the erythrocytic extravasation. In this manner, erythrocytes came out intermittently through the same pin-point holes. The true capillaries with hemorrhagic lesions increased in number with time (TSUCHIYA et al., 1974; OHSAKA, 1976a, b). At a later stage, however, hemorrhage occurred also from the arterioles and venules (OHSAKA et al., 1971b). The extravasated erythrocytic masses varied in size from a few cells, to large numbers of cells forming macroscopically visible petechiae (OHSAKA et al., 1971b). A frequent finding was the segmentally distended endothelial sheath of the venule, inside which a number of erythrocytes had accumulated (OHSAKA et al., 1971b; TSUCHIYA et al., 1974); electron microscopic examinations of this portion of the vessel wall disclosed outward dislocation and marked elongation of the pericyte which enclosed the erythrocytes (TSUCHIYA et al., 1974). Whether or not this phenomenon is related to hemostatic mechanism remains to be determined. Surprisingly, there was no sign of increased vascular permeability, as demonstrated by the use of an indicator dye, prior to the onset of the escape of erythrocytes and even during the course of the events except at the pin-point holes (OHSAKA et al., 1971b). This has been confirmed with purified hemorrhagic principle (HR1) by JUST and his associates (1970), who used ^{125}I-labeled albumin and ^{51}Cr-labeled erythrocytes to distinguish between the increased vascular permeability for albumin and that for erythrocytes (hemorrhage).

Essentially the same results as described above were obtained when rat mesentery was exposed to the hemorrhagic principle, HR1, isolated from this venom (TSUCHIYA et al., 1974).

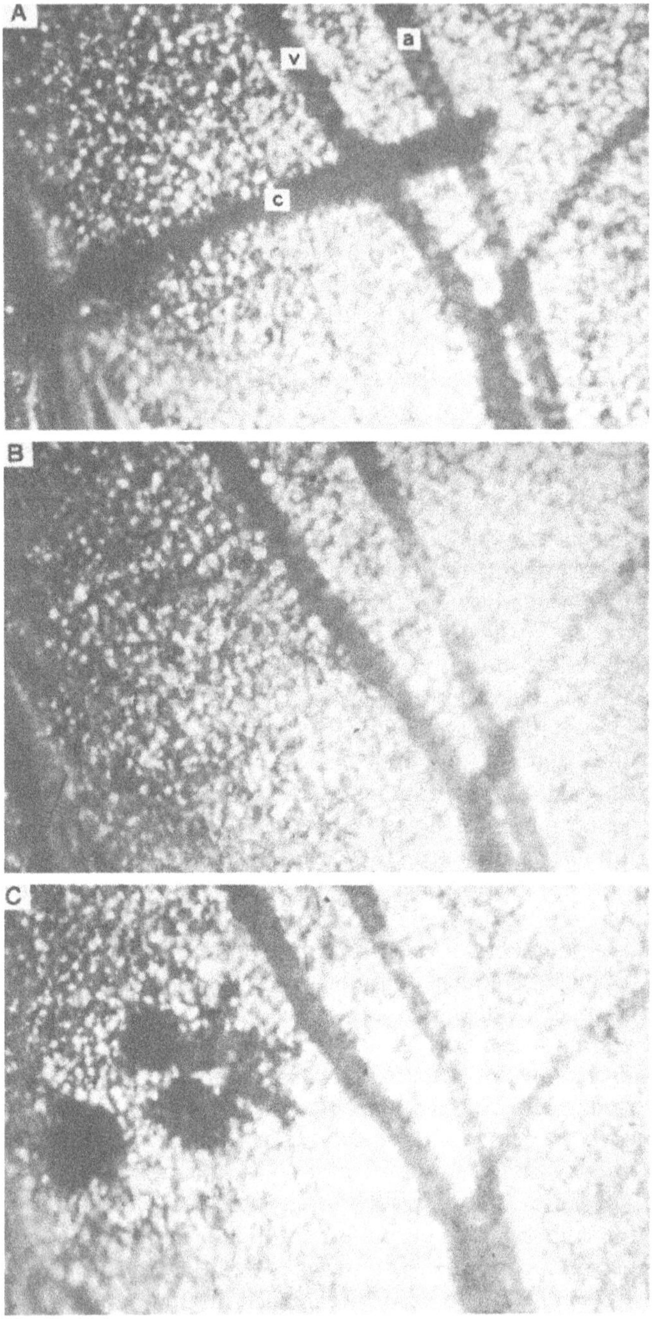

Fig. 10. Vascular effects of *Trimeresurus flavoviridis* venom applied to rat omentum. In A, arteriole (*a*) and venule (*v*), both 300 μm in diameter, are shown before application of 0.25% venom with aid of a cotton fiber (*c*). In B, 3 min after application of venom, severe vasoconstriction is found (40 ×). In C, 7 min after application, hemorrhage is seen in capillary region exposed to venom. Vasoconstriction of arteriole is still seen. All these picture reproduced from a cinephotomicrographic record (OHSAKA et al., 1971 b)

Together with the fact that the venom hemorrhagic principles exert no cytopathic (or cytotoxic) effect on animal cells cultivated in vitro (OHSAKA et al., 1966a; YOSHIKURA et al., 1966; OHSAKA, 1968) and that the purified hemorrhagic principles are either almost (OMORI-SATOH and OHSAKA, 1970) or completely free (TAKAHASHI and OHSAKA, 1970b) of proteolytic activity, the above-described observations at a microscopic level will provide important clues in elucidating the physiological mechanisms involved in hemorrhage (see the later section of this chapter).

V. Action of Hemorrhagic Principles on Smooth Muscles

As described in the preceding section, the early effects of *Trimeresurus flavoviridis* venom or its hemorrhagic principles on the microcirculatory system are characterized by severe vasoconstriction, followed by vasodilatation of larger vessels, especially of arterioles, and subsequent hemorrhage in the capillary bed (OHSAKA et al., 1971b).

In view of the striking vasomotor changes observed, it is of special interest to study the pharmacological actions of the purified hemorrhagic principles on smooth muscles.

Recently ISHIDA et al. (1976) tested the effects of purified hemorrhagic principles (HR1 and HR2) from *Trimeresurus flavoviridis* venom on the isolated smooth muscle, and demonstrated their ability to release vasoactive mediators from the guinea-pig ileum and lung and from the rat peritoneal cells. More details of these observations will be described at this point.

1. Actions of Hemorrhagic Principles (HR1 and HR2) on Isolated Smooth Muscle Preparations

The administration of crude venom in concentrations higher than 10^{-5} g/ml induced contraction of the isolated guinea-pig ileum, but repeated administration produced desensitization (Fig. 11). After the administered crude venom had been washed out thoroughly, the gut showed gradually developing contraction, which was abolished with the antihistamine drug, chlorpheniramine. HR2, depending on its concentration in a range from 10^{-6} to 10^{-5} g/ml, induced contraction of the gut to a graded extent, and the response was not diminished after repetition, whereas neither HR1 nor H_2-proteinase (venom proteinase) at concentrations up to 10^{-4} g/ml produced any contraction of the gut.

It appears that the contractile response of the gut to HR2 is largely due to acetylcholine (ACh) released from the parasympathetic nerves by a neurotropic action of this venom principle, because the contraction induced by HR2 was inhibited in the presence of atropine or tetrodotoxin and potentiated in the presence of eserine (Fig. 12). When added to the bath, after the response of the gut to transmural electrical stimulation had almost disappeared due to tetrodotoxin action, HR2 still produced small and gradual contraction, which could be inhibited by chlorpheniramine (Fig. 13), indicating that such slow contraction is due to histamine release following ACh release from the gut. In a few experiments, some component in the contractile response to HR2 could not be inhibited by administration with both tetrodotoxin and chlorpheniramine, suggesting that the release of a slow-reacting

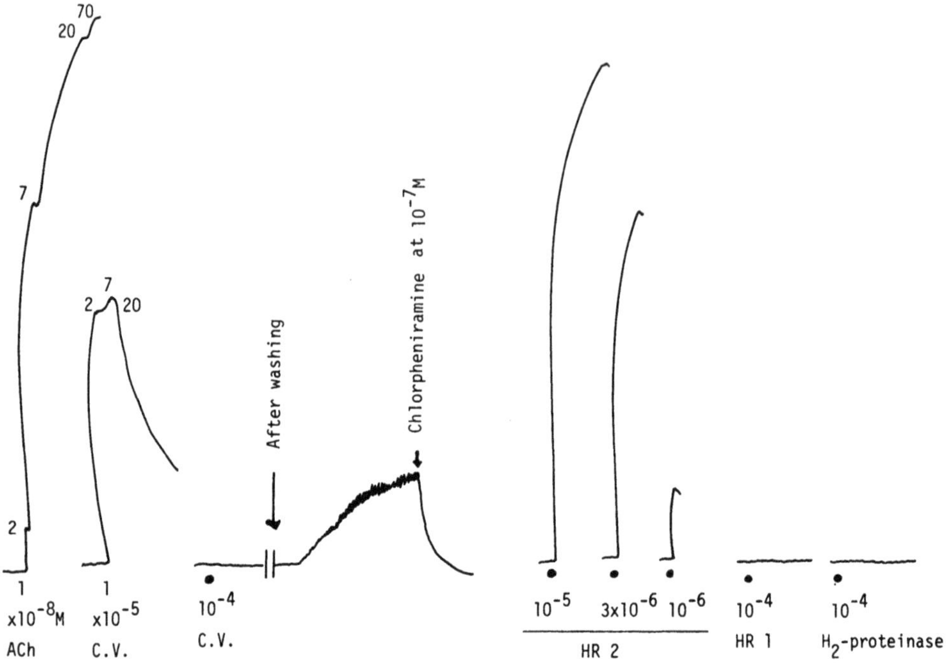

Fig. 11. Actions of crude venom (C.V.), HR1, HR2 and H_2-proteinase (g/ml) on isolated guinea-pig ileum (ISHIDA et al., 1976)

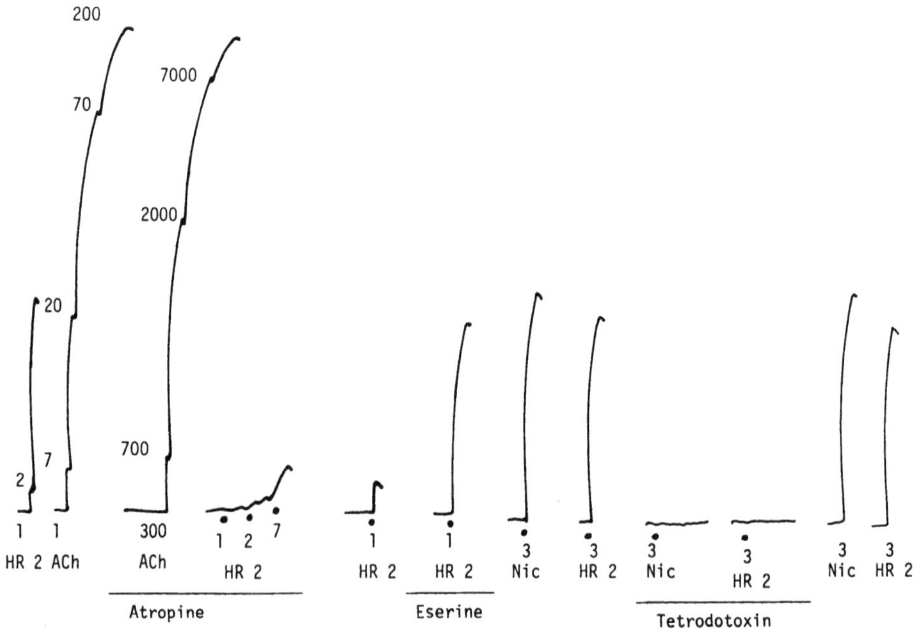

Fig. 12. Contraction of isolated guinea-pig ileum induced by HR2 in presence of atropine at 10^{-8} M, eserine at 10^{-8} M and tetrodotoxin at 3×10^{-8} g/ml. Numbers indicate times of concentration of $\times 10^{-6}$ g/ml for HR2, $\times 10^{-9}$ M for ACh, and $\times 10^{-6}$ M for nicotine (Nic) (ISHIDA et al., 1976)

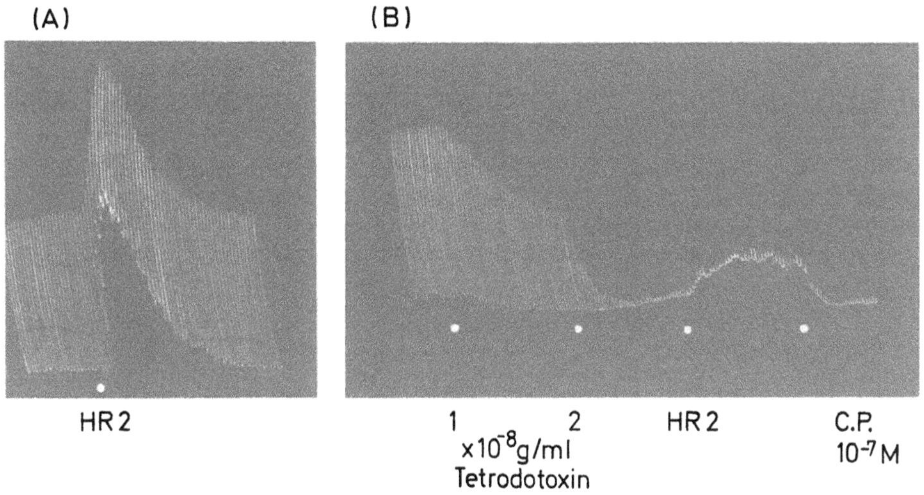

Fig. 13. Effects of HR2 of 10^{-6} g/ml on contraction induced by transmural electrical stimulation (1 ms, 25 V, 0.1 cps) in isolated guinea-pig ileum. (A) HR2 alone; (B) the contraction induced by HR2 after treatment with tetrodotoxin (3×10^{-8} g/ml) is inhibited by chlorpheniramine (C.P.) (ISHIDA et al., 1976)

substance could also be involved in the contractile response. Incidentally, it may be mentioned that HR1 inhibited the contraction of the gut which was induced by transmural electrical stimulation in the presence of chlorpheniramine; the mechanism of this inhibition is unknown.

From these results it was concluded that the contractile response of the guinea-pig ileum to HR2 results from ACh release from the nervous elements in the gut, followed by histamine and/or SRS release. Thus it is apparent that the stimulating effects of HR2 on the smooth muscle are the result of the autopharmacological action (BERALDO and DIAS DA SILVA, 1966; JIMÉNEZ-PORRAS, 1968) of this hemorrhagic principle.

With preparations of other smooth muscles, such as isolated rat uterus and rabbit aortic strip, and also of other tissues, e.g., isolated guinea-pig auricles, rat phrenic nerve-diaphragm, and frog rectus abdominis, neither of the venom principles (HR1 or HR2) displayed any marked effect except when a transient contraction of the isolated rat uterus was induced by crude venom.

2. Mediators Released from Guinea-Pig Lungs and from Rat Peritoneal Cells by the Action of Hemorrhagic Principles (HR1 and HR2)

The media in which the finely chopped guinea-pig lungs had previously been incubated with venom proteins contained different amounts of histamine released from the lung cells. The amounts of histamine released by venom proteins, calculated as histamine base per gram of chopped lungs, were as follows: 2.0–2.8 μg by crude venom (10^{-5} g/ml); 1.1–3.0 μg by HR2 (10^{-5} g/ml); 0.32 μg by HR1 (10^{-5} g/ml); and 0.75 μg by H_2-proteinase (10^{-5} g/ml). The total histamine content of the lungs, as determined after extraction by heating the lungs at 100° C for 15 min, was 9.2–

Table 6. Release of histamine from the rat peritoneal cells induced by crude venom, HR1 and HR2 (ISHIDA et al., 1976)

Venom proteins, g/ml	Released histamine[a], %	Control[a], %
Crude venom of 10^{-4}	59.90 ± 13.43 (4)	3.26 ± 0.22 (4)
HR2 of 3×10^{-5}	52.70 ± 8.25 (5)	7.58 ± 1.26 (4)
HR1 of 3×10^{-5}	12.42 ± 3.18 (5)	5.06 ± 1.08 (5)

[a] Mean ± S.E. Number of experiments in parentheses.

19.0 μg/g. These results demonstrated that the histamine-releasing activities of crude venom and HR 2 are much more potent than those of HR 1 and H_2-proteinase.

The media in which the lungs had been incubated with venom proteins contained, besides histamine, ACh and SRS in small amounts, as demonstrated by the fact that the contractile response of rat ileum to the media in which the lung tissue had been incubated with crude venom was not completely inhibited by chlorpheniramine either alone or in combination with atropine.

The amounts of histamine released from the rat peritoneal cells by the action of venom proteins were determined on the guinea-pig ileum with the results shown in Table 6. The histamine-releasing activity of HR 2 or crude venom is much more potent than that of HR 1 which, though very weak, is still significant.

The medium in which the peritoneal cells had been incubated with crude venom or HR 2 at a concentration of 10^{-4} g/ml induced contraction of the isolated rat uterus; control medium, as well as medium containing HR 1, did not cause any contraction. The contraction of the rat uterus was inhibited by a specific 5-HT antagonist (S-8) (TAKAGI et al., 1969), indicating involvement of 5-HT released from the cells. The amount of 5-HT released into the incubation medium was 0.5 μg with crude venom and 0.13 μg with HR 2.

In summary, crude venom and HR 2 induced the release of mediators such as histamine, 5-HT and slow-reacting substances from chopped guinea-pig lung and rat peritoneal cells; HR 1 released these mediators to a lesser extent. These mediators, if released in vivo, may well open the endothelial cell junctions causing the erythrocytes to come out across the endothelium (OHSAKA, 1973, 1976a, b). However, for the full process of hemorrhage to occur, the basement membrane must also be disrupted by the action of venom hemorrhagic principle and this will be described in Section VI. HR 1, possessing hemorrhagic activity higher than that of HR 2, exerted a weaker effect on the smooth muscle and also induced the release of the mediators to a lesser extent than did HR 2. This contradiction may well be explained by our hypothesis (OHSAKA, 1973, 1976a, b) that these effects, together with other effects of venom principles such as disruption of the basement membrane and inhibition of platelet aggregation, must be involved in the causation of hemorrhage (ISHIDA et al., 1976).

VI. Mechanisms of Action of Hemorrhagic Principles

A minute amount of each of the three hemorrhagic principles, HR 1, HR 2a, and HR 2b, isolated from the venom of *Trimeresurus flavoviridis* in the present author's laboratory (OMORI-SATOH and OHSAKA, 1970; TAKAHASHI and OHSAKA, 1970b; OHSAKA et al., 1971a) induces typical hemorrhage in experimental animals, thereby serving as a model system for bleeding (OHSAKA, 1973, 1976a, b).

As the first step in elucidating the vascular effect of venom hemorrhagic principles, it is of vital importance to reveal the dynamic aspects of the action of venom principles on the microcirculation. Our special interest is focused on where and how the events happen in the microcirculatory unit exposed to venom principles. We demonstrated that the venom hemorrhagic principles act on the microcirculatory system inducing true hemorrhage without a prior increase in vascular permeability (OHSAKA et al., 1971b). The formation of white thrombus (platelet aggregate) is seldom observed at the site of hemorrhage (OHSAKA et al., 1971b; TSUCHIYA et al., 1974).

From these in vivo observations, approaches to the elucidation of the mechanisms of action of the venom hemorrhagic principles have been proposed, as outlined below (OHSAKA, 1973, 1976a, b).

1. The effect of the hemorrhagic principle on vascular permeability for albumin and erythrocytes should be investigated.

2. Those effects on the vessel wall that constitute the primary cause of hemorrhage should be elucidated. In other words, it is necessary to clarify both biochemically and morphologically how the erythrocytes cross the lining of the endothelial cells and also the basement membrane.

3. The inhibitory effects on the hemostatic mechanism constituting the secondary cause of hemorrhage, namely disturbance of blood coagulation and inhibition of platelet aggregation, should be investigated.

The use of venom hemorrhagic principles and also crude venom as analytical tools, has allowed some experimental approaches to the physiological mechanisms involved in hemorrhage (OHSAKA et al., 1971b, 1973a, b, 1975; OHSAKA, 1973, 1976a, b; TSUCHIYA et al., 1974; YAMANAKA et al., 1974; ISHIDA et al., 1976). Some recent information available from the author's own and other laboratories will be presented here in line with this approach.

1. Effect on Vascular Permeability

JUST and his co-workers (1970) were able to divide the increased vascular permeability induced by various vasoactive agents into three types. They injected various agents intracutaneously to rabbits that had been previously injected with ^{125}I-labeled albumin and with ^{51}Cr-labeled erythrocytes to test their vascular effects. Escape of albumin and erythrocytes from the vessels were related to time and to doses of each agent.

Figure 14 shows the effects of bradykinin (JUST et al., 1970); albumin escaped from the vessels, whereas erythrocytes did not. The increased vascular permeability of this type was observed also with histamine.

Figure 15 shows the effects of a venom hemorrhagic principle, HR 1, and of *Clostridium histolyticum* collagenase, which is known to induce hemorrhage (JUST et al., 1970). No increase in vascular permeability for albumin was observed prior to hemorrhage, in agreement with the present author's findings (OHSAKA et al., 1971b). In other words, escape of erythrocytes and that of albumin occurred simultaneously.

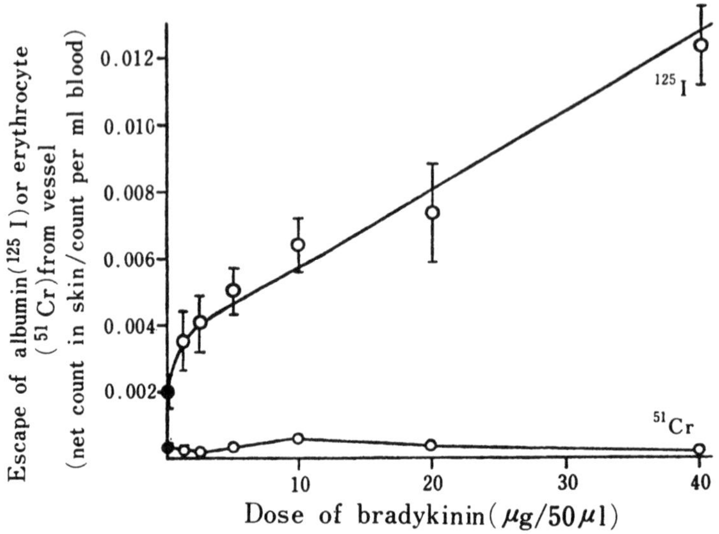

Fig. 14. Increase in vascular permeability caused by bradykinin (JUST et al., 1970). Bradykinin was injected into back skin of rabbits previously injected with ^{125}I-labeled albumin and with ^{51}Cr-labeled erythrocytes. Amounts of albumin and erythrocytes that escaped from vessels into skin were determined by radioactivity measurements. Filled circles represent amounts of ^{125}I and ^{51}Cr that escaped from the vessels when physiological saline was injected (controls)

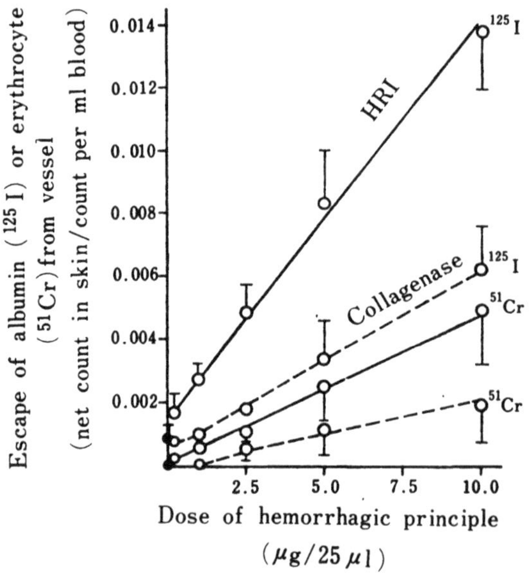

Fig. 15. Increase in vascular permeability caused by hemorrhagic principles (JUST et al., 1970). Snake venom hemorrhagic principle (HR1) or bacterial collagenase was injected into back skin of rabbits previously injected with ^{125}I-labeled albumin and with ^{51}Cr-labeled erythrocytes. Amounts of albumin and erythrocytes that escaped from vessels into skin were determined by radioactivity measurements. Filled circles represent amounts of ^{125}I and ^{51}Cr that escaped from vessels when physiological saline was injected (controls)

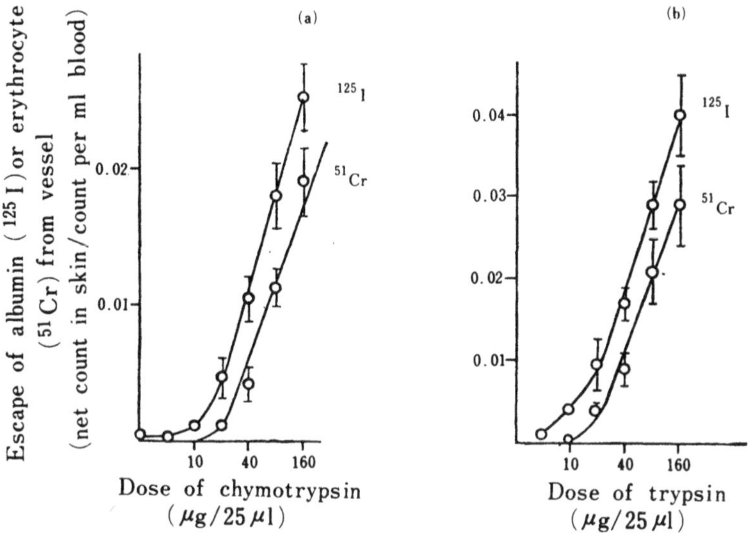

Fig. 16. Increase in vascular permeability caused by proteolytic enzymes (JUST et al., 1970) (a) chymotrypsin; (b) trypsin. Proteolytic enzymes were injected into back skin of rabbits previously injected with ^{125}I-labeled albumin and with ^{51}Cr-labeled erythrocytes. Amounts of albumin and erythrocytes that escaped from vessels into skin were determined by radioactivity measurements

Figure 16 shows the effects of chymotrypsin and of trypsin (JUST et al., 1970). At low doses, these proteolytic enzymes induced an increase in vascular permeability for albumin but not for erythrocytes. At higher doses, however, these enzymes also induced an increase in vascular permeability for erythrocytes.

2. Effect on Vessel Wall

a) Effect on Vascular Endothelium

Figure 17 presents a schematic drawing showing the structure of the vessel wall of muscle-type capillary as revealed by electron microscopy. The vessel wall consists of an endothelial cell lining and a basement membrane surrounding it (FAWCETT, 1963). For hemorrhage to occur, the erythrocytes must cross these two barriers (OHSAKA et al., 1971b; OHSAKA, 1973, 1976a, b). Do the erythrocytes escape through the junction of the endothelial cell lining (Route 1) or do they traverse the cytoplasm of the cell (Route 2)? This question will be answered first.

Figure 18 is an electron micrograph of the vascular endothelial cells treated with *T. flavoviridis* venom (OHSAKA et al., 1975). An erythrocyte in the lumen is just penetrating into a junction (about 0.2 μm wide) by forming a protrusion like the pseudopodium of an ameba; the adjacent basement membrane has been partially disrupted.

Figure 19 is another electron micrograph (OHSAKA et al., 1975). An erythrocyte is escaping from the vessel through an opened junction (about 0.7 μm wide) and the basement membrane has been extensively destroyed. Essentially the same results were obtained with the purified HR 1 (TSUCHIYA et al., 1974) as with crude venom.

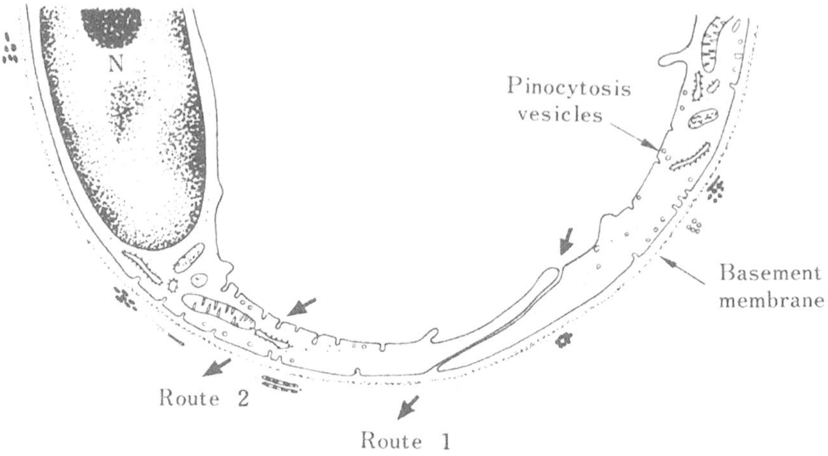

Fig. 17. Schematic drawing showing structure of capillary wall as revealed by electron microscopy. Two possible routes for escape of erythrocytes across endothelium are indicated by arrows (FAWCETT, 1959)

From these observations we conclude that the erythrocyte, changing its shape like an ameba, escapes through an opened junction of the endothelial cell lining, the adjacent basement membrane being disrupted to permit the eventual extravasation of erythrocytes. Our observations are different from those of MCKAY et al. (1970), who claimed that the erythrocytes traverse the cytoplasm of the endothelial cells. While we examined the vascular endothelial cells of the rat's mesentery directly exposed to crotalid venom, MCKAY et al. (1970) injected *Vipera palestinae* venom hemorrhagin subcutaneously to rabbit and investigated the vascular effects at the site of injection. It is possible, therefore, that the discrepancy may be due to the different experimental models used by the two groups.

It remains to be answered how the junction opens. In this connection, it is worth mentioning the observation of ISHIDA et al. (1976) that purified hemorrhagic principles induce release of mediators such as histamine, serotonin, and some other substances from various isolated organs and tissues. Such mediators, if released in vivo, may well open the junction of the endothelial cells to facilitate escape of the erythrocytes across the endothelium (OHSAKA, 1973, 1976a, b).

Figures 18 and 19 also indicate that a small number of platelets gathered at the site of hemorrhage, but they showed no sign of viscous metamorphosis, which is in accordance with previous findings (TSUCHIYA et al., 1974). These results, together with the ability of the venom hemorrhagic principles to inhibit the in vitro aggregation of platelets (YAMANAKA et al., 1974), satisfactorily explain the rare formation of white thrombus at the site of venom-induced hemorrhage (OHSAKA et al., 1971b; TSUCHIYA et al., 1974) (see the later section of this chapter).

b) *Effect on Basement Membrane*

In order to obtain information on the in vivo mode of action of venom hemorrhagic principles, we recently carried out experiments to test the possibility that the venom principles act directly on isolated basement membrane (OHSAKA et al., 1973a, b). For

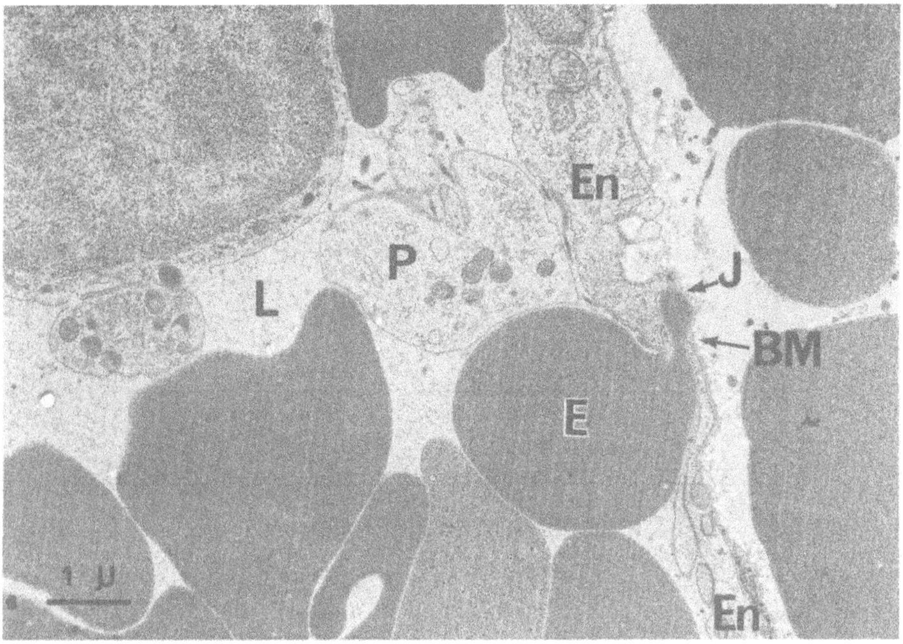

Fig. 18. Electron micrograph showing spurting of an erythrocyte through a junction of vascular endothelium exposed to snake venom. (*E*) erythrocyte; (*L*) vascular lumen; (*J*) junction; (*En*) endothelial cell; (*BM*) basement membrane; (*P*) platelet (OHSAKA et al., 1975)

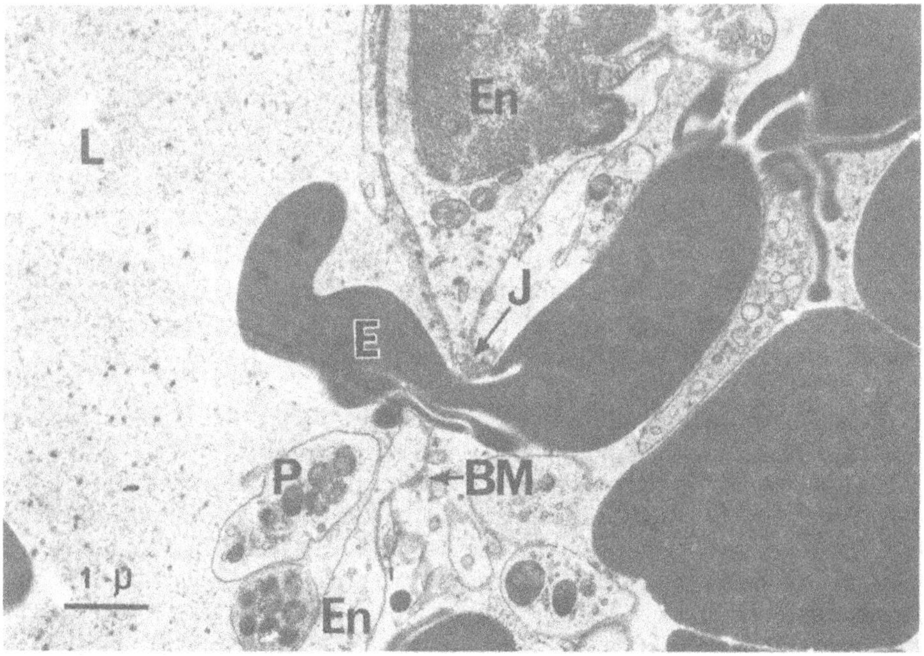

Fig. 19. Electron micrograph showing spurting of an erythrocyte through a junction of vascular endothelium exposed to snake venom. Symbols used are as in Figure 18 (OHSAKA et al., 1975)

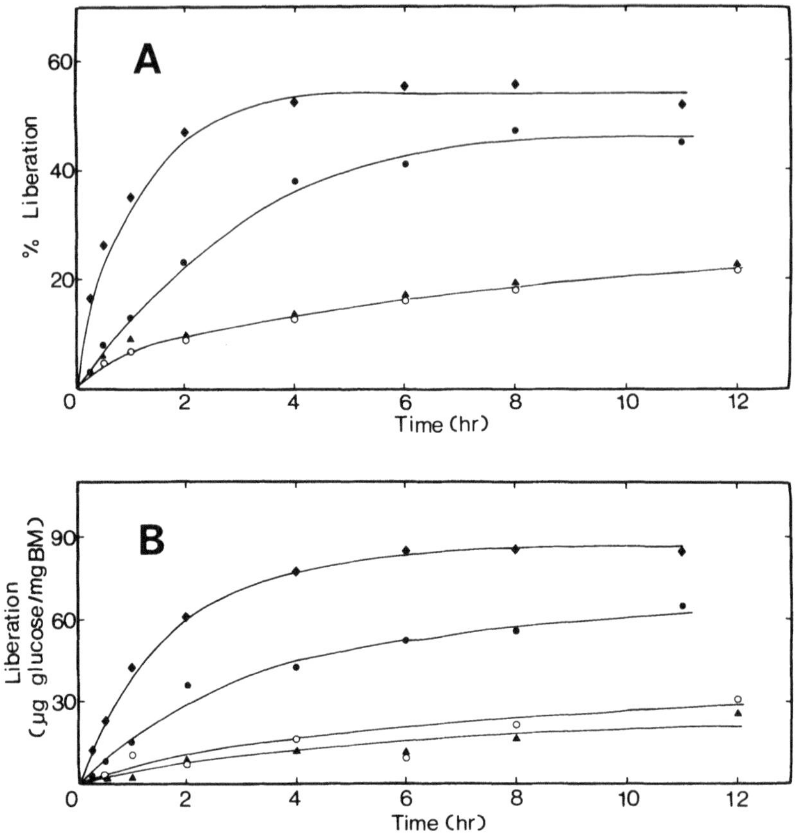

Fig. 20. Time course of liberation of Folin-positive (A) and anthrone-positive (B) material from basement membrane exposed to hemorrhagic principles. Mixture containing 0.5 ml of basement-membrane suspension at pH 7.5 and 0.2 ml of a solution of each hemorrhagic principle at a final concentration of 8.57 μg/ml was incubated at 37° C. ●—●, HR1; ○—○, HR2a; ▲—▲, HR2b; ■—■, collagenase (OHSAKA et al., 1973a)

comparison, the experiments included the use of bacterial collagenase (a mixture of several collagenolytic enzymes) (SEIFTER and HARPER, 1971), which is known to induce hemorrhage (OAKLEY et al., 1948; JUST et al., 1970; KAMEYAMA and AKAMA, 1971).

We demonstrated that all the venom principles disrupt the isolated basement membrane, releasing proteins (or peptides) and carbohydrates.

Figures 20A and 20B show the time course of protein and carbohydrate liberation, respectively, from the basement membrane by venom principles and bacterial collagenase at a given concentration. The bacterial collagenase liberated protein as well as carbohydrate at a much faster rate and to a greater extent than did the venom principles. HR2a and HR2b, showing similar liberation characteristics to each other, acted on the membrane at a much slower rate and to a lesser extent than did collagenase. HR1 showed liberation characteristics intermediate between those of collagenase and HR2a or HR2b.

Table 7. Mean extent of digestion of various preparations of basement membrane after exposure to each hemorrhagic principle under the standard conditions (OHSAKA et al., 1973a). The average protein content of basement membrane in a reaction mixture was 650 ± 195 μg (n=22). Extent of digestion was expressed in terms of Folin-positive and anthrone-positive materials liberated

	Material liberated per mg basement membrane protein	
	μg protein (bovine serum albumin equiv.)	μg carbohydrate (glucose equiv.)
HR1	326 ± 80 (n=10)	43.4 ± 8.7 (n=15)
HR2a	172 ± 53 (n=13)	8.6[a] ± 4.4 (n=11)
HR2b	181 ± 44 (n=13)	9.5[a] ± 2.6 (n=11)
Collagenase	615 ± 110 (n=11)	88.1 ± 13.9 (n= 7)

[a] Just on the level of detection.

Since the liberation of split-product from basement membrane by collagenase reached a maximum in 6 h and the liberation by venom principles went on rather slowly after this period, the incubation of basement membrane with hemorrhagic principles at the specified concentration (8.57 μg/ml) for 6 h at 37° C was designated as standard conditions for preparation of the split-products.

The pH dependence of the liberation of proteins from basement membrane exposed to the venom hemorrhagic principles is relatively steep. Optimal pH values were around 8.0 for all the principles; at pH values lower than 5.0 and higher than 9.0, none of the principles acted on the basement membrane.

Table 7 shows the mean values of the digestion by individual hemorrhagic principles of basement membranes from different batches of tissue. The approximate ratio of proteins liberated by HR2a:HR2b:HR1:collagenase was 1:1:2:4; the corresponding figure for carbohydrate liberated was 0.5:0.5:2:4.

Figures 21–24 show the elution profiles from a Sephadex G-50 column of the split-products of basement membrane incubated with the venom hemorrhagic principles and bacterial collagenase under the standard conditions. The profiles show apparent difference among HR 1, HR 2 (a and b) and collagenase; the major part of the split-product with HR 1 was of high molecular weight (Fig. 21), whereas much of the product with HR2a (Fig. 22) or HR2b (Fig. 23) consisted of low-molecular-weight substances. The product with collagenase was of another type, containing both high- and low-molecular-weight substances at a ratio of roughly 1:2 (Fig. 24).

The above results can be interpreted as indicating that the mode of action of HR2a and HR2b on basement membrane is different from that of HR1 or bacterial collagenase.

Previous reports from this laboratory have demonstrated that EDTA (OMORI-SATOH and OHSAKA, 1970; TAKAHASHI and OHSAKA, 1970b), cysteine (OMORI-SATOH and OHSAKA, 1970; TAKAHASHI and OHSAKA, 1970b), specific antivenin (KONDO et al., 1965b) and the antihemorrhagic factor from snake serum (OMORI-SATOH et al., 1972) inhibit the hemorrhagic activity of the venom hemorrhagic principles. It was of interest, therefore, to study whether or not these hemorrhage inhibi-

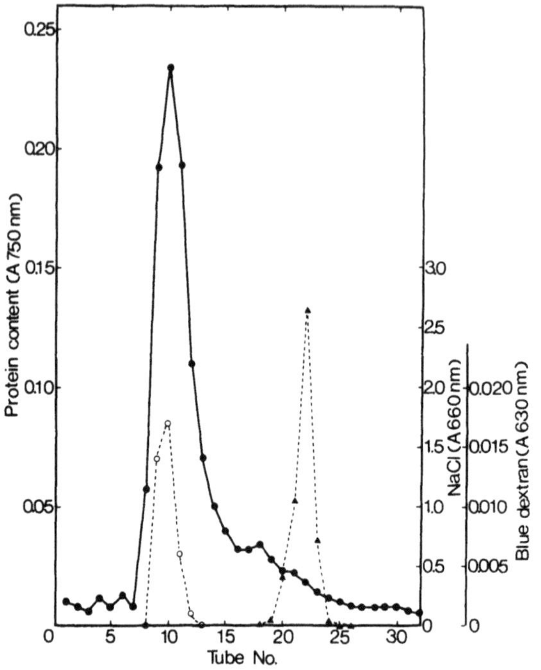

Fig. 21. Gel filtration on Sephadex G-50 of split-product of basement membrane exposed to HR1. Supernatant fluid from reaction mixture, prepared under standard conditions, of HR1 (8.57 μg/ml) and basement membrane was lyophilized; lyophilized material dissolved in water to volume one-fifth that of original supernatant fluid. 200 μl of this solution containing 416 μg bovine serum albumin equivalent was placed on a column (0.6 × 17 cm) of Sephadex G-50 (fine) equilibrated with 0.5% (v/v) acetic acid. Column was eluted with same medium. 300-μl fractions were collected at flow rate of 5–6 ml/h; protein content (●—●) of each fraction was determined. Prior to sample run, void volume had been determined with blue dextran (○- - - - -○) as marker, and emergence of NaCl (▲- - - - -▲) had been detected with $AgNO_3$ solution (OHSAKA et al., 1973a)

tors also inhibit the in vitro reaction between the venom principles and the basement membrane.

As shown in Table 8, the liberation of both proteins (F) and carbohydrates (A) from basement membrane by all the venom principles was inhibited almost completely with 1.0 mM of EDTA, 0.2 mM of cysteine, 50 units/ml of antivenin and 12 units/ml of antihemorrhagic factor. The concentrations of the inhibitors required to abolish the in vitro liberating activity were similar to those for inhibiting the hemorrhagic activity on animal skin (OMORI-SATOH and OHSAKA, 1970; TAKAHASHI and OHSAKA, 1970b).

The results suggest that one and the same entity is responsible for both hemorrhagic and basement membrane-disrupting activities possessed by individual venom principles.

On the basis of the kinetic properties of the in vitro reaction of the venom principles on basement membrane, and of the observed presence of different molecular-weight substances in the split-products brought about by these principles, the

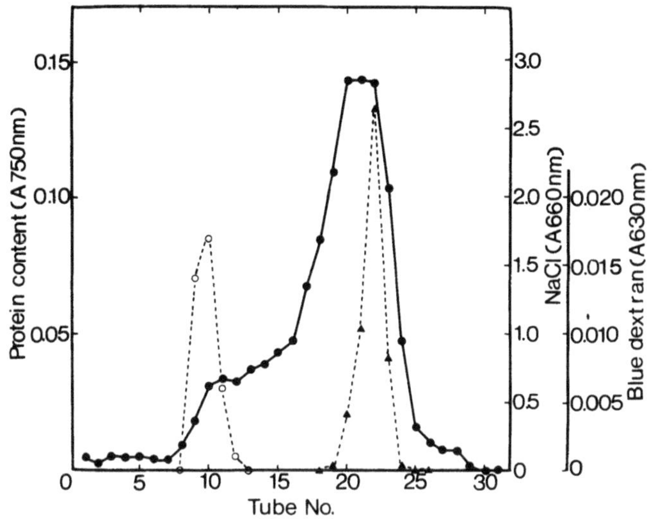

Fig. 22. Gel filtration on Sephadex G-50 of split-product of basement membrane exposed to HR2a. Supernatant fluid from reaction mixture, prepared under standard conditions, of HR2a (8.57 μg/ml) and basement membrane was lyophilized; lyophilized material dissolved in water to volume one-sixteenth that of original supernatant fluid. 200 μl of this solution containing 760 μg bovine serum albumin equivalent was submitted to gel filtration under the same conditions as in Figure 21 (OHSAKA et al., 1973a)

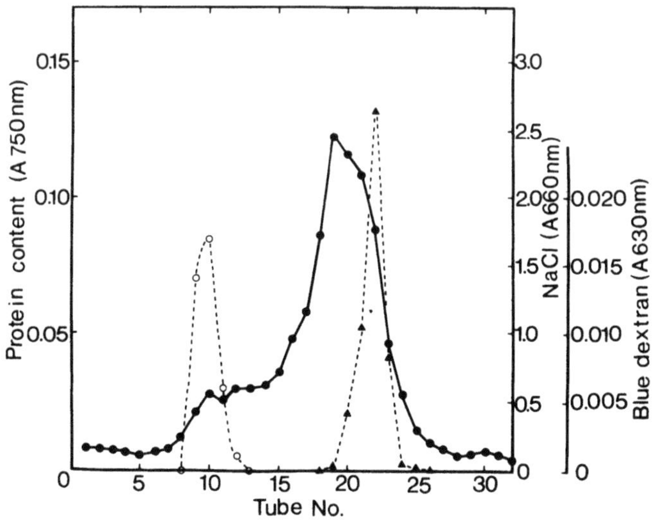

Fig. 23. Gel filtration on Sephadex G-50 of split-product of basement membrane exposed to HR2b. Supernatant fluid from reaction mixture, prepared under standard conditions, of HR2b (8.57 μg/ml) and basement membrane was concentrated as described in Figure 22. 200 μl of this concentrated solution containing 732 μg bovine serum albumin equivalent was submitted to gel filtration under same conditions as in Figure 21 (OHSAKA et al., 1973a)

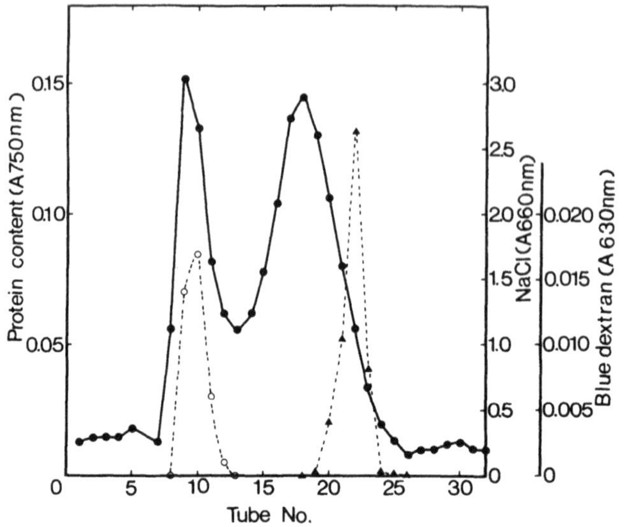

Fig. 24. Gel filtration on Sephadex G-50 of split-product of basement membrane exposed to bacterial collagenase. Supernatant fluid from reaction mixture, prepared under standard conditions, of collagenase (8.57 µg/ml) and basement membrane was lyophilized; lyophilized material dissolved in water to volume three-tenths that of original supernatant fluid. 200 µl of this solution containing 480 µg bovine serum albumin equivalent was submitted to gel filtration under same conditions as in Figure 21 (OHSAKA et al., 1973a)

Table 8. Effect of hemorrhage inhibitors on the liberation of Folin-positive (F) and anthrone-positive (A) materials from basement membrane exposed to hemorrhagic principles (OHSAKA et al., 1973a). Each hemorrhagic principle was allowed to react with the basement membrane under the standard conditions except that the reaction mixture contained a given inhibitor at the indicated final concentration

Inhibitor added		HR1		HR2a		HR2b		Collagenase	
		F[a]	A[b]	F	A	F	A	F	A
None		32	53	16	7	17	9	64	90
EDTA,	0.1 mM	5	13	0	0	0	0	18	—
	1.0 mM	0	0	0	0	0	0	27	—
	10.0 mM	0	0	0	0	0	0	21	—
Cysteine,	0.02 mM	8.4	15.5	8.4	7	9.5	8	61	114
	0.2 mM	0.3	1.6	0	1.2	0.7	0.4	22	22
	2.0 mM	0.8	0	0	0.8	0.8	0	8	0.9
Antivenin,	50 units/ml	0	9.6	0	0	0	0.4	—	—
	100 units/ml	0	1.3	0	0	0	1.7	—	—
Antihemorrhagic factor from snake serum, 12 units/ml		3	0.7	1	0.5	0.3	1.4	75	108

[a] Proteins (bovine serum albumin equiv.) liberated in % of total basement membrane protein.
[b] µg carbohydrates (glucose equiv.) liberated/mg basement membrane protein.

authors concluded that the basement membrane is damaged by enzymatic action of the venom principles. The difference in the ratio of protein to carbohydrate quantities liberated suggests that HR 2a or HR 2b acts on the membrane in a mode of action different from HR 1. Gross comparison of molecular weights among the split-products of the membrane with these principles favors this interpretation.

These results suggest that the hemorrhagic effect of the venom hemorrhagic principles is attributable primarily to enzymatic disruption of the basement membrane with subsequent loss of integrity of the vessel wall (OHSAKA et al., 1973a, b; OHSAKA, 1973, 1976a, b). However, the opening of the endothelial cell junctions occurring at the onset of hemorrhage when the basement membrane has only been partially disrupted may have been due to some unknown mediators released from the tissues by the action of venom hemorrhagic principles (OHSAKA, 1976b).

3. Effect on the Hemostatic Mechanism

It is of interest to test the venom hemorrhagic principles for their inhibitory effects on the hemostatic mechanism. GROTTO et al. (1969) reported that a purified preparation of *Vipera palestinae* hemorrhagin impaired thrombin formation, fibrinogen clottability, fibrin-stabilizing factor activity, platelet clot-retracting activity, ADP- and connective tissue-induced platelet aggregation, and connective tissue-induced platelet-ADP release. However, inactivation of the proteolytic activity contained in this hemorrhagin by treatment with DFP resulted in complete abolition of the first four, and partial inhibition of the last two of the above activities shown by the hemorrhagin, while hemorrhagic activity remained intact. Recently we demonstrated that the purified hemorrhagic principles from *Trimeresurus flavoviridis* venom inhibited ADP-induced platelet aggregation (YAMANAKA et al., 1974), while no appreciable effect on blood coagulation was observed (OHSAKA, unpublished data cited in OHSAKA, 1973, 1976a, b).

Figure 25 shows the effect of HR 1 on ADP-induced platelet aggregation (YAMANAKA et al., 1974). Platelet-rich plasma was preincubated for 5 min with HR 1 at various concentrations. Aggregation reaction was initiated by the addition of ADP. As shown in Figure 25, the maximum inhibition (60%) of platelet aggregation was brought about with HR 1 at a concentration of 6 ng/ml.

Figure 26 shows the effect of HR 2 on ADP-induced platelet aggregation, tested under the same experimental conditions as above (YAMANAKA et al., 1974). HR 2 at 5 or 50 μg/ml inhibits the platelet aggregation by 50%. HR 2 is much less effective than HR 1. A higher concentration of HR 2 is needed to produce an inhibitory effect owing to the slow reactivity of this hemorrhagic principle, as the next figure shows.

Figure 27 shows the inhibitory effect of HR 2 on ADP-induced platelet aggregation as a function of preincubation time (YAMANAKA et al., 1974). The extent of inhibition by HR 2 increases with duration of preincubation; 80-min preincubation resulted in complete inhibition. By contrast, the maximum inhibition with HR 1 is attained by preincubation for 5–10 min.

These results clearly demonstrate the ability of venom hemorrhagic principles to inhibit the in vitro aggregation of platelets. This fact explains the rare formation of thrombus (OHSAKA et al., 1971b; TSUCHIYA et al., 1974) and the lack of viscous

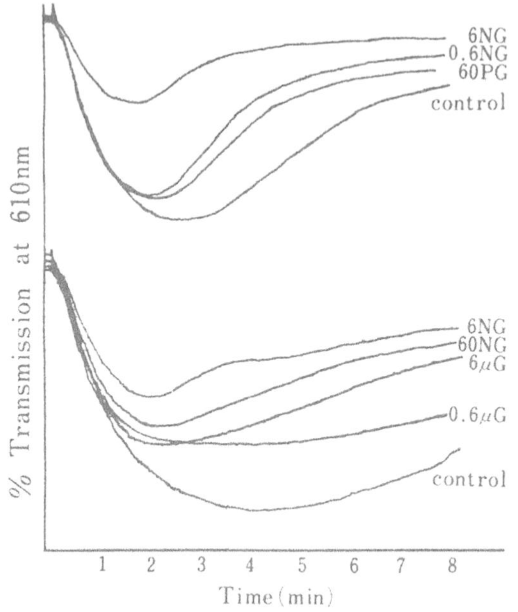

Fig. 25. Effect of HR1 on ADP-induced platelet aggregation (YAMANAKA et al., 1974). Platelet-rich plasma was incubated at room temperature for 5 min with a buffer solution or HR1 at indicated concentrations, prior to addition of ADP. Platelet aggregation was measured by turbidimetry

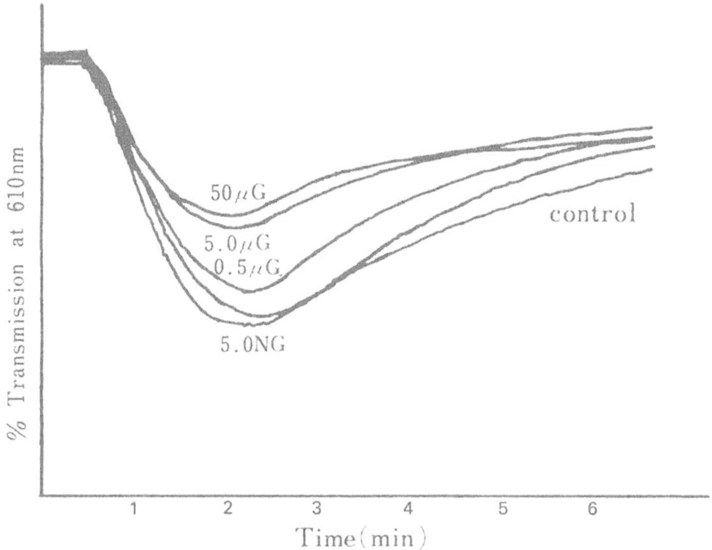

Fig. 26. Effect of HR2 on ADP-induced platelet aggregation (YAMANAKA et al., 1974). Platelet-rich plasma was incubated at room temperature for 5 min with a buffer solution or HR2 at indicated concentrations, prior to addition of ADP. Platelet aggregation was measured by turbidimetry

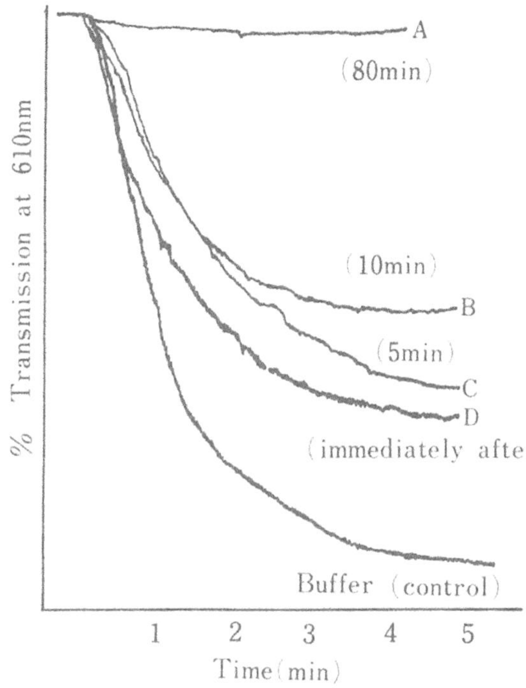

Fig. 27. Inhibitory effect of HR2 on ADP-induced platelet aggregation as a function of preincubation time (YAMANAKA et al., 1974). Platelet-rich plasma was incubated with HR2 (50 μg) at room temperature for periods indicated, prior to addition of ADP. Platelet aggregation was measured by turbidimetry

metamorphosis of platelets (TSUCHIYA et al., 1974; OHSAKA et al., 1975) at the site of venom-induced hemorrhage (see Figs. 18 and 19).

The inhibition of thrombus (platelet aggregate) formation by venom principles may aggravate hemorrhage induced primarily by enzymatic disruption of the basement membrane, thus constituting the secondary cause of hemorrhage (OHSAKA, 1973, 1976a, b).

VII. Involvement of an Endogenous or Exogenous Hemorrhagic Principle in General Physiological Mechanism of Hemorrhage. A Suggestion from Venom Studies

In the course of their studies on the mechanism of venom-induced hemorrhage, the present author and his co-workers have attempted to reveal the general physiological mechanisms involved in hemorrhage. The basement membrane is considered to constitute a solid barrier against erythrocytic escape (OHSAKA, 1973, 1976a, b). From our results, demonstrating that the venom hemorrhagic principles themselves act as the basement membrane-disrupting enzyme (OHSAKA et al., 1973a, b), we have recently put forward the hypothesis that hemorrhage is evoked by either an endogenous or an exogenous hemorrhagic principle of enzymic nature (OHSAKA, 1973, 1976a, b). Snake venom hemorrhagic principles and collagenase from *C. histolyti-*

cum are known examples of such an exogenous hemorrhagic principle. Although no endogenous hemorrhagic principle has yet been shown to exist, or even to be involved, the search for substances with such characteristics as those of the venom hemorrhagic principles (exogenous) at the hemorrhagic site of the Shwartzman reaction (HALPERN, 1964; THOMAS, 1964), the Arthus reaction (THOMAS, 1964), and also the Reilly phenomenon (DECOURT, 1951) may well provide clues that will lead to discovery of the hypothetical endogenous hemorrhagic principle suggested above (OHSAKA, 1973, 1976a, b).

VIII. Antihemorrhagic Factor Present in the Sera of Snakes

It has been frequently observed that venomous and nonvenomous snakes are resistant to the toxic action of snake venoms (NOGUCHI, 1909; CALMETTE, 1908; KELLAWAY, 1937; ESSEX, 1945). Evidence has accumulated to indicate the presence in the blood of certain snakes of a factor(s) that inhibits lethal toxicity (PETERSON and KÕIVASTIK, 1943; BOQUET, 1945; PHILPOT and SMITH, 1950; PHILPOT and DEUTSCH, 1956; DEORAS and MHASALKAR, 1963; ISHII et al., 1970; BONNETT and GUTTMAN, 1971; OMORI-SATOH et al., 1972; OVADIA et al., 1976). Similarly, the hemorrhagic activity (ROSENFELD and GLASS, 1940; OMORI-SATOH et al., 1972; OVADIA et al., 1976), proteolytic activity (BONNETT and GUTTMAN, 1971) and phospholipase A activity (KIHARA, 1976) of snake venoms are also inhibited. It was reported that the serum factor responsible for antilethal activity (PHILPOT and DEUTSCH, 1956; DEORAS and MHASALKAR, 1963; BONNETT and GUTTMAN, 1971; OMORI-SATOH et al., 1972; OVADIA et al., 1976) as well as antiproteolytic activity (PHILPOT and DEUTSCH, 1956; BONNETT and GUTTMAN, 1971) was precipitable with ammonium sulfate.

It is of special interest and importance to purify and characterize such an antihemorrhagic (antitoxic) factor(s), for the following reasons. Firstly, such work may not only give a most plausible explanation for the self-protecting mechanism in the venomous snake but also allow some insight into more complicated self-protecting mechanisms involved in higher animals. Secondly, the antihemorrhagic factor(s), together with EDTA and cysteine, which are known as hemorrhage inhibitors, may be of great help in elucidating the mechanism of action of venom hemorrhagic principles (OMORI-SATOH et al., 1972). There is also the possibility that the antihemorrhagic factor(s) can be put to clinical use.

Recently OMORI-SATOH et al. (1972) succeeded in the extensive purification and physicochemical characterization of an antihemorrhagic (antitoxic) factor in the serum of *Trimeresurus flavoviridis*. OVADIA et al. (1976) reported that the serum of *Vipera palestinae* neutralizes both hemorrhagic and neurotoxic activities of its venom and that the mechanism of the neurotoxin neutralization involves a complex formation between the serum factor and the neurotoxin.

The purification and characterization of an antihemorrhagic factor in the serum of *Trimeresurus flavoviridis* and its inhibitory effects on the hemorrhagic activity of both HR1 and HR2 (a mixture of HR2a and HR2b), and on the lethal toxicity of HR1 known to contain the bulk of the lethal toxicity of the original venom (OMORI-SATOH et al., 1972) will be described here in some detail, as will the mechanism of neutralization of neurotoxin by a similar antitoxic factor present in the serum of *Vipera palestinae* (OVADIA et al., 1976).

1. Purification and Characterization of an Antihemorrhagic Factor from the Serum of Trimeresurus flavoviridis

a) Purification

To 100 ml of snake serum (total absorbance at 280 nm was 5850) solid ammonium sulfate was added to give 35% saturation, and the precipitate formed was removed by centrifugation. To the supernatant fluid, solid ammonium sulfate was added to give 60% saturation, and the mixture was centrifuged. The precipitate was collected and dissolved in 40 ml of distilled water (total absorbance at 280 nm recovered was 2810) and this was dialyzed against the physiological saline. To the dialysis residue (total volume 59 ml) 48 ml of redistilled and chilled ethanol was added. The mixture was kept at $-2°$ C to 0° C for 1 h with constant stirring. The precipitate formed was removed by centrifugation. Then 89 ml of ethanol was added to the supernatant fluid, and this mixture was kept for 1 h at $-2°$ C to 0° C. The precipitate collected was dissolved in 15 ml of the physiological saline. The recovery of total absorbance at 280 nm was 1290. This solution was subjected to gel filtration on Sephadex G-200. After the peak of inert protein had emerged, the antihemorrhagic activity was eluted as a single peak, although the peak of the activity and that of protein did not coincide. The active fractions (fractions No. 68–84) were combined and concentrated to 10 ml (total absorbance at 280 nm recovered was 430). This solution, after dialysis against 0.15 M sodium acetate, was then submitted to chromatography on DEAE-cellulose. The antihemorrhagic activity was eluted as a broad peak. Fractions representing the major part of the antihemorrhagic activity (fractions No. 50–110) were pooled and concentrated to 5 ml. A total absorbance at 280 nm of 120 was recovered. Further purification of the antihemorrhagic factor was achieved by isoelectric focusing with carrier ampholytes, covering a pH range from 3 to 5 in a column of 440 ml (LKB, type 8102). One half of the material from the preceding step, after dialysis against a 1% solution of the carrier ampholytes, was put in the center of the column. The electrolysis was conducted for 48 h at 4° C with an initial power of 4.75 W and a final power of 2.25 W. Fractions (2.5 ml) were collected, and the pH value of each fraction was measured immediately with a 0.1 ml aliquot at room temperature. In order to correct for the ultraviolet absorption due to carrier ampholytes, the A_{280} nm curve of an empty run was subtracted from that of the sample run. The main peak at pH 4.1 was associated with the antihemorrhagic activity. The active fractions were combined and concentrated. A similar run was carried out with the other half of the material from the preceding step.

Table 9 summarizes the purification of the antihemorrhagic factor from the serum of *T. flavoviridis*. The overall purification was 21-fold with an activity yield of 15%.

The Schlieren patterns from a sedimentation velocity experiment indicated a single component in the purified preparation. The sedimentation coefficient ($S_{20,\omega}$) of the purified factor at infinite dilution was found to be 4.05 S.

Upon disc electrophoresis in 7.5% polyacrylamide gel the purified factor migrated as a single band.

Table 9. Purification of antihemorrhagic factor from the serum of *T. flavoviridis* (OMORI-SATOH et al., 1972). The antihemorrhagic activity was determined with HR1 as test toxin

Step	Protein (Total A 280 nm)	Activity (Total units)	Yield (%)	Sp. act. (units/A 280 nm)
Starting material	5850	40000	100	6.85
1. Ammonium sulfate fractionation	2810	25200	63	8.97
2. Ethyl alcohol fractionation	1290	19600	49	15.2
3. Gel filtration on Sephadex G-200	430	10500	26	24.2
4. DEAE-cellulose chromatography	120	7200	18	60.0
5. Isoelectric focusing	40	5800	15	145

Gel filtration of the purified factor on Sephadex G-200 yielded a symmetrical protein peak, the specific antihemorrhagic activity (units/absorbance at 280 nm) being constant throughout the peak.

Isoelectric focusing of the purified preparation in carrier ampholytes covering pH from 3 to 5 in an LKB type 8101 column yielded a single protein peak associated with antihemorrhagic activity. The isoelectric point was estimated to be pH 3.98.

b) *Characterization*

The molecular weight of the antihemorrhagic factor was determined by the ultracentrifugal sedimentation equilibrium method according to YPHANTIS (1960). The partial specific volume of the factor was assumed to be 0.749. From three experiments at various protein concentrations the molecular weight was estimated to be approximately 70000. Ultracentrifugation of the purified factor in sucrose density gradient revealed a symmetrical single peak, which coincided with that of the activity (Fig. 28). Sedimentation patterns of human γ-globulin, bovine serum albumin, ovalbumin, and chymotrypsinogen A, which were used as reference substances, are also shown in the figure. The purified factor sedimented to a position between bovine serum albumin (mol wt 67000) and ovalbumin (mol wt 45000). The discrepancy between the molecular weight values estimated by the sedimentation equilibrium method and by the sedimentation velocity method in sucrose density gradient may be due to the concentration dependence of sedimentation.

The isoelectric point of the purified factor was determined by isoelectric focusing experiments to be approximately 4.

During immunoelectrophoresis in an agarose gel, the purified factor migrated as a single component to a position in the area of albumin and α_1-globulin as judged from the paper electropherogram of the serum of *Agkistrodon rhodostoma* reported by PLAGNOL and VIALARD-GOUDOU (1956). Neither the purified factor nor the crude serum, however, formed a precipitin line with HR 1 or the crude venom.

The antihemorrhagic activity of the crude serum was stable on heating at various temperatures for 3 min and at various pH values between 2 and 11. The serum heated at 56° C for 30 min retained almost all of its antihemorrhagic activity, and approximately 20% of the original activity remained after heating in a boiling water bath for 30 min.

c) *Effects on the Hemorrhagic Activity of HR 1 and HR 2 and on the Lethal Toxicity of HR 1*

It has been demonstrated repeatedly that HR 1 and HR 2 (mixture of HR 2a and 2b) are immunologically distinct; *T. flavoviridis* antivenin contains distinct antibodies to HR 1 and HR 2 (KONDO et al., 1965b; OHSAKA et al., 1966b; OMORI-SATOH et al., 1967; OHSAKA et al., 1971a; OHSAKA, 1976a). The crude serum of this snake, like the antivenin, inhibited the hemorrhagic activity not only of HR 1 but also of HR 2. The antihemorrhagic factor, after extensive purification, inhibited the hemorrhagic activity of both hemorrhagic principles, and the ratio of the antihemorrhagic activities against HR 1 and HR 2 remained constant before and after purification.

Effects of the purified factor as well as of the crude serum on the lethal toxicity of HR 1 were also examined. The crude serum inhibited the lethal toxicity, the antilethal activity of the serum being 31 units per ml. The specific antilethal activity as expressed in units per absorbance at 280 nm, increased approximately 16-fold during purification.

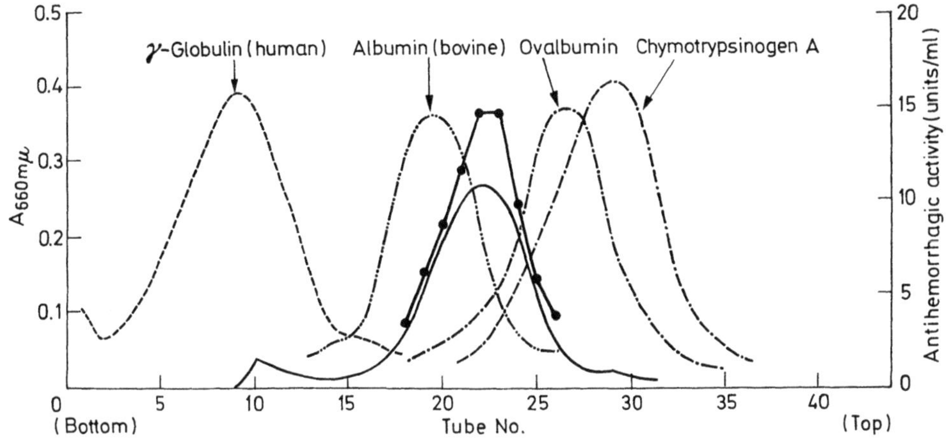

Fig. 28. Sucrose density gradient centrifugation of the purified antihemorrhagic factor. Sucrose density gradients from 10 to 20% in 2.5 mM Tris-HCl buffer (pH 8.5) containing 0.15 M NaCl were prepared in a volume of 5.2 ml. A sample of 150 μg in 0.3 ml of the same buffer was layered on the top of each gradient. Centrifugation was performed in a Beckman Spinco Model L2-65 B ultracentrifuge at 60000 rev./min for 17 h. After the termination of centrifugation, the content of each tube was divided into 42 fractions (about 0.13 ml each). Protein content was determined with a 10-μl aliquot of each fraction by Lowry's Folin reaction. For comparison, runs were made with four reference proteins (OMORI-SATOH et al., 1972)

d) Inhibition of Hemorrhagic Activity of Venoms from Different Species of Snakes

It is interesting to know whether the antihemorrhagic factor from the serum of *Trimeresurus flavoviridis* inhibits the hemorrhagic activity of venoms from different species of snakes. As shown in Table 10, the hemorrhagic activity of all snake venoms tested was more or less inhibited by the serum of *T. flavoviridis* (OMORI-SATOH et al., 1972). The figures in this table are expressed as the hemorrhagic activity in MHD

Table 10. Antihemorrhagic activity of the serum of Habu (*T. flavoviridis*) against various snake venoms (OMORI-SATOH et al., 1972). A dose of 100 MHD of each venom was incubated with varying volumes of the serum in a total volume of 1 ml. 0.2 ml of this mixture was injected into the depilated back skin of rabbits

Snake venom	Hemorrhagic activity (MHD) inhibited by 1 ml of Habu serum
Agkistrodon piscivorus piscivorus	14900
Agkistrodon halys blomhoffii	21000
Bothrops jararaca	1780
Crotalus adamanteus	7450
Crotalus atrox	21000
Trimeresurus flavoviridis	35800
Trimeresurus elegans	29500
Bitis arietans	< 100
Bitis gabonica	500
Vipera ammodytes	2100
Vipera palestinae	< 100
Ophiophagus hannah	600

inhibited per ml of the serum. The hemorrhagic activity of homologous venoms was inhibited more effectively, and that of venoms from snakes belonging to the same family *(Crotalidae)*, except that of *Bothrops jararaca*, was also well inhibited. On the other hand, inhibition of the activity of the venoms from *Viperidae* (*Bitis arietans*, *Bitis gabonica*, *Vipera ammodytes*, and *Vipera palestinae*) and from *Elapidae (Ophiophagus hannah)* was fairly poor. These observations, together with the earlier observations of ROSENFELD and GLASS (1940) that the blood of both a venomous snake, *Crotalus adamanteus* and a nonvenomous snake, *Lampropeltis getulus*, inhibited the hemorrhagic activity of *Bothrops atrox* and *Agkistrodon piscivorus*, led the authors to assume the presence in snake serum of a common mechanism of inhibition of the hemorrhagic activity.

2. Mechanism Involved in the Neutralization by the Serum of Vipera palestinae of a Toxic Fraction of Its Venom

The antitoxic factor from the serum of *Vipera palestinae* was purified by ammonium-sulfate precipitation, DEAE-cellulose chromatography, Sephadex G-75 gel filtration, and hydroxylapatite adsorption (OVADIA et al., 1976). An almost pure protein was obtained, with a 300-fold increase in specific activity. Its molecular weight was approximately 70000 and the isoelectric point approximately 4; it did not form precipitin lines with crude venom in immunodiffusion tests. It is thus clear that the neutralizing protein is of a nonimmunoglobulin nature (OVADIA et al., 1976).

In order to study the mechanism of neutralization by snake serum, OVADIA et al. (1976) examined the following possibilities: (1) the neutralizing factor protects the neurotoxin target sites in vivo, (2) the neutralizing factor destroys the neurotoxin, or (3) the neutralizing factor binds with the neurotoxin to form an inactive complex.

They first established that the neurotoxic fraction of the venom is stable at pH 3 and withstands boiling for 30 min, while antitoxic serum factor alone is inactivated at pH 3 or by heating at 95° C for 5 min. When mixed with the neurotoxic fraction, the antitoxic factor resists boiling for at least 10 min. These results suggested a possible in vitro reaction between the neurotoxic fraction and the antitoxic factor, which apparently form a thermostable complex. This complex, however, could be destroyed at pH 3, the neurotoxic properties then being regained. The reaction between the neutralizing protein and the neurotoxin is accomplished within 30 min; a longer incubation period does not enhance the neutralizing effects.

For a further test of the assumption that the neutralizing mechanism does indeed involve complex formation between the neutralizing protein and neurotoxin, the authors labeled the neurotoxin with ^{131}I. The neurotoxin is a small molecule, which leaves the Sephadex G-75 column in tubes 23–25; the neutralizing protein is a larger molecule and leaves the same column in tubes 13–14 (Fig. 29). After the two were mixed, the labeled neurotoxin emerged in the region of the neutralizing protein (tube 14; Fig. 30), indicating that the two substances were linked to form a stable complex.

During the purification by isoelectrofocusing, the neurotoxin was found to separate into four components, temporarily designated as A, B, C, and D. None of these components, when injected separately even in large amounts, was lethal to mice, although after administration of component A alone, the mice showed some discom-

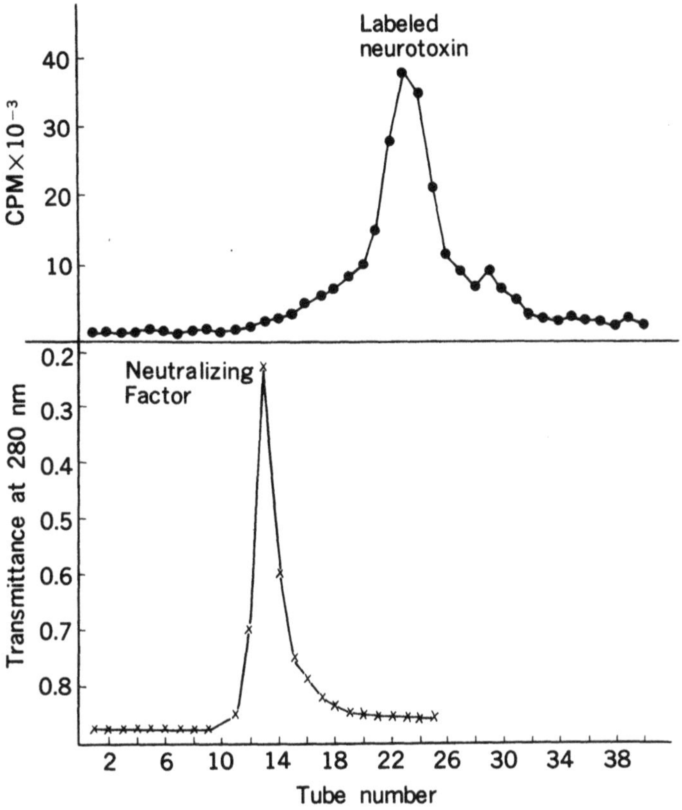

Fig. 29. Sephadex G-75 chromatographies of the venom neurotoxin and of the neutralizing protein. Aliquots of 10 μg of ^{131}I-labeled neurotoxin and 7 mg of the neutralizing protein were run separately on the same column of 2 × 80 cm (OVADIA et al., 1976). ●—●, CPM; ×—×, Transmittance at 280 nm

fort. When injected together, A and D showed the characteristic effects of the whole neurotoxic fraction.

To answer the question as to which of the components A or D is complexing with the neutralizing protein or whether both are involved, OVADIA and his group (1976) labeled the two components separately and incubated each of them with the neutralizing protein. Component A reacted partially with the serum protein, while component D was almost completely bound to it. Moreover, boiled inactive serum protein still reacted with A, but not with D. This binding of the inactive protein with A may indicate that the interaction between the neutralizing protein and component A is not specific and is thus not directly related to the neutralizing mechanism. If this assumption is correct, it leaves the binding between component D and the serum protein as being responsible for the neutralization of the lethal activity of the neurotoxic fraction.

These findings may be considered as a step toward the understanding of the resistance of snakes to snake venoms, and of the mechanisms of neutralization of toxins in higher animals in general.

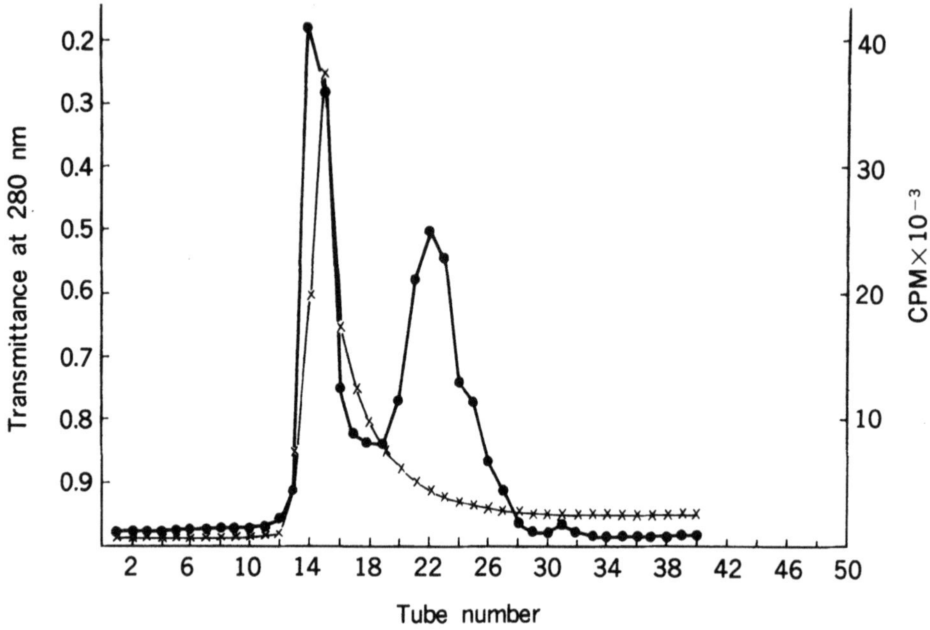

Fig. 30. Sephadex G-75 chromatography of a mixture of ^{131}I-labeled neurotoxin and the neutralizing protein. An aliquot of 10 µg of labeled neurotoxin was incubated with 7 mg of the neutralizing protein and applied to a column of 2 × 80 cm (OVADIA et al., 1976). ●—●, CPM; ×—×, Transmittance at 280 nm

IX. Treatment with Specific Antivenin (Antiserum) and Prophylaxis with Toxoid (Vaccine) of Hemorrhagic Snake Venom Poisoning

1. Neutralization of Hemorrhagic Principles by Specific Antivenin (Antiserum)

Specific antivenin (antiserum) has been widely used for the treatment of envenomation from snakebite. It has been observed that specific antivenin is effective in neutralizing systemic or lethal effects of snake venoms. In many instances, local tissue damage is not prevented by the use of antivenin alone, unless it is administered immediately after envenomation (SAWAI et al., 1962; LIESKE, 1963; REID et al., 1963; STAHNKE, 1966; CHAPMAN, 1968; GITTER and DE VRIES, 1968; REID, 1968). However, there are scant experimental data to confirm this clinical observation.

Hemorrhagic activity of snake venoms is neutralized in vitro by specific antivenin (GITTER et al., 1957; OHSAKA and KONDO, 1960; RECHNIC et al., 1962; KONDO et al., 1965b; OHSAKA et al., 1966b) or antibody fragment (MOROZ et al., 1971). SADAHIRO and his co-workers (unpubl.) have demonstrated that the hemorrhage resulting from the intracutaneous injection of *Trimeresurus flavoviridis* venom into the rabbit skin was prevented by specific antivenin when administered intravenously immediately after the venom injection; antivenin administered 30 min after the venom injection partially prevented the hemorrhage. After this period, however, administration of even a large amount of antivenin failed to prevent the hemorrhage. Similar results were described by HOMMA and TU (1970) for envenomation by South East Asian

Table 11. A model for the mechanism involved in titration of antivenin potency in the rabbit skin in the presence of two hemorrhagic principles and the corresponding antibodies (KONDO et al., 1965b)

	Proportion of the two hemorrhagic principles in test toxin		
	HR1	HR2	
Test toxin	○ ○ ○ ○	● ●	
	Proportion of the two corresponding antibodies in test antivenin		Specific antihemorrhagic activity to be titrated
	Anti-HR1	Anti-HR2	
Antivenin A	◎ ◎ ◎ ◎	◉ ◉ ◉	Anti-HR1
Antivenin B	◎ ◎ ◎ ◎ ◎ ◎	◉ ◉	Anti-HR2

An open circle (○) represents a certain quantity of toxin (HR1) molecules immunologically equivalent to that of the corresponding antibody (anti-HR1) molecules as represented by a double circle (◎). A filled circle (●) for HR2 and a circle with a dark spot (◉) for anti-HR2 represent quantities immunologically equivalent to each other

snakes. These results indicate that even antivenin with a high potency cannot be effective in preventing hemorrhagic snake venom poisoning, once permanent damage due to tissue destruction has been manifested (OHSAKA and KONDO, 1960).

Titration of antihemorrhagic potency in antivenins is not as simple as it would seem, because *Trimeresurus flavoviridis* venom, for example, contains two immunologically-distinct hemorrhagic principles, HR 1 and HR 2 (KONDO et al., 1965b; OHSAKA et al., 1966b; OMORI-SATOH et al., 1967; KONDO et al., 1973; OHSAKA, 1976a) (see Fig. 8). These two hemorrhagic principles are not distinguishable by hemorrhagic action on the rabbit skin (KONDO et al., 1960; OHSAKA et al., 1960a, 1966a). Consequently, antisera prepared against the crude venom contain the corresponding two antibodies, anti-HR 1 and anti-HR 2, in varying proportions (KONDO et al., 1965b; OHSAKA et al., 1966b; OMORI-SATOH et al., 1967).

Should the potency of such an antivenin be titrated against the test toxin containing the two hemorrhagic principles, the question arises as to what the results of such a titration indicate, for example, the potency of only anti-HR 1 or anti-HR 2, or some other implication (OHSAKA and KONDO, 1960; KONDO et al., 1965b; OHSAKA et al., 1966b).

To answer this question a model was proposed (Table 11) for the mechanism involved in titration of the antihemorrhagic potency of an antivenin containing two antibodies, with a test toxin containing two corresponding hemorrhagic principles

Table 12. The neutralization reactions determining the end points of titrations in the rabbit skin predicted from the proposed model (Table 11) (KONDO et al., 1965b)

Section	Test toxin The ratios of HR1 to HR2	Antivenin (and the ratio of anti-HR1 to anti-HR2 in the antivenin)		
		No. 7 (2.73:1)	No. 9 (4.55:1)	No. 23 (14.5:1)
4	60:40 (1.5:1)	HR2[a]	HR2	HR2
5	75:25 (3:1)	HR1[a]	HR2	HR2
6	83:17 (4.9:1)	HR1	HR1	HR2
7	95: 5 (19:1)	HR1	HR1	HR1

[a] HR1 is the abbreviation for the neutralization reaction of HR1 to anti-HR1; HR2 is for that of HR2 to anti-HR2.

(KONDO et al., 1965b; OHSAKA et al., 1966b). In the table, an open circle represents a certain quantity of toxin (HR 1) molecules immunologically equivalent to that of the corresponding antibody (anti-HR 1) molecules, as represented by a double circle. A filled circle for HR 2 and a circle with a dark spot for anti-HR 2 represent quantities immunologically equivalent to each other.

Assume that the ratio of HR 1 to HR 2 in a test toxin is 4:2 and that of anti-HR 1 to anti-HR 2 in an antivenin 4:3 (see antivenin A in Table 11). When HR 1 is neutralized equivalently by anti-HR 1, HR 2 has already been neutralized by the excess amount of anti-HR 2. In this case the end-point of titration in the rabbit skin is entirely dependent on neutralization of HR 1 by anti-HR 1 and only the potency of anti-HR 1 can be determined. On the other hand, with another antivenin having the ratio of anti-HR 1 to anti-HR 2 of 6:2 (see antivenin B), when HR 2 is neutralized equivalently by anti-HR 2, HR 1 has already been neutralized by the excess amount of anti-HR 1. In this case, only the potency of anti-HR 2 can be determined. In other words, either of the two antihemorrhagic activities will be determined depending on the ratio of HR 1 to HR 2 in a test toxin and on that of anti-HR 1 to anti-HR 2 in a test antivenin.

For verification of this model, a series of experiments was conducted. In Table 12, antivenins Nos. 7, 9, and 23 were titrated separately against each of HR 1 and HR 2. The ratios of anti-HR 1 to anti-HR 2 in these antivenins were calculated to be 2.73:1, 4.55:1, and 14.5:1, respectively. When the antihemorrhagic potencies of the three antivenins are titrated against the test toxins containing HR 1 and HR 2 at various ratios, antihemorrhagic activity against either of the hemorrhagic principles should be determined as predicted in Table 12, if the model under discussion (Table 11) is true. The prediction shown in Table 12 was in exact accordance with the actual results of the experiments, except for antivenin No. 23 in Section 7.

From these results the author and his group concluded that the antihemorrhagic potency of the antivenin relative to a standard antivenin can only be determined when the two hemorrhagic principles (HR 1 and HR 2) are used separately as test toxins instead of a crude venom.

To generalize, all the toxic components in a venom indistinguishable in respect to biological action should be separated and each component used as a test toxin

(OHSAKA and KONDO, 1960; KONDO et al., 1965b; OHSAKA et al., 1966b). This general conclusion has been fortified by experiments on the determination of antilethal potency of the antivenin (KONDO et al., 1965a).

The reasoning thus confirmed is applicable to the assay of antitoxic potency of a polyvalent antivenin. Unless each toxic component in venoms is separated and available as a test toxin, monovalent antivenins should not be combined before determining the potencies of the individual antivenins, and immunization with mixed venoms should be avoided (OHSAKA et al., 1966b).

2. Prophylaxis of Envenomation with Toxoids (Vaccines) Prepared from Purified Hemorrhagic Principles

Although it has frequently been shown that antitoxin administration and nonspecific treatments have some therapeutic effects (CHAPMAN, 1968; GITTER and DE VRIES, 1968; REID, 1968), postexposure therapy has its own limitations. Prophylaxis by active immunization with toxoid is needed, therefore, to prevent the effects of envenomation from snake bite.

Attempts have been made by many workers at transforming venom to toxoids by treatment with formalin (RAMON, 1924; YAOI and KAWASHIMA, 1928; KUWAJIMA, 1938; BOQUET, 1941; BOQUET and VENDRELY, 1943; CHRISTENSEN, 1947; WIENER, 1960; MOROZ-PERLMUTTER et al., 1963; KONDO et al., 1970, 1973, 1976; SADAHIRO et al., 1978) or other chemicals (ISHIZAKA, 1907; OKONOGI and HATTORI, 1968; SAWAI and KAWAMURA, 1969), by irradiation with X-ray (FLOWERS, 1963, 1966) or cobalt-60 (MITTELSTAEDT et al., 1973) and by photo-oxidation (KOCHOLATY, 1966; KOCHOLATY and ASHLEY, 1966; KOCHOLATY et al., 1967, 1968). Formalinization, which is in general use for toxoiding bacterial toxins, has often been attempted. All these treatments succeeded in detoxifying venoms completely, but only a few (KONDO et al., 1970, 1973, 1976) of the resulting toxoids were satisfactorily immunogenic.

Numerous fundamental problems have to be solved before a toxoid from a venom with a high immunogenicity can be prepared for human use (KONDO et al., 1973). The optimum conditions for toxoiding must first be established. For this purpose, it is a prerequisite to establish a highly reliable and accurate method for evaluating immunogenicity. This should be satisfied by titrating the circulating antitoxin and expressing the titer in terms of relative potency to a standard toxoid. It is also necessary to correlate the circulating antitoxin titer and the resistance of the immunized animal. Furthermore, purification of each of the multiple toxic principles of a venom involved in envenomation from snakebite is neccessary, so that toxoiding can be performed under optimum conditions and unfavorable side reactions in man to toxoid injection can be minimized.

With these points in mind, the present author and his co-workers studied the toxoiding of *Trimeresurus flavoviridis* venom (KONDO et al., 1970, 1973, 1976; SADAHIRO et al., 1978). Of several toxic principles contained in this venom, the major lethal toxin (OMORI-SATOH and OHSAKA, 1970) and the two hemorrhagic principles, HR 1 (OMORI-SATOH and OHSAKA, 1970) and HR 2 (TAKAHASHI and OHSAKA, 1970b) are known to play the most important role following envenomation by this snake (OHSAKA and KONDO, 1960; KONDO et al., 1965a, b). The major lethal toxin was always associated with the preparation of HR 1 (OHSAKA et al., 1960a; OMORI-

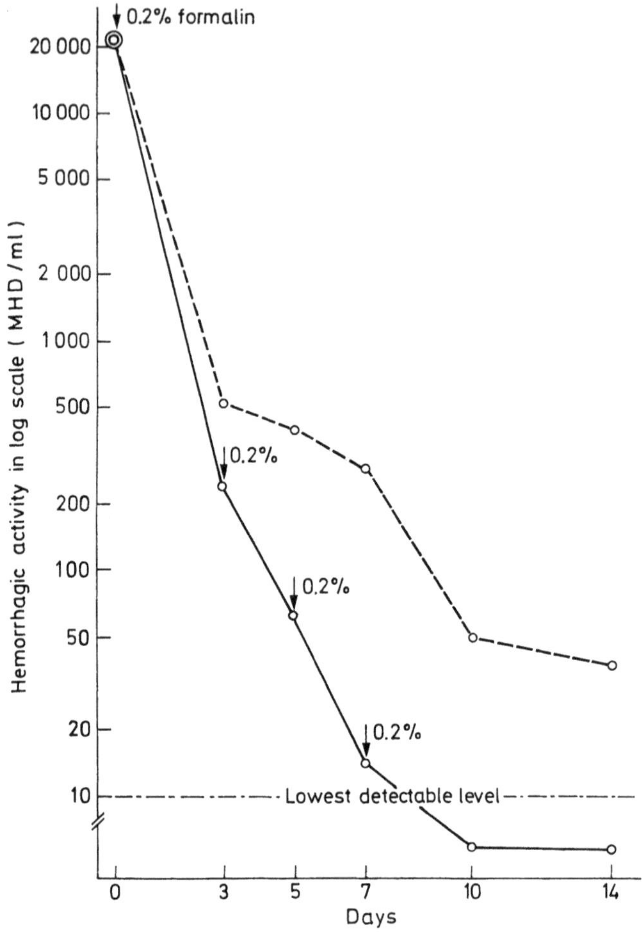

Fig. 31. Time course of inactivation of hemorrhagic activity of *T. flavoviridis* venom with formalin increasing in concentration. 1% crude venom dissolved in M/30 phosphate buffered saline (pH 7.0) was treated at 37° C with formalin at 0.2% (broken line) or at concentrations increased by 0.2% every other day up to 0.8%. Aliquots were withdrawn at various times to determine the minimum hemorrhagic dose (MHD) (KONDO et al., 1973)

SATOH and OHSAKA, 1970). These principles are distinct immunologically from each other (KONDO et al., 1965b; OHSAKA et al., 1966b; OMORI-SATOH et al., 1967; OHSAKA et al., 1971a; OHSAKA, 1976a). The toxoid of this venom, therefore, should stimulate production of antibodies to these toxic principles to certain levels, as otherwise complete protection against envenomation from the snakebite cannot be guaranteed.

Figure 31 shows the time course of detoxification of a 1% solution of crude venom treated with formalin initially at 0.2% and then at concentrations increasing by 0.2% on the 3rd, 5th, and 7th days, in comparison with that of crude venom treated with formalin at a constant concentration of 0.2% (KONDO et al., 1973). The crude venom treated with formalin increasing in concentration to 0.8% became nontoxic

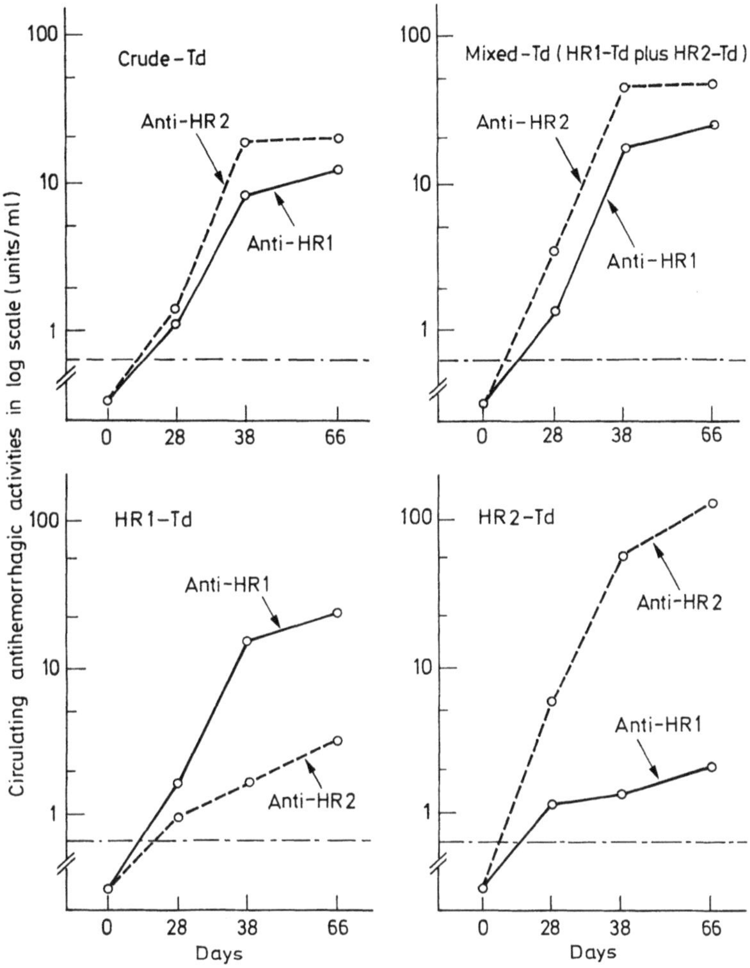

Fig. 32. Immunogenicities for guinea pigs of a formol toxoid prepared from crude venom and those from purified hemorrhagic principles. Each of Crude-Td, HR1-Td, HR2-Td and Mixed-Td was injected subcutaneously into 8 guinea pigs in a 0.5-ml dose three times at 4 weeks' intervals. Each animal was bled four times, prior to and 4 weeks after the 1st injection, and 10 days after the 2nd and the 3rd injections. The circulating anti-HR1 and anti-HR2 titers of each serum were determined. Each point represents the geometric mean of antihemorrhagic titers obtained. –·–·–, lowest detectable level (KONDO et al., 1973)

in 10 days and the immunogenicity was preserved. The purified preparations of HR 1 and HR 2, when treated with formalin, were detoxified in a way essentially similar to the crude venom (KONDO et al., 1973).

The toxoids thus obtained from the crude venom, the purified HR 1, and also the purified HR 2 were dialyzed, and mixed with aluminium phosphate gel ($AlPO_4$). HR 1-toxoid (HR 1-Td) and HR 2-toxoid (HR 2-Td) were mixed to make mixed-toxoid (Mixed-Td). Each toxoid was injected subcutaneously to eight guinea pigs in three doses of 0.5 ml at four-week intervals. The circulating antitoxins were titrated. In Figure 32, the geometric means of antitoxin titers of each group are plotted

Table 13. Resistance of monkeys immunized with *T. flavoviridis* (Habu)-venom toxoid to challenge with crude venom (SADAHIRO et al., 1978)

Toxoid for immunization (Batch No.)	Circulating antitoxin titers (u/ml) Anti-HR1	Anti-HR2	Challenging dose of venom (mg)	Symptoms after challenge
13	4.2	21	5	+
	6.1	16		+
	2	39		±
	14	21		+
	5.2	10		D3
	10	25		±
	3.2	11		±
13-B	6.6	17	5	±
	20	22		D2
	14	9		±
	12	21		±
	3.2	27		D1
	11	15		±
	15	14		±
14	1.8	32	5	−
	2.2	32		++
	1.8	32		−
	3.4	32		D1
	3	32		−
	4.3	28		+
15	4	47	5	−
	2.5	33		±
	4	33		−
	9	28		+
	11	34		+
	5.9	25		−

[a] Monkeys that had received three injections, each of 1 ml of the toxoid were challenged with crude venom administered i.m. 10 or 17 days after the last injection of toxoid. Local symptoms were examined 5 or 8 days after the challenge.
[b] Symbols: ++: Moderate hemorrhage at the injection site only. +: Slight hemorrhage at the injection site only. ±: Doubtful hemorrhage at the injection site only. −: Negative. D3, D2, D1: Died on the date indicated.

(KONDO et al., 1973). In the crude toxoid (Crude-Td)- or Mixed-Td-immunized group, both anti-HR 1 and anti-HR 2 titers increased at similar rates; in the HR 1-Td-immunized group, anti-HR 1 alone developed, with little anti-HR 2; in the HR 2-Td-immunized group, anti-HR 2 alone developed.

It may be mentioned in passing that antilethal activity was below the detectable level in the Crude-Td- and HR 2-Td-immunized groups, whereas in the HR 1-Td- and Mixed-Td-immunized groups, it reached 40–80 U/ml (KONDO et al., 1973).

To test the correlation between the circulating antitoxin titers and the protective capacity of immunized monkeys, the immunized animals were challenged with a dose known to be lethal (5 mg) of crude venom. As shown in Table 13, the immu-

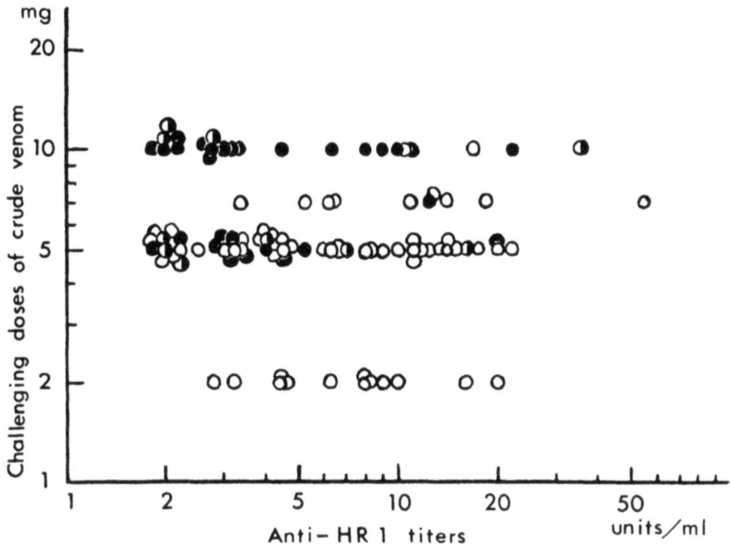

Fig. 33. Relationship between the circulating antitoxin titers and the protective capacity of monkeys immunized with *T. flavoviridis* (Habu)-venom toxoid (SADAHIRO et al., unpublished data). Symbols: ●, animal died; ◑, animal survived with severe symptoms; ○, animal survived with slight, if any, local symptoms

nized animals resisted the challenge fairly well without developing any significant local symptoms (SADAHIRO et al., 1978).

As Figure 33 shows, monkeys having anti-HR 1 titers of about 5 units tolerated a challenge with 7 mg of venom well (SADAHIRO et al., unpublished data). Incidentally, the amount of venom actually ejected by a single bite of this snake was estimated to be 13.2 mg (KONDO et al., 1972). A challenge dose of 10 mg would kill most of the animals, but the survivors would at most show a slight local lesion (SADAHIRO et al., 1978), in good agreement with earlier observations (KONDO et al., 1971). The anti-HR 2 titers were very high in the majority of the immunized animals, being more than 20 units/ml. The level of antilethal activity was below the detectable level (32 U/ml). Experiments with more potent toxoids demonstrated, however, that antilethal activity was detected in some animals having higher anti-HR 1 titers (SADAHIRO et al., 1978).

The immunogenicity of Habu-venom toxoid (Mixed-Td) for man was established by the Committee for Habu-Venom-Toxoid (SOMEYA et al., 1972). A group of volunteers who received two injections of a Mixed-Td produced circulating antitoxin titers of about 2 U/ml for anti-HR 1 and 13 U/ml for anti-HR 2. This anti-HR 1 titer (2 U/ml) was comparable to the calculated titer of circulating antitoxin of patients who received a therapeutic dose of the antivenin. These results indicated that the Mixed-Td is suitable for human use. In field trials, 208 out of 298 persons (69.8%) produced anti-HR 1 titers exceeding 1 U/ml after the basic immunization, and the proportion of persons having such titers increased to 92.1% (140/152) after a booster injection (SADAHIRO et al., 1978).

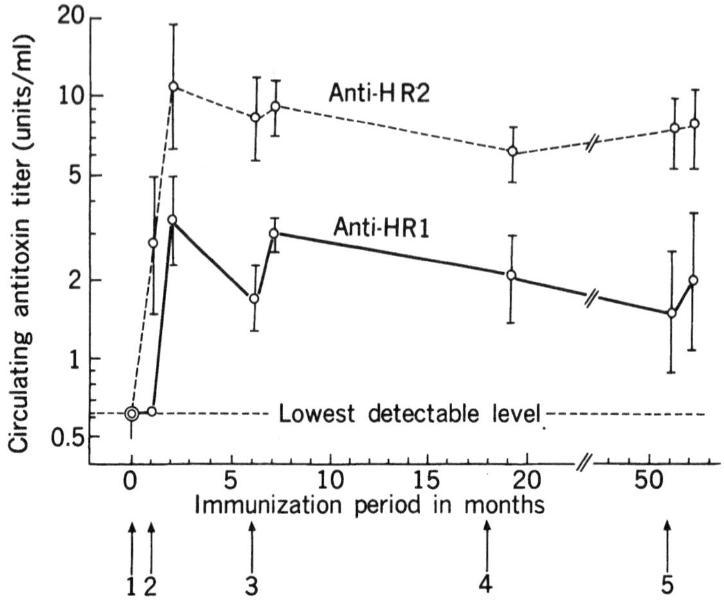

Fig. 34. Immune response of volunteers to *T. flavoviridis* (Habu)-venom toxoid. The arrows indicate the time points at which the toxoid was injected in a dose of 0.5 ml. An open circle represents a logarithmic mean of circulating antitoxin titers with fiducial limits (vertical bars) at a 95% level of probability (SADAHIRO et al., 1978)

The change in antitoxin titers of a group of men immunized with a toxoid preparation was followed up for several years, and the results shown in Figure 34 (SADAHIRO et al., 1978) were obtained. As in monkeys, the rise in antitoxin titers (anti-HR 1 and anti-HR 2) after the booster immunization was not remarkable, though the level of antitoxin titers returned to the level attained after basic immunization. The results obtained with another group showed that the antitoxin titer after booster injection dropped in 10–12 months to half or one-third of the highest value, attained after the basic immunization.

To maintain the antitoxin titer high enough to protect against envenomation over a long period of time, and to enhance the immune response to booster injections, it will be necessary to improve the Mixed-Td preparation, especially the HR 1-Td contained in it, since HR 1 has been shown to be the main toxic principle in this venom and the anti-HR 1 titer in immunized men and animals seems to be closely related to their resistance to the challenge with crude venom (SADAHIRO et al., 1978).

F. Concluding Remarks

Even now, snakebite continues to be a medical problem of considerable magnitude in most parts of the world. Knowledge of snake venoms and of the systemic and local effects they manifest has led to the preparation of antivenins with high potencies and also to the creation of serotherapy and other supportive measures for the rational treatment of cases of snake venom poisoning. Recent success in the isolation of venom hemorrhagic principles has enabled us to prepare venom toxoids for the prophylaxis of hemorrhagic snake venom poisoning.

In addition, snake venoms and their biologically active components are tools of tremendous scientific and medical potential (DINIZ, 1968; ZELLER, 1966; see also Chapter 11). They have been instrumental in the elucidation of such basic physiological process as neuromuscular transmission (LEE and CHANG, 1966; LEE, 1972), blood coagulation (MACFARLANE, 1967; DE VRIES and COHEN, 1969), and release of vasoactive kinins (ROCHA E SILVA et al., 1949). Pharmacological studies on the hemorrhagic principles recently isolated from snake venoms have contributed a great deal to the understanding of the physiological mechanisms involved in hemorrhage (OHSAKA, 1976a, b), and might provide knowledge that would make it possible to develop drugs to prevent bleeding. In all likelihood, snake venoms will become increasingly useful as tools for elucidating the fundamental physiological process involved in both normal and pathophysiological states of human beings.

References

Beraldo, W.T., Dias da Silva, W.: Section A. Release of histamine by animal venoms and bacterial toxins. In: Eichler, O., Farah, A. (Eds.): Handbuch der experimentellen Pharmakologie, Vol. 18, Pt. 1, pp. 334—366. Berlin-Heidelberg-New York: Springer 1966

Bhargava, N., Vargaftig, B.B., Vos, C.J. de, Bonta, I.L., Tijs, T.: Dissociation of oedema provoking factor of *Agkistrodon piscivorus* venom from kininogenase. In: Back, N., Sicuteri, F. (Eds.): Vasopeptides. Chemistry, Pharmacology, and Pathophysiology, pp. 141—148. New York: Plenum 1972

Bhargava, N., Zirinis, P., Bonta, I.L., Vargaftig, B.B.: Comparison of hemorrhagic factors of the venoms of *Naja naja*, *Agkistrodon piscivorus* and *Apis mellifera*. Biochem. Pharmacol. **19**, 2405—2412 (1970)

Bicher, H.I., Roth, M., Gitter, S.: Neurotoxic activity of *Vipera palestinae* venom. Depression of central autonomic vasoregulatory mechanisms. Med. Pharmacol. Exp. **14**, 349—359 (1966)

Bonnett, D.E., Guttman, S.I.: Inhibition of moccasin (*Agkistrodon piscivorus*) venom proteolytic activity by the serum of the Florida king snake (*Lampropeltis getulus floridana*). Toxicon **9**, 417—425 (1971)

Bonta, I.L.: Microvascular lesions as a target of anti-inflammatory and certain other drugs. Acta physiol. pharmacol. neerl. **15**, 188—222 (1969)

Bonta, I.L., Vargaftig, B.B., Bhargava, N., Vos, C.J., de: Method for study of snake venom induced hemorrhage. Toxicon **8**, 3—10 (1970)

Bonta, I.L., Vargaftig, B.B., Vos, C.J., de, Grijsen, H.: Haemorrhagic mechanism of some snake venoms in relation to protection by estriol succinate of blood vessel damage. Life Sci. **8**, 881—888 (1969)

Bonta, I.L., Vos, C.J., de: The effect of estriol-16,17-dihemisuccinate on vascular permeability as evaluated in the rat paw oedema test. Acta endocr. **49**, 403—411 (1965)

Boquet, P.: Rôle du cuivre en quantités infinitésimales dans l'atténuation des venins de *Vipera aspis* et de *Naja tripudians* et d'une toxine végétale, la ricine, par le peroxyde d'hydrogène. Ann. Inst. Pasteur **66**, 379—396 (1941)

Boquet, P.: Sur les propriétés antivenimeuses du sérum de *Vipera aspis*. Ann. Inst. Pasteur **71**, 340—343 (1945)

Boquet, P.: Venins de serpents. I. Physio-pathologie de l'envenimation et propriétés biologiques des venins. Toxicon **2**, 5—41 (1964)

Boquet, P.: Venins de serpents. II. Constitution chimique des venins de serpents et immunité antivenimeuse. Toxicon **3**, 243—279 (1966)

Boquet, P., Vendrely, R.: Influence du pH sur la transformation du venin de cobra en anavenin par l'aldéhyde formique; préparation d'un anavenin solide. C.R. Soc. Biol. (Paris) **137**, 179—180 (1943)

Bücherl, W., Buckley, E. E., Delofeu, V. (Eds.): Venomous Animals and Their Venoms (2 Vols). New York-London: Academic 1968—1971
Calmette, A.: Venoms, Venomous Animals and Antivenomous Serum—Therapeutics. New York: Wood 1908
Chapman, D. S.: The symptomatology, pathology, and treatment of the bites of venomous snakes of Central and Southern Africa. In: Bücherl, W., Buckley, E., Deulofeu, V. (Eds.): Venomous Animals and Their Venoms, Vol. I, pp. 463—527. New York: Academic 1968
Christensen, P. A.: Formol detoxification of Cape cobra *(Naja flava)* venom. S. Afr. J. med. Sci. **12**, 71—75 (1947)
Cohen, I., Zur, M., Kaminsky, E., Vries, A., de: Isolation and characterization of kinin-releasing enzyme of *Echis coloratus* venom. Toxicon **7**, 3—4 (1969)
Coleman, J. E., Vallee, B. L.: Metallocarboxypeptidases: Stability constants and enzymatic characteristics. J. biol. Chem. **236**, 2244—2249 (1961)
Decourt, P.: Études et Documents, Vol. 1. Tanger: Hesperis 1951
Denson, K. W. E.: Coagulant and anticoagulant action of snake venoms. Toxicon **7**, 5—11 (1969)
Deoras, P. J., Mhasalkar, V. B.: Antivenin activity of some snake sera. Toxicon **1**, 89—90 (1963)
Devi, A.: The chemistry, toxicity, biochemistry, and pharmacology of North American snake venoms. In: Bücherl, W., Buckley, E., Deulofeu, V. (Eds.): Venomous Animals and Their Venoms, Vol. II, pp. 175—202. New York: Academic 1971
Diniz, C. R.: Bradykinin formation by snake venoms. In: Bücherl, W., Buckley, E., Deulofeu, V. (Eds.): Venomous Animals and Their Venoms, Vol. I, pp. 217—227. New York: Academic 1968
Djaldetti, M., Joshua, H., Bessler, H., Rosen, M., Gutglas, H., Vries, A., de: Coagulation disturbance in the dog following *Echis colorata* venom inoculation. Hemostase **4**, 323—332 (1964)
Efrati, P., Reif, L.: Clinical and pathological observations on sixty-five cases of viper bite in Israel. Amer. J. trop. Med. Hyg. **2**, 1085—1108 (1953)
Emery, J. A., Russell, F. E.: Lethal and hemorrhagic properties of some North American snake venoms. In: Keagan, H. L., Macfarlane, W. V. (Eds.): Venomous and Poisonous Animals and Noxious Plants of the Pacific Region, pp. 409—413. London: Pergamon 1963
Essex, H. E.: Certain animal venoms and their physiologic action. Physiol. Rev. **25**, 148—170 (1945)
Fawcett, D. W.: The fine structure of capillaries, arterioles and small arteries. In: Reynolds, S. R. M., Zweifach, B. W. (Eds.): The Microcirculation, pp. 1—27. Urbana: The University of Illinois 1959
Fawcett, D. W.: Comparative observations on the fine structure of blood capillaries. In: Orbison, J. L., Smith, D. E. (Eds.): The Peripheral Blood Vessels, pp. 17—44. Baltimore Md: Williams and Wilkins 1963
Fearn, H. J., Smith, C., West, G. B.: Capillary permeability responses to snake venoms. J. Pharm. Pharmacol. **16**, 79—84 (1964)
Flexner, S., Noguchi, H.: The constitution of snake venom and snake sera. J. Path. Bact. **8**, 379—410 (1903)
Flowers, H. H.: The effects of X-irradiation on the biological activity of cottonmouth moccasin *(Ancistrodon piscivorus)* venom. Toxicon **1**, 131—136 (1963)
Flowers, H. H.: Effects of X-irradiation on the antigenic character of *Agkistrodon piscivorus* (cottonmouth moccasin) venom. Toxicon **3**, 301—304 (1966)
Fonseca, F. da: Animais peçonhentos: São Paulo: Inst. Butantan 1949. Cited by Slotta, K.: Progress in Chemistry of Organic Natural Products **12**, 406—465 (1955)
Fulton, G. P., Lutz, B. R., Shulman, M. H., Arendt, K. A.: Moccasin venom as a test for susceptibility to petechial formation in the hamster. In: Buckley, E. E., Porges, N. (Eds.): Venoms, pp. 303—310. Washington, D.C.: American Association for the Advancement of Science 1956
Geh, S. L., Toh, H. T.: The effect of sea snake neurotoxins and a phospholipase fraction on the ultrastructure of mammalian skeletal muscle. Abstract of South-East Asian/Western Pacific Regional Meeting of Pharmacologists, Singapore, May 11—14, 1976
Gennaro, J. F., Ramsey, H. W.: The toxicity of some precipitated fractions of dried moccasin venom *(Ancistrodon piscivorus piscivorus)*. Amer. J. trop. Med. Hyg. **8**, 546—551 (1959)
Gitter, S., Kochwa, S., Vries, A., de, Leffkowitz, M.: Studies on electrophoretic fractions of *Vipera xanthina palestinae* venom. Amer. J. trop. Med. Hyg. **6**, 180—189 (1957)

Gitter, S., Levi, G., Kochwa, S., Vries, A., de, Rechnic, J., Casper, J.: Studies on the venom of *Echis colorata*. Amer. J. trop. Med. Hyg. **9**, 391—399 (1960)
Gitter, S., Moroz-Perlmutter, C., Boss, J. H., Livni, E., Rechnic, J., Goldblum, N., Vries, A., de: Studies on the snake venoms of the Near East: *Walterinnesia aegyptia* and *Pseudocerastes fieldii*. Amer. J. trop. Med. Hyg. **11**, 861—868 (1962)
Gitter, S., Vries, A., de: Symptomatology, pathology, and treatment of bites by Near Eastern, European, and North African snakes. In: Bücherl, W., Buckley, E., Deulofeu, V. (Eds.): Venomous Animals and Their Venoms, Vol. I, pp. 359—401. New York: Academic 1968
Gözsy, B., Kátó, L.: Changes in permeability of the skin capillaries of rats after histamine depletion with 48/80, dextran or egg white. J. Physiol. (Lond.) **139**, 1—9 (1957)
Goucher, C. R., Flowers, H. H.: The chemical modification of necrogenic and proteolytic activities of venom and the use of EDTA to produce *Agkistrodon piscivorus* venom toxoid. Toxicon **2**, 139—147 (1964)
Grotto, L., Jerushalmy, Z., Vries, A., de: Effect of purified *Vipera palestinae* hemorrhagin on blood coagulation and platelet function. Thrombos. Diathes. haemorrh. (Stuttgart) **22**, 482—495 (1969)
Grotto, L., Moroz, C., Vries, A., de, Goldblum, N.: Isolation of *Vipera palestinae* hemorrhagin and distinction between its hemorrhagic and proteolytic activities. Biochim. biophys. Acta (Amst.) **133**, 356—362 (1967)
Habermann, E.: Zur Toxikologie und Pharmakologie des Gasbrandgiftes (*Clostridium welchii* Typ A) und seiner Komponenten. Naunyn-Schmidebergs Arch. exp. Path. Pharmacol. **238**, 502—524 (1960)
Härtel, G.: In vitro studies on the anticoagulant properties of Russell's viper venom. Scand. J. clin. Lab. Invest. **15**, Suppl. 75, 1—86 (1963)
Halpern, B. N.: Inhibition of the local hemorrhagic Shwartzman reaction by a polypeptide possessing potent antiprotease activity. Proc. Soc. exp. Biol. (N.Y.) **115**, 273—276 (1964)
Heyningen, W. E., van: Toxic proteins. In: Neurath, H., Bailey, K. (Eds.): The Proteins, Vol. II, 1st ed., pp. 345—387. New York: Academic 1954
Homma, M., Tu, A. T.: Antivenin for the treatment of local tissue damage due to envenomation by Southeast Asian snakes. Ineffectiveness in the prevention of local tissue damage in mice after envenomation. Amer. J. trop. Med. Hyg. **19**, 880—884 (1970)
Houssay, B. A.: Classification des actions des venins de serpents sur l'organisme animal. C.R. Soc. Biol. Paris **105**, 308—310 (1930)
Ingram, G. I. C.: Syndrômes hémorragiques consécutifs aux morsures de serpent. Hemostase **4**, 311—320 (1964)
Ishida, Y., Yamashita, S., Ohsaka, A., Takahashi, T., Omori-Satoh, T.: Pharmacological studies of the hemorrhagic principles isolated from the venom of *Trimeresurus flavoviridis*, a crotalid. In: Ohsaka, A., Hayashi, K., Sawai, Y. (Eds.): Animal, Plant, and Microbial Toxins, Vol. II, pp. 263—272. New York: Plenum 1976
Ishii, A., Ono, T., Matuhashi, T.: Electrophoretic studies on Habu snake venom (*Trimeresurus flavoviridis*), with special reference to the changes in consecutive venom collection. Japan. J. exp. Med. **40**, 141—149 (1970)
Ishizaka, T.: Studien über das Habuschlangengift. Z. exp. Path. Ther. **4**, 88—117 (1907)
Iwanaga, S., Omori, T., Oshima, G., Suzuki, T.: Studies on snake venoms. XVI. Demonstration of a proteinase with hemorrhagic activity in the venom of *Agkistrodon halys blomhoffii*. J. Biochem. (Tokyo) **57**, 392—401 (1965)
Jiménez-Porras, J. M.: Pharmacology of peptides and proteins in snake venom. Ann. Rev. Pharmacol. **8**, 299—318 (1968)
Jiménez-Porras, J. M.: Biochemistry of snake venoms. Clin. Toxicol. **3**, 389—431 (1970)
Jori, A., Bentivoglio, A. P., Garattini, S.: The mechanism of the local inflammatory reaction induced by compound 48/80 and dextran in rats. J. Pharm. Pharmacol. **13**, 617—619 (1961)
Just, D., Urbanitz, D., Habermann, E.: Pharmakologische Charakterisierung der vasculären Schrankenfunktion gegenüber Erythrocyten und Albumin. Naunyn-Schmiedebergs Arch. Pharmakol. **267**, 399—420 (1970)
Kaiser, E. (Ed.): Animal and Plant Toxins. Munich: Goldmann 1973
Kaiser, E., Michl, H.: In: Die Biochemie der tierischen Gifte, 1st ed., pp. 134—222. Vienna: Deuticke 1958

Kameyama, S., Akama, K.: Purification and some properties of kappa toxin of *Clostridium perfringens*. Japan J. med. Sci. Biol. **24**, 9—23 (1971)
Kellaway, C. H.: Snake venoms. III. Immunity. Bull. Johns Hopkins Hosp. **60**, 159—177 (1937)
Kellaway, C. H.: Animal poisons. Ann. Rev. Biochem. **8**, 541—556 (1939)
Kihara, H.: Studies on phospholipase A in *Trimeresurus flavoviridis* venom. III. Purification and some properties of phospholipase A inhibitor in Habu serum. J. Biochem. (Tokyo) **80**, 341—349 (1976)
Klemmer, K.: Liste der rezenten Giftschlangen. *Elapidae, Hydropheidae, Viperidae* und *Crotalidae*. In: Die Giftschlangen der Erde. Wirkung und Antigenität der Gifte. Therapie von Giftschlangenbissen. Behringwerk-Mitteilungen, pp. 255—464. Marburg/Lahn: Elwert 1963
Klobusitzky, D. von: Coagulant and anticoagulant agents in snake venoms. Amer. J. med. Sci. **242**, 147—163 (1961)
Kocholaty, W. F.: Detoxification of *Crotalus atrox* venom by photooxidation in the presence of methylene blue. Toxicon **3**, 175—186 (1966)
Kocholaty, W. F., Ashley, B. D.: Detoxification of Russell's viper *(Vipera russellii)* and water moccasin *(Agkistrodon piscivorus)* venom by photooxidation. Toxicon **3**, 187—194 (1966)
Kocholaty, W. F., Ashley, B. D., Billings, T. A.: An immune serum against the North American coral snake *(Micrurus fulvius fulvius)* venom obtained by photooxidative detoxification. Toxicon **5**, 43—46 (1967)
Kocholaty, W. F., Goetz, J. C., Ashley, B. D., Billings, T. A., Ledford, E. B.: Immunogenic response of the venom fer-de-lance, *Bothrops atrox asper*, and la cascabella, *Crotalus durissus durissus* following photooxidative detoxification. Toxicon **5**, 153—158 (1968)
Kochwa, S., Perlmutter, C., Gitter, S., Rechnic, J., Vries, A., de: Studies on *Vipera palestinae* venom. Fractionation by ion exchange chromatography. Amer. J. trop. Med. Hyg. **9**, 374—380 (1960)
Kondo, H., Kondo, S., Ikezawa, H., Murata, R., Ohsaka, A.: Studies on the quantitative method for the determination of hemorrhagic activity of Habu snake venom. Japan. J. med. Sci. Biol. **13**, 43—51 (1960)
Kondo, H., Kondo, S., Sadahiro, S., Yamauchi, K., Murata, R.: Standardization of *Trimeresurus flavoviridis* (Habu) antivenin. Japan. J. med. Sci. Biol. **24**, 323—327 (1971)
Kondo, H., Kondo, S., Sadahiro, S., Yamauchi, K., Ohsaka, A., Murata, R.: Standardization of antivenine. I. A method for determination of antilethal potency of Habu antivenine. Japan. J. med. Sci. Biol. **18**, 101—110 (1965a)
Kondo, H., Kondo, S., Sadahiro, S., Yamauchi, K., Ohsaka, A., Murata, R.: Standardization of antivenine. II. A method for determination of antihemorrhagic potency of Habu antivenine in the presence of two hemorrhagic principles and their antibodies. Japan. J. med. Sci. Biol. **18**, 127—141 (1965b)
Kondo, H., Kondo, S., Sadahiro, S., Yamauchi, K., Ohsaka, A., Murata, R., Hokama, Z., Yamakawa, M.: Estimation by a new method of the amount of venom ejected by a single bite of *Trimeresurus* species. Japan. J. med. Sci. Biol. **25**, 123—131 (1972)
Kondo, H., Kondo, S., Sadahiro, S., Yamauchi, K., Ohsaka, A., Murata, R.: Preparation and immunogenicity of Habu *(Trimeresurus flavoviridis)* toxoid. In: Vries, A., de, Kochva, E. (Eds.): Toxins of Animal and Plant Origin, Vol. III, pp. 845—862. London: Gordon and Breach 1973
Kondo, H., Sadahiro, S., Kondo, S., Yamauchi, K., Honjo, S., Cho, F., Ohsaka, A., Murata, R.: Immunogenicity in monkeys of a combined toxoid from the main toxic principles separated from Habu snake venom. Japan. J. med. Sci. Biol. **23**, 413—418 (1970)
Kondo, S., Sadahiro, S., Murata, R.: Relationship between the amount of Habu toxoid injected into the monkey and the resulting antitoxin titer in the circulation. In: Ohsaka, A., Hayashi, K., Sawai, Y. (Eds.): Animal, Plant, and Microbial Toxins, Vol. II, pp. 431—438. New York: Plenum 1976
Kurashige, S., Hara, Y., Kawakami, M., Mitsuhashi, S.: Studies on Habu snake venom. VII. Heat-stable myolytic factor and development of its activity by addition of phospholipase A. Japan. J. Microbiol. **10**, 23—31 (1966)
Kuwajima, Y.: Studies on immunization with snake venoms (I) [in Japanese]. Jikken Igaku Zasshi (J. exp. Med.) **22**, 1170—1190 (1938)

Lai, M. K., Wen, C. Y., Lee, C. Y.: Local lesions caused by cardiotoxin isolated from Formosan cobra venom. J. Formosan med. Ass. **71**, 328—332 (1972)

Lancker, J. L., van: In: Molecular and Cellular Mechanisms in Diseases, Vol. 2, pp. 607—1116. Berlin-Heidelberg-New York: Springer 1976

Lee, C. Y.: Chemistry and pharmacology of polypeptide toxins in snake venoms. Ann. Rev. Pharmacol. **12**, 265—286 (1972)

Lee, C. Y., Chang, C. C.: Modes of actions of purified toxins from elapid venoms on neuromuscular transmission. Mem. Inst. Butantan, Simp. Internac. **33**, 555—572 (1966)

Lee, C. Y., Chang, C. C., Chiu, T. H., Chiu, P. J. S., Tseng, T. C., Lee, S. Y.: Pharmacological properties of cardiotoxin isolated from Formosan cobra venom. Naunyn-Schmiedebergs Arch. Pharmakol. exp. Pathol. **259**, 360—374 (1968)

Lieske, H.: Symptomatik und Therapie von Giftschlangenbissen. In: Die Giftschlangen der Erde. Wirkungen und Antigenität der Gifte. Therapie von Giftschlangenbissen. Behringwerk-Mitteilungen, pp. 121—160. Marburg/Lahn: Elwert 1963

MacFarlane, R. G.: Russell's viper venom, 1934—64. Brit. J. Haematol. **13**, 437—451 (1967)

Maeno, H.: Biochemical analysis of pathological lesions caused by Habu snake venom with special reference to hemorrhage. J. Biochem. (Tokyo) **52**, 343—350 (1962)

Maeno, H., Mitsuhashi, S.: Studies of Hβ-proteinase of Habu snake venom, with special reference to substrate specificity and inhibitory effect of serum. J. Biochem. (Tokyo) **50**, 330—336 (1961)

Maeno, H., Mitsuhashi, S., Sato, R.: Studies on Habu snake venom. 2c. Studies on Hβ-proteinase of Habu venom. Japan. J. Microbiol. **4**, 173—180 (1960)

Maeno, H., Mitsuhashi, S., Okonogi, T., Hoshi, S., Homma, M.: Studies on Habu snake venom. V. Myolysis caused by phospholipase A in Habu snake venom. Japan. J. exp. Med. **32**, 55—64 (1962)

Maeno, H., Mitsuhashi, S., Sawai, Y., Okonogi, T.: Studies on Habu snake venom. 2a. Enzymic studies on the proteinase of Habu snake venom. Japan. J. Microbiol. **3**, 131—138 (1959a)

Maeno, H., Morimura, M., Mitsuhashi, S., Sawai, Y., Okonogi, T.: Studies on Habu snake venom. 2b. Further purification and enzymic and biological activities of Hα-proteinase. Japan. J. Microbiol. **3**, 277—284 (1959b)

Mandelbaum, F. R., Reichl, A. P., Assakura, M. T.: Some physical and biochemical characteristics of HF_2, one of the hemorrhagic factors in the venom of *Bothrops jararaca*. In: Ohsaka, A., Hayashi, K., Sawai, Y. (Eds.): Animal, Plant, and Microbial Toxins, Vol. I, pp. 111—121. New York: Plenum 1976

Marsten, J. L., Kok-Ewe, C., Ankeney, J. L., Botti, R. E.: Antithrombotic effect of Malayan pit viper venom on experimental thrombosis of the inferior vena cava produced by a new method. Circulat. Res. **19**, 514—519 (1966)

McCollough, N. C., Gennaro, J. F., Jr.: Coral snake bites in the United States. J. Florida med. Ass. **49**, 968—972 (1963)

McCollough, N. C., Gennaro, J. G.: The diagnosis, symptoms, treatment and sequelae of envenomation by *Crotalus adamanteus* and genus *Agkistrodon*. Mem. Inst. Butantan, Simp. Internac. **33**, 175—178 (1966)

McKay, D. G., Moroz, C., Vries, A., de, Csavossy, I., Cruse, V.: The action of hemorrhagin and phospholipase derived from *Vipera palestinae* venom on the microcirculation. Lab. Invest. **22**, 387—399 (1970)

Meaume, J.: Les venins de serpents agents modificateurs de la coagulation sanguine. Toxicon **4**, 25—58 (1966)

Meldrum, B. S.: The actions of snake venoms on nerve and muscle. The pharmacology of phospholipase A and of polypeptide toxins. Pharmacol. Rev. **17**, 393—445 (1965)

Minton, S. A., Jr.: Some properties of North American pit viper venoms and their correlation with phylogeny. In: Buckley, E. E., Porges, N. (Eds.): Venoms, pp. 145—151. Washington, D.C.: American Association for the Advancement of Science 1956

Mitchell, S. W.: Researches upon the Venom of the Rattlesnake. Washington, D.C.: Smithsonian Institution 1860

Mitchell, S. W., Reichert, E. T.: Researches upon the Venoms of Poisonous Serpents. Washington, D. C.: Smithsonian Institution 1886

Mitsuhashi,S., Maeno,H., Kawakami,M., Hashimoto,H., Sawai,Y., Miyazaki,S., Makino,M., Kobayashi,M., Okonogi,T., Yamaguchi,K.: Studies on Habu snake venom. I. Comparison of several biological activities of fresh and dried Habu snake venom. Japan. J. Microbiol. **3**, 95—103 (1959)

Mittelstaedt,J.S., Shaw,S.M., Tiffany,L.W.: The detoxifying effect of cobalt-60 radiation on the venom of the hooded cobra, *Naja naja*. In: Vries,A.,de, Kochva,E. (Eds.): Toxins of Animal and Plant Origin, Vol. III, pp. 889—896. London: Gordon and Breach 1973

Moroz,C., Hahn,J., Vries,A.de: Neutralization of *Vipera palestinae* hemorrhagin by antibody fragments. Toxicon **9**, 57—62 (1971)

Moroz-Perlmutter,C., Goldblum,N., Vries,A.,de, Gitter,S.: Detoxification of snake venoms and venom fractions by formaldehyde. Proc. Soc. exp. Biol. (N.Y.) **112**, 595—598 (1963)

Noguchi,H.: Snake venoms. An investigation of Venomous Snakes with Special Reference to the Phenomena of Their Venoms. Washington, D.C.: Carnegie Institution of Washington 1909

Oakley,C.L., Warrack,G.H., Warren,M.E.: The kappa and lambda antigens of *Clostridium welchii*. J. Path. Bact. **60**, 495—503 (1948)

Ohsaka,A.: Fractionation of Habu snake venom by chromatography on CM-cellulose with special reference to biological activities. Japan. J. med. Sci. Biol. **13**, 199—205 (1960a)

Ohsaka,A.: Proteolytic activities of Habu snake venom and their separation from lethal toxicity. Japan. J. med. Sci. Biol. **13**, 33—41 (1960b)

Ohsaka,A.: Hemorrhagic principles and hemolysins of bacterial and animal origin — their chemical nature and biological functions [in Japanese]. Protein, Nucleic Acid, Enzyme **13**, 1007—1025 (1968)

Ohsaka,A.: An approach to the mechanism of hemorrhage: Hemorrhagic principles isolated from snake venom as a useful analytical tool [in Japanese]. Seitainokagaku (Life Science) **24**, 266—293 (1973)

Ohsaka,A.: An approach to the physiological mechanisms involved in hemorrhage: Snake venom hemorrhagic principles as a useful analytical tool. In: Ohsaka,A., Hayashi,K., Sawai,Y. (Eds.): Animal, Plant, and Microbial Toxins, Vol. I, pp. 123—136. New York: Plenum 1976a

Ohsaka,A.: Biochemical aspect of increased vascular permeability for proteins and erythrocytes with special reference to the mechanism of hemorrhage [in Japanese]. J. Japan. biochem. Soc. **48**, 308—331 (1976b)

Ohsaka,A., Hayashi,K., Sawai,Y. (Eds.): Animal, Plant, and Microbial Toxins (2 Vols.). New York: Plenum 1976

Ohsaka,A., Ikezawa,H., Kondo,H., Kondo,S.: Two hemorrhagic principles derived from Habu snake venom and their difference in zone electrophoretical mobility. Japan. J. med. Sci. Biol. **13**, 73—76 (1960b)

Ohsaka,A., Ikezawa,H., Kondo,H., Kondo,S., Uchida,N.: Haemorrhagic activities of Habu snake venom, and their relations to lethal toxicity, proteolytic activities and other pathological activities. Brit. J. exp. Path. **41**, 478—486 (1960a)

Ohsaka,A., Just,M., Habermann,E.: Action of snake venom hemorrhagic principles on isolated glomerular basement membrane. Biochim. biophys. Acta (Amst.) **323**, 415—438 (1973a)

Ohsaka,A., Just,M., Habermann,E.: Action of snake venom hemorrhagic principles on isolated glomerular basement membrane. In: Kaiser,E. (Ed.): Animal and Plant Toxins, pp. 93—97. Munich: Goldmann 1973b

Ohsaka,A., Kondo,H.: Biochemistry of snake venoms. In: Recent Advances in Medical Science and Biology, Vol. I, pp. 269—322 [in Japanese]. Tokyo: Igaku Seibutsugaku Kenkyu Shórei-kai 1960

Ohsaka,A., Kondo,H., Kondo,S., Kurokawa,M., Murata,R.: Problems in determination of antihemorrhagic potency of Habu (*Trimeresurus flavoviridis*) antivenine in the presence of multiple hemorrhagic principles and their antibodies. Mem. Inst. Butantan, Simp. Internac. **33**, 331—337 (1966b)

Ohsaka,A., Ohashi,M., Tsuchiya,M., Kamisaka,Y., Fujishiro,Y.: Action of *Trimeresurus flavoviridis* venom on the microcirculatory system of rat; dynamic aspects as revealed by cinephotomicrographic recording. Japan. J. med. Sci. Biol. **24**, 34—39 (1971b)

Ohsaka, A., Omori-Satoh, T., Kondo, H., Kondo, S., Murata, R.: Biochemical and pathological aspects of hemorrhagic principles in snake venoms with special reference to Habu (*Trimeresurus flavoviridis*) venom. Mem. Inst. Butantan, Simp. Internac. **33**, 193—205 (1966a)
Ohsaka, A., Suzuki, K., Ohashi, M.: The spurting of erythrocytes through junctions of the vascular endothelium treated with snake venom. Microvasc. Res. **10**, 208—213 (1975)
Ohsaka, A., Takahashi, T., Omori-Satoh, T., Murata, R.: Purification and characterization of the hemorrhagic principles in the venom of *Trimeresurus flavoviridis*. In: Vries, A., de, Kochva, E. (Eds.): Toxins of Animal and Plant Origin, Vol. I, pp. 369—399. London: Gordon and Breach 1971a
Okonogi, T., Hattori, Z.: Attenuation of Habu-snake (*Trimeresurus flavoviridis*) venom by treatment with alcohol and its effect as immunizing antigen [in Japanese]. Nihon Saikingaku Zasshi (Japan. J. Bacteriol.) **23**, 137—144 (1968)
Omori, T., Iwanaga, S., Suzuki, T.: The relationship between the hemorrhagic and lethal activities of Japanese Mamushi (*Agkistrodon halys blomhoffii*) venom. Toxicon **2**, 1—4 (1964)
Omori-Satoh, T., Ohsaka, A.: Purification and some properties of hemorrhagic principle 1 in the venom of *Trimeresurus flavoviridis*. Biochim. biophys. Acta (Amst.) **207**, 432—444 (1970)
Omori-Satoh, T., Ohsaka, A., Kondo, S., Kondo, H.: A simple and rapid method for separating two hemorrhagic principles in the venom of *Trimeresurus flavoviridis*. Toxicon **5**, 17—24 (1967)
Omori-Satoh, T., Sadahiro, S., Ohsaka, A., Murata, R.: Purification and characterization of an antihemorrhagic factor in the serum of *Trimeresurus flavoviridis*, a crotalid. Biochim. biophys. Acta (Amst.) **285**, 414—426 (1972)
Oshima, G., Iwanaga, S., Suzuki, T.: Studies on snake venoms. XVIII. An improved method for purification of the proteinase b from the venom of *Agkistrodon halys blomhoffii* and its physicochemical properties. J. Biochem. (Tokyo) **64**, 215—225 (1968)
Oshima, G., Iwanaga, S., Suzuki, T.: Some properties of proteinase b in the venom of *Agkistrodon halys blomhoffii*. Biochim. biophys. Acta (Amst.) **250**, 416—427 (1971)
Oshima, G., Omori-Satoh, T., Iwanaga, S., Suzuki, T.: Studies on snake venom hemorrhagic factor I (HR-I) in the venom of *Agkistrodon halys blomhoffii*. Its purification and biological properties. J. Biochem. (Tokyo) **72**, 1483—1494 (1972)
Ouchterlony, Ö.: In vitro method for testing the toxin-producing capacity of diphtheria bacteria. Acta pathol. microbiol. scand. **25**, 186—191 (1948)
Ovadia, M., Moav, B., Kochva, E.: Factors in the blood serum of *Vipera palestinae* neutralizing toxic fractions of its venom. In: Ohsaka, A., Hayashi, K., Sawai, Y. (Eds.): Animal, Plant, and Microbial Toxins, Vol. I, pp. 137—142. New York: Plenum 1976
Ownby, C. L., Cameron, D., Tu, A. T.: Isolation of myotoxic component from rattlesnake (*Crotalus viridis viridis*) venom. Electron microscopic analysis of muscle damage. Amer. J. Pathol. **85**, 149—166 (1976)
Park, J. H., Meriwether, B. P., Clodfelder, P., Cunningham, L. W.: The hydrolysis of p-nitrophenyl acetate catalyzed by 3-phosphoglyceraldehyde dehydrogenase. J. biol. Chem. **236**, 136—141 (1961)
Parratt, J. R., West, G. B.: 5-Hydroxytryptamine and the anaphylactoid reaction in the rat. J. Physiol. (Lond.) **139**, 27—41 (1957)
Peterson, H., Kõivastik, T.: Von der Toxität des Kreuzottern-(*Vipera berus berus*)-Serums und seinen antitoxischen Eigenschaften bezüglich homologer und heterologer Schlangengifte. Z. Immun.-Forsch. **102**, 324—331 (1943)
Phillips, G. B., Bachner, P., McKay, D. G.: Tissue effects of lysolecithin injected subcutaneously in mice. Proc. exp. Biol. (N.Y.) **119**, 846—850 (1965)
Philpot, V. B., Jr., Deutsch, H. F.: Inhibition and activation of venom proteases. Biochim. biophys. Acta (Amst.) **21**, 524—530 (1956)
Philpot, V. B., Smith, R. G.: Neutralization of pit viper venom by king snake serum. Proc. Soc. exp. Biol. (N.Y.) **74**, 521—523 (1950)
Plagnol, H., Vialard-Goudou, A.: Électrophorèse sur papier du sérum de différents serpents. Ann. Inst. Pasteur **90**, 276—281 (1956)
Poller, L. (Ed.): Recent Advances in Blood Coagulation. London: Churchill 1969
Porath, J., Bennich, H.: Recycling chromatography. Arch. Biochem. Biophys. Suppl. **1**, 152—156 (1962)

Porges, N.: Snake venoms, their biochemistry and mode of action. Science **117**, 47—51 (1953)

Ramon, G.: Des anatoxines. C.R. Acad. Sci. **178**, 1436—1439 (1924)

Rašková, H. (Ed.): Pharmacology of Naturally Occurring Toxins, Vol. 1. Oxford: Pergamon 1971

Rechnic, J., Trachtenberg, P., Casper, J., Moroz, C., Vries, A., de: Afibrinogenemia and thrombocytopenia in guinea pigs following injection of *Echis colorata* venom. Blood **20**, 735—749 (1962)

Rechnic, J., Vries, A., de, Perlmutter, C., Levi, G., Kochwa, S., Gitter, S.: Coagulation factors in the venoms of *Vipera palestinae* and *Echis colorata*. Bull. Res. Council Israel **8 E**, 81—86 (1960)

Reid, H. A.: Cobra-bites. Brit. med. J. **1964 II**, 540—545

Reid, H. A.: Defibrination by *Agkistrodon rhodostoma* venom. In: Russell, F. E., Saunders, P. R. (Eds.): Animal Toxins, pp. 323—335. Oxford: Pergamon 1967

Reid, H. A.: Symptomatology, pathology, and treatment of land snake bite in India and Southeast Asia. In: Bücherl, W., Buckley, E., Deulofeu, V. (Eds.): Venomous Animals and Their Venoms, Vol. I, pp. 611—642. New York: Academic 1968

Reid, H. A., Thean, P. C., Martin, W. J.: Specific antivenine and predonisone in viper-bite poisoning; controlled trial. Brit. med. J. **1963 II**, 1378—1380

Rocha e Silva, M., Beraldo, W. T., Rosenfeld, G.: Bradykinin, a hypotensive and smooth muscle stimulating factor released from plasma globulin by snake venoms and by trypsin. Amer. J. Physiol. **156**, 261—273 (1949)

Rosenfeld, G.: Unfälle durch Giftschlangen. In: Die Giftschlangen der Erde. Wirkung und Antigenität der Gifte. Therapie von Giftschlangenbissen. Behringwerk-Mitteilungen, pp. 161—202. Marburg/Lahn: Elwert 1963

Rosenfeld, G.: Fibrinolysis by snake venoms. Sangre (Barcelona), **9**, 352—354 (1964)

Rosenfeld, G.: Symptomatology, pathology, and treatment of snake bites in South America. In: Bücherl, W., Buckley, E., Deulofeu, V. (Eds.): Venomous Animals and Their Venoms, Vol. II, pp. 345—384. New York: Academic 1971

Rosenfeld, S., Glass, S.: The inhibiting effect of snake bloods upon the hemorrhagic action of viper venoms on mice. Amer. J. med. Sci. **199**, 482—486 (1940)

Rowley, D. A., Benditt, E. P.: 5-Hydroxytryptamine and histamine as mediators of the vascular injury produced by agents which damage mast cells in rats. J. exp. Med. **103**, 399—412 (1956)

Russell, F. E.: Rattlesnake bites in Southern California. Amer. J. med. Sci. **239**, 51—60 (1960)

Sadahiro, S., Kondo, S., Kondo, H., Ohsaka, A., Fukushima, H., Murata, R.: Standardization of Habu (*Trimeresurus flavoviridis*) snake-venom toxoid. Toxicon **16**, 275—282 (1978)

Sagara, Y.: Studies on the effect of *Trimeresurus* venom on peripheral vessels [in Japanese]. J. Kagoshima Medical School **12**, 1064—1077 (1960)

Sarkar, N. K., Devi, A.: Enzymes in snake venoms. In: Bücherl, W., Buckley, E., Deulofeu, V. (Eds.): Venomous Animals and Their Venoms, Vol. I, pp. 167—216. New York: Academic 1968

Sato, T., Iwanaga, S., Mizushima, Y., Suzuki, T.: Studies on snake venoms. XV. Separation of arginine ester hydrolase of *Agkistrodon halys blomhoffii* venom into three enzymatic entities: "Bradykinin releasing", "clotting", and "permeability increasing". J. Biochem. (Tokyo) **57**, 380—391 (1965)

Sawai, Y., Kawamura, Y.: Study on the toxoids against the venoms of certain Asian snakes. Toxicon **7**, 19—24 (1969)

Sawai, Y., Makino, M., Tateno, I., Okonogi, T., Mitsuhashi, S.: Studies on the improvement of treatment of Habu snake (*Trimeresurus flavoviridis*) bite. 3. Clinical analysis and medical treatment of Habu snake bite on the Amami Islands. Japan. J. exp. Med. **32**, 117—138 (1962)

Seifter, S., Harper, E.: The collagenases. In: Boyer, P. D. (Ed.): The Enzymes, Vol. III, 3rd Ed., pp. 649—697. London: Academic 1971

Slotta, K. H.: Chemistry and biochemistry of snake venoms. Progress in Chemistry of Organic Natural Products **12**, 406—465 (1955)

Somani, P.: Changes in permeability of the skin capillaries of rats by *Echis carinatus* (saw-scaled viper) venom, and its modification by promethazine, LSD_{25} and reserpine pretreatment. Int. Arch. Allergy **21**, 186—192 (1962)

Somani, P., Arora, R. B.: Effect of hydrocortisone on capillary permeability changes induced by *Echis carinatus* (saw-scaled viper) venom in the rat. J. Pharm. Pharmacol. **14**, 535—537 (1962)

Someya, S., Murata, R., Sawai, Y., Kondo, H., Ishii, A.: Active immunization of man with toxoid of Habu (*Trimeresurus flavoviridis*) venom. Japan. J. med. Sci. Biol. **25**, 47—51 (1972)

Spector, W.G.: Substances which affect capillary permeability. Pharmacol. Rev. **10**, 473—505 (1958)

Stahnke, H.L.: The Treatment of Venomous Bites and Stings. Tempe: Arizona State University 1966

Suzuki, T.: Pharmacologically and biochemically active components of Japanese ophidian venoms. Mem. Inst. Butantan, Simp. Internac. **33**, 519—521 (1966a)

Suzuki, T.: Separation methods of animal venoms constituents. Mem. Inst. Butantan, Simp. Internac. **33**, 389—409 (1966b)

Suzuki, T., Tamiya, N., Funatsu, M., Murata, R., Ohsaka, A., Ohashi, M. (Eds.): Protein Toxins, Vol. 2. Tokyo: Kōdansha Scientific 1971

Swaroop, S., Grab, B.: Snakebite mortality in the world. Bull. Wld. Hlth. Org. **10**, 35—76 (1954)

Swaroop, S., Grab, B.: The snakebite mortality problem in the world. In: Buckley, E.E., Porges, N. (Eds.): Venoms, 1st Ed., pp. 439—446. Washington: American Association for the Advancement of Science 1956

Táborská, E.: Intraspecies variability of the venom of *Echis carinatus*. Physiol. Bohemoslov. **20**, 307—318 (1971)

Takagi, K., Takayanagi, I., Irikura, T., Nishino, K., Ito, M., Ohkubo, H., Ichinoseki, N.: A potent competitive inhibitor of 5-hydroxytryptamine: 3-(2'-benzylaminoethyl)-5-methoxyindol hydrochloride. Japan. J. Pharmacol. **19**, 234—239 (1969)

Takahashi, T., Ohsaka, A.: Purification and characterization of a proteinase in the venom of *Trimeresurus flavoviridis*. Complete separation of the enzyme from hemorrhagic activity. Biochim. biophys. Acta (Amst.) **198**, 293—307 (1970a)

Takahashi, T., Ohsaka, A.: Purification and some properties of two hemorrhagic principles (HR2a and HR2b) in the venom of *Trimeresurus flavoviridis*; complete separation of the principles from proteolytic activity. Biochim. biophys. Acta (Amst.) **207**, 65—75 (1970b)

Taube, H.N., Essex, H.E.: Pathologic changes in the tissues of the dog following injections of rattlesnake venom. Arch. Path. **24**, 43—51 (1937)

Thomas, L.: Possible role of leucocyte granules in the Shwartzman and Arthus reactions. Proc. Soc. exp. Biol. (N.Y.) **115**, 235—240 (1964)

Toom, P.M., Squire, P.G., Tu, A.T.: Characterization of the enzymatic and biological activities of snake venoms by isoelectric focusing. Biochim. biophys. Acta (Amst.) **181**, 339—341 (1969)

Tsuchiya, M., Ohshio, C., Ohashi, M., Ohsaka, A., Suzuki, K., Fujishiro, Y.: Cinematographic and electron microscopic analyses of the hemorrhage induced by the main hemorrhagic principle, HR 1, isolated from the venom of *Trimeresurus flavoviridis*. In: Didisheim, P., Shimamoto, T., Yamazaki, H. (Eds.): Platelets, Thrombosis, Inhibitors, pp. 439—446. Stuttgart: Schattauer 1974

Tu, A.T., Homma, M., Hong, B.-S.: Hemorrhagic, myonecrotic, thrombotic, and proteolytic activities of viper venoms. Toxicon **6**, 175—178 (1969)

Tu, A.T., Passey, R.B.: Phospholipase A from sea snake venom and its biological properties. In: Vries, A., de, Kochva, E. (Eds.): Toxins of Animal and Plant Origin, Vol. I, pp. 419—436. London: Gordon and Breach 1971

Tu, A.T., Toom, P.M., Ganthavorn, S.: Hemorrhagic and proteolytic activities of Thailand snake venoms. Biochem. Pharmacol. **16**, 2125—2130 (1967)

Vesterberg, O., Svensson, H.: Isoelectric fractionation, analysis, and characterization of ampholytes in natural pH gradients. IV. Further studies on the resolving power in connection with separation of myoglobins. Acta chem. scand. **20**, 820—834 (1966)

Vick, J.A., Blanchard, R.J., Perry, J.F., Jr.: Effects of epsilon amino caproic acid on pulmonary vascular changes produced by snake venom. Proc. exp. Biol. (N.Y.) **113**, 841—844 (1963)

Vries, A., de, Cohen, I.: Hemorrhagic and blood coagulation disturbing action of snake venoms. In: Poller, L. (Ed.): Recent Advances in Blood Coagulation, pp. 277—297. London: Churchill 1969

Vries, A., de, Condrea, E., Klibansky, C., Rechnic, J., Moroz, C., Kirschmann, C.: Hematological effects of the venoms of two Near Eastern snakes: *Vipera palestinae* and *Echis colorata*. New Istanbul Contrib. clin. Sci. **5**, 151—169 (1962)

Vries, A., de, Kochva, E. (Eds.): Toxins of Animal and Plant Origin (3 Vols.). London: Gordon and Breach 1971—1973

Watt, C. H., Jr., Gennaro, J. F., Jr.: Pit viper bites in south Georgia and north Florida. Trans. Southern Surg. Ass. **77**, 378—386 (1966)

West, G. B.: Chemical nature and possible role of mediators in allergic reactions. Int. Arch. Allergy **18**, 56—61 (1961)

Wiener, S.: Active immunization of man against the venom of the Australian tiger snake *(Notechis scutatus)*. Amer. J. trop. Med. Hyg. **9**, 284—292 (1960)

Yamakawa, M., Nozaki, M., Hokama, Z.: Fractionation of Sakishima-habu *(Trimeresurus elegans)* venom and lethal, hemorrhagic, and edema-forming activities of the fractions. In: Ohsaka, A., Hayashi, K., Sawai, Y. (Eds.): Animal, Plant, and Microbial Toxins, Vol. I, pp. 97—109. New York: Plenum 1976

Yamanaka, M., Matsuda, M., Isobe, J., Ohsaka, A., Takahashi, T., Omori-Satoh, T.: Effect of purified hemorrhagic principles from Habu snake venom on platelet aggregation. In: Didisheim, P., Shimamoto, T., Yamazaki, H. (Eds.): Platelets, Thrombosis, and Inhibitors, pp. 335—344. Stuttgart: Schattauer 1974

Yaoi, H., Kawashima, S.: Effective immunization with anatoxins from bacterial toxins and snake venoms [in Japanese]. Nihon Densenbyo Gakkai Zasshi (Japan. J. infect. Dis.) **2**, 1141—1151 (1928)

Yoshikura, H., Ogawa, H., Ohsaka, A., Omori-Satoh, T.: Action of *Trimeresurus flavoviridis* venom and the partially purified hemorrhagic principles on animal cells cultivated in vitro. Toxicon **4**, 183—190 (1966)

Yphantis, D. A.: Rapid determination of molecular weights of peptides and proteins. Ann. N.Y. Acad. Sci. **88**, 586—601 (1960)

Zeller, E. A.: Enzymes of snake venoms and their biological significance. Advanc. Enzymol. **8**, 459—495 (1948)

Zeller, E. A.: Enzymes as essential components of toxins. In: Sumner, J. B., Myrbäck, K. (Eds.): The Enyzmes, Vol. I, Part 2, pp. 986—1013. New York: Academic 1951

Zeller, E. A.: Enzymes of snake venoms as tools in biochemical research. Mem. Inst. Butantan, Simp. Internac. **33**, 349—357 (1966)

CHAPTER 15

Cardiovascular Effects of Snake Venoms

C. Y. LEE and S. Y. LEE

Introduction

Snake venoms have a variety of deleterious effects on almost every organ system. In most cases of snake venom poisoning, circulatory disturbance is one of the most frequently encountered events. Since a single snake venom contains a variety of enzymes as well as nonenzymatic components of different biologic activities, it is not difficult to appreciate the complexity of cardiovascular changes produced by different snake venoms.

Some attempts have been made to define the relationships between the direct effects of snake venoms on the cardiovascular system and those which may be caused by autopharmacological substances liberated from the tissues by the venom. During recent years, attempts have also been made to determine which component or components of snake venoms are responsible for these effects. In the course of these investigations, many important data, which indicated the complexity of the vascular response, have been obtained. This review was undertaken to provide a survey of the literature on the circulatory effects produced by snake venoms and their components.

Cardiovascular Effects of Crotalid and Viperid Venoms

Crotalid venoms are characterized by the richest source of overall enzymatic activities among snake venoms: proteolytic enzyme activity in crotalid venoms has been shown to be the most potent among snake venoms so far examined. The viperid venoms have lesser amounts of proteinases, while the elapid and sea snake venoms either have very little or no proteolytic enzyme activity (KOCHOLATY et al., 1971). Venoms that are rich in proteinases produce marked tissue destruction and also deleterious effects on the cardiovascular system. However, what role the proteinases play in these deleterious effects is still not fully understood. The autopharmacologic substances released by snake venom enzymes could contribute towards the circulatory shock produced by crotalid and viperid venoms. These substances include bradykinin, histamine, 5-hydroxytryptamine, and prostaglandins (see Chap. 16). Again, to what extent each of these substances may be responsible for the cardiovascular changes produced by different venoms is still an unsolved problem. In addition, some of viperid and crotalid venoms contain coagulant or procoagulant enzymes (see Chap. 18), which may produce intravascular clotting and thus contribute to the cardiovascular changes, even leading to sudden death. Apart from such enzyme activities, the crotalid and viperid venoms may contain some toxic principles which affect the cardiovascular system either directly or through central regulatory mechanisms.

A. Hemodynamic Effects of Crotalid Venoms

I. Rattlesnake (Crotalus) Venoms

1. C. horridus (Timber Rattlesnake) and C. atrox (Western Diamondback Rattlesnake) Venoms

The most conspicuous hemodynamic effect produced by rattlesnake venoms in general is an immediate and profound fall in systemic blood pressure. Intravenous injection of "crotalin" (*C. horridus* or *C. atrox* venom) in dogs produced a precipitous fall in arterial blood pressure after a latent period of 15–30 s (ESSEX and MARKOWITZ, 1930a). The level to which it fell was roughly proportional to the amount of venom given. A dose of 0.07 ml of 2% crotalin caused a decided fall, but such small doses were followed by spontaneous recovery. Larger doses caused a fall to low levels, with little tendency toward recovery, and eventually the animal died. A certain degree of tachyphylaxis was observed following the first injection. After an initial fall to a low level, subsequent larger doses either failed to produce any immediate response or produced only a slight fall in the blood pressure. Histamine (1–2 mg) also failed to produce any depressor action after the crotalin had taken effect. The condition of desensitization was temporary, so that after 24 h the same dose of venom produced practically the same fall in blood pressure.

The condition of crotalin shock was analogous to that of surgical shock in the response of blood pressure to intravenous administration of fluid (e.g., a 5% solution of gum acacia or a 7% solution of gelatine). Subcutaneous injection of crotalin produced the characteristic hypotension seen with intravenous doses, but larger doses were needed and the effect was delayed.

Following intravenous injection of crotalin, there was invariably a slight rise in pulmonary pressure, followed by a fall which was probably dependent on a deficient return flow of blood to the right side of the heart. Lymph flow from the thoracic duct rose approximately twofold immediately following administration of crotalin; it returned to control values within a few minutes. Using plethysmography, an increase in volume in the hind leg, accompanying the depressor action of crotalin, was invariably observed. However, the spleen, kidney, liver, and intestine first decreased in volume, and then, within a variable length of time, the splanchnic viscera all increased profoundly in volume. ESSEX and MARKOWITZ (1930c) also noted a consistent rise in hematocrit after injection of crotalin, as well as a marked increase in the volume of the erythrocytes. They demonstrated that the rise in hematocrit was due to the swelling of the red blood cells, but not to the loss of plasma from the circulation. Hemolysis from rattlesnake venom was concluded to be due to the expansion of the erythrocytes, with accompanying injury to their membrane.

BALDES et al. (1931) observed a marked increase in viscosity in blood removed from dogs immediately after injections of crotalin and also in blood in which the venom was added in vitro, contrary to their expectation. Under normal conditions, such marked increase in the viscosity of the blood should raise the peripheral resistance, thus causing an increase in blood pressure. Viscosity increased until hemolysis occurred, after which it decreased. They attributed the increased viscosity of blood to the swelling of the erythrocytes.

In order to simulate the slow continuous absorption of subcutaneously deposited venom, effects of slow intravenous infusions of *Crotalus* venoms have been studied (WITHAM et al., 1953; HALMAGYI et al., 1965; WHIGHAM et al., 1973; CARLSON et al., 1975). Very shortly after the infusion with *C. horridus* venom in dogs, the arterial pressure fell sharply and the heart rate accelerated (WITHAM et al., 1953). Since the arterial pressure fall was accompanied by an increase in cardiac output, the calculated resistance was decreased. These changes were the expected result for a potent vasodilator, and it was presumed that the venom acted directly upon the arterioles. Oxygen consumption was increased. Usually the right atrial pressure was reduced. If the infusion was interrupted at any point in the initial phase, the blood pressure and heart rate returned slowly to preinjection levels. If it was continued, the arterial pressure and cardiac output fell slowly. When the dosage level reached 0.3–0.7 mg/kg, a new set of signs appeared and an irreversible stage was reached; respiratory movements became jerky, intercostal participation failed, and salivation and some vomiting occurred. Intestinal activity was increased, sometimes with defecation. Urination occurred and petechial hemorrhages appeared at the margins of the gums and eyelids. Recovery never occurred once these signs appeared. An increase in hematocrit was observed in the initial stage: the hemoconcentration reached its maximum in about 10 min, and usually showed little further change. However, when the spleen was removed prior to venom administration, hemoconcentration was not seen, suggesting that splenic contraction might be responsible for the increase in cell/blood ratio. In vivo hemolysis was sometimes present, but not to a large degree. At the time of the secondary phase, blood samples would no longer clot. At autopsy, petechial hemorrhages were present on serosal or mucosal membranes, particularly in the omentum, the mesenteries, and the heart. Visceral congestion, especially engorgement of the mucosa of the lower intestine, was evident. Blood volume determination disclosed that a total loss of about 20 ml/kg of blood volume occurred by the time of death. It was concluded that the venom had a potent vasodilator action and that myocardial weakness, oligemia, and biochemical changes in the blood also contributed in variable amounts to the total collapse (WITHAM et al., 1953).

RUSSELL et al. (1961, 1962) studied the effects of *C. atrox* venom in cats and other animals. The most rapid and severe fall in arterial pressure appears to occur in the cat; it is slightly less pronounced in the rabbit, sometimes delayed in the dog, and least severe in the monkey. The change of heart rate in cats was variable; in 10 out of 15 cats injected with 0.75 mg/kg, heart rate decreased. In most cats the electrocardiograms were essentially normal until after the initial hypotensive response. An increase in pulmonary artery pressure, accompanied by a decrease in pressure and flow from the left heart, was observed in almost all preparations. In the isolated lung preparation, an accumulation of fluid was evident within 40 s. Portal vein pressure remained unchanged initially, but then increased, and an increase in hematocrit was also observed. Cisternal cerebrospinal fluid pressure increased initially and then fell slowly. Apnea often occurred for periods of 5–30 s, followed by an increased respiratory rate.

Cardiovascular effects of *C. atrox* venom were also studied by slow infusion in sheep (HALMAGYI et al., 1965). The venom (60–600 μg/kg) infusion was titrated to maintain a systemic arterial pressure of about 40 mm Hg. This "stop-and-go" procedure was repeated several times until the arterial pressure was stable and would not spontaneously recover for 4–6 h. The shocked animals demonstrated a significant fall in cardiac output, systemic vascular resistance, and total serum proteins, and a rise in hemoglobin content. Abnormal electrocardiograms were rarely seen and usually consisted only of low voltage. Right atrial pressure, plasma sodium and potassium concentrations remained normal. The changes were compatible with the assumption that plasma loss, secondary to venom-induced increase in capillary permeability, initiated circulatory failure. Occasional onset of pulmonary hypertension was not related to direct pulmonary vascular effects of the venom, but rather to the production of thromboembolism in the pulmonary vascular bed. *Crotalus* venom frequently produced initial and transient hypercoagulability of the blood. In contrast to hyperventilation characteristic of other types of shock, alveolar hypoventilation was observed in most animals, except those with superimposed lung embolism. Continuous intravenous infusion of isoproterenol improved alveolar ventilation and restored spontaneous breathing in some cases of crotalin-induced respiratory arrest. Administration of antivenin in the shocked animals proved to be ineffective. Dextran infusion restored cardiac output, but accentuated respiratory depression. Death occurred during the shock; one was due to cardiac arrest, but all others were a result of respiratory failure. Postmortem findings in the lung consisted mainly of multiple atelectasis, subpleural petecchiae, and increased secretions in the airways. Contrary to the findings in dogs (ESSEX and MARKOWITZ, 1930b) and cats (RUSSELL et al., 1962), gross lung edema was observed in two animals only. Mean lung weight for the entire group was not significantly different from that of normal sheep. Multiple thromboemboli were found in the pulmonary vascular bed in animals with pulmonary hypertension and were invariably absent in the other sheep (HALMAGYI et al., 1965).

2. C. adamanteus (Eastern Diamond Rattlesnake) Venom

Intravenous injection of *C. adamanteus* venom (0.5 mg/kg) in dogs produced a precipitous fall in arterial blood pressure and a decrease in the pulse pressure (VICK et al., 1967). This was followed at 8–10 min by partial recovery of blood pressure to near normal levels and an increase in pulse pressure. Just prior to death, arterial pressure once again decreased sharply, terminating with cardiac arrest. Respiration appeared unaffected during the first 2–5 min after injection; then an abrupt cessation in ventilation occurred. EKG showed depression of the S–T segment, inversion of the T wave, and finally, overwhelming cardiac hypoxia. This venom produced an immediate and marked bradycardia which became progressively severe until just prior to death. Bilateral vagotomy did not prevent the fall in blood pressure but did allow for an increase in heart rate. Evisceration for the most part prevented the sharp fall in arterial blood pressure and the decrease in heart rate observed in the intact dog; rather, blood pressure decreased moderately and heart rate increased. However, with the venom of *C. atrox*, these authors found that evisceration only partially prevented the initial fall in arterial blood pressure. Therefore, they postulated that the fall in arterial blood pressure produced by these rattlesnake venoms is most probably due to pooling of blood in the pulmonary tissues as well as in the hepatosplanchnic bed.

3. C. viridis helleri (Southern Pacific Rattlesnake) Venom

Hemodynamic effects of the venom of *C. viridis helleri* were studied in rats (WHIGHAM et al., 1973; CARLSON et al., 1975; SCHAEFFER et al., 1978a) and dogs (SCHAEFFER, 1973; SCHAEFFER et al., 1978b). The intravenous infusion of a lethal dose of the venom into rats produced an immediate fall in arterial pressure, a striking increase in hematocrit, and a slight increase in oxygen consumption. This was followed by a progressive decline in hematocrit and oxygen consumption, a profound increase in arterial blood lactate, and metabolic acidosis. No significant change in heart rate was observed. Death occurred after 3–18 h (WHIGHAM et al., 1973). The most sensitive indicators of the severity of poisoning were the magnitude and duration of lactacidemia and hemoconcentration. Ventilation was little affected until just prior to death. Significant reductions in plasma volume and red cell mass were observed, and were attributed to an increase in vascular permeability and hemorrhage (CARLSON et al., 1975; SCHAEFFER et al., 1978a). In dogs, within 15 s of the intravenous injection of the venom (50 μg/kg), abdominal aortic pressure fell precipitously, accompanied simultaneously by an increase in ascending aortic flow. Arterial pressure reached its lowest value at 30 s after injection and remained depressed for 60 min. Ascending aortic flow reached a maximum at 30 s after injection and remained increased for 2–5 min, then progressively declined. Flow in the subclavian artery increased concurrently with ascending aortic flow; it reached a maximum of 50% above the initial value after 30 s. Femoral artery flow remained unchanged for the initial 25 s, but thereafter increased to 130% of the initial value. Subsequent changes in flow of the femoral and subclavian arteries mirrored those in the ascending aorta. Flow in the superior mesenteric artery decreased 20 s after injection. Systemic, subclavian, and femoral artery resistances were markedly reduced during the initial 5 min while superior mesenteric resistance was not significantly affected during this interval. However, by 10 min all resistances were markedly elevated. Pulmonary artery, pulmonary artery wedge, and left ventricular end-diastolic pressures changed little. Pulmonary vascular resistance was reduced for 2–5 min, but then gradually increased. Heart rate and EKG were not significantly altered during the initial 10 min following venom injection. Portal vein and right atrial pressures also changed little. Lactacidemia and hemoconcentration developed within 1 min after injection and remained elevated throughout the monitoring period. It was concluded that the initial hypotensive crisis is due to a profound decrease in vascular resistance. The vasculature supplying skeletal muscle appears to be the site of the rapid decrease in peripheral vascular resistance. After these initial changes, venom shock is characterized by prolonged hypotension, a decrease in cardiac output, and hemoconcentration (SCHAEFFER, 1973; SCHAEFFER et al., 1978b).

4. C. durissus terrificus (Tropical Rattlesnake) Venom

The venom of *C. durissus terrificus* is unique among rattlesnake venoms in containing a potent neurotoxic component called crotoxin (SLOTTA and FRAENKEL-CONRAT, 1938). The cause of death due to envenomation by this rattlesnake is respiratory paralysis rather than circulatory failure. Besides, the venom of this snake produces far less tissue destruction and almost no hemorrhage.

Cardiovascular effects of this venom were first studied in rabbits by ARTHUS (1913). He observed a triple response, i.e., a transient and abrupt fall in arterial blood pressure which was followed by a hypertensive period of short duration and a subsequent progressive hypotension. However, VELLARD and HUIDOBRO (1941) reported that the venom of *C. durissus terrificus* from some geographical regions produces only depression of blood pressure, a finding confirmed by VITAL BRAZIL (1954) with venom of the same species from Santiago del Estero, Argentina. The triple effect was not suppressed in dogs, (i) injected with atropine, (ii) with their central nervous system destroyed, (iii) with their autonomic ganglia blocked by hexamethonium, and (iv) with their α-adrenergic receptors blocked by dibenamine or chlorpromazine (VITAL BRAZIL, 1954). MARKWARDT et al. (1966) showed that in rabbits the intravenous administration of "the amine releasing component" (AFK) of *C. durissus terrificus* venom was able to produce a triphasic blood pressure change, which was reproduced in part by 5-hydroxytryptamine.

Crotoxin, a crystalline neurotoxin, was first isolated from the venom of *C. durissus terrificus* by SLOTTA and FRAENKEL-CONRAT (1938). Recent studies have shown crotoxin to be a complex of an acidic protein and a basic phospholipase A (see Chap. 5). The effect of crotoxin on the neuromuscular transmission is discussed in detail in Chapter 10.

The acute effects produced by crotoxin on blood pressure, hematocrit value, and respiration were compared with those produced by *C. d. terrificus* venom in dogs (VITAL BRAZIL et al., 1966). The venom used in this study belonged to the variety devoid of crotamine. Crotoxin produced a rather gradual blood pressure fall which began to appear 2–3 min after its administration. The hypotensive effect elicited by crotoxin (0.25 mg/kg) was always reversible; the blood pressure usually attained its initial level less than 2 h after its administration. However, with the crude venom, an abrupt and transient fall in blood pressure appeared within 30 s and was followed by a pressor effect of 1–2 min duration. Thereafter a less abrupt and prolonged fall occurred in all experiments. The striking differences in the effects elicited by crotoxin and crude venom were also revealed by injecting them in the same dog. The venom caused the usual triple effect on blood pressure after the dog was made irresponsive (tachyphylactic) to the hypotensive action of crotoxin. Respiration was not acutely modified by crotoxin. The venom, on the other hand, caused an intense and transient increase in the frequency and amplitude of the respiratory movements within a few seconds, followed by a brief period of apnea, and then tachypnea which persisted for more than 1 h. Crotoxin was also much less active than crude venom in increasing the hematocrit value. VITAL BRAZIL et al. (1966) concluded that the acute disturbances produced by the venom on circulation and respiration cannot be due to crotoxin or to crotamine. There are other venom components whose pharmacological actions must play an important role in *C. d. terrificus* envenomation, especially in the genesis of shock.

5. C. scutulatus (Mojave Rattlesnake) Venom and Mojave Toxin

An acidic protein toxin, "Mojave toxin", has recently been isolated from *C. scutulatus* (Mojave rattlesnake) venom (BIEBER et al., 1975). The Mojave toxin was claimed to be an acidic cardiotoxin, but both the chemical and pharmacological properties of this toxin are apparently different from those of cobra cardiotoxins. After intravenous injection of Mojave toxin (1 mg/kg) in the rabbit, a fall in arterial pressure began immediately and reached its lowest level within 2 min. About 30–40 min after injection, the pulse pressure increased, and the respiratory rate gradually decreased. The EKG showed a decrease in amplitude of the P wave, an increase in the R/S ratio, and an increase in the voltage of the QRS complex and bradycardia during this period. Between 70 and 120 min after injection, the blood pressure gradually declined and respiration was markedly impaired. Finally, cardiovascular collapse and respiratory failure occurred simultaneously; artificial respiration could not restore the blood pressure. From these results, the authors concluded that Mojave toxin has remarkable cardiotoxic effects.

The effects of crude venom on the circulatory system were somewhat different from those of Mojave toxin. The intravenous administration of 1 mg/kg of crude venom induced a fall in the blood pressure followed by a restoration to the preinjection value within 60 min. An increase in the pulse pressure was observed for a few minutes after injection. Apnea of 5–10 s duration appeared immediately after injection. The fairly constant findings in the EKG were increased T wave voltage followed by a decrease of the voltage of the QRS complex and very tall, slender, peaked T waves (BIEBER et al., 1975).

6. Basic Protein Toxins from Rattlesnake Venoms

There has been a widely held misconception that the venom secretions from all species of rattlesnakes are similar. Small molecular weight basic protein toxins have been isolated from venoms of four North American rattlesnakes (*C. adamanteus*, *C. h. horridus*, *C. v. viridus*, and *C. h. atricaudatus*). However, these toxins are absent in most other rattlesnake venoms so far studied (BONILLA and FIERO, 1971). Although all of these basic protein toxins have a marked effect on the neuromuscular transmission (LEE et al., 1973), two of them (*C. adamanteus* and *C. h. atricaudatus*) have been shown to cause death by inducing a pronounced ischemia and subsequent myocardial failure (BONILLA et al., 1971; BONILLA, 1972; ABEL et al., 1973). Single, sublethal injections of these two toxins elicited dose-dependent rises in serum glutamic-oxaloacetic transaminase (SGOT), creatine phosphokinase (CPK), hydroxybutyric dehydrogenase (α-HBD), and aldolase in mice. No changes in the level of alkaline phosphatase, hematocrit, or total serum protein were observed. The increase of serum enzymes is consistent with myocardial necrosis and similar to that induced by isoproterenol, a β-adrenergic agonist (BONILLA et al., 1971). They concluded that the basic protein toxins exerted their lethal action by producing myocardial failure in animals. ABEL et al. (1973) used both light and electron microscopes to evaluate myocardial damage induced in cats by the basic protein toxin from *C. adamanteus* venom. After intravenous injection of the toxin in two cats at a dose of 14.4 mg/kg, the animals were allowed to die and a complete necropsy was carried out. Light microscopic examinations of the myocardial tissue when stained with hematoxylin and eosin revealed little sign of ischemia. There was no leukocytic infiltration or myocardial degeneration in the cat living four days. However, they observed lesions suggestive of early myocardial ischemia in the wall of the left ventricle stained with basic fuchsin. They believed that ultrastructural changes produced by the basic protein toxin in myocardium, such as depletion of glycogen granules, accumulation of lipid droplets, and changes in mitochondrial fine structure, were similar to those induced by isoproterenol, and suggested that some final common factor, possibly anoxia, was responsible for the heart failure.

A similar protein, called myocardial depressor protein (MDP) was recently isolated from the venom of *C. atrox* (BONILLA and RAMMEL, 1976). Intravenous injection of MDP (0.5 mg/kg) to experimental animals (dogs and cats) produced an immediate and profound decrease in the cardiac output, mean aortic arterial pressure, and left ventricular systolic pressure. The maximal velocity of contractile element shortening of left ventricular muscle was significantly decreased. EKG changes included R wave depression, atrial fibrillation, S–T segment elevation or depression, paroxysmal ventricular tachycardia, and interference dissociation. Both systemic and pulmonary vascular resistances became elevated. There was a rise in serum CPK, GOT, GPT, and arterial lactate concentrations following the administration of MDP (BONILLA and SKOGLUND, unpublished). The minimal molecular weight for MDP was estimated to be approximately 10000 daltons. BONILLA and RAMMEL (1976) reported that MDP is devoid of the phospholipase A and the proteolytic and esterolytic activities known to exist in the crude venom of *C. atrox*. However, a recent study on MDP revealed that it possesses the phospholipase A activity comparable to that of the Formosan cobra venom (LIN SHIAU et al., 1977).

Another potent hypotensive peptide, "hypotensin," has also been isolated from the same venom (BONILLA, 1976). It consists of approximately 20 amino-acid residues, with leucine at N-terminus and serine at C-terminus. Intravenous injection of the purified hypotensive peptide (1.0 mg/kg) produced an immediate and profound decrease in systemic arterial pressure which lasted for 2 h or longer in anesthetized dogs. Hypotensin does not appear to be destroyed by lung peptidases as judged by the duration of hypotensive response in intact dogs. It is, likewise, not destroyed by gastrointestinal peptidases since when administered orally it induces a dose-dependent hypotention in normal and spontaneously hypertensive rats (BONILLA, unpublished). The mechanism of action of hypotensin has not been elucidated.

II. Other Crotalid Venoms

1. Agkistrodon Venoms

ESSEX (1932) reported that the venom of the water moccasin (*Agkistrodon piscivorus*) produced an almost identical response to that previously described for rattlesnake venom. Although BROWN (1941) also noted that all the dogs in his experiments with the water moccasin venom exhibited a precipitous fall in blood pressure, he concluded that poisoning by this venom was partially due to the "neurotoxic" action which produced respiratory and vasomotor depression, since 55% of the animals died of respiratory paralysis, accompanied by an asphyxial rise in blood pressure; persistently low blood pressure and the hemorrhagic vascular effects were responsible for the mortality of the rest of the animals. The phrenic nerve was apparently unaffected, and he found no evidence that the venom had a curarelike effect. However, since the respiratory failure was always preceded by a sharp fall in arterial blood pressure, it could be secondary to the circulatory failure. The contention that crotalid venom poisoning is due to central neurotoxic action has also been questioned by HADIDIAN (1956).

VICK et al. (1967) studied the circulatory effects of venoms from three *Agkistrodon* species. A dose of 1.0 mg/kg of *A. piscivorus* venom produced a precipitous fall in arterial pressure with increased pulse pressure. This was followed by partial recovery at 3–5 min and a subsequent decline in both arterial and pulse pressures. Just prior to death, a marked increase in both arterial and pulse pressures occurred, apparently because of respiratory depression and generalized hypoxia. No significant changes in EKG were noted until severe respiratory depression became apparent. Evisceration did not prevent the precipitous decrease in blood pressure or the bradycardia produced by this venom. An 1.25 mg/kg dose of northern copperhead *(A. contortrix mokeson)* venom or a 0.5 mg/kg dose of southern copperhead *(A. c. contortrix)* venom produced similar changes as described for *A. piscivorus venom.* Since evisceration did not modify the initial fall in blood pressure observed in the intact dogs, VICK et al. (1967) concluded that pulmonary vascular pooling per se occurred with these venoms.

The hemodynamic effect of the Malayan pit viper *(Agkistrodon rhodostoma)* venom was studied in dogs (MARSHALL and ESNOUF, 1968). The venom was given intravenously to 14 dogs in a dose of 50 μg/kg which was sufficient to make the blood incoagulable within 20 min. Systemic blood pressure and lung function were not affected, and no blood clot was found in the lungs or systemic vessels at autopsy. A transient slight rise in pulmonary arterial pressure and resistance occurred in some of the dogs, but the pressure usually remained within normal limits and returned to the initial level within 1–2 h after the venom was given. However, a dose of venom four times the usual dose produced death by extensive thrombosis in the right heart and pulmonary arteries.

2. Trimeresurus Venoms

ISHIZAKA (1907) reported that Habu (*Trimeresurus riukiuanus*, probably identical with *T. flavoviridis*) venom produces a precipitous fall in blood pressure in rabbits and dogs following intravenous application, and he attributed the blood pressure change to impairment of the heart. On the other hand, MIYAZAKI (1921) observed that the venom of *Trimeresurus flavoviridis* produces a rise in the pulmonary arterial blood pressure concurrent with a fall in systemic pressure in rabbits, and that the impairment of heart takes place only in the late stage of venom action. PENG (1951 b) studied the effects of the venom of Taiwan habu *(Trimeresurus mucrosquamatus)* in rabbits. The venom (0.05–1.0 mg/kg) produced an immediate fall in arterial blood pressure, which recovered gradually in 20–50 min. Bradycardia was noted and the amplitude of the heart beats decreased. With a lethal dose (5 mg/kg), irregular pulsations took place and no recovery was observed. Artificial respiration failed to restore normal blood pressure. With small doses (0.05–0.1 mg/kg), the pulmonary arterial pressure decreased slightly as the systemic blood pressure fell, whereas with higher doses (0.5–1.0 mg/kg) a transient rise in the pulmonary arterial pressure was observed. Both the intestinal and kidney volumes decreased while the volume of the hind limb increased. Both the portal and jugular venous pressures decreased. Atropinization, cutting of the vagi, and elimination of the brain circulation did not alter the circulatory effects of the venom. Elimination of the carotid sinus nerves and cutting of the depressor nerves also failed to alter the venom action. PENG (1951b) concluded that the fall in blood pressure induced by the habu venom is not central in origin and is due to vasodilatation in the skin and muscles as well as cardiac impediment.

3. Bothrops Venoms

The *Bothrops* venoms show necrotizing and blood-coagulating effects and may induce death in a few minutes with massive intravascular clotting following the inoculation of sufficiently high doses (ROSENFELD, 1971). ROCHA E SILVA et al. (1949) first demonstrated that when plasma globulins are exposed to the venom of *Bothrops jararaca*, a substance, which they named bradykinin, is formed having a marked ability to decrease blood pressure. They attributed the fall in blood pressure produced by *Bothrops* venom to the formation of bradykinin rather than histamine release. However, bradykinin effects are very brief since this substance is rapidly destroyed in the blood stream and tissues. FERREIRA (1965) has found a bradykinin-potentiating factor (BPF) in the venom of *Bothrops jararaca*, which effectively increases the hemodynamic action of bradykinin (AMORIM et al., 1967). More recently, ROTHSCHILD and ALMEIDA (1972) have studied the role of kinin release in the fatal shock induced by *Bothrops jararaca* venom in rats and found that even a massive release of bradykinin by the venom can be tolerated by rats, provided that intravascular coagulation is prevented by a preliminary treatment with heparin or cellulose sulfate. Heparin did not prevent the breakdown of plasma bradykinin precursor (bradykininogen) by the venom, but effectively counteracted its hypercoagulative action. Cellulose sulfate caused extensive plasma bradykininogen consumption, did not alter blood coagulation time, but led to marked fibrinogenopenia. This effect is probably the cause of the protection afforded by this sulfopolysaccharide.

III. Thrombinlike Enzymes from Crotalid Venoms

The effect of Arvin, a thrombinlike enzyme purified from the Malayan pit viper (*Agkistrodon rhodostoma*) venom, on cardiac function was investigated in dogs (KLEIN et al., 1969). A slow infusion of Arvin in a dose varying from 1.4 to 2.0 μg/kg body weight over 30 min did not cause any significant changes in left ventricular function, both tension-generating and velocity-shortening attributes remaining unchanged. Within 30–60 min fibrinogen levels declined to nondetectable levels, remaining so for more than 24 h. No excessive external bleeding was noticed in any of the animals.

The influence of Arvin on the flow properties of blood was studied in 12 patients suffering from peripheral arterial arteriosclerosis (EHRLY, 1973). Arvin therapy led to a defibrinogenation of blood and to a consequent decrease in the viscosity of blood and plasma. The aggregation of erythrocytes was drastically reduced. Decrease in blood viscosity was most pronounced at low rates of shear (structural viscosity). According to Hagen-Poiseuille's law, this improvement of the flow properties of blood by Arvin therapy in man would tend to increase the blood flow in the large vessels, and plethysmographic measurements indeed indicated an increased blood flow (EHRLY, 1972).

Hemodynamic effects of slow and rapid defibrination induced by administration of "defibrizyme," the thrombinlike enzyme from the venom of *C. h. horridus* (timber rattlesnake), were also studied in dogs (BONILLA et al., 1975). While induction of defibrination by slow intravenous infusion did not cause significant hemodynamic alterations, there was a significant drop in cardiac output, stroke volume, and mean aortic arterial pressure immediately after rapid (bolus) intravenous administration of defibrizyme at dose levels of 0.5 and 0.83 mg/kg of body weight. There was a decrease in heart rate and mean left ventricular end-diastolic pressure was essentially unchanged. Cardiac and minute work indexes dropped and pulmonary artery pressure increased. Pulmonary capillary wedge, mean right ventricular, and central venous pressure were unaltered. The calculated systemic and pulmonary vascular resistances were drastically increased, whereas arterial Po_2, Pco_2, and pH were unaffected. BONILLA et al. (1975) attributed these changes to the rapid decline in plasma fibrinogen concentration and/or blood viscosity. However, they did not rule out the possibility of pulmonary thromboembolism that might occur due to rapid (bolus) intravenous administration of the defibrinating enzyme (see MARSHALL and ESNOUF, 1968).

B. Mechanism of the Depressor Action of Crotalid Venoms

I. Site of Action

ESSEX and MARKOWITZ (1930a) considered that rattlesnake (*C. horridus* and *C. atrox*) venoms do not kill as a result of universal muscular paralysis, because artificial respiration had no influence on the toxicity of these venoms, and a curarized dog responded to crotalin in a similar manner. Nevertheless, HALMAGYI et al. (1965) reported that respiratory failure was the most frequent cause of death in their studies of shock due to rattlesnake (*C. atrox*) venom in sheep. They observed that the administration of agents that improved circulation further depressed respiratory function in the shocked animals; elevation of arterial pressure during norepinephrine infusion was accompanied by further fall in arterial oxygen saturation, while dextran infusion that fully restored cardiac output further accentuated hypoventilation. Therefore, they suggested that the respiratory effect of *Crotalus* venom may be dominant in determining its physiological action.

However, since *Crotalus* venoms manifest their usual effect in the decapitated or decerebrated animal, the fall in blood pressure obviously is not central and therefore must be either cardiac or peripheral in nature (ESSEX and MARKOWITZ, 1930a; RUSSELL et al., 1962). The initial fall in blood pressure from most crotalid venoms is not cardiac in origin, since there is no evidence of any significant cardiac depression during this period. In most cases no EKG alterations are found until a later stage (RUSSELL et al., 1962; SCHAEFFER, 1973; SCHAEFFER et al., 1978b); cardiac output is usually increased during the initial stage (WITHAM et al., 1953; SCHAEFFER, 1973; SCHAEFFER et al., 1978b). However, WITHAM et al. (1953) observed a depression of the S–T segment and an increased T wave amplitude at the small dosage level. RUSSELL et al. (1962) also noted EKG changes following large doses of venom; ectopic ventricular rhythms were observed within 15 s following injection. Using the isolated trabeculae carnae preparation, a negative inotropic effect was demonstrated with large doses (1–5 mg/ml of bath media) of venom. BROWN (1940) described similar effects with *Agkistrodon piscivorus* venom in the isolated frog heart, and ESSEX and MARKOWITZ (1930b) also reported a negative inotropic effect of crotalin in the isolated rabbit heart. However, all of these studies utilized relatively large doses of venom. Likewise, in an in vivo study, ABEL et al. (1973) used a massive dose (14.4 mg/kg) of a purified basic protein toxin from *C. adamanteus* venom to produce histologically demonstrable myocardial damage.

Since eviscerated or dehepatized animals also showed the typical response to crotalin, ESSEX and MARKOWITZ (1930a) concluded that the initial fall in blood pressure was not dependent on spasm of the hepatic veins or congestion in the splanchnic viscera, as had been supposed by some investigators to be the case in anaphylactic shock. On the other hand, VICK et al. (1967) observed that evisceration partially prevented the decrease in arterial blood pressure produced by either *C. adamanteus* or *C. atrox* venom, while it did not modify the initial drop in blood pressure produced by three *Agkistrodon* venoms. Therefore, they concluded that *Crotalus* venoms produce pooling of blood in both the pulmonary tissues and the hepatosplanchnic bed, while pulmonary vascular pooling per se occurs with *Agkistrodon* venoms they studied. RUSSELL et al. (1962) also reported that the pooling occurred in the major blood vessels of the chest and in the lungs during the fall in systemic arterial pressure produced by *C. atrox* venom. They observed a decrease in pressure and flow from the left heart and an increase in pulmonary artery pressure. RUSSELL (1967a, b) suggested that these changes might be due to an increase in resistance in the postcapillary veins, possibly in the smaller venules in the lungs. On the other hand, HALMAGYI et al. (1965) observed that occasional onset of pulmonary hypertension was associated with the production of thromboembolism in the pulmonary vascular bed. Although RUSSELL (1962) himself described that multiple pulmonary emboli are frequently found in patients receiving a fatal rattlesnake bite, and are one of the changes that can lead to death, he believes that it seems unlikely that thromboembolism is responsible for the immediate circulatory changes (RUSSELL, 1967a, b). ESSEX and MARKOWITZ (1930a) also did not believe that intravascular thrombosis was the cause of the venom's effect on blood pressure, since in defibrinated or heparinized dogs crotalin still produced the typical fall in blood pressure. It may be true that crotalid venoms can produce immediate circulatory changes without causing thromboembolism. However, it is also possible that some of the circulatory changes, e.g., pulmonary hypertension, might be due to intravascular clotting. Actually, pulmonary hypertension appears not to be a constant finding (HALMAGYI et al., 1965). SCHAEFFER (1973) and SCHAEFFER et al. (1978b) reported that they did not observe a significant change in pulmonary artery pressure in dogs injected with *C. viridis helleri* venom.

The initial arterial hypotension appears to be due to a profound vasodilatation leading to a decline in peripheral resistance (WITHAM et al., 1953; HALMAGYI et al., 1965). The finding that the initial hypotension is associated with a concomitant increase in ascending aortic flow provides evidence that venous return and myocardial competence may be increased (SCHAEFFER, 1973; SCHAEFFER et al., 1978b). It has been suggested that the site of initial decrease in peripheral resistance is the skeletal muscle vasculature (ESSEX and MARKOWITZ, 1930a; PENG, 1951b; SCHAEFFER, 1973; SCHAEFFER et al., 1978b), rather than the splanchnic circulation as suggested by VICK et al. (1963). ESSEX and MARKOWITZ (1930a) demonstrated an increase in hind limb volume within 1 min of intravenous injection of crotalin in the dog, and PENG (1951 b) obtained a similar result with *T. mucrosquamatus* venom in the rabbit. SCHAEFFER et al. (1978 b) observed that superior mesenteric artery flow and resistance decreased as abdominal aortic pressure fell, while ascending aortic and femoral artery flow increased; portal vein pressure was unchanged. Based on these data, they concluded that the splanchnic circulation does not participate in the active decrease in peripheral resistance associated with the initial hypotension. Their conclusion is also supported by the observations of ESSEX and MARKOWITZ (1930a, b) in which plethysmographic studies of splanchnic organs showed a decline in volume following crotalin administration.

The decrease in peripheral resistance does not appear to primarily involve neurogenic mechanisms since vasomotor center ablation and vagotomy do not alter the hemodynamic effects of these venoms (ESSEX and MARKOWITZ, 1930a; PENG, 1951 b; RUSSELL et al., 1962). Elimination of the carotid sinus nerves and cutting of the depressor nerves also do not alter the venom action (PENG, 1951 b). The increase in heart rate concomitant with the systemic arterial hypotension in most cases also suggests that the baroreceptors of the carotid sinus and their pathways are not impaired by the venom (SCHAEFFER, 1973).

On the other hand, hypovolemia and hemoconcentration may play a significant role in the later stage of circulatory failure. The reductions in left ventricular end-diastolic, pulmonary artery, and right atrial pressures as well as tachycardia are consistent with hypovolemia and a decrease in venous return (SCHAEFFER et al., 1978 b). A marked rise in Hb content and a fall in plasma protein level are constant features of *Crotalus* venom-induced shock. These changes are compatible with the assumption that plasma loss, secondary to venom-induced increase in capillary permeability, initiated circulatory failure (WITHAM et al., 1953; HALMAGYI et al., 1965). The development of widespread petechial hemorrhages, visceral congestion, and frank hemorrhage into the lumen of the lower intestine may also contribute to the reduction in total blood volume (WITHAM et al., 1953). A decline in cardiac output may result from cardiac damage, either primary or secondary, as reflected electrocardiographically by a depression in S–T segment and conduction disturbances (WITHAM et al., 1953; RUSSELL et al., 1962; VICK et al., 1967). In addition, changes induced by venom in the rheological properties of blood (BALDES et al., 1931) may also influence the hemodynamic alterations. The marked increase in hematocrit (ESSEX and MARKOWITZ, 1930c; WITHAM et al., 1953; SCHAEFFER, 1973; SCHAEFFER et al., 1978 b) may also contribute to the decrease in cardiac output. The hemoconcentration may adversely affect microcirculatory flow and further compromise oxygen delivery to the tissues.

II. Venom Components Responsible for the Depressor Action

Knowledge about the exact mechanism of depressor action of crotalid venoms is still limited. The peripheral vasodilatation and increase in capillary permeability could be due to either the direct action of some venom component(s), the release of autopharmacological substances, or both.

Only a limited number of investigations of purified toxins from crotalid venoms have been made due to the great complexity of crotalid venoms, which makes isolation of pure toxins rather difficult. Some of the small molecular weight basic protein toxins isolated from venoms of four species of rattlesnakes (BONILLA and FIERO, 1971), the myocardial depressor protein (MDP) from *C. atrox* venom (BONILLA and RAMMEL, 1976), and the Mojave toxin from *C. scutulatus* venom (BIEBER et al., 1975), all produce myocardial depression or failure and thus contribute to the overall circulatory collapse produced by the respective venom. However, none of these toxins appear to be responsible for the initial fall in arterial blood pressure produced by the crude venom, since the cardiac function is usually unaffected until the later stage, as described in the previous section. The only toxin so far isolated from rattlesnake venoms, which may be responsible for the initial fall in arterial blood pressure, is "hypotensin" isolated from *C. atrox* venom (BONILLA, 1976). However, since the mechanism of action of "hypotensin" has not been elucidated, it is not known to what extent this toxin is responsible for the overall circulatory effect of the crude venom. It is also not known whether all rattlesnake venoms contain such a toxin as the common component.

Some enzyme components of crotalid venoms have been tested for their role in producing hypotension. The ophio-L-amino acid oxidase of *Crotalus* venoms was found not to contribute to the profound fall in systemic arterial pressure produced by the crude venom (RUSSELL et al., 1963b). Phosphodiesterase isolated from venoms of *C. atrox*, *C. adamanteus*, *C. viridis helleri*, and *C. h. horridus* produced an immediate and profound fall in the systemic arterial pressure of cats after its intravenous injection (RUSSELL et al., 1963a). Unfortunately, the same phosphodiesterase was shown to be composed of several fractions on disc electrophoresis. Therefore, the hypotensive action, while it may be due to the enzyme, might also be caused by some other substance separated with the enzyme (RUSSELL, 1972).

Many investigators have related the hemodynamic alterations induced by crotalid venoms to the release of autopharmacological substances (FELDBERG and KELLAWAY, 1937c; ROCHA E SILVA and ESSEX, 1942; ROCHA E SILVA et al., 1949; VICK et al., 1963; MARGOLIS et al., 1965; RUSSELL, 1965; KAISER and RAAB, 1966), including histamine, 5-hydroxytryptamine, bradykinin, and slow-reacting substances (see Chap. 16).

The remarkable similarity between reactions to crotalin and histamine was first noted by ESSEX and MARKOWITZ (1930a, d), and the release of histamine from the perfused lungs of guinea pigs by snake venoms (*N. naja* and *C. atrox*) was reported by FELDBERG and KELLAWAY (1937c). The latter authors postulated that lysolecithin generated by the action of phospholipase A present in snake venoms damages cellular histamine depot sites, causing the release of the amine (FELDBERG and KELLAWAY, 1938). The presence of a histamine-releasing protein component unrelated to phospholipase A, possibly of proteolytic enzyme nature, has also been demonstrated in the venom of the Brazilian rattlesnake (*C. durissus terrificus*) (ROTHSCHILD, 1966; MARKWARDT et al., 1966). Nevertheless, since premedication with antihistamines fails to modify the effect of crotalid venoms (DRAGSTEDT et al., 1938; SCHÖTTLER, 1954; HALMAGYI et al., 1965), it is generally considered that the release of histamine plays only a minor role in the crotalid venom-induced circulatory failure.

ROCHA E SILVA et al. (1949) were the first to demonstrate that bradykinin, a hypotensive and smooth muscle stimulating polypeptide, was released from plasma globulin by the venom of *Bothrops jararaca* and by trypsin. Subsequent studies have shown that kinin-forming enzymes, kininogenases, are widely distributed among crotalid and viperid venoms (DEUTSCH and DINIZ, 1955; OSHIMA et al., 1969; MEBS, 1970). Kinins produce relaxation of vascular smooth muscle as well as an increase in capillary permeability in the microcirculation of mesentery and other tissues (see HADDY et al., 1970). Intravenous infusion of bradykinin produces a fall in systemic arterial pressure and resistance which is very similar to that produced by rattlesnake venoms (HARRISON et al., 1968). Decreased amounts or even complete disappearance of circulatory kininogen have been observed in both experimental and clinical studies of rattlesnake envenomation (MARGOLIS et al., 1965; RUSSELL, 1965). These findings suggest that bradykinin probably plays a role in the acute hypotension produced by crotalid and viperid venoms. However, the persistence or recurrence of shock with larger or repeated doses of venom after plasma kininogen stores had been exhausted suggests that the release of bradykinin into the circulation is not the sole source of hypotension (MARGOLIS et al., 1965).

KAISER and RAAB (1966) reported that pretreatment with antihistamines or antiserotonins did not show any significant influence on survival time following injection of a lethal dose of *Agkistrodon piscivorus* venom (20 mg/kg i.v.) in mice. However, after administration of a combined antihistamine-antiserotonin substance (cyproheptadine), a longer survival time was found. In several animals rapid death due to anaphylactoid shock was prevented. Optimal results were obtained with a combined antihistamine-antiserotonin-antikinin substance (WA-335, Dr. Karl Thomas, Germany). Pretreatment with this substance (15 min before injection of the venom) not only prolonged the survival time, but the lethal dose of the venom was tolerated by a number of mice. KAISER and RAAB (1966) suggested that the high antikinin activity might exert a direct antitoxic effect by neutralizing toxic fractions of the venom.

C. Hemodynamic Effects of Viperid Venoms

I. Russell's Viper (Vipera russellii) Venom

The action of Russell's viper venom on the circulatory system was extensively studied by CHOPRA and CHOWHAN (1934). A small dose of the venom (0.05–0.1 mg/kg) injected intravenously into a cat produced a slight initial rise in blood pressure followed by a gradual fall amounting to 20–30 mm Hg. With larger doses (0.2–0.5 mg/kg), the fall was more pronounced and the blood pressure remained permanently at a lower level. Rapid administration of large doses produced a sudden fall in blood pressure and the animal sometimes died suddenly of convulsions and heart failure. Using heparin and other anticoagulants, LEE (1944) proved that the sudden death produced by Russell's viper venom is due to intravascular clotting. The same conclusion was also reached by AHUJA et al. (1946a). If the dose of the venom was gradually increased, the animals developed a sort of tolerance to it. Once the blood pressure had reached its lowest level after a dose of the venom, further administration of much larger doses did not produce any effect on the blood pressure (CHOPRA and CHOWHAN, 1934). These authors summarized their experimental results as follows:

In case of viper venom the haemorrhagic phenomena appear at the outset of the poisoning and are very extensive in character. Death is preceded by spasmodic and irregular respiration, convulsions and asphyxia indicating the involvement of the vagal centre owing to deficient blood supply.

Daboia (Russell's viper) venom has a marked tendency to produce thrombosis and gangrene at the site of the bite and death is due to secondary shock. The systemic blood vessels, especially the peripheral ones, are found to be contracted and those of the splanchnic area are widely dilated as in histamine shock. That the nervous centres are not much affected is shown by the fact that in decerebrated animals exactly the same results are produced.

The symptoms of shock in daboia poisoning are not due to reflex impulses but are due to the local dilatation of the capillaries of the splanchnic area. There is enormous engorgement of the abdominal viscera and that the collapse goes hand in hand with hyperaemia of the splanchnic area (chiefly the gut) is shown by the fact that if the mesenteric arteries are clamped, quite large doses of the venom do not produce any marked effect in the blood pressure.

The paralytic action of the venom seems to be confined to the capillaries only. In the perfusion experiment it was observed that the veins and arteries are not dilated, on the other hand, they show a tendency to constrict. The paralytic action of the venom on the capillaries was observed to be similar to that of histamine since the venom does not give any fall of blood pressure after large doses of histamine and vice versa. Drugs like ether and chloroform which depress the capillaries, potentiate the action of the venom. Under the microscope, fine capillaries of the frog's omentum were seen to dilate widely when exposed to the action of daboia venom. Adrenalin and pituitrin, which tone up the capillaries, and glucose, gelatine and gum-saline, which increase the total volume and the viscosity of the blood, tend to revive the blood pressure. The haemorrhagic tendency and enormous leakage of the plasma from the capillaries is further supported by the fact that the coagulation time is increased and the red cell count is also increased after large doses of the venom. From the above data we are justified in concluding that the venom has a paralytic action on the capillaries which increases the leakage, thus producing symptoms similar to that of shock. Death is secondary to shock and life can be saved if the shock can be overcome early.

VICK et al. (1967) also reported that a lethal dose (0.5 mg/kg, i.v.) of Russell's viper venom produced an immediate and irreversible decline in arterial blood pressure. Pulse pressure narrowed and heart rate decreased as arterial pressure fell. No terminal signs of hypoxia were exhibited with this venom. Respiration was not affected during the initial postinjection period, but after approximately 10 min respiratory movements ceased abruptly, and profound bradycardia was noted. Progressive hypoxia-induced changes in EKG were noted and at time of death electrical disassociation leading to cardiac arrest was seen. Evisceration prevented the initial hypotension and bradycardia. A rather slow progressive decline in arterial blood pressure occurred over a 15–30 min period. Vagotomy did not prevent the sharp fall in arterial blood pressure noted in the intact animal; however, bradycardia was prevented and a significant increase in heart rate occurred. Since surgical removal of the viscera prior to envenomation prevented the initial fall in blood pressure, VICK et al. (1967) concluded that Russell's viper venom produces a pooling of blood in the hepato-splanchnic bed of the dog. Apparently, these authors did not consider the possibility of intravascular clotting by this venom.

The circulatory action of the venom of *V. russellii formosensis*, a subspecies of Russell's viper, was studied in rabbits (LEE, 1948). This venom, like Indian daboia venom, has a coagulant action and produces intravascular clotting upon intravenous administration. When a sublethal dose (0.05–0.1 mg/kg) was injected into rabbits intravenously, an immediate fall in mean arterial blood pressure and an increase in heart rate were observed. Subsequent injection of the same dose did not produce significant changes in either blood pressure or heart rate. However, after a dose of 0.5 mg/kg, the blood pressure fell suddenly to the zero line within a few minutes and no recovery was observed. Injection of adrenaline, transfusion of normal saline, or artificial respiration failed to restore the blood pressure. Section of both vagi and atropinization did not in any way alter the venom action (LEE, 1948). On the other hand, in the animals pretreated with heparin (25 mg/kg), no sudden death was observed even with 5 mg/kg of the venom. The arterial blood pressure fell to a very low level and finally the animals died of circulatory failure after several hours (LEE, 1944).

The hemodynamic effects of this venom were further studied after heat treatment (at 80° C, for 30 min) which destroyed the coagulant and most other enzyme activities of the venom (LEE, 1948). The heated venom did not produce sudden death even at large doses (5–10 mg/kg); as in the heparin-pretreated animals, it produced an immediate and irreversible fall in the arterial blood pressure and the animals died of circulatory failure within several hours. The hypotensive action of the venom was not affected by the heat treatment; a dose as small as 0.05 mg/kg of the heated venom still produced a transient fall in the arterial blood pressure. With 0.1–1.0 mg/kg, the hypotensive effect was more pronounced and long lasting; the heart rate increased as the blood pressure fell. However, with lethal doses (5–10 mg/kg) bradycardia took place and arrhythmia appeared prior to cardiac arrest. With small doses (0.5–1.0 mg/kg), the pulmonary arterial pressure decreased slightly as the systemic blood pressure fell, whereas with large doses (5–10 mg/kg) a transient and slight rise followed by a fall was observed. Regardless of whether a small or large dose was administered, the volume of the small intestine was markedly increased when the blood pressure fell. The liver volume also increased slightly, whereas the kidney volume showed a decrease followed by an increase. The limb volume decreased after a transient increase. The portal vein pressure decreased and, in some cases, was followed by an increase. Intracisternal injection of 0.1 mg/kg of the heated venom caused a rise in the systemic blood pressure. With 1.0 mg/kg, the rise in blood pressure was followed by a gradual decline to the zero line. Neither elimination of the brain circulation nor cutting of the carotid sinus and depressor nerves altered the hypotensive effects of the heated venom. It was concluded that the cause of death by the Russell's viper venom is at least twofold: (1) the coagulant enzyme is responsible for the acute sudden death due to intravascular clotting, and (2) the thermostable vasculotoxin produces a sustained hypotension leading to delayed circulatory failure (LEE, 1944). The cause of hypotension by the vasculotoxin is not central in origin and is due to peripheral vasodilatation, especially in the splanchnic area (LEE, 1948).

II. Other Viper Venoms

1. Vipera ammodytes Venom

Intravenous injection of *Vipera ammodytes* venom (4.5 mg/kg) in rats produced a rapid fall in the arterial blood pressure followed by respiratory failure (SKET et al., 1973). Severe cardiac disturbances did not appear until the animal was in hypoxia. A basic protein fraction from *V. ammodytes* venom produced similar effects, but it required a larger dose (22.5 mg/kg, i.v.). After injection of a smaller dose, the initially depressed arterial blood pressure recovered to the normal level, but after a certain delay coma and death followed. By isoelectric focusing and preparative disc electrophoresis, this basic fraction yielded three homogeneous proteins (SKET et al., 1973). In the rat neither the crude venom nor the basic protein fraction (both in the concentration of 100 μg/ml) produced neuromuscular block after prolonged stimulation. Since no labeled crude venom and only traces of the basic protein fraction were found in the brain, the respiratory depression could be caused by anoxia of the central nervous system due to the arterial hypotension (SKET et al., 1973), although it had been claimed that this venom contained a neurotoxic fraction which was devoid of hemorrhagic activity, but produced paralysis of extremities and respiratory failure in mice (MUIĆ and PIANTANIDA, 1955).

2. Vipera palestinae Venom

Intravenous injection of a maximum sublethal dose of *Vipera palestinae* venom or its separated neurotoxic fraction, viperotoxin (MOROZ et al., 1966), into cats, produced an immediate and sharp fall in blood pressure (BICHER et al., 1966; KRUPNICK et al., 1968). This reduction in blood pressure continued throughout the duration of the experiment in most of the animals and was associated with progressive peripheral vasodilation. The pulse pressure diminished progressively to a very low amplitude. The action potentials of the cervical sympathetic chain disappeared completely within 30 s of injection. The voltage of electrocorticograms was also diminished in all leads, and sometimes entirely abolished for short periods 3 min after the injection of venom or neurotoxin. The neurotoxin showed no cardiotoxic or ganglionic-blocking action. When administered to spinal cats, it produced a slight transient rise in blood pressure, probably due to a moderate vasoconstriction. From these results the authors concluded that the primary circulatory shock produced by *V. palestinae* venom is correlated with its neurotoxic components, which cause depression of the central autonomic vasoregulatory mechanism. The hemorrhagic component of *V. palestinae* venom does not produce circulatory shock and has no influence on the sympathetic nerve potentials. This fraction produces bleeding in experimental animals, which eventually leads to death (BICHER et al., 1966).

3. Echis carinatus and Echis coloratus Venoms

The circulatory effects of *Echis carinatus* (saw-scaled viper) venom are similar to those of Russell's viper venom (CHOPRA et al., 1935). A slight initial rise followed by a gradual but marked fall in blood pressure was produced by a dose of 0.2 mg/kg of *Echis* venom injected intravenously into a cat. When larger doses (0.5–1.0 mg/kg) were administered, a marked and permanent fall in blood pressure was observed. The volumes of the intestines, spleen, and the kidneys were definitely increased, while the limb vessels remained unaffected or even contracted. The fall in blood pressure does not appear to be central as it was obtained in decerebrated and despinated animals. It is not cardiac in origin as the venom did not produce any marked effect on the heart. The fall is almost entirely due to the dilatation of the blood vessels of the abdominal viscera, since in eviscerated animals or when the splanchnic circulation had been excluded there was hardly any fall in blood pressure. The *Echis* venom is rich in hemorrhagins which are at least ten times stronger than those of the Indian doboia venom, and it also has a strong coagulant action (MASTER and RAO, 1963). These authors, as well as KORNALIK and PUDLAK (1962), attributed the cause of death to the effect on clotting mechanism. AHUJA et al. (1946b) studied the action of heparin on this venom injected in rabbits and stated: (1) that comparatively a much larger quantity of heparin is required to counteract the toxic effect of *Echis* venom than that of Russell's viper venom, and (2) that when the dose of *Echis* venom injected is increased to 20 times the minimal lethal dose, some of the animals show paralysis of the limbs and respiratory failure, as against the convulsive seizures seen with smaller doses. They felt that with higher doses, toxic fractions other than the one responsible for intravascular coagulation increase from sublethal to lethal dose, against which heparin is ineffective. Using columns of Sephadex G 100, ZAKI et al. (1970) have separated five protein fractions from *Echis carinatus* venom. One of these fractions (Fraction 4) is lethal to mice. In rabbits, this fraction increased capillary permeability and caused a fall in blood pressure followed by death. The effects of this fraction could be completely abolished by the antihistaminic drug, promethazine. The circulatory shock caused by the whole venom was delayed to a great extent by the antihistaminic drug and to a greater extent by the antihistaminic drug together with an antiserotonin drug.

As in envenomation by *Echis carinatus*, hemorrhage associated with intravascular clotting is a prominent feature of *Echis coloratus* envenomation. Injection of *E. coloratus* venom into mice or guinea pigs caused widespread hemorrhage, afibrinogenemia, and severe thrombocytopenia (RECHNIC et al., 1962). Neurotoxic activities were also observed in association with a diffuse breakdown of the blood-brain barrier (SANDBANK and DJALDETTI, 1966).

The effect of *E. coloratus* venom on the brain capillaries of the mouse was further studied electron microscopically using horseradish peroxidase as a tracer (SANDBANK et al., 1974). It was demonstrated that the envenomation resulted in breakdown of the blood-brain barrier manifested by leakage of the peroxidase through the capillary wall. The peroxidase penetrated both by endothelial pinocytosis and through opened tight junctions between the endothelial cells. The envenomated mice showed hemorrhages and intravascular fibrin clots in the lungs and kidneys, but not in the brain. Although neurologic manifestations were observed in the absence of bleeding in the brain, fractionation of this venom by column chromatography did not yield a separate neurotoxin (GITTER et al., 1960).

4. Bitis arietans Venom

Intravenous injection of the venom of *Bitis arietans* (puff adder) in doses of 0.05–0.3 mg/kg produced after a latent period of 10–20 s a gradual and marked fall in the blood pressure of cats that persisted for 30 min or more and then returned to near-normal levels. Repeating the injection of the venom caused a further fall in blood pressure that reached a very low level and resulted in circulatory shock and death (OSMAN and GUMAA, 1974). The crude venom was fractionated on Sephadex G-100 into five main fractions, of which only fraction 1 was lethal to mice in a dose of 1 μg/g i.p., producing hemorrhagic lesions in both the lungs and kidneys. Fractions 1 and 2 produced hypotension when injected in doses of 25–50 μg/kg in cats. Other fractions did not produce any significant effect on the blood pressure. When equal concentrations were used, fraction 1 was the most powerful depressant of the isolated rabbit heart, while fraction 2 was the most potent in increasing capillary permeability and producing hypotension. The hypotensive effect of the venom or its fractions was not antagonized by pretreatment with hexamethonium, cyproheptadine, propranolol, atropine, indomethacin, or trasylol. The authors concluded that at least three factors contribute to the circulatory shock caused by the venom: (1) a direct inhibitory effect of the vascular smooth muscles resulting in vasodilation of the arterioles; (2) a direct depressant action on the myocardium; and (3) an extensive increase in vascular permeability that was also unmodified by pretreatment with antihistamines, anti-serotoninergics, or agents which inhibit kinins or prostaglandins. VICK et al. (1967), using dogs, showed that evisceration did not prevent the hypotensive effect of *Bitis arietans* venom, but eliminated the bradycardia. They suggested that the venom did not produce a marked pooling of blood in the hepato-splanchnic bed; however, pulmonary pooling might be responsible for the hypotension.

D. Mechanism of the Depressor Action of Viperid Venoms

I. Mode of Hypotensive Action

Viperid venoms in general have a pronounced hemorrhagic activity and some of them are also blood-coagulating agents. Clinically, hypovolemic shock may be caused by extravasation of blood into soft tissues and various internal organs. Circulatory failure or bleeding is the frequent cause of death in viper bites (see Chap. 26). Although clear evidence of disseminated intravascular clotting (D.I.C.) was rarely found in clinical cases of viper bites, intravascular clotting has been proven to be the cause of sudden death of animals following innoculation of sufficiently high doses of these so-called coagulating venoms (LEE, 1944; AHUJA et al., 1946a, b).

Like crotalid venoms, most viperid venoms do not kill the animals as a result of central or peripheral neurotoxic effects. Certain viperid venoms (SCHÖTTLER, 1938; CÉSARI and BOQUET, 1939; GITTER et al., 1960) or their partially purified protein fractions (GHOSH et al., 1937; KOCHWA et al., 1960; MASTER and RAO, 1961) have been claimed to contain proteins with neurotropic action. However, direct evidence to show the distribution of such a neurotoxic protein in the central nervous system after envenomation is still lacking. Most claims that certain "neurotoxins" are present in certain viperid venoms were usually based only on the signs and symptoms manifested by the envenomated animals. Moreover, there is no clear-cut evidence that "curarizing" toxins are present in certain viperid venoms (see Chap. 10). It is possible that the venoms affect the central nervous system indirectly as a consequence of anoxia resulting from the arterial hypotension (MELDRUM, 1965; SKET et al., 1973). Alternatively, the neurotoxic effects may be attributed to hemorrhages in the brain. However, in the absence of the latter, the breakdown of the blood-brain barrier due to damage of the capillary basement membrane may be responsible for the neurotoxic action of venoms of certain vipers, such as *Echis coloratus* (SANDBANK and DJALDETTI, 1966). On the other hand, the venom of *Vipera palestinae* and its purified neurotoxic protein, viperotoxin, have been claimed to act primarily on medullary vasopressor centers leading to lethal circulatory failure (BICHER et al.,

1966; KRUPNICK et al., 1968). However, it remains to be proven that such a basic protein can pass through the blood-brain barrier in sufficient quantity to produce such central effects.

The fall in blood pressure produced by most viperid venoms is not central in origin, since in decerebrated or despinated animals (CHOPRA and CHOWHAN, 1934; CHOPRA et al., 1935), or after elimination of the brain circulation (LEE, 1948), exactly the same results are produced. As in the case of most crotalid venoms, the cardiac function is not significantly affected until the later stage (CHOPRA and CHOWHAN, 1934; CHOPRA et al., 1935; LEE, 1948; VICK et al., 1967; SKET et al., 1973). The initial arterial hypotension appears to be due to peripheral vasodilatation, especially capillary dilatation in the splanchnic area, since the volume of the intestines is markedly increased, while the limb vessels remain unaffected or even contracted (CHOPRA and CHOWHAN, 1934; CHOPRA et al., 1935; LEE, 1948). That the blood accumulated in the abdominal viscera has also been shown by the fact that in the eviscerated animals or when the splanchnic circulation has been excluded, injection of Russell viper's venom, as well as of *Echis carinatus* venom, produces little or no fall in blood pressure (CHOPRA and CHOWHAN, 1934; CHOPRA et al., 1935; VICK et al., 1967). As described previously (B. I), the site of initial decrease in peripheral resistance produced by most crotalid venoms appears to occur in the skeletal muscle vasculature rather than in the splanchnic circulation. There is so far no explanation for such differences between venoms of these two groups.

II. Venom Components Responsible for the Hypotensive Action

So far no purified toxin responsible for the hypotensive action has been isolated from viper venoms, except viperotoxin from *Vipera palestinae* venom (MOROZ et al., 1966). A basic protein fraction, which produces a rapid fall in the arterial blood pressure, has been isolated from *Vipera ammodytes* venom (SKET et al., 1973), but this fraction is a mixture of three proteins and is less active than the crude venom.

The role played by kinin-releasing enzymes (kininogenases) in the hypotensive effect of viperid venoms is apparently much less important as compared with crotalid venoms, since viperid venoms have in general much lower kinin-forming activity than crotalid venoms (see Chap. 16). In line with this contention is the finding that heat treatment (80° C for 30 min) did not appreciably affect the hypotensive activity of Russell's viper venom (LEE, 1944, 1948). Apparently this venom contains a heatstable toxin which may act on the capillary vascular bed, especially in the splanchnic area.

Cardiovascular Effects of Elapid and Sea Snake Venoms

Although the primary cause of death in envenomation by elapid and sea snakes has been shown to be peripheral respiratory paralysis in many species of animals (see LEE, 1972), these venoms also produce cardiovascular changes. Since the elapid and sea snake venoms have either very little or no proteolytic enzyme activity, the cardiovascular changes produced by these venoms are in general not as profound as those produced by crotalid or viperid venoms. Moreover, because of the presence of highly neurotoxic components, it is generally overlooked that circulatory collapse may be also a cause of death in some elapid envenomations. For instance, cats poisoned with cobra venom may die of cardiac failure rather than respiratory paralysis (EPSTEIN, 1930; LEE and PENG, 1961) and the venom of spitting cobra *(Naja nigricollis)* invariably causes a profound cardiovascular depression predominating over its paralytic action on envenomated animals (CHEYMOL et al., 1966).

A. Cobra (Naja) Venoms

I. Action on the Heart

One of the earliest studies done on the pharmacologic action of cobra venom was that by BRUNTON and FAYRER (1873). They considered that cobra venom acted on the cerebro-spinal nerve centers, and in large doses it also acted on the ganglia of the heart, causing arrest of cardiac action; little stress was laid on the role played by circulatory failure. They were unable to come to any definite conclusion as to the exact influence of the venom on the heart, but they thought that the heart's arrest in systole, which they at times observed, was due to "... some action on the cardiac ganglia." RAGOTZI (1890) observed that large doses of cobra venom stopped the frog heart in systole. In the mammal, strong doses of venom lessened the amount of the heart's movements, while smaller doses increased it. To kill the heart in diastole, small doses, subcutaneously given, were required. He surmised that "systolic death" must be due to a direct action of the venom on the heart muscle, and that "diastolic death" is to be attributed to paralysis of the "intracardiac ganglia." However, VOLLMER (1893) found that the venom also produced systolic arrest after subcutaneous application. ELLIOT (1905) found that cobra venom acted directly on the isolated frog ventricle, killing it in a position of firm systole if the solution was concentrated, and stimulating it if a weaker strength was employed. He compared this action of cobra venom with that of strophanthin, a glucoside of the digitalis group, finding that its action was more rapid than that of strophanthin, and was not inferior to it in strength. Atropine and cobra venom, when acting in the same solution, intensified each other's action; the total effect was greater than one would have anticipated. He also found that cobra venom powerfully affected the isolated mammalian (cat and rabbit) heart when solutions of it were perfused through the coronary circulation. With strong solutions, he found an irregular and extreme excitation of the heart, followed by early death in a position of systolic tone. If the concentration was less, the early stage of excitement yielded to a prolonged phase, in which the tonic action of the venom on the heart was most pronounced; the beat became regular, steady, and strong. CUSHNY and YAGI (1918), in agreement with ELLIOTT (1905), also observed that cobra venom produced a transient augmentation of the amplitude of ventricular contractions, followed by progressive diminution in the isolated frog heart as well as in the rabbit heart in situ. MANWARING and WILLIAMS (1923) observed that cobra venom produces decreased myocardial contractions, occasionally preceded by a preliminary period of increased contractions in the perfused rabbit heart. The depressant effect is progressive, ending in complete cessation of heart beats, usually first in the left ventricle, somewhat later in the right ventricle and, after a delay of several minutes, in the atria. The myocardial tone is progressively increased, leading to systolic contracture. These authors further observed seasonal variations in cardiac resistance to cobra venom; the isolated rabbit heart showed a distinct resistance during the summer months, but a hypersusceptibility during the winter months. EPSTEIN (1930) reported that large doses of Cape cobra venom produced systolic arrest of frog heart in vivo as well as in vitro, and that smaller lethal doses caused the ventricle to cease in diastole. In the isolated frog heart, the amplitude showed a slight preliminary increase, soon followed by a marked diminution, chiefly the result of a lessened relaxation, and the ventricle finally ceased in systole. An increase in tone of the muscle was produced. Changes in the rate were not marked and irregularities in rhythm were seldom observed. Similar results were obtained in the isolated mammalian heart, but the heart of the cat was about four times more resistant toward Cape cobra venom than the heart of the rabbit. GUNN and HEATHCOTE (1921) had reported a similar result. CHOPRA and ISWARIAH (1931) studied the effect of the Indian cobra venom on the hearts of kittens and rabbits and also found that the isolated heart of the kitten was more resistant to the Indian cobra venom than the heart of the rabbit. In neither species did any concentration of the venom, high or low, produce any definite stimulation of the heart either by its action on the sympathetic nervous system or direct action on the myocardium. With lethal doses given intravenously, the heart stopped in a short time, the atria and the ventricles at first beating slowly and irregularly and finally stopping in a condition of partial systole. IWASE (1933) also could not find any stimulatory effect of the Formosan cobra venom on the isolated rabbit heart, although he, cf. NAKAMURA (1933), observed a pronounced stimulation of the isolated frog heart with low concentrations of this venom. However, GAUTRELET et al. (1934) observed that intravenous injection of the Indian cobra venom (0.2 mg/kg) in a dog caused a marked augmentation of the amplitude of ventricular contraction with some extrasystoles. GOTTDENKER and WACHSTEIN (1940) confirmed the findings of earlier workers that cobra venom causes enfeeblement of the contractions, leading to systolic contracture in the isolated frog heart. Immediately after the addition of the venom to the perfusion fluid there was occasionally some augmentation of the contractions, followed by a diminution of diastole, and finally the heart passed into a systolic contracture. The atria remained dilated, but later on also passed into systolic contracture. In the absence of calcium ions in the perfusion fluid, the cardiac muscle became less sensitive to the venom, which produced stoppage of beat without signs of systolic contracture. They also observed that cobra venom caused systolic standstill of the atrial strip of the rabbit's and guinea-pig's heart and of the fiber of Purkinje of the dog's heart. The systolic contracture was irreversible even when the bath fluid was repeatedly changed to venom free salt solution with or without adrenaline. Weaker concentrations of venom (up to 1 in 10 millions) caused an initial diminution of the contractions, followed by great augmentation without any change in frequency in the atrial strip preparation. PENG (1951 a) reported that the venom of *Naja naja atra* as well as its cardiotoxic fraction (D' fraction) caused an initial augmentation of frog heart contractions, followed by a diminution of diastole and sometimes arrhythmia. The ventricle finally stopped in systole while the atria continued beating for some time. ZAKI et al. (1967) also found that *Naja naja* venom caused an initial augmentation of toad heart contractions, followed by gradual paralysis leading to complete stoppage of the heart in systole. These authors suggested that the initial augmentation of the heart contractions might be due to cholinesterase, while cardiotoxin caused the inhibition of heart contraction leading to complete and irreversible paralysis.

In the rabbit, GUNN and HEATHCOTE (1921) obtained strong constriction of the coronary vessels when the isolated heart was perfused with salt solution containing venom in a concentration of 1 in 600000. In similar experiments on the cat's heart the venom caused vasodilatation. FELDBERG and KELLAWAY (1938) also obtained mainly vasodilator effects when large doses of venom were injected into the cat's heart perfused with salt solution, although with a large initial coronary flow the venom usually caused vasoconstriction. GOTTDENKER and WACHSTEIN (1940) found that in the heart lung preparation of the dog, the injection of cobra venom (60 μg) produced long-lasting dilatation of the coronary vessels, which could readily be desensitized against the venom by first injecting a subthreshold dose. The action of venom on the coronary vessels resembles that of histamine, which also constricts the coronary vessels in the rabbit and dilates those in the cat and dog. The similarity might be due to the fact that the venom acts on the coronary vessels by releasing histamine (FELDBERG and KELLAWAY, 1937a, b, c, 1938; FELDEBERG et al., 1938), or it might only indicate that in these animals the coronary vessels respond to a variety of stimuli in the same manner (GOTTDENKER and WACHSTEIN, 1940).

Electrocardiographic studies on the effect of cobra venom were made by several workers. GAUTRELET et al. (1934) observed that intravenous injection of 0.2 mg/kg of cobra venom in the dog is followed by the appearance of extrasystoles. BEERENS and CUYPERS (1935) described the following changes in the rabbit and guinea-pig heart after intravenous injection of nonlethal doses of cobra venom: sinus bradycardia, T wave changes, S–T segment depression, atrial flutter, extrasystoles, ventricular bigeminy, slow ventricular rhythm, and A–V dissociation. FELDBERG and KELLAWAY (1937b) analysed the electrocardiographic changes produced by intravenous injection of large doses (1.5–2 mg/kg) of cobra venom in dogs. Their results are summarized as follows: The first changes to be noted, occurring within a minute or two of the injection, are in the form of the T wave. Next, the P–R interval becomes progressively longer and the ventricular complexes wider. The development of aberrant ventricular complexes may follow, sometimes preceded by a great diminution in the voltage of the ventricular complexes, or an abrupt onset of heart block occurs. This may originally be partial, 2:1 or 3:1, but usually becomes complete. Ventricular tachycardia and fibrillation may also occur. The toxic effects of the venom on the atria are longer delayed than those on the conducting tissues and on the ventricles. In the late stage the P waves are reduced in voltage and sometimes disappear altogether. AMUCHASTEGUI (1940) reported similar results in dogs. KELLAWAY and TRETHEWIE (1940) observed the following changes in the rabbit heart: bradycardia, increased P–R interval, S–T deviation, and terminal heart block. In cats, they observed increased heart rate, inversion of T wave, prominent P wave, extrasystoles, increased P–R interval, aberrant QRS–T complex resembling bundle branch block, and ventricular fibrillation. LEE et al. (1971) found similar electrocardiographic changes in cats after intravenous injection of the Formosan cobra venom. Thus, although the changes in the electrocardiograms are somewhat different from one species to another, they all show impairment of conduction and myocardial damage as the dominant features of the action of the venom.

II. Cardiotoxin and its Action on the Heart

GHOSH et al. (1941) isolated from the Indian cobra venom various enzymes together with neurotoxin and hemolysin (phospholipase A), and the effects of neurotoxin, hemolysin, and choline-esterase on heart, blood pressure, and respiration were studied by SARKAR et al. (1942). Their results are summarized as follows: Cobra venom in small doses stimulates the perfused toad's heart, after large doses stimulation is followed by depression, irregularities, and eventual stoppage in systole. Purified neurotoxin acts similarly, except that its does not cause stoppage even when administered in large doses. In rabbits neurotoxin has little effect on blood pressure, but eventually paralyzes respiration. Purified hemolysin produces augmentation in the toad heart followed by depression and irregularity, but no cardiac failure; large doses in rabbits and guinea-pigs cause both circulatory and respiratory failure. Large amounts of choline esterase stimulate the toad heart slightly, but have little effect on the blood pressure and respiration of rabbits. Apparently the neurotoxin and hemolysin purified by these authors were incompletely separated from the cardiotoxic component, since more recent studies by TSENG (1964) and LEE et al. (1968) demonstrated that neither cobra neurotoxin nor phospholipase A separated from the venom of *Naja naja atra* produced any cardiotoxic effects on the frog heart with concentrations of up to 10^{-4} g/ml. In addition to the neurotoxin, hemolysin, and choline esterase, a new principle, "cardiotoxin," responsible for the cardiac failure was separated from Indian cobra venom by fractional precipitation (SARKAR, 1947a). SARKAR (1947b) estimated its molecular weight to be about 46200 by a diffusion method, but it was subsequently shown to be not a single protein (RAUDONAT and HOLLER, 1958; TSENG, 1964). Using gradient chromatography on a CM-Sephadex column, three cardiotoxic fractions were separated from the venom of *Naja naja atra* (LO et al., 1966; LEE et al., 1968), together constituting more than 50% of the venom protein. After repeated rechromatography on a CM-cellulose column, the major cardiotoxic fraction was found to be free from phospholipase A activity, and its homogeneity was verified by disc gel electrophoresis, sedimentation velocity, amino acids analysis, and end group analysis. Molecular weight of this cardiotoxin was estimated to be about 6000 by sedimentation equilibrium method and its amino acid sequence was determined (NARITA and LEE, 1970). Subsequently, more than 20 homologous toxins have been isolated from venoms of various cobra species, ringhals, and mambas (see Chap. 5).

The action of cardiotoxins on the isolated frog heart resembles that of crude cobra venom. They cause augmentation of systole at low concentrations and systolic contracture at high concentrations (SARKAR, 1951; DEVI and SARKAR, 1966; LEE et al., 1968). It has been suggested that cardiotoxin has a digitalislike action (SARKAR, 1951). However, in the rat atrium, the positive inotropic effect of cardiotoxin is quite transient and soon followed by depression. In cats, neither consistent enhancement of contractility of the heart nor a shortening of Q–T interval is observed with cardiotoxin (LEE et al., 1968). Electrophysiological studies by LEE and CHIU (1971) and HO et al. (1975) show that the transmembrane potential of myocardial cells is irreversibly decreased by cardiotoxin. The decrease in maximum diastolic repolarization of the pacemaker type cells occurs much later and to a much lesser extent. Associated with the decrease of resting potential, the magnitude and rate of rise of the action potential, the overshoot, the time to 80% repolarization, and the spike ionic conductance are also decreased. The effect of the toxin on the membrane potential is not altered by either tetrodotoxin or sodium removal, but is inhibited by high calcium (HO et al., 1975). TAZIEFF-DEPIERRE and TRETHEWIE (1975) also found that $CaCl_2$ decreased the cardiotoxicity in the rat of the purified γ-toxin (cardiotoxin) isolated from the venom of *Naja nigricollis*. Injection of γ-toxin (1 mg/kg) into rats caused arrhythmia followed by death several minutes later. Pretreatment with $CaCl_2$ (10 or 20 mg/kg) prevented the subsequent cardiotoxic effects of even up to four doses of the toxin. When $CaCl_2$ was injected after the toxin, but before appearance of arrhythmia, the induced cardiac disorders were only transient. When $CaCl_2$ was injected later, the animal survived, but arrhythmia were severe and long lasting.

III. Hemodynamic Effects

The old literatures on the hemodynamic effects of various cobra venoms are numerous and sometimes conflicting (see LEE, 1971). The most prominent and constant hemodynamic change produced by crude cobra venom in general is a fall in systemic arterial pressure, sometimes preceded by an initial transient rise if the venom is administered intravenously. The animals may die of cardiac failure within several minutes if the dose is large enough, or the blood pressure may recover to its previous level and remain steady until an asphyxial rise in blood pressure occurs immediately before respiratory arrest. This secondary rise in arterial pressure, accompanied by marked bradycardia, progresses gradually and parallel with the development of respiratory paralysis. Soon after the complete cessation of respiratory movements, the blood pressure falls again abruptly and the heart usually continues to beat for many minutes. If asphyxia is prevented by artificial respiration, the blood pressure may be maintained for hours in most animal species except the cat and then gradually fall until the animal expires due to cardiac failure.

1. Pressor Effect

ELLIOT (1905) observed in rabbits that when the dose of cobra venom was a low one and gradually given, the blood pressure rose steadily from the beginning, and sometimes attained very high levels. He concluded that the high level of blood pressure was due to: (1) the direct action of the circulating venom on the muscular tissue of the arterioles, causing a constriction of these vessels; (2) the increased force of the heart beat as the outcome of the direct stimulating action of the venom on the myocardium; and (3) the stimulation of the vasomotor center as a result of the steadily increasing venosity of the blood. The last factor may be responsible for the asphyxial increase in blood pressure before respiratory arrest, but certainly not for the immediate initial rise in blood pressure. CUSHNY and YAGI (1918) reported that with the blood vessels of frogs and rabbits there was marked constriction of the vessels when the venom was added to the Ringer's solution perfused through them, and that the venom acted more peripherally than adrenaline on the muscle walls, since the addition of ergotoxine to the perfusing fluid abolished the action of adrenaline on the vessels while leaving the action of the venom unchanged. The action of the venom, therefore, appears to be directly upon the muscle itself, resulting in the tonic contraction of the muscle. EPSTEIN (1930) also reported that a slight rise in blood pressure was usually observed in cats and rabbits, after small intravenous doses (e.g., 0.1 mg/kg) of the Cape cobra *(Naja nivea)* venom. He also found vasoconstriction of the frog's blood vessels perfused with solutions of 1–40000 cobra venom. CHOPRA and ISWARIAH (1931) reported that the Indian cobra venom sometimes caused a fall and sometimes a rise of blood pressure in cats anesthetized with urethane. A dose of 0.3–0.7 mg of venom invariably produced a small rise in blood pressure. Up to a certain point the blood pressure rose in proportion to the dose. The rise in blood pressure after injections of sublethal doses of the venom was not due to any stimulant action on the accelerator mechanism of the heart or on the myocardium. They attributed it to the stimulation of the vasomotor center in the medulla, as it was absent in decerebrated animals. VENTAKACHALAM and RATNAGIRISWARAN (1934) stated that only certain samples of the Indian cobra venom, and at some undetermined stage of their keeping, were observed to produce the marked rise in blood pressure. They suggested that this rise was due to the combined effects of the venom in causing stimulation of the myocardium, asphyxia consequent to the narrowing of the lumen of the bronchi, and general vascular constriction. GOTTDENKER and WACHSTEIN (1940) reported that in cats and rabbits the intravenous injection of a small dose of Indian cobra venom caused a long-lasting rise in arterial blood pressure, occasionally preceded by an evanescent depressor effect. They used exceedingly minute doses (6–9 μg/kg) which were considered to be subeffective doses by most other workers. Since weak concentrations of venom caused vasoconstriction in the rabbit's ear perfused with physiological salt solution, they were in favor of a direct peripheral vasoconstriction as the cause of the rise in pressure. FELDBERG and KELLAWAY (1937b) also concluded that the vasoconstriction observed in the ileum and hind limb after the arterial injection of cobra venom suffices to explain both the initial transient pressor response preceding the main fall in systemic arterial pressure caused by the intravenous injection of a first large dose of venom, and the more pronounced pressor effect of a second dose. The results of experiments in which the animals were desensitized against the vasodilator action of the venom and responded by vasoconstriction to a second large dose suggest that the constrictor actions of this venom may be caused by the presence of an active principle distinct from that which causes vasodilatation. More recently LEE et al. (1971) have compared the hemodynamic effects of cardiotoxin purified from the venom of *Naja naja atra* (LEE et al., 1968) with those of the crude venom. They observed that the purified cardiotoxin (1.0 mg/kg i.v.) produced a transient rise in systemic arterial pressure followed by a progressive decline leading to cardiac arrest in cats, whereas the crude venom (0.5–1.0 mg/kg) caused a precipitous fall without an initial rise in arterial pressure. However, a pressor effect was also observed with the crude venom when a second larger dose was given after the depressor effect of the previous injection of a smaller dose had subsided. They concluded that the pressor response was due to peripheral vasoconstriction caused by cardiotoxin, since total peripheral resistance was increased and cardiac output decreased by cardiotoxin. No other fraction from cobra venom has been found to produce a pressor effect in cats (LEE, CHIU and LEE, unpublished).

2. Depressor Effect

a) Analysis of the Initial Depressor Effect

The primary hypotensive effect of cobra venom is peripheral in nature (GAUTRELET et al., 1934; PENG, 1952; BHANGANADA and PERRY, 1963), although some early authors attributed it either partly or entirely to a central action (ELLIOT, 1905; CHOPRA and ISWARIAH, 1931). ELLIOT (1905) suggested that the early fall produced by cobra venom in large doses was due to inhibition of the heart, which was mainly brought about by the direct action of the venom on the vagal centers, whereas CHOPRA and ISWARIAH (1931) claimed that the fall in blood pressure with large doses was mainly due to paralysis of the vasomotor center, since in decerebrated animals kept alive with artificial respiration, the venom produced no fall in blood pressure. However, ELLIOT (1905) tested the activity of the vasomotor center in the rabbit by stimulating in turn the depressor and sciatic nerves in animals which were in various stages of cobraism and found that a marked response was elicited in both cases until death. Therefore, he concluded that the vasomotor center was not markedly affected by cobra venom, confirming the early work by RAGOTZI (1890) who also found that the vasomotor center remained active until the end stage of cobraism. ELLIOT (1905), while suggesting the central vagal effect of cobra venom, also stated that the cutting off of central vagal impulses from the heart, either by the severance of the vagi or by the use of atropine, did not stop the progress of inhibition, though greatly retarded it; the heart rate still declined, and the blood pressure fell in spite of these measures. GAUTRELET et al. (1934) also found that in dogs, section of vago-sympathetics or atropine pretreatment did not prevent the hypotensive effect of cobra venom. Using the crossed cephalic circulation technique, they observed that perfusion of the cranial circulation of the recipient dog with venom-containing blood of the donor dog caused no change in arterial pressure in the rest of the body of the recipient dog. BHANGANADA and PERRY (1963) made a similar observation. PENG (1952) reported that cobra venom injected into the cerebellomedullary cistern caused a rise, instead of a fall, in the arterial blood pressure. All of these findings indicate that the mechanism of the initial fall in blood pressure is not central in origin. Moreover, neither the carotid sinus reflex nor the aortic reflex plays a role in the mechanism of hypotensive action of cobra venom, since destruction of both carotid sinuses and cutting of the depressor nerves do not alter the hypotensive action of the venom (GAUTRELET et al., 1934; PENG, 1952).

The initial precipitous fall in arterial pressure produced by cobra venom has been attributed to: (1) vasodilatation in the periphery (GAUTRELET et al., 1934; PENG, 1952; BHANGANADA and PERRY, 1963), combined with constriction of the hepatic veins, especially in dogs (FELDBERG and KELLAWAY, 1937b); (2) a pronounced pulmonary vasoconstriction, especially in cats (YONEGAWA, 1926; FELDBERG and KELLAWAY, 1937a; CHIU et al., 1968; LEE et al., 1971), or (3) a direct venom action on the heart (ELLIOT, 1905; AMUCHASTEGUI, 1940; DEVI and SARKAR, 1966; PHILLIPS, 1972).

Apparently, there are some species differences in vascular response to cobra venom. In cats, the immediate steep fall in systemic blood pressure produced by cobra venom can be accounted for by constriction of the pulmonary vessels without the participation of hepatic obstruction, peripheral vasodilatation, or heart failure (YONEGAWA, 1926; FELDBERG and KELLAWAY, 1937a; LEE et al., 1971). In dogs, the lung vessels are not constricted by cobra venom, and the fall in arterial pressure results from peripheral vasodilatation (GAUTRELET et al., 1934; FELDBERG and KELLAWAY, 1937b; BHANGANADA and PERRY, 1963) being accentuated by constriction of the hepatic veins (FELDBERG and KELLAWAY, 1937b). According to FELDBERG and KELLAWAY (1937a, b), in both species the depressor effect is accompanied by loss of fluid from circulation, but whereas in cats, part of the fluid loss is accounted for by edema of the lungs, in dogs, edema of the lungs is absent, and the whole of the fluid loss must be attributed to changes in the permeability of the capillaries of the general circulation. Despite the differences between the circulatory effects of cobra venom in the cat and dog, there are many points of resemblance. In both animals, the venom has a powerful toxic action upon the heart which may prove fatal after large doses. In both, a first dose of the venom has a desensitizing action, and a second large dose causes a rise instead of a fall in blood pressure. In both, the capillaries are dilated by the venom, and an increase in their permeability is indicated by the fluid loss from circulation. Although the venous outflow from the cat's limb was decreased and that from the dog's limb was increased after arterial injections of small doses of venom, the capillaries may have been dilated in both, and the difference is accounted for by reactions on the arterial side of the vascular tree, which is constricted in the cat and dilated in the dog. Even in the dog, large doses of venom decrease the venous outflow from the limb. Differences in the reactions of the arterial side of the vascular tree are therefore in part quantitative rather than qualitative (FELDBERG and KELLAWAY, 1937b). This interpretation of the vascular effects of the venom has much in common with that given for histamine, which constricts the arterioles in the cat and dilates them in the dog, but causes dilatation of the capillaries in both species (DALE and RICHARDS, 1918).

In rabbits, the Formosan cobra venom also caused a rise in pulmonary arterial blood pressure, but the rise was usually preceded by a preliminary fall which was apparently due to a fall in the systemic blood pressure. In the splanchnic area the venom caused an increase of the liver volume, a rise in the portal pressure, an increase of the intestinal volume, and a decrease of the kidney volume. The limb vessels showed a transient dilatation. From these findings, PENG (1952) concluded that the fall in blood pressure in rabbits injected with the Formosan cobra venom was chiefly due to vasodilatation in the splanchnic area as well as in the skin and muscles, since the time course of pulmonary constriction observed in this animal species did not correspond to that of the fall in systemic arterial blood pressure.

The vascular effect of cobra venom has been largely explained by a liberation of histamine in the body by the action of phospholipase A present in the venom (FELDBERG and KELLAWAY, 1938; FELDBERG et al., 1938; HÖGBERG and UVNÄS, 1960; WESTERMANN and KLAPPER, 1960), but there is evidence that not only phospholipase A but also the direct lytic factor (cardiotoxin) of cobra venom can release histamine (KAISER et al., 1972; DAMERAU et al., 1975). Moreover, besides histamine, other vasoactive principles such as serotonin and "slow reacting substance" (SRS-C), consisting mainly of prostaglandins, are also released from tissues by cobra venom (see Chap. 16). However, unlike crotalid and viperid venoms, cobra and other elapid venoms do not release bradykinin, since they have either very low or no kinin-forming activity (MEBS, 1968, 1970; OSHIMA et al., 1969).

b) Venom Components Responsible for the Initial Depressor Effect

Only a few investigations of the circulatory effects of purified components from cobra venoms have been reported. Cobra neurotoxin has been found to be devoid of any appreciable effect on systemic blood pressure, except for the asphyxial rise before respiratory arrest (SARKAR et al., 1942; LEE, 1965). Cardiotoxin isolated from the Formosan cobra venom was first found to cause a fall in systemic arterial blood pressure and various EKG changes, leading to cardiac failure in cats (LEE et al., 1968). Later experiments with more purified cardiotoxin, free from traces of phospholipase A activity, revealed that cardiotoxin (1 mg/kg) caused an initial rise in systemic blood pressure followed by a more sustained decline leading to cardiac arrest. Whereas the pulmonary artery pressure was markedly increased by cobra venom, it was increased only slightly by cardiotoxin (CHIU et al., 1968; LEE et al., 1971). In search of the component(s) responsible for the initial depressor action of cobra venom, LEE, CHIU and LEE (unpublished) compared the hemodynamic effects of purified cardiotoxin and phospholipase A with those of the whole cobra venom in cats. As summarized in Table 1, the hemodynamic effects of phospholipase A were in general more similar to those of the whole cobra venom as compared with cardiotoxin, although phospholipase A was less toxic than either the whole venom or cardiotoxin. However, apparently neither phospholipase A nor cardiotoxin alone is responsible for the initial hemodynamic effect of cobra venom. Probably, the combined action of phospholipase A and cardiotoxin is responsible for the initial depressor action. In line with this contention is the finding that phospholipase A and cardiotoxin are synergistic in releasing histamine (DAMERAU et al., 1975).

Table 1. Comparison of hemodynamic effects of Fromosan cobra venom and its components (1 mg/kg) within 1 min after i. v. injection

	Mean % changes (± S.E.)		
	Whole venom	Cardiotoxin	Phospholipase A
Carotid arterial pressure	− 42.3± 5.7 (n=14)	+24.1± 9.5 (n=13)	− 21.4± 1.3 (n=8)
Heart rate	+ 9.9± 2.8 (n= 6) − 14.9± 4.0 (n= 8)	− 5.4± 3.5 (n=13)	− 2.0± 2.3 (n=8)
Cardiac output	− 49.3±11.6 (n= 6)	−25.6± 7.0 (n= 6)	− 38.0± 0.8 (n=5)
Stroke volume	− 44.7±13.0 (n= 6)	−22.8± 5.7 (n= 6)	− 37.0± 0.7 (n=5)
Pulmonary arterial pressure	+123.5±16.9 (n=10)	+22.6±10.7 (n= 6)	+ 57.6± 1.1 (n=8)
Pulmonary vascular resistance	+286.2±89.4 (n= 4)	+37.0±10.7 (n= 5)	+192.2± 1.3 (n=5)
Femoral artery flow	− 54.0± 0.6 (n= 4)	−32.9± 1.3 (n= 3)	− 26.7± 1.0 (n=3)
Total peripheral resistance	+ 51.8± 1.8 (n= 4) − 25.1± 1.1 (n= 2)	+32.3±11.9 (n= 6)	+ 24.8± 1.6 (n=5)
Death time (min)	30.7± 9.9 (n= 9)	36.3±11.1 (n= 9)	79.2±14.1 (n=5)[a]

+ Increase
− Decrease.
[a] Five out of eight cats died within 2 h.
Figures in parentheses denote the number of experiments.
LEE, C. Y., CHIU, T. H. and LEE, S. Y. (unpublished data).

B. Other Elapid Venoms

I. Krait (Bungarus) Venoms

ROGERS (1905) reported that the venom of banded krait *(Bungarus fasciatus)* produces a marked fall in blood pressure very shortly after intravenous injection of the venom in both rabbits and cats, whereas only a slight fall in blood pressure is observed with the venom of *Bungarus caeruleus*. As in the case of cobra venom, the blood pressure always rises during the asphyxial stage following the cessation of respiration and subsequently falls again at the time of death. However, in contrast to the cases of most elapid venoms, artificial respiration after the cessation of natural breathing failed to keep the circulation going in the case of *Bungarus fasciatus* venom. Heating the venom to 90° C for 30 s (or 73–75° C for 30 min) had the effect of greatly lessening the action of the venom in causing a fall in blood pressure, while it did not reduce its action on respiration. In the experiment with the heated venom, artificial respiration had a much more marked effect in maintaining the blood pressure than in the experiment with unheated venom. Based on these findings, ROGERS (1905) concluded that the venom of *Bungarus fasciatus* contains a mixture of viperine and colubrine (elapid) elements, the former being much more readily destroyed by heat, and thus closely resembles the venom of the Australian snake, *Pseudechis porphyracus*, as reported by MARTIN (1895). The so-called viperine element might be identical with the cardiotoxic principle, recently isolated from this venom by LIN SHIAU et al. (1972, 1975). LEE and PENG (1961) observed that the venom of *Bungarus multicinctus* causes a sharp fall in arterial blood pressure in dogs and cats, followed by a period of partial recovery and then an asphyxial rise immediately before respiratory arrest. Under artificial respiration, the blood pressure can be maintained for many hours in both animal species. Neither α- nor β-bungarotoxins isolated from this venom (CHANG and LEE, 1963; LEE et al., 1972) produce any circulatory effects under artificial respiration (LEE and TSAI, unpublished data). The fall in blood pressure produced by these *Bungarus* venoms is probably due to phospholipase A; it has also been demonstrated that these venoms are capable of liberating histamine from the tissues (DUTTA and NARAYANA, 1954; CHIANG et al., 1964).

II. Mamba (Dendroaspis) Venoms

PETKOVIC et al. (1971) reported that an intravenous injection of 0.5 mg/kg of the black mamba *(Dendroaspis polylepis)* venom caused a triphasic response in rabbits. There was a sudden fall in arterial blood pressure followed in 15–20 s by a rapid recovery and a rise in the pressure above the original level. This rise in blood pressure lasted for about 15 s, and then there was a gradual and continuous fall in blood pressure. These changes could not be prevented by atropine or antihistamines. These authors also observed that the black mamba venom had a depressant effect on both the mammalian and frog hearts: it produced a reduction in the amplitude and rate of contractions. High concentrations of the venom caused stoppage of the heart in diastole. The effect of this venom on the heart was not irreversible as there was always recovery after washing. OSMAN et al. (1973) have studied circulatory effects of the green mamba *(Dendroaspis angusticeps)* venom. In doses of 0.05–0.2 mg/kg it produced an immediate sharp fall in the arterial blood pressure of cats, which returned only partially toward the normal level within 1–2 min, and remained at this level for more than 30 min. The hypotensive effect of the crude venom was largely due to acetylcholine since it was blocked by atropine. WELSH (1967) reported that the green mamba venom contains exceptionally large amounts of acetylcholine. The dialysed and desalted venom which contains little or no acetylcholine produced only a slight hypotension, but markedly potentiated the effect of subsequent doses of acetylcholine. It appears that the green mamba venom contains component(s) which potentiate and prolong the action of acetylcholine present in this venom. These authors also observed that the green mamba venom in large doses produced a direct depression of the isolated rabbit and guinea-pig hearts which was not mediated through cholinergic receptors. TELANG et al. (1976b) reported that intravenous injection of the venom of *Dendroaspis jamesoni* in a dose of 1 mg into the cat produced a steep fall in blood pressure within 1 min and was accompanied by bradycardia, while administration of 0.1 mg of venom did not produce any perceptible change in blood pressure or heart rate. Although the blood pressure recovered partially, it did not return to normal levels even after 60 min. Intravenous administration of the venom (1 mg) in cats 1 h after pretreatment with propantheline produced only a small fall in blood pressure and heart rate. Propantheline is a quaternary ammonium compound with powerful antimuscarinic actions; it does not readily penetrate the blood-brain barrier. Thus, the attenuation of cardiovascular response to intravenous injection of the venom must be due to blockade of muscarinic sites in the heart and blood vessels by propantheline. The venom itself has been found to contain acetylcholine or an acetylcholinelike material (TELANG et al., 1976a) besides neurotoxins and cytotoxins (cardiotoxins) (see Chap. 5). TELANG et al. (1976a) also observed that lateral ventricular administration of the venom (100 μg) in cats produced a persistent fall in blood pressure and bradycardia, which returned gradually to normal levels after about 1 h. No hypotension or bradycardia occurred after the perfusate was tapped through the caudal end of the aqueduct of Sylvius. The cardiovascular response was again observed after injecting venom into the third ventricle and tapping the perfusate through the cisterna magna. Injection of venom directly into the cisterna magna did not produce any cardiovascular response. Thus, the site of action of the venom appeared to be on the floor of the fourth ventricle, possibly the vasomotor center. These authors suggested that a small portion of the intravenously administered venom may penetrate the blood-brain barrier to reach the crucial sites in the central nervous system, since injection of the venom into the vertebral artery produced hypotension and bradycardia in a dose one-tenth of that required to produce the same effect by the intravenous route. On the other hand, from the results obtained after bilateral vagotomy, removal of both stellate ganglia, and transection of the spinal cord (C-2), they also concluded that the efferent nervous pathway for the central cardiovascular effects of the venom is the sympathetic nervous system. If so, the cardiovascular effects of the venom by the intravenous route should be peripheral rather than central in origin, since these effects were mostly blocked by propantheline which does not readily penetrate the blood-brain barrier.

III. Coral Snake (Micrurus) Venoms

WEIS and MCISAAC (1971) reported that the venom of the eastern coral snake (*Micrurus fulvius*) produced a rapid fall in blood pressure followed by a gradual recovery toward the normal level, but cats supported by artificial respiration died eventually through cardiac depression. The electrocardiogram showed elevation of S-T segments, biphasic T waves, and low voltage, as seen in myocardial injury or myocarditis, 1–2 h after the start of the venom infusion. They also observed that ventricular muscle strips cut from rat hearts were readily depressed by the venom with a time course similar to skeletal muscle depression. Thus, *Micrurus fulvius* venom appears to contain, besides the curarimimetic toxin, a fraction which acts in a fashion anologous in some respects to the cardiotoxin portion of cobra venom. RAMSEY et al. (1972) studied hemodynamic changes following infusion of lethal doses of *Micrurus f. fulvius* venom into dogs. Intravenous venom injection produced a precipitous fall in aortic pressure concurrent with a marked reduction in cardiac output and elevation of hepatic and portal vein and pulmonary artery pressures. The onset of the pressure changes occurred within 30 s after injection and was maximal by 5–8 min following which the pressures and cardiac outputs returned toward control values. The amplitude of myocardial contraction initially increased within 5 min of venom injection, then progressively declined with eventual systolic arrest. Hind limb resistance was initially reduced following envenomation, but by 5 min hind limb resistance recovered to above the control level and remained elevated for the rest of the observation period. These alterations were followed by interference with myocardial contraction resulting in death despite controlled ventilation. These authors concluded that the initial profound decreases in cardiac output and aortic pressure occur secondary to sequestration of venous return in the hepatosplanchnic bed. The increase in pulmonary artery pressure may serve as a contributory factor in the initial sequestration of blood and subsequent reduction in cardiac output.

IV. Australian Elapid Venoms

Although most of the Australian snake venoms, like tiger snake *(Notechis scutatus)*, taipan *(Oxyuranus scutellatus)*, death adder *(Acanthophis antarcticus)*, and brown snake *(Demansia textilis)*, are powerfully neurotoxic, some of them also produce profound cardiovascular effects. MARTIN (1895) first reported that the venom of the Australian black snake *(Pseudechis porphyriacus)* produces a sudden great fall in the arterial blood pressure in dogs following the intravenous injection. The initial fall in blood pressure may be only temporary, and in the course of a few minutes to 1 h may rise again to nearly the normal level. However, this recovery does not last long if a fatal dose is injected; the pressure declines again until the animal dies. This fatal fall in blood pressure also invariably occurs in those cases where artificial respiration is maintained. Since, in dogs with severed cervical cord, the venom produced precisely similar results to those obtained with normal dogs, and the fall in blood pressure was accompanied by a simultaneous and equally abrupt diminution in the volume of the spleen and kidney, MARTIN (1895) concluded that the fall in blood pressure is mainly due to a direct action of the venom upon the heart. On the other hand, he also observed that the venom produces intravascular clotting when injected intravenously into the dog. Therefore, the sudden fall in blood pressure might be explained at least partly in this way, as in the case of Russell's viper venom. However, TRETHEWIE and DAY (1948) showed that in heparinized cats, the black snake venom still produced a fall in systemic blood pressure, though less pronounced than in nonheparinized cats. Apparently, the venom contains some other constituent(s) which also produce hypotensive effect either directly or by release of pharmacologically active substances from the tissues. It has been demonstrated that histamine and SRS are liberated from the lung of the dog by the powerfully hemolytic black snake venom (TRETHEWIE, 1939).

KELLAWAY and LE MESSURIER (1936) reported that the fall in blood pressure caused by intravenous injection of the venom of Australian copperhead *(Denisonia superba)* is chiefly due to peripheral vasodilation, although lung edema and weakening of heart action may be contributory factors. FELDBERG and KELLAWAY (1937d) further showed that this venom produced a primary shock, followed by a recuperation period and a subsequent phase of secondary shock in cats. The primary shock was characterized by a sharp fall in the systemic blood pressure within 1 min of venom administration. During the recuperation period, blood pressure rose to a high level within 10–30 min, where the pressure remained for 1–2 h before the phase of secondary shock set in. These authors pointed out that this picture reproduced entirely that observed in the dog after the administration of histamine. They also observed that the response of pulmonary artery to venom injection depended upon the dose. Higher doses caused a fall in the pulmonary arterial blood pressure, while smaller doses had the opposite effect. The sensitivity of pulmonary arterial blood pressure to venom action was also found to be correlated with the histamine content of the lungs. A 30–60% increase in hematocrit was found in cats injected with the venom; this venom-induced effect, like the corresponding histamine-induced hemoconcentration, seemed to be due to loss of fluid from the circulation, since a marked lung edema was also found in these experiments. On the other hand, TRETHEWIE and DAY (1948) observed that the rise in pulmonary arterial blood pressure, as well as the fall in systemic pressure, following intravenous injection of the black snake venom in the heparinized cat, was neither abolished nor even reduced by antihistamine, and therefore they concluded that it is unlikely that these effects are due to histamine. Nevertheless, it had been shown that the release of histamine and SRS-C by the powerfully hemolytic black snake venom and the feebly hemolytic death adder *(Acanthophis antarcticus)* venom was proportional to the hemolytic power of the respective venom for the red cells of the dog (TRETHEWIE, 1939). This is considered to lend force to the suggestion that the release of histamine and SRS-C is due to the formation of lysolecithin by phospholipase A, found in all these venoms, which damages the cells and thereby effects their release. The release of histamine was considered in the case of black snake venom to be a contributory cause of death, since it was found that when the clotting effect and the histamine effect were concurrently inhibited, the mortality rate was greatly reduced (TRETHEWIE and DAY, 1948).

C. Sea Snake Venoms

Sea snake venoms are in general highly toxic and produce muscular paralysis and respiratory failure in animals, like venoms of land elapid snakes. These effects have been attributed to neurotoxic components, especially curarimimetic toxins, present in these venoms (see Chap. 5), and besides neurotoxic symptoms, muscle pain, myoglobinuria, and necrosis of skeletal muscle have been reported in human victims bitten by some species of sea snakes (see Chap. 25). Unlike cobra and some other elapid venoms, no cardiotoxin (cytotoxin)-like component has been found in sea snake venoms.

The cardiovascular changes produced by sea snake venoms are in general not pronounced, but the victim may succumb from hyperkalemic cardiac arrest or acute renal failure in protracted poisoning (see Chap. 25). Tu (1967) reported that intravenous injection of 0.1–0.2 mg/kg of *Laticauda laticaudata* venom into rabbits produced a transient fall followed by a gradual rise in arterial blood pressure along with the advance of respiratory depression. The blood pressure fell again after respiration had completely ceased. Cutting of the vagi and administration of atropine prior to venom injection did not alter the venom action. In the isolated frog heart, the venom produced an augmentation of the ventricular contraction. No inhibitory effect was found in cases of perfusion of up to 0.01% of venom solution. The rabbit heart was not affected by the venom. Phillips (1972) also showed that *Laticauda semifasciata* venom (1.0 mg/kg) essentially caused no immediate hemodynamic changes other than an initial blood pressure fall in dogs. Yang and Lee (1978) also obtained similar results with the venom of *Hydrophis cyanocinctus* in rats and cats. While most sea snake venoms so far studied have produced an initial fall in systemic arterial pressure following intravenous administration, the venom of *Pelamis platurus* did not produce any changes in blood pressure, heart rate, and electrocardiogram until asphyxia became apparent when respiration was severely depressed (Tu et al., 1976). The cause of such differences has not been identified but may be related to the content of some constituent of the venom, such as phospholipase A (Lee, 1971).

Summary and Conclusions

A. Crotalid and Viperid Venoms

Circulatory shock with internal hemorrhage is the frequent cause of death in viper bites. In experiments on animals, administration of crotalid and viperid venoms produces a precipitous fall in systemic blood pressure, followed by a partial recovery, but eventually the pressure falls again, terminating with cardiac arrest. Artificial respiration fails to maintain the blood pressure.

The initial hypotensive crisis after crotalid and viperid envenomations is not primarily cardiac in origin, but mainly due to vasodilatation leading to a profound decrease in peripheral vascular resistance. Although opinions of different authors conflict, the site of initial decrease in peripheral resistance produced by most crotalid venoms appears to lie mainly in the skeletal muscle vasculature, whereas most viperid venoms produce capillary dilatation in the splanchnic area rather than in the skeletal muscle. So far no explanation for such differences has been produced.

Although disseminated intravascular clotting is rarely found in viper bites, intravascular clotting has been proved to be the cause of sudden death of animals following injection of high doses of "coagulating venoms." Occasional onset of pulmonary hypertension may be related to the production of thromboembolism in the pulmonary vascular bed.

After the initial changes, venom shock is characterized by prolonged hypotension, decrease in cardiac output, hypovolemia, and hemoconcentration. This secondary shock may be caused by extravasation of plasma or blood into soft tissues and various internal organs. So far, no single component has been identified that may be responsible for the circulatory changes produced by the crude venom. The basic protein toxins isolated from venoms of certain species of rattlesnakes, including the myocardial depressor protein (MDP) from *C. atrox* venom, produce myocardial depression and thus contribute to the overall circulatory collapse produced by these venoms.

The autopharmacologic substances (bradykinin, histamine, serotonin, prostaglandins, etc.) released by venom enzymes, such as proteinases and phospholipase A, could also contribute toward the circulatory changes produced by crotalid and viperid venoms. However, to what extent each of these substances may be responsible for the circulatory changes produced by different venoms is an unsolved problem. The peripheral vasodilatation and increase in capillary permeability could be due to the combined effects of these autopharmacologic substances.

Crotalus durissus terrificus venom is unique among crotalid venoms in containing a potent neurotoxin (crotoxin) which produces respiratory paralysis rather than circulatory failure.

Viperotoxin isolated from *Vipera palestinae* venom has been claimed to act primarily on medullary vasopressor centers leading to circulatory failure. It remains to be proven that viperotoxin can pass through the blood-brain barrier in sufficient amounts to produce such central effects.

B. Elapid and Sea Snake Venoms

Cardiovascular changes produced by elapid and sea snake venoms are in general not as profound as those produced by crotalid or viperid venoms. However, circulatory failure may be also a cause of death in certain animal species (e.g., cats) poisoned with cobra and some other elapid venoms, which contain cardiotoxic components besides neurotoxins, phospholipases A, and other enzymes.

The most prominent circulatory change produced by elapid or sea snake venoms is an immediate fall in systemic blood pressure if the venom is administered intravenously. The pressure may return to normal and remain steady until an asphyxial rise in blood pressure and marked bradycardia occur immediately before respiratory arrest. Soon after the complete cessation of respiration, the blood pressure falls again abruptly. Under artificial respiration, the blood pressure can be maintained for a long period in most elapid and sea snake envenomation. However, with cobra, mamba, and coral snake venoms, which contain cardiotoxic components, the animal may eventually die of cardiac failure even under artificial respiration.

The pressor effect often observed immediately after injection of cobra venom is attributable to cardiotoxin which causes peripheral vasoconstriction besides cardiotoxic effects.

The initial fall in systemic blood pressure produced by cobra venom can be attributed either to peripheral vasodilatation, accentuated by constriction of the hepatic veins, especially in dogs, or to a pronounced pulmonary vasoconstriction, especially in cats. A direct action on the heart by cardiotoxin is considered to be a contributory factor. Neither phospholipase A nor cardiotoxin alone, but the combined effect of these two components, appears to be responsible for the overall circulatory changes produced by cobra venom.

The depressor effect of other elapid and sea snake venoms, which are devoid of cardiotoxic components, is probably due to phospholipase A which liberates histamine, serotonin, and prostaglandins from tissues. Unlike crotalid and viperid venoms, elapid and sea snake venoms do not release bradykinin, since they contain either very little or no kininogenases.

Venoms of certain species of mamba *(Dendroaspis)* contain exceptionally large amounts of acetylcholine, which is largely responsible for the initial hypotensive effect of these venoms.

Acknowledgements. To a large extent this review was prepared during the tenure of the Scholar-in-Residence, Fogarty International Center, National Institutes of Health, USA from July 1976 to February 1977. We wish to express our appreciation to the staff of the Fogarty International Center for their assistance during the writing of this article. We are also indebted to Dr. SHARON, L. VALLEY, National Library of Medicine, Bethesda, Md., USA, for her help in search of literature performed on the Toxline (Medlars II).

References

Abel, J. H., Jr., Nelson, A. W., Bonilla, C. A.: *Crotalus adamanteus* basic protein toxin: Electron microscopic evaluation of myocardial damage. Toxicon **11**, 59—63 (1973)

Ahuja, M. L., Brooks, A. G., Veeraraghavan, N., Menon, I. G. K.: A note on the action of heparin on Russell's viper venom. Indian J. med. Res. **34**, 317—322 (1946a)

Ahuja, M. L., Veeraraghavan, N., Menon, I. G. K.: Action of heparin on the venom of *Echis carinatus.* Nature (Lond.) **158**, 878 (1946b)

Amorim, D. S., Ferreira, S. H., Manco, J. C., Tanaka, A., Sader, A. A., Cardoso, S.: Potentiation of circulatory effects of bradykinin by a factor contained in the *Bothrops jararaca* venom. Cardiologia (Basel) **50**, 23—32 (1967)

Amuchastegui, S. R.: Action du venin de cobra *(Naja tripudians)* sur le coeur et la dynamique circulatoire. C.R. Soc. Biol. (Paris) **133**, 318—319 (1940)

Arthus, M.: Recherches experimentales sur les phenomenes vasomoteurs produits par quelques venins. Arch. int. Physiol. **13**, 329—332, 395—414 (1913)

Baldes, E. J., Essex, H. E., Markowitz, J.: The physiologic action of rattlesnake venom (crotalin). X. Influence of crotalin on the viscosity of blood. Amer. J. Physiol. **97**, 26—31 (1931)

Beerens, J., Cuypers, H.: Action du venin de cobra sur la circulation. Brux.-med. **15**, 757—771 (1935)

Bhanganada, K., Perry, J. F.: Cardiovascular effects of cobra venom. J. Amer. med. Ass. **183**, 257—259 (1963)

Bicher, H. I., Roth, M., Gitter, S.: Neurotoxic activity of *Vipera palestinae* venom. Depression of central autonomic vasoregulatory mechanisms. Med. Pharmacol. Exp. **14**, 349—359 (1966)

Bieber, A. L., Tu, T., Tu, A. T.: Studies of an acidic cardiotoxin isolated from the venom of Mojave rattlesnake *(Crotalus scutulatus).* Biochim. Biophys. Acta (Amst.) **400**, 178—188 (1975)

Bonilla, C. A.: Rattlesnake venom protein toxins: their use in the development of a new experimental model to investigate acute myocardial infarction. In: Advance in Automated Analysis. The Technicon International Congress, New York, 1972

Bonilla, C. A.: Hypotensin-a hypotensive peptide isolated from *Crotalus atrox* venom: Purification, amino acid composition and terminal amino acid residues. FEBS Letters **68**, 297—302 (1976)

Bonilla, C. A., Diclementi, D., MacCarter, D. J.: Hemodynamic effects of slow and rapid defibrination with defibrizyme, the thrombin-like enzyme from venom of the timber rattlesnake. Amer. Heart J. **90**, 43—49 (1975)

Bonilla, C. A., Fiero, M. K.: Comparative biochemistry and pharmacology of salivary gland secretions. II. Chromatographic separation of the basic proteins from some North American rattlesnake venoms. J. Chromatogr. **56**, 253—263 (1971)

Bonilla, C. A., Fiero, M. K., Novak, J.: Serum enzyme activities following administration of purified basic proteins from rattlesnake venoms. Chem.-Biol. Interact. **4**, 1—10 (1971)
Bonilla, C. A., Rammel, O. J.: Comparative biochemistry and pharmacology of salivary gland secretions. III. Chromatographic isolation of a myocardial depressor protein (MDP) from the venom of *Crotalus atrox*. J. Chromatogr. **124**, 303—314 (1976)
Brown, R. V.: The action of water moccasin venom on the isolated frog heart. Amer. J. Physiol. **130**, 613—619 (1940)
Brown, R. V.: The effects of water moccasin venom on dogs. Amer. J. Physiol. **134**, 202—207 (1941)
Brunton, T. L., Fayrer, J.: On the nature and physiological action of the poison of *Naja tripudians* and other Indian venomous snakes, pt. 1, Proc. R. Soc. London **21**, 358—374 (1873)
Carlson, R. W., Schaeffer, R. C., Jr., Whigham, H., Michaels, S., Russell, F. E., Weil, M. H.: Rattlesnake venom shock in the rat: Development of a method. Amer. J. Physiol. **229**, 1668—1674 (1975)
Césari, E., Boquet, P.: Etude sur le venin blanc de *Vipera aspis*. Ann. Inst. Pasteur **63**, 592—599 (1939)
Chang, C. C., Lee, C. Y.: Isolation of neurotoxins from the venom of *Bungarus multicinctus* and their modes of neuromuscular blocking action. Arch. int. Pharmacodyn. **144**, 241—257 (1963)
Cheymol, J., Bourillet, F., Roch-Arveiller, M.: Action neuromusculaire des venin de quelques Crotalidae, Elapidae et Hydrophiidae. Mem. Inst. Butantan **33**, 541—554 (1966)
Chiang, T. S., Ho, K. J., Lee, C. Y.: Release of histamine from the rat diaphragm preparation by Formosan snake venoms. J. Formosan med. Ass. **63**, 127—132 (1964)
Chiu, T. H., Lee, C. Y., Lee, S. Y.: Hemodynamic effects of cardiotoxin isolated from Formosan cobra venom. J. Formosan med. Ass. **67**, 557 (abstract) (1968)
Chopra, R. N., Chowhan, J. S.: Action of the Indian Dobia (*Vipera russellii*) venom on the circulatory system. Indian J. med. Res. **21**, 493—506 (1934)
Chopra, R. N., Chowhan, J. S., De, N. N.: An experimental investigation into the action of the venom of *Echis carinata*. Indian J. med. Res. **23**, 391—405 (1935)
Chopra, R. N., Iswariah, V.: An experimental investigation into the action of the venom of the Indian cobra—*Naia naia vel tripudians*. Indian J. med. Res. **18**, 1113—1125 (1931)
Cushny, A. R., Yagi, S.: On the action of cobra venom. Phil. Trans. B **208**, 1—36 (1918)
Dale, H. H., Richards, A. N.: The vasodilator action of histamine and of some other substances. J. Physiol. (Lond.) **52**, 110—165 (1918)
Damerau, B., Lege, L., Oldigs, H.-D., Vogt, W.: Histamine release, formation of prostaglandin-like activity (SRS-C) and mast cell degranulation by the direct lytic factor (DLF) and phospholipase A of cobra venom. Naunyn-Schmiedebergs Arch. Pharmacol. **287**, 141—156 (1975)
Deutsch, H. F., Diniz, C. R.: Some proteolytic activities of snake venoms. J. biol. Chem. **216**, 17—26 (1955)
Devi, A., Sarkar, N. K.: Cardiotoxic and cardiostimulating factors in cobra venom. Mem. Inst. Butantan **33**, 573—582 (1966)
Dragstedt, C. A., Mead, F. B., Eyer, S. W.: Role of histamine in circulatory effects of rattlesnake venom (Crotalin). Proc. Soc. exp. Biol. (N.Y.) **37**, 709—710 (1938)
Dutta, N. K., Narayana, K. G. A.: Release of histamine from skeletal muscle by snake venoms. Brit. J. Pharmacol. **9**, 408—412 (1954)
Ehrly, A. M.: Increased blood flow by improvement of the flow properties of blood: A new concept in the treatment of vascular diseases. 18th Int. Cong. of Angiology, Rio de Janeiro, 1972
Ehrly, A. M.: Influence of Arvin on the flow properties of blood. Biorheology **10**, 453—456 (1973)
Elliot, R. H.: A contribution to the study of the action of Indian cobra venom. Phil. Trans. B **197**, 361—406 (1905)
Epstein, D.: The pharmacology of the venom of the Cape cobra (*Naja flava*). Quart. J. exp. Physiol. **20**, 7—19 (1930)
Essex, H. E.: Physiologic action of venom of the water moccasin (*Agkistrodon piscivorus*). Amer. J. Physiol. **99**, 681—684 (1932)
Essex, H. E., Markowitz, J.: The physiologic action of rattlesnake venom (crotalin). I. Effect on blood pressure: symptoms and post-mortem observations. Amer. J. Physiol. **92**, 317—328 (1930a)

Essex, H. E., Markowitz, J.: The physiologic action of rattlesnake venom (crotalin). II. The effect of crotalin on surviving organs. Amer. J. Physiol. **92**, 329—334 (1930b)

Essex, H. E., Markowitz, J.: The physiologic action of rattlesnake venom (crotalin). III. The influence of crotalin on blood in vitro and in vivo. Amer. J. Physiol. **92**, 335—341 (1930c)

Essex, H. E., Markowitz, J.: The physiological action of rattlesnake venom (crotalin). VII. The similarity of crotalin shock and anaphylactic shock. Amer. J. Physiol. **92**, 698—704 (1930d)

Feldberg, W., Holden, H. F., Kellaway, C. H.: The formation of lysocithin and of a muscle-stimulating substance by snake venoms. J. Physiol. (Lond.) **94**, 232—248 (1938)

Feldberg, W., Kellaway, C. H.: Circulatory effects of the venom of the Indian cobra *(Naja naja)* in cats. Aust. J. exp. Biol. med. Sci. **15**, 159—172 (1937a)

Feldberg, W., Kellaway, C. H.: Circulatory effects of the venom of the Indian cobra *(Naja naja)* in dogs. Aust. J. exp. Biol. med. Sci. **15**, 441—460 (1937b)

Feldberg, W., Kellaway, C. H.: Liberation of histamine from the perfused lung by snake venoms. J. Physiol. (Lond.) **90**, 257—279 (1937c)

Feldberg, W., Kellaway, C. H.: Circulatory and pulmonary effects of venom of Australian copperhead, *Denisonia superba* (comparison with histamine). Aust. J. exp. Biol. med. Sci. **15**, 81—95 (1937d)

Feldberg, W., Kellaway, C. H.: Liberation of histamine and formation of lysolecithin-like substance by cobra venom. J. Physiol. (Lond.) **94**, 187—226 (1938)

Ferreira, S. H.: A bradykinin-potentiating factor (BPF) present in the venom of *Bothrops jararaca*. Brit. J. Pharmacol. **24**, 163—169 (1965)

Gautrelet, J., Halpern, N., Corteggiani, E.: Du mechanisme d'action des doses physiologiques de venin de cobra sur la circulation, la respiration et l'excitabilite neuro-musculaire. Arch. int. Physiol. **38**, 293—352 (1934)

Ghosh, B. N., De, S. S., Bhathacharjee, D. P.: Partial separation of the neurotoxin of Russell viper venom. Sci. Cult. **3**, 298 (abstract) (1937)

Ghosh, B. N., De, S. S., Chaudhuri, D. K.: Separation of the neurotoxin from the crude cobra venom and study of the action of a number of reducing agents on it. Indian J. med. Res. **29**, 367—373 (1941)

Gitter, S., Levi, G., Kochwa, S., de Vries, A., Rechnic, J., Casper, J.: Studies on the venom of *Echis colorata*. Amer. J. trop. Med. **9**, 391—399 (1960)

Gottdenker, F., Wachstein, M.: Circulatory effects of the venom of the Indian cobra *(Naja naja)*. J. Pharmacol. **69**, 117—127 (1940)

Gunn, J. A., Heathcote, R. St. A.: Cellular immunity: observation on natural and acquired immunity to cobra venom. Proc. roy. Soc. B **92**, 81—101 (1921)

Haddy, F. J., Emerson, T. E., Jr., Scott, J. B., Daugherty, N. M., Jr.: The effect of the kinins on the cardiovascular system. In: Handb. Exp. Pharmacol. Bradykinin, Kallidin, and Kallikrein, Vol. XXV. Berlin-Heidelberg-New York: Springer 1970

Hadidian, Z.: Proteolytic activity and physiologic and pharmacologic actions of *Agkistrodon piscivorus* venom. In: Buckley, E. E., Porges, N. (Eds.): Venoms, pp. 205—215, Publicat. No. 44. Washington, D.C.: Am. Assoc. Adv. Sci. 1956

Halmagyi, D. F. J., Starzecki, B., Horner, G. J.: Mechanism and pharmacology of shock due to rattlesnake venom in sheep. J. appl. Physiol. **20**, 709—718 (1965)

Harrison, D. C., Henry, W. L., Paaso, B., Miller, H. A.: Circulatory response to bradykinin before and after autonomic nervous system blockade. Amer. J. Physiol. **214**, 1035—1040 (1968)

Ho, C. L., Lee, C. Y., Lu, H. H.: Electrophysiological effects of cobra cardiotoxin on rabbit heart cells. Toxicon **13**, 437—446 (1975)

Högberg, B., Uvnäs, B.: Further observation on the disruption of rat mesentery mast cells caused by compound 48/80, antigen-antibody-reaction, lecithinase A and decylamine. Acta physiol. scand. **48**, 133—145 (1960)

Ishizaka, T.: Studien über das Habuschlangengift. Z. exp. Pathol. Ther. **4**, 88—117 (1907)

Iwase, Y.: Über die toxikologischen Wirkungen des *Naja naja atra* Giftes. J. Formosan med. Ass. **32**, 57—59 (abstract) 624—638 (in Japanese) (1933)

Kaiser, E., Kramer, R., Lambrechter, R.: The action of direct lytic agents from animal venoms on cells and isolated cell fractions. In: Toxin of Animal and Plant Origin, Vol. 2, pp. 675—682. New York-London-Paris: Gordon and Breach 1972

Kaiser, E., Raab, W.: Liberation of pharmacological active substances from mast cells by animal venoms. Mem. Inst. Butantan **33**, 461—466 (1966)

Kellaway, C. H., Le Messurier, D. H.: The vasodepressant action of the venom of the Australian copperhead *(Denisonia superba)*. Aust. J. exp. Biol. med. Sci. **14**, 57—76 (1936)

Kellaway, C. H., Trethewie, E. R.: The liberation of adenyl compounds from perfused organs by cobra venom. Aust. J. exp. Biol. med. Sci. **18**, 63—88 (1940)

Klein, M. D., Bell, W., Nejad, N., Lown, B.: Effect of Arvin upon cardiac function. Proc. Soc. exp. Biol. (N.Y.) **132**, 1123—1126 (1969)

Kocholaty, W. F., Ledford, E. B., Daly, J. G., Billings, T. A.: Toxicity and some enzymatic properties and activities in the venoms of *Crotalidae*, *Elapidae*, and *Viperidae*. Toxicon **9**, 131—138 (1971)

Kochwa, S., Moroz-Perlmutter, C., Gitter, S., Rechnic, J., de Vries, A.: Studies on *Vipera palestinae* venom, fractionation by ion exchange chromatography. Amer. J. trop. Med. **9**, 374—380 (1960)

Kornalik, F., Pudlak, P.: Coagulation defect following nontoxic doses of *Echis* viper venom. Experientia (Basel) **18**, 381—382 (1962)

Krupnick, J., Bicher, H. I., Gitter, S.: Central neurotoxic effects of the venoms of *Naja naja* and *Vipera palestinae*. Toxicon **6**, 11—15 (1968)

Lee, C. Y.: Toxicological studies on the venom of *Vipera russellii formosensis*. IV. On the cause of death in rabbits. Folia pharmacol. jap. **40**, 53—54 (abstract in Japanese) (1944)

Lee, C. Y.: Toxicological studies on the venom of *Vipera russellii formosensis*. V. Circulatory effects in rabbits. J. Formosan med. Ass. **47**, 14 (abstract in Chinese) (1948)

Lee, C. Y.: Studies on the neurotoxins isolated from the elapine venoms. J. Showa med. Ass. **23**, 221—229 (in Japanese) (1965)

Lee, C. Y.: Mode of action of cobra venom and its purified toxins. In: Simpson, L. L. (Ed.): Neuropoisons, Vol. 1, pp. 21—70. New York: Plenum Press 1971

Lee, C. Y.: Chemistry and pharmacology of polypeptide toxins in snake venoms. Ann. Rev. Pharmacol. **12**, 265—286 (1972)

Lee, C. Y., Chang, C. C., Chiu, T. H., Chiu, P. J. S., Tseng, T. C., Lee, S. Y.: Pharmacological properties of cardiotoxin isolated from Formosan cobra venom. Naunyn-Schmiedebergs Arch.-Pharmak. exp. Path. **259**, 360—374 (1968)

Lee, C. Y., Chang, S. L., Kau, S. T., Luh, S. H.: Chromatographic separation of the venom of *Bungarus multicinctus* and characterization of its components. J. Chromatogr. **72**, 71—82 (1972)

Lee, C. Y., Chiu, T. H.: Studies on cardiotoxin isolated from cobra venom. I. Effects of cardiotoxin on contractility, absolute refractory period, and action potentials of cardiac muscle. Ann. Rep., U.S. Army Res. Dev. Group, Far East, Rep. No. FE-369-4, pp. 1—5 (1971)

Lee, C. Y., Chiu, T. H., Lee, S. Y.: Studies on cardiotoxin and vaso-active substance releasing component(s) of cobra venom: Comparison of hemodynamic effects of cardiotoxin with those of cobra venom. Ann. Rep., U.S. Army Res. Dev. Group, Far East, Rep. No. FE-369-2, 1—11 (1971)

Lee, C. Y., Huang, M. C., Bonilla, C. A.: Mode of action of purified basic proteins from three rattlesnake venoms on neuromuscular junctions of the chick biventer cervicis muscle. In: Kaiser, E. (Ed.): Animal and Plant Toxins, pp. 173—178. München: Whilhelm Goldmann 1973

Lee, C. Y., Peng, M. T.: An analysis of the respiratory failure produced by the Formosan elapid venoms. Arch. int. Pharmacodyn. **133**, 180—192 (1961)

Lin Shiau, S. Y., Huang, M.-C., Lee, C. Y.: Isolation of cardiotoxic and neurotoxic principles from the venom of *Bungarus fasciatus*. J. Formosan med. Ass. **71**, 350—357 (1972)

Lin Shiau, S.-Y., Huang, M.-C., Lee, C. Y.: A study of cardiotoxic principles from the venom of *Bungarus fasciatus* (Schneider). Toxicon **13**, 189—196 (1975)

Lin Shiau, S. Y., Huang, C. W., Lee, C. Y.: Comparison of biological activities of acidic and basic phospholipase A, myocardial depressor protein and β-bungarotoxin. J. Chin. biochem. Soc. **6**, 8 p. (abstract) (1977)

Lo, T. B., Chen, Y. H., Lee, C. Y.: Chemical studies of Formosan cobra *(Naja naja atra)* venom. Part 1. Chromatographic separation of crude venom on CM-Sephadex and preliminary characterization of its components. J. Chin. chem. Soc. **13**, 25—37 (1966)

Manwaring, W. H., Williams, T. B.: Physiological adaptations of fixed-tissues in anaphylaxis and immunity. I. Reactions of the isolated rabbit heart to cobra venom. J. Immunol. **8**, 75—81 (1923)
Margolis, J., Bruch, S., Starzecki, B., Horner, G. J., Halmagyi, D. F.: Release of bradykinin-like substance (BKLS) in sheep by venom of *Crotalus atrox*. Aust. J. exp. Biol. med. Sci. **43**, 237—244 (1965)
Markwardt, F., Barthel, W., Glusa, E., Hoffmann, A.: Über die Freisetzung biogener Amine aus Blutplättchen durch tierische Gifte. Naunyn-Schmiedebergs Arch. Pharmak. exp. Path. **252**, 297—304 (1966)
Marshall, R., Esnouf, M. P.: The effect of *Ancistrodon rhodostoma* venom in the dog. Clin. Sci. **35**, 251—259 (1968)
Martin, C. J.: On the physiological action of the venom of the Australian black snake *(Pseudechis porphyriacus)*. Proc. roy. Soc. New South Wales (Sydney) **29**, 146—277 (1895)
Master, R. W. P., Rao, S. S.: Identification of enzymes and toxins in the venoms of Indian cobra and Russell's viper after starch gel electrophoresis. J. biol. Chem. **236**, 1986—1990 (1961)
Master, R. W. P., Rao, S. S.: Starch-gel electrophoresis of venoms of Indian krait and saw-scaled viper and identification of enzymes and toxins. Biochim. Biophys. Acta (Amst.) **71**, 416—421 (1963)
Mebs, D.: Vergleichende Enzymuntersuchungen an Schlangengiften unter besonderer Berücksichtigung ihrer caseinspaltenden Proteasen. Hoppe-Seylers Z. physiol. Chem. **349**, 1115—1125 (1968)
Mebs, D.: A comparative study of enzyme activities in snake venoms. Int. J. Biochem. **1**, 335—342 (1970)
Meldrum, B. S.: The action of snake venoms on nerve and muscle. The pharmacology of phospholipase A and polypeptide toxins. Pharmacol. Rev. **17**, 393—445 (1965)
Miyazaki, S.: A study on circulatory and respiratory effects of Habu venom. Keio Igaku **1**, 1001—1022 (in Japanese) (1921)
Moroz, C., de Vries, A., Sela, M.: Isolation and characterization of a neurotoxin from *Vipera palestinae* venom. Biochim. Biophys. Acta (Amst.) **124**, 136—146 (1966)
Muić, N., Piantanida, M.: Zur Kenntnis des Sandottergiftes: Elektrophoretische und chemische Charakterisierung der Hauptfraktionen. Z. physiol. Chem. **299**, 6—14 (1955)
Nakamura, T.: Über die Wirkung des Giftes von *Naja naja atra* auf isolierte Froschherzen. J. med. Ass. Formosa **32**, 33 (abstract), 424—430 (in Japanese) (1933)
Narita, K., Lee, C. Y.: The amino acid sequence of cardiotoxin from Formosan cobra *(Naja naja atra)* venom. Biochem. biophys. Res. Commun. **41**, 339—343 (1970)
Oshima, G., Sato-Omori, T., Suzuki, T.: Distribution of proteinase, arginine ester hydrolase and kinin releasing enzyme in various kinds of snake venoms. Toxicon 7, 229—233 (1969)
Osman, O. H., Gumaa, K. A.: Pharmacological studies of snake *(Bitis arientans)* venom. Toxicon **12**, 569—575 (1974)
Osman, O. H., Ismail, L., El-Asmart, M. F.: Pharmacological studies of snake *(Dendroaspis angusticeps)* venom. Toxicon **11**, 185—192 (1973)
Peng, M. T.: A toxicological study on the fractionated venom of *Naja naja atra*. Mem. Fac. Med. Nat. Taiwan Univ. **1**, 200—213 (1951 a)
Peng, M. T.: Action of the venom of *Trimeresurus mucrosquamatus* on circulation and respiration. Mem. Fac. Med. Nat. Taiwan Univ. **1**, 215—222 (1951 b)
Peng, M. T.: Action of the venom of *Naja naja atra* on respiration and circulation. Mem. Fac. Med. Nat. Taiwan Univ. **2**, 170—183 (1952)
Petkovic, D., Khogali, A., Abdel Rahman, Y., Zaki, O. A.: Cardiovascular and respiratory changes caused by black mamba *(Dendroaspis polylepis)* venom. Iugoslav. Physiol. Pharmacol. Acta 7, 375—383 (1971)
Phillips, S. J.: The effect of snake and bee venoms on cardiovascular hemodynamics and function. In: de Vries, A., Kochva, E. (Eds.): Toxins of animal and plant origin, Vol. 2, pp. 683—701. New York: Gordon and Breach 1972
Ragotzi, V.: Über die Wirkung des Giftes der *Naja tripudians*. Virchows Arch. path. Anat. **122**, 201—234 (1890)
Ramsey, H. W., Taylor, W. J., Boruchow, I. B., Snyder, G. K.: Mechanism of shock produced by an elapid snake *(Micrurus f. fulvius)* venom in dogs. Amer. J. Physiol. **222**, 782—786 (1972)

Raudonat, H. W., Holler, B.: Über die herzwirksame Komponente des Kobragiftes (cardiotoxin). Naunyn-Schmiedebergs Arch. exp. Path. Pharmak. **233**, 431—437 (1958)
Rechnic, J., Trachtenberg, P., Casper, J., Moroz, C., de Vries, A.: Afibrinogenemia and thrombocytopenia in guinea-pigs following injection of *Echis colorata* venom. Blood **20**, 735—749 (1962)
Rocha e Silva, M., Beraldo, W. T., Rosenfeld, G.: Bradykinin, a hypotensive and smooth muscle stimulating factor released from plasma globulin by snake venoms and by trypsin. Amer. J. Physiol. **156**, 261—273 (1949)
Rocha e Silva, M., Essex, H. E.: The effect of animal poisons (rattlesnake venom and trypsin) on the blood histamine of guinea pigs and rabbits. Amer. J. Physiol. **135**, 372—377 (1942)
Rogers, L.: The physiological action and antidotes of colubrine and viperine snake venoms. Phil. Trans. B **197**, 123—191 (1905)
Rosenfeld, G.: Symptomatology, pathology, and treatment of snake bites in South America. In: Bücherl, W., Buckley, E. E. (Eds.): Venomous Animals and Their Venoms, Vol. II, pp. 345—384. New York-London: Academic Press 1971
Rothschild, A. M.: Mechanism of histamine release by animal venoms. Mem. Inst. Butantan **33**, 467—475 (1966)
Rothschild, A. M., Almeida, J. A.: Role of bradykinin in the fatal shock induced by *Bothrops jararaca* venom in the rat. In: de Vries, A., Kochva, E. (Eds.): Toxins of Animal and Plant Origin, Vol. 2, pp. 721—728. New York-London: Gordon and Breach 1972
Russell, F. E.: Snake venom poisoning. In: Piersol, G. M. (Ed.): Cyclopedia of medicine, surgery and the specialities, Vol. II, pp. 199—210. Philadelphia: F. A. Davis 1962
Russell, F. E.: Bradykininogen levels following *Crotalus* envenomation. Toxicon **2**, 277—279 (1965)
Russell, F. E.: Pharmacology of animal venoms. Clin. Pharmacol. Ther. **8**, 849—873 (1967a)
Russell, F. E.: Comparative pharmacology of some animal toxins. Fed. Proc. **26**, 1206—1224 (1967b)
Russell, F. E.: The biochemistry and pharmacology of snake venoms. In: de Vries, A., Kochva, E. (Eds.): Toxins of Animal and Plant Origin, Vol. II, pp. 643—654. New York-London: Gordon and Breach 1972
Russell, F. E., Buess, F. W., Strassberg, J.: Cardiovascular response to *Crotalus* venom. Toxicon **1**, 5—18 (1962)
Russell, F. E., Buess, F. W., Woo, M. Y.: Zootoxicological properties of venom phosphodiesterase. Toxicon **1**, 99—108 (1963a)
Russell, F. E., Buess, F. W., Woo, M. Y., Eventov, R.: Zootoxicological properties of venom L-amino acid oxidase. Toxicon **1**, 229—234 (1963b)
Russell, F. E., Michaelis, B. A., Buess, F. W.: Some physiopharmacological properties of rattlesnake venom. Proc. West Pharmacol. Soc. **4**, 27—31 (1961)
Sandbank, K. U., Djaldetti, M.: Effect of *Echis colorata* venom inoculation on the nervous system of the dog and guinea pig. Acta Neuropath. **6**, 61—69 (1966)
Sandbank, K. U., Jerushalmy, Z., Ben-David, E., de Vries, A.: Effect of *Echis coloratus* venom on brain vessel. Toxicon **12**, 267—271 (1974)
Sarkar, B. B., Maitra, S. R., Ghosh, B. N.: The effect of neurotoxin, haemolysin, and choline esterase isolated from cobra venom on heart, blood pressure and respiration. Indian J. med. Res. **30**, 453—466 (1942)
Sarkar, N. K.: Isolation of cardiotoxin from cobra venom (*Naja tripudians* monocellate variety). J. Indian chem. Soc. **24**, 227—232 (1947a)
Sarkar, N. K.: Determination of molecular weight of cardiotoxin by a diffusion method. J. Indian chem. Soc. **24**, 61—64 (1947b)
Sarkar, N. K.: Action mechanism of cobra venom, cardiotoxin, and allied substances on muscle contraction. Proc. Soc. exp. Biol. (N.Y.) **78**, 469—471 (1951)
Schaeffer, R. C., Jr.: The hemodynamic properties of Southern Pacific rattlesnake, *Crotalus viridis helleri*, venom and the histochemistry of the snake's venom apparatus. Ph.D. dissertation, Univ. South. Calif. USA (1973)
Schaeffer, R. C., Jr., Pattabhiraman, T. R., Russell, F. E., Carlson, R. W., Weil, M. H.: Pharmacologic properties of some fractions of the venom of the southern pacific rattlesnake (*Crotalus viridis helleri*). Submitted to Toxicon (1978a)

Schaeffer, R. C., Jr., Carlson, R. W., Wigham, H., Weil, M. H., Russell, F. E.: Acute hemodynamic effects of rattlesnake *(Crotalus viridis helleri)* venom. In: Rosenberg, P. (Ed.): Toxins: Animal, Plant, and Microbial. Oxford-New York: Pergamon 1978b

Schöttler, W. H. A.: Die Gifte von *Vipera latasti* und *V. lebetina*. Z. Hyg. Infekt.-Kr. **120**, 408—434 (1938)

Schöttler, W. H. A.: Antihistamine, ACTH, cortisone, hydrocortisone, and anesthetics in snake bite. Amer. J. trop. Med. **3**, 1083—1091 (1954)

Sket, D., Gubensek, F., Adamic, S., Lebez, D.: Action of a partially purified basic protein fraction from *Vipera ammodytes* venom. Toxicon **11**, 47—53 (1973)

Slotta, K. H., Fraenkel-Conrat, H. L.: Schlangengifte. III. Reinigung und Krystallisation des Klapperschlangengiftes. Ber. dtsch. Chem. Ges. **71**, 1076—1081 (1938)

Tazieff-Depierre, F., Trethewie, E. R.: Action du chlorure de calcium sur la cardiotoxicite chez le rat de la toxine γ, purifiée, isolée du venin de *Naja nigricollis*. C.R. Acad. Sci. (Paris) (D) **280**, 137—140 (1975)

Telang, B. V., Galzigna, L., Mainna, G., Ngángá, J. N.: Mechanism of action of Jameson's mamba venom on the superior cervical ganglion of cat. Toxicon **14**, 15—26 (1976a)

Telang, B. V., Lutunya, R. J. M., Njoroge, D.: Studies on the central vasomotor reflexes in cats after intraventricular administration of whole venom of *Dendroaspis jamesoni*. Toxicon **14**, 133—138 (1976b)

Trethewie, E. R.: Comparison of haemolysis and liberation of histamine by two Australian snake venoms. Aust. J. exp. Biol. med. Sci. **17**, 145—155 (1939)

Trethewie, E. R., Day, A. J.: New therapy of ophidiasis. Aust. J. exp. Biol. med. Sci. **26**, 153—161 (1948)

Tseng, T. C.: A study on cardiotoxin isolated from Formosan cobra venom. M.S. thesis, Nat. Taiwan Univ. (1964)

Tu, T.: Toxicological studies on the venom of the sea snake *Laticauda laticaudata affinis*. In.: Russell, F. E., Saunders, P. R. (Eds.): Animal Toxins, pp. 245—248. Oxford: Pergamon Press 1967

Tu, T., Tu, A. T., Lin, T.: Some pharmacological properties of the venom, venom fractions, and pure toxin of the Yellow-bellied sea snake *Pelamis platurus*. J. Pharm. Pharmacol. **28**, 139—145 (1976)

Vellard, J., Huidobro, F.: Acción comparada de diversos venenos de ofidios sobre la presión arterial. Rev. Soc. Argent. Biol. **17**, 72 (1941)

Ventakachalam, K., Ratnagiriswaran, A. M.: Some experimental observations on the venom of the Indian cobra. Indian J. med. Res. **22**, 289—294 (1934)

Vick, J. A., Blanchard, R. J., Perry, J. F., Jr.: Effects of epsilon amino caproic acid on pulmonary vascular changes produced by snake venoms. Proc. Soc. exp. Biol. (N.Y.) **113**, 841—844 (1963)

Vick, J. A.: Ciuchta, H. P., Manthei, J. H.: Pathophysiological studies of ten snake venoms: In: Russell, F. E., Saunders, P. R. (Eds.): Animal Toxin, pp. 269—282. Oxford: Pergamon 1967

Vital Brazil, O.: Hiperpiese provocada pela peconha da *Crotalus terrificus terrificus*. Ann. Fac. Med. Univ. S. Paulo **29**, 159—174 (1954)

Vital Brazil, O., Farina, R., Yoshida, L., de Oliverira, V. A.: Pharmacology of crystalline crotoxin. III. Cardiovascular and respiratory effects of crotoxin and *Crotalus durissus terrificus* venom. Mem. Inst. Butantan **33**, 993—1000 (1966)

Vollmer, E.: Über die Wirkung des Brillenschlangengiftes. Naunyn-Schmiedebergs Arch. exp. Path. Pharm. **31**, 1—14 (1893)

Weis, R., McIsaak, R. J.: Cardiovascular and muscular effects of venom from coral snake, *Micrurus fulvius*, Toxicon **9**, 219—228 (1971)

Welsh, J. H.: Acetylcholine in snake venoms. In: Russell, F. E., Saunders, P. R. (Eds.): Animal Toxins, pp. 363—368. Oxford: Pergamon Press 1967

Westermann, E., Klapper, W.: Untersuchungen über die Kreislaufwirkung des Kobragiftes. Naunyn-Schmiedebergs Arch. exp. Pathol. Pharmacol. **239**, 68—80 (1960)

Whigham, H., Russell, F. E., Weil, M. H.: Circulatory and metabolic alterations in rats following intravenous infusion of rattlesnake *(Crotalus viridis helleri)* venom. Proc. West. Pharmacol. Soc. **16**, 223—225 (1973)

Witham, A. C., Remington, J. W., Lombard, E. A.: Cardiovascular response to rattlesnake venoms. Amer. J. Physiol. **173**, 535—541 (1953)
Yang, T. Y., Lee, C. Y.: Pharmacological studies on the venom of a sea snake *Hydrophis cyanocinctus*. In: Rosenberg, P. (Ed.): Toxins: Anim. Plant and Microbiol., pp. 415—428. Oxford-New York: Pergamon 1978
Yonegawa, M.: On the effects of cobra venom. Keio Igaku **6**, 1349—1365 (in Japanese) (1926)
Zaki, O. A., Khogali, A., Abdel-Rahman, Y., El-Nagdi, S.: Circulatory shock caused by a toxic fraction from *Echis carinatus* venom. Ain Shams med. J. **21**, 647—655 (1970)
Zaki, O. A., Khogali, A., Petkovic, D., Ibrahim, S. A.: The effect of whole cobra venom *(Naja naja)* and its fractions on the heart. Toxicon **5**, 91—95 (1967)

CHAPTER 16

Liberation of Pharmacologically Active Substances by Snake Venoms

A. M. ROTHSCHILD and Z. ROTHSCHILD

General Introduction

Indirect effects of snake venoms due to the release or formation of pharmacologically highly active autacoids (DOUGLAS, 1975) are an important aspect of snake venom pharmacology. Autacoids like histamine, kinins, slow-reacting substances (SRS), 5-hydroxytryptamine, and anaphylatoxins have been associated with a great number of pathologic processes ranging in severity from mild allergy to anaphylactic or septic shock. However, considerable mystery still surrounds the origin and contribution of each of these compounds to such pathologic reactions. This statement also holds true for many symptoms of snake venom poisoning. Nevertheless, considerable inroads into the field of autopharmacology, especially in its relation to pathology, have resulted from snake venom research and further progress is to be expected. The recognition of the sensitivity of labile histamine reservoirs in tissues to cytolytic agents (FELDBERG and KELLAWAY, 1937b), of the ability of tissues and blood to generate "slow-reacting" smooth muscle stimulants (FELDBERG and KELLAWAY, 1938; ROCHA E SILVA et al., 1949), of the relationship of kinins to the kallikrein system (WERLE et al., 1950), and of the biochemical relationships of anaphylatoxin-generating venoms (VOGT and SCHMIDT, 1964) to the complement system (MÜLLER-EBERHARD, 1967) are outstanding examples of the contributions which snake venom research has brought to basic biology.

In the following pages, we have endeavored to unite in a possible orderly manner the often quite fragmentary information on the existence, mechanism, and possible pathologic significance of processes leading to the release or formation of pharmacologically active substances by snake venoms. It is hoped that this assembled data will yield a broadened starting point for future studies in a still promising field of pharmacology.

A. Histamine

I. Introduction

DALE and LAIDLAW in 1910 were among the first to study the pharmacologic actions of histamine: knowledge about the subject has been accumulating ever since. It has been the object of many reviews, the most recent and extensive of which appeared in Volume XVIII of this Handbook (ROCHA E SILVA, 1966). Almost apace with interest in the pharmacology of histamine, knowledge grew about the many stimuli through which this amine can be released from tissues to exert its fugacious and potentially toxic effects on blood pressure, pulmonary function, vascular permeability, visceral smooth muscle tone, and gastric secretion. Methods used to test histamine release by snake venoms or other agents have not substantially changed during the last decade. They have been reviewed in detail by BERALDO and DIAS DA SILVA (1966).

II. Survey of the Histamine-Releasing Activity of Snake Venoms

Table 1 shows that the ability to release histamine from animal tissues is widespread among snake venoms. It is found in elapid and in both viperid (true viper) and crotalid (pit viper) venoms. The diversity of animal structures and techniques employed by different authors for the assessment of this activity is large and renders comparisons of relative potencies somewhat difficult. An extensive comparative survey of histamine-releasing activity among snake venoms has been presented by MARKWARDT et al. (1966a). Its main features are reproduced in Table 2, which shows the relative ability to release histamine and 5-hydroxytryptamine (serotonin) from isolated rabbit platelets, of venoms from seven elapid, five viperid and 17 crotalid species. However, when results obtained with venoms from the same species, shown in Tables 1 and 2 respectively, are compared, discrepancies concerning the histamine-releasing activity of certain viperid and crotalid venoms become apparent. Thus, the venom of *Echis carinatus*, the saw-scaled viper, released histamine in the intact dog, rabbit, or rat (MOHAMED et al., 1968; SOMANI and ARORA, 1964) and in the isolated rat diaphragm; yet, it failed to act on rabbit platelets (MARKWARDT et al., 1966a). Venoms of snakes from the genus *Vipera* were ineffective releasers of histamine in rabbit platelets (Table 2). ROTHSCHILD and ROTHSCHILD (1971), however, showed *V. palestinae* venom to have pronounced activity on the histamine stores of isolated rat peritoneal fluid mast cells and to produce typical degranulation of rat mesentery mast cells in vitro. The venom of *Crotalus adamanteus* was inactive on isolated rabbit platelets (Table 2), yet released histamine in the intact guinea-pig or rabbit. *C. atrox* venom, a histamine releaser, although relatively weak but definitely active, when perfused through the isolated guinea-pig lung (FELDBERG and KELLAWAY, 1937b) or when injected into the dog (DRAGSTEDT et al., 1932), was inactive on rabbit platelets. These differences emphasize that evidence of histamine-releasing capacity of a venom in one species or tissue does not imply that such a result will also be found in assays performed on tissues from the same or another species of experimental animals.

III. Mechanistic Aspects

1. Phospholipase A Activity and Histamine Release

FELDBERG and KELLAWAY (1938) pioneered in studies on the mechanism by which animal venoms release histamine from tissues. Their view was that lysophosphatides (lysolecithin, lysocephalin) generated by the action of phospholipase A, an enzyme present in most snake venoms, damage cellular histamine depot sites, causing the release and eventual distribution of the amine over the victim's body. This opinion, corroborated by findings of TRETHEWIE (1939), CHIANG et al. (1964), and OUYANG and SHIAU (1970), is correct but incomplete: it fails to account for histamine-

Table 1. Histamine (H)-releasing ability of snake venoms

Species	Test animal	Biologic structure	Experimental evidence	Reference
Elapidae				
Acanthopis antarcticus	Dog	Lung, liver (perf.)	H. release	Trethewie (1939)
Bungarus multicinctus	Rat	Diaphragm, in vitro	H. release	Chiang et al. (1964)
Denisonia superba	Cat	Whole animal	Hemoconcentration; hypotension; lung vessel hypertension and congestion; pulmonary edema	Feldberg and Kellaway (1937a)
Denisonia superba	Guinea pig	Lung (perf.)	H. release	Feldberg and Kellaway (1937b)
Denisonia superba	Guinea pig	Ileum, in vitro	H. release	Rocha e Silva (1949)
Naja naja	Cat	Whole animal	Hypotension; lung vessel obstruction and congestion	Feldberg and Kellaway (1937c)
Naja naja	Cat	Whole animal	Increased histaminemia	Westermann and Klapper (1960)
Naja naja	Dog	Whole animal	Hemoconcentration; hypotension; liver and duodenum congestion; portal hypertension; hepatic vein constriction	Feldberg and Kellaway (1937d)
Naja naja	Dog	Lung, liver (perf.)	H. release	Feldberg and Kellaway (1938)
Naja naja	Guinea pig	Lung (perf.)	H. release	Feldberg and Kellaway (1937b)
Naja naja	Guinea pig	Lung (slices)	H. release	Damerau et al. (1975)
Naja naja	Guinea pig	Diaphragm, heart, ileum, kidney, lung, uterus	H. release in vitro	Middleton and Phillips (1964)
Naja naja	Guinea pig	Brain, liver, spleen	No H. release in vitro	Middleton and Phillips (1964)
Naja naja	Guinea pig	Whole animal	Increased histaminemia	May et al. (1967)
Naja naja	Guinea pig	Mesentery, in vitro	H. release	May et al. (1967)
Naja naja	Monkey (*Rhesus*)	Lung (perf.)	H. release	Feldberg and Kellaway (1938)
Naja naja	Monkey (*Rhesus*)	Liver (perf.)	No H. release	Feldberg and Kellaway (1938)
Naja naja	Rat	Diaphragm, in vitro	H. release	Dutta and Narayaman (1952)
Naja naja	Rat	Peritoneal fluid mast cells, in vitro	H. release	May et al. (1967) Kaiser et al. (1972) Damerau et al. (1975)
Naja naja	Rat	Whole animal	Increased histaminemia	May et al. (1967)

Table 1 (continued)

Species	Test animal	Biologic structure	Experimental evidence	Reference
Naja naja atra	Rat	Diaphragm, in vitro	H. release	CHIANG et al. (1964)
Naja nigricollis	Dog	Whole animal	Increased histaminemia	MOHAMED et al. (1971)
Naja nigricollis	Rat	Diaphragm, in vitro	H. release	MOHAMED et al. (1971)
Pseudechis porphyriacus	Dog	Lung, liver (perf.)	H. release	TRETHEWIE (1939)
Walterinnesia aegyptia	Dog	Whole animal	Increased histaminemia	MOHAMED and ZAKI (1957a)
Walterinnesia aegyptia	Rat	Diaphragm, in vitro	H. release	MOHAMED and ZAKI (1957b)
Tiperidae				
Bitis arietans	Cat	Whole animal	Blood pressure changes not affected by antihistaminic drug	OSMAN and GUMAA (1974)
Bitis arietans	Rabbit	Skin	Increased vascular permeability not affected by antihistaminic	OSMAN and GUMAA (1974)
Cerastes cerastes	Dog	Whole animal	Increased histaminemia	MOHAMED and KHALED (1969)
Cerastes cerastes	Rat	Diaphragm, in vitro	H. release	MOHAMED and KHALED (1969)
Echis carinatus	Cat	Whole animal	Hypotension; capillary vasodilation; visceral vascular congestion	CHOPRA et al. (1935)
Echis carinatus	Dog	Whole animal	Increased histaminemia	MOHAMED et al. (1968)
Echis carinatus	Rabbit	Leg	Increased vascular permeability sensitive to antihistaminic	MOHAMED et al. (1968)
Echis carinatus	Rat	Skin	Increased vascular permeability sensitive to antihistaminic	SOMANI and ARORA (1964)
Echis carinatus	Rat	Diaphragm, in vitro	H. release	MOHAMED et al. (1968)
Vipera palestinae	Guinea pig	Ileum, in vitro	H. release	ROSEN et al. (1964)
Vipera palestinae	Rat	Peritoneal fluid mast cells, in vitro	H. release	ROTHSCHILD and ROTHSCHILD (1971)
Vipera palestinae	Rat	Mesentery, in vitro	Mast cell degranulation	ROTHSCHILD (unpubl.)
Vipera russellii	Cat	Whole animal	Tachyphylactic hypotension; visceral vascular congestion; increased vascular permeability	CHOPRA and CHOWHAN (1934)

Table 1 (continued)

Species	Test animal	Biologic structure	Experimental evidence	Reference
Crotaliae				
Agkistrodon acutus	Rat	Diaphragm, in vitro	H. release	CHIANG et al. (1964)
Bothrops atrox	Guinea pig	Ileum, in vitro	H. release	ROCHA E SILVA (1949)
Bothrops atrox	Guinea pig	Ileum, in vitro	H. release	ROCHA E SILVA (1949)
Bothrops atrox		Whole animal	Decreased vascular effects after antihistaminic	SEBA (1949)
Crotalus adamanteus	Guinea pig	Whole animal	Lung emphysema	ROCHA E SILVA and ESSEX (1942)
Crotalus adamanteus	Rabbit	Whole animal	Decreased histaminemia	ROCHA E SILVA and ESSEX (1942)
Crotalus adamanteus	Rat	Mesentery, in vitro	Mast cell degranulation	HÖGBERG and ÜVNAS (1957)
Crotalus atrox	Dog	Whole animal	Increased histaminemia	DRAGSTEDT et al. (1938)
Crotalus atrox	Guinea pig	Lung (perf.)	H. release	FELDBERG and KELLAWAY (1937b)
Crotalus atrox	Rat	Mesentery, in vitro	Mast cell degranulation	HÖGBERG and ÜVNAS (1957)
Crotalus horridus	Rabbit	Whole animal	Decreased histaminemia	CHUTE and WATERS (1941)
Crotalus terrificus	Guinea pig	Ileum, in vitro	H. release	ROCHA E SILVA (1949)
Crotalus terrificus	Rabbit	Blood platelets, in vitro	H. release	MARKWARDT et al. (1966a)
Crotalus terrificus	Rat	Skin	Increased vascular permeability	MOURA GONCALVES (1956)
Crotalus terrificus	Rat	Peritoneal fluid mast cells, in vitro	H. release	ROTHSCHILD (1966a)
Crotalus terrificus	Rat	Mesentery, in vitro	Mast cell degranulation	HÖGBERG and ÜVNAS (1957)
Trimeresurus flavoviridis	Guinea pig	Ileum	Histaminic contraction	ISHIDA et al. (1974)
Trimeresurus flavoviridis	Guinea pig	Lung, in vitro	H. release	ISHIDA et al. (1974)
Trimeresurus flavoviridis	Rabbit	Blood platelets, in vitro	H. release	ISHIDA et al. (1974)
Trimeresurus flavoviridis	Rat	Peritoneal fluid mast cells, in vitro	H. release	ISHIDA et al. (1974)
Trimeresurus gramineus	Rat	Diaphragm, in vitro	H. release	CHIANG et al. (1964)
Trimeresurus gramineus	Rat	Peritoneal fluid mast cells, in vitro	H. release	OUYANG and SHIAU (1970)
Trimeresurus gramineus	Rat	Skin	Increased vascular permeability	OUYANG and SHIAU (1970)
Trimeresurus mucrosquamatus	Rat	Diaphragm, in vitro	H. release	CHIANG et al. (1964)

Table 2. Effect of venoms from different species of snakes on the histamine (H) and serotonin (S) content of isolated rabbit platelets. (According to MARKWARDT et al., 1966a)

Venom	Concentration µg/ml	Effect[a] H	Effect[a] S
Naja flava, N. haje	100	0	0
N. naja, N. n. oxiana, N. nigricollis	100	++	++
Bungarus fasciatus	100	0	0
Dendroaspis viridis	100	0	0
Bitis arietans	100	0	0
Echis carinatus	100	0	0
Vipera ammodytes, V. berus, V. russellii	100	0	0
Agkistrodon piscivorus	100	0	0
A. contortrix	100	+	0
Bothrops alternata	100	0	0
B. neuwiedii	100	0	0
B. cotiara, B. insularis	10	+	0
B. jararacussu	10	+	+
B. jararaca	10	++	+
Crotalus adamanteus C. atrox, C. viridis, Lachesis muta	100	0	0
Sistrurus catenatus	100	++	++
Crotalus horridus	10	++	++
C. horridus	1	+	+
C. durissus terrificus	10	++	++
C. durissus terrificus	1	+	+
C. durissus terrificus	0.1	+	+

[a] 0 = no release; ++ = over 50% release; + = less than 50% release.

releasing principles other than phospholipase A which, as discussed in the following pages, have been shown to be contained in certain snake venoms. Mast cells, the major depots of histamine in skin and other organs rich in connective tissue, release histamine when acted upon by lysolecithin in vitro (HÖGBERG and UVNÄS, 1957; KELLER, 1964; ROTHSCHILD, 1965, 1966b; FREDHOLM and HAEGERMARK, 1967). Observations by the last three groups of authors, as well as by MARKWARDT et al. (1966b) and DAMERAU et al. (1975), have shown, however, that neither mast cells harvested from the peritoneal cavity of rats nor platelets isolated from rabbit blood release more than minimal amounts of histamine following exposure to purified bee or rattlesnake venom phospholipase A. Apparently, such cells cannot produce cytolytic phosphatides, being either shielded from, insensitive to, or acted upon by phospholipase A in a manner not leading to the production of cytolytic compounds (ROTHSCHILD, 1965; DAMERAU et al., 1975). Since, however, bee venom phospholipase A is clearly able to release histamine from rat skin in vivo or in vitro, it can be concluded that the enzyme does act as a histamine releaser albeit in an indirect way, mediated by lysophosphatides generated from nonmast cell sources (ROTHSCHILD, 1965). In view of the wide distribution of phospholipase A, this process may be expected to contribute, to a greater or lesser extent, to the release of histamine occurring in the body of all victims of poisonous snake bites.

2. Histamine Release by Snake Venom Components Other Than Phospholipase A

Crotamine, a basic myotoxic (CHEYMOL et al., 1972; VITAL BRAZIL et al., 1972) polypeptide (mol wt 4880), whose primary structure has been recently elucidated (LAURE, 1975), was first detected and described by MOURA GONÇALVES (1956) in the venom of some Brazilian rattlesnakes *(Crotalus durissus terrificus)*. Its ability to release histamine from the perfused hindquarters of the rat was reported by MOURA GONÇALVES and ROCHA E SILVA (1958) and confirmed in a more direct way by ROTHSCHILD (1966a), who demonstrated that crotamine could release histamine from isolated rat peritoneal fluid mast cells. This activity was, however, considerably smaller than that of crude rattlesnake venom. This result, as well as observations showing that venoms of Brazilian rattlesnakes originating from northern and central regions of the country which contain no free crotamine (SCHENBERG, 1959) and were nevertheless quite active in releasing histamine from isolated rat peritoneal fluid mast cells, led to a search for other histamine-releasing principles present in such venoms (ROTHSCHILD, 1963, 1966a, 1967).

Figure 1 presents the results of a chromatographic analysis on an ion-exchange resin (Amberlite CG-50) of "crotamine-negative" rattlesnake venom. The presence of a nonphospholipase A component, highly active on rat mast cell histamine, could be clearly demonstrated. Table 3 presents a survey of some of its properties in comparison to those of crotamine and the amine-liberating protein (ALP) isolated from the same venom, at approximately the same time, by MARKWARDT et al. (1966b).

Unlike crotamine, the histamine-releasing substances isolated by ROTHSCHILD and by MARKWARDT appear to be high molecular weight, neutral proteins, possibly of proteolytic enzyme nature; they may be chemically identic. Both fail to release histamine from mast cells or platelets pretreated with metabolic inhibitors. Histamine release by lysolecithin is not affected in this way (ROTHSCHILD, 1965, 1966a); lysolecithin probably acts in a nonspecific, cytolytic manner. The "direct" histamine-releasing principle of rattlesnake venom, in contrast, seems to stimulate merocrine secretory activity of mast cells (SMITH, 1958). This indicates that certain snake venoms possess the same ability as immunologic mediators (review by KALINER and AUSTEN, 1973), basic compounds (ROTHSCHILD, 1966b, 1970; GOTH and JOHNSON, 1975), or chymotrypsin (SAEKI, 1964; SASAKI, 1975) to mobilize the biochemically complex sequence of events which lead to granule extrusion and active histamine secretion from mast cells.

The presence of a heat-labile, histamine-releasing protein component unrelated to phospholipase A has also been demonstrated in *Vipera palestinae* venom (ROTHSCHILD and ROTHSCHILD, 1971). Chromatographic fractionation of this venom on DEAE cellulose according to KOCHWA et al. (1960) resulted in the separation of four fractions (Fig. 2). Table 4 shows the major pharmacologic activities associated with each one. It can be seen that fraction I contained most of the histamine-releasing activity of the venom but was practically devoid of phospholipase A. In contrast, fraction III, which contained the bulk of the venom's phospholipolytic enzyme, was practically inactive in releasing histamine from the isolated rat peritoneal fluid mast

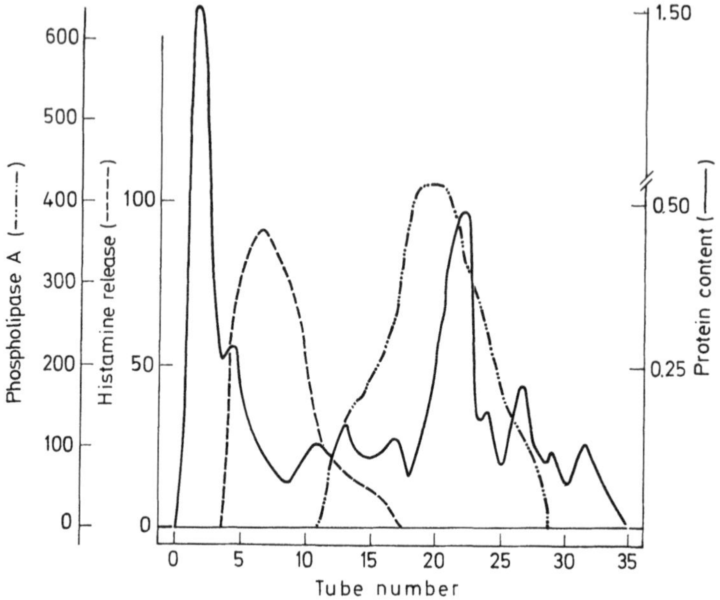

Fig. 1. Chromatographic fractionation of *Crotalus durissus terrificus* venom on Amberlite CG-50 (XE-64), ion-exchange resin (ROTHSCHILD, 1967). Phospholipase A: μg crude venom equivalents/ml effluent. Histamine release: percent of total amine in rat peritoneal fluid suspension, released after 10 min at 37° C with 1 μg fraction sample protein/ml. Protein: total absorbancy at 280 nm/sample

Table 3. Biochemical characteristics of histamine-releasing components other than phospholipase A, obtained from rattlesnake (*C. durissus terrificus*) venom by ROTHSCHILD (1966, 1967) and MARKWARDT et al. (1966b)

Characteristic	ROTHSCHILD		MARKWARDT et al.
	Crotamine	Noncrotamine component	ALP
Electrophoretic mobility (pH 8.0)	Fast cationic	Slow anionic	Slow anionic
Histamine release tested on:	Isolated rat peritoneal fluid mast cells		Isolated rabbit platelets
Concentration for maximal release (μg/ml)	25	0.25	0.1
Loss of activity upon:			
Heating	No	Yes	Yes
Dialysis	Yes	No	No
Digestion by trypsin		Yes	
DFP treatment			Yes
SH reagent treatment			No
Treatment of mast cells or platelets with metabolic inhibitors	Partial	Yes	Yes
Proteolytic activity on:		Bradykinin	Insulin (β-chain)

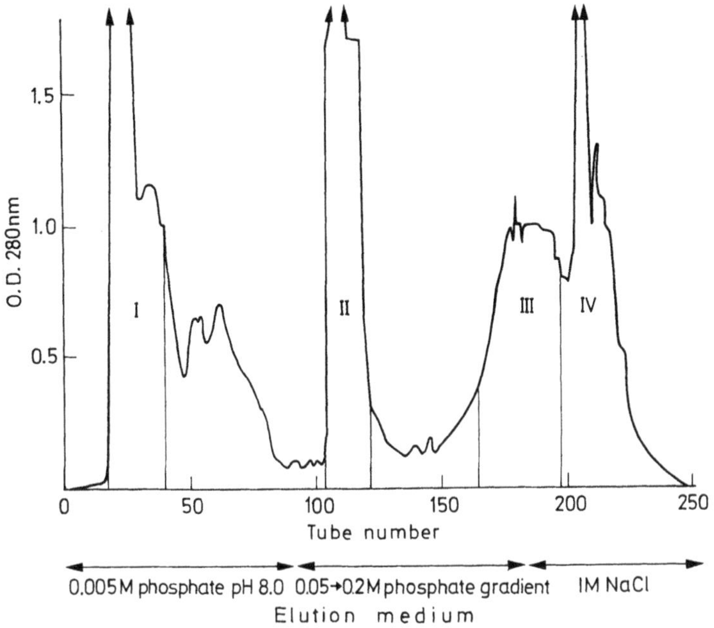

Fig. 2. Chromatographic analysis of *Vipera palestinae* venom on a DEAE-cellulose column (ROTHSCHILD and ROTHSCHILD, 1971). Roman numerals refer to pooled eluates whose pharmacologic activity is described in Table 4

Table 4. Pharmacologic and enzymic properties of fractions obtained after chromatographic separation of *Vipera palestinae* venom on a DEAE-cellulose column. (ROTHSCHILD and ROTHSCHILD, 1971)

Fraction[a]	Activity						
	Histamine release	Brady-kinin formation	Brady-kinin destruction	TAME esterase	Phospho-lipase A	Vascular perme-ability increasing	Hyaluroni-dase
I	+	+	−	+	−	+	+
II	−	−	−	+	−	−	−
III	−	−	−	−	+	−	−
IV	±	−	+	+	±	±	−

[a] Obtained as described in Figure 2.

cells. Like the rattlesnake venom factor (described in Table 3), the histamine-releasing component of *Vipera palestinae* venom did not act on mast cells pretreated with a metabolic inhibitor, 2-4-dinitrophenol (unpublished result).

The direct lytic factor (DLF) is a basic polypeptide present in the Indian cobra (*Naja naja*) venom which markedly potentiates the hemolytic activity of phospholipase A (CONDREA et al., 1964). KAISER et al. (1972), as well as DAMERAU et al. (1975), reported histamine release from rat peritoneal fluid mast cell suspensions by DLF.

This is not unexpected in view of the basic, bulky nature of the compound; such substances are usually good histamine liberators in the rat and occasionally in man (PATON, 1957; ROTHSCHILD, 1966b). KAISER et al. (1972), as well as DAMERAU et al. (1975), looked for a synergism between the histamine-releasing action of cobra venom phospholipase A and DLF. Two biologic structures were used in their investigations: isolated rat peritoneal fluid mast cell suspensions (KAISER et al., 1972; DAMERAU et al., 1975) and the perfused guinea-pig lung (DAMERAU et al., 1975). The results obtained showed that DLF and phospholipase A did not influence each other's action on rat mast cells; in contrast, in the guinea-pig lung, they were definitely synergistic. Rat and guinea-pig mast cells vary greatly in their sensitivity to basic histamine releasers which have compound 48/80 as their prototype (ROTHSCHILD, 1966b). Those of guinea-pig lung, for instance, require nearly 100 times higher concentrations of 48/80 than those of rat lung to present the same degree of histamine release (MOTA, 1966; ROTHSCHILD, 1970). Qualitative differences also exist: guinea-pig mast cells cannot be stimulated to release histamine by the metabolically linked, secretory process involving granule exocytosis (DOUGLAS, 1968), which characterizes the rat mast cell's response to compound 48/80. ROTHSCHILD (1970) postulated a nonspecific ion-exchange process as the mechanism by which 48/80 releases histamine from guinea-pig tissue.

In partial agreement with this finding, DAMERAU et al. (1975), have concluded that DLF has two mechanisms of action: 1) as a basic compound, it may attack the highly sensitive mast cells of the rat in the manner of compound 48/80 and in concentrations too small to potentiate the effect of phospholipase A, and 2) the less sensitive mast cells of guinea-pigs may be damaged by a cytolytic, nonspecific process, involving the potentiation of phospholipase A in the manner described by CONDREA et al. (1964) for the synergistically hemolytic action of DLF and phospholipase A on erythrocytes.

IV. Contribution of Histamine Toward Toxic Effects of Snake Venoms

The contribution of histamine-releasing factors toward the toxic effects of a snake bite is, like that of other pharmacologically active components of venoms, difficult to evaluate. As pointed out many years ago by CHOPRA et al. (1935), and reemphasized by HALMAGYI et al. (1965), the effects of intravenous injections of high doses of venoms, or the results of experiments employing perfusion or incubation of isolated tissues or cells with pharmacologically active quantities of venom (Table 1), may represent an overly magnified picture of the consequences of the slow absorption and distribution over the body of venom innoculated by a snake into its victim. Nevertheless, histamine release following a poisonous snake bite may, on occasion, give rise to serious disturbances. EFRATI (1966) has described the gastrointestinal distress (nausea, abdominal pain, diarrhea), peripheral shock, and angioneurotic (Quinke) edema of tongue, lips, glottis, and even brain, observed in some victims by *Vipera palestinae* who, for technical reasons, could not be given specific antivenin therapy. These symptoms closely resemble those of anaphylactic shock (ROCHA E SILVA, 1966) and are probably due to generalized histamine release. It is interesting to note that such symptomatology may also arise after a snakebite, not only because of the action of histamine-releasing components present in venom, but also as a consequence of true anaphylactic shock occurring in individuals previously sensitized to snake venom proteins (MINTON, 1974).

It is usually considered that snake venoms owe only a minor part of their systemic toxicity to histamine release. This conclusion first brought forth by DRAGSTEDT et al. (1938) has been restated by SCHÖTTLER (1954), LEFRON and MICHAUD (1956), SNYDER (1962), DEVI and SARKAR (1966), and others, who based their claim on the inefficacy of antihistamine therapy to prevent death of experimentally envenomed animals. Even strong histamine-releasing venoms like those of the elapids *Denisonia superba* and *Naja naja* (FELDBERG and KELLAWAY, 1938), or the crotalid *Crotalus durissus terrificus* (MARKWARDT et al., 1966b), would then owe little of their systemic toxicity to histamine. While neurotoxins and/or cardiotoxins existing in such venoms are certainly to be blamed for their major toxic effects, it is our view that further experimental evaluation of histamine's contribution to systemic and, especially, local toxicity of snake venoms is desirable. BLACK et al. (1972) have recently shown that some of the circulatory symptoms evoked by histamine cannot be fully inhibited by classic H_1 histamine-receptor antagonists but require, in addition, treatment with H_2-type antihistaminics. The recorded inability of antihistamines to influence snake venom toxicity should be reexamined in the light of these newer findings. Evidence of the partial involvement of histamine in the vascular permeability-increasing effect of *V. palestinae* venom is discussed in Section C.IV.3.

Histamine release by purified snake venom fractions has been comparatively little investigated in vivo. WESTERMAN and KLAPPER (1960), using a simple dialysis procedure, separated the venom of *Naja naja* into two mixtures made up of, respectively, low (ND) and high (NR) molecular weight components. The ND mixture produced a threefold rise in plasma histamine following intravenous injection into cats; a maximal effect, occurring 4 min after the injection, was accompanied by a corresponding fall of blood pressure. The association between the two phenomena was also demonstrated in antihistamine-pretreated cats, which failed to present the hypotensive response. NR, the nondialyzable, presumably enzymatic components of the venom, also produced a hypotensive response in the cat; this, however, was unaffected by antihistaminics. DAMERAU et al. (1975) assigned to DLF (CONDREA et al., 1964) the major responsibility for the histamine-releasing activity of cobra venom. This factor is presumably the active component of the dialysate ND. Yet, using the same fractionation procedure as WESTERMAN and KLAPPER (1960), MAY et al. (1967) showed that the ND fraction failed to release histamine in guinea-pigs or rats which, however, responded to NR, the phospholipase A-containing, high molecular weight fraction of the venom. These discrepancies indicate that species-linked variations in sensitivity to the different histamine-releasing components of a snake venom should be expected in work with different experimental animal species.

B. 5-Hydroxytryptamine

I. Survey of 5-Hydroxytryptamine-Releasing Activity of Snake Venoms

Evidence on the 5-hydroxytryptamine (5-HT, serotonin)-releasing activity of snake venoms is slight. Practically the only systematic survey on this subject is that of MARKWARDT et al. (1966), who used rabbit platelets suspended in rabbit plasma or in buffer as sources of the amine. Their results, reproduced in abridged form in Table 2, show that histamine- and 5-HT-releasing activity of all venoms tested are closely paralleled. Rabbit platelets are an adequate source for such studies, since rabbits are unique among laboratory animals in having large amounts of both 5-HT and histamine in circulating platelets. It would be hazardous, however, to expect the same pattern of relative activities shown in Table 2 to occur in other tissues or species. No studies on the effect of snake venoms on mast cell 5-HT have been reported. Since histamine and 5-HT are released together from rat mast cells exposed to compound 48/80 or antigen (MORAN et al., 1962), it would be of interest to know whether snake venoms cause a similar parallel pattern of amine release when incubated with isolated rat mast cells. In species other than rat, hamster, or mouse, 5-HT is not stored in mast cells (ERSPAMER, 1966). Even in the rat skin which is particularly rich in 5-HT and histamine, nonmast cell storage of 5-HT has been described (PARRAT and WEST, 1957; SMITH and LEWIS, 1961). Nonrodents contain 5-HT only in the enterochromaffin cells of the gut, in blood platelets, and in certain areas (mainly brain stem, rhinencephalon, and neostriatum) of the central nervous system (ERSPAMER, 1966). These would be the sites to look for evidence of 5-HT release in future studies on the role of 5-HT in snake venom pharmacology.

II. Systemic Effects

The only evidence of the release of 5-HT by a purified snake venom component has been presented by MARKWARDT et al. (1966b). They showed that the intravenous administration to rabbits of the ALP of rattlesnake *(Crotalus durissus terrificus)* venom (see Table 3) was able to produce a triphasic blood pressure change, of strong tachyphylactic character, reproduced in part by 5-HT. The amounts of the amine injected were approximately equal to those found to be lost from the blood of the rabbit as a consequence of the injection of the active fraction. The injection of ALP was well-tolerated both by rabbits and mice. The latter were asymptomatic after the injection of ALP in amounts equivalent, on a weight basis, to a rapidly lethal dose of crude rattlesnake venom. The contribution of 5-HT toward serious systemic symptoms of *Crotalus d. terrificus* envenomation thus appears to be negligible in experimental animals. According to the evidence presented in Table 2, histamine must have been released together with 5-HT. In their explanation of the blood pressure changes evoked by ALP, the contribution of histamine was apparently not taken into account by MARKWARDT et al. (1966). This does not seem to be justified, since histamine is a potent vasodepressor agent in the urethane-anesthetized rabbit (FELDBERG, 1927).

III. Local Effects

With the exception of the rat, experimental animals present only weak vascular permeability changes to the intradermal injection of doses of 5-HT equal or even higher than those expected to be released at the site of a snakebite. The importance of serotonin as a mediator of the vascular permeability change caused by *Vipera russellii* and *Echis carinatus* venoms (FEARN et al., 1964) should be restricted to the rat and closely related rodents.

C. Bradykinin

I. Introduction

ROCHA E SILVA et al. (1949) were the first to demonstrate that a snake venom, that of *Bothrops jararaca*, was able to release a smooth muscle-stimulating, powerfully hypotensive polypeptide, termed bradykinin, from plasma globulin, a physiologically abundant substrate. Subsequent studies, reviewed by BRECHER and BROBMAN (1970), HADDY et al. (1970), HILTON (1970), SCHACHTER (1970), WALASZEK (1970), and ARMSTRONG (1970), have extended the range of pharmacodynamic activities of bradykinin and related kinins to include, among others, effects on vascular tone, vascular permeability and the production of localized pain. Since these symptoms are also caused by many poisonous snakes and since kinin-forming enzymes, kininogenases, are widely distributed among viperid and crotalid snake venoms, a relatively large amount of information on the release and possible role of bradykinin in snake venom toxicity has been gathered.

II. Survey of the Kinin-Forming Capacity of Snake Venoms

Table 5 shows the results of surveys, made by different authors, of the bradykinin-forming capacity of venoms from 50 species of poisonous snakes. Although each group of authors worked under somewhat different experimental conditions, their results were compared in order to present, as far as possible, a uniform picture of the field. With the exception of *Dendroaspis angusticeps* (OSHIMA et al., 1969), elapid snake venoms have either very low or no kinin-forming activity. Among viperids, relatively high kinin-releasing activity was found in *Bitis gabonica* and *Vipera ammodytes* venoms (OSHIMA et al., 1969; MEBS, 1970). *Vipera palestinae* venom was found to be an active kinin-releasing agent both by OSHIMA et al. (1969) and ROTHSCHILD and ROTHSCHILD (1971). Opinions agree in placing crotalid venoms among the most active of the kinin-forming venoms. *Crotalus viridis viridis* is outstanding in this respect, followed in effectiveness by the venoms of *Crotalus horridus*, *Sistrurus miliaris*, and *Agkistrodon piscivorus* (MEBS, 1970), or, according to OSHIMA et al. (1969), the venoms of *C. atrox*, *T. gramineus*, and *A. contortrix contortrix*. DEUTSCH and DINIZ (1955) showed *A. contortrix contortrix* venom as the most active kinin-releasing agent of their series, followed by the venoms of *C. atrox*, *Lachesis muta*, *C. adamanteus*, and *C. horridus*. The venom of *L. muta* has recently been further purified (MAGALHÃES et al., 1973); its kinin-releasing component was found to be at least twice as active as crystalline trypsin when tested on a partly purified dog plasma kininogen substrate.

The comparison of the kinin-forming potencies of the venoms studied by DEUTSCH and DINIZ (1955) with those by OSHIMA et al. (1969) is not directly possible because, in contrast to DEUTSCH and DINIZ, the Japanese workers employed venoms whose kinin-destroying (kininase) activities had been blocked by pretreatment with ethylenediaminetetraacetate (EDTA). Kininase action, although usually appreciably slower than that of the kinin-releasing enzymes of snake venoms, can decrease kinin yield even after short incubation periods. Since, however, DEUTSCH and DINIZ (1955) presented data on the intrinsic, kinin-destroying activity of the venoms examined, it

Table 5. Kinin-forming activity of snake venoms according to different authors

Species	Activity units[a]			
	DEUTSCH and DINIZ (1955)	MEBS (1968, 1970)	OSHIMA et al. (1969a)	Others
Elapidae				
Naja naja	—	0	—	
N. naja atra	—	0	3.9	
N. melanoleuca	—	—	0	
N. nivea	—	0	—	
N. nigricollis	—	0	0.3	
Hemachatus haemachatus	—	0	0.2	
Dendroaspis angusticeps	—	0	15.6	
Ophiophagus hannah	—	0	0	
Bungarus fasciatus	—	0	0.1	
B. multicinctus	—	0	0	
Pseudechis collettii	—	0	—	
Colubridae				
Leptodeira annulata	—	0	—	
Viperidae				
Bitis arietans	—	0	6.57	+[d]
B. gabonica	—	4	215.0	
B. nasicornis	—	15	—	
Echis carinatus	—	1	9.6	2.5[b]
E. coloratus	—	2.5	—	
Cerastes cerastes	—	0	—	
Causus rhombeatus	—	0	6.6	
Vipera ammodytes	—	6	107.8	+[d]
V. berus	—	—	—	+[d]
V. palestinae	—	—	40.0	4.2[c]
V. russellii	—	0	1.3	0[d]
V. lebetina	—	—	—	0.25[b]
V. ursini	—	—	—	0.61[b]
Crotalidae				0.61[b]
Agkistrodon acutus	—	—	0.5	
A. bilineatus	—	0	0	
A. contortrix mokeson	—	—	38.6	
A. contortrix contortrix	26.5	5	72.6	
A. halys blomhoffii	—	3	25.2	
A. p. piscivorus	6.8	7.5	28.0	5.5[b]
Bothrops alternata	0.3	0	—	
B. atrox	1.9	0	5.0	
B. cotiara	1.3	7	—	
B. jararaca	8.6	1.5	10.4	
B. jararacussu	—	0	—	2.1[b]
B. insularis	0.70	0	—	
B. neuwidii	0.45	0	—	
B. numifera	—	2.5	—	
B. picadoi	—	3.5	—	
Lachesis muta	20.5	—	—	
Crotalus adamanteus	18.1	2.5	20.4	
C. atrox	23.1	6	124.3	
C. basilicus	—	—	24.5	
C. durissus terrificus	1.3	0	56.5	

Table 5 (continued)

Species	Activity units[a]			
	DEUTSCH and DINIZ (1955)	MEBS (1968, 1970)	OSHIMA et al. (1969a)	Others
C. horridus	15.6	12	—	
C. viridis viridis	—	31	233.5	
Sistrurus catenatus	—	5	—	
S. miliaris	—	10	—	
Trimeresurus flavoviridis	—	0	3.0	
T. gramineus	—	—	54.4	
T. mucrosquamatus	—	—	28.6	
T. okinavensis	—	2.5	4.3	

[a] 0: no activity; –: not tested; +: qualitative evidence of activity. Units: DEUTSCH and DINIZ (1955): units (1 U = 0.5 μg synthetic bradykinin) of kinin formed per mg of venom per min at 37° C, from bovine serum pseudo globulin substrate; MEBS (1968, 1970): 1 mg venom contains 1 U when it releases 1 μg bradykinin per min at 37° C, equine plasma; OSHIMA et al. (1969): 1 mg venom contains 1 U when it releases 1 μg bradykinin per min at 37° C, from purified bovine kininogen, in the presence of EDTA.
[b] According to HENRIQUES and EVSEEVA (1969).
[c] According to ROTHSCHILD and ROTHSCHILD (1971).
[d] According to WERLE et al. (1950).

Table 6. Kinin-releasing (KR) and kinin-destroying (KD) activities of some snake venoms

Species	Untreated venom[a]				EDTA-treated venom[b] KR	
	KR		KD			
	Units	Relative activity	Units	Relative activity	Units	Relative activity
Agkistrodon contortrix	26.5	(100)	0	(0)	72.6	(100)
Crotalus atrox	23.1	(87)	5.6	(100)	124.3	(171)
Crotalus adamanteus	18.1	(68)	0.03	(0.5)	20.4	(28)
Bothrops jararaca	8.6	(32)	0.36	(6)	10.4	(14)
Agkistrodon piscivorus	6.8	(25)	0	(0)	28.0	(38)
Bothrops atrox	1.9	(7)	0.25	(4)	5.0	(7)
C. durissus terrificus	1.7	(6)	0.30	(5)	56.5	(78)

[a] According to DEUTSCH and DINIZ (1955).
[b] According to OSHIMA et al. (1969); it is assumed that kinin-destroying activity is fully inhibited by EDTA.

became possible, by assigning a value of 100 to the most active member of each author's series, placing the remaining values on scales of decreasing potencies and using kininase data to explain major discrepancies, to obtain a useful comparison between the results of these groups of workers (Table 6). Thus, the venoms from *A. contortrix* and *A. piscivorus* had approximately the same relative activities regardless of the presence of EDTA, a finding explainable by their absolute lack of kinin-destroying activity. In contrast, the venoms of *C. atrox* and *C. durissus terrificus* became relatively much more active after EDTA treatment, an expected consequence of the removal of their high kininase activity. No clear correlations could be established between EDTA treatment and the kinin-forming capacities of *B. jararaca* and *B. atrox* venoms. Although containing comparable amounts of kinin-destroying activity, these venoms showed, respectively, a lessened and unchanged relative kinin-forming activity after EDTA treatment. Such discrepancies, which may have been due to methodologic differences, presence of activators, kinin-releasing cofactors, or other causes, reflect both the challenge and the complexity of quantitative snake venom pharmacology.

III. Mechanistic Aspects

1. Arginine Ester Hydrolase Activity and Kinin Release

HAMBERG and ROCHA E SILVA (1957) showed that the kininogenase activity of *Bothrops jararaca* venom was due to part of its benzoylarginine methyl ester hydrolase content. Subsequent work (HABERMANN, 1961; IWANAGA et al., 1965; MEBS, 1968; ROTHSCHILD and ROTHSCHILD, 1971) extended these observations to other snake species and showed that indeed only some of the snake venom's arginine esterases is responsible for kinin-releasing action. OSHIMA et al. (1969) have examined, respectively, kinin-releasing and TAME-hydrolyzing activities in the venoms of 23 species of vipers and concluded that no parallelism exists between them. MEBS (1968) even showed that the elapid *Ophiophagus hannah's* venom had fair BAEE esterase activity but no ability to form kinin. OSHIMA et al. (1969) have made an opposite observation: the venom from *Dendroaspis angusticeps* was able to release kinin but surprisingly had no detectable activity on p-tosylarginine methyl ester (TAME). TU et al. (1965), as well as KOCHOLATY et al. (1971), confirmed inactivity of this venom on TAME but did not investigate its kinin-releasing effect. Nevertheless, no purified snake venom kininogenase has as yet been shown to be exempt of arginine ester hydrolase activity (SUZUKI and IWANAGA, 1970).

2. Substrate Requirements

Presently available synthetic arginine esters lack sufficient specific susceptibility to be useful substrates for the assay of snake venom kininogenases. Thus, they cannot be employed in the manner recommended for some mammalian kininogenases by TRAUTSCHOLD (1970), and the evaluation of a venom's kinin-forming ability must still be performed using kininogen, its natural protein substrate.

There is only scant evidence (HAMBERG and ROCHA E SILVA, 1957) to suggest that snake venoms can act indirectly on plasma kininogen via the activation of a plasma kallikrein precursor in the manner demonstrated by WERLE et al. (1955) for trypsin. Most snake venoms are, therefore, to be considered true kininogenases in the sense described by the Committee on Nomenclature for Hypotensive Peptides (WEBSTER, 1970). Since kinin-destroying enzymes of plasma lose their activity after heating, while kininogen retains it (ERDÖS and YANG, 1970), heated whole plasma of different origins has been used as the substrate for the assay of snake venom kininogenase

(HENRIQUES and EVSEEVA, 1969; COHEN et al., 1970; HABERMANN, 1970; ROTHSCHILD and ROTHSCHILD, 1971). Another preferred substrate (DEUTSCH and DINIZ, 1955; MEBS, 1968; HENRIQUES et al., 1962) has been the ammonium sulfate-precipitated globulin fraction of bovine or canine plasma; it contains the bulk of the kinin precursor reserves of animal plasma and little or none of its kinin-destroying enzymes (ROCHA E SILVA et al., 1949).

3. Kinin Peptides Released by Snake Venoms

There is little evidence to suggest that snake venoms release kinins other than bradykinin (kinin-9). HABERMANN (1963), as well as WEBSTER and PIERCE (1963), have shown that the venoms of *Vipera ammodytes*, *Crotalus adamanteus*, *Bothrops jararaca*, *Agkistrodon contortrix*, and *A. piscivorus* release only bradykinin from whole plasma. In this respect, they resemble trypsin but not glandular kallikrein or plasmin which besides bradykinin release other kinin peptides from whole plasma (WEBSTER and PIERCE, 1963; HENRIQUES et al., 1969).

4. Inhibition of Kinin-Releasing Activity

Venoms from *B. jararaca*, *V. ammodytes*, *C. adamanteus*, and *A. halys blomhoffii* are inhibited in over 95% of their kinin-releasing activity by pretreatment with diisopropylfluorophosphate (DFP), a specific reactant of the serine group of the active center of many esterases (HABERMANN, 1961; IWANAGA et al., 1965). Both HABERMANN (1961), working with the crude venom of *B. jararaca*, *C. adamanteus*, and *V. ammodytes*, and COHEN et al. (1970), working with a purified kininogenase from *Echis colorata* venom, showed inhibition of kinin release by the arginine hydrolase substrate, TAME or BAEE. In contrast, none of these venoms nor the kininogenase from *E. colorata* was inhibited by benzoylargininamide (BAA), a typical amidase substrate. The absence of an amidase character of the kinin-releasing enzyme in *B. jararaca* venom has been reported by HENRIQUES et al. (1960) and in *A. halys blomhoffii* venom by SATO et al. (1965).

With the exception of the kininogenase from *Vipera lebetina*, which was sensitive to the trypsin inhibitor from soybeans (SBTI), (HENRIQUES and EVSEEVA, 1969) and the kinin-releasing enzyme from *A. halys blomhoffii*, which was sensitive to the kallikrein inhibitor from bovine tissues, trasylol (IWANAGA, 1965), no other venom has as yet been reported to be inhibited in its kinin-releasing activity by proteinase inhibitors of plant or animal origin (WERLE et al., 1950; DEUTSCH and DINIZ, 1955; HENRIQUES and EVSEEVA, 1969; COHEN et al., 1970).

IV. Contribution of Bradykinin Toward Systemic and Local Effects of Snake Venoms

1. Hypotension

The release of large amounts of bradykinin into the circulation can be expected to lead to transient hypotension, since this is the predominant effect observed after intravenous administration of the polypeptide to most mammalian species. It is the consequence of the action of bradykinin on peripheral arterioles, producing vasodilatation (HADDY et al., 1970). Most viperid and crotalid venoms contain bradykinin-releasing enzymes; together with histamine, they certainly could contribute toward the circulatory shock observed when doses of venom high enough to cause generalized kinin release reach the circulation within a sufficiently short time. This can occur when a snakebite is so placed that an appreciable amount of venom is innoculated directly into a major blood vessel of the victim. MINTON (1974) has suggested that the sudden release of large amounts of kinin could be responsible for hypotension severe enough to cause the transient loss of consciousness observed after bites by large vipers. EFRATI (1966) reported peripheral shock in some victims of bites by *Vipera palestinae*, a species whose venom is known to contain, besides histamine-releasing, kinin-forming activity (ROSEN et al., 1964; ROTHSCHILD and ROTHSCHILD, 1971).

WERLE et al. (1950) reported that venoms from *B. jararaca* and *V. ammodytes*, although able to release kinin in vitro, were only weakly hypotensive in the intact animal. These results were not confirmed. ROTHSCHILD and ALMEIDA (1972) have shown that 0.5–2.0 mg/kg of *B. jararaca* venom caused rapid disappearance of circulatory kininogen, accompanied by intense but transitory hypotension, in rats protected from the venom's lethal intravascular clotting effect by heparin. OSHIMA et al. (1969) have analyzed the effects of venoms from four species of crotalid snakes in the dog. They showed that while venoms from *Agkistrodon halys blomhoffii* and *Trimeresurus gramineus* were capable of inducing both kinin release and hypotension, those from *A. acutus* and *T. flavoviridis* were weakly hypotensive and poor kinin-releasing agents. MARGOLIS et al. (1965) have studied the relationship between kininogen stores and the hypotensive action of *Crotalus atrox* venom in sheep. They found kinin precursor to be completely exhausted by a continuous, 30–60 min infusion of 1.5–2 μg/kg/min of venom, which, after 10 min also caused a reversible fall in femoral artery blood pressure, roughly equivalent to that elicited by a 4-min infusion of 2 μg of synthetic bradykinin per kg. Thus, kinin probably plays a role in the acute hypotension which follows the injection of *Crotalus atrox* venom into sheep. However, as observed by MARGOLIS et al. (1965), the persistence or recurrence of shock with larger or repeated doses of venom after $^1/_2$–1 h, i.e., after plasma kininogen stores had been exhausted, suggests that the release of kinin into the circulation was not the sole source of hypotension. It is worth noting that *Crotalus atrox* has weak but definite histamine-releasing ability (FELDBERG and KELLAWAY, 1937b; DRAGSTEDT et al., 1938). Since tissue histamine stores are only slowly depleted in envenomed animals (FELDBERG and KELLAWAY, 1937b), histamine may become the major hypotensive factor in envenomed, plasma kininogen-depleted animals. It would, however, also be important to assess the contribution toward such delayed snake venom toxicity, of nonhumoral kinin, which exists in the kininogen stores, shown by WERLE and ZACH (1970) to occur in most animal organs. HABERMANN (1961) demonstrated that electrophoretically separated fractions from *V. ammodytes*, *B. jararaca*, and *C. adamanteus* venoms are able both to lower blood pressure and to release kinin in rabbits. Crude *V. ammodytes* venom evoked a hypotensive response, characterized by a rapid intense initial fall followed, within 1 min, by a secondary hypotensive phase of a slightly slower character, irreversible for at least 1 h. The first response was apparently unchanged when venom preincubated for 30 min with DFP was used; the second response was abolished. A different picture was shown when venoms from *B. jararaca* and *C. adamanteus* were tested. Although a biphasic hypotensive response was again obtained, it was now the first phase which was abolished, when venoms pretreated with DFP were employed. Interpretation of these data is difficult, because other experiments (HABERMANN, 1961) showed that activity after DFP treatment was not only quantitatively but also qualitatively different according to the dose of venom injected into the animal. However, it becomes clear that DFP, preincubated with each of these venoms, was able to substantially reduce one or more phases of the hypotensive response evoked in the rabbit. Since DFP was also able to inhibit the in vitro kinin-releasing activity of these venoms, such results indicate the importance of kinin in the shock which may follow envenomation by true or pit vipers. However, the participation of other factors, whose activity may also be sensitive to DFP, must be taken into account. One such factor is histamine which, under the conditions employed by HABERMANN (1961), e.g., urethane-chloralose anesthesia, can be expected to cause hypotension in the rabbit (FELDBERG, 1927). It seems that real knowledge about the manner by which pharmacologically complex mixtures like viper venoms induce hypotension will only be gained when their pure constituents, prepared with utmost refinements of protein fractionation technique, will be assayed in the experimental animal, adequately combined to reproduce the whole venom's pharmacologic effects. This goal may not be reached for quite some time.

2. Lethality

HABERMANN (1961) has pointed out that although DFP pretreatment of *B. jararaca* venom blocks its kinin-releasing activity in rabbits, it fails to change its lethality in mice. ROTHSCHILD and ALMEIDA (1972) depleted rats of 50% of their plasma kininogen stores by treating them with cellulose sulfate, a potent activator of plasma kininogenase (ROTHSCHILD, 1968). Such rats presented lower lethality after *Bothrops jararaca* venom (Table 7). This result led at first to the conclusion that kinin release was of major importance in causing death by *B. jararaca* venom in the rat. Further experimentation, however, showed this not to be so. Heparin was as efficient an inhibitor of the venom's lethality as cellulose sulfate, yet failed to inhibit the hypotensive response (Fig. 3) or plasma kininogen consumption (Table 7) evoked by the venom.

Confirming previous findings by GRASSET and SCHWARTZ (1954) that rabbits present lethal intravascular clotting during *B. jararaca* envenomation, ROTHSCHILD and ALMEIDA (1972) showed that heparin, as well as cellulose sulfate, prevented death by inhibiting venom-induced hypercoagulation of the blood. The former acts by inhibiting activation of endogenous thrombin caused by the venom's procoagulant action (HOLTZ and RAUDONAT, 1956; DE VRIES et al., 1963), whereas the latter, by causing extensive consumption of circulating fibrinogen (ROSA et al., 1972), an essential component of the blood clotting system (Table 7). Autopsies confirmed these conclusions: control *Bothrops* envenomed rats presented extensive intravascular clotting in the splanchnic area, while cellulose sulfate or heparin-pretreated animals were free of this symptom. If one permits oneself a teleologic digression, this result could perhaps mean that production of hypotension rather than death, resulting from massive kinin release, was destined by nature to aid a snake in immobilizing its

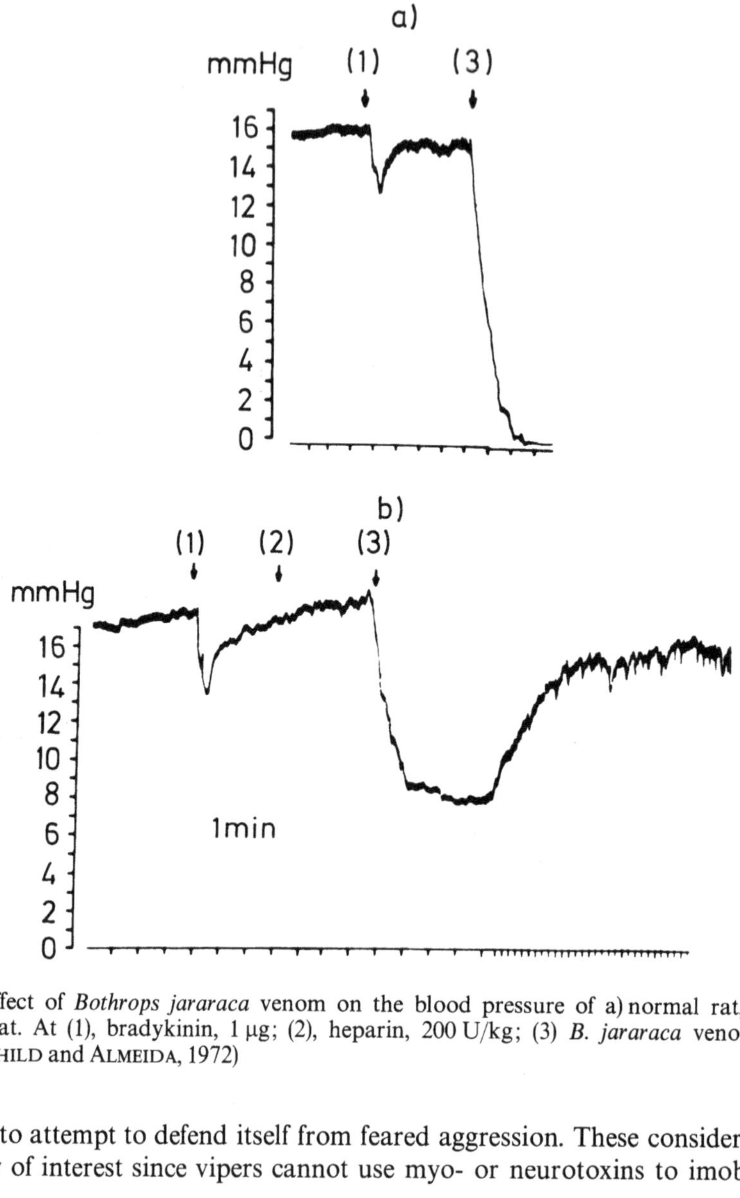

Fig. 3. Effect of *Bothrops jararaca* venom on the blood pressure of a) normal rat, b) heparin treated rat. At (1), bradykinin, 1 μg; (2), heparin, 200 U/kg; (3) *B. jararaca* venom, 2 mg/kg (ROTHSCHILD and ALMEIDA, 1972)

prey or to attempt to defend itself from feared aggression. These considerations are possibly of interest since vipers cannot use myo- or neurotoxins to imobilize their victims.

3. Increased Vascular Permeability and Pain

MINTON (1974) presented vivid descriptions of the intense, spreading edema and acute pain arising at the site of a viper's bite. These symptoms recall the strong vascular permeability-enhancing and algogenic properties of bradykinin, possibly the most powerful natural agonist of these effects in experimental animals and man (WILHLEM, 1962; COLLIER and LEE, 1963; KEELE and ARMSTRONG, 1964; ARMSTRONG, 1970). In contrast to viperids and crotalids, elapid snakes are, in general

Table 7. Effect of heparin (Hep) and cellulose sulfate (CS) on mortality, plasma bradykininogen (BKG), clotting time, and fibrinogen content of the blood of rats injected with *B. jararaca* venom (Vb). (From ROTHSCHILD and ALMEIDA, 1972)

Treatment mg/kg, i.v.	Survival time	BKG[a] %	Clotting time (LEE-WHITE)	Fibrinogen (mg %)
Saline		100	60 s	238
Vb, 0.5	> 7 days	65	15 s[ly]	0
Vb, 1.0	14 min	40	10 s[ly]	0
Vb, 2.0	3 min	33	10 s[ly]	0
Hep, 1.0		100	> 2 h	225
Hep, 2.0		100	> 2 h	230
Hep, 1.0; after 15'Vb, 2.0	8 min	35	10 s	0
Hep, 2.0; after 15'Vb, 2.0	> 7 days	35	> 2 h	26
CS, 1.0	> 7 days	53	62 s	57
Cs, 1.0; after 15'Vb, 2.0	> 7 days	21	2 h	0

[a] Det. 3–5 min after treatment; controls had 2.4±0.1 μg BKG/ml. 1y indicates clotting followed by rapid lysis. Each result is the average of 3–6 experiments.

unable to release bradykinin although certain *Naja* species liberate histamine (Table 1) and anaphylatoxin (p. 618). It is perhaps a testimony of the importance of kinin for the local effects of snake venoms that such symptoms are usually slight after elapid snakebites (MINTON, 1974). Nevertheless, clear-cut evidence to implicate kinin in the etiology of these effects has been far from clear. One of the reasons for this is undoubtedly the unavailability of specific antagonists of bradykinin (SCHRÖDER, 1970). Another reason is the awareness that, at the site of innoculation of a venom, bradykinin, histamine, and probably other, not fully known mediators contribute in a synergistic manner toward vascular and painful symptoms. Identification of a single mediator's contribution to such local reactions should be an extremely complex task. Attempts in this direction have been made, but seem to have gone further in discrediting than in proving the participation of a given mediator in such reactions. SATO et al. (1965) separated the venom of *Agkistrodon halys blomhoffii* into several chromatographically purified components. One of these, capable of inducing increased vascular permeability when injected into a rabbit's skin, did not release kinin from bovine plasma globulin substrate. Another component had opposite properties; it was a strong kinin releasing agent but failed to increase vascular permeability. The same dissociation between kinin-releasing action and vascular permeability-increasing activity was observed by BHARGAVA et al. (1972), with fractions obtained from the venom of *Agkistrodon piscivorus*. ROTHSCHILD and ROTHSCHILD (unpublished) have recently partly separated and analyzed the histamine-liberating, kinin-forming, and vascular permeability-increasing properties of the basic fraction of *Vipera palestinae* venom, isolated according to KOCHWA et al. (1960).

After chromatography on Sephadex G-100, two pharmacologically active components could be demonstrated (Fig. 4). One released histamine from isolated rat peritoneal fluid mast cells, raised vascular permeability in the rat skin, and exhibited strong hydrolytic activity on benzoylarginine ethyl ester (BAEE); the other formed bradykinin in heated equine plasma, had no effect on vascular permeability, and a

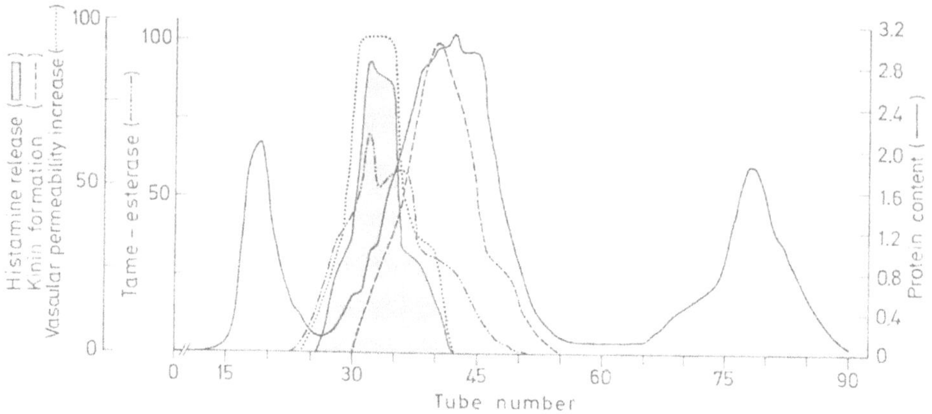

Fig. 4. Chromatographic fractionation on Sephadex G-100 of histamine-releasing, kinin-forming, rat skin vascular permeability-increasing, and p-TAME hydrolyzing activities contained in the basic fraction (Fig. 2) of *Vipera palestinae* venom. Column: 105 × 20 cm; 49 mg protein, 0.1 M, pH 8.0 phosphate buffer eluent at 9 ml/h, room temperature. Protein: total absorbancy at 280 nm/sample. Histamine release: percent of total amine in rat peritoneal fluid suspension, released after 10 min at 37° C with 10 µg fraction sample protein/ml. TAME esterase: µmoles of 20 mM substrate hydrolyzed per mg protein per min at 37° C (ROTHSCHILD, 1968). Vascular permeability increase: percent of the blued area evoked by 200 µg crude venom, caused by 200 µg fraction sample protein/site

relatively modest activity on BAEE. The overlapping of histamine-releasing and vascular permeability-increasing activity, as well as the separation between the latter and the kinin-forming activity, became apparent. In the rat skin, both histamine and serotonin are contained in mast cells (PARRAT and WEST, 1957), released together, and active on vascular permeability (WILHELM, 1962). It seemed, therefore, that histamine and serotonin were the mediators of *V. palestinae* venom's action on vascular permeability. However, tests employing specific inhibitors of the vascular effects of these amines indicated a more complex mechanism.

As shown in Table 8, the effects of the most active fractions of the vascular permeability-increasing component (No. 31 and 32, electrophoretically homogeneous) were only partially inhibited by antihistaminic plus antiserotoninic treatment. Control experiments (Table 8) showed that these inhibitors were able to prevent the vascular permeability-increasing action of compound 48/80, a powerful histamine and serotonin-releasing agent in the rat but failed to affect the action of bradykinin on vascular permeability. It had to be concluded that, besides histamine and serotonin, other factors released by the vasoactive component of *V. palestinae* venom must be contributing toward its vascular permeability-increasing effect in the rat skin. As in the case of an equivalent component of *A. halys blomhoffii* venom (SATO et al., 1965), its mechanism of action remains unknown. It is worth remarking, however, that an alternative cause for its activity, not involving histamine and serotonin, could be the formation of bradykinin not directly from kininogen but indirectly through the activation of the victim's kininogenase system. In order to substantiate such an hypothesis, proof of the existence of a prekallikrein activator (prokininogenase) in snake venoms, equivalent to that described in human or animal plasma (RATNOFF

Table 8. Effect of the histamine and serotonin antagonists, mepyramine and bromolysergic acid diethylamide (BOL), on the responses of vascular rat skin to compound 48/80, bradykinin (BK), and a vascular permeability-increasing component obtained from *Vipera palestinae* venom. (ROTHSCHILD and ROTHSCHILD, 1971)

Compound	Treatment	
	Controls Area of lesion (mm^2)	BOL + Mepyramine[a] Area of lesion (mm^2)
48/80, 50 μg	76 (2)	0 (2)
BK, 5 μg	44 (2)	56 (2)
V. palestinae component (Fractions 31 and 32, Fig. 4)	72 (8)	45 (8)

[a] Drugs were dissolved in saline either in the presence of or without 2 μg each BOL and mepyramine; 0.05 ml of each mixture were injected contralaterally (controls vs. treated) into the ventral skin of rats, previously given an i.v. injection of Evans blue. Responses were read on the everted skin of animals decapitated 20 min after treatment; they are expressed as the product of perpendicular diameters of the blued areas. Figures within parentheses refer to the number of experimental animals employed.

and MILES, 1964; SCHOENMAKERS et al., 1965; KAPLAN and AUSTEN, 1970; TRELOAR et al., 1972; BAGDASARIAN et al., 1973), would, however, have to be provided. Such activators are usually unable to activate kallikrein in heated plasma. Since ROTHSCHILD and ROTHSCHILD (1971) employed such a substrate in their studies, a prekallikrein activator, if present in the vascular permeability-enhancing chromatographic fraction of *V. palestinae* venom, could have escaped detection. We wish to recall in this connection that, working with *Bothrops jararaca* venom, HAMBERG and ROCHA E SILVA (1957) did demonstrate the existence of a kinin-generating mechanism which was only active on unheated bovine plasma. The possible significance of this finding has been generally overlooked.

4. Potentiation of Bradykinin Effects

In most clinical situations, the distribution within the body of the enzymes released from the bitten site is a gradual process in which, among other factors, the hyaluronidase (spreading factor) content of the venom, as well as inflammatory reactions partly due to infection leading to alterations in blood and lymph flow barriers (EDERY and LEWIS, 1963), may play a part. A continuous, perhaps small, but potentially insiduous outpouring of toxic factors from the bitten site occurs, leading to local and systemic edema and pain (EFRATI, 1966; MINTON, 1974). Histamine and kinin may participate in these reactions; in the case of kinin, it is well to recall that nature has provided snakes with means of amplifying their activity. The presence of "bradykinin-potentiating factors" in the venom of *B. jararaca* (FERREIRA, 1965), *A. halys blomhoffii* (SUZUKI and IWANAGA, 1970), *Vipera palestinae* (ROTHSCHILD and ROTHSCHILD, 1971), and some other *Bothrops* and *Crotalus* species (FERREIRA, personal communication) has been reported. Such factors effectively increase both local and systemic actions of kinins (FERREIRA, 1965; AMORIM et al., 1967; ARMSTRONG, 1970).

D. Slow-Reacting Substances, Prostaglandins, and Lysophosphatides

I. Background

Slow-reacting substances (SRS) have been described by VOGT (1969) as substances which slowly contract the guinea-pig ileum, released from tissues or cells but not from plasma, following injurious or potentially injurious stimulation. Being lipids, SRS are easily dissolved in organic solvents; this property distinguishes them from the highly polar kinin polypeptides, which are much more soluble in water than in lipid solvents.

The first clear demonstration that a smooth muscle-contracting principle different from histamine arises during the contact of snake venoms with animal tissues was supplied by FELDBERG and KELLAWAY (1937b, 1938). They showed that venoms from *Denisonia superba*, *Naja naja*, and *Crotalus atrox* perfused through the lung or liver of guinea-pigs, cats, dogs, or rhesus monkeys led to the progressive increase of the perfusing fluid's ability to cause a delayed, slowly developing contraction of the guinea-pig jejunum. Unlike histamine, the slowly acting gut stimulant was not preformed in the tissue but arose as a consequence of an enzymic attack of the venom on proper substrates present in tissues. In further studies which, judging from the state of knowledge at that time and the complexity of the subject, are masterworks of clarity, FELDBERG and KELLAWAY (1938) and FELDBERG et al. (1938) presented evidence that at least two pharmacologically active groups of substances arose after contact of animal tissues with cobra venom. One, termed "lysocithin," was a mixture of lysophosphatides arising from the action of cobra venom's powerful phospholipase A on phospholipids. It could be selectively precipitated by ethyl ether and was demonstrated not to be responsible for the gut-stimulating activity of envenomed organ extracts. Lysophosphatides actually had a definite depressant activity on the intestine; of course, they also showed a strong direct hemolytic activity. The ether-soluble portions of envenomed organ or egg yolk extracts contained the gut-stimulating activity; they were only weakly hemolytic and already at that time considered to be unsaturated fatty acids. Chromatographic separations of the products of the contact of cobra venom with egg yolk (VOGT, 1957) revealed their pharmacologic similarity to products arising from the envenomed guinea-pig lung tissue (SCHÜTZ and VOGT, 1961), confirming earlier conclusions of FELDBERG et al. (1938).

According to SCHÜTZ and VOGT (1961), the spasmogenic agonists are conveniently assayed on the antihistamine-treated guinea-pig ileum; it should be noted that they sensitize this structure toward other spasmogens. The type of contraction which they elicited caused them to be named slow-reacting substances (SRS), in analogy with apparently similar principles, SRS-A, found to arise in sensitized, antigen-stimulated tissues (KELLAWAY and TRETHEWIE, 1940; CHAKRAVARTY and UVNÄS, 1960; BROCKLEHURST, 1960; ORANGE et al., 1973). Chromatographic analysis of active principles formed in cobra venom-perfused guinea-pig lung (SRS-C) showed them to be hydroxylated, unsaturated fatty acids belonging to the prostaglandin family (PGF) (VOGT et al., 1969b). More highly oxidized derivatives, presumably fatty acid peroxides produced by autoxidation, were also found in the active lung effluents (VOGT et al., 1969b). The high bronchoconstrictor and pulmonary vasoconstrictor activity of prostaglandin PGF_2 (KADOWITZ et al., 1975) suggests that, in future interpretations of pulmonary symptoms of cobra venom poisoning, the contribution of prostaglandins might have to be taken into account.

II. Mechanistic Aspect

DAMERAU et al. (1975) have shown that the DLF from cobra venom is able to promote the release of SRS-C from both rat peritoneal fluid cells and the perfused guinea-pig lung. It also markedly potentiated the SRS-C-releasing effect of cobra venom phospholipase A in lung. It is believed that DLF activates endogenous phospholipase A to cleave cellular phospholipids by partial hydrolysis, producing lysophosphatides and free fatty acids (VAN DEENEM and DE HAAS, 1966), which in turn, under the action of tissue prostaglandin synthetase (BERGSTRÖM et al., 1964; VAN DORP et al., 1964; FLOWER, 1974), yield the slow-reacting substances (prostaglandins).

III. Sites of Formation

1. Tissues

The relative ability of guinea-pig tissues to form SRS-C following contact with cobra venom has been examined by MIDDLETON and PHILIPS (1964). They found that, after 20 min incubation of 100 mg/ml of chopped tissues with 0.5 mg/ml of cobra venom at 37° C, only the lung gave rise to substantial amounts of SRS-C; small amounts were produced by envenomed aorta, spleen, and ileum and none by heart, liver, uterus, trachea, brain, and diaphragm. This difference may be due to the higher prostaglandin synthetase activity of lung as compared with that of most other organs (FLOWER, 1974). Histamine release by cobra venom in vitro, a process which does not appear to require prostaglandin synthesis, did not run parallel to the SRS-C-forming capacity in guinea-pig tissues (MIDDLETON and PHILLIPS, 1964). The organ extracts used by these authors suffered no purification other than a 15 min boiling period to destroy direct gut-stimulating activity of contaminating cobra venom components. Such extracts must have contained unknown amounts of lysolecithin (FELDBERG and KELLAWAY, 1938; HABERMANN and NEUMANN, 1954; VOGT, 1957), which could have decreased the guinea-pig ileum's sensitivity and led to errors in the estimation of both histamine and SRS-C.

2. Cells

DAMERAU et al. (1975) have shown that loose cell suspensions harvested from the peritoneal cavity of rats yield SRS-C upon incubation with cobra venom. When analyzed in the light of data furnished by PADAWER and GORDON (1956) and ROTHSCHILD et al. (1974), such cell suspensions should contain lymphocytes, eosinophils, mast cells, traces of erythrocytes, but no polymorphonuclear leukocytes nor platelets. Although no details on the composition of their cell suspensions were given, DAMERAU et al. (1975) believe that mast cells are more active in forming SRS-C than other cells. Since SRS-C formation was also observed in the leukocyte fraction of whole rat blood which does not contain mast cells, it seems that SRS-C can also arise from nonmast cell sources, which remain to be identified. It appears that although released concomitantly during envenomation (FELDBERG and KELLAWAY, 1938), SRS-C and histamine do not necessarily originate from the same cells.

IV. Contribution Toward Toxic Effects of Venoms

1. Lysophosphatides

Up to now, available data have implicated only elapid venoms (*Naja* species, *Pseudechis* species) (FELDBERG and KELLAWAY, 1938; FELDBERG et al., 1938; SCHÜTZ and VOGT, 1961; VOGT et al., 1969b) as originators of SRS-C in animal tissues. According to what has been previously discussed, the formation of lysophosphatides must accompany the appearance of prostaglandin (SRS-C) activity during elapid envenomation; both groups of substances result from the action of phospholipase A on tissue phospholipids (FELDBERG and KELLAWAY, 1938; VOGT, 1957). SLOTTA et al. (1972) have stated that lysophosphatides do not contribute toward the toxicity of elapid venoms, because such substances are rapidly neutralized by plasma cholesterol. Since they did not present data on the actual absence of systemic effects of injected lysolecithin, this view conflicts with the data of FELDBERG et al. (1938) on pharmacologic effects and toxicity of "lysocithin," the ether-insoluble portion of methanolic extracts of incubates of egg yolk with the elapid *Pseudechis porphyriacus* venom. The intravenous injection of 6–12 mg/kg of this preparation caused a steep fall of systemic arterial blood pressure in cats or dogs; in the former, this was associated with a rise of pressure in the pulmonary artery and hemorrhagic edema of the lung. High doses caused death within a few minutes. Dogs responded to lysocythin with a rise in pressure in the portal vein, a relatively short-lasting effect which, together with peripheral vasodilatation, seemed to account for the fall of systemic blood pressure. It was the opinion of the authors that the strong histamine-releasing capacity of envenomed egg yolk preparations accounted for most of these effects. In order to reconcile these observations with the lack of systemic toxicity of lysolecithin proposed by SLOTTA et al. (1972), one must admit that the lysocythin preparation of FELDBERG et al. (1938) may have been contaminated with other histamine-releasing components, most likely DLF, presumed to be present in *P. porphyriacus* venom as in that of other elapid snakes (CONDREA et al., 1964). This conclusion poses a problem. Should one altogether reject the idea of a histamine-releasing activity of lysolecithin in vivo? It would seem that if one admits that lysolecithin arising within envenomed tissue acts on histamine-containing cells and adrenomedullary cells (see Sect. E), prior to its binding to plasma or tissue factors, the postulated role of lysophospholipids mediating the release of pharmacologically active products by most snake venoms (FELDBERG et al., 1938; KELLER, 1964; ROTHSCHILD, 1965; FREDHOLM and HAEGERMARK, 1967; DAMERAU et al., 1975) should be maintained. The elegant observations reported by ROSENBERG (1972), showing that extrinsic lysophospholipids are the mediators of the disruption of the axonal conduction mechanism evoked in squid giant axons by phospholipase A-containing snake venoms, lend indirect support to this postulate.

2. Prostaglandins

No data on the SRS-C-(prostaglandin) releasing activity in animals of venoms other than those from snakes of the elapid genus *Naja* are available (FELDBERG and KELLAWAY, 1938; FELDBERG et al., 1938; SCHÜTZ and VOGT, 1961; VOGT et al., 1969; VARGAFTIG and DAO, 1970, 1972). Presumably, in cases of accidents due to such snakes, the major contribution of SRS-C would be exerted on pulmonary smooth muscle, which is highly sensitive to prostaglandins (BERGSTRÖM et al., 1968; WEEKS, 1972; KADOWITZ et al., 1975). Their action could lead to increased resistance to ventilation due to bronchiolar smooth muscle constriction, increased pulmonary vascular resistance, and lung edema resulting from permeability changes at lung vessel walls. Like those of other autopharmacologic principles arising in a victim's body, these effects may be of very minor significance in the face of hemodynamic changes due to cardiotoxic components of cobra venom. VARGAFTIG(1972) has indicated that venoms from *Vipera berus* and from the crotalids *C. durissus terrificus*, *C. adamanteus*, *Agkistrodon piscivorus*, *Bothrops jararaca*, *B. atrox*, and from the sea snake *Laticauda semifasciata*, release a hypotensive factor from crude egg yolk or from pure lecithin, considered to be SRS-C. The activity of the venom-egg yolk incubates was apparently removed by lipid extraction and retained after postincubation addition of specific antivenin to block contaminating, native venom components. It was exerted not only on blood pressure (rabbits, dogs, monkeys) but also on bronchial muscle tone of guinea-pigs. It remains to be seen whether prostaglandins play a role in the toxicity of viperid and crotalid snake venoms which do not contain strong neurotoxic principles. Since these venoms do, as a rule, contain phospholipases A, they would be potentially able to generate SRS (prostaglandins) in the animal body.

According to VOGT (1969) and DAMERAU et al. (1975), snake venoms supply the enzyme (phospholipase A) required for the first step of the prostaglandin forming process by releasing unsaturated fatty acids from tissue phospholipids; tissue enzymes, in a secondary phase, transform them into pharmacologically active prostaglandins. The relationship between this process and the formation of SRS-C in venom-egg yolk or venom-lecithin incubates, which presumably lack the secondary, prostaglandin-synthesizing enzyme, awaits clarification.

E. Catecholamines

Adrenaline

Virtually the only complete report on the catecholamine-releasing activity of snake venoms is that of FELDBERG (1940), describing the effects of the perfusion of the cat's adrenal gland with cobra *(Naja naja)* venom. Like his other work on snake venom pharmacology (FELDBERG and KELLAWAY, 1937a, b, c, d, 1938; FELDBERG et al., 1938), it is of outstanding clarity and completeness. It showed that in cats, cobra venom caused a long-lasting output of adrenaline from the adrenals, if injected into the central stump of the coeliac artery after evisceration. This effect was attributed to phospholipase-induced formation of lysolecithin in the adrenals; the latter was found to cause an output of adrenaline similar to that produced by the venom, associated with a diminished adrenaline content of the adrenals. After repeated large doses of venom or of lysolecithin, adrenomedullary cells became irresponsive to secretory stimuli. The increase in arterial blood pressure evoked by cobra venom or by lysolecithin injected into the central stump of the coeliac artery of eviscerated, pithed cats was entirely due to adrenaline discharge from the adrenal gland. Removal of these glands prevented hypertension. The long-lasting output of adrenaline caused by lysolecithin was regarded as a response of the medullary cells to injury and was contrasted to the strong but evanescent output produced by acetylcholine or by splanchnic nerve stimulation. At the later stages of injury, the medullary cells ceased to secrete and became irresponsive to renewed stimulation either by its nerve or lysolecithin. The injury, however, was not intense or widespread enough to produce changes in the cells visible on histologic examination.

In the rabbit, cobra venom or lysolecithin caused, upon intravenous injection, a steep fall in arterial blood pressure, usually resulting in death. This effect was associated with a rise of pressure in the pulmonary artery and was probably mainly due to pulmonary vasoconstriction. In contrast to the effect observed in cats, venom or lysolecithin had only a slight and inconstant effect on the secretory activity of the adrenal medulla in rabbits. Although not discussed in his paper, it is quite probable that a massive discharge of histamine and 5-HT from the rabbit's platelets caused the observed vasomotor changes.

F. Anaphylatoxin

I. Background

We know now that the importance of the early observations of FRIEDBERGER et al. (1913) on the generation of anaphylatoxins during incubation of cobra *(Naja naja)* venom with animal sera lay less in their toxicologic significance than in the insights which the study of this reaction, mainly in recent years, has brought toward an understanding of the mechanism and role of complement inactivation in immunology and pathology. The participation of the complement inactivating factor from cobra venom (CVF) in the generation of the pharmacologically highly active anaphylatoxins, complement fragments C3a and C5a, has been recently reviewed in great detail (VOGT, 1974; MÜLLER-EBERHARD, 1975). Its main points will be described.

VOGT and SCHMIDT (1964), KLEIN and WELLENSIECK (1965), MÜLLER-EBERHARD (1967), BALLOW and COCHRANE (1969), KLEINE et al. (1970), COCHRANE et al. (1970), GÖTZE and MÜLLER-EBERHARD (1971), MÜLLER-EBERHARD and FJELLSTRÖM (1971), RUDDY et al. (1972), HUNSICKER et al. (1973), VOGT et al. (1974), and others cleared the way toward an understanding of the mechanism by which cobra venom and, by extension, other immunologic and nonimmunologic stimuli produce anaphylatoxins in animal blood. In conjunction with these investigations, studies on the reactivity of CVF-treated animals to certain noxious stimuli (MAILLARD and ZARCO, 1968; HENSON and COCHRANE, 1969; PICKERING et al., 1969; COCHRANE et al., 1970; FONG and GOOD, 1971; HENSON, 1971; GEWURZ et al., 1971) significantly contributed toward knowledge about the role of complement in the generation of disease.

CVF is a 6.7 S, 144000 molecular weight protein of low toxicity when injected into laboratory animals. Its major effect is the depletion of the C3 and C5 complement components of the circulatory system leading to near disappearance of the animal's ability to participate in complement-requiring immune hemolysis. CVF initiates this action by combining with a glycine-rich β-glycoprotein (GBG, or B factor), a component of the alternate (properdin) pathway of complement activation. The resulting vulnerable complex, CVF-GBG, is changed into CVF-GGG, a glycine-rich γ-glycoprotein. This transformation is controlled by Mg^{2+} and an enzyme, variously named C3PA convertase, GBG convertase or factor D of the properdin pathway. CVF-GGG, also named C3 activator (C3A), cleaves the C3 component of plasma complement, giving rise to the pharmacologically active peptide C3a (mol wt 8900) and the immunochemically, but not pharmacologically reactive, bulkier protein C3b (mol wt 171000); CVF also affects the C5 anaphylatoxin precursor. While in the form of the C3A and in the presence of factor E of the properdin pathway, it converts C5 into the pharmacologically very active C5a anaphylatoxin (mol wt 16500) and a remaining bulky protein C5b.

Anaphylatoxins C3a and C5a have the ability to release histamine from either human or guinea-pig mast cells; C5a is nearly 2000 times more active than C3a in eliciting the wheal and flare response in human skin, a histamine-mediated phenomenon. On rat mast cells, C5a is inactive; C3a, on the other hand, produces degranulation and histamine release from such cells (DIAS DA SILVA and LEPOW, 1967; COCHRANE and MÜLLER-EBERHARD, 1968; JOHNSON et al., 1975). Both agents can be conveniently assayed on the isolated guinea-pig ileum which they contract in a partly antihistamine-sensitive (VOGT et al., 1969a), strongly tachyphylactic manner (ROTHSCHILD and ROCHA E SILVA, 1954; ROCHA E SILVA and ROTHSCHILD, 1956). C5a is, on a molar basis, nearly ten times more active on this structure than C3a (MÜLLER-EBERHARD and VALLOTA, 1971).

While C5a anaphylatoxins generated by CVF in human, guinea-pig, rat, rabbit, pig, or mouse sera are immunochemically identic, they differ from human C3a. Human C5a can be demonstrated in a system of pure complement components but not in human plasma. Carboxypeptidase B (CPB) an enzyme which removes the terminal arginine group from this anaphylatoxin, causes very rapid disappearance of its histamine-releasing and spasmogenic activity; C5a's ability to induce chemotaxis (see below), is less rapidly destroyed. Epsilon aminocaproic acid (EACA) protects human C5a and C3a from CPB (VALLOTA and MÜLLER-EBERHARD, 1973). C5a anaphylatoxin, generated in rat or guinea-pig plasma by CVF, antigen-antibody aggregates, or polysaccharides (inulin, agar, zymosan), is shielded from CPB.

The ability to attract polymorphonuclear leucocytes, eosinophils, and monocytes, termed chemotaxis, is a crucial component of the inflammatory reaction; it may be the most important function of anaphylatoxin. The C5a peptide seems to be considerably more active in this respect; this difference, however, is still a matter of controversy (VOGT, 1974).

The dramatic ability of purified anaphylatoxin (BODAMMER and VOGT, 1967) to cause severe, often fatal bronchoconstriction and lung emphysema in the guinea-pig (see review by GIERTZ and HAHN, 1966) has apparently not been studied with the pure anaphylatoxin peptides in other species.

The injection of pure CVF does not cause serious symptoms in experimental animals even though C5a anaphylatoxin is generated in large amounts. This has been an important argument for those who believe that anaphylatoxins play no role in systemic anaphylaxis (VOGT, 1974).

II. Contribution Toward Toxic Effects of Elapid Snake Venoms

In spite of its high, histamine-mediated wheal and flare-producing activity, it is unlikely that anaphylatoxin contributes to the local effects of cobra venom. Human anaphylatoxin is very rapidly inactivated by serum CPB; very minor amounts of it would accumulate at a bitten site, unless considerable local pooling of blood occurs. Based on the data of RUDDY et al. (1972), it can be predicted that the maximal amounts of either C 3a or C 5a supplied by one ml of the victim's plasma would be well below the amounts required for threshold wheal and flare responses of the human skin (MÜLLER-EBERHARD and VALLOTA, 1971). It is probable that the powerful, comparatively stable DLF of cobra venom, acting alone or in conjunction with venom phospholipase A (DAMERAU et al., 1975), is the major responsible factor for the histamine-dependent symptoms of cobra venom poisoning. The same arguments could probably be extended to other local and systemic pharmacologic effects of anaphylatoxin in man, whose morphologic aspects have been described by LEPOW et al. (1970). Judging from experiments in animals, such effects could include: stimulation of mast cell secretory activity (MOTA, 1957), bronchoconstriction (BODAMMER and VOGT, 1967; GIERTZ, 1969), hypotension (BODAMMER, 1969), adrenergic hypertension (BODAMMER and VOGT, 1967; MAHLER et al., 1975), and intestinal smooth muscle contraction (KLEINE et al., 1970).

A more significant role of anaphylatoxin in envenomation may be the induction of chemotaxis, i.e., the accumulation of polymorphonuclear leukocytes over the bitten area. In practice, this activity would probably be overshadowed by the much more intense release of chemotactic factors due to stimuli arising from bacterial contamination and other phlogogenic mediators (WARD, 1971; WARD et al., 1973) brought to or released at the site of a snakebite.

BIRDSEY et al. (1971) have measured the action of 32 snake venoms on guinea-pig serum complement in vitro. Certain patterns of selective consumption of complement components could be established among elapid, viperid, and crotalid venoms. No data on the anaphylatoxin-forming activity of the venoms were presented; it is noteworthy, however, that 14 of the species tested had the ability to consume C3–C9 components of the complement system. Since the C3 precursor of anaphylatoxin is included among them, it is to be expected that such venoms would also be able to produce this mediator at a bitten site.

Sustained, systemic hemolytic complement consumption in guinea-pigs given purified anticomplementary fractions from *Naja haje*, *Agkistrodon rhodostoma*, *Bitis arietans*, *Bothrops atrox*, *B. jararaca*, and *Lachesis muta* venoms, could only be obtained in animals given the *N. haje* venom derivative. This species is closely related to *N. naja*, the "classic" producer of CVF. The possibility of a pharmacologically meaningful local anaphylatoxin-forming activity on the part of C3-consuming venoms awaits experimental evaluation.

References

Amorim, D. S., Manço, J. C., Ferreira, S. H., Tanaka, A., Cardoso, S. S.: Hemodynamic effects of bradykinin potentiated by a factor contained in the *Bothrops jararaca* venom. Comparative results with eledoisin. Acta physiol. lat.-amer. **17**, 258—261 (1967)

Armstrong, D.: Pain. In: Handb. Exp. Pharmacol. Bradykinin, Kallidin, and Kallikrein, Vol. XXV. Berlin-Heidelberg-New York: Springer 1970

Bagdasarian, A., Talamo, R. C., Colman, R. W.: Isolation of high molecular weight activators of human plasma prekallikrein. J. biol. Chem. **248**, 3456—3463 (1973)

Ballow, M., Cochrane, G. G.: Two anticomplementary factors in cobra venom: hemolysis of guinea pig erythrocytes by one of them. J. Immunol. **103**, 944—952 (1969)

Beraldo, W.T., Dias da Silva, W.: Release of histamine by animal venoms and bacterial toxins. In: Handb. Exp. Pharmacol. Histamine. Its Chemistry Metabolism and Physiological and Pharmacological Actions, Vol. XVIII. Berlin-Heidelberg-New York: Springer 1966
Bergström, S., Carlson, L.A., Weeks, J.R.: The prostaglandins: a family of biologically active lipids. Pharmacol. Rev. **20**, 1—48 (1968)
Bergström, S., Danielsson, H., Samuelsson, B.: The enzymatic formation of prostaglandin E_2 from arachidonic acid. Biochim. biophys. Acta (Amst.) **90**, 207—210 (1964)
Bhargava, N., Vargaftig, B.B., Vos, C.J., de, Bonta, I.L., Tijs, T.: Dissociation of oedema provoking factor of *Agkistrodon piscivorus* venom from kininogenase. In: Back, N., Sicuteri, I. (Eds.): Vasopeptides. Chemistry, Pharmacology, and Pathophysiology. New York-London: Plenum Press 1972
Birdsey, V., Lindorfer, J., Gewurz, H.: Interaction of toxic venoms with the complement system. Immunology **21**, 299—310 (1971)
Black, J.W., Duncan, W.A.M., Durant, C.J., Ganellin, C.R., Parsons, E.M.: Definition and antagonism of histamine H_2-receptors. Nature (Lond.) New Biol. **236**, 358—390 (1972)
Bodammer, G.: Untersuchungen über den Mechanismus der Blutdruckwirkung des Anaphylatoxins bei Katzen und Meerschweinchen. Naunyn-Schmiedebergs Arch.-Pharmak. exp. Path. **262**, 197—207 (1969)
Bodammer, G., Vogt, W.: Actions of anaphylatoxin on circulation and respiration of the guinea pig. Int. Arch. Allergy **32**, 417—428 (1967)
Brecher, G.A., Brobmann, G.F.: Effect of kallikrein on the cardiovascular system. In: Handb. Exp. Pharmacol., Vol. XXV. Bradykinin, Kallidin, and Kallikrein. Berlin-Heidelberg-New York: Springer 1970
Brocklehurst, W.E.: The release of histamine and formation of a slow reacting substance (SRS-A) during anaphylactic shock. J. Physiol. (Lond.) **151**, 416—435 (1960)
Chakravarty, N., Uvnäs, B.: Histamine and a lipid-soluble smooth-muscle stimulating principle ("SRS") in anaphylactic reaction. Acta physiol. scand. **48**, 302—314 (1960)
Cheymol, J., Bourillet, F., Roch-Arveiller, M.: Actions neuromusculaires de venins de serpents. In: Vries, A., de, Kochva, E. (Eds.): Toxins of Animal and Plant Origin, Vol. II. New York-London-Paris: Gordon and Breach 1972
Chiang, T.S., Ho, K.J., Lee, C.Y.: Release of histamine from the rat diaphragm preparation by Formosan snake venoms. J. Formosan med. Ass. **63**, 127—132 (1964)
Chopra, R.N., Chowhan, J.S.: Action of the Indian daboia (*Vipera russellii*) venom on the circulatory system. Indian J. med. Res. **21**, 493—506 (1934)
Chopra, R.N., Chowhan, J.S., De, N.N.: An experimental investigation into the action of the venom of *E. carinata*. Indian J. med. Res. **23**, 391—405 (1935)
Chute, A.L., Waters, E.T.: Effect of rattlesnake venom (Crotalin) on plasma histamine of the rabbit. Amer. J. Physiol. **132**, 552—554 (1941)
Cochrane, C.G., Müller-Eberhard, H.J.: The derivation of two distinct anaphylatoxin activities from the third and fifth components of human complement. J. exp. Med. **127**, 371—386 (1968)
Cochrane, C.G., Müller-Eberhard, H.J., Aikin, B.S.: Depletion of plasma complement in vivo by a protein of cobra venom: its effect on various immunologic reactions. J. Immunol. **105**, 55 (1970)
Cohen, I., Zur, M., Kaminsky, E., Vries, A. de: Isolation and characterization of kinin-releasing enzyme of *Echis coloratus* venom. Biochem. Pharmacol. **19**, 785—793 (1970)
Collier, H.O., Lee, I.R.: Nocioceptive responses of guinea-pigs to intradermal injections of bradykinin and kallidin-10. Brit. J. Pharmacol. **21**, 155—164 (1963)
Condrea, E., Vries, A. de, Mager, J.: Hemolysis and splitting of human erythrocyte phospholipids by snake venoms. Biochim. biophys. Acta (Amst.) **84**, 60—73 (1964)
Dale, H.H., Laidlaw, P.P.: The physiological action of β-imidazolylethylamine. J. Physiol. (Lond.) **41**, 318—344 (1910)
Damerau, B., Lege, L., Oldigs, H.-D., Vogt, W.: Histamine release, formation of prostaglandin-like activity (SRS-C) and mast cell degranulation by the direct lytic factor (DLF) and phospholipase A of cobra venom. Naunyn-Schmiedebergs Arch. Pharmacol. **287**, 141—156 (1975)
Deenen, L.L.M. van, Haas, G.H. de: Phosphoglycerides and phospholipases. Ann. Rev. Biochem. **35**, 157—194 (1966)

Dorp, D. A. van, Beerthius, R. K., Nugteren, D. H., Vonkeman, H.: The biosynthesis of prostaglandins. Biochim. biophys. Acta (Amst.) **90**, 204—207 (1964)

Deutsch, H. F., Diniz, C. R.: Some proteolytic activities of snake venoms. J. biol. Chem. **216**, 17—25 (1955)

Devi, A., Sarkar, N. K.: Cardiotoxic and cardio-stimulating factors in cobra venom. Mem. Inst. Butantan **33**, 573—582 (1966)

Dias da Silva, W., Lepow, I. H.: Complement as a mediator of inflammation. II. Biological properties of anaphylatoxin prepared with purified component of human complement. J. exp. Med. **125**, 921—946 (1967)

Douglas, W. W.: Stimulus-secretion coupling: the concept and clues from chromaffin and other cells. Brit. J. Pharmacol. **34**, 451—474 (1968)

Douglas, W. W.: Autacoids. In: The Pharmacological Basis of Therapeutics, 5th Ed. New York: Collier MacMillan 1975

Dragstedt, C. A., Mead, F. B., Eyer, S. W.: Role of histamine in circulatory effects of rattlesnake venom. Proc. Soc. exp. Biol. (N.Y.) **37**, 709—710 (1938)

Dutta, N. K., Naranyan, K. G. A.: Release of histamine from rat diaphragm by cobra venom. Nature (Lond.) **169**, 1064—1065 (1952)

Edery, H., Lewis, G. P.: Kinin-forming activity and histamine in lymph after tissue injury. J. Physiol. (Lond.) **169**, 568—583 (1963)

Efrati, P.: Clinical manifestations of snake bite by *Vipera xanthina palestinae* (Werner) and their pathophysiological basis. Mem. Inst. Butantan **33**, 189—191 (1966)

Erdös, E. G., Yang, H. Y. T.: Kininases. In: Handb. Exp. Pharmacol. Bradykinin, Kallidin, and Kallikrein, Vol. XXV. Berlin-Heidelberg-New York: Springer 1970

Erspamer, V.: Occurrence of indolealkylamines in nature. In: Handb. Exp. Pharmacol. 5-Hydroxytryptamine and Related Indolealkylamines, Vol. XIX. Berlin-Heidelberg-New York: Springer 1966

Fearn, H. J., Smith, C., West, G. B.: Capillary permeability responses to snake venoms. J. Pharm. Pharmacol. **16**, 79—84 (1964)

Feldberg, W.: The action of histamine on the blood vessels of the rabbit. J. Physiol. (Lond.) **63**, 211—216 (1927)

Feldberg, W.: The action of bee venom, cobra venom and lysolecithin on the adrenal medulla. J. Physiol. (Lond.) **99**, 104—118 (1940)

Feldberg, W., Holden, H. F., Kellaway, C. H.: The formation of lysocithin and of a muscle-stimulating substance by snake venoms. J. Physiol. (Lond.) **94**, 232—248 (1938)

Feldberg, W., Kellaway, C. H.: The circulatory and pulmonary effects of the venom of the Australian copperhead *(Denisonia superba)*. Aust. J. Biol. med. Sci. **15**, 81—95 (1937a)

Feldberg, W., Kellaway, C. H.: Liberation of histamine from the perfused lung by snake venoms. J. Physiol. (Lond.) **90**, 257—279 (1937b)

Feldberg, W., Kellaway, C. H.: Circulatory effects of the venom of the Indian cobra *(N. naja)* in cats. Aust. J. Biol. med. Sci. **15**, 159—172 (1937c)

Feldberg, W., Kellaway, C. H.: Circulatory effects of the venom of the Indian cobra *(N. naja)* in dogs. Aust. J. Biol. med. Sci. **15**, 441—460 (1937d)

Feldberg, W., Kellaway, C.H.: Liberation of histamine and formation of lysolecithin-like substances by Cobra venom. J. Physiol. (Lond.) **94**, 187—226 (1938)

Ferreira, S. H.: A bradykinin-potentiating factor (BPF) present in the venom of *Bothrops jararaca*. Brit. J. Pharmacol. **24**, 163—169 (1965)

Flower, R. J.: Drugs which inhibit prostaglandin biosynthesis. Pharmacol. Rev. **26**, 33—67 (1974)

Fong, J. S. C., Good, R. A.: Prevention of the localized and generalized Schwartzman reaction by an anticomplementary agent, cobra venom factor. J. exp. Med. **134**, 642—655 (1971)

Fredholm, B., Haegermark, Ö.: Histamine release from rat mast cells induced by a mast cell degranulating factor in bee venom. Acta physiol. scand. **69**, 304—1312 (1967)

Friedberger, E., Mita, S., Kumagai, T.: Die Bildung eines akutwirkenden Giftes (Anaphylatoxin) aus Toxinen (Tetanus, Diphterie, Schlangengift). Z. Immun.-Forsch. **17**, 506—538 (1913)

Gewurz, H., Pickering, R. J., Day, N. K., Good, R. A.: Cobra venom factor-induced activation of the complement system: Developmental, experimental and clinical considerations. Int. Arch. Allergy **40**, 47—58 (1971)

Giertz, H.: Pharmacology of anaphylatoxin. In: Movat, H. Z. (Ed.): Cellular and Humoral Mechanisms in Anaphylaxis and Allergy. Basel-New York: Karger 1969

Giertz, H., Hahn, F.: Makromolekulare Histaminliberatoren. C. Das Anaphylatoxin. In: Handb. Exp. Pharmacol., Vol. XVIII. Berlin-Heidelberg-New York: Springer 1966
Götze, O., Müller-Eberhard, H. J.: The C3-activator system: an alternate pathway of complement activation. J. exp. Med. **134**, 905—108 (1971)
Goth, A., Johnson, A. R.: Current concepts on the secretory function of mast cells. Life Sci. **16**, 1201—1214 (1975)
Grasset, E., Schwartz, D. E.: Inhibition des principes coagulants de venins de serpents par le sulfate de dextran. Rev. Suisse Pathol. Bacteriol. **17**, 38—45 (1954)
Habermann, E.: Zuordnung pharmakologischer und enzymatischer Wirkungen von Kallikrein und Schlangengiften mittels Diisoprophylfluorophosphat und Elektrophorese. Naunyn-Schmiedebergs Arch. Exp. Pharmakol. **240**, 552—572 (1961)
Habermann, E.: Fortschritte auf dem Gebiet der Plasmakinine. Naunyn-Schmiedebergs Arch. exp. Path. Pharmak. **245**, 230—253 (1963)
Habermann, E.: Kininogens. In: Handb. Exp. Pharmacol. Bradykinin, Kallidin, and Kallikrein, Vol. XXV. Berlin-Heidelberg-New York: Springer 1970
Habermann, E., Neumann, W.: Die Hemmung der Hitzekoagulation von Eigelb durch Bienengift, ein Phospholipase-Effect. Hoppe-Seylers Z. physiol. Chem. **297**, 179—189 (1954)
Haddy, F. J., Emerson, T. E., Jr., Scott, J. B., Daugherty, N. M., Jr.: The effect of the kinins on the cardiovascular system. In: Handb. Exp. Pharmacol. Bradykinin, Kallidin, and Kallikrein, Vol. XXV. Berlin-Heidelberg-New York: Springer 1970
Halmagyi, D. F. J., Starzecki, B., Horner, G. J.: Mechanism and pharmacology of shock due to rattlesnake venom in sheep. J. appl. Physiol. **20**, 709—718 (1965)
Hamberg, U., Rocha e Silva, M.: On the release of bradykinin by trypsin and snake venoms. Arch. int. Pharmacodyn. Ther. **110**, 222—238 (1957)
Henriques, O. B., Evseeva, L.: Proteolytic, esterase, and kinin-releasing activities of some soviet snake venoms. Toxicon **6**, 205—209 (1969)
Henriques, O. B., Fichman, M., Beraldo, W. T.: Bradykinin-releasing factor from *Bothrops jararaca* venom. Nature (Lond.) **187**, 414—415 (1960)
Henriques, O. B., Gapanhuk, E., Kauritcheva, A., Budnitskaya, B.: Methionyl-lysyl bradykinin release from plasma kininogen by plasmin. Biochem. Pharmacol. **18**, 1788—1790 (1969)
Henriques, O. B., Picarelli, Z. P., Ferraz de Oliveira, M. C.: Partial purification of the plasma substrate for the bradykinin-releasing enzyme from the venom of *Bothrops jararaca.* Biochem. Pharmacol. **11**, 707—713 (1962)
Henson, P. M.: Interaction of cells with immune complexes, adherence, release of constituents, and tissue injury. J. exp. Med. **134**, 114s—135s (1971)
Henson, P. M., Cochrane, C. G.: Antigen-antibody complexes, platelets, and increased vascular permeability. In: Movat, H. Z. (Ed.): Cellular and Humoral Mechanisms of Anaphylaxis and Allergy. Basel: Karger 1969
Hilton, S. M.: The physiological role of glandular kallikreins. In: Handb. Exp. Pharmacol., Vol. XXV. Bradykinin, Kallidin, and Kallikrein. Berlin-Heidelberg-New York: Springer 1970
Högberg, B., Uvnäs, B.: The mechanism of the disruption of mast cells produced by compound 48/80. Acta physiol. scand. **41**, 345—369 (1957)
Holtz, P., Raudonat, H. W.: Über Beziehungen zwischen proteolytischer Aktivität und blutcoagulierender sowie bradykinin-freisetzender Wirkung von Schlangengiften. Naunyn-Schmiedebergs Arch. exp. Path. Pharmak. **229**, 113—122 (1956)
Hunsicker, L. G., Ruddy, S., Austen, K. F.: Alternate complement pathway factors involved in cobra venom factor (CVF) activation of the 3rd component of complement (C3). J. Immunol. **11**, 128 (1973)
Ishida, Y., Yamashita, S., Ohsaka, A., Takahashi, T., Omori-Satoh, T.: Abstracts 4th International Symposium on Animal, Plant, and Microbial Toxins. Tokyo 1974
Iwanaga, S., Sato, T., Mizushina, Y., Suzuki, T.: Studies on snake venoms. XVII. Properties of the bradykinin releasing enzyme in the venom of *Agkistrodon halys blomhoffii.* J. Biochem. (Tokyo) **58**, 123—129 (1965)
Johnson, A. R., Hugli, T. E., Müller-Eberhard, H. J.: Release of histamine from rat mast cells by the complement peptides C3a and C5a. Immunology **28**, 1067—1080 (1975)
Kadowitz, P. J., Joiner, P. D., Hyman, A. L.: Physiological and pharmacological roles of prostaglandins. Ann. Rev. Pharmacol. **15**, 285—306 (1975)

Kaiser, E., Kramer, R., Lambrechter, R.: The action of direct lytic agents from animal venoms on cells and isolated cell fractions. In: de Vries, A., Kochva, E. (Eds.): Toxins of Animal and Plant Origin, Vol. II. New York-London-Paris: Gordon and Breach 1972
Kaliner, M., Austen, K. F.: A sequence of biochemical events in the antigen-induced release of chemical mediators from sensitized human lung tissue. J. exp. Med. **138**, 1077—1094 (1973)
Kaplan, A. P., Austen, K. F.: A prealbumin activator of prekallikrein. J. Immunol. **105**, 802—812 (1970)
Keele, C. A., Armstrong, D.: Substances Producing Pain and Itch. London: Edward Arnold 1964
Kellaway, C.H., Trethewie, E.R.: The liberation of a show-reacting smooth-muscle-stimulating substance in anaphylaxis. Quast. J. exptl. Physiol. **30**, 121—145 (1970)
Keller, R.: Voraussetzungen für das Zustandekommen eines zytolysierenden Effektes durch Phosphatidase A. Helv. physiol. pharmacol. Acta **22**, 76 C—78 C (1964)
Klein, P. G., Wellensiek, H. J.: Multiple nature of the third component of guinea pig complement. I. Separation and characterization of three factors a, b, and c, essential for hemolysis. Immunology **8**, 590—603 (1965)
Kleine, I., Poppe, B., Vogt, W.: Functional identity of anaphylatoxin preparations obtained from different sources and by different activation procedures. I. Pharmacological experiments. Europ. J. Pharmacol. **10**, 398—403 (1970)
Kocholaty, W. F., Ledford, E. B., Daly, J. G., Billings, T. A.: Toxicity and some enzymatic properties and activities in the venoms of crotalidae, elapidae, and viperidae. Toxicon **9**, 131—138 (1971)
Kochwa, S., Perlmutter, C., Gitter, S., Rechnic, J., Vries, A. de: Studies on *Vipera palestinae* venom. Fractionation by ion exchange chromatography. Amer. J. trop. Med. **9**, 374—380 (1960)
Laure, J. C.: Die Primärstruktur des Crotamins. Hoppe-Seylers Z. physiol. Chem. **356**, 213—215 (1975)
Lefron, G., Michaud, V.: Contribution a l'étude de l'action des antihistaminiques dans le traitement des envenimations par mordures de serpents. Bull. Soc. Path. Exot. **49**, 936—946 (1956)
Lepow, I. H., Willms-Kretschmer, K., Patrick, R. A., Rosen, F. S.: Gross and ultrastructural observation on lesions produced by intradermal injection of human C3a in man. Amer. J. Path. **61**, 13—24 (1970)
Magalhães, A., Souza, G. J., Diniz, C. R.: Proteases de serpentes brasilieras. I. Separação de enzima coagulante (Clotase) do veneno de *Lachesis mutus*. Symposium: Application of Snake Venom in Pharmacology and Cell Biochemistry. Biological Society of Ribeirão Preto 1972. Ciência Cultura **25**, 863—874 (1973)
Mahler, F., Intaglietta, M., Hugli, T. E., Johnson, A. R.: Influences of C3a anaphylatoxin compared to other vasoactive agents on the microcirculation of the rabbit omentum. Microvasc. Res. **9**, 345—356 (1975)
Maillard, J. L., Zarco, R. M.: Decomplémentation par un facteur extrait du venin de cobra. Effect sur plusieurs reactions immunes des cobayes et du rat. Ann. Inst. Pasteur (Paris) **114**, 756—774 (1968)
Margolis, J., Bruce, S., Starzecki, B., Horner, G. J., Halmagyi, D. F. J.: Release of bradykinin-like substance (BKLS) in sheep by venom of *Crotalus atrox*. Aust. J. exp. Biol. med. Sci. **43**, 237—245 (1965)
Markwardt, F., Barthel, W., Glusa, E., Hoffmann, A.: Über die Freisetzung biogener Amine aus Blutplättchen durch tierische Gifte. Naunyn-Schmiedebergs Arch. exp. Path. Pharmak. **252**, 297—304 (1966 a)
Markwardt, F., Barthel, W., Glusa, E., Hoffmann, A., Walsmann, P.: Über eine aminfreisetzende Komponente des *Crotalus terrificus*-Giftes. Biochem. Z. **346**, 351—356 (1966 b)
May, B., Holler, C., Westermann, E.: Über die Bedeutung der Phospholipase A für die histaminfreisetzende Wirkung des Cobragiftes. Naunyn-Schmiedebergs Arch.-Pharmak. exp. Path. **256**, 237—256 (1967)
Mebs, D.: Vergleichende Enzymuntersuchungen an Schlangengiften unter besonderer Berücksichtigung ihrer caseinspaltenden Proteasen. Hoppe-Seylers Z. physiol. Chem. **349**, 1115—1125 (1968)
Mebs, D.: A comparative study of enzyme activities in snake venoms. Int. J. Biochem. **1**, 335—342 (1970)
Middleton, E. Jr., Phillips, G. B.: Distribution and properties of anaphylactic and venom-induced slow-reacting substance and histamine in guinea pigs. J. Immunol. **93**, 220—227 (1964)

Minton, S. A. Jr.: Venom Diseases. Springfield: Thomas 1974

Mohamed, A. H., El-Serougi, M. S., Hamed, R. M.: Effects of *Naja nigricollis* venom on blood and tissue histamine. Toxicon **9**, 169—172 (1971)

Mohamed, A. H., Kamel, A., Ayobe, M. H.: Effects of *Echis carinatus* venom on tissue and blood histamine and their relations to local tissue reactions and eosinophil changes. Toxicon **6**, 51—54 (1968)

Mohamed, A. H., Khaled, L. Z.: Effect of *Cerastes cerastes* venom on blood and tissue histamine and on arterial blood pressure. Toxicon **6**, 221—223 (1969)

Mohamed, A. H., Zaki, O.: Effect of Egyptian black snake toxin on histamine of blood and its relation to blood eosinophils. Amer. J. Physiol. **190**, 113—116 (1957 a)

Mohamed, A. H., Zaki, O.: The Walterinnesia toxin as a liberator of histamine from tissues. J. trop. Med. Hyg. **60**, 275—280 (1957 b)

Moran, N. C., Uvnäs, B., Westerholm, B.: Release of 5-hydroxytryptamine and histamine from rat mast cells. Acta physiol. scand. **56**, 26—41 (1962)

Mota, I.: The mechanism of action of anaphylatoxin: its effect of guinea pig mast cells. Immunology **2**, 403—413 (1959)

Mota, I.: Release of histamine from mast cells. In: Handb. Exp. Pharmacol. Histamine. Its Chemistry, Metabolism and Physiological and Pharmacological Actions, Vol. XVIII. Berlin-Heidelberg-New York: Springer 1966

Moura Gonçalves, J.: Purification and properties of crotamine. In: Buckley, E. E., Porges, N. (Eds.): Venoms, p. 261. Washington, D.C.: Amer. Ass. Advanc. Science 1956

Moura Gonçalves, J., Rocha e Silva, M.: Fator de permeabilidade capilar no veneno de *Crotalus terrificus crotaminicus*. Ciência Cultura (Brazil) **10**, 163 (1958)

Müller-Eberhard, H. J.: Mechanism of inactivation of the third component of human complement (C'3) by cobra venom. Fed. Proc. **26**, 744 (1967)

Müller-Eberhard, H. J.: Complement. Ann. Rev. Biochem. **44**, 697—724 (1975)

Müller-Eberhard, H. J., Fjellström, K. E.: Isolation of the anticomplementary protein from cobra venom and its mode of action on C3. J. Immunol. **107**, 1666—1672 (1972)

Müller-Eberhard, H. J., Vallota, E. H.: In: Austen, K. F., Becker, E. L. (Eds.): Biochemistry of the Acute Allergic Reactions. Oxford: Blackwell 1971

Orange, R. P., Murphy, R. C., Karnovsky, M. L., Austen, K. F.: The physiochemical characteristics and purification of slow-reacting substance of anaphylaxis. J. Immunol. **110**, 760—770 (1973)

Oshima, G., Sato Omori, T., Suzuki, T.: Distribution of proteinase, arginine ester hydrolase and kinin releasing enzyme in various kinds of snake venoms. Toxicon **7**, 229—233 (1969)

Osman, O. H., Gumaa, K. A.: Pharmacological studies of snake *(Bitis arietans)* venom. Toxicon **12**, 569—575 (1974)

Ouyang, C. H., Shiau, S. Y.: Relationship between pharmacological actions and enzymatic activities of the venom of *Trimeresurus gramineus*. Toxicon **8**, 183—191 (1970)

Padawer, J., Gordon, A. S.: Cellular elements in the peritoneal fluid of some mammals. Anat. Rec. **124**, 209—222 (1956)

Parrat, J. R., West, G. B.: 5-Hydroxytryptamine and tissue mast cells. J. Physiol. (Lond.) **137**, 169—178 (1957)

Paton, W. D. M.: Histamine release by compounds of simple chemical structure. Pharmacol. Rev. **9**, 269—328 (1957)

Pickering, R. J., Wolfrom, M. R., Good, R. A., Gewurz, H.: Passive hemolysis by serum and cobra factor: a new mechanism inducing membrane damage by complement. Proc. nat. Acad. Sci. (Wash.) **62**, 521—527 (1969)

Ratnoff, O., Miles, A. A.: The induction of permeability-increasing activity in human plasma by activated Hageman factor. Brit. J. exp. Path. **45**, 328—338 (1964)

Rocha e Silva, M.: Autofarmacologia e venenos animais. Arq. Inst. Biol. (Sao Paulo) **19**, 1—22 (1949)

Rocha e Silva, M.: Action of histamine upon the circulatory apparatus. In: Handb. Exp. Pharmacol. Histamine. Its Chemistry, Metabolism and Physiological and Pharmacological Actions, Vol. XVIII. Berlin-Heidelberg-New York: Springer 1966

Rocha e Silva, M., Beraldo, W. T., Rosenfeld, G.: Bradykinin, a hypotensive and smooth muscle stimulating principle released from plasma globulin by snake venoms and by trypsin. Amer. J. Physiol. **156**, 261—273 (1949)

Rocha e Silva, M., Essex, H. E.: The effects of animal poisons (rattle-snake venom and trypsin) on blood histamine of guinea pigs and rabbits. Amer. J. Physiol. **135**, 372—377 (1942)
Rocha e Silva, M., Rothschild, A. M.: Experimental design for bioassay of a material inducing strong tachyphylactic effect (anaphylatoxin). Brit. J. Pharmacol. **11**, 252—263 (1956)
Rosa, A. T., Rothschild, Z., Rothschild, A. M.: Fibrinolytic activity evoked in the plasma of normal and adrenalectomized rats by cellulose sulphate. Brit. J. Pharmacol. **45**, 470—475 (1972)
Rosen, M., Gitter, S., Edery, H.: Histamine release and formation of a bradykinin-like substance by *Vipera palestinae* snake venom. Harokeach Haivri **10**, 333 (1964)
Rosenberg, P.: Use of phospholipases in studying nerve structure and function. In: Vries, A. de, Kochva, E. (Eds.): Toxins of Animal and Plant Origin, Vol. I. New York-London-Paris: Gordon and Breach 1972
Rothschild, A. M.: Fatores liberadores de histamina de venenos crotálico e de abelha. Ciência Cultura **15**, 278—279 (1963)
Rothschild, A. M.: Histamine release by bee venom phospholipase A and melittin in the rat. Brit. J. Pharmacol. **25**, 59—66 (1965)
Rothschild, A. M.: Mechanism of histamine release by animal venoms. Mem. Inst. Butantan **33**, 467—476 (1966a)
Rothschild, A. M.: Histamine release by basic compounds. In: Handb. Exp. Pharmacol. Histamine. Its Chemistry, Metabolism and Physiological and Pharmacological Actions, Vol. XVIII. Berlin-Heidelberg-New York: Springer 1966b
Rothschild, A. M.: Chromatographic separation of phospholipase A from a histamine releasing component of Brazilian rattlesnake venom. Experientia (Basel) **23**, 741—742 (1967)
Rothschild, A. M.: Pharmacodynamic properties of cellulose sulfate, a bradykininogen-depleting agent in the rat. Brit. J. Pharm. **33**, 501—511 (1968)
Rothschild, A. M.: Mechanisms of histamine release by compound 48/80. Brit. J. Pharmacol. **38**, 253—262 (1970)
Rothschild, A. M., Almeida, J. A.: Role of bradykinin in the fatal shock induced by *Bothrops jararaca* venom in the rat. In: Vries, A. de, Kochva, E. (Eds.): Toxins of Animal and Plant Origin, Vol. II. New York-London-Paris: Gordon and Breach 1972
Rothschild, A. M., Cordeiro, R. S. B., Castania, A.: Lowering of kininogen in rat blood by catecholamines. Involvement of non-eosinophil granulocytes and selective inhibition by Trasylol. Naunyn-Schmiedebergs Arch. Pharmacol. **282**, 323—327 (1974)
Rothschild, A. M., Rocha e Silva, M.: Activation of a histamine-releasing agent (anaphylatoxin) in normal rat plasma. Brit. J. exp. Path. **35**, 507—518 (1954)
Rothschild, A. M., Rothschild, Z.: Enzimas proteolíticas e liberação de histamina. Ciência Cultura **23**, 481—485 (1971)
Ruddy, S., Gigli, I., Austen, K. F.: The complement system of man. New Engl. J. Med. **287**, 489—495 (1972)
Saeki, K.: Effects of compound 48/80, chymotrypsin and anti-serum on isolated mast cells under aerobic and anaerobic conditions. Jap. J. Pharmacol. **14**, 375—390 (1964)
Sasaki, J.: Mechanism of histamine release by α-chymotrypsin from isolated rat mast cells. Jap. J. Pharmacol. **25**, 311—324 (1975)
Sato, T., Iwanaga, S., Mizushima, Y., Suzuki, T.: Studies on Snake Venoms. XV. Separation of arginine ester hydrolase of *Agkistrodon halys blomhoffii* venom into three enzymatic entities: bradykinin-releasing, clotting, and permeability-increasing. J. Biochem. (Tokyo) **57**, 380—391 (1965)
Schachter, M.: Vasodilatation in the submaxillary gland of the cat, rabbit, sheep. In: Handb. Exp. Pharmacol. Bradykinin, Kallidin, and Kallikrein, Vol. XXV. Berlin-Heidelberg-New York: Springer 1970
Schenberg, S.: Geographical pattern of crotamine distribution in the same rattlesnake species. Science **129**, 1361—1363 (1959)
Schoenmakers, J. G. G., Matze, R., Haanen, C., Zilliken, F.: Hageman factor, a novel sialoglycoprotein with esterase activity. Biochem. biophys. Acta (Amst.) **101**, 166—173 (1965)
Schöttler, W. H. A.: Antihistamine, ACTH, cortisone, hydrocortisone, and anesthetics in snake bites. Amer. J. trop. Med. **3**, 1083—1091 (1954)
Schröder, E.: Structure-activity relationships of kinins. In: Handb. Exp. Pharmacol. Bradykinin, Kallidin, and Kallikrein, Vol. XXV. Berlin-Heidelberg-New York: Springer 1970

Schütz, R. M., Vogt, W.: Über die Natur der durch Cobragift in durchströmten Meerschweinchenlungen freigesetzten "Slow Reacting Substance". Naunyn-Schmiedebergs Arch. exp. Path. Pharmak. **240**, 540—513 (1961)

Seba, R. A.: Efeitos vasculares do veneno de *B. atrox*: sua inibição pela rutina e um antihistamínico. Rev. Flumin. Med. **14**, 179—188 (1949)

Slotta, K. H., Vick, J. A., Ginsberg, N. J.: Enzymatic and toxic activity of phospholipase A. In: Vries, A. de, Kochva, E. (Eds.): Toxins of Animal and Plant Origin, Vol. I. New York-London-Paris: Gordon and Breach 1972

Smith, D. E.: Nature of secretory activity of the mast cell. Amer. J. Physiol. **193**, 573—580 (1958)

Smith, D. E., Lewis, Y. S.: Preparation and effects of an anti-mast cell serum. J. exp. Med. **113**, 683—692 (1961)

Snyder, R.: Snake bite. Am. J. Dis. Child. **103**, 85—96 (1962)

Somani, P., Arora, R. B.: Mechanism of increased capillary permeability induced by saw scaled viper *(E. carinatus)* venom. A possible new approach to the treatment of viperine snake poisoning. J. Pharm. Pharmacol. **14**, 394—395 (1964)

Suzuki, T., Iwanaga, S.: Snake Venoms. In: Handb. Exp. Pharmacol. Bradykinin, Kallidin, and Kallikrein, Vol. XXV. Berlin-Heidelberg-New York: Springer 1970

Trautschold, I.: Assay methods in the kinin system. In: Handb. Exp. Pharmacol. Bradykinin, Kallidin, and Kallikrein, Vol. XXV. Berlin-Heidelberg-New York: Springer 1970

Treloar, M. P., Pyle, H. A., Fuller, P. J., Movat, H. Z.: Guinea pig prekallikrein activator. In: Back, N., Sicuteri, F. (Eds.): Vasopeptides, Chemistry, Pharmacology, and Pathophysiology. New York-London: Plenum Press 1972

Trethewie, E. R.: Comparison of hemolysis and liberation of histamine by two Australian snake venoms. Aust. J. exp. Biol. med. Sci. **17**, 145—156 (1939)

Tu, A. T., James, G. P., Chua, A.: Some biochemical evidence in support of the classification of venomous snakes. Toxicon **3**, 5—8 (1965)

Vallota, E. H., Müller-Eberhard, H. J.: Formation of C3a and C5a anaphylatoxins in whole human serum after inhibition of the anaphylatoxin inactivator. J. exp. Med. **137**, 1109—1123 (1973)

Vargaftig, B. B.: Search for common mechanism underlying the various effects of putative inflammatory mediators. In: Ramwell, P. W. (Ed.): The Prostaglandins, Vol. II. New York-London: Plenum Press 1972

Vargaftig, B. B., Dao, N.: Antagonism by anti-inflammatory drugs of tissue slow reacting substance C. Pharmacol. Res. Commun. **2**, 149—157 (1970)

Vargaftig, B. B., Dao, N.: Inhibition by sulfhydryl reagents of the effects of bradykinin, arachidonic acid and "slow reacting substance C". In: Back, N., Sicuteri, F. (Eds.): Vasopeptides. Chemistry, Pharmacology, and Pathophysiology. New York-London: Plenum Press 1972

Vital Brazil, O., Prado-Franceschi, J., Laure, J. C.: On the nature of some effects caused by crotamine on skeletal muscle. Abstr. Comm. V. Intern. Congr. Pharmacol., S. Francisco, 1972, p. 243

Vogt, W.: Pharmacologically active substances formed in egg yolk by cobra venom. J. Physiol. (Lond.) **136**, 131—147 (1957)

Vogt, W.: Slow reacting substances. In: Movat, H. Z. (Ed.): Cellular and Humoral Mechanisms in Anaphylaxis and Allergy, pp. 187—195. Basel-New York: Karger 1969

Vogt, W.: Activation, activities, and pharmacologically active products of complement. Pharmacol. Rev. **26**, 125—169 (1974)

Vogt, W., Dieminger, L., Lynen, R., Schmidt, G.: Alternate pathway to complement activation in human serum: formation and composition of the complex with cobra venom factor which cleaves the third component of complement. Hoppe-Seylers Z. physiol. Chem. **355**, 171—183 (1974)

Vogt, W., Meyer, U., Kunze, H., Luft, E., Babilli, S.: Entstehung von SRS-C in der durchströmten Meerschweinchenlunge durch Phospholipase A. Identifizierung mit Prostaglandin. Naunyn-Schmiedebergs Arch. Pharmak. exp. Path. **262**, 124—134 (1969 b)

Vogt, W., Schmidt, G.: Abtrennung des anaphylatoxin-bildenden Prinzips aus Cobragift von anderen Giftkomponenten. Experientia (Basel) **20**, 207—208 (1964)

Vogt, W., Zeman, N., Garbe, G.: Histaminunabhängige Wirkungen von Anaphylatoxin auf glatte Muskulatur isolierter Organe. Naunyn-Schmiedebergs Arch.-Pharmak. exp. Path. **262**, 399—404 (1969a)
Vries, A. de, Rechnic, Y., Moroz, Ch., Moav, B.: Prevention of *Echis colorata* venom-induced afibrinogenemia by heparin. Toxicon **1**, 241—242 (1963)
Vugman, I., Rocha e Silva, M.: Biological determination of histamine in living tissues and body fluids. In: Handb. Exp. Pharmacol. Histamine. Its Chemistry, Metabolism, and Physiological and Pharmacological Actions, Vol. XVIII. Berlin-Heidelberg-New York: Springer 1966
Walaszek, E. J.: The effect of bradykinin and kallidin on smooth muscle. In: Handb. Exp. Pharmacol. Bradykinin, Kallidin, and Kallikrein, Vol. XXV. Berlin-Heidelberg-New York: Springer 1970
Ward, P. A.: Chemotactic factors for neutrophils, eosinophils, mononuclear cells and lymphocytes. In: Austen, K. F., Becker, E. L. (Eds.): Biochemistry of the Acute Allergic Reactions. Oxford: Blackwell 1971
Ward, P. A., Chapitis, J., Conroy, M. C., Lepow, I. H.: Generation by bacterial proteinases of leukotactic factors from human serum and human C3 and C5. J. Immunol. **110**, 1003—1013 (1973)
Webster, M. E.: Recommendations for Nomenclature and Units. In: Handb. Exp. Pharmacol. Bradykinin, Kallidin, and Kallikrein, Vol. XXV. Berlin-Heidelberg-New York: Springer 1970
Webster, M. E., Pierce, J. V.: The nature of the kallidins released from human plasma by kallikreins and other enzymes. Ann. N.Y. Acad. Sci. **104**, 91—107 (1963)
Weeks, J. R.: Prostaglandins. Ann. Rev. Pharmacol. **12**, 317—336 (1972)
Werle, E., Forrel, M. M., Maier, L.: Zur Kenntnis der blutdrucksenkenden Wirkung des Trypsins. Naunyn-Schmiedebergs Arch. exp. Path. Pharmak. **225**, 369—380 (1955)
Werle, E., Kehl, R., Koebke, K.: Über Bradykinin, Kallidin und Hypertensin. Biochem. Z. **320**, 372—383 (1950)
Werle, E., Zach, P.: Verteilung von Kininogen in Serum und Geweben bei Ratten und anderen Säugetieren. Z. klin. Chem. klin. Biochem. **8**, 186—189 (1970)
Westermann, E., Klapper, W.: Untersuchungen über die Kreislaufwirkung des Kobragiftes. Naunyn-Schmiedebergs Arch. exp. Path. Pharmak. **239**, 68—80 (1960)
Wilhelm, D. L.: The mediation of increased vascular permeability in inflammation. Pharmacol. Rev. **14**, 251—280 (1962)

CHAPTER 17

Snake Venoms as an Experimental Tool to Induce and Study Models of Microvessel Damage*

I. L. BONTA, B. B. VARGAFTIG and G. M. BÖHM

"Experimental model of a disease is an ideal test object for potentially curative drugs and for the analysis of disease producing mechanisms."
H. Selye

A. Introduction

I. By Way of Speculating About Disease Models

The catchwords of this chapter came from a scientist whose significant work covers two fields: pharmacology and experimental pathology. The above motto (SELYE, 1964) is thus a true reflection of his doublefold preoccupation, recognizing hereby that basic problems of medicine demand an integral approach from angles of more than one discipline. As two authors of this chapter are pharmacologists and the third an experimental pathologist, the symbolic connection to the above is evident. An even more important bridge between the motto and this chapter is the subject proper to be dealt with: experimental disease models of vascular conditions. It will be shown that a number of snake venoms and purified components thereof can, under specified circumstances, induce vascular changes which in morphology, biochemical pathogenesis, and pharmacologic responsiveness represent models of early phases of tissue injury conditions. The purpose of this article is to describe and discuss several aspects of such models. At the outset, however, it appears useful to briefly speculate on what the characteristics of disease models in general are. Let us start with the realization that a model is never a perfect replica of the original. This is an inherent truism, valid for every model, because if it were not so the model would be identic with the original disease and not its model. Certain models show a phenomenologic resemblance to disease conditions. The danger of such models is that this resemblance may hide the underlying mechanism, thus leading to misinterpretation. In fact, this happened with one of the models discussed in this article: its macroscopic appearance and pharmacologic responsiveness led to its interpretation in terms of hemorrhagic disorders, whereas microscopic studies unmasked it as being an inflammatory-condition model with an unconventional pharmacologic profile.

Until approximately the first half of this century, experimental medicine was foremostly limited to static analysis of abnormalities (macroscopic and microscopic morphology, chemical composition of structures, etc.). For a variety of complex

* This work is devoted to Professor Hans Selye (Montreal, Canada), on the occasion of his 70th anniversary.

syndromes, many of which are dynamic processes rather than stationary conditions, the static approach obviously proved unsatisfactory. Inflammation is a good example, because the injured tissue site undergoes continuous changes, and there is neither a single theory to explain nor a single drug to control all phases of the inflammatory reaction. Obvious as it is that the study of complex conditions demands complex models, it is equally evident that excessive complexity may create problems of identic magnitude with the model as with the natural condition. The ideal is a balance between functional resemblance and feasibility to solve problems. To this end, it is appropriate to design models representing one or the other particular phase of the disease. Remaining at the example of inflammation, it is conventional to divide it into the acute and the chronic phase. In accordance with this, most of the accepted models have bearing on one or the other of these phases. In some of the acute models, the inducing noxa causes the release of inflammatory mediators and they are therefore, suitable for studying the release process as such as well as drug interactions either with the release or the effect of mediators. In other cases, a recognized mediator serves as an inducing agent proper. One of the objectives of this article is to discuss the evidence—partially still circumstantial—that some components of snake venoms can, without participation of endogenous mediator release, produce in lung tissue such inflammatory vascular changes which under nonartificial conditions are caused by intervention of mediators. In this context, the venom components in question replace the mediators and as such may be considered to be functional models of the latter. While inflammatory mediators cause a multiplicity of effects, the venom components to be dealt with do not necessarily produce all of them.

There is a gradual transition between rather simple and very complex model situations. The fact that the venom-induced vascular conditions reach their peak within a few minutes eliminates the problem of chronicity, the latter being the usual component which determines complexity of pathologic models. On the other hand, as certain biochemical and pharmacologic properties of endogenous mediators are mimicked by the venom components, the latter can be considered to be model substances of the former. Hence, we are faced with the undesired circumstance that both the inducing factor and the condition induced are imitations of disease elements, hereby creating a doublefold model situation. All this is put forward *by way of defense to anticipate* the discussion that our model, while probably useful to approach the solution of some older problems, raised an at least equal number of new problems, the majority of which have as yet remained unanswered.

II. Venoms as Stores of Vasculotoxic Materials

The term vasculotoxicity is somewhat elusive and it appears important to define how it will be used in this article. Within one organism, several kinds of vessels exist, largely differing from each other in structure, biochemistry, innervation, and function. The changes to occur after pharmacologic challenge will depend greatly on which kind of vessel and which parameter of it is influenced. The gross changes in hemodynamics (blood pressure and flow, cardiovascular reflexes, generalized edema) resulting from alterations in arteries and veins will not be considered in this work, thus limiting it to effects on arterioles, venules, and capillaries. While these limitations seemingly restrict the field to the vessel wall as a membrane, this structure is functionally interwoven with some blood components (erythrocytes, platelets) to such extent that changes in the latter will inevitably be treated. The main vascular alterations to be considered will be hyperemia, stasis, and leakage. The experimental conditions from which several conclusions of this work were drawn did not on many occasions allow a discrimination of these changes. Whenever this was the case, the vague general term of *vascular lesion* will be used.

Microvessels are very vulnerable and thus injured during tissue damage whatever the noxa be. This occurs not only because many noxious agents have a *direct* deleterious effect on small vessels but also because of the *indirect* effect exerted through various endogenous materials (enzymes and mediators). In view of this and since a single snake venom usually is composed of 5–15 enzymes, 3–12 nonenzymic proteins and peptides, and an additional half dozen other substances (RUSSEL and PUFFER, 1970), it is easy to appreciate that such venoms are exceptionally rich sources of materials which in one way or another disturb the integrity of vessels. The reader interested in the present status of knowledge on the chemistry and pharmacology of snake venoms is directed to recent exhaustive reviews (JIMÉNEZ-PORRAS, 1968; JIMÉNEZ-PORRAS, 1970; LEE, 1971; LEE, 1972; LEE, 1973; RUSSEL and PUFFER, 1970; ZLOTKIN, 1973) in addition to Chap. 4, 5, and 7 of this Handbook. Instead of going through all the well-defined venom components and discussing which of them is a putative vasculotoxin—a task beyond the scope of this article—a brief account will be given of those which can be considered prototypes for comparison with those actually investigated by us.

The enzymes will be considered first. Amongst them, phospholipase A_2 is of paramount importance for the following reasons. The products of its hydrolytic action are pharmacologically very active, both lysophosphatides and unsaturated fatty acids being membrane damagers and the latter precursors of prostaglandins and slow-reacting substance C as well. In addition, phospholipase A_2 is a mast cell-degranulating agent, thus yielding histamine and serotonin, the latter in the case of rodents. The presence of phospholipase A_2 renders all snake and bee venoms candidate vasculotoxins. The pharmacologically unknown phospholipase B, however, which splits lysolecithin to a fatty acid and glycerophosphorylcholine, is present in *Naja naja* venom but not in *Hemachatus haemachatus* venom (Ringhals cobra). Phospholipase C acts on phosphotidylcholine to yield a diglyceride and choline phosphate and is present in *N. naja* venom but absent in *Naja naja atra* venom (LEE, 1971). This enzyme is hemolytic and increases vessel permeability (HABERMANN, 1960).

Proteases and nonproteolytic arginine esterases are ubiquitary in crotalid and viperid venoms, but elapid venoms do not contain them in significant amounts. These enzymes are recognized releasers of bradykinin, a vasoactive tissue injury mediator of primary importance. The coagulant activity of the two groups of venoms is also attributed to the presence of the mentioned enzymes.

All snake venoms, with the exception of *Naja nigricollis* (ZWISLER, 1966), contain hyaluronidase which depolymerizes hyaluronic acid. The latter, an acid mucopolysaccharide, is a constituent of the kit material in the vascular basement membrane.

Collagenase activity has recently been shown with the venom of *Trimeresurus flavoviridis* (Habu snake), a crotalid (OHSAKA et al., 1973). The possibility that small peptides, split by collagenase from basement membrane collagen components, serve as tissue injury mediators, has to be considered when vasotoxicity of venoms is analyzed. Evidence in favor of this will be presented in Sect. D.II.2.

From the group of nonenzymic components of venoms, the hemorrhagins are *eo ipso* destructive to the vessels. Several hemorrhagins, some of which are proteolytic, have been reported. Crotalid and viperid venoms have a time-honored reputation of being rich in these substances.

Abundant constituents of cobra (elapid snake) venoms are those cationic peptides which appear in the literature under different names: cardiotoxin, direct lytic factor (DLF), cobramines A and B, toxin γ, and cytotoxin [1]. Chemically and pharmacologically they differ from each other in subordinate points. It has even been proposed that these substances are identic to each other (LEE, 1971; LEE et al., 1970). *In vitro* on erythrocyte lysis, they are mutually synergistic with phospholipase A_2, a property which, since the work of DE VRIES and associates (CONDREA, 1964), was studied in great detail in several systems but still remains poorly understood. This group of substances is also known to cause local tissue injury (LEE et al., 1968; LAI et al., 1972), thus rendering them candidate vasculotoxins. Section C.II.1 will provide evidence for this. Several properties of DLF are, at least qualitatively, shared by melittin, the strongly basic peptide of bee venom. The latter also contains phospholipase A_2 and apamin, which was shown to increase capillary permeability (HABERMANN, 1965), three reasons to expect vessel lesions by bee venom.

Some genuine neurotoxins have additional properties by which they can cause vessel lesions. One example is crotactin, an acidic, nonenzymic fraction of *Crotalus terrificus* venom, reported to release histamine and increase vessel permeability (HABERMANN and NEUMANN, 1956). The latter effect was also shown with the neurotoxic fraction A of *Notechis scutatus* (Australian tiger snake) venom (DOERY, 1958).

From the brief enumeration above, it should be clear that practically all snake venom was intradermally administered (EMERY and RUSSELL, 1963). Yet this venom is devoid of significant vascular hemorrhagic effect when applied topically to lung including those containing abundant amounts of highly active substances which cause vessel damage, is greatly dependent on the experimental conditions. While this sounds like a pharmacologic banality, it can nevertheless easily be overlooked. The venom of the Eastern diamondback rattlesnake *(Crotalus adamanteus)* is classified as strongly hemorrhagic (JIMÉNEZ-PORRAS, 1970), based on experiments in which the venom was intradermally administered (EMERY and RUSSEL, 1963). Yet this venom is devoid of significant vascular hemorrhagic effect when applied topically to lung tissue (BONTA et al., 1969). The venom of *Agkistrodon piscivorus*, however, while strongly hemorrhagic on pulmonary vessels (BONTA et al., 1969), is considerably less destructive than *C. adamanteus* venom on skin vessels (EMERY and RUSSELL, 1963). The sensitivity of vessels toward the challenging material largely depends on the type of vessels, as will be shown in *Sect. B.II* of this Chapter. The surrounding tissue in which the vessel is inbedded might be another determining factor, particularly if the

[1] Note on nomenclature: A variety of descriptive terms, such as "direct lytic factor," "hemolysins," "neurotoxins," "cardiotoxins," etc., are used in this Chapter. The authors are aware of the increasing criticism among toxinologists concerning use of such phenomenologic nomenclature. Lack of a generally accepted classification and nomenclature of toxic factors, based on molecular characteristics, led us to this use. Progress in this area should hopefully allow replacement of such terms by more scientific and rational ones.

vessel lesion is not caused directly by the venom component but through a mediator liberated from the tissue. It has little sense, therefore, to question whether a particular venom is a vasculotoxin. It was stated earlier that all snake venoms be considered capable of producing changes in any organ system (RUSSELL and PUFFER, 1970). The art is rather to select those components of the venoms which produce changes considered characteristic models for disorders of specified organs. In this sense, the snake venoms, along with bee venom, are definitely valuable as will be discussed in *Section* C.II. It will be also shown, however, that the same venom (component) may serve to create different vascular condition models even in the same organism, the determining factor being the type and location of the vessels. It now appears appropriate to describe the morphologic aspects of some of the vascular beds we shall study before describing the methods used.

B. Morphology, Methodology, and Phenomenology of Venom-Induced Vessel Lesion

I. Comparative Morphology of Lung and Cremaster Vessels

The structure of vessels differs greatly according to the species of animals and the kind of tissues to which they belong. This fact is too frequently forgotten in microcirculation research. A survey of the literature on inflammatory processes, for example, leaves the impression that there is only one vascular reaction pattern but, in reality, there are probably as many patterns as morphologic variations of the vessels.

In 1959, BENNETT et al. proposed a simple three-digit classification of vertebrate blood capillaries based on the presence or absence of continuous basement membrane (presence type = A, absence = B), the nature of the endothelial cell (without fenestrations or perforations = 1, with intracellular fenestrations or perforations = 2, with intercellular fenestrations or gaps = 3), and on the presence or absence of a complete investment of pericapillary cells (presence = β, absence = α). This classification is only for capillaries and it should be remembered that in most injuries the venules and arterioles participate in the vascular response and that these vessels also do not show structural uniformity. Since in our investigations we mostly used lungs and cremasters, a brief description of the vessels of these tissues follows.

1. Capillaries

The cremaster capillaries, as those from striated muscle, skin, and connective tissue, belong to the type A.1.α and may be designated as systemic capillaries. The dermal capillaries have a thin endothelial layer. The systemic capillaries have been reviewed by MAJNO (1965) and LUFT (1973). The pulmonary capillaries are classified as type A.1.β and WEIBEL'S (1973) paper deals thoroughly with their description.

The endothelium is similar in lung and cremaster capillaries. Opposite to the nucleus, it is approximately 200 nm thick in the cremaster and 100–200 nm in the lung. The pulmonary endothelium is thinned down to about 20 nm in some regions of the air-blood barrier, mainly in small mammals (WEIBEL, 1973). The intercellular junctions are similar in both types of vessels and the narrowest portion of the gap measures 4.0–4.5 nm (SCHNEEBERGER and KARNOVSKY, 1971; LUFT, 1973). Functionally, there is good evidence that the pulmonary endothelial junctions are less permeable than those of systemic vessels, both under physiologic and pathologic conditions (PIETRA et al., 1971b; GABBIANI et al., 1972; STAUB, 1974; MACHADO et al., 1976).

The basement membrane of the capillary is easily observed under the electron microscope as a continuous, 50 nm thick, fibrillar layer in the cremaster. This is not the case in lung capillaries. Although they are also completely surrounded by a basement membrane, as is evident in pulmonary edema (BÖHM et al., 1973), under normal conditions the basement membrane cannot be distingushed from that of the alveolar cell at the level of the airblood barrier. Fusion of the two membranes is generally accepted, but the possibility of a real structural differentiation should be considered, in which case, splitting of the membrane by interstitial edema could be the "artifact" instead of the fusion.

External to systemic capillaries there are pericytes forming an incomplete layer around the vessels. These cells are considered to be embedded in the basement membrane of the capillary (MAJNO, 1965). The presence of pericytes in pulmonary capillaries was disputed until WEIBEL (1973) demonstrated their existence in the thicker portion of the alveolar interstitium. Furthermore, he concluded that they are rarer and less densely branched than in the systemic capillaries.

The most distinctive feature of lung capillaries is the presence of a complete pericapillary layer, 100–200 nm thick, formed by the squamous alveolar cells (squamous epithelial cells or pneumocytes type I). It is accepted that the intercellular junctions of the alveolar epithelium are less permeable to fluids and proteins than those of the endothelium (PIETRA et al., 1971b; STAUB, 1974).

2. Arterioles and Venules

The differences between cremaster and pulmonary arterioles and venules are difficult to establish and cannot be generalized. For example, the distribution of elastic and muscle layers in the pulmonary arteries varies greatly with the animal species (FERENCZ, 1969). In small mammals, the pulmonary veins and venules are surrounded by cardiac muscle (ALMEIDA et al., 1975). In the rat, the endothelium of these vessels is similar, but the middle layer of pulmonary arterioles and venules is thinner than that of the cremaster. The distribution of elastic tissue is also peculiar. In contrast to systemic vessels, in the lungs the internal elastic layer is thicker in the venules than in the arterioles (MACHADO et al., 1976). Cardiac fibers and cushions of smooth muscle cells which are not seen in the cremaster are present in the veins and greater venules of rat lungs (ALMEIDA et al., 1975).

Two important functional differences have been shown. First, the well-known leakage through systemic venules in the early phase of inflammatory reaction (MAJNO et al., 1961) is not found in the pulmonary vessels. There are structural changes and permeability alterations in the pulmonary venules, but opening of intercellular junctions is seldom seen. Thus, biphasic sequence of permeability, first venular and next capillary, has not been observed in lungs (BÖHM, 1966; MACHADO et al., 1976). Second, in rats the pulmonary arterioles participate intensely in the permeability alterations (BÖHM, 1973a; BÖHM et al., 1976), which is not the case in the cremaster.

II. Methodology and Phenomenology of Vessel Lesions in Different Tissues

Before entering the more technical parts of this section, a few introductory comments seem appropriate. Speaking in terms of gross generalization—inevitable when reviews are written—the two main groups of abnormalities in which microvessels are involved are thrombohemorrhagic and inflammatory changes. Characteristics for the thrombohemorrhagic phenomena are:

1. By definition of the phenomena, the vessel lesion always reaches the degree to permit extravasation of whole blood.
2. The vessel lesion is unexceptionally accompanied by markedly altered coagulation and to pinpoint the primary disturbance is difficult. The latter is a consequence of the functional entity formed between the intraluminar surface of the vessel endothelium and blood elements, e.g., the platelets.

Regarding the inflammatory condition:

1. Changes in the barrier function of the vessels are mostly restricted to the extent that massive erythrocyte extravasation does not occur.
2. Coagulation disturbances, if present, are mostly of subordinate magnitude. There is a doublefold connecting link between the two kinds of abnormalities. First, the membrane function of the microvessels is disturbed, whatever the magnitude, including the graduality of the changes. Second, there occurs in both conditions a massive endogenous release of a variety of humoral mediators, all of which have effects pertinent to both conditions.

It is customary to interpret disturbances in the barrier function of microvessels as due to increased permeability of the capillaries. This concept remained beyond the range of challenge after the discovery that tissue damage is accompanied by increased vascular permeability (COHNHEIM, 1973). It has been shown, however, that histamine and serotonin exert their specific effect, manifested as vessel leakage, on the venular side of the vascular tree (MAJNO et al., 1961). The same site of action was more recently shown for other humoral mediators of acute vascular injury (KALEY and WEINER, 1971; ROCHA E SILVA, 1972). Such findings indicate that caution should be exercised when describing and interpreting the effect of substances on vascular permeability, since capillaries are unlikely to be their only direct target. Moreover, it should be remembered that increased permeability and release of vasoactive mediators interact doublefold; mediator release necessarily results in permeability changes, whereas the latter may in turn create a situation which leads to activation of another mediator. Thus, histamine release, causing plasma extravasation, will result in the appearance of bradykinin due to activation of the diluting factor.

Keeping the above considerations in mind, the methodologic aspects of investigating vascular effects of venoms will be discussed.

1. Pulmonary Vessels

The pre- and postcapillary end branches, and obviously the capillaries proper of lungs, are directly under the transparent cell monolayer of the visceral pleura. This circumstance offers two advantages. First, the venom (for that matter any other substance) has easy access to the microvessels after topical application on the pleural surface. Second, manifestations of vascular lesions are directly observable due to the transparency of the pleura. These two factors prompted us to work out the pulmonary surface method. It has two variants, each of them having its own merits and disadvantages.

a) Canine Lung Surface Test

The original variant consists of topical testing on dog lungs; however, any large laboratory animal (cat, rabbit) can serve the purpose. Under anesthesia and artificial respiration, the thorax is opened, thus exposing the lungs. Filter paper disks are soaked with the solution of the venom or separate components thereof and applied to the lung surface for a few minutes. The application time can be chosen freely, provided it is kept constant during each particular experiment, because the effect is directly correlated with the length of the time during which the tissue is in contact with the venom. After removal of the filter paper, the site of application is observed with the unaided eye. The time elapsing between the removal of the filter paper and the distinct appearance of a microvascular event (blanching, redness, hemorrhage) is assessed to the nearest minute. The intensity of the lesion is rated on a nonparametric scale. The inherent subjective element in nonparametric rating can be easily circumvented by performing the experiment under "blind" conditions, i.e., keeping the observer unaware of the test material. This will only occasionally be necessary, because with some practice, the differences are readily distinguishable. A skilled experimentor can perform the testing of up to six samples simultaneously (Figs. 1a and 1b), comparing them for potency and differences in the macroscopic appearance of the lesions. The surface of the canine lung permits the investigation of 10–20 samples within one animal. For any other technical detail of this design, the reader is referred to the original papers (BONTA et al., 1965; BONTA et al., 1969; BONTA et al., 1970c).

Macroscopically, two main types of vascular lesions were observed in the above situation. Diffuse redness of the pulmonary surface, strictly localized to the site of application, is characteristic for the lesion produced by *N. naja* venom. At the peak of intensity (mostly some 10 min after onset), the lesion has cherry red color and strongly suggests the presence of a confluent hemorrhage. In a number of earlier papers (BONTA et al., 1965; BONTA et al., 1969; BONTA et al., 1970c; BONTA et al., 1971; BONTA et al., 1970b; BHARGAVA et al., 1970a; BONTA et al., 1972; VINCENT et al., 1971), these lesions were indeed denoted as hemorrhages. More recent histologic studies (GREGORIO et al., 1977) unmasked that this was an erratic interpretation, the lesions de facto reflecting vascular congestion and edema (see also Sect. C.I.1).

The other type of lesion is characteristically produced by *A. piscivorus* venom. This damage starts with petechial dots, which soon become confluent and display dark red areas, resembling clots, in the center of the lesion. Histology verified the frank hemorrhagic nature of this phenomenon (GREGORIO, 1977; Sect. D.I.1). The sharp difference between the two lesions is shown in Figures 2 and 3, which also demonstrates that both phenomena are clearly dose dependent.

Diffuse lesions, qualitatively not distinguishable from those of *N. naja* venom, can be produced by other elapid snake venoms (*N. nigricollis*, *N. n. siamensis*, *Hemachatus haemachatus*) and by venom of the bee (*Apis mellifera*) (BONTA et al., 1969;

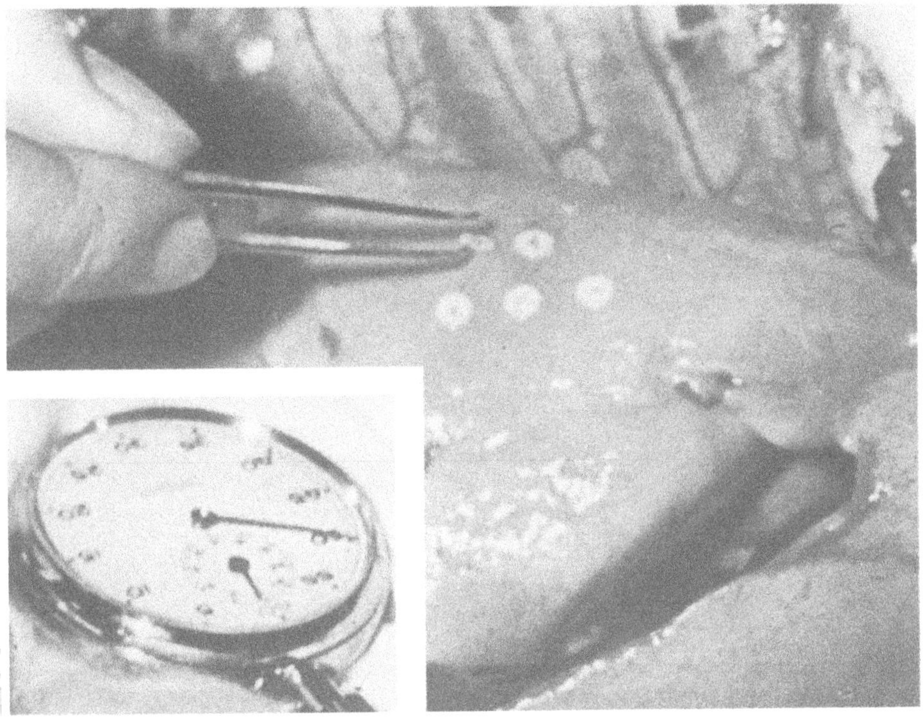

a

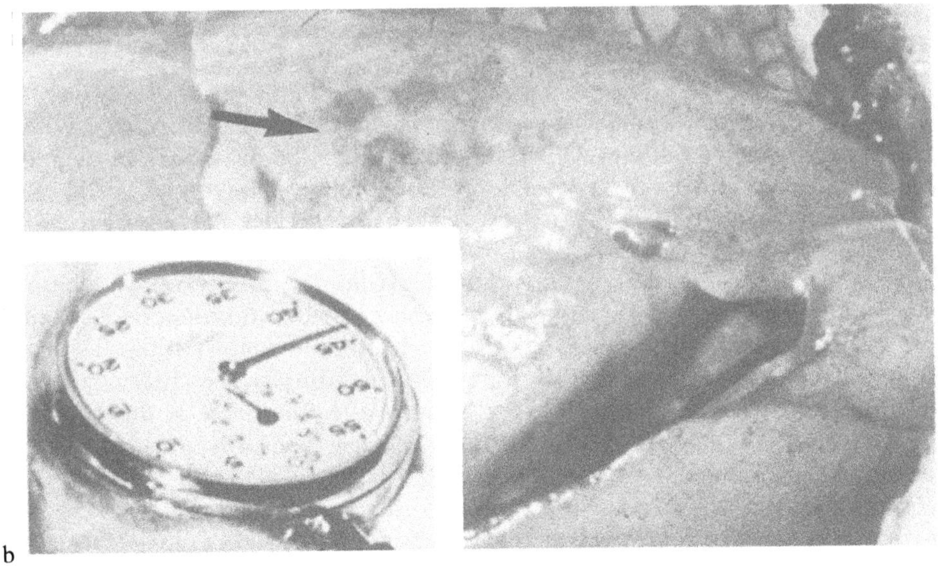

b

Fig. 1a and b. The canine lung surface test. Panel a: on the surface of the exposed lung of an anesthetized dog filter paper disks, which were soaked with venom solutions, are applied. At the same time, a stopwatch is started to monitor the onset of the lesions. Panel b: stopwatch shows that this photo was made 14 min after the application of the filter papers, which were removed after 3 min contact with the lung surface. Arrow indicates the lesions

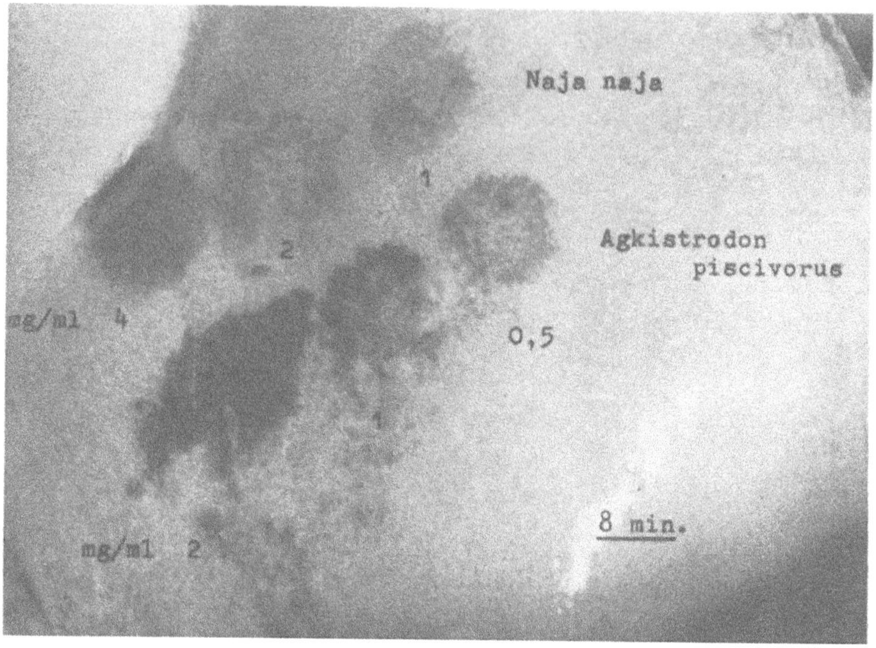

Fig. 2. Macroscopic appearance of pulmonary lesions produced by three concentrations of *Naja naja* and *Agkistrodon piscivorus* venoms. Lesions by *N. naja* venom are diffuse, while those by *A. piscivorus* are dotted. Note the dose-dependent intensity of the lesions. Photograph was taken 8 min after removal of the filter paper disks from the lung surface

BHARGAVA et al., 1970a; BONTA et al., 1976; BONTA and VARGAFTIG, 1976). The potency of bee venom is somewhat lower as compared to that of *N. naja* venom (BONTA et al., 1971). In Section C.II.1, the evidence will be discussed that peptides identic or related to DLF are responsible for this type of local injury.

The hemorrhagic type of pulmonary damage can, besides *A. piscivorus* venom, also be produced by venoms of *Bothrops jararaca* (VARGAFTIG et al., 1974) and *Lachesis mutus* (Bushmaster) (E. GREGORIO, G. M. BÖHM, I. L. BONTA, unpublished observation). There are some qualitative differences between these lesions. The outer area of the *B. jararaca* lesion displays a large hyperemic zone (VARGAFTIG et al., 1974), usually not present in that of *A. piscivorus*. Lesions by the latter commence with petechiae, which appear only a few minutes after the onset of the injury by *L. mutus* venom. No early vasculotoxicity in pulmonary tissue was observed with the venoms of *C. adamanteus* (VARGAFTIG et al., 1974; BONTA et al., 1969) and *C. durissus terrificus* (VARGAFTIG et al., 1974) although these rattlesnake venoms produce marked hemorrhages in skin vessels (EMERY and RUSSELL, 1963; VARGAFTIG et al., 1974). The gross differences between the hemorrhagic profile of these venoms shows a high specificity toward vascular beds from various regions.

When the onset of lesion was taken as a measure, a direct comparison indicated *N. naja* venom to be three times less potent than *A. piscivorus* venom on canine pulmonary tissue (BONTA et al., 1970c; BONTA et al., 1971). This was confirmed more recently (G. M. BÖHM, E. GREGORIO, unpublished data).

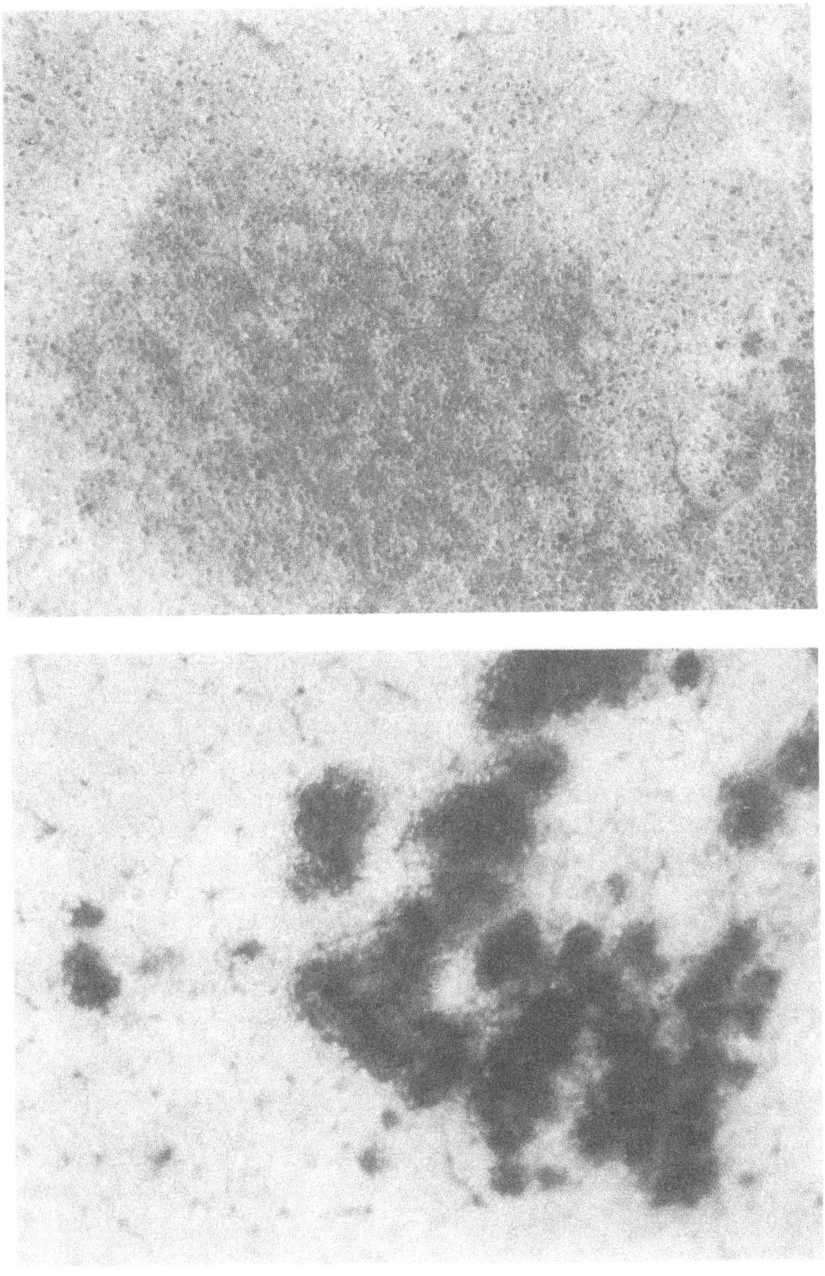

a

b

Fig. 3a and b. High magnification (40) photo of lesions produced by two snake venoms on dog lung surface. Panel a: *Naja naja* venom. Panel b: *Agkistrodon piscivorus* venom

b) Rodent Intrathoracic Test

The method of topical application of venoms to the pulmonary pleural surface in open-chest preparations of anesthetized dogs is particularly convenient for the assessment of direct vascular effects, but it does not provide a possibility for determining the contribution of the vessel-damaging property to the lethal effect of the venom. Therefore, a variant of the method was developed, essentially consisting of intrathoracic administration—i.e., between the parietal and visceral pleura to conscious mice (BONTA et al., 1970b; BONTA et al., 1971). More recently, small modifications allowed us to also adapt this method for rats (ALMEIDA et al., 1976). The survival time is measured, the type of vessel damage assessed by *post-mortem* inspection, and a lung weight index calculated to determine the extent of pulmonary edema as a quantitative parameter of vascular leakage.

The venoms of *Elapidae* (*N. naja* and *N. nigricollis*) and the bee produce, by intrathoracic application in mice and rats, the same picture as in dogs, diffusely reddish and seemingly hemorrhagic appearance of the lungs (BONTA et al., 1970b; BONTA et al., 1971; ALMEIDA, 1975; ALMEIDA et al., 1976). Histology in mice showed erythrocyte extravasation (BONTA et al., 1972a). Repeated intramuscular administration of sublethal doses of *N. nigricollis* venom in mice was also reported to cause pulmonary hemorrhages (MOHAMED et al., 1973). More recent studies with intrathoracic administration in rats (ALMEIDA, 1975; ALMEIDA et al., 1976) indicated that the lesions were foremostly restricted to congestion associated with plasma leakage (see also Sect. C.I.1). There was a marked increase in lung weight, which in succumbing animals was nearly double as compared to mice without venom treatment. With *N. naja* venom, however, the vasculotoxic component contributed only to a small extent to lethality, the main lethal factor apparently being the neurotoxin component of the venom. Within the dose range studied, *N. naja* venom-treated mice invariably succumbed within 10 min, but with an equieffective vasculotoxic dose of bee venom—not containing neurotoxin—most animals survived as long as 60 min (BONTA et al., 1971). In rats pretreated with the mast cell depleter, compound 48/80, the effect of *N. naja* venom was by no means diminished (ALMEIDA et al., 1976). This again shows that histamine release does not contribute to the pulmonary vasculotoxic effect of this venom. Regarding the intrathoracic route of administration, *N. naja* venom proved approximately twice as potent in mice than in rats (O. P. ALMEIDA, G. M. BÖHM, I. L. BONTA, unpublished observation).

Crotalid venoms studied with the intrathoracic administration included those of *A. piscivorus* (BONTA et al., 1971; ALMEIDA et al., 1976) and *B. jararaca* (see Sect. D.II). Macroscopic inspection in mice and rats revealed the presence of scattered hemorrhagic spots on the lung surface of animals sacrificed 10–15 min after the venom administration. Diffusely dark reddish lungs were observed in mice sacrificed 30 min after administration of *B. jararaca* venom. With the latter, the hemorrhagic effect was possibly followed by massive thrombosis. However, this diffuse dark reddish appearance of the lungs was never observed in *A. piscivorus*-treated animals, which after a dose causing markedly increased lung weight can survive as long as 60 min. It is pertinent to mention that mice treated with a chromatographically isolated hemorrhagic fraction of *A. piscivorus* venom survived as long as 2h despite the presence of massive vascular lesion in the lungs (BONTA et al., 1971). Again this shows that pulmonary vessel lesion per se does not cause rapid lethality, confirming the results obtained with *N. naja* venom and bee venoms. The macroscopic phenomenology of crotalid venoms causing hemorrhagic alterations when intrathoracically injected to rats was confirmed by histology (Sect. D.I.1).

N. naja venom is approximately three times as potent as the venom of *A. piscivorus* (ALMEIDA et al., 1976), when the minimal dose required to cause vascular lesion in rats was measured. This shows reversed sensitivity toward these venoms as compared to lung tissue vessels of dogs.

2. Cremaster Vessels

The cremaster vessels of rats have originally been used to study the effects of histamine and serotonin on the vascular tree (MAJNO et al., 1961). The method makes use of the anatomic relationships of the cremaster muscle which forms a pouch containing one testis. This pouch can be easily separated and stretched to become a membrane which can be mounted on a glass slide as a tissue section. The vessels of the cremaster are embedded between the two very thin muscular layers and are relatively independent from the vascular supply of the overlying skin. Local administration of the substances and colloidal carbon labeling of the vessels makes it possible to observe the site of action of a vessel-damaging material. For more technical details, reference is made to the original paper (MAJNO et al., 1961).

Two venoms were studied on cremaster vessels (ALMEIDA et al., 1976). The effect of *N. naja* venom was confined to the venules, whereas *A. piscivorus* venom also inflicted the capillaries and caused hemorrhages. The cremaster vessels display equal sensitivity toward the two venoms, the microscopic findings being discussed in Sections C.I.2 and D.I.2, respectively.

3. Rat Paw Edema

Any influence, whatever its mechanism is, which causes vessel lesion with increased permeability leads to plasma exudation manifested as local edema. On the other hand, a disturbance in the colloid osmotic pressure of blood (e.g., massive plasma protein loss due to renal disorder or prolonged starvation) can lead to plasma extravasation in the absence of vessel lesion. Provided that colloid osmotic imbalance is excluded, a local edema is indicative of abnormal vascular permeability increase. Amongst the methods used to study local edema, the induction of fluid accumulation in the peritoneal or pleural cavity suffers from the disadvantage that to measure the event quantitatively the animal has to be sacrificed, and a large number of animals is required to monitor the process at one time. The edematous swelling of an extremity is devoid of this drawback, because the increment in size of the extremity can be assessed without killing or even anesthetizing the animal. Thus, since rats can easily develop edema in the loose connective tissue of their legs, the rat hind paw edema is much preferred for the study of tissue damage—thus including vascular injury—and pharmacologic influences on it. Omitting a discussion on the technical aspects of measuring the rat paw edema, it is recalled that the results to be reported in this article were obtained by determining the thickness of the paws as described previously (BONTA and NOORDHOEK, 1973).

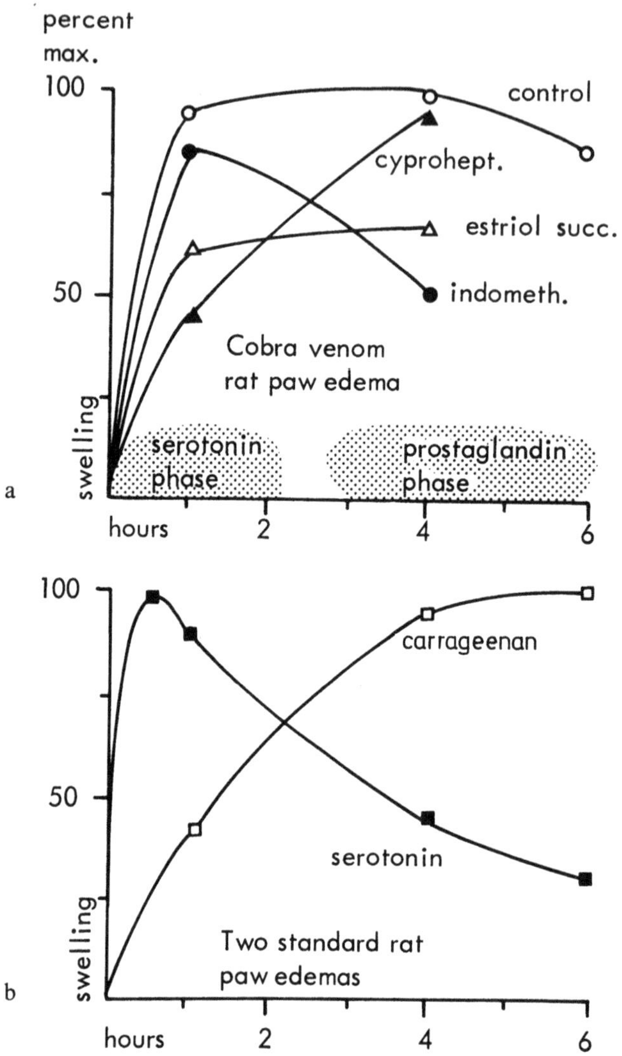

Fig. 4a and b. Development of rat paw edema plotted against time after subplantar injection of the inducing agent. Panel a: time-course and intensity of swelling induced by 1 µg *N. naja* venom (control). In cypropheptadine (1 mg/kg p.o.) treated animals, the early phase of the swelling is suppressed. Pretreatment by indomethacin (5 mg/kg p.o.) has no influence on the early phase, but suppresses the delayed phase. Estriol succinate (200 mg/kg i.v.) equally suppresses the early and delayed phases. Panel b: prototype rat paw edemas induced either by serotonin or carrageenan

A rat paw edema can be provoked by subplantar injection of a large variety of substances, including nonspecific irritants leading to simultaneous release of several mediators, specific activators of one particular mediator system, and the mediators proper. Depending on the provoking substances, the hind limb edema displays characteristic profiles of time-course and shows different sensitivity toward inhibitory influences by drugs. Much work was devoted to correlate the latter two parameters with the conceivable mechanisms involved in the hind limb edema. The bulk of evidence (for original data and survey of literature, see BONTA, 1969; DI ROSA et al., 1971; VINEGAR et al., 1974; FERREIRA et al., 1974; BONTA et al., 1974) shows that there are two main types of rat paw swelling (Fig. 4). The short type displays a rapid onset swelling with a peak within $^1/_2$–1 h and declining thereafter. In this case, the release of amines (mainly serotonin and to some extent histamine) subsequent to mast cell degranulation plays an important role, and antiserotonin agents are effective antagonists. In the delayed type of edema, the peak of swelling is usually observed within 4–6 h, and resolution starts approximately 8–10 h after the subplantar injection. Invasion of neutrophils and release of prostaglandins and bradykinin are involved in such edemas; circumstantial evidence points to the participation of complement as well (DI ROSA et al., 1971). Kaolin and carrageenan are prototype agents for the delayed type of edema. Drugs which interfere with the release of the mentioned mediators can counteract the delayed rat paw swelling.

Three snake venoms have been studied in the rat paw swelling design. Crude *N. naja* venom in a dose of 1 μg produces an edema that reaches its maximum at 1 h. This level is unchanged for up to 4 h and then slowly declines (BONTA and DE VOS, 1965). Regarding its time-course, cobra venom thus induces a mixed type of edema combining the characteristics of the two main types as described above. The dose of 10 μg of cobra venom causes a marked purple-reddish appearance of the rat paw (unpublished observation). Considering the composition of *N. naja* venom, results with the use of individual venom components to induce swelling (Sect. C.I.1) and its pharmacologic inhibition pattern (BONTA, 1969; BONTA and DE VOS, 1965), it is likely that rat paw edema by cobra venom results from a combination of the amine phase and of the so-called prostaglandin phase (Fig. 4). This question will be discussed in detail more in Section C.II.3.

A rat paw edema similar in onset and duration to the above was also observed with *Bothrops jararaca* venom (VARGAFTIG, unpublished). It will be shown later that collagenase activity of this venom is likely to be involved in this effect. The venom of another crotalid, *A. piscivorus*, produces a rat paw swelling of the rapid and transient type, since it reaches a maximum as early as 30 min, thereafter declining and being completely resolved within 4 h (BHARGAVA et al., 1970b). Though *A. piscivorus* venom is a recognized releaser of bradykinin (ROCHA E SILVA et al., 1969), its rat paw edema-inducing effect is rather due to a component causing hemorrhages in lung vessels than to kinin release (BHARGAVA et al., 1970b).

The above examples show that the time-courses of venom-induced rat paw edemas are unpredictable, as are the mechanisms involved.

4. Skin Vascular Lesions

The potential agonists can also be injected by the intradermal route to the shaved skin of animals, particularly rats. Observations with the unaided eye permit the assessment of gross hemorrhages, whereas observation of leakage of plasma components requires the prior administration of an albumin-bound dye or of labeled albumin. In this case, if plasma leaks to the extravascular skin compartment, either the dye that accompanies albumin can be visualized and extracted for quantitative determinations of permeability extent or counts can be performed of the radioactive label. Rats show such skin vascular increased permeability reactions to injections of histamine, serotonin, and their releasing agents, such as compound 48/80 or polymixin B (HALPERN et al., 1959). These effects are totally suppressed by antihistaminic/antiserotonin agents. In contrast with what occurs in rat paw edema tests, where bradykinin is a mild agent, in the case of skin its effects are relatively marked. Moreover, and this represents a major difference between the skin permeability tests and rat paw edema, carrageenan has a very low activity on the skin, and delayed responses equivalent to those occurring in the rat paw are more easily obtained by challenging the skin with specific antigens or antibodies in appropriately prepared animals or after UV irradiation (LOGAN and WILHELM, 1963). Failure to respond with a delayed permeability increase, as shown in the paw, is not due to lack of responsiveness of skin vessels to potential mediators such as prostaglandins, since the latter are capable of inducing direct permeability effects (CRUNKHORN and WILLIS, 1971), and in fact, are more active on the skin than on the rat paw. Moreover, differences between the skin permeability and edema tests are not due to lack of precursors of prostaglandins (GREAVES and MCDONALD-GIBSON, 1972). These differences may be due to different patterns of cell invasion of injured tissues particularly by leukocytes that carry prostaglandin synthetase (HIGGS and YOULTEN, 1972) and kininogenases (GREENBAUM and KIM, 1967). A similar difference will be found for venom effects on skin tests, as seen below.

5. Miscellaneous Vascular Beds

Topical application of *N. naja* venom solution to the everted mesenterium of rats immediately causes gross vasoconstriction of the arteries (Fig. 5). This is probably due to the venom's content of basic polypeptides (DLF-type) known to induce arterial vasoconstriction (LEE et al., 1968). *A. piscivorus* venom produced petechial hemorrhages when applied to the mesoappendix of rats with immunothrombocytopenic purpura (SPACT, 1952). The same venom causes arteriolar vasoconstriction after topical application to the everted transilluminated cheek pouch of hamsters (FULTON, 1956), accompanied by petechiae which mostly occur at venous junctions (SPACT, 1952; ARENDT et al., 1953; FULTON et al., 1956).

C. Elapid Snake and Bee Venoms

I. Morphologic Aspects of Elapid Venom Effects on Lung and Cremaster

1. Lung Effects

The histologic and ultrastructural methods that have been used are described elsewhere (ALMEIDA et al., 1976; GREGORIO, 1977). It is noteworthy that morphologic changes can be induced simply by opening the thoracic cavity of the dog and that some of these changes may overlap with those of the experiments.

When *N. naja* venom is applied to the canine lung surface at a concentration of 4 mg/ml, the lesion appears within 1–2 min after removing the filter paper. It starts as a uniform reddish area changing to cherry-red color, and after 30 min, a regular dark-red depression with sharp boundaries is formed. This "late" lesion is due to

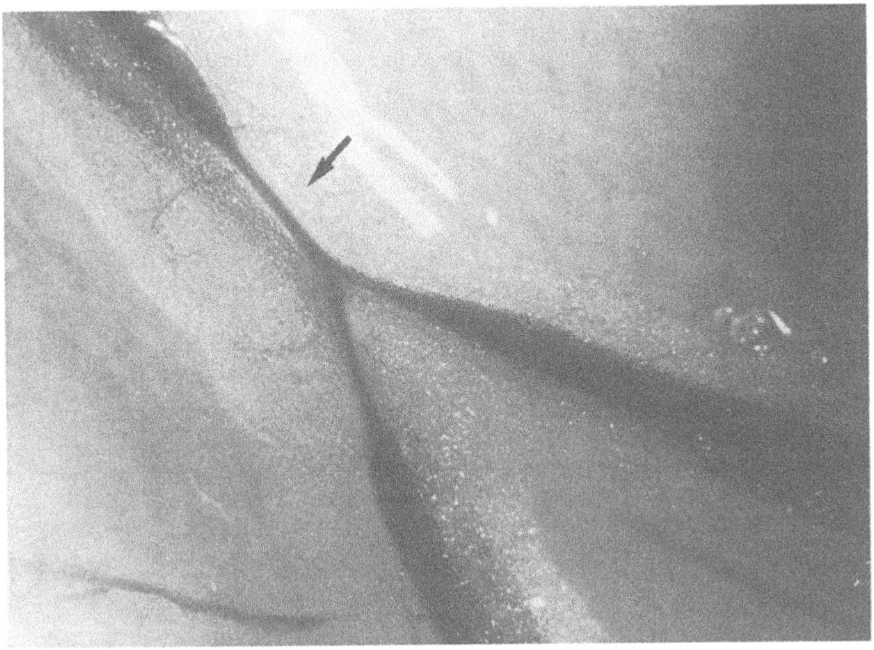

Fig. 5. Rat mesenterial artery after the topical application of *N. naja* venom solution (1 mg/ml). Arrow indicates that at the site where the venom was applied, marked vasoconstriction occurs

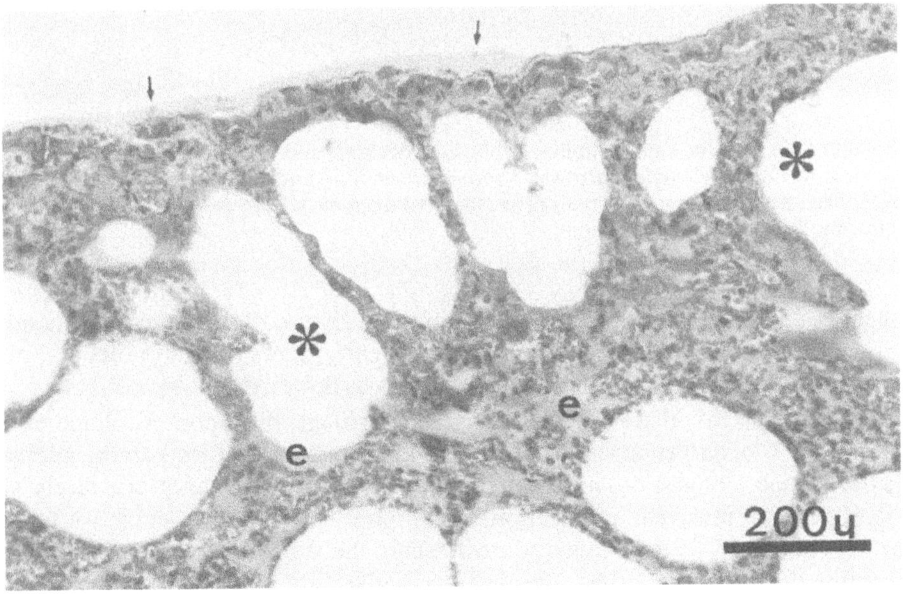

Fig. 6. Photomicrograph of canine lung treated with *N. naja* venom. Pleural Interstitial and alveolar edema (*e*) appear 10 min after application of the venom and some erythrocytes are noticeable in the fluid (arrows). The alveolar spaces (asterisks) are distended. 5μ-thick section stained with hematoxylin and eosin

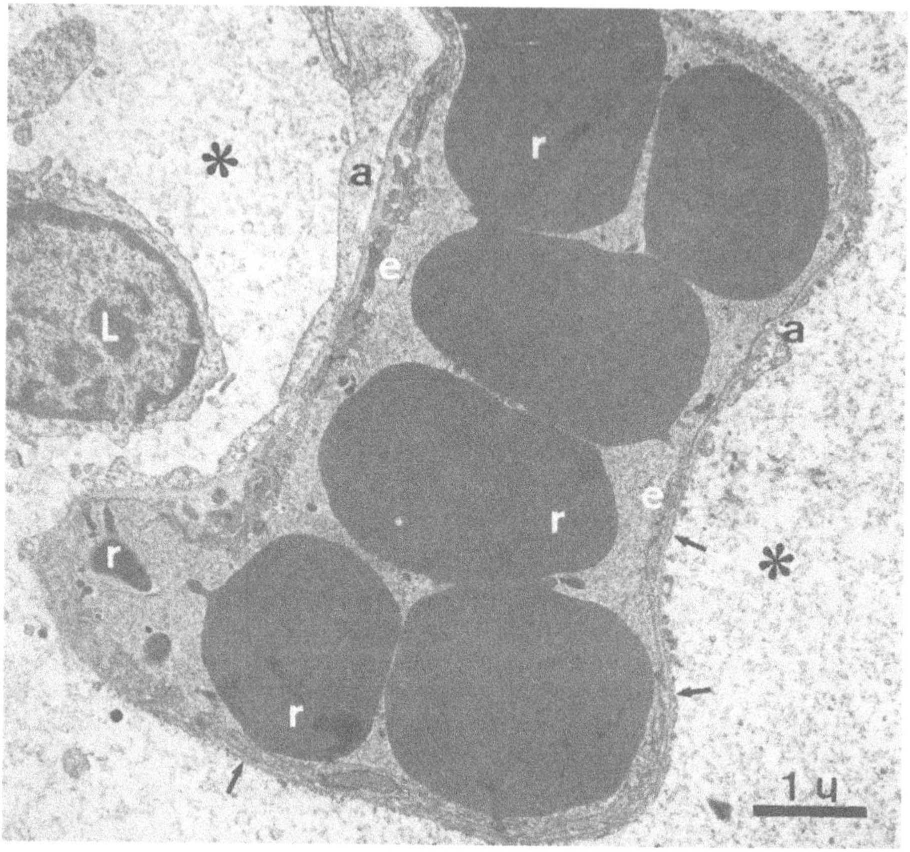

Fig. 7. EM of pulmonary capillary of rat treated with *N. naja* venom. The epithelium is much more damaged than the endothelium (*e*), showing edema (*a*) and severe degeneration leaving the basement membrane denuded (arrows). There is edema fluid and a leukocyte (*L*) in the alveolar space. The red cells (*r*) present small projections which detach from the cell body (erythrocytic fragmentation)

collapse of the alveolar spaces and is a common response of the pulmonary tissue to many injuries. Here we shall deal only with the early, acute lesion. In rats and mice, the whole lung surface is homogeneously altered, as described above.

Macroscopically, these aspects suggest hemorrhage, but upon histologic examination, the *N. naja* venom-induced lesions are characterized by pleural and subpleural edema, congestion, and signs of hemolysis. Hemorrhages are rarely seen (Fig. 6). In rats, intravenous injection of colloidal carbon—a vascular tracer with particles about 25–35 nm—labels almost evenly the subpleural capillaries and only exceptionally the larger vessels. The deeper circulation of lung parenchyma does not retain carbon.

Electron microscopy shows degenerative changes of mesothelial cells and lesions of the subpleural capillaries. The most striking alterations are those of the epithelium. The squamous alveolar cells (type I) present vacuolation, cytoplasmic edema, or even severe fragmentation leaving a denuded basement membrane. The endothelial damage is similar but less intense. Larger vessels, with 20 μm diameter or more, generally only show interstitial edema. Erythrocytic fragmentation is a common finding; the red cells present small projections which detach from the cell body and assume a spheric form. These small spherules have a density similar to erythrocytes and are limited by a typical plasma membrane (Fig. 7). Many capillaries are occluded by platelet and leukocytic thrombi. Besides the damage of the mesothelium, seeping of erythrocytes through the pleura is observed. This phenomenon is also seen in control tissue—possibly a preparation artifact—but in *N. naja* venom-treated pleura, it is definitively more intense (Fig. 8).

2. Cremaster Effects

The venom was injected in one side of the scrotum and the opposite side was used as control. For a typical lesion, 0.05 ml of a 0.25–0.50 mg/ml solution is recommended.

The colloid carbon technique shows the classic picture of acute vascular response to histamine: the carbon particles are predominantly retained by venules. Hemorrhages and blackening of arterioles are not seen. Close to the vessels, extrusion of granules by mast cells may be observed. The carbon tests are positive even with venom solutions as diluted as 0.05 mg/ml.

Under electron microscopy, the typical alterations of an early inflammatory response may be detected: extravasation of carbon particles through open endothelial junctions, adherence and diapedesis of leukocytes, and intense congestion. Erythrocytic fragmentation, as described in the lungs, are present. It seems that there are no degenerative changes of endothelial cells or pericytes.

II. Pharmacologic Aspects

1. Individual Venom Components: Role of Various Polypeptides and Phospholipase A_2

The macroscopic phenomenology of pulmonary vessel lesions produced by elapid or bee venoms are undistinguishable from each other. Therefore, a common denominator was sought to pinpoint the components responsible for this type of vessel damage. These venoms are recognized mast cell-degranulating agents, but the participation of histamine and/or serotonin release was excluded on the basis of the following reasons. Other histamine releasers, including trypsin, polymyxin B, and compound 48/80, when applied to the pleural surface of dog lungs did not produce the alterations characteristically caused by the venoms (BONTA et al., 1969). Also, the mast cell-degranulating (MCD) peptide of bee venom (BREITHAUPT and HABERMANN, 1968) had no effect in this situation (BONTA, unpublished). Lesions could not be produced by topical application of histamine itself; furthermore, antihistamines failed to prevent the injury (see also Sect. C.II.2). Hyaluronidase-mediated destruction of the kit material in the vessel basement membrane was also ruled out; first, because *N. nigricollis* venom does not contain hyaluronidase (ZWISLER, 1966), a fact we have confirmed (Fig. 9)—this venom did produce lesions identic to those due to *N. naja* venom (BONTA et al., 1969)—and second, because hyaluronidase itself proved unable to produce the lesion (BONTA et al., 1969). Phospholipase A_2, though present in all

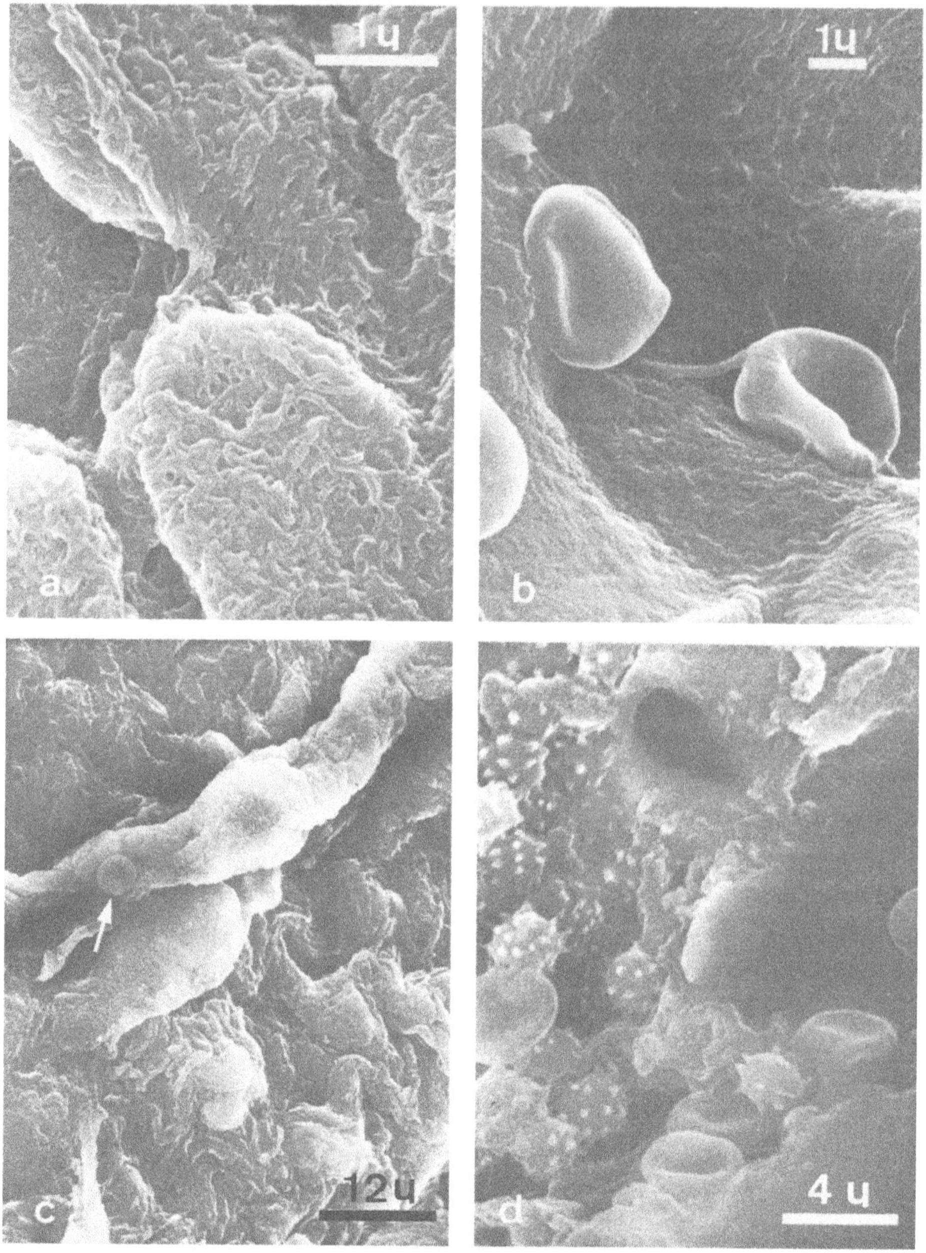

Fig. 8a–d. Scanning EM of normal mesothelial cells (a). Scanning of canine pleura treated with *N. naja* venom. In mildly affected areas, red cells are found on mesothelial cells which can be identified although their microvilli are blurred (b). Same as in b. In the typical lesion a serofibrinous exsudate covers the pleura and the mesothelial cells cannot be seen. The arrow points to an erythrocyte (c). Scanning EM of canine pleura treated with *A. piscivorus* venom. The mesothelium is covered by a hemorrhagic exsudate. The majority of the red cells is crenated (d)

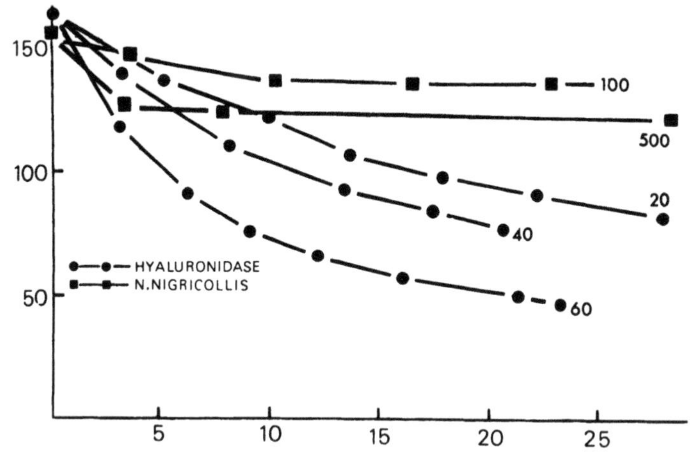

Fig. 9. Inability of crude *N. nigricollis* venom to reduce viscosity of hyaluronic acid. Specific viscosity (vertical axis) of hyaluronic acid from umbelical cord in NaCl-phosphate buffer (pH 6.2) was determined with an Ostwald viscosimeter after incubation for different time intervals (horizontal axis) with crude *N. nigricollis* venom (■–■) or with testicular hyaluronidase (●–●). Amounts of enzyme are indicated as μg per 6 ml of total volume of reaction. Original method of MADINAVEITIA and QUIBELL (Biochem. J. **34**, 625, 1940) as modified by G. J. M. SPROKEL (Thesis, Utrecht, 1952). Observe time and concentration-related degradation of hyaluronic acid by hyaluronidase and absence of clear activity of *N. nigricollis* venom

venoms, was excluded since it lacked the property to induce the lesion (BONTA et al., 1969). The latter observation was confirmed in subsequent studies (BONTA et al., 1972b; BONTA et al., 1972a; BONTA et al., 1976).

When heparin was added to the venoms *in vitro* their vessel-damaging property was entirely abolished, whether assessed by the canine lung surface test (BHARGAVA et al., 1970a; BONTA et al., 1969; BONTA et al., 1970c) or by the mouse intrathoracic test (BONTA et al., 1970b; BONTA et al., 1971). In the latter situation, heparin treatment of *N. naja* venom did not only prevent the pulmonary vessel lesion but in addition prolonged the survival of mice, although the death of the animals was not prevented. This observation obviously shows that the vascular damage and subsequent pulmonary edema is a contributory factor to the lethal effect of intrathoracically administered cobra venom (BONTA et al., 1971). The vessel-damaging property of *N. naja* venom can also be abolished when dextran sulfate (500000 mol wt) is added *in vitro*, although incubation with dextran sulfate (5000000 mol wt) proved in this respect ineffective (BONTA, unpublished observation). Polyanions had earlier been shown to abolish the hemolytic effect of elapid venoms (CONDREA et al., 1964) and to destroy a number of other activities due to DLF or to its "isotoxin" analogues (LEE et al., 1970). The DLF group of strongly cationic polypeptide components of cobra venoms is heat stable at acid pH but is destroyed when heated at alkaline pH (LARSEN and WOLFF, 1968). A similar heat stability profile was also found with respect to the vasculotoxic effect of *N. naja* venom (BONTA et al., 1970c; BONTA et al., 1971). The two coincidental observations, annihilation by polyanions and heat stability profile, led to the proposal that the pulmonary vasculotoxicity of elapid venoms is due to DLF (BONTA et al., 1969; BONTA et al., 1970c). The evidence was delivered by demonstrating that from ten chromatographically separated fractions of *N. naja* venom the DLF fraction was the only one which in the dog lung surface test produced vessel lesion qualitatively identic to that due to the full venom (BONTA et al., 1972). This type of pulmonary vessel lesion—microscopically representing acute inflammatory changes—can also be caused by topical application of DLF from *Hemachatus haemachatus* (BONTA et al., 1976) and γ-toxin of *N. nigricollis* (Fig. 10). Furthermore, the bee venom polypeptide melittin—also a cationic material, pharmacologically somewhat resembling DLF—was also shown to produce this type of vessel lesion in mice (BONTA et al., 1971) and more recently in dogs (BONTA, unpublished). It is easy to appreciate that the identic vessel lesions produced by elapid venoms and bee venom can be explained by their content of DLF and mellitin, respectively.

Considering that DLF amounts on a dry weight basis to 25–50% of the total constitution of cobra venom (LEE, 1972; LEE et al., 1968), it might have been expected that if the vessel-damaging effect of e.g. *N. naja* venom was entirely attributable to DLF, the latter alone should on weight basis be several times more active than the full venom. In fact, the opposite is true. When identic amounts of full *N. naja* venom and purified DLF were tested on the dog lung surface, the effect of DLF—though undistinguishable in appearance—was considerably less than that of whole venom (BONTA et al., 1972). The total vasculotoxic activity of the whole venom was retrieved only when a chromatographic fraction containing the venom's phospholipase A_2 was applied before, simultaneously, or after DLF (BONTA et al., 1972a). However, it should be emphasized that in all these experiments, phospholipase A_2 alone was devoid of any visible effect, an observation made earlier (BHARGAVA et al., 1970; BONTA et al., 1969) and mentioned above. Not only phospholipase A_2 of venom origin but also pancreatic phospholipase A_2 enhanced the effect of DLF (BONTA et al., 1972a). Phospholipase A_2 can sensitize the tissue to such an extent that the activity of subsequently administered DLF occasionally surpasses the effect of the full venom (BONTA et al., 1976), even though DLF alone usually does not produce more than half the vasculotoxicity of the whole venom.

The synergism of phospholipase A_2 with DLF is by itself not a new phenomenon. Thus, it was known that phospholipase A_2 produces lytic compounds (e.g., lysolecithin) by plasma phospholipid hydrolysis but by itself is unable to attack the erythrocytes directly. DLF, which is moderately lytic per se, enables the venom phospholipase A_2 to hydrolyze phospholipids in the erythrocyte membrane, resulting in marked hydrolysis (CONDREA et al., 1964a). Subsequently, the synergism was the subject of many studies and speculations (CONDREA et al., 1965; CONDREA and DE VRIES, 1965; CONDREA et al., 1970; CONDREA et al., 1972a; KLIBANSKY et al., 1968; KAISER et al., 1972; SCHROETER et al., 1973; SLOTTA et al., 1967).

Based on such studies, it is currently believed that the positive charge of the cationic peptide DLF is responsible for attachment to the negatively charged cell membrane, whereas the orientation of the lipophilic groups—characteristic for DLF peptides (FRYKLUND and EAKER, 1973)—is involved in the facilitation of the approach of the phospholipase A_2 to the phospholipid substrates situated inside the membrane. This concept is mainly based on observations concerning cell lysis.

It is, however, at least questionable, if not unlikely, whether the vascular lesion described by us is *de facto* correlated with events of cell lysis. A number of vessel

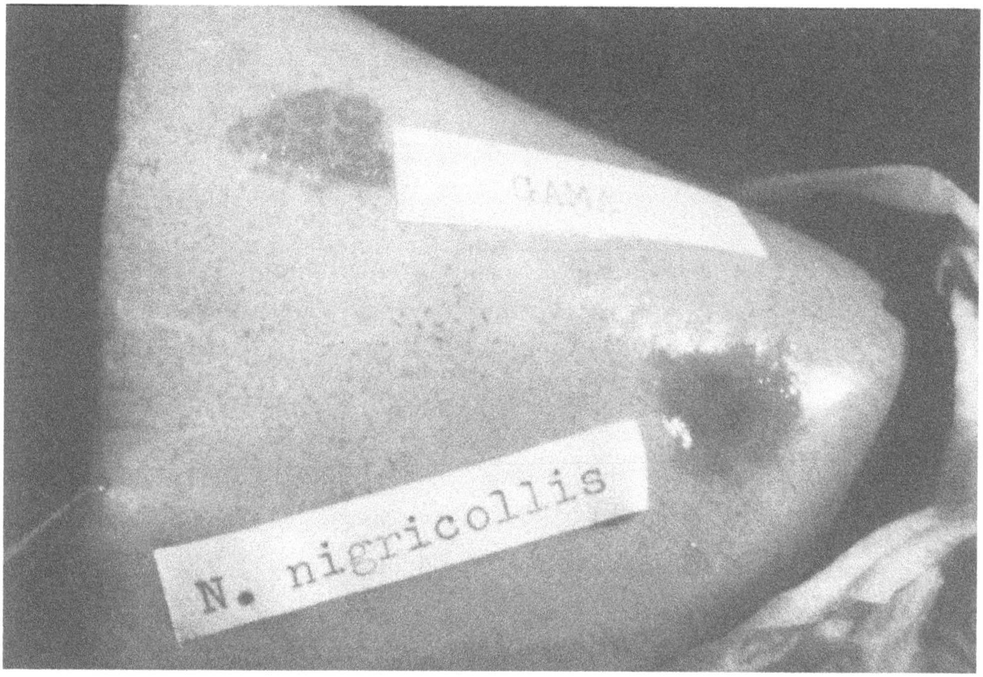

Fig. 10. Canine pulmonary lung lesion induced by γ-toxin and *N. nigricollis* venom. Both materials were applied in the concentration of 1 mg/ml. Note that γ-toxin induces a lesion which is similar in appearance but of weaker intensity than the lesion produced by the full venom

lesion-producing substances (DLF of *N. naja* and of Ringhals venoms, bee venom, melittin) are hemolytic. Histology also revealed the presence of hemolysis in lung tissue exposed to *N. naja* venom. Nevertheless, there are arguments against the possibility that the vessel-damaging and hemolytic properties of the substances are correlated. First, a hemolytic fraction of *N. naja* venom was not found to produce pulmonary vessel lesion (BHARGAVA et al., 1970). Second, bee venom (and for that matter melittin) is considerably more hemolytic but slightly less potent in producing pulmonary vessel lesion than is *N. naja* venom. Third, γ-toxin of *N. nigricollis* (IZARD et al., 1969a) can produce the vessel lesion (Fig. 10), although its hemolytic effect is debatable (IZARD et al., 1969b) and displays detergent properties on rabbit platelets (VARGAFTIG, unpublished). Fourth, lysolecithin is strongly hemolytic, but is not vasculotoxic when applied on the lung surface (BONTA et al., 1969). It appears, thus, that vasculotoxicity and hemolytic activity, though each being a property of DLF, do not necessarily parallel each other.

In an attempt to understand the potentiation of DLF by phospholipase A_2 in the pulmonary vessel lesion phenomenon, we were guided by the following train of thoughts. The lipid-splitting enzyme may act in two different, though simultaneously occurring ways. Besides producing lysolecithin, phospholipase A_2 also liberates unsaturated fatty acids, which are precursors in the biosynthesis of prostaglandins. Activation of cellular phospholipase A_2 is *de facto* considered as the primary trigger in the formation of prostaglandins (KUNZE and VOGT, 1971). Characteristic for

Table 1. Prostaglandin biosynthesis inhibitors on pulmonary vessel lesion (venom or venom components 4 mg/ml; intensity score mean ± SEM)

PG biosynthesis inhibitor 10 mg/ml[a]	*N. naja* full venom	DLF	Phospholipase A + DLF
—	17.5 ± 1.2	8.25 ± 0.75	17.5 ± 1.5
Indomethacin	17.5 ± 1.5	12 ± 1.5	16.5 ± 1.8
TYA	19 ± 1.5	n.t.	n.t.

[a] Pretreatment 10 min. Results from observations in three dogs.

Table 2. Prostaglandin antagonists on pulmonary vessel damage induced by venoms

Venom	Antagonist	Onset min	Intensity score
N. naja 4 mg/ml	—	0.75 ± 0.25	19.5 ± 1
	Polyphloretin phosphate	1.9 ± 0.30[a]	12.7 ± 0.5[a]
	SC-1920	0.7 ± 0.25	19 ± 1.5
A. piscivorus 2 mg/ml	—	1.0 ± 0.25	17.5 ± 1.5
	Polyphloretin phosphate	2.0 ± 0.75[b]	14 ± 0.6[b]

[a] $p<0.01$
[b] $p<0.05$

lysolecithin is the altering of membrane permeability. Prostaglandins are known to enhance vascular permeability (KALEY and WEINER, 1971). We tested the possible involvement of the above mechanisms by trying to mimic the potentiation of DLF by phospholipase A_2 by replacing the enzyme with lysolecithin on the one hand and prostaglandins on the other. Both agents, though each being devoid of a visible effect by its own virtue, did enhance the activity of DLF (BONTA et al., 1976). In each case, however, the extent of potentiation was clearly less than when the tissue was exposed to phospholipase A_2. The vasculotoxic effect of DLF is not only potentiated by PGE_1 but also by PGE_2, while a third prostaglandin, $PGF_{2\alpha}$ proved inactive (BONTA et al., 1976). It is easily appreciable that if prostaglandin formation is involved in the potentiating effect of phospholipase A_2, one would expect that the vasculotoxic effect of full *N. naja* venom—containing phospholipase A *and* DLF—should be partially counteracted either by an inhibitor of prostaglandin biosynthesis or by some antagonist of the effect of prostaglandins. Indomethacin and tetraynoic acid (TYA), which are established prostaglandin synthesis inhibitors, failed to counteract the vasculotoxic effect of *N. naja* venom on dog lung surface (BONTA and VARGAFTIG, 1976). Indomethacin also proved ineffective when, instead of the full venom, a combination of phospholipase A_2 and DLF were used to produce the vessel lesion (Table 1). Two antagonists of prostaglandins were also studied in this situation. Compound SC-19220 (SANNER, 1969) proved inactive against the vessel lesion due to *N. naja* venom. Polyphloretin phosphate (PPP) on the other hand counteracted the effect of cobra venom on the pulmonary surface (Table 2) as well as that of other agents (Fig. 11). This profile of PPP is understandable since it is a

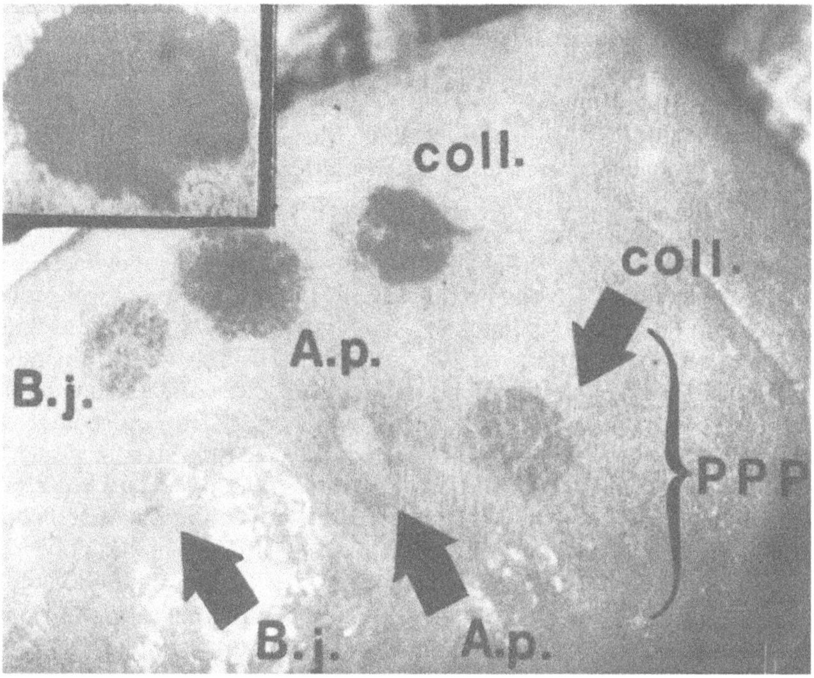

Fig. 11. Canine pulmonary lesions produced by venoms of *B. jararaca*, *A. piscivorus*, and collagenase, without and after local pretreatment of the tissue with polyphloretin phosphate (PPP, 10 mg/ml). Note that collagenase suppresses all three lesions. Insert shows the lesion by collagenase at higher magnification

nonspecific inhibitor of vascular permeability rather than a specific antagonist of prostaglandins (EAKINS et al., 1971; FRIES, 1960). The above results thus show that while the vasculotoxic effect of DLF is to some extent potentiated by E-type prostaglandins, the endogenous release of these mediators is not involved in the phospholipase A_2-induced sensitization of the pulmonary vessels towards DLF. Furthermore, it appears that endogenous prostaglandins do not participate in the mechanism by which cobra venom produces vessel lesion in lung tissue (see C.II.2.b).

It is appropriate to briefly mention that in the pulmonary vessel-damaging effect of cobra venoms and/or DLF not only the participation of endogenous histamine release (see introductory paragraph of this section) and prostaglandin release can be ruled out, but the primary involvement of still another mediator, viz. bradykinin is unlikely as well. First, because elapid venoms do not contain proteases and arginine esterases which split kinins from kininogen. Second, because kallikrein and trypsin—which are releasers of bradykinin—were unable to produce the vessel lesion in lung tissue (BONTA et al., 1969). Third, because incubation of the cobra venom with Trasylol—an inhibitor of plasmatic and glandular kininogenases—was unable to inhibit the vessel-damaging effect (BONTA et al., 1970a). Nevertheless, it is possible that plasma leakage, due to the vessel damage caused primarily by the venom, leads to kinin release which might reinforce the vascular injury, although bradykinin by itself had no effect on the lung index when used at 0.9 mg/kg intrathoracically

(J. LEFORT, B. B. VARGAFTIG, unpublished). Finally, application of the kininase inhibitor $BPP_{9\alpha}$ to the lung surface did not increase the subsequent effect of *N. naja* venom. Potentiation of this effect would be expected if bradykinin were involved, since it would be spared from catabolism by kininase inhibition.

There is no doubt that the strongly cationic character of DLF is of importance in attachment to biomembranes. This is also valid for the lytic polypeptide melittin (SESSA et al., 1969). Positively charged substances may mimic some effects of DLF. Thus, protamine imitates the effect of DLF on some enzymes of the erythrocyte membrane (CONDREA et al., 1972b). A few synthetic cationic copolymers are more potent lytic agents than DLF and promoted phospholipid splitting by phospholipase A_2 (KLIBANSKY et al., 1968). Pulmonary vessel lesions similar to those produced by DLF are induced by melittin (BONTA et al., 1971). Histones of calf thymus origin were, however, scarcely able to imitate the vascular effect of DLF on canine lung. Since a high content of lysine is characteristic for the amino acid composition of DLF (LEE, 1972) one might have expected that a lysine-rich histone would display DLF-like effects. However, it failed to do this, unless the tissue had been sensitized with phospholipase A, even though, under the latter condition, the effect of the lysine-rich histone was not impressive (BONTA et al., 1976). Finally, polylysine was unable to imitate the effect of DLF on lung vessels (I. L. BONTA, unpublished).

We may conclude that in vessel injury due to topical application of elapid venoms, participation of endogenous inflammatory mediators is unlikely and is apparently replaced by DLF itself. This is reflected in the pharmacologic antagonistic profile, as will be discussed in Section C.II.2. It is appropriate to emphasize that under alternative conditions, the vessel lesion-inducing effect of elapid venoms is definitely exerted through mediator release, the rat paw edema caused by *N. naja* venom being a good example for the later case (Sect. B.II.3).

2. Pharmacologic Influences on Venom-Induced Vessel Injury

Administration of pharmacologic agents in model conditions may serve several purposes. An obvious one is to obtain indications regarding the therapeutic use of a drug. In cases, however, when uncertainty exists as to which human condition is the model correlated—we might call this a "cryptic" model—drugs with a recognized mode of action may help to a better understanding of the model proper. The arguments will be discussed now to show that the use of several classes of drugs led us to propose that elapid venoms can induce two kinds of vascular inflammatory models: the pulmonary vessel model in which the venom or DLF replaces the mediators and the rat paw edema situation in which the venom acts through release of mediators.

The results on lung vessels as discussed below were mostly obtained with the canine lung surface test, in which case the drugs were applied topically before exposing the tissue to elapid venom or DLF. Some conclusions are also derived from the rodent intrathoracic test, in which the drugs were topically injected before or together with the venom. In the rat paw edema test, the venom was administered into the subplantar tissue of the hind leg, but the putative antagonists were given orally or intravenously. Some results have been published earlier (BONTA and VARGAFTIG, 1976) but will be given now in more detail, accompanied by as yet unpublished data.

Table 3. Histamine and antihistamines on pulmonary vessel lesion, by *N. naja* venom

Compound 10 mg/ml	Onset min	Intensity score
—	0.8 ± 0.2	18 ± 1.2
Mepyramine (H_1 block)	1.1 ± 0.3	17.5 ± 1.5
Burimamide (H_2 block)	0.9 ± 0.4	18.5 ± 1
Mepyr. + Burim.	0.9 ± 0.2	17.5 ± 0.8

a) Antihistamines

As described in Section C.II.1, MCD agents (polymyxin B, compound 48/80) and histamine itself were unable to imitate the elapid venom-induced vessel injury in the canine lung surface model. Pretreatment of rats with compound 48/80 did not attenuate the effect of the venom when administered intrathoracically. Such results render the participation of endogenous histamine unlikely. Support for this assumption was obtained by showing that topical application of the antihistamines mepyramine (blocker of H_1-type histamine receptor) and burimamide (blocker of H_2-type receptor), either alone or jointly with each other, failed to counteract the venom effect on lung tissue (Table 3). In fact, occasionally, application of histamine itself on the lung surface before *N. naja* venom or DLF considerably delayed the appearance of the injury. The mechanism by which histamine may have acted is not understood.

In contrast, H_1 antihistamines clearly inhibit the early (1 h) part of the cobra venom-induced rat paw edema, although they fail to counteract the delayed (4 h) phase (BONTA and DE VOS, 1965). This is interpreted in terms that the rat paw swelling by cobra venom starts with release of amines from the mast cells, whereas this process is apparently not involved in the delayed phase of this inflammation. H_1-type antihistamines also inhibit the rat paw edema induced by melittin; in the latter case, however, inhibition lasted up to 4 h (FORMANEK and KREIL, 1975), suggesting the involvement of different mechanisms in the rat paw swelling provoked by cobra venom and melittin, respectively.

b) Nonsteroid (Acidic) Anti-Inflammatory Drugs (NSAID)

It was observed earlier that in the canine lung surface test aminopyrine and phenylbutazone were unable to counteract the effect of *N. naja* venom (BONTA, 1969). Similar results were more recently obtained with indomethacin, irrespective of whether this drug was topically applied to the pleural surface or administered intravenously (5 mg/kg) before challenging the pulmonary vessels with the venom (see also Table 1). NSAID inhibit the biosynthesis of prostaglandins (VANE, 1971) and there is a bulk of evidence to show that inhibition of the synthesis of prostaglandins is a major mechanism in the acute anti-inflammatory action of NSAID in general, and of indomethacin in particular (FERREIRA and VANE, 1971). Indomethacin does not inhibit lipoxigenase, the enzyme responsible for the biotransformation of arachidonic acid into lipid peroxides which are not prostaglandin precursors (FLOWER, 1974). TYA inhibits cycloxigenase and lipoxigenase (FLOWER, 1974) and proved ineffective in counteracting the pulmonary vessel lesion. These results can be considered strong arguments against the possibility that the tissue release of lipid (endo)-

peroxides is involved in the mechanism by which elapid venoms cause vessel injury when applied to the lung surface.

In the venom-induced rat paw swelling situation, however, phenylbutazone (BONTA and VE VOS, 1965) and indomethacin (BONTA, 1969) inhibit the delayed phase, though the early phase was unaffected. While there is no direct evidence that prostaglandin release indeed occurs and significantly contributes to the delayed phase of edema when *N. naja* venom is injected into the hind paw, this is the most probable explanation of the effect of NSAIDs.

c) Corticosteroids

In the canine lung surface test, cortisol hemisuccinate and dexamethasone phosphate failed entirely to diminish the effect of *N. naja* venom (DE VOS and BONTA, unpublished).

The delayed phase of the rat paw edema was, however, suppressed by dexamethasone, which did not inhibit the early phase (BONTA, 1969; CHRISPIJN and BONTA, unpublished). A discussion on the variety of mechanisms underlying the anti-inflammatory effect of corticosteroids would go beyond the scope of this article. Inhibition by dexamethasone of venom-induced rat paw swelling is in good agreement with those results which show that in the hind paw edema the antagonistic profile of corticosteroids and NSAID parallel each other (VINEGAR et al., 1974).

d) Protease Inhibitors

When applied together with the venom, Trasylol failed to inhibit the pulmonary vessel lesion (BONTA et al., 1970a), in which case bradykinin is unlikely to be primarily involved.

In the rat paw edema, some protection in the early phase was observed with Trasylol, whereas soybean trypsin inhibitor inhibited both the early and delayed phases (H. CHRISPIJN and I. L. BONTA, unpublished). Soybean trypsin inhibitor is a nonspecific inhibitor of kininogenase and accordingly may counteract the release of plasma kinins. Bradykinin is supposed to participate in a variety of rat paw edemas, including rapid and delayed ones (FERREIRA et al., 1974; BONTA and DE VOS, 1967; for other references, see ROCHA E SILVA and GARCIA-LEME, 1972).

e) Estrogens

Estrogens have some reputation as beneficially influencing hemorrhagic conditions, and it is believed that these compounds do not exert their effect through the blood clotting system, but rather by protecting the wall of the microvessels (LUDWIG, 1966; RONA, 1963; for other references, see VINCENT et al., 1971). This clinical claim and the early macroscopic impression that the pulmonary lesions induced by elapid venoms represent hemorrhages prompted the study of estrogens in the canine lung surface test (BONTA et al., 1965). In two subsequent papers, the effect of estrogens on the lesions by elapid venoms has been erroneously interpreted as an antihemorrhagic action (BONTA et al., 1969; VINCENT et al., 1970). Although histology demonstrated (see Sect. C.I.1) that elapid venoms do not induce hemorrhages but acute inflammatory changes in the vessels, the effect of estrogens is of considerable interest. First, because very few compounds provided some protection of the vessels towards the

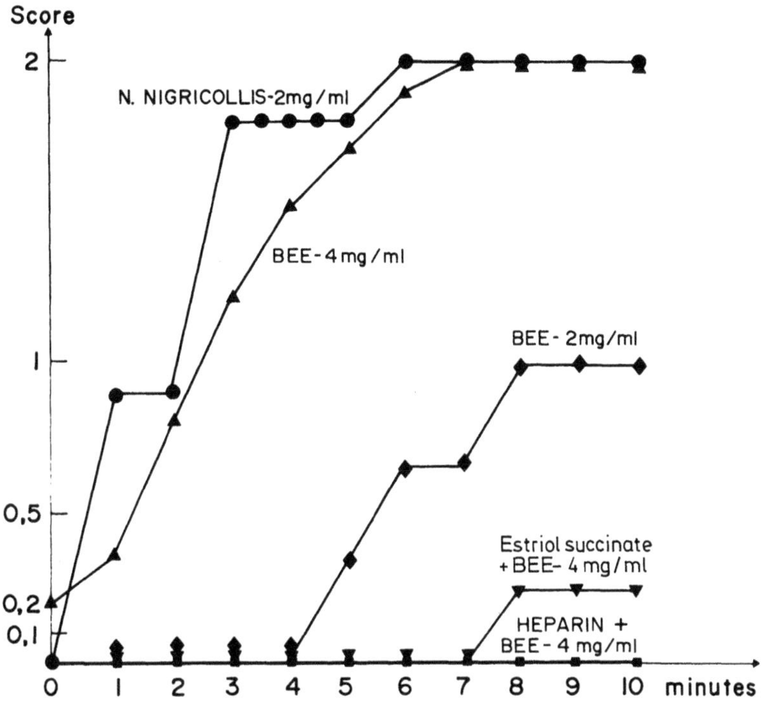

Fig. 12. Intensity of pulmonary lesions as plotted against the time after the onset. *N. nigricollis* venom at 2 mg/ml is approximately equieffective with bee venom at 4 mg/ml concentration. Local pretreatment of the tissue with estriol succinate markedly suppressed the effect of bee venom. Incubation of bee venom with heparin completely abolished the effect of the venom

venom. Second, because more recently estrogens have also in other situations been shown to exert acute anti-inflammatory effect (ISHIOKA et al., 1969; BONTA and DE VOS, 1965; HEMPEL et al., 1970; PERSELLIN and PERRY, 1972; WEISSMANN and RITA, 1972; LERNER et al., 1975). Therefore, the influence of estrogens on the venom-induced vessel injury will be discussed in some detail. Originally, it was shown that estriol succinate delayed the onset and reduced the intensity of the vessel injury caused by *N. naja* venom but was without effect on the hemorrhagic lesion produced by crotalid venom (BONTA et al., 1965; BONTA et al., 1969). The effect of estriol succinate on lesions by elapid venoms was confirmed using *N. nigricollis* and bee venoms (Fig. 12). Subsequently, it was shown that stilbestrol—a nonsteroid estrogen—displayed a similar profile (VINCENT et al., 1970). More recently, such results were also obtained with the steroid OK-63, which is a diethylamino ethylester of estriol (Fig. 13). OK-63 is devoid of the usual effects of estrogen hormones on female sex organs. The inhibitory effect of OK-63 on the vessel lesions (Table 4) confirms the earlier impression (BONTA et al., 1965; VINCENT et al., 1970) that the vessel-protecting and endocrine property of estrogens are two unrelated activities. Estriol succinate also prevents the increased vascular permeability provoked by bradykinin (ISHIOKA et al., 1969). In the latter case, the effect of estriol succinate is not dose dependent. Lack of dose dependency is also valid for the vessel-protecting activity of estriol

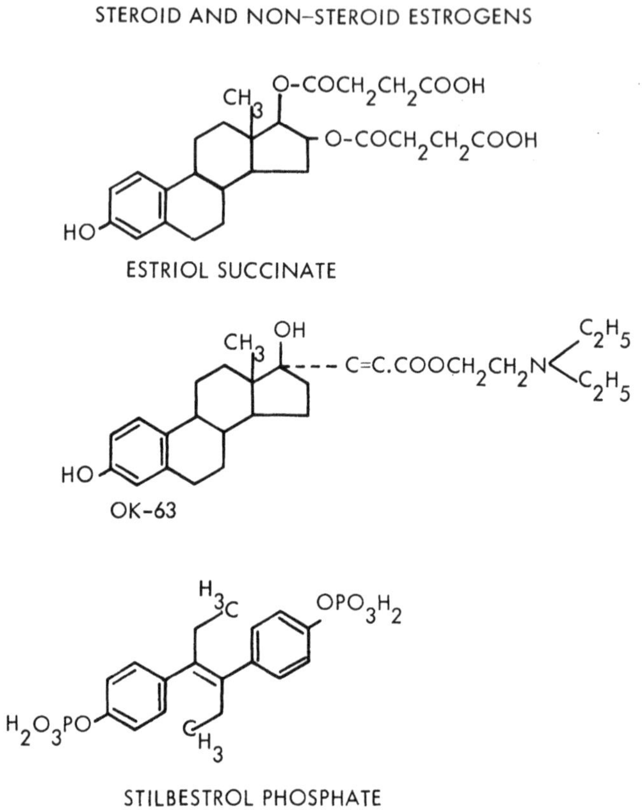

Fig. 13. Chemical structure of two steroid and one nonsteroid estrogen. Estriol succinate and OK-63 (17α-carboxy-ethinyl-(2′-diethyl-aminoethylester)-Δ 1,3,5 (10)-estratriene-3,17β-diol) have very feeble estrogen effect in the Allen-Doisy vaginal cornification test in mice. In the latter test, stilbestrol is highly estrogenic

Table 4. Estrogens on pulmonary vessel damage induced by cobra venom

Estrogen 10 mg/ml	Onset min	Intensity score
—	0.6 ± 0.15	19.2 ± 0.8
Estriol succinate	1.5 ± 0.25[a]	15.1 ± 1.2[b]
OK63	1.6 ± 0.3[a]	16 ± 1.3[b]
Stilbestrol phosphate	3.1 ± 0.55[a]	11 ± 0.75[a]

[a] $p < 0.001$.
[b] $p < 0.01$.

succinate toward the elapid venom-induced lesion (Fig. 4). However, this is not a general property of estrogens as vessel-protecting agents, since a dose-dependent effect was observed with OK-63 (Fig. 14). The vessel-protecting effect of estrogens can also be demonstrated in the rodent intrathoracic test, in which case its topical administration can prolong the survival and diminish the pulmonary edema induced by *N. naja* venom in mice (Figs. 15a and 15b).

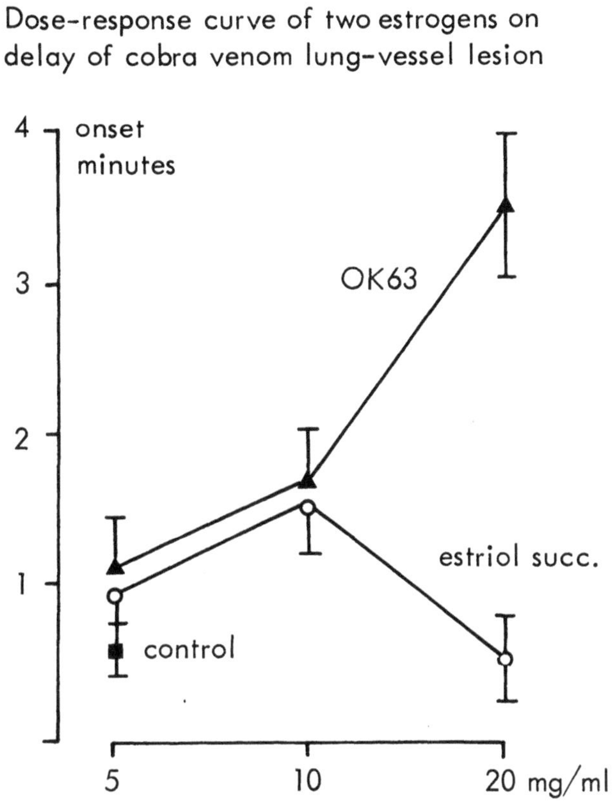

Fig. 14. Delay of onset of *N. naja* venom induced pulmonary vessel lesion after topical pretreatment of the tissue with estrogens. Horizontal scale shows the concentrations of the estrogens. Control point shows the onset of lesion without pretreatment by estrogen. Note that the delaying effect of estriol succinate is not dose related but a clearly dose-dependent delay was observed after OK-63

Estriol succinate also inhibits both the early and delayed phases of the rat paw edema induced by cobra venom (BONTA and DE VOS, 1965), differing in this respect from the antihistamines and NSAID which selectively inhibit one of these phases only. This effect of the estrogens indicates that they do not interfere with either the action or the release of one particular mediator but exert direct protecting effect on the microvessels, the latter being the final target organs of the inflammatory rat paw edema. This interpretation is in agreement with results showing the antipermeability effect of estrogens on skin vessels (ISHIOKA et al., 1969). Their membrane-stabilizing effect has also been shown on liposomes (WEISSMANN and RITA, 1972), which are artificial membrane models akin to lysosomes. In line with this, estrogens also counteract the release of lysosomal enzymes (HEMPEL et al., 1970; PERSELLIN and PERRY, 1972). Some inhibition of prostaglandin biosynthesis has been described with nonsteroid estrogens recently (LERNER et al., 1975). Anti-inflammatory activity of estrogens was also shown in models of chronic inflammation (GLENN, 1966; MUELLER and KAPPAS, 1964; TOIVANEN et al., 1967). Finally, estrogens have been reported to

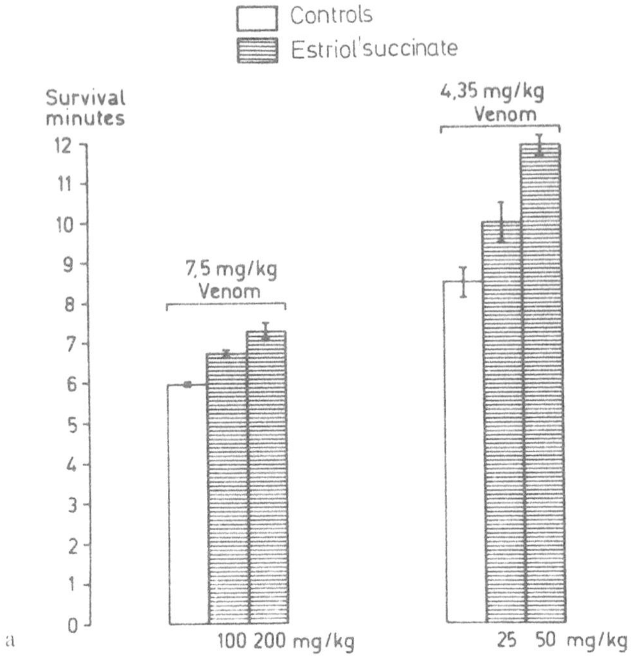

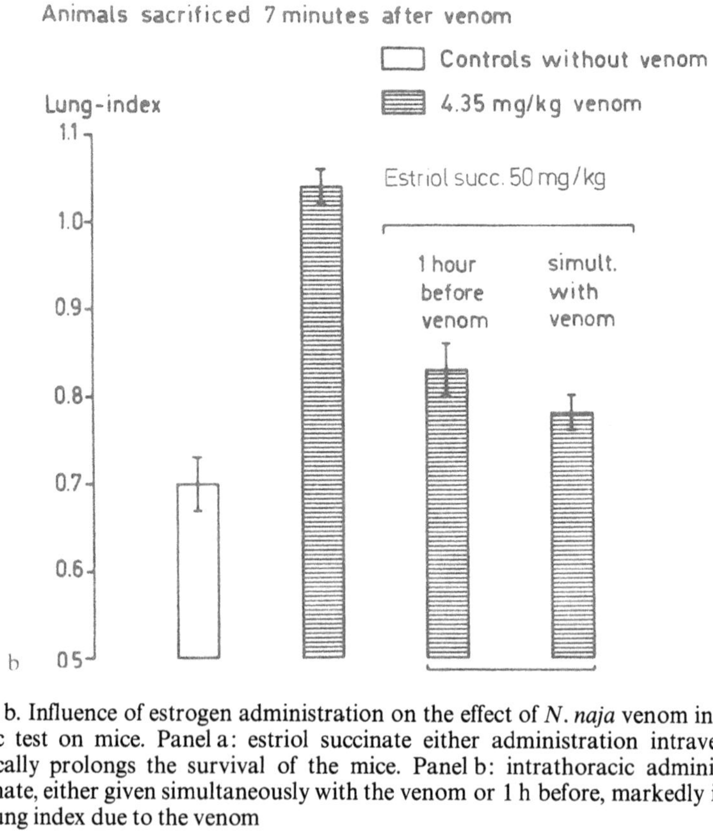

Fig. 15a and b. Influence of estrogen administration on the effect of *N. naja* venom in the rodent intrathoracic test on mice. Panel a: estriol succinate either administration intravenously, or intrathoracically prolongs the survival of the mice. Panel b: intrathoracic administration of estriol succinate, either given simultaneously with the venom or 1 h before, markedly inhibits the increase of lung index due to the venom benefit some cases of human inflammatory rheumatoid arthritis (SPANGLER et al., 1969).

Several observations thus indicate that estrogens delay the capacity of tissues to react to inflammatory stimuli. But the closer mechanism of this "tissue-protecting" effect is poorly understood as yet. Nevertheless, it is of some interest that the pulmonary vessel lesion, provoked by elapid and bee venoms, provides a model in which the acute component of the tissue-protecting anti-inflammatory effect of estrogens can be demonstrated.

f) Flavonoids

The flavonoids represent a class of compounds which are chemically related yellow pigments and share the property of vitamin P to decrease the permeability of capillaries (GOODMAN and GILMAN, 1975). Moreover, chalkones (which are flavonoids) have been shown to display estrogen activity (SHARMA et al., 1972). Three flavonoids, viz. venoruton, morin, and trihydroxychalcon, when applied topically to the lung surface, slightly delayed the onset and reduced the intensity of the vascular injury provoked by *N. naja* venom (BONTA, unpublished observation). Quercetin, another flavonoid, however, failed to protect the vessels.

The inhibitory effect of vitamin P (rutin) in the rat paw edema test was suggested earlier to be due to a reduction of microvessel permeability (VOGEL and MAREK, 1961). In accordance, vitamin P inhibits both the early and delayed phases of the rat paw edema induced by *N. naja* venom (BONTA, 1969).

g) Polyphloretin Phosphate

Although polyphloretin phosphate has been described as antagonizing some effects of prostaglandins, it is also an inhibitor of hyaluronidase and appears to be a nonspecific inhibitor of vascular permeability (FRIES, 1960; EAKINS et al., 1971). Apparently due to the latter property, polyphloretin phosphate provided protection toward the vessel lesion induced by *N. naja* venom (see Sect. D.II). The compound SC-19220, which is also a prostaglandin antagonist (SANNER, 1969), failed to counteract the effect of *N. naja* venom on pulmonary vessels. This suggests that specific antagonism toward prostaglandins is not involved with the effect of polyphloretin phosphate.

h) Heparin

As discussed in Section C.II.1, incubation of *N. naja* venom with the polyanion heparin results in abolition of the vessel-damaging property of the venom, because heparin forms an inactive complex with the cationic peptide DLF which is responsible for the vascular injury by the venom. In the rodent intrathoracic test, it was shown, however, that the vessel-damaging effect of *N. naja* venom was also counteracted when heparin was administered *in vivo* into the pleural cavity of mice (BONTA et al., 1970b). On the basis of arguments found in the original paper, it is reasonable to assume that heparin protects the integrity of microvessels. The effect of heparin on connective tissue (GASTPAR, 1965) and on vascular permeability (NAZAROV and PETRISCHEV, 1968) has been demonstrated. Incorporation of heparin into the intercellular ground substance, and activation of fibrinolysis have been suggested as the mechanism of action. To which extent such mechanisms contribute to the effect of heparin leading to an increased resistance of the vessels toward the damaging influence of elapid venom is poorly understood.

i) Cyclic Adenosine Monophosphate (cAMP)

The combined administration of dibutyryl cAMP and of the phosphodiesterase inhibitor theophylline resulted in some protection toward the vessel injury due to *N. naja* venom in the canine lung surface test (VINCENT et al., 1970). In the latter publication, this observation was brought in connection with the vessel-protecting effect of estrogens, which acutely elevate the level of cAMP, at least in the uterine tissue (SZEGO and DAVIS, 1967). This has not been shown, to our knowledge, in the vascular tissue. An elevated level of cAMP has been recently shown to correlate with protection toward inflammatory stimuli (ICHIKAWA et al., 1972; IGNARRO and GEORGE, 1974). The current view is that cAMP controls the release of lysosomal enzymes, thereby counteracting inflammation (IGNARRO and GEORGE, 1974). The mechanism by which cAMP partially inhibits the vessel lesion provoked by elapid venom is unknown.

3. Rat Paw Edema and Permeability Increase Due to Elapid and Bee Venoms

Although results obtained with the rat paw edema test have been mentioned in the above section, it is pertinent at this stage to review other aspects of the problem.

a) Rat Paw Edema

The venom components responsible for the various phases of the edema (Sect. B.II.3 and B.II.4) have not been identified, but it has been shown that cardiotoxin (DLF) induces rat paw edema (LEE et al., 1968) with a similar time-course as the crude *N. naja* venom (H. CHRISPIJN and I. L. BONTA, unpublished).

Three components of bee venom are known to induce mast cell degranulation and thus to release edema-inducing serotonin and histamine. These are phospholipase A_2, melittin, and a MCD peptide (HÖGBERG and UVNÄS, 1958; UVNÄS et al., 1962; HABERMANN and BREITHAUPT, 1968; BREITHAUPT and HABERMANN, 1968). Moreover, since addition of heparin to bee venom reduces its cytolytic and toxic activities (HIGGINBOTHAM and KARNELLA, 1971) and its ability to induce lung hemorrhages (Sect. C.II.1), the contribution of hemolytic basic peptides to the whole range of pharmacologic effects of bee venom—which is devoid of neuromuscular blocking neurotoxins—appears to be very large.

The delayed phase of rat paw edema due to *N. naja* venom is inhibited by NSAID, but not by antihistaminic/antiserotonin agents (BONTA and DE VOS, 1965). This suggests that prostaglandins may be involved in this delayed edema, since NSAID inhibit their generation (VANE, 1971). Other explanations could be evoked, but it is tempting to think that prostaglandins are formed after release of their precursor, namely arachidonic acid from phospholipids by the venom phospholipase A_2 (ROTHSCHILD, 1965). This would require that pure phospholipase A_2 should also induce an aspirin-sensitive rat paw edema. In fact, the edema-inducing effect of *N. naja* phospholipase A_2 was exceedingly feeble (J. NOORDHOEK, unpublished). The situation is thus more complex, since phospholipase A_2 from different animal venoms may vary in their ability to split membrane phospholipids from isolated cells, as in the case of platelets (KIRSCHMAN et al., 1964).

Moreover, purified bee venom phospholipase A_2 only induces an increase in vascular permeability, attributable to mast cell degranulation, when tested *in vivo*, presumably because lysolecithin and fatty acids are released from plasma phospholipids, whereas isolated mast cells resist this activity, unless exogenous phospholipid substrates for the added phospholipase A_2 are included in the experimental setup (ROTHSCHILD, 1965). As discussed above (Sect. B.II.4), the situation may be quite different when venoms are injected into the skin of the back of a rat. In this case, no delayed effect can be visualized, suggesting that mast cell products are fully responsible for the effects. In contrast, the delayed phase of rat paw edema, which is resistant to antiserotonin/antihistamine treatment and is inhibited by NSAID, is a more complex situation where prostaglandins may play a role. This has been shown by using a partially purified phospholipase A_2 preparation (Fraction III, BOQUET et al., 1967) which had no major effect on the lung surface but which induced rat paw edema. Intraplantar injection of 2.5 μg of this fraction induced a $25 \pm 3\%$ increase in paw thickness within 30 min and $35.5 \pm 11\%$ within 4 h, i.e., both the immediate and the delayed edema, respectively. The standard antiserotonin and antihistaminic agent cyproheptadine inhibited 80% of the early edema, whereas the delayed one was blocked by only 44%. In contrast, the standard NSAID indomethacin inhibited 20% of the early edema, and 45% of the delayed one. Since Fraction III is contaminated, although to a slight extent only, by amine-releasing basic polypeptides, a combination of both cyproheptadine and indomethacin would certainly inhibit both edema phases to a larger extent than either alone.

b) *Skin Vascular Permeability*

The effects of *N. naja*, *N. nigricollis*, and bee venoms on skin vascular permeability after intradermal injections resemble those of compound 48/80, since vascular permeability increases rapidly and declines within $^1/_2$–1 h. These effects are fully inhibited by cyproheptadine and a mixture of the antihistaminic mepyramine and the antiserotonin methysergide. Nonsteroid anti-inflammatory agents, anti-inflammatory steroids, and the antiallergic substance cromoglycate, when administered systemically, fail to suppress those effects of venoms or of compound 48/80. It has been reported (FORMANEK and KREIL, 1975) that cromoglycate, when administered together with the basic polypeptide melittin, which accounts for one-third of the weight of bee venom, does not inhibit the rat paw edema induced by it but inhibits edema resulting from a decapeptide melittin fragment. This indicates that this fragment releases rat skin histamine and/or serotonin by a mechanism resembling that of cutaneous anaphylaxis (FORMANEK and KREIL, 1975), which is the experimental setup in which cromoglycate acts the best. Since cromoglycate also inhibits histamine release by phospholipase A_2 (ORR and COX, 1969), a sort of vicious circle may be operative in which melittin activates mast cell phospholipase A_2, thus triggering amine release. In fact, melittin is a highly surface active substance and it might be anticipated that its cell-damaging effect would result from a direct physical interaction with the membrane, unlikely to be inhibited by pharmacologic agents (FREDHOLM and HAEGERMARK, 1967).

D. Crotalid Venoms and Enzymes Simulating Their Effects

I. Morphologic Aspects of Crotalid Venom Effects on Lung and Cremaster

1. Lung Effects

A 1 mg/ml solution of *A. piscivorus* venom produces on the canine lung surface an effect of the same intensity as the 4 mg/ml *N. naja* venom, but there is a macroscopic difference. Small hemorrhagic dots appear on the pleura 1–2 min after removal of the filter paper. It may be seen with a magnifying glass that these petechiae are under and not above the mesothelial layer. The hemorrhagic dots increase, become confluent, and within approximately 10 min, the area covered by the venom is dark red, and a hemorrhagic exudate is seen on the pleura. Rats and mice are less sensitive to *A. piscivorus* venom than dogs, since higher amounts of venom are required to obtain a typical lesion. In this case, hemorrhagic fluid in the pleural cavity and petechiae on the pulmonary surface are found.

Light and electron microscopies confirm the hemorrhagic features of the pulmonary alterations (Fig. 16). The hemorrhages are pleural and subpleural and do not occur in the depth of the lung tissue. Edema and erythrocyte fragmentation are present. The ultrastructural picture of *A. piscivorus* lesion is more pronounced than that of *N. naja* venom. Usually, complete destruction of mesothelial cells and of the capillary walls is observed (Fig. 17).

The colloidal carbon test gives a surprisingly negative result in rats treated with *A. piscivorus* venom, since only the hemorrhagic areas are blackened by carbon particles.

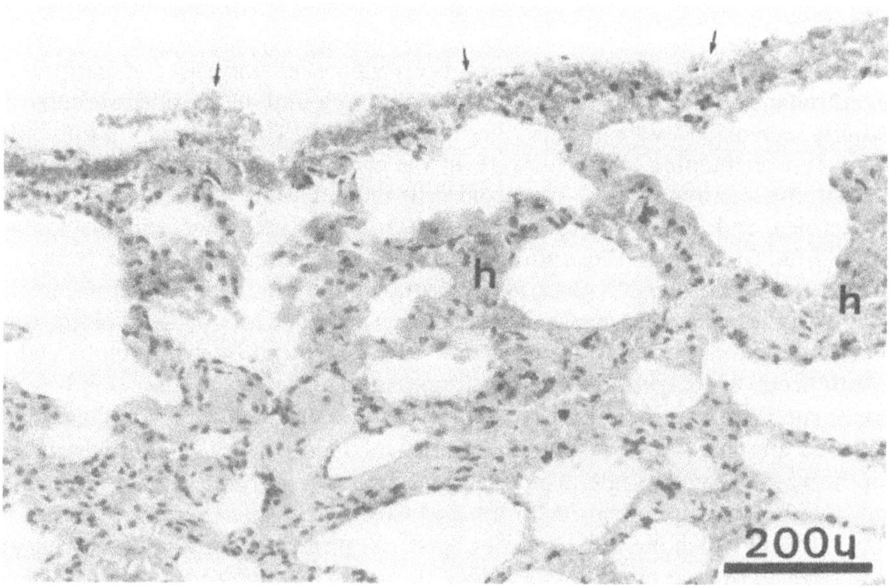

Fig. 16. Photomicrograph of canine lung treated with *A. piscivorus* venom. These hemorrhages (h and arrows) were observed 2 min after the removal of the filter paper soaked in the venom. 5 µ-thick section stained with hematoxylin and eosin

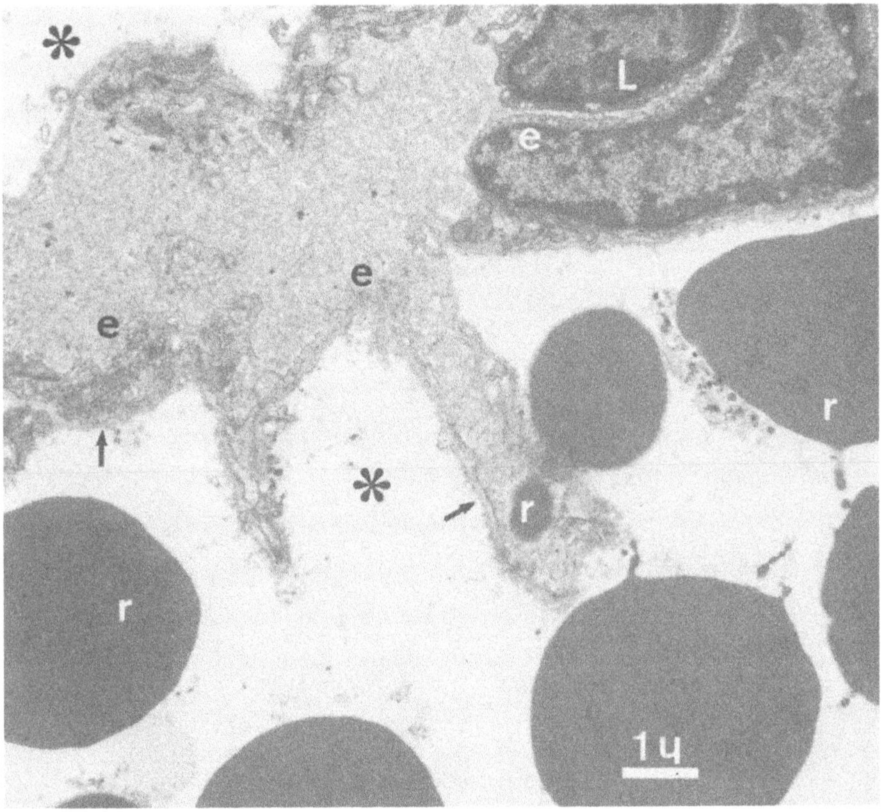

Fig. 17. EM of pulmonary capillary of rat treated with *A. piscivorus* venom. Advanced endothelial and epithelial lesions may be observed. The basement membrane is almost completely exposed (arrows). One erythrocyte is half in and half out of the vessel in a badly damaged region. In the alveolar space (asterisks) there are some red cells (*r*) showing "fragmentation"

2. Cremaster Effects

A. piscivorus venom administered in the same dose as *N. naja* venom causes bleeding in the cremaster muscle of rats and carbon particles label both capillaries and venules in the affected region. Vascular rupture is frequently observed, besides events of early inflammatory response. Electron microscopy also shows endothelial degeneration in otherwise normal vessels. Capillary and venular thromboses are common (Fig. 18).

II. Pharmacologic Aspects

1. Similarities and Differences Between Effects of Some Crotalid Snake Venoms

When the first description of lung injury with animal venoms was provided, morphologic and biochemical evidence allowed us to distinguish lesions by bee or elapid venoms from those due to a crotalid venom, namely that of *A. piscivorus* (BONTA et

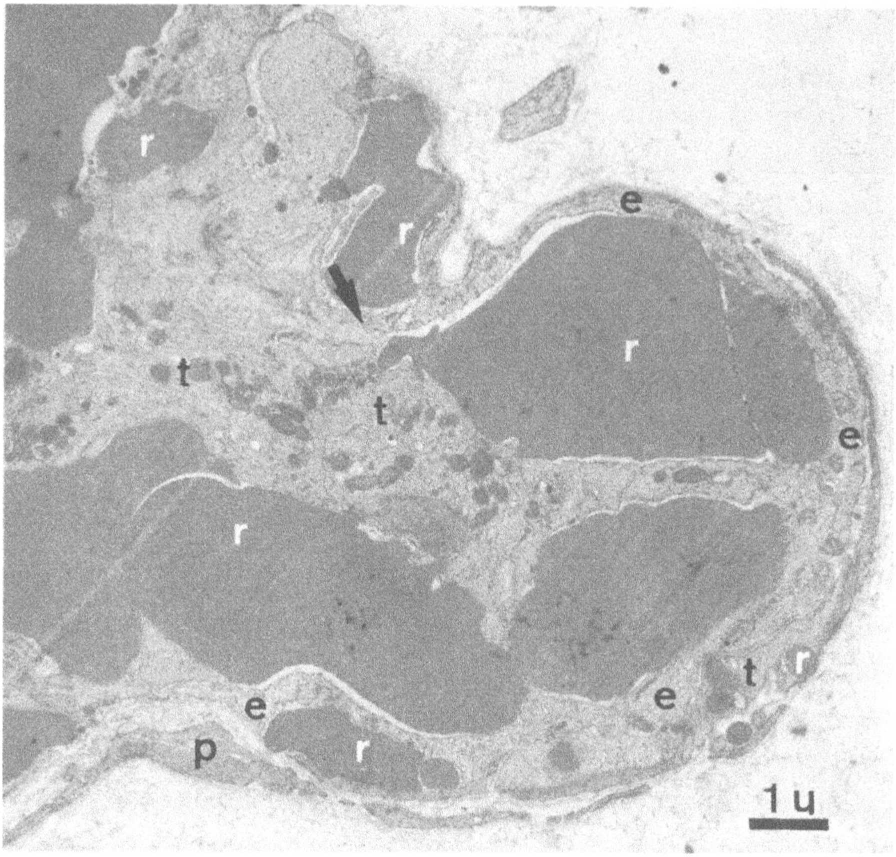

Fig. 18. EM of cremaster capillary of rat treated with *A. piscivorus* venom. The vessel is distended by a thrombus containing red cells (*r*) and platelets (*t*). After the arrow, in the upper left corner, the endothelium (*e*) is destroyed and red cells mixed with cytoplasmic rests lay free in the interstitium. Erythrocytic fragmentation is present and some of the small erythrocytic spherulae may be observed between the endothelium and the pericytes (*p*)

al., 1971). Bee and elapid snake venoms induced the nonpetechial lesions described above, whereas the venom from *A. piscivorus* induced petechial spots, particularly when submaximal amounts of venom were used (Figs. 2 and 3).

Lesions induced by venoms from the two snake families can also be distinguished on pharmacologic grounds. Heparin inhibits the lesions by elapid and bee venoms, whereas the lesions by crotalid venom as well as those due to collagenase are either unaffected or even increased.

Not much biochemical work has been performed to identify the precise venom fractions responsible for the effects of *A. piscivorus* venom. The hemorrhagic activity was found in a low (<10000) molecular weight fraction (BHARGAVA et al., 1970a), which proved nonhemolytic, free from kinin-releasing enzymes, but contaminated with phospholipase A_2 activity. However, phospholipase A_2 does not induce hemorrhagic lesions (Sect. C.II.1). Since *A. piscivorus* is a feeble coagulant venom, direct clotting was discarded as explanation of its local damaging effect, whereas this activity could account for the activity of *B. jararaca* venom (NAHAS et al., 1964). Partially purified fractions of the latter (VARGAFTIG et al., 1974) have been tested for clotting properties and hemorrhagic activity found in two fractions, one with and the other without clotting activity. The fraction free from this activity (BJ G 50 II, VARGAFTIG et al., 1974) had phospholipase A_2 and esterase activities and was thus still a mixture of various enzymes. It is, nevertheless, important to note that hemorrhages can be induced by a *B. jararaca* fraction devoid of clotting properties. This could be anticipated, since *A. piscivorus* venom has a marked damaging activity on lung vessels but is not coagulant (DAVEY and LÜSCHER, 1967). Moreover, trypsin, *C. adamanteus*, and *C. terrificus* venoms which do not damage lung vessels are powerful coagulant agents. This demonstrates that thrombin-like and vessel-damaging activities are not necessarily associated. Nevertheless, once blood leaks from the vessels, if the venom contains coagulant factors, extravasated blood will eventually coagulate. A vascular lesion is the *sine qua non* condition for crotalid venom-induced hemorrhages on the lung, but other associated venom factors may interfere and thus aggravate the condition. Another possible mechanism of action for hemorrhages by crotalid snake venoms would be through their collagenolytic activity. The subject has been exhaustively investigated by OHSAKA (see Chap. 14 of this handbook), and will only be discussed here for the sake of comparison. In early publications (see OSHAKA et al., 1972), the proteolytic activity of *T. flavoviridis* (Habu snake) venom was found to be completely distinct from the hemorrhagic components. In further work (TAKAHASHI and OHSAKA, 1970), it was demonstrated that two hemorrhagic factors effective on the rabbit skin were not able to dissolve reconstituted collagen fibers. They speculated, nevertheless, that the hemorrhagic factors might attack the collagen layers on the blood vessels. This indicated that snake venom hemorrhagic factors lacking caseinolytic activities could still be proteases, inasmuch as they might hydrolyze collagen in an organized vascular structure. It was demonstrated later that hemorrhagic principles from *T. flavoviridis* release proteins and carbohydrates from isolated glomerular basement membranes. Bacterial collagenase has a similar effect qualitatively and is even more potent than the venom factors (OHSAKA et al., 1973). Hemorrhagic activities and the ability to split basement membranes were inhibited by incubating the fractions with EDTA or with cysteine. These two reagents inhibit the pulmonary hemorrhagic effect of *Crotalidae* venoms and of bacterial collagenase (VARGAFTIG et al., 1976). The overall conclusion was that *T. flavoviridis* hemorrhagic principles might be proteolytic enzymes with high specificity with respect to substrate, particularly organized collagen. These principles have not been tested on pulmonary vessels, but on the basis of the above data, a damaging effect can reasonably be anticipated. Lung hemorrhages by *Crotalidae* venoms differ from those by bacterial collagenase (see Sect. D.II) in that the latter does not induce petechiae, whereas venoms of both *A. piscivorus* and *B. jararaca* evoke the appearance of petechial hemorrhages. If collagenolytic enzymes account for the crotalid venom-induced hemorrhagic activity, clotting and perhaps even petechiae may be additional events, produced by noncollagenolytic components of crude or only partially purified snake fractions. Furthermore, one might anticipate that those snake venoms that induce true hemorrhages, but not those from elapids or the bee, should split collagen fibers. This is indeed the case and results similar to those in Figure 19 have been

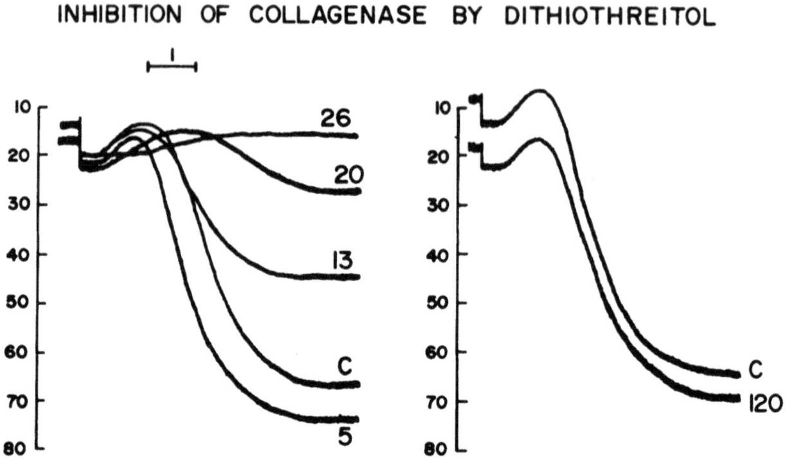

Fig. 19. Inhibition by dithiothreitol of the property of collagen to induce platelet aggregation. Platelet-rich plasma prepared from citrated rabbit blood was stirred at 1100 rpm at 37° C in an aggregometer. Aggregation was started by adding to the platelet preparation 20 μl of a collagen suspension. The aggregation curves are superimposed. C stands for control aggregation by collagen, whereas the figures indicate time intervals during which an equivalent volume of collagen was incubated with bacterial collagenase, which by itself had no platelet effect. The property of collagen to induce aggregation is gradually reduced, after an initial increase, and at 20–26 min has totally disappeared. Collagenase preincubated with dithiothreitol loses the ability to disrupt collagen, since even after a 120 min incubation, collagen is intact and aggregates the platelets. Details in VARGAFTIG et al. (1976)

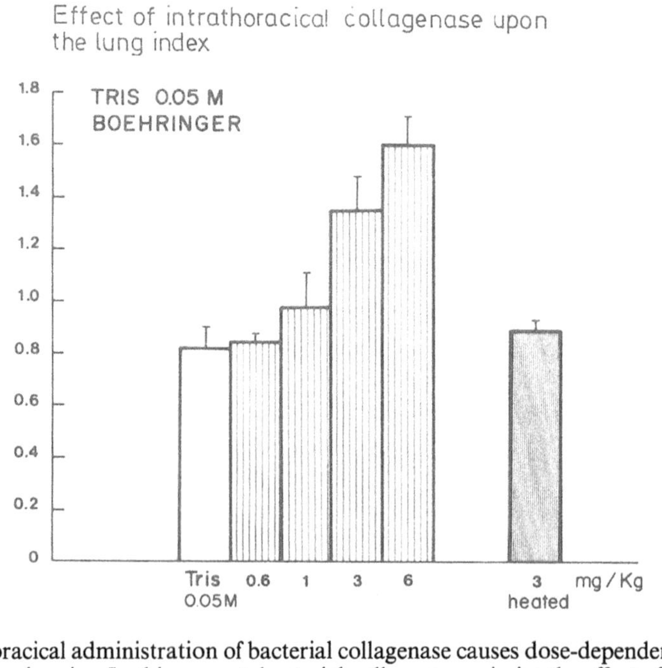

Fig. 20. Intrathoracical administration of bacterial collagenase causes dose-dependent increase of lung weight index in mice. In this respect, bacterial collagenase mimics the effect of vasculotoxic snake venoms. Heated collagenase is ineffective

obtained with *B. jararaca* venom. No data are available for *A. piscivorus* venom. It is noteworthy that *B. jararaca* and *A. piscivorus* venoms have no detectable activity on a synthetic pentapeptide substrate for collagenase, under conditions where crude bacterial collagenase did show this type of activity (E. L. GIROUX, personal communication). Lack of activity of crotalid snake venoms on synthetic collagenase substrates has been reported by MURATA et al. (1963). The collagenolytic activity of *B. jararaca*, as well as that of collagenase, was abolished when incubated with cysteine or with Na_2 EDTA before testing (Fig. 19).

2. Lung Effects of Collagenase and Other Proteolytic Enzymes

Bacterial *(Clostridium histolyticum)* collagenase has a powerful local effect on the dog lung, which differs from that due to crotalid snake venoms because petechiae are not visible, although blood leakage can be seen macroscopically and microscopically (Fig. 11) (VARGAFTIG et al., 1976; VARGAFTIG, 1976). A further difference between crotalid snake venoms and collagenase consists in that the latter does not increase vascular permeability in the skin, whereas the former do so (HABERMANN, 1974). It is interesting to note that *T. flavoviridis* venom, whose hemorrhagic activity may be explained by its collagenolytic activity (Sect. B.II.4) is also devoid of vascular permeability-increasing effects of rat mesenteric vessels (OHSAKA et al., 1971). The activity of collagenase can also be shown in the rodent intrathoracic test, hemorrhages and massive clots being present (Fig. 20).

III. Pharmacologic Influences on Crotalid Snake Venoms and Collagenase-Induced Hemorrhagic Effects

1. In Vitro Inactivation of Vasculotoxic Materials

Incubation of *B. jararaca* venom with Na_2 EDTA, dithiothreitol, penicillamine, and cysteine resulted in loss of lung hemorrhagic activity and of collagenolytic activity as measured in the bioassay (Fig. 19) or on the pentapeptide synthetic substrate (E. L. GIROUX, personal communication). Na_2 EDTA also suppressed the hemorrhagic activity of *A. piscivorus*, the other reagents not having been tested. Furthermore, Na_2 EDTA also abolished the vasculotoxic effect of elapid snake venoms (BONTA et al., 1970). The following materials failed to block the effects of *B. jararaca* and of *A. piscivorus* venoms: Trasylol (BHARGAVA et al., 1970a; VARGAFTIG et al., 1976) and heparin (BHARGAVA et al., 1970a). Soybean trypsin inhibitor, and p-chloromercuribenzoate, a thiol group scavenger, failed to affect the activities of *B. jararaca* venom and bacterial collagenase. Phenylbutazone, indomethacin, and aspirin which inhibit collagenase from another source (WOJTECKA-LUKASIK and DANCEWICZ, 1974) failed to interfere with the hemorrhagic activity of *B. jararaca* venom and collagenase (J. LEFORT, personal communication).

2. Local Application of Putative Inhibitors to the Tissue

The following drugs failed to inhibit the effects of collagenase and of *B. jararaca* venom on the dog lung surface: estriol succinate, ε-amino caproic acid (250 mg/ml), dexamethasone phosphate (4 mg/ml), prostaglandin E_1 (0.1 mg/ml), $MgCl_2$ and

$CaCl_2$ (0.1 M of either), and dibutyryl cAMP (20 mM). The only drugs that inhibited the effects of hemorrhagic enzymes on the lung surface were Na_2 EDTA, presumably by a similar mechanism that accounts for inhibition of enzyme activity upon incubation, i.e., metal chelation, and polyphloretin phosphate. The latter is an enzyme inhibitor that also prevents some effects of prostaglandins (Sect. C.II.2). It blocked unspecifically the effects of bacterial collagenase, *B. jararaca* and *A. piscivorus* venoms, as well as those of nonhemorrhagic venoms (*N. nigricollis*, *N. naja*, and bee) (Fig. 19).

3. Intravenous Administration of Putative Inhibitors

Intravenous treatment with the following drugs (doses in mg/kg) failed to block the subsequent collagenase and *B. jararaca* venom-induced lung hemorrhages on the dog: heparin (5), dexamethasone (2), aspirin (100), phenylbutazone (5), and antiplatelet serum raised in rabbits and administered at an amount that reduced the platelet counts to nil (VARGAFTIG et al., 1976).

4. Effects of Collagenase in the Rodent Intrathoracic Test

Results obtained in mice injected with collagenase provided results somewhat different, indicating that in this model processes other than hemorrhages occur, which is understandable since collagenase comes in contact with a closed cavity, the thorax, whereas in the dog model it has a strictly local effect. Moreover, the end point in the dog model is a figure to quantitate extent of hemorrhage to the naked eye, whereas in the mice model, the measured parameter is lung weight. Under those conditions, not only will the hemorrhages be measured but lung edema as well. The protein protease inhibitors Iniprol and Zymofren, when incubated with collagenase for 1 h and then injected intrathoracically, reduced the extent of increase of the lung index, as compared to control animals only injected with collagenase (VARGAFTIG et al., 1976). Since hemorrhages were not inhibited, which is in accordance with lack of inhibition on the lung surface of the dog, it is probable that in mice other effects resulting from hemorrhages, or directly induced by collagenase, are inhibited. Since the bradykinin-potentiating peptide BBP9 failed to display any effect on the lung, release of kinins appears as irrelevant under those conditions. It is interesting to note that the same protease inhibitors, as well as soybean trypsin inhibitor and polyarginine, when injected i.v. 5 min before intrathoracical collagenase, rather increased its effects. This may indicate that systemic inhibition of proteases inhibits removal of clots from the lungs, thus increasing their weight, and as a consequence, increasing the lung index.

IV. Effects of Different Enzymes on the Lung Surface Vessels

The following enzymes failed to induce local hemorrhages, when tested on the lung surface; chymotrypsin, trypsin, thrombin, pancreatic kallikrein, pure phospholipase A_2, hyaluronidase, and elastase. The latter displays a peculiar effect, since it induces the appearance of a bula on the lung surface, which is more evident during inspiration. If collagenase is assayed on top of this bula, or if mixtures of collagenase and elastase are tested, the hemorrhagic effect is markedly increased (Table 5) (VARGAFTIG, 1976; VARGAFTIG et al., 1976). Nevertheless, elastase does not increase rat paw

Table 5. Potentiation by elastase of the hemorrhagic effect of bacterial collagenase on the lung surface of the dog

Tested agent	µg/spot	Total score ± SD
Dog 1		
Elastase	3	0.29 ± 0.75
	10	4.35 ± 0.84
Collagenase	3	1.75 ± 2.05
	10	9.67 ± 0.67
Elastase + collagenase	3 + 3	5.57 ± 1.20[a]
	10 + 10	19.40 ± 4.00[a]
Dog 2		
Elastase	3	0.80 ± 1.5
	10	7.70 ± 2.0
Collagenase	3	1.7 ± 1.5
	10	11.0 ± 2.0
Elastase + collagenase	3 + 3	7.30 ± 2.5[a]
	10 + 10	21.00 ± 2.8[a]

[a] $p < 0.001$.

edema nor the effect of collagenase on the mice lung, indicating the presence of an elastase-degradable barrier, most probably the visceral pleura, that prevents collagenase from reaching the vessels. This barrier is absent from rat paws and less effective in the case of intrathoracical injections to mice, thus explaining the ineffectiveness of elastase in these two models.

Another interesting enzyme for local lung activity is papain, which has been used as an emphysema-inducing substance, when administered to animals by forced inhalation (GROSS et al., 1965). Papain had a marked hemorrhagic activity by itself on the lung surface, much alike that due to collagenase; when it lost its activity with time, it still retained the ability to potentiate collagenase, i.e., to mimic elastase. Papain-induced hemorrhages and the increase of the rat skin vascular permeability are not inhibited by antiserotonin and antihistamine treatment. In contrast (Sect. D.II.2) collagenase has no permeability-increasing activity and only induces hemorrhages.

V. Rat Paw Edema Due to Crotalid Snake Venoms

Edema due to crotalid snake venoms can be distinguished from that due to elapid and bee venoms, since the lesions become hemorrhagic eventually. This makes it difficult to evaluate quantitatively the activity of putative inhibitors, because hemorrhages may overshadow the inhibition of the underlying, more specific mediator-induced swelling. Heating of *B. jararaca* venom for a few minutes up to 86° C destroys the coagulant factors (HAMBERG and ROCHA E SILVA, 1957), as well as the ability of the venom to induce lung hemorrhages (VARGAFTIG et al., 1974). The kinin-releasing activity, as well as the ability to induce rat paw edema, remain unaffected by this procedure. Since phospholipase A_2 is thermoresistant as well (CONDREA and DE VRIES, 1965), the edema-inducing activity of *B. jararaca* venom may thus result from a combined activity of kinins and prostaglandins released by kininogenases and

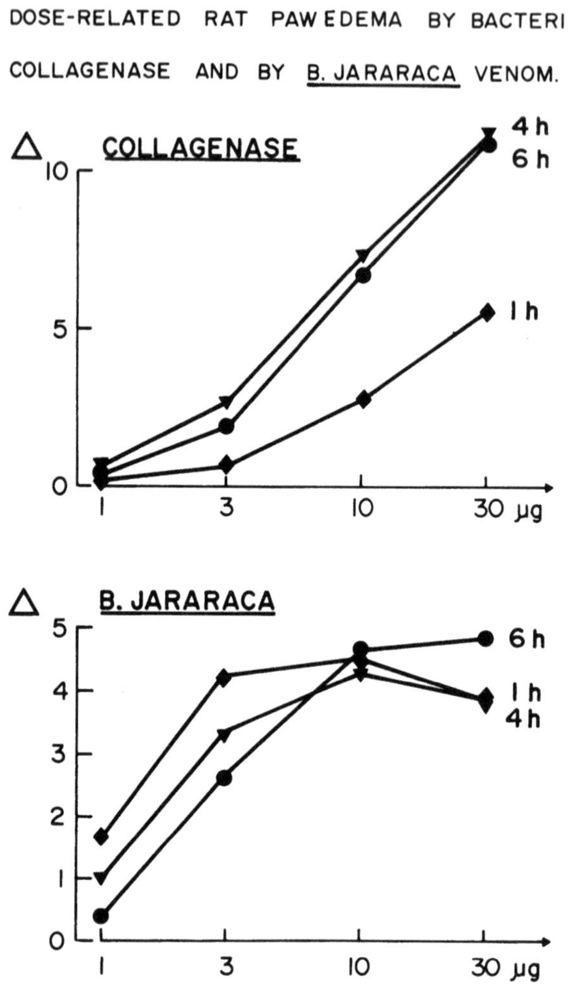

Fig. 21. Rat paw edema induced by bacterial collagenase and *B. jararaca* venom. Bacterial collagenase and *B. jararaca* venom were injected at the indicated amounts in 0.1 ml of 0.9% NaCl into the rat paw, and thickness was measured after 1, 4, and 6 h, as indicated. Observe dose-related effect of collagenase up to 30 μg at all time intervals. Edema by *B. jararaca* is self-limiting and ceils at 10 μg. Scale is the difference between venom or collagenase-injected paws and saline-injected paws of a control weight-paired group of rats, in arbitrary scale difference (Δ)

phospholipase A_2, respectively. This combination of activity is expected to display effects beyond those induced by each agonist itself, since a mutual potentiating activity has been described between the kininogenase kallikrein and phospholipase A_2 (AMUNDSEN et al., 1969). A moderate heating of crude *B. jararaca* venom (56° C, pH 7.6) results, already within 1 min, in a marked enhancement of the edema-inducing ability, of around 50%, which is noticeable both for the early (30 min) and for the delayed (4 h) readings. This enhanced venom effect is maximal within 5 min after start of heating, decreases within 7.5–10 min, and is again very marked at 30 min, both for early and for late readings. Since the local hemorrhagic effect is completely suppressed for heating longer than 10 min, it is reasonable to assume that the hemorrhagic effect is not involved and that a venom component responsible for limiting the edema is heat-sensitive. A good candidate is kininase which, by destroying kinins as soon as the venom kininogenase releases them from kininogen, would suppress one edema-inducing factor, namely bradykinin. Moreover, edema is maximal for doses of *B. jararaca* up to 10 μg per paw (Fig. 21), whereas overt hemorrhages are only apparent at doses above 30 μg, again dissociating the capability of the venom to induce edema from hemorrhagic activity. The following drugs were unable to inhibit the *B. jararaca* induced rat paw edema: mepyramine, cyproheptadine, indomethacin, aspirin, and phenylbutazone (VARGAFTIG, unpublished).

VI. Rat Paw Edema and Skin Vascular Permeability Effects of Bacterial Collagenase

Since bacterial collagenase has been used as a model for lung hemorrhages, it is useful to summarize its other effects. Collagenase free from both kinin-releasing and kinin-destroying factors induces rat paw edema (Fig. 21) which is accompanied, for doses above 10 μg, by overt hemorrhages. Edema resembles that due to carrageenan, insomuch as an early phase (within 30 min after intraplantar injection) is inhibited by the standard antiserotonin and antihistaminic agent cyproheptadine, whereas a late edema (around 3–5 h) is partially, but significantly, inhibited by NSAID and dexamethasone (VINEGAR et al., 1974; VARGAFTIG et al., 1976). Hemorrhages by collagenase are unaffected by these inhibitors, which probably explains why inhibition of swelling is partial and the dose-effect curve for inhibition rather shallow.

Permeability assays with bacterial collagenase allow a better understanding of the different time-related effects obtained with venoms or with other agonists on skin or paws. Collagenase has no specific effect on skin vascular permeability other than that of inducing hemorrhages and no blueing reaction, as found in dye-injected animals challenged with specific permeability-increasing drugs (serotonin, compound 48/80, snake venoms), can be visualized (HABERMANN, 1974; VARGAFTIG et al., 1976). Hemorrhages are thus produced when blood leaks from damaged vessels, but no specific capillary or venular effect is present, in contrast to what occurs in the case of nonhemorrhagic elapid and bee venoms.

VII. Increase in Skin Vascular Permeability Due to Crotalid Snake Venoms

The mechanism of action underlying the marked effect upon skin vascular permeability displayed by the various crotalid snake venoms is not homogeneous. This is clear from the study of crude venoms themselves. Thus *A. piscivorus* venom induces leakage of labeled albumin from vessels to extravascular spaces by releasing amines, as do the elapid and bee venoms. This effect is inhibited by antiserotonin and antihistaminic agents, whereas a similar effect, when induced by *B. jararaca* venom, appears to involve other factors, since antiamine agents do not prevent it. Moreover, "bradykinin-releasing enzyme" extracted from *B. jararaca* venom imitates its effect on the skin, which is unaffected by cyproheptadine at doses that fully prevent the effects of serotonin, histamine, or of compound 48/80. The coagulant factors present in *B. jararaca* venom are not involved directly with the skin permeability effect, since heating of the venom suppresses all coagulant (and local hemorrhagic activity) but has no effect on the increase in vascular permeability (VARGAFTIG et al., 1974).

Fractions extracted from *B. jararaca* venom have been described as inducing skin hemorrhages (MANDELBAUM et al., 1972) and evidence has been provided that those fractions are metalloproteins. No data were given on permeability of vessels at doses lower than those required for inducing blood leakage or for rat paw edema. It is noteworthy that those hemorrhagic factors do not release bradykinin, whereas a kinin-releasing enzyme, extracted from *B. jararaca* venom, as well as *Bothrops* protease A, has been shown not to affect the dog lung surface (VARGAFTIG et al., 1974). Moreover, the lung hemorrhagic effect of *B. jararaca* venom (see Section D.II.1) is also inhibited by the reagents chosen to demonstrate metal involvement in enzyme activity of skin hemorrhagic factors, pointing to similar substances.

A clear-cut dissociation between the permeability-increasing and the hemorrhagic effect can be provided by studies with *C. adamanteus* venom, since hemorrhages are visualized when the venom is injected i.d. to rats, without prior i.v. administration of Evans blue dye. When the latter is given, a blue spot will hide the blood-colored lesion, but the latter will again appear if the animals are pretreated with cyproheptadine to suppress the effects resulting from amine release in the skin. Bacterial collagenase can be contrasted to this venom, since on the contrary it only induces hemorrhages and in no instance a blue spot can be produced (VARGAFTIG et al., 1976).

E. General Conclusions: Interrelationships Between Morphology and Function

Lung and cremaster microcirculations react differently to *N. naja* and *A. piscivorus* venoms. The elapid venom produces increased vascular permeability and hemolysis, which are alterations induced by many animal venoms (DANON et al., 1961; DE VRIES et al., 1962; KLIBANSKY et al., 1966; VINCENT et al., 1971). The microscopic picture of the colloidal carbon test and the finding of degranulated mast cells in the neighborhood of altered venules in the cremaster suggest the participation of histamine in the *N. naja* lesion in this tissue. It is likely that this is valid as well for skin vessels. The participation of histamine for the lung vasculotoxic effect of *N. naja* venom is unlikely on the basis of pharmacologic evidence. Nevertheless, morphologically these lesions resemble those produced by histamine, although the subject is poorly known.

Phospholipase A_2 and DLF synergism clearly seen on lung tissue was studied on cremasters with inconclusive results. The electron microscopy did not help to elucidate the potentiating effect of phospholipase A_2 or the protecting action of estrogens, despite our efforts to observe alterations of the ground substance which is the most likely place to look for morphologic evidence of these effects (PORGES, 1953; SCHIFF and BURN, 1961). However, usually more is expected from electron microscopy than the instrument actually can offer and disillusions are frequent. This happens, for example, in pulmonary edema where the pathways of fluids and proteins are still unknown (STAUB, 1974) and, what is worse, the likelihood of seeing them is very small statistically (KARNOVSKY, 1970).

Hemorrhages are the dominant feature of crotalid venom-induced vascular lesions. This is the case with *C. atrox* (OWNBY et al., 1974), *T. flavoviridis* hemorrhagic principle (TSUCHIYA et al., 1974), and other snake venoms (HOMMA and TU, 1971), including *V. palestinae* (MCKAY et al., 1970). The mechanism of bleeding in snake envenomation has been described as a direct distructive action on the capillaries and oozing of red cells through ruptured vessels (MCKAY et al., 1970), as well as an exudation of erythrocytes through interendothelial gaps (TSUCHIYA et al., 1974). In our experiments with *A. piscivorus* venom, complete destruction of the microcirculation was frequently observed, but convincing evidence for an interendothelial pathway was not found. Even so, we do not support the transcytoplasmatic escape of red cells as the only possible route. In our experience with electron microscopy of blood vessels, it is exceptionally rare to observe the passage of an erythrocyte in the intercellular junctions. It must be almost an "explosive" phenomenon with immediate closure of the gap. The complexity of red cell escape from the circulation is well-illustrated in the lung, where erythrocytes are commonly found in hydrostatic edema fluid but not in certain cases of toxic pulmonary edema in which the vessels are severely damaged (COTTRELL et al., 1967).

There is a good correlation between the presence of thrombi in cremasters treated with *A. piscivorus* venom and their absence in the case of *Naja naja* venom. Most crotalid venoms are coagulants, whereas most elapid venoms are not. Despite this, the finding of platelet thrombi in pulmonary vessels treated with *N. naja* venom is not unexpected, since intravascular clots occur very frequently in animals that undergo thoracotomy and unavoidable manipulation as in the experiments now reported. Therefore, the absence of thrombi in the cremaster treated with *N. naja* venom is more significant than their presence in the pulmonary circulation.

ROCHA E SILVA et al. (1969) demonstrated liberation of kinins by *A. piscivorus* venom. It is possible that the effect of this venom on the microcirculation is not due exclusively to a direct action on the vessels but also to chemical mediators. However, the colloidal carbon technique, which is very sensitive (BÖHM, 1973b), failed to demonstrate an indirect action, at least in rat lungs. The generalized carbon retention in subpleural capillaries of *N. naja*-venom injected animals and the accumulation of carbon particles only at the proximity of the hemorrhagic areas provoked by *A. piscivorus* venom suggest involvement of chemical mediators or materials imitating them in the case of the former but not of the latter. The colloidal carbon tests also suggest that both venoms act only locally, because no permeability alterations were shown in the microcirculation distantly to the topical application of the venoms. Thus, no parallels can be drawn with pulmonary edema-inducing agents, such as ammonium salts, α-naphthyl-thiourea and others as shown by BÖHM (1966) and BÖHM et al. (1973).

The pulmonary vessels of rats and mice are more sensitive to *N. naja* venom and less so to *A. piscivorus* venom than the camine lung vessels. Rat pulmonary and systemic vessels also differ in sensitivity to both venoms, the cremaster vessels being more reactive than those of the lung. These species and tissue differences have also been observed for other snake venoms: *B. jararaca* (AMORIM et al., 1961), *C. adamanteus* (VARGAFTIG et al., 1974), and *Echis coloratus* (SANDBANK et al., 1974). The structural variation of the vessels, shown in the beginning of this review, is possibly the main explanation for these discrepancies.

F. Speculations on the Significance of Venom-Induced Inflammation of Microvessels

From the evidence presented in this chapter, the picture emerges that when elapid venoms or DLF are applied to the lung surface, vascular injury without intervention of known mediator follows. In this situation, the venom material proper seems to *replace* the mediators and accordingly can be considered as a model thereof. Cationic proteins and polypeptides released from leukocytes and platelets under inflammatory stimuli have been shown to increase vascular permeability (NACHMAN and WEKSLER, 1972). In this respect, these substances resemble the elapid venom materials responsible for their respective vasculotoxic effects. Both materials, released from mammal cells and those found in elapid venoms, can cause an inflammatory type of vascular lesion. The latter differ fundamentally from hemorrhages as produced by crotalid venoms and bacterial collagenase. It is attractive to speculate that the vasculotoxic cationic polypeptides of the elapid venoms are indeed a model of, and a tool for a naturally occurring inflammatory material released from cells and pertinent to tissue injury. The mechanism by which the venom materials referred to cause vessel injury is incompletely understood, just as little is known about drug mechanisms to provide inhibition toward this lesion. Injected into the rat hind paw or into the skin, venoms apparently trigger the *release* of several mediators (serotonin, histamine, bradykinin, prostaglandins) which are recognized to participate in the acute inflammatory reaction. Any pharmacologic interference with the mediators—either inhibition of the release or blockade of the receptor—obviously suppresses the effect of venom materials in the rat paw. It is easy to appreciate that drugs acting at the target organ (e.g., the microvessels) of the inflammatory mediators also inhibit the rat paw edema provoked by venom materials.

Obvious as it is, the above image is an oversimplified view of reality. But for that matter, every model is necessarily an oversimplification. Nevertheless, such models may serve as conceivable blueprints to help understand the far more complicated natural events.

Acknowledgements. A number of colleagues have been involved in various stages of the work summarized in this Chapter. We particularly wish to acknowledge the stimulating discussions held with Drs. E.L. GIROUX, J. NOORDHOEK, N. BHARGAVA, J.E. VINCENT, O.P. ALMEIDA, E.A. GREGORIO, Mrs. J. LEFORT, and C.J. DE VOS, as well as the authorization to use as yet unpublished information. Experimental work performed on morphologic aspects of *N. naja* and *A. piscivorus* lung lesions were supported by grant 73/1122 of Fundaçao de Amparo à Pesquisa do Estado de S. Paulo, Brazil. The competent secretarial assistance of Miss A. MUHL is gratefully acknowledged.

References

Almeida, M. R. H.: Fatores hemorrágicos da peçonha de *Bothrops jararaca:* separação em coluna de hidroxiapatita e electroforese em papel, Thesis, Botucatu, 1973

Almeida, O. P.: Alteracões morfologicas causadas pelos venenos das cobras *Naja naja* e *Agkistrodon piscivorus* no pulmão e cremaster de rato. Thesis, Ribeirao Preto, 1975

Almeida, O. P., Böhm, G. M., Bonta, I. L.: Morphological study of lesions induced by snake venoms (*Naja naja* and *Agkistrodon piscivorus*) in the lung and cremaster vessels of rats. J. Path. Bact. **121**, 169—176 (1977)

Almeida, O. P., Böhm, G. M., Carvalho, M. P., Carvalho, A. P.: The cardiac muscle in the pulmonary vein of the rat: A morphological and electrophysiological study. J. Morph. **145**, 409—434 (1975)

Amorim, M. F., Mello, R. F., Saliba, F.: Envenenamento Botrópico e Crotálico—contribuição para o estudo experimental das lesões. Mem. Inst. Butantan **23**, 63—108 (1951)

Amundsen, E., Ofstad, E., Hagen, P.-O.: Histamine release induced by synergistic action of kallikrein and phospholipase A. Arch. int. Pharmacodyn. **178**, 104—114 (1969)

Arendt, K. A., Shulman, M. H., Fulton, G. P., Lutz, B. R.: Post-irradiation petechiae and the mechanism of formation with snake venom. Anat. Rec. **117**, 595 (1953)

Bennett, H. S., Luft, J. H., Hampton, J. C.: Morphological classifications of vertebrate blood capillaries. Amer. J. Physiol. **196**, 381—390 (1959)

Bhargava, N., Vargaftig, B. B., Vos, C. J. de, Bonta, I. L., Tijs, T.: Dissociation of oedema provoking factor of *Agkistrodon piscivorus* venom from kininogenase. In: Back, N., Sicuteri, F. (Eds.): Vasopeptides. New York: Plenum Press 1970b

Bhargava, N., Zirinis, P., Bonta, I. L., Vargaftig, B. B.: Comparison of hemorrhagic factors of the venoms of *Naja naja*, *Agkistrodon piscivorus* and *Apis mellifera*. Biochem. Pharmacol. **19**, 2405—2412 (1970a)

Böhm, G. M.: Vascular permeability changes during experimentally produced pulmonary oedema in rats. J. Path. Bact. **92**, 151—161 (1966)

Böhm. G. M.: Changes in lung arterioles in pulmonary oedema induced in rats by alpha-naphthylthiourea. J. Path. Bact. **110**, 343—345 (1973a)

Böhm, G. M.: The sensitivity of the colloidal carbon technique in measuring pulmonary vascular permeability changes. J. Path. Bact. **111**, 47—51 (1973b)

Böhm, G. M.: Ultrastructural aspects of lung vessel permeability alterations in experimental conditions. Agents Actions **6**, 283—284 (1976)

Böhm, G. M., Machado, D. C., Padovan, P. A.: Ultrastructural changes in rat lung arterioles in conditions of altered permeability. J. Path. Bact. (in press) (1977)

Böhm, G. M., Vugman, I., Valeri, V., Sarti, W., Carvalho, I. F., Laus-Filho, J. A.: Ultrastructural alterations to pulmonary blood vessels in acute immunological lung lesions in rats, mice, and guinea-pigs. J. Path. Bact. **111**, 95—101 (1973)

Bonta, I. L.: Microvascular lesions as a target of anti-inflammatory and certain other drugs. Acta physiol. pharmacol. neerl. **15**, 188—222 (1969)

Bonta, I. L., Bhargava, N., Vargaftig, B. B.: Hemorrhagic snake venoms and kallikrein inhibitors as tools to study factors determining the integrity of the vessel wall. In: Sicuteri, F., Rocha e Silva, M., Back, N. (Eds.): Bradikinin and related kinins. Cardiovasc. Biochem. and Neural Actions. Adv. in Expt. Medicine and Biol., Vol. 8, pp. 191—199. New York: Plenum Press 1970a

Bonta, I.L., Bhargava, N., Vargaftig, B.B.: Dissociation between hemorrhagic, enzymatic and lethal activity of some snake venoms and of bee venom as studied in a new model. In: Vries, A. de, Kochva, E. (Eds.): Toxins of Animal and Plant Origin, Vol. II. New York: Gordon and Breach 1971

Bonta, I. L., Chrispijn, H., Noordhoek, J., Vincent, J. E.: Reduction of prostaglandin phase in hind paw inflammation and partial failure of indomethacin to exert anti-inflammatory effect in rats on essential fatty acid deficient diet. Prostaglandins **5**, 495—503 (1974)

Bonta, I. L., Dijk, M. van, Noordhoek, J., Vincent, J. E.: Enhancement of the cobra venom direct lytic factor by prostaglandins and related synergistic phenomena on pulmonary microvascular events. In: Ohsaka, A., Hayashi, K., Sawai, Y. (Eds.): Animal, Plant, and Microbial Toxins, Vol. II, pp. 217—227. New York: Plenum Press 1976

Bonta, I. L., Noordhoek, J.: Anti-inflammatory mechanism of inflamed-tissue factor. Agents Actions **3**, 348—356 (1973)

Bonta, I. L., Vargaftig, B. B.: Cobra venom induced pulmonary vessel lesion: an unconventional model of acute inflammation. Bull. Inst. Pasteur Lille **74**, 131—136 (1976)

Bonta, I. L., Vargaftig, B. B., Bhargava, N., Vos, C. J. de: Method for study of snake venom induced hemorrhages. Toxicon **8**, 3—10 (1970c)

Bonta, I. L., Vargaftig, B. B., Vos, C. J. de, Grijsen, H.: Haemorrhagic mechanisms of some snake venoms in relation to protection by estriol succinate of blood vessel damage. Life Sci. **8**, 881—888 (1969)

Bonta, I. L., Vincent, J. E., Noordhoek, J.: The role of direct lytic factor (DLF) and phospholipase-A in the local hemorrhagic effect of *Naja naja* venom. J. Formosan med. Ass. **71**, 333—335 (1972b)

Bonta, I. L., Vincent, J. E., Noordhoek, J., Wielinga, G.: Vascular hemorrhagic effect of *Naja naja* venom: participation of phospholipase-A and DLF. Toxicon **10**, 523—538 (1972a)

Bonta, I. L., Vos, C. J de: The effect of estriol-16-17-dihemisuccinate on vascular permeability as evaluated in the rat paw oedema test. Acta Endocrinol. (Kbh.) **49**, 403—411 (1965)

Bonta, I. L., Vos, C. J. de: The significance of the kinin system in the rat paw oedema and drug effects on it. Europ. J. Pharmacol. **1**, 222—225 (1967)

Bonta, I. L., Vos, C. J. de Delver, A.: Inhibitory effects of estriol-16-17-disodium succinate on local haemorrhages induced by snake venom in canine heart-lung preparations. Acta endocrinol. (Kbh.) **48**, 137—146 (1965)

Bonta, I. L., Vries-Kragt, K. de, Vos, C. J. de, Bhargava, N.: Preventive effect of local heparin administration on microvascular pulmonary hemorrhages induced by cobra venom in mice. Europ. J. Pharmacol. **13**, 97—102 (1970b)

Boquet, P., Izard, Y., Meaune, J., Jouannet, M.: Recherches biochimiques et immunologiques sur le venin des serpents. Ann. Inst. Pasteur **112**, 213—235 (1967)

Breithaupt, H., Habermann, E.: Mastzelldegranulierendes Peptid (MCD-Peptid) aus Bienengift: Isolierung, biochemische und pharmakologische Eigenschaften. Naunyn-Schmiedebergs Arch. Pharmak. exp. Path. **261**, 252—270 (1968)

Cohnheim, J.: Neue Untersuchungen über die Entzündung. Berlin: A. Hirschwald 1973

Condrea, E., Barzilay, M., Mager, J.: Role of cobra venom direct lytic factor and Ca^{2+} in promoting the activity of snake venom phospholipase A. Biochim. biophys. Acta (Amst.) **210**, 65—73 (1970)

Condrea, E., Barzilay, M., Vries, A. de: Cobra basic polypeptide as a mediator in the hydrolysis of membranal phospholipids by phospholipase-A. In: Vries, A. de, Kochva, E. (Eds.): Toxins of Animal and Plant Origin, Vol. I. New York: Gordon and Breach 1972a

Condrea, E., Fajnholc, N., Vries, A. de: Activation of enzymes in red blood cell membranes by a basic protein isolated from cobra venom (Abstract). Toxicon **10**, 526 (1972b)

Condrea, A., Kendzersky, I., Vries, A. de: Binding of Ringhals venom direct hemolytic factor to erythrocytes and osmotic ghosts of various animal species. Experientia (Basel) **21**, 461—462 (1965)

Condrea, E., Mammon, Z., Aloof, S., Vries, A. de: Susceptibility of erythrocytes of various animal species to the hemolytic and phospholipid splitting action of snake venom. Biochim. biophys. Acta (Amst.) **84**, 365—375 (1964b)

Condrea, E., Vries, A. de: Venom phospholipase A: a review. Toxicon **2**, 261—273 (1965)

Condrea, E., Vries, A. de, Mager, J.: Hemolysis and splitting of human erythrocyte phospholipids by snake venom. Biochim. biophys. Acta (Amst.) **84**, 60—73 (1964a)

Cottrell, T. S., Levine, O. R., Senior, R. M., Wieber, J., Spiro, D., Fishman, A. P.: Electron microscopic alterations at the alveolar level in pulmonary edema. Circulation Res. **21**, 783—798 (1967)

Crunkhorn, P., Willis, A. L.: Cutaneous reactions to intradermal prostaglandins. Brit. J. Pharmacol. **41**, 49—56 (1971)

Danon, D., Gitter, S., Rosen, M.: Deformation of red cell shape induced by *Vipera palestinae* venom in vivo. Nature (Lond.) **189**, 320—321 (1961)

Davey, M. G., Lüscher, E. F.: Actions of thrombin and other coagulant and proteolytic enzymes on blood platelets. Nature (Lond.) **216**, 857—858 (1967)

Doery, H. M.: The separation and properties of the neurotoxins from the venom of the tiger snake *Notechis scutatus scutatus*. Biochem. J. **70**, 535—543 (1958)

Eakins, K. E., Miller, J. D., Karim, S. M. M.: The nature of the prostaglandin-blocking activity of polyphloretin phosphate. J. Pharmacol. exp. Ther. **176**, 441—447 (1971)

Emery, J. A., Russell, F. E.: Lethal and hemorrhagic properties of some North American snake venoms. In: Keegan, H. L., Macfarlane, W. V. (Eds.): Venomous and Poisonous Animals and Noxious Plants of the Pacific Area. Oxford-London-New York-Paris: Pergamon Press 1963

Ferencz, C.: Pulmonary arterial design in mammals. Johns Hopk. med. J. **125**, 207—222 (1969)

Ferreira, S. H., Moncada, S., Parsons, M., Vane, J. R.: The concomitant release of bradykinin and prostaglandin in the inflammatory response to carrageenin. Brit. J. Pharmacol. **52**, 1081—1097 (1974)

Ferreira, S. H., Vane, J. R.: New aspects of the mode of action of nonsteroid anti-inflammatory drugs. Ann. Rev. Pharmacol. **14**, 57—73 (1974)

Flower, R. J.: Drugs which inhibit prostaglandin biosynthesis. Pharmacol. Rev. **26**, 33—67 (1974)

Formanek, K., Kreil, G.: Charakterisierung der entzündungserregenden Wirkung des Melittins, seines C-terminalen Fragments und einiger basischer Peptide an Rattenpfoten. Arzneimittel-Forsch. **25**, 1783—1786 (1975)

Fredholm, B., Haegermark, Ö.: Histamine release from rat mast cell granules induced by bee venom fractions. Acta physiol. scand. **71**, 357—367 (1967)

Fries, B.: The edema-inhibiting action of polyphloretin phosphate (PPP) in some type of capillary damage. An experimental investigation. Acta chir. scand. **119**, 1—7 (1960)

Fryklund, L., Eaker, D.: Complete amino acid sequence of a non-neurotoxic hemolytic protein from the venom of *Hemachatus haemachatus* (African Ringhals cobra). Biochemistry **12**, 661—667 (1973)

Fulton, G.P., Lutz, B.R., Shulman, M.H., Arendt, K.A.: Moccasin venom as a test for susceptibility to petechial formation in the hamster. In.: Buckley, E. E., Porges, N. (Eds.): Venoms, Vol. 44. Washington, D.C.: Publ. Am. Assoc. Adv. Sci. 1956

Gabbiani, G., Badonnel, M. C., Gervasoni, C., Portmann, B., Majno, G.: Carbon deposition in bronchial and pulmonary vessels in response to vasoactive compounds. Proc. Soc. exp. Biol. (N.Y.) **140**, 958—962 (1972)

Gastpar, H.: Heparin: Physiologische Bedeutung und pharmakologische Wirkungen des Heparins. In: Thrombosis et Diathesis Haemorrhagica, Suppl. 16. Stuttgart: Schattauer Verlag 1965

Glenn, M. E.: Adjuvant-induced arthritis: Effects of certain drugs on incidence clinical severity and biochemical changes. Am. J. Vet. Res. **27**, 339—352 (1966)

Goodman, L. S., Gilman, A.: The Pharmacological Basis of Therapeutics, 4th Ed. New York: MacMillan 1975

Greaves, M. W., McDonald-Gibson, W.: Inhibition of prostaglandin biosynthesis by corticosteroids. Brit. med. J. **1972 II**, 83—84

Greenbaum, L. M., Kim, K. S.: The kinin-forming and kininase activities of rabbit polymorphonuclear leucocytes. Brit. J. Pharmacol. **29**, 238—247 (1967)

Gregorio, E. A., Ação dos venenos de cobras *Naja naja* e *Agkistrodon piscivorus* e de alguns de seus componentes purificados sobre a microcirculação pulmonar do cão. Thesis. Ribeirao Preto (SP), Brazil, 1977

Gross, P., Pfitzer, E. A., Tolker, E., Babyak, M. A., Kaschak, M.: Experimental emphysema. Arch. environm. Hlth. **11**, 50—58 (1965)

Habermann, E.: Zur Toxicologie und Pharmakologie des Gasbrandgiftes (*Clostridium welchii* Type A) und seine Componenten. Naunyn-Schmiedebergs Arch. exp. Path. Pharmak. **238**, 502—524 (1960)

Habermann, E.: Recent studies on *Hymenopfera* venoms. In: Randonat, H. W. (Ed.): Recent Advances in the Pharmacology of Toxins. Oxford: Pergamon Press 1965

Habermann, E.: Über Gefäßpermeabilität und Hämorrhagie: Mechanismen und potentielle Mediatoren. Med. Welt **25**, 25—28 (1974)

Habermann, E., Breithaupt, H.: MCL-Peptide, a selectively mastocytolytic factor isolated from bee venom. Naunyn-Schmiedebergs Arch. Pharmak. exp. Path. **260**, 127—128 (1968)

Habermann, E., Neumann, W. P.: Crotactin, ein neues pharmakologisches Wirkprinzip aus dem Gift von *Crotalus terrificus*. Naunyn-Schmiedebergs Arch. exp. Path. Pharmak. **228**, 217—219 (1956)

Halpern, B. N., Liacopoulos, P., Liacopoulos-Briot, M.: Recherches sur les substances exogènes et endogènes agissant sur la perméabilité capillaire et leurs antagonistes. Arch. int. Pharmacodyn. **119**, 56—101 (1959)

Hamberg, U., Rocha e Silva, M.: Release of bradykinin as related to the esterase activity of trypsin and of venom of *B. jararaca*. Experientia (Basel) **13**, 489—490 (1957)

Hempel, K. H., Fernandez, L. A., Persellin, R. H.: Effect of pregnancy sera on isolated lysosomes. Nature (Lond.) **225**, 955—956 (1970)

Higginbotham, R. D., Karnella, S.: The significance of the mast cell response to bee venom. J. Immunol. **106**, 233—240 (1971)

Higgs, G. A., Youlten, L. J. F.: Prostaglandin production by rabbit peritoneal polymorphonuclear leucocytes in vitro. Brit. J. Pharmacol. **44**, 330 p (1972)

Högberg, B., Üvnas, B.: Inhibitory action of allicin on degranulation of mast cells produced by compound 48/80, histamine liberator from Ascaris, lecithinase A, and antigen. Acta physiol. scand. **44**, 157—162 (1958)

Homma, M., Tu, A. T.: Morphology of local tissue damage in experimental snake envenomation. Brit. J. exp. Path. **52**, 538—542 (1971)

Ichikawa, A., Nagasaki, M., Umezu, K., Hayashi, H., Tomita, K.: Effect of cyclic 3',5'-monophosphate on oedema and granuloma induced by carrageenin. Biochem. Pharmacol. **21**, 2615—2626 (1972)

Ignarro, L. J., George, W. J.: Hormonal control of lysosomal enzyme release from human neutrophils. Elevation of cyclic nucleotide levels by autonomic neurohormones. Proc. nat. Acad. Sci. (Wash.) **71**, 2027—2031 (1974)

Ishioka, T., Honda, Y., Sagara, A., Shimamoto, T.: The effect of oestrogens on blueing lesions by bradykinine and histamine. Acta endocr. (Kbh.) **60**, 177—183 (1969)

Izard, Y., Boquet, P., Golemi, E., Goupil, D.: La toxins *gamma* n'est pas le facteur lytique direct du venin de *Naja nigricollis*. C.R. Acad. Sci. (Paris) **269**, 666—667 (1969 b)

Izard, Y., Boquet, M., Ronsseray, A. M., Boquet, P.: Isolement d'une protéine toxique du venin de *Naja nigricollis*: la toxine *gamma*. C.R. Acad. Sci [D] (Paris) **269**, 96—97 (1969 a)

Jiménez-Porras, J. M.: Pharmacology of peptides and proteins in snake venoms. Ann. Rev. Pharmacol. **8**, 299—318 (1968)

Jiménez-Porras, J. M.: Biochemistry of snake venoms (Review). Clin. Toxicol. **3**, 389—431 (1970)

Kaiser, E., Kramar, L., Lambrechter, R.: The action of direct lytic agents from animal venoms on cells and isolated cell fractions. In: Vries, A. de, Kochva, E. (Eds.): Toxins of Animal and Plant Origin, Vol. II. New York: Gordon and Breach 1972

Kaley, G., Weiner, R.: Prostaglandin E_1: A potential mediator of the inflammatory response. Ann. N.Y. Acad. Sci. **180**, 338—349 (1971)

Karnovsky, M. J.: Morphology of capillaries with special reference to muscle capillaries. In: Crome, C., Lassen, N. A. (Eds.): Capillary Permeability, pp. 341—350. New York: Academic Press 1970

Klibansky, C., London, Y., Frenkel, A., Vries, A. de: Enhancing action of synthetic and natural basic polypeptides on erythrocyte-ghost phospholipid hydrolysis by phospholipase-A. Biochim. biophys. Acta (Amst.) **150**, 15—23 (1968)

Klibansky, Ch., Özcan, E., Joshua, H., Djaldetti, M.: Intravascular hemolysis in dogs induced by *Echis coloratus* venom. Toxicon **3**, 213—221 (1966)

Kirschmann, Ch., Condrea, E., Moav, N., Aloof, S., Vries, A. de: Action of snake venom on human platelet phospholipids. Arch. int. Pharmacodyn. **150**, 372—378 (1964)

Kunze, H., Vogt, W.: Significance of phospholipase-A for prostaglandin formation. Ann. N.Y. Acad. Sci. **180**, 123—125 (1971)

Lai, M. K., Wen, C. Y., Lee, C. Y.: Local lesions caused by cardiotoxin isolated from Formosan cobra venom. J. Formosan med. Ass. **71**, 328—332 (1972)

Larsen, P. R., Wolff, J.: The basic proteins of cobra venom. J. biol. Chem. **243**, 1283—1289 (1968)

Lee, C.Y.: Mode of action of cobra venom and its purified toxins. In: Simpson, L. (Ed.): Neuropoisons: Their Pathophysiological Actions, Vol. I. New York: Plenum Press 1971

Lee, C. Y.: Chemistry and pharmacology of polypeptide toxins in snake venoms. Ann. Rev. Pharmacol. **12**, 265—286 (1972)

Lee, C. Y.: Chemistry and pharmacology of purified toxins from elapid and sea snake venoms. Pharmacology and the Future of Man. Proc. 5th Int. Congr. Pharmacol., San Francisco, 1972, Vol. II, pp. 210—232. Basel: Karger 1973

Lee, C. Y., Chang, C. C., Chiu, T. H., Chiu, P. S., Tseng, T. C., Lee, S. Y.: Pharmacological properties of cardiotoxin isolated from Formosan cobra venom. Naunyn-Schmiedebergs Arch. Pharmak. exp. Path. **259**, 360—374 (1968)

Lee, C. Y., Lin, J. S., Wei, J. W.: Identification of cardiotoxin with cobramine B, DLF, Toxin γ, and cobra venom cytotoxin. In: Vries, A. de, Kochva, E. (Eds.): Toxins of Animal and Plant Origin, pp. 307—318. New York: Gordon and Breach 1970

Lerner, L. J., Carminati, P., Schiatti, P.: Correlation of anti-inflammatory activity with inhibition of prostaglandin synthesis activity of non-steroidal anti-estrogens and estrogens. Proc. Soc. exp. Biol. (N.Y.) **148**, 329—332 (1975)

Lewis, G. P., Piper, P. J.: Inhibition of release of prostaglandins as an explanation of some of the actions of anti-inflammatory corticosteroids. Nature (Lond.) **254**, 308—311 (1975)

Logan, G., Wilhelm, D. L.: Ultra-violet injury as an experimental model of the inflammatory reaction. Nature (Lond.) **198**, 968—969 (1963)

Ludwig, H.: Weibliche Hormone-Oestrogene und Haemostase. Thrombos. Diathes. haemorrh. (Stuttg.) (Suppl.) **19**, 223 (1966)

Luft, J. H.: Capillary permeability I. Structural considerations. In: Zweifach, B. W., Grand, L., McClusky, R. T. (Eds.): The Inflammatory Process, Vol. II. New York-London: Academic Press 1973

Machado, D. C., Böhm, G. M., Padovan, P. A.: Comparative study of the ultrastructural alterations of vessels of the pulmonary circulation of rats treated with alpha-naphthyl-thiourea (ANTU) and ammonium sulphate. J. Path. Bact. **121**, 205—211 (1977)

McKay, D. G., Moroz, C., Vries, A. de, Csavosay, I., Crusa, V.: The action of hemorrhagin and phospholipase derived from *Vipera palestinae* venom on the microcirculation. Lab. Invest. **22**, 387—399 (1970)

Majno, G.: Ultrastructure of the vascular membrane. In: Hamilton, H. E. (Ed.): Handbook of Physiology, Vol. III. Baltimore: Williams and Wilkins 1965

Majno, G., Palade, G. E., Schoefel, G. I.: Studies on inflammation. II. The site of action of histamine and serotonin along the vascular tree: a topographic study. J. biophys. biochem. Cytol. **11**, 607—626 (1961)

Mandelbaum, F. R.: Isolamento e caracterizção de dois fatores hemorrágicos do veneno de *Bothrops jararaca*, Thesis, Escola Paulista de Medicina, São Paulo, 1976

Mandelbaum, F. R., Castro, T. A. M., Assakura, M. T., Aldred, N.: Biochemical aspects of hemorrhagic factors isolated from *Bothrops jararaca* venom. Proc. 5th Intern. Congr. of Pharmacology. San Francisco, p. 148, 1972

Mohamed, A. H., Nawar, N. N. Y., Mohamed, F. A.: Effects of hydrocortisone and polyvalent antivenin on the histological changes in the lung after *Naja nigricollis* envenomation. Toxicon **11**, 181—183 (1973)

Mueller, M. N., Kappas, A.: Estrogen pharmacology II. Suppression of experimental immune polyarthritis. Proc. Soc. exp. Biol. (N.Y.) **117**, 845—847 (1964)

Murata, Y., Satake, M., Suzuki, T.: Studies on snake venom. XII. Distribution of proteinase activities among Japanese and Formosan snake venoms. J. Biochem. (Tokyo) **53**, 431—437 (1963)

Nachman, R. L., Weksler, B.: The platelet as an inflammatory cell. Ann. N.Y. Acad. Sci. **201**, 131—137 (1972)

Nahas, L., Denson, K. W. E., Macfarlane, R. G.: A study of the coagulant action of eight snake venoms. Thrombos. Diathes. haemorrh. (Stuttg.) **12**, 355—367 (1964)

Nazarov, G. F., Petrischev, N. N.: The influence of heparin on the vascular permeability disturbed by histamine. Byull. éksp. Biol. Med. **65**, 58—60 (in Russian) (1968)

Ohsaka, A., Just, M., Habermann, E.: Action of snake venom hemorrhagic principles on isolated glomerular basement membrane. Biochim. biphys. Acta (Amst.) **323**, 415—428 (1973)

Ohsaka, A., Ohashi, M., Tsuchiya, M., Kamisaka, Y., Fujishiro, Y.: Action of *Trimeresurus flavoviridis* venom on the microcirculatory system of rat; dynamic aspects as revealed by cinephotomicrographic recording. Jap. J. med. Sci. Biol. **24**, 34—39 (1971)

Ohsaka, A., Takahashi, T., Omori-Satoh, T., Murata, R.: Purification and characterization of the hemorrhagic principles in the venom of *Trimeresurus flavoviridis*. In: Toxins of Animal and Plant Origin, Vol. I, Paper III-12. London: Gordon and Breach 1972

Orr, T. S. C., Cox, J. S. G.: Disodium cromoglycate, an inhibitor of mast cell degranulation and histamine release induced by phospholipase A. Nature (Lond.) **223**, 197—198 (1969)

Ownby, C. L., Kainer, R. A., Tu, A. T.: Pathogenesis of hemorrhage induced by rattlesnake venom. Amer. J. Path. **76**, 401—414 (1974)

Persellin, R. H., Perry, A.: Effect of pregnancy serum on experimental inflammation. Clin. Res. **20**, 49 (1972)

Pietra, G. G., Szidon, J. P., Leventhal, M. M., Fishman, A. P.: Histamine and interstitial pulmonary edema in the dog. Circulation Res. **29**, 323—337 (1971)

Porges, N.: Snake venoms, their biochemistry and mode of action. Science **117**, 47—51 (1953)

Rocha e Silva, M.: The possible kinin function in the acute inflammatory reaction. Pharmacology and the future of man. Proc. 5th Int. Congr. Pharmacol. San Francisco Vol. **V**, pp. 320—327, Basel: Karger 1973

Rocha e Silva, M., Cavalcanti, R. G., Reis, M. L.: Anti-inflammatory action of sulphated polysaccharides. Biochem. Pharmacol. **18**, 1285—1295 (1969)

Rocha e Silva, M., Garcia-Leme, J.: Chemical Mediators of the Acute Inflammatory Reaction. New York: Pergamon Press 1972

Rona, G.: The role of vascular mucopolysaccharides in the hemostatic action of oestrogens. Amer. J. Obstet. Gynec. **87**, 434—444 (1963)

Rosa, M., di, Giroud, J. P., Willoughby, D. A.: Studies of the mediators of the acute inflammatory response induced in rats in different sites by carrageenan and turpentine. J. Path. Bact. **104**, 15—29 (1971)

Rothschild, A. M.: Histamine release by bee venom phospholipase A and melittin in the rat. Brit. J. Pharmacol. **25**, 59—66 (1965)

Russell, F. E., Puffer, H. W.: Pharmacology of snake venoms. Clin. Toxicol. **3**, 433—444 (1970)

Sandbank, U., Jerushalmy, Z., Ben-David, E., Vries, A. de: Effect of *Echis coloratus* venom on brain vessels. Toxicon **12**, 267—271 (1974)

Sanner, J. H.: Antagonism of prostaglandin-E_2 by 1-acetyl-2-(8-chloro-10,11-dihydrodibenz b,f oxazepine-10-carbonyl) hydrazine (SC-19220). Arch. int. Pharmacodyn. **180**, 46—56 (1969)

Schiff, M., Burn, H. F.: The effect of intravenous estrogens on ground substance. Arch. Otolaryng. **73**, 43—51 (1961)

Schneeberger, E., Karnovsky, M. J.: The influence of intravascular fluid volume on the permeability of newborn and adult mouse lung to ultrastructural protein tracers. J. Cell Biol. **49**, 319—334 (1971)

Schroeter, R., Damerau, B., Vogt, W.: Differences in binding of the direct lytic factor (DLF) of cobra venom *Naja naja*) to intact red cells and ghosts. Naunyn-Schmiedebergs Arch. Pharmacol. **280**, 201—207 (1973)

Selye, H.: From Dream to Discovery: On Being a Scientist, p. 223. New York: McGraw-Hill 1964

Sessa, G., Freer, J. H., Colacicco, G., Weissmann, G.: Interaction of a lytic polypeptide, melittin, with lipid membrane systems. J. biol. Chem. **244**, 3575—3582 (1969)

Sharma, R. C., Gupta, S. K., Gupta, L.: Oestrogenic activity of some chalkone epoxides and formyldeoxybenzoins in mice and their structure activity relationship. Indian J. exp. Biol. **10**, 455—456 (1972)

Slotta, K. H., Gonzales, J. D., Roth, S. C.: The direct and indirect hemolytic factors from animal venoms. In: Russell, F. E., Sanders, P. R. (Eds.): Animal Toxins. Oxford: Pergamon Press 1967

Spact, T. H.: Microscopic studies on blood vessels of rats with experimental purpose. Amer. J. Physiol. **170**, 333 (1952)

Spangler, A. S., Antoniades, H. N., Slotman, S. L.: Enhancement of the anti-inflammatory action of hydrocortisone by estrogen. J. clin. Endocr. **29**, 650—655 (1969)

Staub, N. C.: Pulmonary edema. Physiol. Rev. **54**, 678—811 (1974)

Suzuki, T.: Pharmacologically and biochemically active components of Japanese ophidian venoms. Mem. Inst. Butantan Simp. Intern. **33**(2), 519—522 (1966)

Szego, C. M., Davis, J. S.: Adenosine 3′5′ monophosphate in rat uterus. Acute elevation by estrogen. Proc. nat. Acad. Sci. (Wash.) **58**, 1711—1718 (1967)

Takahashi, T., Ohsaka, A.: Purification and some properties of two hemorrhagic principles (HR_{2a} and HR_{2b}) in the venom of *Trimeresurus flavoviridis;* complete separation of the principles from proteolytic activity. Biochim. biophys. Acta (Amst.) **207**, 65—75 (1970)

Toivanen, P., Maatta, K., Suolanen, R., Tykkylainen, R.: Effect of estrone and progesterone on adjuvant arthritis in rats. Med. Pharmacol. **17**, 33—42 (1967)

Tsuchiya, M., Ohshio, C., Ohashi, M., Ohsaka, A., Suzuki, K., Fujishiro, Y.: Cinematographic and electron microscopic analyses of the hemorrhage induced by the main hemorrhagic principle, HR 1, isolated from the venom of *Trimeresurus flavoviridis*. In: Didishum, P., Shimamoto, T., Yamasaki, H. (Eds.): Platelets, Thrombosis, and Inhibitors, pp. 439—446. Stuttgart-New York: F. K. Schattauer Verlag 1974

Üvnas, B., Diamant, B., Högberg, B.: Trigger action of phospholipase A on mast cells. Arch. int. Pharmacodyn. **140**, 577—580 (1962)

Vane, J. R.: Inhibition of prostaglandin synthesis as a mechanism of action for aspirin-like drugs. Nature (Lond.) New Biol. **231**, 232—235 (1971)

Vargaftig, B. B.: Aspects of release of pharmacologically active substances from the lungs by chemical stimuli. Agents Actions **6**, 551—557 (1976)

Vargaftig, B. B., Bhargava, N., Bonta, I. L.: Haemorrhagic and permeability increasing effects of *Bothrops jararaca* and other Crotalidae venoms as related to amine or kinin release. Agents Actions **4**, 163—168 (1974)

Vargaftig, B. B., Lefort, J., Giroux, E. L.: Haemorrhagic and inflammatory properties of collagenase from *C. histolyticum*. Agents Actions **6**, 627—635 (1976)

Vincent, J. E., Bonta, I. L., Noordhoek, J.: Some effects of guinea pig serum and heparin on hemolysis induced by *Naja naja*, *Agkistrodon piscivorus*, and *Apis mellifera* venom. Toxicon **10**, 415—417 (1972)

Vincent, J. E., Bonta, I. L., Vries-Kragt, K. de, Bhargava, N.: L'influence des oestrogènes sur la perméabilité de la paroi vasculaire. Steroidologia **1**, 367—377 (1971)

Vinegar, R., Macklin, A. W., Truax, J. F., Selph, J. L.; Formation of pedal edema in normal and granulocytopenic rats. In: Arman, G. G. van (Ed.): White Cells in Inflammation, pp. 111—138. Springfield: Charles C. Thomas 1974

Vogel, G., Marek, M. L.: On the inhibition of various rat paw edemas by serotonin antogonists. Arzneimittel-Forsch. **11**, 356 (1961)

Vries, A. de, Kirschmann, Ch., Klibansky, Ch., Condrea, E., Gitter, S.: Hemolytic action of indirect lytic snake venom in vivo. Toxicon **1**, 19—23 (1962)

Weibel, E. R.: Morphological basis of alveolar-capillary gas exchange. Physiol. Rev. **53**, 419—495 (1973)

Weissmann, G., Rita, G. A.: Molecular basis of gouty inflammation. Interaction of monosodium urate crystals with lysosomes and liposomes. Nature (Lond.) New Biol. **240**, 167—172 (1972)

Wojtecka-Lukasik, E., Dancewicz, A. M.: Inhibition of human leucocyte collagenase by some drugs used in the therapy of rheumatic diseases. Biochem. Pharmac. **23**, 2077—2081 (1974)

Zlotkin, E.: Chemistry of animal venoms. Experientia (Basel) **29**, 1453—1466 (1973)

Zwisler, O.: The role of enzymes in the processes responsible for the toxicity of snake venoms (an immunological study). Mem. Inst. Butantan Simp. Intern. **33**(1), 281—289 (1966)

CHAPTER 18

Snake Venoms and Blood Coagulation

W. H. SEEGERS and C. OUYANG

A. Blood Coagulation Mechanisms

Certain snake venoms modify the blood coagulation system as well as the physiology of hemostasis. Our knowledge in this field of study has advanced appreciably so that deleterious effects of venoms can often be abated, and, in addition, venoms have been used as therapeutic agents. Furthermore, in the development of our knowledge of blood coagulation, venoms proved to be useful agents for clarifying some basic concepts. Thus, EAGLE (1937) used venoms for obtaining data used as a basis for emphasizing that blood coagulation is primarily a function involving enzymes. It is clear from reading some of the older general presentations such as the ones by BOQUET (1964), MEAUME (1966), JIMÉNEZ-PORRAS (1968, 1970), DENSON (1969), and others that an understanding of the blood coagulation system is a prerequisite to an account of the effects of snake venoms in that system. With due allowance for the limitations of facts related to blood coagulation, we shall first make a survey of the nature of the basic chemistry. Since even minimal coverage of literature references would require numerous pages, only a few are cited as convenient introductions to the vast literature. Some general ones follow: GULLIVER (1846), QUICK (1942), JORPES (1946), OWREN (1947), SEEGERS and SHARP (1948), DEUTSCH (1955), HEILBRUN (1956), SCHERAGA and LASKOWSKI (1957), MORAWITZ (1958), RATNOFF (1960), JOHNSON et al. (1961), MACMILLAN and MUSTARD (1961), DOUGLAS (1962), SEEGERS (1962), HOUGIE (1963), VON KAULLA (1963), TOCANTINS and KAZAL (1964), FEARNLEY (1965), HARDISTY and INGRAM (1965), HECHT (1965), JOHNSON and GREENWALT (1965), MARCUS and ZUCKER (1965), MCKAY (1965), SAWYER (1965), BIGGS and MACFARLANE (1966), HARDAWAY (1966), SELYE (1966), SEEGERS (1967a, b), HAGEN et al. (1968), LAKI (1968), SEEGERS et al. (1968), HEMKER et al. (1969), JOHNSON and GUEST (1969), MAUPIN (1969), OWEN et al. (1969), POLLER (1969), SEEGERS (1969), BANG et al. (1971), BOWIE et al. (1971), BRINKHOUS and SHERMER (1971), JOHNSON (1971), BIGGS (1972), SEEGERS (1973a, b), BALDINI and EBBE (1974), MURANO (1974), SHERRY and SCRIABINE (1974), WINTROBE (1974), BRADSHAW and WESSLER (1975), DAVIE and FUJIKAWA (1975), LORAND and ROBBINS (1975), and SEEGERS et al. (1975).

I. Blood Coagulation Nomenclature

Each speciality in scientific work practically has its own language and in the field of blood coagulation, plasma components have been given Roman numerals to serve as an equivalent to diverse common names. Platelet factors are given Arabic numbers.

Quite possibly, in due course, the numbers will drop as a common name becomes well-recognized and advanced through repetitive use. Even now fibrinogen is rarely called Factor I, while prothrombin was named many decades before Factor II became a new name for it, and why call calcium ions Factor IV? Thus, the list below is given for purposes of convenience.

Factor I	Fibrinogen
Factor II	Prothrombin
Factor III	Thromboplastin, tissue factor
Factor IV	Calcium ions
Factor V	Ac-globulin, labile factor, proaccelerin
Factor VI	Not verified
Factor VII	Cothromboplastin, stable factor, proconvertin, serum prothrombin conversion accelerator (SPCA)
Factor VIII	Antihemophilic factor or globulin, platelet Cofactor I, hemophilia A factor, thromboplastinogen
Factor IX	Antihemophilia B factor, autoprothrombin II, Christmas factor, platelet Cofactor II
Factor X	Autoprothrombin III, Auto-III, Stuart-Prower factor, prothrombokinase
Factor XI	Plasma thromboplastin antecedent (PTA), antihemophilic factor C
Factor XII	Hageman factor, glass factor, contact factor
Factor XIII	Fibrinoligase, plasma transglutaminase, fibrinstabilizing factor
Factor XIV	Protein C, autoprothrombin II-A

The above system has been expanded to designate active enzymes as follows: Factor IIa (thrombin), Factor IXa, Factor Xa (autoprothrombin C, thrombokinase), and variants have been indicated. For example, Factor Xa^{Cit} means activity was generated in 25% sodium citrate solution. Other active forms are Factor XIa and Factor XIIIa. It is not correct to write Factor Va because no enzyme activation occurs when thrombin potentiates the activity of Factor V, and the same seems to be true for Factor VIIIa.

II. Three Basic Reactions of Blood Coagulation

Blood coagulation can be regarded as a cybernetic system. Some of the controlling components consist of positive and negative feedback, retarded chain reactions, multiple enzyme involvement, apparent stoichiometric reactions, and integration with organ function. It is convenient to consider inhibitors last, and begin by dividing the system into three basic events or reactions as follows:

1. the formation of autoprothrombin C (Factor Xa);
2. the formation of thrombin;
3. the formation of fibrin.

These reactions, in which fibrin forms and the activity of two enzymes develops, most likely occur in sequence with each successive one depending upon the preceding one as follows:

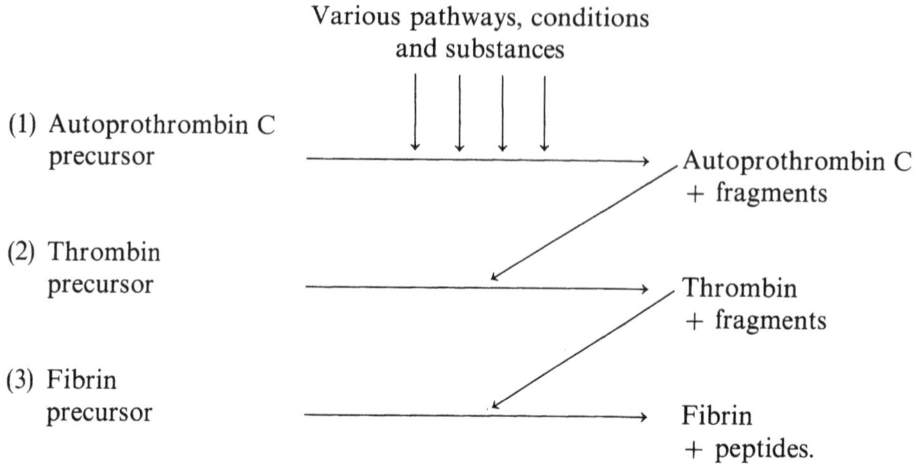

III. Formation of Fibrin

The fibrinogen of plasma, with a molecular weight near 340000 and having three distinct polypeptide chains, undergoes limited proteolysis by thrombin. The process removes fibrinopeptide A (or two variants AY, AP) and fibrinopeptide B from each fibrinogen molecule, which amounts to about 3% of the large molecule. The fibrinopeptides are removed from the $A\alpha$- and $B\beta$-chains of fibrinogen, but nothing is removed from the γ-chain (BLOMBÄCK and YAMASHINA, 1958). Each one of the three chains of fibrinogen is duplicated in the fibrinogen molecule. The work of thrombin can thus be represented by a diagram (Fig. 1) and as follows:

$$(A\alpha \cdot B\beta \cdot \gamma)_2 \xrightarrow{\text{Thrombin}} (\alpha \cdot \beta \cdot \gamma)_2 + 2A + 2B$$
$$\downarrow$$
$$[(\alpha \cdot \beta \cdot \gamma)_2]_n .$$

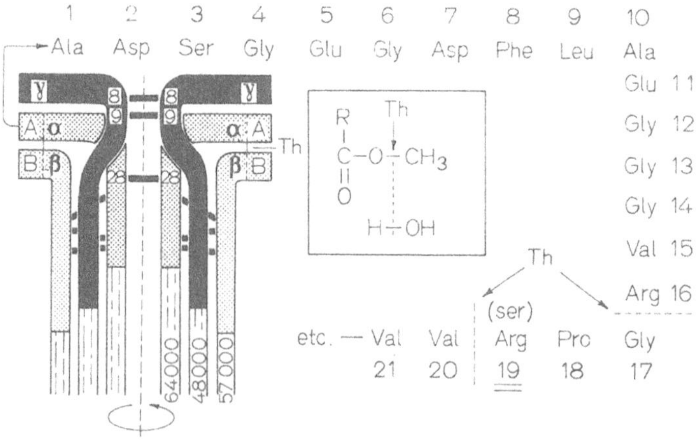

Fig. 1. Illustrating three chains of fibrinogen linked by disulfide bonds. Removal of fibrinopeptides A and B is indicated. Primary structure of peptide A is given plus the residues of interest in fibrinogen Detroit. In that dysfibrinogenemia there is an amino acid substitution at position 19. Model based on work of BLOMBÄCK

The fibrinogen, without fibrinopeptides, is referred to as a fibrin monomer and by a process of self-assembly, the monomer forms polymers. The molecules align end-to-end and side-to-side, and the fibrin has interconnecting branches. The resulting gel is of variable strength and consistency depending primarily upon the concentration of the protein and pH of the reaction. The rate of fibrin formation is dependent on pH, ionic strength of the medium, fibrinogen concentration, thrombin concentration, calcium ion concentration, temperature, and many other variables (SEEGERS and SMITH, 1942). All of these, except thrombin, are held more or less constant in the physiologic environment. Consequently, thrombin concentration is the main determinant for rate of fibrin formation, the highest concentrations being associated with the most rapid clotting. Calcium ions accelerate the clotting of fibrinogen but are not necessary. Platelets contain a substance known as platelet Factor 2 (WARE et al., 1948) which has the property of shortening the clotting time of plasma or fibrinogen. It is apparently a proteolytic enzyme. Thrombin tends to adsorb on fibrin, and fibrinogen decomposition products resulting from fibrinolysis not only retard the formation of fibrin, but an abnormal fibrin forms because of the random incorporation of some of the decomposition products.

IV. Cross-Linking of Fibrin

Artificial fibrin obtained by clotting purified fibrinogen with purified thrombin has several characteristics that distinguish it from the true or genuine fibrin obtained from whole blood clots (ROBBINS, 1944). The main property generally featured is solubility in urea as a characteristic of fibrin from purified systems (fibrin-*s*) and

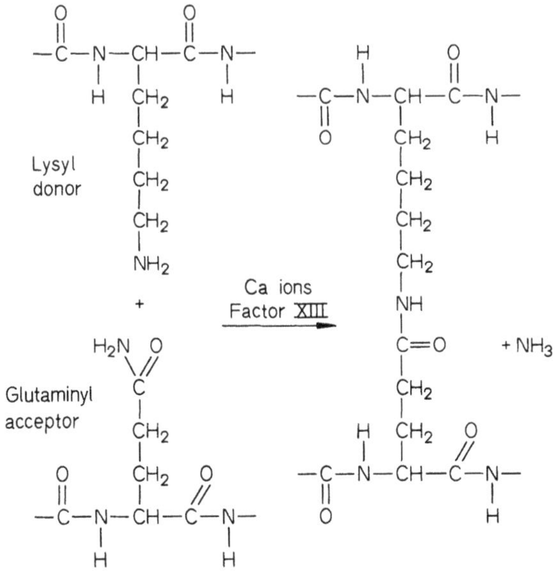

Fig. 2. The cross-linking reaction by activated Factor XIII consists of the formation of a peptide bond involving lysine residues as donors and glutamine residues as acceptors. Free ammonia forms

insolubility for the fibrin (fibrin-*i*) from the natural clot. The conversion of fibrin-*s* to fibrin-*i* is brought about by the cross-linking enzyme of plasma (LAKI and LORAND, 1948). It functions after it has been converted by thrombin and/or autoprothrombin C to its active form (Factor XIIIa). The enzyme forms peptide bonds between preferred glutamic acid and lysine residues (Fig. 2). Platelets also contain fibrinoligase in the inactive form, and crystals of this enzyme precursor have been obtained from platelet sources. The concentration of the enzyme in serum is low for reasons not clearly delineated. In clot retraction, for which whole platelets are necessary, the cross-linked fibrin retracts less readily than the other. The formation of cross-linked fibrin can be indicated as follows:

$$\begin{array}{c}\text{Factor XIII}\\ \downarrow \text{Thrombin}\end{array}$$

$$[(\alpha \cdot \beta \cdot \gamma)_2]_n \xrightarrow{\text{Factor XIIIa}} [(\alpha \cdot \beta \cdot \gamma)_2]_n^x + NH_3 .$$

Plasma Factor XIII, with a molecular weight of 340000, is composed of two pairs of nonidentical polypeptide chains A and B. The respective molecular weights are 75000 and 88000. The formula for the tetramer can be written as A_2B_2. The A chains contain the catalytic function and are the only chains found in the crystalline protein obtained from platelets. Activation occurs in two steps as follows:

$$A_2B_2 \xrightarrow{\text{Thrombin}} \begin{array}{c}A'_2B_2\\ +\\ \text{2 Peptides}\end{array} \xrightarrow{Ca^{2+}} \begin{array}{c}A'_2\\ +\\ B_2 .\end{array}$$

The A'_2B_2 structure is not active, but dissociation occurs in the presence of calcium ions. An active center A'—SH is unmasked to give the active protein while the B chains then no longer serve as carriers.

V. Formation of Thrombin

About half of the prothrombin molecule is needed for the thrombin structure (SEEGERS et al., 1950). For many years, data completely supported the view that the formation of thrombin is a process in which prothrombin is degraded. It was only recently, however, that functions for the nonthrombin portion of prothrombin were found. It is the region where phospholipids, calcium ions, and Ac-globulin bind to form complexes, and thus make the activation process efficient. The binding sites in the prothrombin molecule are primarily provided by the recently discovered γ-carboxyglutamic acid residues at the NH_2 terminal region (STENFLO et al., 1974; MAGNUSSON et al., 1974; NELSESTUEN et al., 1974). Without vitamin K, an incomplete prothrombin is produced in which the corresponding residues are glutamic acid. Among the degradation fragments of prothrombin conversion to thrombin are accelerators (ESMON et al., 1974) and inhibitors (SEEGERS et al., 1974). The profragment 2 region is essential for the accelerator function of Ac-globulin (ESMON et al., 1974). Profragment 2 depresses the clotting function of thrombin, but enhances the esterase activity. Profragment 1 has the calcium binding sites of prothrombin and inhibits prothrombin activation. In the case of converting purified prethrombin 1 to

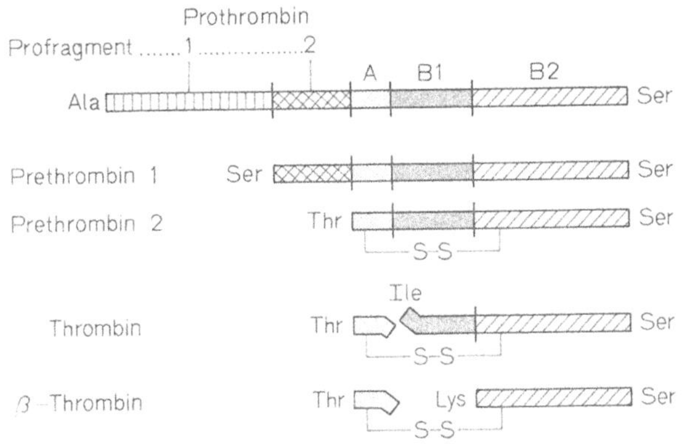

Fig. 3. The prothrombin molecule is represented as a single straight chain polypeptide divided into profragment 1, profragment 2, A, B 1, and B 2 segments. As drawn, the length of each segment is proportional to its molecular weight. Prothrombin is about 73000 and thrombin 38000. Profragment 1 segment is most easily removed from bovine prothrombin with thrombin. Profragment 2 is removed by autoprothrombin C. The latter enzyme breaks the Arg-Ile bond of prethrombin 1 to produce classic thrombin. By autolysis, involving loss of B 1 fragment from the B chain, thrombin E (β-thrombin) is formed. Thrombin has esterase and proteolytic activity while prethrombin 2 is inactive. Thrombin E has only esterase activity. In the literature, profragment 1·2 has been called PRO piece, fragment 1·2, F_x, C fragment, and nonthrombin portion. Profragment 1 has been called PR fragment, fragment 1, F_A, NH_2 terminal fragment, and intermediate 3. Profragment 2 has also been referred to as 0 fragment, fragment 2, F_B, inner fragment, intermediate 4, and 3·6 protein. The term prethrombin was introduced and used in this laboratory about a decade ago. This has been revised and expanded to prethrombin 1 and prethrombin 2

thrombin, the profragment 1 serves as an accelerator. It, therefore, functions just as well when separated from prothrombin as when attached. Depending upon species, profragment 1 accelerates or retards the clotting of whole blood.

Many years ago, it was incorrectly proposed that in addition to thrombin, Factors VII a, IX a, and X a were degradation products of a single molecule called prothrombin (SEEGERS, 1962). Today, there is evidence that Factors II, VII, IX, XIV, and X arose from a common ancestral gene by divergence, and in modern times, each one of the factors can be isolated separately from the prothrombin complex of plasma. Prothrombin has a higher molecular weight than Factors VII, IX, XIV, and X because of a partial gene duplication which took place after the five factors arose by divergence (HEWETT-EMMETT et al., 1974). Evidence has recently been presented for a sixth vitamin K-dependent protein.

Prothrombin is a single-chain polypeptide (mol wt = 73000) while thrombin is a two-chain structure in which the chains are connected by a disulfide bond. The systematic degradation of prothrombin is presented as a diagram (Fig. 3). Profragment 1 is removed by thrombin leaving prethrombin 1. Autoprothrombin C, but not thrombin, can remove profragment 2 leaving prethrombin 2. Alternatively, conditions can be arranged so that autoprothrombin C removes Fragment 1·2 directly to leave prethrombin 2, and this could very well be a main event when thrombin forms naturally. Prethrombin 2 is a single-chain structure with an amino acid composition and molecular weight equal to thrombin (Fig. 3). It is inactive. Between the 49th and 50th residues of the prethrombin 2 molecule is an Arg-Ile peptide bond that is broken by autoprothrombin C (Factor Xa) to yield thrombin. After breaking the Arg-Ile bond, the 49 amino acid residues remain bound to the longer polypeptide chain (B chain) by a disulfide bond. This structure is classic thrombin with esterase and coagulant activity and was first crystallized only recently (TSERNOGLOU et al., 1972). The A chain of human thrombin is 13 amino acid residues shorter at the NH_2 terminal end than the A chain of the bovine enzyme.

Thrombin slowly undergoes autolysis in an alkaline medium. This process is associated with a break in the B chain resulting in the loss of the B1 chain (73 amino acid residues). The B2 chain remains bound to the A chain by the disulfide bond. After autolysis of thrombin, only traces of coagulant activity remain (Fig. 3), while esterase activity exceeds that found before autolysis. The enzyme with only esterase activity is called thrombin E or β-thrombin.

For the conversion of prothrombin to classical thrombin, only autoprothrombin C (Factor Xa) is essential. The powerful enzyme is, nevertheless, not sufficiently active nor present in high enough concentration under physiologic conditions to function adequately. To compensate for this and to introduce control mechanisms, support is supplied from accessories; namely, plasma Ac-globulin (Factor V), calcium ions, and platelet phospholipids and/or protein-bound platelet phospholipids. A condensed equation for thrombin formation, recorded in two nomenclatures, follows:

$$\text{Prothrombin} \xrightarrow{\begin{array}{l}\text{Calcium ions}\\ \text{Platelet Factor 3}\\ \text{Ac-globulin}\\ \text{Autoprothrombin C}\end{array}} \text{Thrombin} + \text{Peptides}$$

$$\text{Factor II} \xrightarrow{\begin{array}{l}\text{Ca}^{2+}\\ \text{PF-3}\\ \text{Factor V}\\ \text{Factor Xa}\end{array}} \text{Factor IIa} + \text{Peptides.}$$

As an example, the system for studying the generation of thrombin activity was composed of purified components (SEEGERS et al., 1972a). These were entirely of bovine origin and consisted of purified prothrombin as substrate, purified autoprothrombin C as enzyme, purified Ac-globulin as determiner protein, a platelet factor 3 preparation, and calcium ions as follows:

Substance	*Concentration*	*Moles*[1]
Prothrombin	1000 U/ml	195
Autoprothrombin C	12 U/ml	1.00
Ac-globulin	50 U/ml	0.109
Phosphatidylserine	0.3 mg/ml	$7{,}86 \times 10^6$
Calcium ions	0.01 M	

[1] At half maximum velocity and these are tentative estimates.

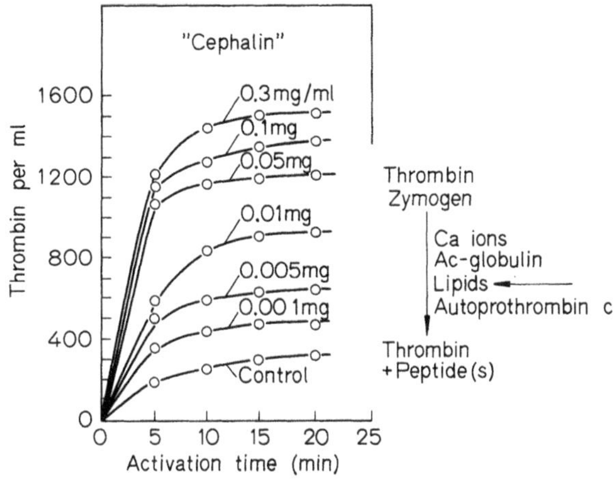

Fig. 4. Formation of thrombin from purified prothrombin with purified autoprothrombin C ($F = Xa_1$), purified Ac-globulin, and crude "cephalin." The latter can be replaced with platelet factor 3 preparations, released platelet factor 3, purified PI or PS, or certain bile salts. Note apparent stoichiometric effect associated with decrease in lipid concentration. The same effect is produced if any one of the "activator" components is reduced in concentration including calcium ions and prothrombin. This depicts the basis for quantitative analysis of all components in the reaction. Data of SEEGERS et al. (1972a)

The five-component system outlined above yielded all of the thrombin which was possible from the selected amount of prothrombin (Fig. 4). By reducing the concentration of platelet Factor 3 stepwise, the yield of thrombin was reduced. In like manner, every other component was studied. Reducing the prothrombin, autoprothrombin C, Ac-globulin, or calcium ion concentration stepwise was associated with a correspondingly reduced yield of thrombin. Thrombin initially makes Ac-globulin more active, but that is not a prerequisite for the function of Ac-globulin. On the basis of this complex way to obtain thrombin, at least five different deficiencies in thrombin formation are clearly possible; namely, a deficiency for prothrombin, for autoprothrombin III, for Ac-globulin, for platelet Factor 3, and for calcium ions. In addition, the apparent stoichiometric nature of the reaction is the basis for buffering the generation of thrombin activity.

Under physiologic conditions, platelets and/or thromboplastin are the source of phospholipids (protein-bound phospholipids or phospholipoproteins) and for physiologic purposes are essential, but experimental platelet substitution is quite possible for the generation of thrombin activity. The requirements are fulfilled by phosphatidylinositol and phosphatidyl-L-serine, but not very satisfactorily by phosphatidylethanolamine (β-γ-dipalmitoyl-DL-α-phosphatidylethanolamine) or phosphatidylcholine (BARTHELS and SEEGERS, 1969). Preparations of platelet as well as red cell membranes are effective (SEEGERS et al., 1972a). Certain bile salts are also effective at a concentration where micelles form. The approximate activity from highest to lowest was conjugated sodium salt of taurocholic acid, sodium cholate, sodium deoxycholate. Sodium dehydrocholate was ineffective. This highlights the importance of surfaces, charged surfaces, and colloidal particles. The degree of phospholipid dispersion is important.

The amount of phospholipid needed depends upon the nature of the thrombin zymogen substrate. By a factor of ten, purified prothrombin required less phospholipid than prethrombin 1. This is probably in some way related to the fact that prethrombin 1 does not have calcium and/or phospholipid binding sites found in prothrombin. The requirement can, however, be satisfied by supplying purified profragment 1. The same quantitative difference between prethrombin 1 and prothrombin was found for bile salts as with lipids. The maximum rate of conversion of prothrombin to thrombin by autoprothrombin C and accessory substances is an order of magnitude 120 times greater than for prethrombin 1.

Important facts for thrombin generation can be summarized: prothrombin is a substrate which is degraded by autoprothrombin C as enzyme. The enzyme can function by itself, but far more effectively when Ac-globulin serves as determiner protein and when phospholipids from platelets are present. Lipids form complexes and serve as a surface on which the molecular interactions take place. Calcium ions presumably enable the formation of complexes involving calcium binding sites on prothrombin (HENRIKSEN and JACKSON, 1975). Ac-globulin binds at the profragment 2 area in prothrombin and prethrombin 1. Lipids bind directly to prothrombin, but apparently not efficiently to prethrombin 1 which does not have the special γ-carboxyglutamic acid binding sites for calcium ions. As a consequence, prethrombin 1 requires more autoprothrombin C and different proportion of accessories than prothrombin, and for that reason is probably not an intermediate in thrombin formation. The most likely intermediate is prethrombin 2 which becomes thrombin rapidly if profragment 1·2 of prothrombin is present as an accelerator (ESMON et al., 1974). In the case of bovine blood, prethrombin 1, prothrombin fragment 1, and prothrombin fragment 2 have been identified in plasma by immunologic technics. Additionally, a protein which could be either prethrombin 2 or thrombin has been found. Some of the prothrombin fragment 2 is bound to Ac-globulin. These factors support the conclusion that prothrombin degradation is a continuous process subject to acceleration in emergencies.

VI. Formation of Autoprothrombin C (Factor Xa)

The formation of autoprothrombin C occurs under a variety of conditions and with the support of several different substances. Based on their origin, at least four main classifications of substances can be made; namely, as follows:

1. Extrinsic Group
   a) Calcium ions
   b) Tissue thromboplastin
   c) Factor VII (cothromboplastin).
2. Intrinsic Group
   a) Calcium ions
   b) Platelet cofactor (Factor VIII)
   c) Platelet Factor 3
   d) Autoprothrombin II (Factor IXa).
3. Autocatalysis.
4. Enzymes and Enzymes from Snake Venoms
   a) Trypsin, papain, cathepsin C
   b) Russell's viper, *Echis carinatus*, etc.

The usual isolated form of Factor X consists of two chains connected by a disulfide bond. Isolation of a single-chain polypeptide (MATTOCK and ESNOUF, 1973) has not been confirmed. Bovine autoprothrombin III has a molecular weight of 55000, and during activation, this is reduced to about 44000 by the removal of a carbohydrate-rich polypeptide from the NH_2 terminal end of the heavy chain. The COOH terminal end of the heavy chain may or may not be degraded. It has been found that the structure of the Factor Xa depends to a certain extent upon the enzyme and/or set of conditions by which it is produced (DOMBROSE and SEEGERS, 1973), but similar enzymes have been found following use of four different activation conditions (RADCLIFFE and BARTON, 1973).

The *autocatalytic* formation of autoprothrombin C from purified autoprothrombin III occurs most rapidly in strong salt solutions such as 25% sodium citrate solution. It also occurs in physiologic saline solutions.

The yield of autoprothrombin C by the "*extrinsic*" and "*intrinsic*" groups of procoagulants is usually less than with snake venoms such as Russell's viper venom. As a consequence, the sera of most species contain appreciable amounts of residual or unactivated autoprothrombin III (RENO and SEEGERS, 1967). Thromboplastin of the extrinsic system is structurally and functionally different from PF-3 of the intrinsic system. When the two systems are in operation at the same time, the result is a synergistic function.

The mechanics of autoprothrombin C formation by the intrinsic system are similar to thrombin formation. In both cases, an enzyme creates an active enzyme in the presence of accessory substances. A reduction in concentration of a reactant from its optimum concentration limits the yield of active enzyme. In the case of autoprothrombin C formation, Factor IXa, platelet Factor 3, Factor VIII, and calcium ions are involved. The requirements for intrinsic autoprothrombin C formation are stated in two nomenclatures as follows:

Calcium ions
Platelet Factor 3
Antihemophilic Factor A
Antihemophilic Factor B
Autoprothrombin III ⟶ Autoprothrombin C + Peptide(s)

$$\text{Factor X} \xrightarrow[]{\substack{\text{Factor IV}\\ \text{PF-3}\\ \text{Factor VIII}\\ \text{Factor IXa}}} \text{Factor Xa} + \text{Peptide(s)}.$$

Under conditions of extrinsic autoprothrombin C formation, only four components are involved; namely, the substrate (autoprothrombin III), tissue thromboplastin, Factor VII (OWEN and BOLLMAN, 1948), and calcium ions. Presumably, Factor VII is the enzyme. As stated by RADCLIFFE and NEMERSON (1975): "Single chain Factor VII is rapidly hydrolyzed by Factor Xa in the presence of calcium ions and phospholipids, and by thrombin, to a two-chain form which possesses at least 85 times the Factor VII clotting activity of the single chain species. The two-chain form of the enzyme requires tissue factor in order to activate Factor X." Tissue thromboplastin consists of phospholipid-bound to protein (LIU and MCCOY, 1975a, b). An equation is given in two nomenclatures:

$$\text{Autoprothrombin III} \xrightarrow[]{\substack{\text{Calcium ions}\\ \text{Cothromboplastin}\\ \text{Thromboplastin}}} \text{Autoprothrombin C} + \text{Peptide(s)}$$

$$\text{Factor X} \xrightarrow{\substack{\text{Factor IV}\\ \text{Factor VII}\\ \text{Factor III}}} \text{Factor Xa} + \text{Peptide(s)}$$

Some of the molecular changes associated with the autoprothrombin III molecule during activation are known (Fig. 5). If the purified protein is digested with thrombin, a modified form (autoprothrombin III*m*) is obtained, because thrombin removes a peptide from the COOH terminal end of the heavy chain. The autoprothrombin III*m* is not readily converted to autoprothrombin C*m*, except with Russell's viper venom and is an inhibitor of autoprothrombin III activation. The structure of autoprothrombin C differs from autoprothrombin C*m* because the latter does not contain the peptide removed by thrombin. The structure is the same whether the peptide is removed from autoprothrombin III or from autoprothrombin C. In case a preparation of autoprothrombin C is free of thrombin, it spontaneously converts to the modified form referred to as autoprothrombin C*m* or Factor Xaβ.

One view, which seems to have become dogma, accounts for the formation of Factor IXa (WINTROBE, 1974). Hageman factor becomes activated upon contact with certain surfaces and then produces Factor XIa from its precursor, in the presence of high molecular weight kininogen (FITZGERALD Factor) (COLMAN et al., 1975; KAPLAN et al., 1976). Calcium ions and phospholipids also have a role in these mechanisms. Since Hageman factor deficiency is clinically asymptomatic in terms of blood coagulation, we must assume that there are other pathways to account for the formation of active Factor IXa. Factor IXa obtained by activation of Factor IX with thrombin has been purified and characterized (HARMISON and SEEGERS, 1962).

Much more must, however, be ascribed to Factor XII. As a surface-sensitive protein it is activated by collagen, phospholipids, and kallikrein (active Fletcher factor) (COCHRANE et al., 1973). Factor XIIa itself converts prekallikrein to kallikrein and the latter converts high molecular weight kininogen (Fitzgerald factor) to active kinin (bradykinin, etc.) (KAPLAN and AUSTEN, 1970; KAPLAN et al., 1976). At one time, bradykinin was called vascularin (GUEST et al., 1947a). The active kinins are associated with the production of pain, inflammatory states, leukocyte migration, increased vascular permeability, and smooth muscle contraction.

Factor XIIa also functions in fibrinolysis; namely, as follows:

$$\text{Proactivator} \xrightarrow{\text{F-XIIa}} \text{Activator}$$

$$\text{Plasminogen} \xrightarrow{\text{Activator}} \text{Plasmin}$$

$$\text{Fibrinogen and/or fibrin} \xrightarrow{\text{Plasmin}} \text{Digestion products.}$$

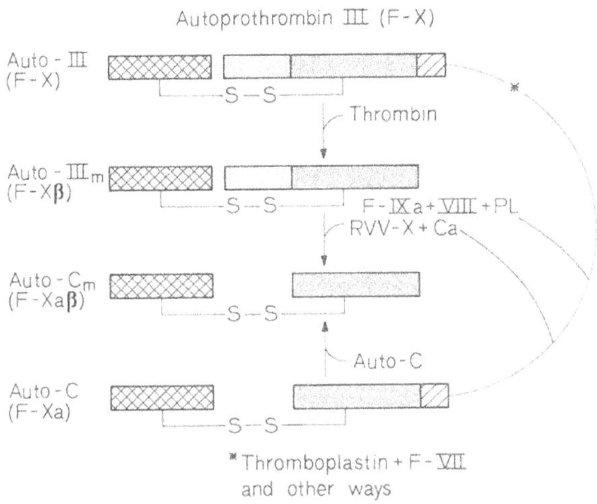

Fig. 5. Activation of autoprothrombin III. Disulfide bonds are arbitrarily positioned. Chain lengths are drawn to scale. Transformation of Auto-III (55000 daltons) to a peptide (4500 daltons) and Auto-III*m* with purified thrombin. Auto-III*m* forms Auto-C*m* (Factor Xa_{β}) with RVV-X. Auto-III transforms to a peptide (11500 daltons) and Auto-C under multiple conditions, including thromboplastin + Factor VII and calcium ions, Factor IXa + Factor VIII + phospholipid + calcium ions, and RVV-X. Most likely, also with *Echis carinatus* venom, cream, uroplastin, cathepsin, trypsin, papain, autocatalysis, etc. Auto-C ultimately transforms to Auto-C*m* + peptide by autolysis and more rapidly, if phospholipid is also present. Presumably, Auto-C is also transformed to Auto-C*m* by thrombin. The peptides removed from the heavy chain of Auto-III contain the carbohydrate of the proenzyme

In the above equations, proactivator is very likely the same as prekallikrein. It should be realized that the proteolytic enzyme, plasmin, has multiple functions. It not only digests fibrinogen and fibrin but also Ac-globulin, Factor VIII, and Factor IX, as well as purified prothrombin. In addition, plasmin directly activates the first and third components of complement.

Before considering broader ramifications, or adding more complicated aspects of blood coagulation, it is helpful to review the three basic reactions (Fig. 6). The diagram to illustrate these is carried into the more elaborate one (Fig. 7). The approach is to proceed from first principles, then consider the earlier phases, and lastly important inhibitors.

Throughout the literature of the past decades, there appears a desire to find that which "triggers blood coagulation," to find "the substance that leads to clot formation," or to describe the "early phases of coagulation," or to decide which theory most nearly describes the "chain reaction," or the "cascade of events." It is altogether too easy to see a fibrin clot and be distracted from what is constantly in operation at levels that do not produce a fibrin gel or at levels that follow gel formation. As a consequence of these restricted ways of progressing, it is innovative to point out that a biocybernetic system is involved (Fig. 7). The built-in components and/or factors of this system read their own performance and adjust accordingly. Dominant facts are that the resources are obtained from distinct anatomic compartments such as platelets, plasma, and tissues. For example, platelets alone or even their materials produce

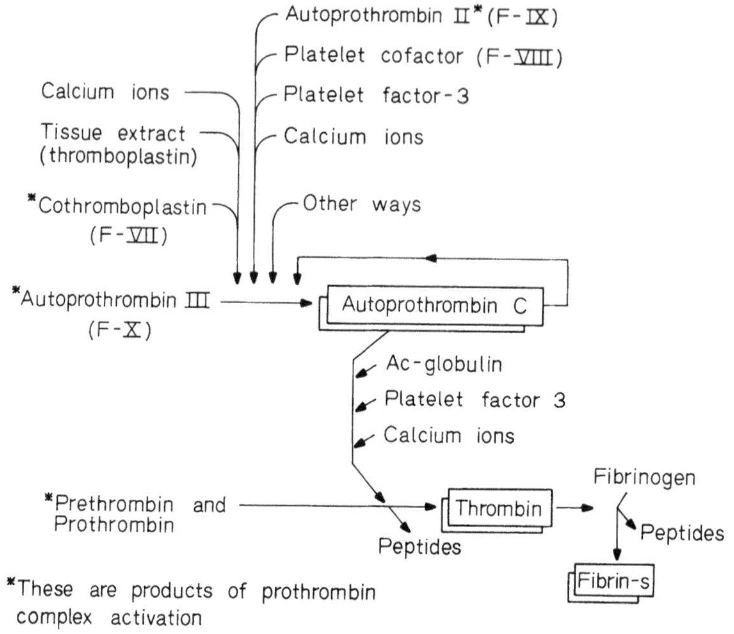

Fig. 6. Three basic reactions of blood coagulation. a) Formation of autoprothrombin C in four different ways. These can function synergistically. b) Formation of thrombin by autoprothrombin C, assisted by accessory factors including platelet factor 3. c) Formation of fibrin. Autoprothrombin II (Factor IXa) is presumably formed by Factor XIa. Prethrombin 1 requires more procoagulant materials than prothrombin for the formation of thrombin. Note that inhibitors have not been taken into account. For that aspect, see Figure 7

limited perturbation without active plasma components. No one factor or component is sufficient to accelerate the system even though removal of a single factor can conspicuously retard normal functioning. Acceleration of continuous operation of this biocybernetic system occurs when materials from more than one anatomic compartment participate. Mechanical injury is one means for fulfilling that requirement.

Purified Factor VIII has only recently become available in suitable form for chemical studies (IRWIN, 1975). It is a glycoprotein with a molecular weight near a million. Upon reduction, subunits, similar or perhaps identic, with a molecular weight of 200000 are obtained. Dissociation of the large molecule occurs in a medium of high ionic strength and is reversible. Along with the Factor VIII preparation, a platelet aggregating agent (von Willebrand factor) is isolated. For the present, the chemical relationship of one of these factors to the other requires further investigation. Most likely, the platelet aggregating component is distinctly different from the procoagulant component.

Factor IX (autoprothrombin II), with a molecular weight near 55000, is a single-chain polypeptide rich in carbohydrate and shows much amino acid sequence homology with prothrombin and the light chain of Factor X (FUJIKAWA et al., 1974). During activation, the single chain polypeptide is degraded in two steps. A break in the chain produces an intermediate consisting of light and heavy chains bound by a

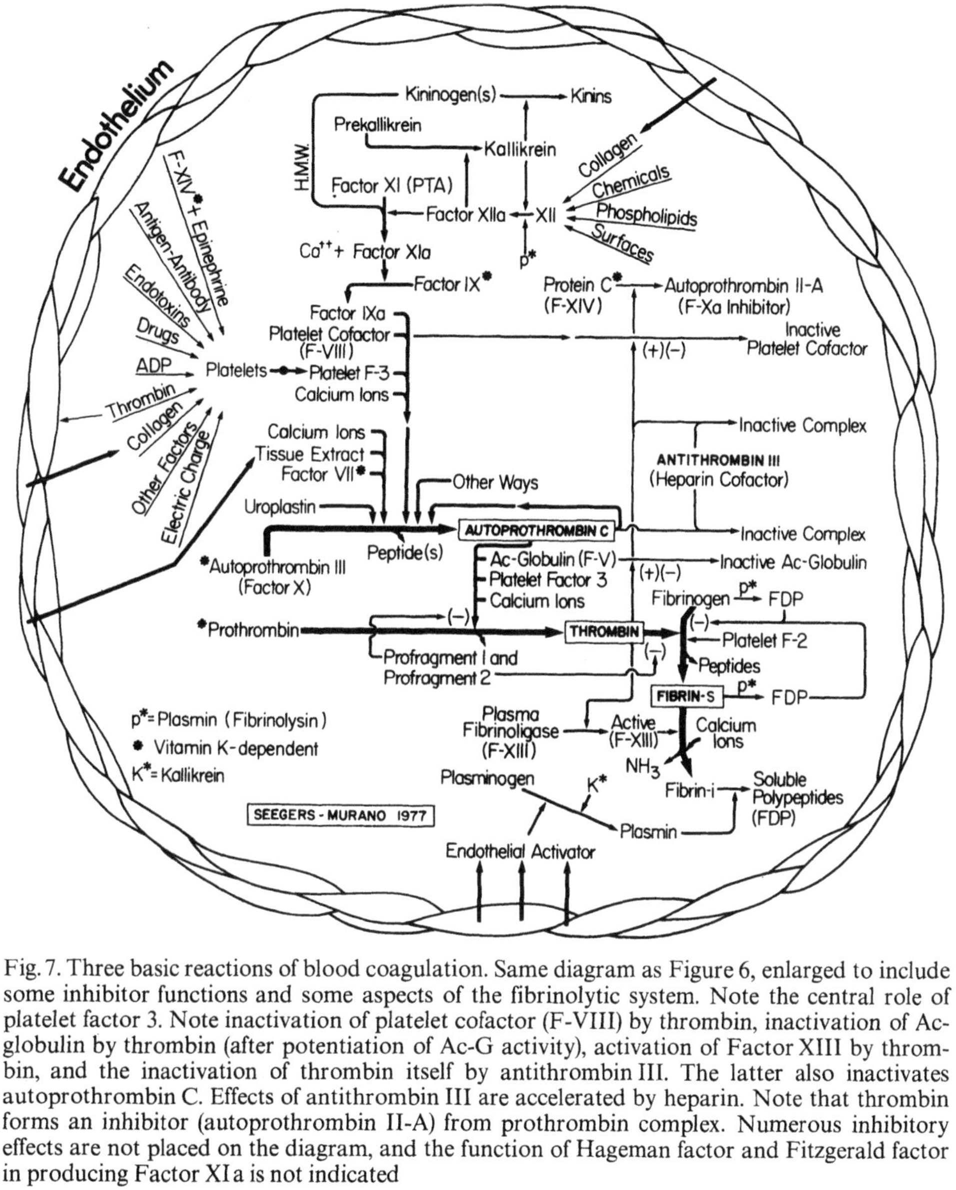

Fig. 7. Three basic reactions of blood coagulation. Same diagram as Figure 6, enlarged to include some inhibitor functions and some aspects of the fibrinolytic system. Note the central role of platelet factor 3. Note inactivation of platelet cofactor (F-VIII) by thrombin, inactivation of Ac-globulin by thrombin (after potentiation of Ac-G activity), activation of Factor XIII by thrombin, and the inactivation of thrombin itself by antithrombin III. The latter also inactivates autoprothrombin C. Effects of antithrombin III are accelerated by heparin. Note that thrombin forms an inhibitor (autoprothrombin II-A) from prothrombin complex. Numerous inhibitory effects are not placed on the diagram, and the function of Hageman factor and Fitzgerald factor in producing Factor XIa is not indicated

disulfide bridge. This structure becomes active when a peptide (9000 daltons) is split from the NH_2 terminal end of its heavy chain.

VII. General Procoagulant Effects

Enzymes such as trypsin, papain, cathepsin, etc. have various procoagulant effects which lead to the formation of fibrin, but it is not a part of this discussion to elaborate. However, a few points are mentioned. Venom enzymes sometimes have their effectiveness augmented by platelet materials and by Ac-globulin. Procoagulant effects of bacteria are also discussed extensively in the literature. Perhaps the best known procoagulant is staphylocoagulase which produces an unusual thrombin from prothrombin known as coagulase thrombin (TAGER and DRUMMOND, 1970). This thrombin is not sensitive to antithrombin III, heparin, and hirudin but removes peptides A and B from fibrinogen (JOSSO et al., 1968). In contemporary experiments, it was found that prothrombin and staphylocoagulase form a 1:1 stoichiometric product with procoagulant properties. No peptide bonds seem to be split from prothrombin by the bacterial protein.

Complement-activating agents initiate blood coagulation. These agents do not function if the C6 component is absent. Such a deficient state was found in a certain strain of rabbits. Small amounts of purified C6 component, when added to the deficient plasma, normalized the plasma so that it would again clot rapidly upon using complement-activating agents such as inulin, endotoxin, and lipopolysaccharide (ZIMMERMAN and MÜLLER-EBERHARD, 1971; ZIMMERMAN et al., 1971). In the C6 component-deficient blood, whole blood clotting times are prolonged and prothrombin consumption is decreased.

VIII. Inhibition of Procoagulants

If blood coagulation is considered only in terms of the procoagulants, the three basic reactions are easily summarized by means of a diagram (Fig. 6). That, however, is about half of what is involved. The equally important inhibitors function in various ways and must be taken into account in order to complete a description of a cybernetic system recognized as blood coagulation. Without negative feedback aspects, the system would operate completely out of control, and there would be no way to survive thrombosis. Consequently, there are numerous ways in which the overall procoagulant forces are checked.

1. Nature of Anticoagulant Systems

The blood anticoagulation system contains specific inhibitors that inhibit the main procoagulant components. In certain cases, the inhibitors are made more powerful by accessory compounds. In addition, there is product inhibition. There are apparent stoichiometric reactions, mutual depletion systems, and substrates that are converted to less reactive substrates by partial degradation. As considered earlier in this discussion, there are multiple pathways for the development of procoagulant activity. Analogously, the same is true for the retarding mechanisms of the system. The whole is integrated with metabolic functions which involve synthesis of components, their subsequent degradation and, in certain cases, their removal, degradation, and elimination by the reticuloendothelial system. The fibrinolytic system, though directed primarily at the dissolution of fibrin, is essentially in balance with the coagulation system (SEEGERS, 1973b).

2. Fibrinogen and Fibrin Degradation Products (FDP)

Allowing for exceptions, these are generally inhibitors of blood coagulation. They have an antithrombin effect and form complexes with fibrinogen that coagulate slowly, and the fibrin may be structurally abnormal (TRIANTAPHYLLOPOULOS and TRIANTAPHYLLOPOULOS, 1966; BANG and CHANG, 1974). FDP may impair platelet function. Certain fibrin degradation products can function as accessory protein in thrombin formation.

3. Prothrombin Derivatives

Profragment 1 (PR fragment, fragment 1, F_A, intermediate 3, NH_2 terminal fragment), which is the NH_2 terminal end of prothrombin, binds calcium and phospholipids. Consequently, when it is separated from prothrombin, the remaining zymogen (prethrombin 1) requires more procoagulant material to form thrombin than is required by prothrombin. Profragment 2 (0 fragment, fragment 2, inner fragment, intermediate 4) from the center of the prothrombin molecule is also active. It enhances the esterase activity of thrombin but strongly inhibits its limited proteolysis of fibrinogen. In opposition to this effect of profragment 2 on thrombin is the binding of Ac-globulin to profragment 2. When bound in that way, profragment 2 has no effect on thrombin. Profragment 2 also has another procoagulant effect in purified systems. The main example is its role in the conversion of prethrombin 2 to thrombin. This substrate has no profragment 2; thus, Ac-globulin cannot function efficiently unless profragment 2 is added in purified form (ESMON and JACKSON, 1974). Alternatively, the generation of thrombin from prethrombin 2 can be enhanced by adding profragment 2 without separating it from profragment 1·2 (ESMON et al., 1974). Profragment 1 is an inhibitor of thrombin generation from prothrombin in the five-component system. On the other hand, profragment 1 serves as an accelerator when prethrombin 1 is converted to thrombin in the five-component system.

4. Antithrombin III

This plasma protein inactivates autoprothrombin C and thrombin (SEEGERS, 1962). A mutual depletion system is involved. In the case of thrombin, the active serine center is required as well as arginine residues of the inhibitor. The process is accelerated by heparin, and for that function, lysyl residues of the inhibitor probably serve as binding sites for heparin (ROSENBERG and DAMUS, 1973). In both cases of inhibition, the activity of antithrombin III is also diminished because complexes form which represent enzyme plus inhibitor. Antithrombin III also reduces the activity of plasmin (HIGHSMITH and ROSENBERG, 1974) and Factor IXa, as well as Factor VII, but only limited information about these inhibitions is available. The fact that a deficiency of antithrombin III is accompanied by a thrombosing tendency is evidence that it is one of the most important inhibitors of thrombin and autoprothrombin C.

5. Other Plasma Inhibitors

α_1-antitrypsin also inactivates thrombin but does not function to neutralize nearly as much thrombin as is inactivated by antithrombin III. Purified α_2-macroglobulin neutralizes only the proteolytic (clotting) property of thrombin leaving the esterolytic function active (SEEGERS, 1969).

6. Thrombin

Considering this enzyme from the viewpoint of its contribution to anticoagulation was a slowly developing process, probably because everyone knew so very well that thrombin clots blood and is the essential procoagulant. However, under suitable conditions, it has a procoagulant function followed by an anticoagulant effect. Thrombin has the dual effect of first potentiating the activity of Ac-globulin and later inactivating the protein (WARE and SEEGERS, 1948). Apparently, this is a proteolytic process because acetylated thrombin, which does not clot fibrinogen, does not produce the effect. In like manner, thrombin first augments the activity of Factor VIII and subsequently inactivates it. Contrary to what has frequently been written and placed into diagrams, it is not essential for thrombin to activate Factor VIII because it functions very well in the absence of thrombin (IRWIN et al., 1975).

Autoprothrombin II-A is an inhibitor produced by thrombin. It was discovered when purified prothrombin complex was activated by small amounts of purified thrombin. Instead of the expected generation of thrombin by autocatalysis, an inhibitor was produced (MAMMEN et al., 1960). It is a competitive inhibitor of autoprothrombin C. It is composed of two polypeptide chains with apparent molecular mass of 40000 and 22000 daltons (SEEGERS et al., 1972b). Its origin remained uncertain until protein C was isolated (STENFLO, 1976) and designated as a new vitamin K-dependent protein. Protein C is the precursor of autoprothrombin II-A (SEEGERS et al., 1976).

Another interesting fact is that autoprothrombin II-A serves to induce fibrinolysis in addition to its anticoagulant function. It is thus a unique protein, with more than one function. The molecular basis for its function in fibrinolysis is only to a minor degree due to activation of profibrinolysin (plasminogen). The major portion of the induced fibrinolysis is due to the suppression of inhibitors of fibrinolysis (ZOLTON and SEEGERS, 1973). In this connection, it is interesting that at one time small amounts of thrombin were infused intravenously in the interest of treating thrombosis (BRAMBEL, 1957). The small amounts of thrombin produced fibrinolysis. One possibility is that the thrombin functioned indirectly by producing autoprothrombin II-A. Purified thrombin does not activate purified plasminogen. An attempt has been made to represent, by means of a diagram (Fig. 7), a view of blood coagulation as a cybernetic system.

IX. Clot Retraction

A well-illustrated description of clot retraction has been presented by BALLERINI and SEEGERS (1959). The extent of clot retraction is dependent on numerous variables such as temperature, cell volume, surface contact, pH, fibrinogen, thrombin, calcium ion, and platelet concentrations. Thrombin strongly induces clot retraction, and platelets are essential. This quality of platelets is lost by such treatment as dialysis, exposure to ultrasonic waves, storage, and freezing. In the latter case, there is some protection in glycerol solutions. Plasma contains dialyzable material concerned with clot retraction. This includes glucose, phosphorus compounds, and perhaps other substances. Moreover, plasma contains one or more proteins of interest in clot retraction, and this protein(s) can be adsorbed on barium carbonate and subsequently eluted with sodium citrate solution. There may be clot retraction without the dialyzable material of plasma if the nondialyzable protein(s) is present and vice versa. An actomyosin-like protein has been obtained from platelets (BETTEX-GALLAND and LÜSCHER, 1965). When it is mixed with fibrinogen, ATP, and thrombin, "retraction" follows. Glucose is a source of energy for clot retraction as well as for the synthesis of ATP of platelets.

In the mechanics of clot retraction, the platelets accumulate at junctions where fibers cross. Pseudopods from the platelets reach adjoining fibers and upon contraction, as the result of the work of actomyosin, the clots diminish in volume. The force of this retraction is relatively weak. Consequently, the lumen of the blood vessel is not closed by the retraction as might be supposed. Additionally, the force of contraction of the blood vessel wall is not sufficient to compress the gel. Consequently, the reduction in size of the clot, by retraction, enables the blood vessel wall to follow by its own contractile activity.

X. Fibrinolytic System

In fibrinolysis, an enzyme alternatively called profibrinolysin or plasminogen becomes converted to the active form, respectively fibrinolysin and plasmin. Upon degradation of fibrin by plasmin, a solution replaces the solid fibrin mass while degradation of fibrinogen leaves the protein in a state that will not polymerize (remains in solution) upon adding thrombin. For practical purposes, the fibrin and fibrinogen degradation products are virtually the same (SEEGERS et al., 1945). Sometimes a double meaning is conveyed by using the term "fibrin(ogen)" degradation products. The main ones of those which appear during the later stages of lysis are now designated fragment E and fragment D.

The formation of plasmin from its precursor occurs in several ways. The best known substances that bring it about are staphylokinase, tissue activator, activated plasma proactivator, streptokinase, and urokinase. The latter two have been used as therapeutic agents in selected cases of thrombosis. As an example, depletion of fibrinogen and plasminogen to below 5% of preinfusion level can take place within 30 min after the infusion of purified streptokinase. The material derived from bacteria functions together with plasminogen to form a plasminogen-streptokinase complex which functions as activator of plasminogen. Urokinase, on the other hand, has direct activator qualities by itself.

Inhibitors in plasma can neutralize the enzyme. Plasmin forms complexes with α_1-antitrypsin and α_2-macroglobulin. One theory holds that much of the potential fibrinolytic pool resides in such complexes (NORMAN and HILL, 1958). In the case of autoprothrombin II-A, induction of fibrinolysis is largely due to depression of plasmin inhibitors. Antiplasmin concentration increases when chickens are on a pteroylglutamic acid-deficient diet (GUEST et al., 1947 b).

Factor XII is also concerned with the activation of plasminogen (KAPLAN and AUSTEN, 1972). This is only one of the functions ascribed to Factor XIIa, the others being activation of coagulation, activation of a kinin system, and activation of the complement system. Factor XII deficiency is described as an asymptomatic condition. Consequently, there remains the perplexing question about its necessity in the several roles it can have in these complicated mechanisms. For fibrinolysis, Factor XII a functions in terms of a plasma proactivator which is converted to activator, and the latter generates plasmin from its precursor. The main role attributed to Factor XII a in fibrinolysis can be indicated as follows:

$$\begin{array}{c}\text{Plasma proactivator}\\ \downarrow \text{Factor XIIa}\\ \text{Plasminogen} \xrightarrow{\text{Plasma activator}} \text{Plasmin}\end{array}$$

As already mentioned, the decomposition of fibrinogen by plasmin and the decomposition of fibrin by plasmin yield nearly the same split products (SEEGERS et al., 1945). With few exceptions, it is, therefore, not customary to refer to fibrinogenolysis and fibrinolysis. The latter term is used with a dual meaning. In the same way, the terms fibrin split products (FSP) or fibrin degradation products (FDP) imply the possibility of identic degradation products from fibrin and fibrinogen. Fibrin degradation products form soluble complexes with fibrin monomer, inhibit formation of fibrin by thrombin, and contribute to the formation of a modified fibrin structure. Retarded platelet aggregation is also a function of FDP and probably mainly of the small dialyzable fractions (STACHURSKA, 1970). For any one of these functions, each one of the several FDP classes of molecules has different activity from the other.

B. Physiology of Hemostasis

To comprehend some of the situations encountered with snake venoms, it is essential to have foremost in mind that blood coagulation and hemostasis are not synonymous. Hemostasis is the arrest of bleeding or holding the blood in blood vessels. Descriptions of some of the main features of hemostasis have appeared from time to time. A quotation from one of these is given (HENRY and STEIMAN, 1968):

> Today, although the exact mechanisms are still undetermined, there is almost complete agreement that the principal roles in hemostasis are played by the blood platelets, the coagulation of the blood, and the blood vessels. When these three component mechanisms of hemostasis are present and active, we believe the cessation of bleeding occurs in the following way:
>
> When a blood vessel is injured to the point where blood loss occurs there is an exposure of connective tissue underlying the endothelium. Platelets begin to adhere to the collagen of connective tissue resulting in a release of ADP and catecholamines. The catecholamines together with local stimulants (unknown) and perhaps local neurogenic responses bring about vascular smooth muscle contraction. The vascular smooth muscle contraction enhances the ability of platelets to plug the site of injury by reducing the diameter of the blood vessels at the point of injury. Less cohesion of platelets is then necessary to form a plug large enough to stop blood loss. If this initial platelet plug is still in a reversible form and vascular smooth muscle relaxation occurs, the platelet plug will be lost resulting in a resumption of bleeding. If, together, the platelets and the vascular smooth muscle can stop blood loss long enough for secondary reactions to occur (that is, release of platelet factor 3, platelet factor 4, and further release of ADP) due to the effects of ADP and the catecholamines or traces of thrombin, then coagulation mechanisms come into play to form a more stable hemostatic mass. Platelets having undergone such changes can no longer disaggregate and fibrin forms a meshwork spanning from the vessel walls and into the platelet plug. The coagulation mechanisms, then, are necessary for permanent hemostasis. Prolongation of the clotting time prolongs the time the initial plug needs to be held in place by platelet aggregation and smooth muscle contraction. Without platelet aggregation it would be necessary for the vascular smooth muscle along with tissue pressures (increased by blood loss into the tissues) or externally applied pressure to stop blood loss long enough for the clotting

mechanisms to form a fibrin based plug. Without vascular smooth muscle function, more time is needed for a platelet mass to form which is large enough to plug the opening.

As anticipated, removal of any two components of hemostasis resulted in continuous bleeding, indicating that one functioning component was unable to initiate even temporary hemostasis. Therefore, a loss of, or damage to, the hemostatic function of the vascular smooth muscle and the platelets, the vascular smooth muscle and the clotting mechanism, or the platelets and the clotting mechanism resulted in continuous bleeding from each wounded blood vessel in the scarified area of a rat's tail.

The hemostatic possibilities for the topical application of snake venoms were explored many years ago (MACFARLANE and BARNETT, 1934). They continue to be used and typical examples can suffice (STACHER and BÖHNEL, 1959; DURANTE et al., 1962). Meanwhile, it became possible to produce thrombin on a large scale (SEEGERS and SHARP, 1948), and it was introduced as an hemostatic agent (SEEGERS et al., 1939; WARNER et al., 1939; TIDRICK et al., 1943). It has been used extensively and in association with absorbable surgical sponges (SEEGERS and SHARP, 1948). In addition to producing fibrin, thrombin activates Factor XIII, promotes the platelet release reaction, promotes clot retraction, increases the activity of Factors V and VIII, and probably promotes wound healing.

C. Snake Venoms and Blood Coagulation

I. Introductory Remarks

The literature contains much evidence of enthusiasm for the use of snake venoms for the purpose of elucidating the nature of the blood coagulation mechanisms as well as for the need to understand snake venoms more fully. Apparently, the main attraction for investigators in the field of hemostasis and thrombosis has been the utility of venoms and venom materials in practical laboratory tests, in clinical uses, and, more recently, for applications in theoretic studies.

Which one of the venoms has either one or some combination of procoagulant, anticoagulant, fibrinolytic, hemorrhagic, or other qualities has been documented to a certain extent, and is not taken as being within the scope of our task for comment (EAGLE, 1937; BOQUET, 1964; NAHAS et al., 1964; MEAUME, 1966; BÜCHERL et al., 1968; DEVI, 1968; ROSENFELD et al., 1968; DENSON, 1969; DE VRIES and COHEN, 1969; BELL and PITNEY, 1970; JIMÉNEZ-PORRAS, 1970; PITNEY, 1970; REID, 1970; BELL, 1971; BLOMBÄCK et al., 1971; HENRIQUES and HENRIQUES, 1971; KWAAN and BARLOW, 1971a, b; SHARP, 1971; COPLEY et al., 1973; RUSSELL et al., 1975). An attempt is made to consider those aspects which are concerned at the molecular level of observation. Since blood coagulation phenomena naturally fall within the scope of three basic reactions, snake venoms can also be studied in terms of their place within the sphere of these three basic reactions.

II. Snake Venoms and Fibrinogen

The clotting of fibrinogen by venoms was recognized at the beginning of this century and most likely earlier (MELLANBY, 1909; HOUSSAY and SORDELLA, 1919). A recent survey included 43 species of four families of snakes (COPLEY et al., 1973). Thrombin-like activity was found in most of the *Crotalidae* group of venoms. None was found

Table 1. Snake venoms containing thrombin-like enzymes[a]

Agkistrodon acutus; OUYANG et al. (1971a)
Agkistrodon rhodostoma; ESNOUF and TUNNAH (1967)
Agkistrodon contortrix contortrix; HERZIG et al. (1970)
Agkistrodon bilineatus; DENSON et al. (1972)
Agkistrodon contortrix mokeson; DENSON et al. (1972)
Bitis gabonica; MARSH and WHALER (1974)
Bothrops alternatus; STOCKER et al. (1974)
Bothrops asper; Stocker et al. (1974)
Bothrops cotiara; STOCKER et al. (1974)
Bothrops jararaca; STOCKER et al. (1974)
Bothrops jararacussu; STOCKER et al. (1974)
Bothrops lanceolatus; STOCKER et al. (1974)
Bothrops neuwiedii; STOCKER et al. (1974)
Bothrops marajoensis; STOCKER et al. (1974)
Bothrops moojeni; STOCKER et al. (1974)
Crotalus adamanteus; MARKLAND and DAMUS (1971)
Crotalus h. atricaudatus; BONILLA (1975)
Crotalus durissus durissus; DENSON et al. (1972)
Crotalus terrificus; DENSON (1969)
Crotalus viridis helleri; DENSON et al. (1972)
Crotalus horridus; DENSON (1969)
Trimeresurus erythrurus; MITRAKUL (1973)
Trimeresurus popeorum; MITRAKUL (1973)
Trimeresurus okinavensis; ANDERSSON (1972)
Trimeresurus flavoviridis; DENSON et al. (1972)
Trimeresurus purpureomaculata; DENSON (1969)
Trimeresurus gramineus; OUYANG and YANG (1974)

[a] This list of reported snake venoms which contain thrombin-like enzymes was arranged by GRANT H. BARLOW for the ICTH task force on venoms. The references cited are the most accessible for each entry; they do not necessarily indicate the source most deserving of credit.

in the venoms of the *Elapidae* and *Hydrophidae* groups of snakes. Only one *(Vipera ammodytes)* was found in the *Viperidae* group. A list of snake venoms containing thrombin-like enzymes has been arranged (Table 1). It was suggested that the thrombin-like activity be called *thromboserpentin* activity (COPLEY et al., 1973). This appears to be an excellent suggestion and might be found useful.

It is difficult to follow the precise meaning of terms in the literature. Trade names are used as well as the thrombin-like designation. We have made an attempt to account for the development of puzzling details (Table 2). Differences in trademark regulations from one country to another account for several names for one product. Otherwise, ambiguities are perhaps no more prevalent than in any other literature.

The thrombin time of plasma is defined as the time required for the clotting of plasmas by a standardized preparation of purified thrombin. One of the active principles of *Bothrops atrox* (Reptilase) venom produces coagulation by directly modifying fibrinogen. So one can prepare a standard solution of Reptilase and determine the reptilase time of plasma. By comparing the results with the thrombin time, useful information is obtained (FUNK et al., 1971). Thrombin time is prolonged with plasma where there is hypofibrinogenemia, dysfibrinogenemia (abnormal

Table 2. Nomenclature of some coagulant snake venom enzyme preparations[a]

Intended or established use	Scientific description	Registered trade mark	Trade mark owner	Generic name
Hemostatic drug (on the market in Europe and Asia since 1954)	Coagulant fraction of *Bothrops atrox* venom containing a thrombin-like enzyme as well as a F-X activator which requires phospholipid	Reptilase (Europe, etc.) Hemostase (USA)	Pentapharm Ltd. Basel	Haemocoagulase Klobusitzky (not approved by WHO)
Reagent for laboratory use (on the market since 1970)	Purified thromboserpentin enzyme of venom of *B. atrox* (proposed subspecies *B. marajoensis*) free from F-X activator	Reptilase-Reagent Reptilase-R	Pentapharm Ltd. Basel	Batroxobin (approved by WHO)
Defibrinogenating agent for human use (registration pending/registered in Poland)	Purified thromboserpentin enzyme of venom of *B. atrox* (proposed subspecies B. moojeni) free of F-X activator	Defibrase (CH, GFR, etc.) Defibrol (S, N, DK, etc.) D-Fibrol (UK, etc.)	Pentapharm Ltd. Basel	Batroxobin (approved by WHO)
Defibrinogenating agent (registration pending/ on the market in UK and GFR)	Purified thrombin-like enzyme from *Agkistrodon rhodostoma* venom	Arvin (UK and others) Arwin (GFR and others)	Twyford Pharm. Services (England) Knoll AG (GFR)	Ancrod (approved by WHO?)
Defibrinogenating agent	Purified thromboserpentin from *A. rhodostoma*	Venacil (USA)	Abbott, North Chicago	Ancrod

[a] We owe special thanks to Dr. KURT STOCKER of Pentapharm Ltd., Basel, for most of the information assembled and also to Dr. GRANT H. BARLOW at the Abbott Laboratories for his helpful comments. Crotalase is the name used for the enzyme from *Crotalus adamanteus*. Bothropase is a trade name for an enzyme produced in Brazil. In the case of Ancrod, Arvin, Arwin, and Venacil, each company does its own manufacturing. Apparently, National Research Corporation, London, holds patents for the fractionation of *A. rhodostoma* venom.

Due to different national trade mark regulations it is almost impossible to register one single internationally valid trade mark for a product; therefore Defibrase = Defibrol and D-Fibrol in some countries and Arvin = Arwin and Venacil. Pentapharm is the producer of Reptilase, Reptilase-Reagent and Defibrase and is the owner of the respective registered trade marks. The said products are internationally distributed unter licenses (in some cases, sublicenses) by different sales organizations. Thus, Reptilase in Taiwan is available from Nan-Fong Co., Taipei, a sublicensee of Solco, Basel, a company to which Pentapharm has licensed Reptilase for quite a number of countries. Arvin, originating from Twyford, is distributed and/or manufactured in cooperation between Twyford Pharmaceutical Services, Knoll AG, and Abbott Laboratories.

fibrinogen molecule), heparin, or one or more fibrinogen derivatives. The reptilase time is normal in the presence of heparin, only slightly prolonged in the presence of fibrinogen split products, and strongly prolonged in association with abnormal fibrinogen molecules (LATALLO and TEISSEYRE, 1971). The information obtained by the comparative tests can be supplemented. If the plasma is presumed to contain heparin, the latter can be neutralized to normalize the plasma; if removal of hypothetic heparin leaves the thrombin time prolonged, the fibrinogen split products are probably present. Stability of thrombin is important in all studies, and it is helpful to appreciate that thrombin is stable for more than a year near pH 5 and at 4° C (SEEGERS and McCOY, 1972). At alkaline pH, it is not stable; thus, one cannot say categorically that thrombin solutions are not stable (FUNK et al., 1971).

In the assay for antithrombin III, it is essential to remove fibrinogen so that there is no adsorption of thrombin on fibrin. Defibrinogenation is achieved by heating the plasma at 56° C for 3 min (SEEGERS et al., 1952). The fibrinogen can be removed more conveniently by using a small amount of ancrod (HOWIE et al., 1973).

Purification of the thrombin-like enzyme from various venoms has served to reduce confusion with inhibitors, fibrinolysins, other procoagulant enzymes, and the like. Most of the purification procedures have involved use of modern reagents and equipment now used in protein chemistry. Owing to the importance of such work, we have, in most instances, quoted directly the author's own summary. The amino acid composition of some thrombin-like enzymes is given (Table 3).

One of the first thromboserpentins to be isolated was from the venom of the Malayan pit viper, *Agkistrodon rhodostoma* (ESNOUF and TUNNAH, 1967). The molecular weight was found to be near 30000. It did not alter other coagulation factors. As compared with the thrombin used in the experiments, thromboserpentin hydrolyzed *p*-nitrophenyl esters of various amino acids more readily, as well as some benzoyl arginine ethyl ester and *p*-toluenesulfonyl-L-arginine methyl ester. The thrombin-like enzyme was a little more resistant to DFP and toluenesulfonyl fluoride than thrombin. It was not inhibited by heparin, hirudin, or soybean trypsin inhibitor when the test substrate was fibrinogen. Thrombin is, incidentally, also not inhibited by soybean trypsin inhibitor.

Procedures have been developed for obtaining pure batroxobin (STOCKER and BARLOW, 1975a, b). The enzyme was isolated from three different *Bothrops* species; namely, *B. asper*, *B. marajoensis*, and *B. moojeni*. Some properties of the latter two are outlined (Table 4). Antibodies to either one neutralized the clotting activity and amidolytic activity on benzoylphenylalanyl-valyl-arginyl-*p*-nitroanilide of the venoms from *B. asper*, *B. atrox columbiensis*, *B. atrox venezolensis*, *B. marajoensis*, *B. moojeni*, and *B. pradoi*. The antibodies did not, however, neutralize the clotting activity of *Agkistrodon rhodostoma*. It is generally found in the literature that batroxobin activates Factor XIII, but the enzyme from *B. marajoensis* was found to be an exception.

There are species preferences for fibrinogen (WIK et al., 1972). As an example, the coagulation of rabbit fibrinogen takes ten times longer than human fibrinogen for an equal amount of batroxobin. This is an involved topic on which there is much information from which it is difficult to synthesize a generalization.

In a preliminary work, the anticoagulant principle(s) and procoagulant protein were separated from the venom of the Hundred-pace snake, *Agkistrodon acutus*

Table 3. Amino acid composition of the thrombin-like enzymes of the venoms of *A. rhodostoma*, *A. acutus*, *T. gramineus*, *C. h. horridus*, *C. adamanteus*, *T. okinavensis*, and bovine thrombin

Amino acid	(1)[a]	(2)[b]	(3)[c]	(4)[d]	(5)[e]	(6)[f]	(7)[g]
Lysine	11	15	7	7	11	12	24
Histidine	6	10	6	4	9	8	7
Arginine	18	10	7	4	12	16	22
Aspartic acid	30	24	27	22	31	39	29
Threonine	7	9	11	7	14	20	13
Serine	9	7	11	12	16	21	12
Glutamic acid	14	18	14	15	23	23	34
Proline	12	10	10	5	22	23	17
Glycine	16	10	17	10	20	25	25
Alanine	11	7	12	8	11	12	15
Half-cystine	13	15	16	5	14	10	8
Valine	8	7	10	9	17	19	21
Methionine	5	5	3	1	2	4	5
Isoleucine	17	8	11	5	18	17	15
Leucine	14	11	12	8	21	27	28
Tyrosine	6	14	7	6	7	10	11
Phenylalanine	6	7	6	6	13	10	12
Tryptophan	ND	ND	2	5	6	5	10
Total	203	187	189	139	267	301	308

[a] *A. rhodostoma*, ESNOUF and TUNNAH (1967).
[b] *A. acutus*, OUYANG et al. (1971a).
[c] *T. gramineus*, OUYANG and YANG (1974).
[d] *C. h. horridus*, BONILLA (1975).
[e] *C. adamanteus*, MARKLAND and DAMUS (1971).
[f] *T. okinavensis*, ANDERSSON (1972).
[g] Bovine thrombin, SEEGERS et al. (1974).

Table 4. Properties of thrombin-like enzymes from venoms of *B. marajoensis* and *B. moojeni*[a]

	B. marajoensis	*B. moojeni*
Mol wt, SDS gel		
Reduction prevented	43000	36000
Reduced and alkylated	41600	35800
Electrophoretic mobility in 7.5% polyacrylamide/pH 2.5	0.77	1.0
Neutral carbohydrate	10%	6%
Peptide A released	Yes	Yes
Peptide B released	No	No
Inhibition by heparin	No	No
Activation of F-XIII	No	Yes
Clot solubility 5 M urea[b]	Yes	No
Clot retraction	No	No
Specific activity	1900[c]	500[c]
NH_2 terminal amino acid	VAL	VAL

[a] Modified from STOCKER and BARLOW (1975a).
[b] Prothrombin-free human plasma plus calcium ions.
[c] Plasma clotting units/mg.

(CHENG and OUYANG, 1967). The thromboserpentin was later obtained in the same laboratory in purified form and the work was summarized as given below (OUYANG et al., 1971 a):

By means of DEAE-Sephadex column chromatography, *Agkistrodon acutus* venom was separated into 12 fractions. The thrombin-like activity was concentrated in Fr. 10. This fraction was rechromatographed on Sephadex G-200. A single band was found on microzone electrophoresis at pH 7.4. A single boundary with $S^0_{20,w}$ of 3.82 S, which was almost symmetrical, was observed by ultracentrifugation. The estimated molecular weight is 33 500. The chemical analysis shows that the thrombin-like principle of the venom is a glycoprotein. The specific activity is 13 times higher than that of the crude venom. The optimal pH value of the thrombin-like principle (pH 7.5) of the venom is almost identical with that of the bovine thrombin (pH 7.2). The thrombin-like principle of the venom is not affected by heparin, while the clotting activity of the bovine thrombin is inhibited by heparin. The thrombin-like principle of the venom is much more heat stable than the bovine thrombin. No clot retraction was found with the thrombin-like principle of the venom, while the marked clot retraction occurred after plasma was coagulated with thrombin. Thrombin can activate Factor XIII (fibrin stabilizing factor), while the thrombin-like principle can not.

The carbohydrate analysis was as follows: neutral sugars 8.0%, sialic acid 4.0%, and hexosamine 1.2%.

Inhibition of the thrombin-like enzyme from the Hundred-pace snake *(Agkistrodon acutus)* by various inhibitors was studied (OUYANG and HONG, 1974). Most of the reagents that inhibit thrombin (CALDWELL and SEEGERS, 1965), including DFP, were found to inhibit the purified thromboserpentin. Perhaps the most interesting was the failure of N-α-tosyl-L-lysine-chloromethylketone (TLCK) to inhibit. This compound inhibits thrombin, but there is an interesting peculiarity. Thrombin undergoes autolysis at alkaline pH. In that process, a portion of the NH_2 terminal end of the B chain is lost. The modified thrombin is called thrombin E or β-thrombin. The B 1 chain lost during autolysis carries the active histidine with which the TLCK reacts. Loss of B 1 chain destroys the fibrinogen clotting power but not the capacity to hydrolyze TAME (SEEGERS and ANDARY, 1974). The special active histidine is apparently not needed by thromboserpentin and only for the proteolytic function of thrombin. Thrombin E, mentioned above, is inhibited by antithrombin III and by DFP.

Another thromboserpentin has been isolated from the venom of the Eastern diamondback rattlesnake, *Crotalus adamanteus* (MARKLAND and DAMUS, 1971). The summary follows:

A thrombin-like enzyme has been purified to homogeneity from the venom of *Crotalus adamanteus* (Eastern diamondback rattlesnake). The enzyme acts directly on fibrinogen in vivo (and in vitro) apparently without affecting any of the other proteins involved in blood coagulation. The enzyme has esterase activity on basic amino acid esters and *p*-nitrophenyl esters of various N-carbobenzoxy amino acids. It exhibits no activity with a variety of N-benzoyl or N-methyl amino acid amides. Physicochemical studies indicated that the enzyme is a glycoprotein with a molecular weight of 32 700. Additionally, sedimentation equilibrium in guanidine β-mercaptoethanol showed that the enzyme contains a single polypeptide chain. The protein contains approximately 267 residues with a relatively high content of cystine. The enzyme is optimally active near pH 8 and is stable to neutral and alkaline pH; however, it loses activity upon exposure to acid pH. Both clotting and esterase activities are inhibited by diisopropyl phosphofluoridate, showing that the enzyme, like thrombin, is a serine esterase. Furthermore, the chloromethyl ketone of tosyl-L-lysine, a specific inhibitor of trypsin and thrombin, inhibits the venom enzyme indicating that a histidine residue is necessary for the activity of this enzyme. The chloromethyl ketone of tosyl-L-phenylalanine is not an inhibitor of the venom enzyme. Nitration of the enzyme with tetranitromethane causes loss of clotting activity with little effect on esterase activity suggesting that 1 or more tyrosine residues may be involved in the binding site for large substrates. Finally, the importance of disulfide bridges to the structural integrity of the venom enzyme was indicated by the rapid loss of activity in the presence of β-mercaptoethanol.

The venom of the Bamboo snake *(Trimeresurus gramineus)* was divided into several fractions. One of these contained much thromboserpentin, while another contained anticoagulant (SHIAU and OUYANG, 1965). The purification of the coagulant was described later (OUYANG and YANG, 1974), and the summary of that presentation was approximately as follows:

By means of Sephadex G-100 column chromatography, *Trimeresurus gramineus* venom was separated into five fractions. The thrombin-like activity was concentrated in Fraction I. This fraction was rechromatographed on Sephadex G-100 and CM-cellulose, and a single peak was obtained. The patterns of microzone and disc electrophoresis also showed a single band. A single, symmetrical boundary with a value of 3.22 S was obtained by ultracentrifugation. The estimated molecular weight was 29500. The isoelectric point was pH 3.5. The chemical analysis showed that the *T. gramineus* thrombin-like enzyme was a glycoprotein. The specific activity was eleven times higher than that of the crude venom. The optimal pH value of *T. gramineus* thrombin-like enzyme (pH 7.3) was identical with that of the bovine thrombin (pH 7.3). *T. gramineus* thrombin-like enzyme was not affected by heparin. No clot retraction was found with *T. gramineus* thrombin-like enzyme, while the marked clot retraction occurred after plasma was coagulated with thrombin. Thrombin could activate Factor XIII (fibrin stabilizing factor), while the thrombin-like enzyme could not.

The enzyme was unusually heat resistant and contained much carbohydrate; namely, 14.3% neutral sugars and 10.7% sialic acid.

A thrombin-like enzyme was isolated from the Timber rattlesnake *(C.h. horridus)* venom (BONILLA, 1975). Part of the summary is given:

A defibrinating (thrombin-like) enzyme, isolated from Timber rattlesnake *(C.h. horridus)* venom by gel filtration, ion exchange and adsorption chromatography was found to be homogeneous by (i) analytical ultracentrifugation, (ii) electrophoresis in highly cross-linked (12.8%), acidic, 6 M urea polyacrylamide gels. The molecular weight was 19610 based on amino acid composition, 19500 by sedimentation velocity and 19500 by sedimentation equilibrium. The enzyme is specific for the fibrinogen-fibrin conversion and does not affect other blood clotting factors; it exhibits an unusually high stability to acid pH and high temperature and it is partially inhibited by heparin only in very high concentrations.

The purified material did not activate fibrinoligase. The same fractionation procedure was applied to *C. adamanteus* venom thromboserpentin with equal molecular weight and amino acid composition was obtained. Since this differs from other results (MARKLAND and DAMUS, 1971), it could be that there are two kinds of thromboserpentin obtainable from *C. adamanteus* venom, one with molecular mass 32700 and another with 20000 daltons.

The amino acid composition of purified thrombin-like enzyme from *Trimeresurus okinavensis* venom has been determined (ANDERSSON, 1972) and like other thrombin-like enzymes is low in tryptophan, phenylalanine, tyrosine, methionine, and histidine. It seems likely that much homology will be found for these enzymes when the primary structure is determined. It is a glycoprotein with a molecular weight near 35000.

Another thrombin-like enzyme was isolated from the venom of the Gaboon viper *(Bitis gabonica)* (MARSH et al., 1975). The preparation had no plasminogen activator activity and no proteolytic activity on casein and fibrin. Two active fractions were obtained, but the purified material was a single component with a molecular weight in the range of 40000. This thrombin-like enzyme removed both fibrinopeptides A and B and activated Factor XIII.

III. Formation of Fibrin

The difference between the formation of fibrin with thrombin-like enzymes, as compared with thrombin, is repeatedly referred to in the literature. Consider thrombin first. Its substrate, fibrinogen (mol wt 340000), is composed of three polypeptide chains bound by disulfide bridges. The chains are named Aα, Bβ, and γ. Each one of these occurs as a dimer in fibrinogen. Thrombin removes peptide A rapidly and peptide B more slowly. Peptide A in the human begins with Ala-Asp-Ser and has variants known as AP in which serine is phosphorylated. Another variant is AY which does not have the Ala residue. The remaining protein is the fibrin monomer which, by a process of self-assembly, forms the fibrin polymer recognized as a gel.

The resulting fibrin polymer is soluble in such reagents as concentrated urea solution and again forms a gel if the urea is removed. To account for the fact that normal clots are *not* soluble, it has been found that Factor XIII is activated by thrombin. The resulting Factor XIIIa produces peptide bonds between preferred ε-amino groups of lysine and glutamine. Such cross-linked fibrin is not soluble in 5 M urea solutions. The fibrin is commonly designated as fibrin-*i* or $[(\alpha\cdot\beta\cdot\gamma)_2]_n^x$ as compared with the soluble fibrin-*s* or $[(\alpha\cdot\beta\cdot\gamma)_2]_n$. In the fibrin polymer, the molecules are aligned end-to-end and side-to-side (BLOMBÄCK, 1958; LAURENT and BLOMBÄCK, 1958).

In the case of ancrod[1] and batroxobin[1] only fibrinopeptide A and the variants are released (BLOMBÄCK et al., 1957; BLOMBÄCK, 1958; BLOMBÄCK and LAURENT, 1958; BLOMBÄCK and YAMASHINA, 1958; HOLLEMAN and COEN, 1970; EWART et al., 1970). As a consequence, the fibrin polymer has the composition $[(\alpha\cdot B\beta\cdot\gamma)_2]_n$ and is structured mainly end-to-end. In addition, ancrod and batroxobin slowly release other peptides, and even small amounts of fibrinopeptide B (HESSEL and BLOMBÄCK, 1971), but the two enzymes have different specificities. Southern copperhead (*Agkistrodon contortrix contortrix*) snake venom releases peptide B preferentially and is thus unusual (HERZIG et al., 1970). The polymer can be designated $[(A\alpha\cdot\beta\cdot\gamma)_2]_n$ and does not form a visible gel. To have gel formation requires a significant release of peptide A. The thromboserpentin was completely inhibited by PMSF and a human pancreatic trypsin inhibitor but not by lima bean trypsin inhibitor.

In addition to the limited or rapid digestion of fibrinogen by ancrod or batroxobin, a slower degradation follows. The disulfide knot, which is the NH_2 terminal dimeric portion of the fibrinogen molecule obtained by treatment of fibrinogen with cyanogen bromide, is digested by ancrod as well as batroxobin. Each enzyme, including thrombin, produces slightly different digestion products (HESSEL and BLOMBÄCK, 1971). Ancrod digested the Aα chain of human fibrinogen to produce a polypeptide of mol wt = 39000. This was bound within the clot. A free polypeptide of mol wt = 31000 was in the supernatant solution and was further digested. In higher enzyme concentration, α-polymers of cross-linked fibrin were digested (EDGAR and PRENTICE, 1973). The authors further state:

[1] In this context, it is convenient to use generic designations (Table 2).

Digestion of the separated Aα, Bβ, and γ chains of S-carboxymethyl fibrinogen by ancrod showed the Aα chain to be the most susceptible to proteolysis and that the same digestion products were formed as from the intact fibrinogen molecule. Additionally, limited proteolytic digestion of the separated γ chain was observed.

In the fibrinogen molecule, γ-chain digestion was not observed.

In the investigations of PIZZO et al. (1972), it was found that ancrod extensively digested α-chains of fibrin monomers at different sites than plasmin. Batroxobin or thrombin did not do this. The fibrin formed by ancrod was strikingly more vulnerable to plasmin digestion than fibrin formed with batroxobin or thrombin. Fibrin formed with ancrod has degraded α-chains.

At this juncture, it appears helpful to record a generalization which seems to be upheld quite well. In plasmin digestion of fibrinogen, the Aα chain is preferred, then Bβ, while the γ-chain is most resistant (MURANO et al., 1972). The earliest plasmin degradation products of fibrinogen are from the C terminal portion of the Aα-chain. For cross-linking, the preferred location is near the C terminal ends of the γ-chains (DOOLITTLE et al., 1972), followed by α- and lastly the β-chain. Fibrin is more readily cross-linked than fibrinogen because removal of fibrinopeptides makes the cross-linking sites more accessible to fibrinoligase. Noncross-linked fibrin is more susceptible to lysis by plasmin than the cross-linked variety (BRUNER-LORAND et al., 1966; MCDONAGH et al., 1971; FEDDERSEN and GORMSEN, 1971). Urokinase was used to induce plasminogen activation and thrombin-activated Factor XIII was found to render clots more resistant to fibrinolysis. The same could be inferred from previous work (GORMSEN et al., 1967). A general discussion of the topic has been written (FINLAYSON, 1974).

Concanavalin A (Con-A) prolongs the thrombin clotting time of plasma or purified fibrinogen. This is because Con-A binds to carbohydrate on the thrombin molecule. The prolongation of the clotting time is prevented by α-methyl-D-mannoside which also binds to Con-A thus protecting the binding site(s) on thrombin (KARPATKIN and KARPATKIN, 1974). Batroxobin and the thrombin-like enzyme in the venom of *Agkistrodon c. contortrix* (releases fibrinopeptide B initially) are not retarded by Con-A. Batroxobin, like thrombin, also contains carbohydrate, but it probably is not suitable for binding to Con-A or if there is binding, this does not result in an interference with the activity.

Effects of purified thrombin-like and anticoagulant principles of *Agkistrodon acutus* were studied by OUYANG and TENG (1976a). They state:

The effects of the purified thrombin-like and anticoagulant principles of the snake venom of *Agkistrodon acutus* on blood coagulation of rabbits in vivo were studied. The thrombin-like principle caused a marked prolongation of whole blood coagulation time and one-stage plasma prothrombin time and a marked decrease of the fibrinogen concentration, while no significant change in the two-stage plasma prothrombin level was detected. It is concluded that the retardation of blood clotting by the thrombin-like principle was chiefly due to the decrease of plasma fibrinogen level. The anticoagulant principle caused a marked, but transient prolongation of whole blood coagulation time and one-stage plasma prothrombin time with no significant change in the two-stage plasma prothrombin level or plasma fibrinogen level. Combining these results with our previous in vitro findings, it is concluded that the retardation of blood clotting by the anticoagulant principle might be due to the interference in the interaction between prothrombin and its activation factors.

Similar results were obtained respectively with the purified thrombin-like and anticoagulant principles of *Trimeresurus gramineus* venom (OUYANG and YANG, 1976).

IV. Thrombin-Like Enzymes and Cross-Linking of Fibrin

Ancrod does not activate Factor XIII and, consequently, clots that form with this enzyme are not cross-linked (CHAN et al., 1965; BARLOW et al., 1970; EWART et al., 1970). On the other hand, batroxobin activates Factor XIII (KOPEĆ et al., 1969; DVILANSKY et al., 1970; HARDER and STRAUB, 1972; EGBERG et al., 1971; BLOMBÄCK and EGBERG, 1975). In the article of DVILANSKY et al. (1970), it is pointed out that the normal range of fibrinoligase concentration in plasma is wide. Aged serum contains about 12% of that in plasma. Fresh plasma and outdated bank blood have the same concentration. In another report (PIZZO et al., 1972), it is stated that ancrod did not produce active fibrinoligase, whereas batroxobin and thrombin did.

V. Platelets and Thrombin-like Enzymes

Apparently all authors who have taken it into account report that there is no change in platelet count associated with the infusion of thrombin-like enzymes. The situation may be quite different when the whole venom is used (DAVEY and LÜSCHER, 1965). In that case, some venoms are powerful aggregating agents.

Older methods of clot retraction have been improved and now excellent recording systems for measuring the strength of retraction can be used. The thrombin-like enzyme of the Southern copperhead *(Agkistrodon c. contortrix)* venom did not aggregate rabbit platelets (TANGEN et al., 1973). Batroxobin clotting was not followed by retraction nor the development of mechanical strength unless additional substances were used (DE GAETANO et al., 1974). Adenosine 5′-diphosphate (ADP) in a final concentration 4×10^{-6}–4×10^{-5} M was added to a clot of platelet-rich plasma. The strength of the retraction increased progressively for about 40 min. If the ADP was washed out of the bath around the clot, the development of mechanic strength continued. Prostaglandin E_1 (PGE_1) added at any time before maximal contraction reversed the activity with the retraction falling to the original base line. PGE_1 inhibition was reversible, for it could be washed out and retraction followed upon a second addition of ADP. Platelet-poor plasma responded to neither ADP nor PGE_1.

In an earlier paper than the one discussed above, DE GAETANO et al. (1973) reported additional details about retraction of platelet-rich batroxobin clots. In addition to ADP, they found that collagen, adrenaline or thrombofax (a partial thromboplastin reagent) served as "cofactors" to induce retraction and probably alter platelet membrane function. Neither ancrod nor batroxobin induces the platelet release reaction and, therefore, these enzymes alone are not sufficient for clot retraction. As inhibitors PGE_1, methylxanthines, dipyridamole, and congeners were effective. This was interpreted to mean interference with activation of the contractile system. The anti-inflammatory drugs function at the level of extrusion of specific platelet compounds. Acetylsalicylic acid and indomethacin had no inhibitory effect comparable to PGE_1 etc. The three functional levels are membrane alteration (ADP, collagen, adrenaline, thrombofax and thrombin), activation of contractile system (inhibited by PGE_1 etc.) and extrusion of platelet components (anti-inflammatory compounds).

In the enthusiasm for the use of thromboserpentin, it has been stated that the adhesion-aggregation reaction cannot be evaluated when clotting is elicited with thrombin because thrombin itself provokes this reaction. This does not account for information obtained with the use of purified thrombin and purified fibrinogen. It was clearly shown (BALLERINI and SEEGERS, 1959) that a combination of purified fibrinogen + platelets + purified thrombin + calcium ions would not retract. Retraction was induced if a plasma dialysate was also added or if a protein fraction, obtained from plasma by adsorption on barium carbonate and subsequent fractionation, was added.

Platelets interact with polymerizing fibrin when produced by batroxobin (NIEWIAROWSKI et al., 1972). The venom enzyme did not initiate the platelet release reaction. Others independently came to the same conclusion (BROWN et al., 1972) with the use of ancrod. Human platelets incubated with ancrod did not aggregate but aggregated when subsequently treated with purified thrombin.

VI. Animal and Clinical Work

The idea to use thromboserpentin as an agent for treating certain types of thrombosis evidently developed from reports on the effects of snake bites. The main facts were that victims frequently had incoagulable blood and, nevertheless, did not bleed extensively (REID, 1963). Fibrinogen was generally depleted by coagulation and associated fibrinolysis was observed (REID et al., 1963a, b). In the latter article, much historic information appears. The paradox of using a coagulant with the intention of achieving anticoagulation was clearly appreciated (REID and CHAN, 1968). In nine patients, defibrination[1] was produced with ancrod (BELL et al., 1968a). Plasma fibrinogen levels were brought to less than 40 mg/100 ml, remained low during therapy, and slowly returned to normal 2 or more weeks after therapy. Fibrinogen-fibrin decomposition products were evident the first 36 h. There were no hemorrhages including two cases during the menstrual cycle. In seven cases of venous thrombosis, there was rapid resolution of signs and symptoms. Three patients had thrombosis for 5 weeks, failing to respond to conventional therapy. Two developed thrombosis during oral anticoagulant therapy and responded to ancrod.

In somewhat similar pioneer clinical applications (SHARP et al., 1968), ancrod was given every 12 h. Much of the ancrod appeared unaltered in the urine. There were some difficulties with bleeding from surgical wounds, from a small bowel lesion, but an absence of spontaneous bleeding from normal tissues. The procedure was highly recommended where drastic lifesaving anticoagulation is required. In further clinical work (BELL et al., 1968b), it was observed that no changes were produced in blood coagulation Factors V, VIII, IX, or X, but there was some loss of VII. The ancrod was given slowly every 6, and later, 12 h. Upon cessation, the fibrinogen concentration returned to normal over a period of about 5 days. Along the same lines of investigation (CHAN et al., 1965), coagulation with ancrod was not retarded by heparin, there was no clot retraction, and some plasmas apparently retarded the venom activity. In recent clinical work, the enzyme was administered subcutaneously (EHRLY, 1975a). As compared with the i.v. route, the defibrination progressed slowly, was less dangerous, simpler, and required less of the material.

[1] Some authors use the term defibrinogenation, which is most accurate, while many shorten this to defibrination. We use the latter or the most common designation.

Ancrod is an effective anticoagulant for hemodialysis but is not recommended as a substitute for heparin (HALL et al., 1970).

Ancrod was used as a defibrinating agent in sickle cell crisis but without benefit to the patients (MANN et al., 1972). Management of priapism met with success (BELL and PITNEY, 1969), and there are comments on historic developments (PITNEY et al., 1970) of a general nature.

A comparative study was made of the value of heparin, streptokinase, or ancrod for patients with deep vein thrombosis of the legs of less than 4 h duration (KAKKAR et al., 1969a, b). They state: "We conclude that if deep vein thrombosis can be diagnosed within 36 h of onset, thrombi can be dissolved completely and valvular function preserved." Streptokinase was found to be the most effective thrombolytic agent—the best therapeutic agent for the patient. The work was carefully monitored by infusing ^{125}I-labeled fibrinogen and observing by repeated phlebography. In a study with 30 patients with *established* deep vein thrombosis of the leg, heparin and ancrod were compared. There were no serious side-effects, but neither substance had a significant effect on the resolution of thrombosis in the deep leg veins (DAVIES et al., 1972).

In experimental work with dogs (MARSTEN et al., 1966), a segment of tape was fixed across the lumen of the inferior vena cava without interfering with blood flow. It was possible to reduce the extent of experimental thrombosis by first defibrinating with the use of Malayan pit viper venom. During the defibrination, the platelet counts remained up and fibrinolysis was accelerated by "nonspecific" and as yet unexplained manner. Working with *A. rhodostoma* venom (ESNOUF and MARSHALL, 1968; MARSHALL and ESNOUF, 1968), defibrination was achieved with only a transient rise in pulmonary pressure. No blood clots were found in the lungs or systemic vessels at autopsy. With high doses (higher than needed for therapeutic purposes), death followed and clots were observed in the right heart and pulmonary vessels. From experiments in which the reticuloendothelial system (RES) and liver circulation were manipulated, it was decided that the RES is likely not to be a factor of importance for effects of the venom. On the other hand, others found a strong stimulation of RES by ancrod (ASHFORD and BUNN, 1970) when rabbits were used as experimental animals. Ancrod itself is taken up and metabolized by RES (REGOECZI and BELL, 1969). ASHFORD et al. (1968) reported that there were no changes in EKG or in systemic blood pressure when ancrod was used in a clinically defibrinating dose in animal experiments involving rabbits, cats, dogs, and rats.

In additional experiments with dogs, OLSSON et al. (1973) were motivated by the fact that surgery on deep veins is hazardous because a thrombus is likely to form at the site of vessel injury and conventional anticoagulation is likely to promote bleeding. Surgery immediately after treatment with batroxobin was associated with dangerous bleeding due to the high concentration of fibrinogen decomposition products which interfered with some fibrin formation and perhaps also platelet function (PRENTICE et al., 1969; KOWALSKI et al., 1965). It has, however, also been reported that there is no reduction in platelet adhesiveness (MARTIN and MARTIN, 1975). Defibrinogenation 2 days before surgery made it possible to perform surgery. This has been confirmed (BROWSE, 1975). There were no deaths due to bleeding. There was some impairment of wound healing.

Experimental work with dogs involved chemical injury to a short segment of the femoral vein (RAHIMTOOLA et al., 1970). This clearly produced thrombosis. The thrombus organized, and collateral circulation was established. Prophylactic treatment of the dogs with ancrod to produce defibrination immediately after the operation to produce chemical injury of the vein segment prevented thrombus formation. The injured section of the vein formed a new endothelial lining. A small percentage of the dogs was lost due to bleeding. The use of heparin instead of ancrod did not prevent thrombosis and the incidences of bleeding were greater. With the administration of the thrombin-like enzyme in the presence of performed thrombi, there was no lysis of the thrombus even though it was less than 24 h old. Heparin also was of no value in the treatment of the experimental thrombosis and, in fact, contributed to morbidity and bleeding. In another report, it was suggested that more experiments ought to be done on streptokinase therapy followed by ancrod in the treatment of deep vein thrombosis (PITNEY et al., 1971). In experimental pulmonary embolism, beneficial effects were produced with ancrod (SHARMA et al., 1973; OLSEN and PITNEY, 1969).

Ancrod infusion (rabbits) developed hypofibrinogenemia and induced the formation of circulating fibrin monomer complexes, but microthrombi were not detected in the glomerular capillaries unless endotoxin was also injected (MÜLLER-BERGHAUS and HOCKE, 1973). The formation of microthrombi in the kidney could not be prevented with heparin; thus, there was no activation of the coagulation system to produce thrombi. Possibly the endotoxin stimulated the α-adrenergic receptor sites and/or released basic proteins from platelets and/or leukocytes. The basic proteins would precipitate fibrin monomer complexes.

A comprehensive discussion, based on original experiments, covers many of the points referred to in this review (EGBERG, 1973).

After completing their own experimental work, PIZZO et al. (1972) state an overall perspective as follows:

On the basis of our data and results from other studies, it is possible to postulate the following sequence of events to account for the anticoagulant effect of ancrod in vivo: (a) the administration of ancrod results in the formation of fibrin clots in the microcirculation, particularly in the kidney, lungs, liver, and bone marrow; (b) these clots, however, contain non-crosslinked fibrin and furthermore become defective as the α chains continue to be significantly degraded by ancrod; (c) the activation of plasminogen to plasmin occurs in a manner analogous to that observed when intravascular clotting occurs as a result of thrombin generation; (d) the resultant high level of plasmin then digests ancrod-formed fibrin at a much more rapid rate than thrombin-formed fibrin, and this can be attributed to the fact that such fibrin is non-crosslinked and in addition, has already been significantly degraded by ancrod; (e) the generation of fibrin split products as well as the fibrinogenopenia produces a hypocoagulable state. In general, the results of clinical studies support these mechanisms. In such studies, patients receiving ancrod showed a marked decrease in plasminogen concentration, which often approached zero after about 10 h from the onset of ancrod administration. Also at this time, these investigators found that fibrin degradation products had usually reached a peak value. While the mechanism by which the fibrinolytic system becomes activated is not understood, it is clear that ancrod does not activate plasminogen as has been shown in this study by direct observations of ancrod action on purified plasminogen. Despite what mechanism may be invoked to explain the rapid activation of plasminogen to plasmin during intravascular clotting, it is apparent that ancrod clots are strikingly susceptible to plasmin degradation ... Besides digestion of plasmin, phagocytosis of fibrin by the reticuloendothelial system represents a second important method by which fibrin is removed from the microcirculation. However, whether or not the defective, non-crosslinked fibrin formed by ancrod is more susceptible to phagocytosis by the reticuloendothelial system is conjectural and must await further study.

KWAAN et al. (1973) came to the conclusion that noncross-linking of ancrod fibrin is not the basis for its susceptibility to lysis. Structural differences are suggested as a possible reason. They also found fibrin degradation products of smaller size than with thrombin clots appear rather early during the fibrinolytic process.

VII. Autoprothrombin II-A and Fibrinolysis

Thromboserpentin defibrination, with its distinct differences from thrombin defibrination, has, nevertheless, many similarities. Even good therapeutic results were reported at one time with the use of thrombin infusion (BRAMBEL, 1957). This practice was probably abandoned because any infusion of thrombin is presumed to be dangerous. In the same way, one is also confronted with a paradox with snake venoms where a procoagulant is used as an anticoagulant. Fibrinolysis is essential for survival. In the case of thrombin, one explanation for the associated fibrinolysis has been given. It occurs through generation of autoprothrombin II-A activity from prothrombin complex by small amounts of thrombin (MAMMEN et al., 1960; SEEGERS and ULUTIN, 1961). Autoprothrombin II-A is a competitive inhibitor of autoprothrombin C (Factor Xa) (MURANO et al., 1974; MARCINIAK et al., 1967). This inhibition of coagulation is thus in addition to the formation of fibrinogen degradation products (KOWALSKI et al., 1965). The inhibitor was also produced in rabbits (WETMORE and GUREWICH, 1974). Autoprothrombin II-A has been isolated and obtained in purified form (SEEGERS et al., 1972b). The purified material, in addition to functioning as an anticoagulant, induced fibrinolysis (SEEGERS et al., 1972b). This mechanism proved to involve only minimal direct activation of plasminogen with the main fibrinolysis being due to a substantial depression of inhibitors of fibrinolysis (ZOLTON and SEEGERS, 1973). Autoprothrombin II-A also depressed the activity of soybean trypsin inhibitor. It is quite likely that autoprothrombin II-A has an important role to contribute to our physiology as an anticoagulant and as an agent that promotes fibrinolysis. So far, apparently no one has tried to see whether autoprothrombin II-A activity can be produced with thromboserpentin. At the time of this writing, experiments on autoprothrombin II-A are in progress at Wayne State University. As in the early work (MAMMEN et al., 1960), it appears that autoprothrombin II-A is derived from Factor XIV (protein C) by activation with thrombin (SEEGERS et al., 1976).

VIII. Defibrination and Fibrinolysis with Acetylated Thrombin

Thrombin was acetylated and infused experimentally with the hope of inducing fibrinolysis and overcoming the natural objection to producing a coagulum or disseminated fibrin. Acetylation destroyed most of the proteolytic activity of thrombin with retention of esterase function (LANDABURU and SEEGERS, 1959). It was not possible to remove all coagulant thrombin. At best, about 1 unit remained for every 25000 esterase units, nor was it possible to be certain that regeneration of activity did not occur in vivo. Infusion of such material (SEEGERS et al., 1960a, b; LANDABURU et al., 1968; PECHET et al., 1968) induced fibrinolysis in dogs. Early during the intravenous infusion, the plasminogen concentration and fibrinogen concentration were reduced to the 30% range. There was a shortening of the euglobulin lysis time. Fibrin split products appeared early in plasma (RIDDLE and BARNHART, 1969). Platelet counts remained normal as well as heart rate and respiration. With large quantities of infused acetylated thrombin, it was possible to produce elevated heart rate, to increase the right ventricular pressure and to reduce aortic flow due to intravascular clots. In the lower ranges of infusion rates, animals had microvascular thrombosis in the kidneys. This fibrin remained only temporarily and animals survived without ill effects (BROERSMA et al., 1971). To produce platelet aggregation in vitro, large amounts of acetylated thrombin were required (SEEGERS et al., 1970) and, depending upon dosage, the process reversed itself in a short time. Others also have found that acetylated thrombin does not aggregate platelets (TANGEN and BYGDEMAN, 1972).

The fibrinolysis induced in dogs with acetylated thrombin was not blocked by epsilon aminocaproic acid (EACA) or aprotinin (trasylol). If plasmin was involved in the traditional sense, EACA as well as aprotinin should have blocked the lysis. Heparin was also without effect. The eosinophilic leukocyte count was reduced and presumably their fibrinolysin content was utilized. One dog was pretreated, before acetylated thrombin infusion, with Coumadin to decrease the prothrombin complex concentration of plasma. There was no temporary decrease in platelet count in that animal (MCCOY et al., 1971). Possibly, here is a relationship to the observation that retraction of purified fibrin clots requires a factor that is adsorbed from plasma on, and eluted from, barium carbonate (BALLERINI and SEEGERS, 1959).

The similarity in the responses to the infusion of thromboserpentin, thrombin in small amounts, or acetylated thrombin is extensive. It is important to note that this occurs in vivo and not so strikingly in test tubes. It remains to be determined whether acetylated thrombin activates Factor XIII or whether the clots that form in vivo after acetylated thrombin infusion are the result of fibrinopeptide A or B removal or both. It remains to be determined whether thrombin-like enzymes reduce eosinophilic leukocyte counts as occurs with thrombin. These cells contain plasminogen. There is more than one way to account for the fibrinolysis that follows the infusion of thrombin-like enzymes, acetylated thrombin, or thrombin itself. We can assume a common feature. Autoprothrombin II-A has already been mentioned as a likely factor, but apparently no one has tried to see whether thrombin-like enzymes convert protein C to autoprothrombin II-A. Hypoxia could be another "cause" as well as the accumulation of metabolic products due to a diminished flow rate. Perhaps some tissue activator is released. Possibly there is direct or indirect activation of prekallikrein with subsequent activation of plasminogen. Whether the fibrinolytic process is induced with acetylated thrombin or thromboserpentin, it is difficult, in either case, to delay it with EACA or aprotinin (trasylol).

IX. Miscellaneous Aspects

1. Units of Activity

The ancrod unit of clotting activity has been compared with thrombin activity. The clotting of fibrinogen by thrombin can be of short duration such as a few seconds. As the thrombin is diluted, clotting times are progressively prolonged (SEEGERS and SMITH, 1942). The original unit of thrombin (Iowa unit) was defined as the amount which would clot 1 ml of standardized fibrinogen solution in 15 sec. It requires

1.2 Iowa units for 1 NIH unit. The ancrod unit was intended to match 1 NIH unit, but is about one-third of an NIH unit (BARLOW and DEVINE, 1974). The above holds for proteolytic or "clotting" units when fibrinogen is the substrate. The regression curves obtained with thrombin and the thrombin-like enzymes in determining the fibrin coagulation time are not the same (BARLOW and DEVINE, 1974; VINAZZER, 1975). As has already been mentioned (LANDABURU and SEEGERS, 1959), thrombin esterase units and clotting units are only equivalent under specified conditions and by definition (SEEGERS, 1962). The claim that esterase and clotting activities of *B. atrox* venom belong to different molecules (DEVI et al., 1972) is really not based on sufficient evidence. One molecule can have both functions (EGBERG, 1974). In the case of thrombin, esterase and clotting activities are the property of one molecule; that same molecule can be degraded so that there is only esterase activity (SEEGERS et al., 1974). Furthermore, a substance such as profragment 2 can enhance esterase activity while proteolytic activity is depressed at the same time. It is interesting to compare the potency of thrombin and ancrod. The latter, as a highly purified preparation, was found to have 100 NIH units (EGBERG, 1974), or in reality, 33.3 units. Purified bovine thrombin had 7770 NIH units/mg dry weight (SEEGERS et al., 1974). With more precise figures or simultaneous comparisons, only approximations are possible. Thrombin might be about 235 times more active on fibrinogen than ancrod.

2. Elimination of Thrombin-Like Enzyme

Attempts have been made to account for the metabolism of infused thromboserpentin. In one study, ancrod was labeled with radioactive iodine (EGBERG, 1974). More or less, 10–25% of the radioactivity was associated with plasma protein. The half-life of the enzyme was estimated to be near the duration of the defibrinating effect of the enzyme, namely, 3–10 h. Effects are, however, much longer. The labeled enzyme was slowly excreted in the urine in an inactive form. A slow turnover was earlier reported (EGBERG, 1972). The batroxobin used formed a complex with plasma α_2-macroglobulin, as well as with purified α_2-macroglobulin. The complex had very little proteolytic activity but, like thrombin, retained its hydrolytic activity on small substrates. This complex was dissociated by dialysis against water and freeze-drying. Ancrod was also found to complex with α_2-macroglobulin (PITNEY and REGOECZI, 1970). There seems to be no clear answer as to whether antithrombin III neutralizes the activity.

In the discussion of other literature (EGBERG, 1974), it is pointed out that the enzyme may be taken up by the reticuloendothelial cells, degraded, liberated to the circulation, and excreted in the urine. In the case of plasmin, complexes formed with plasma constituents have proteolytic activity and serve as a reservoir of enzyme activity. This mechanism probably does not apply to thromboserpentin. The elimination of the enzyme appears to be independent of the fibrinogen level (STRAUB et al., 1975). In the case of trypsin, α_2-macroglobulin-trypsin complexes are rapidly eliminated by the RES.

3. Inhibitors

The amount of thromboserpentin inhibitor(s) in plasma can be measured quantitatively (STOCKER and YEH, 1975). A fibrinogen solution is placed in small glass tubes

(4×60 mm). This is overlayered by the venom or purified thrombin-like enzyme solution. A clot forms and the thromboserpentin diffuses into the fibrinogen. An inhibitor in the fibrinogen solution reduces the velocity of clot propagation. By this method, there was inhibition by antiserum to ancrod and batroxobin and heparinized serum but not by heparin alone or plasma-containing fibrinogen split products. In this connection, it is interesting that thrombin does not propagate or diffuse progressively because it is adsorbed onto fibrin (SEEGERS, 1962). By investigations with radioactive materials and immunologic techniques (EGBERG, 1972), a precipitation arc representing α_2-macroglobulin was the only line with radioactivity. There was none corresponding to antithrombin III or α_1-antitrypsin. This evidence is against the latter two as having any reaction with batroxobin. Antibodies to ancrod are distinctly different from antibodies to batroxobin, and no cross-reactions were observed (BARLOW et al., 1973a). The venom of the Malayan pit viper apparently produced antibodies in sheep (ROBERTSON SMITH and MORAG, 1972). Resistance to infused venom developed in about 21 days.

4. Hemostasis

Earlier in this review, we considered that the requirements for hemostasis involved three functions; namely, a) hemostatic function of the vascular smooth muscle, b) hemostatic function of the platelets, and c) hemostatic function of blood coagulation. Any single one is dispensable, enabling the remaining two to function adequately or at least temporarily. This approximation holds for the hemostasis which can be achieved if the blood coagulation mechanisms are drastically impaired by the infusion of thromboserpentin. If platelet function is additionally interfered with, a bleeding tendency develops. With a dog as experimental model, thromboserpentin was given to simulate therapeutic conditions (OLSSON and JOHNSSON, 1972), and bleeding was measured. It was not extensive in the controls. It was significantly increased by acetylsalicylic acid, heparin, and by fibrinogen decomposition products. The authors presume that the effect of heparin was due to indirect impaired function of remaining fibrinogen. The other two substances impaired the function of platelets. Bleeding appeared to be prolonged during the defibrination period (EGBERG and JOHNSSON, 1972) when fibrinogen concentration was low and FDP products were in high concentration.

Surgery is possible in states of defibrinogenation (OLSSON et al., 1971), and the following was concluded on the basis of experiments with animals and observations of one patient:

> Dogs were defibrinogenated with Reptilase. The bleeding tendency measured on the third day of the Reptilase treatment was found to be moderate. Administration of acetylsalicylic acid or heparin enhanced the bleeding. Defibrinogenated dogs had the inferior vena cava replaced with dacron grafts. The defibrinogenation was maintained for 1 week postoperatively. All dogs survived and the graft remained patent. Grafts in control animals were all occluded. One patient had thrombi removed from the inferior vena cava and left iliac vein under Reptilase treatment. Four months postoperatively the veins were patent.

From time to time, snake venoms have been used systemically and for topical applications. Evaluation is difficult and the topic will not be discussed further. An example of the problem of evaluation is the work of KOEHNLEIN (1972). An evaluation of thrombin for topical application has been made (SEEGERS and SHARP, 1948).

It is suggested that infusion of thrombin-like enzymes in hemophiliacs should be studied in further detail (HARDER et al., 1972).

5. Rheology

Under treatment with ancrod, a physiologically significant reduction in blood viscosity occurs and, as a consequence, blood flow is increased (EHRINGER et al., 1975). One of the benefits is rise in blood oxygenation and oxygen supply and a change in nonoxygen-consuming metabolism (KÖHLER, 1975). This is without hemodilution. The membrane properties of erythrocytes are not affected (EHRLY, 1975b). In certain cases, beneficial effects of batroxobin in deep vein thrombosis could be demonstrated with phlebograms (DIENER, 1975). In animal experiments (OLSON, 1975), controlled production of thrombin proved that there is a substantial difference between the carotid artery and the jugular vein. On the arterial side, localized adherence and aggregation of platelets seems necessary for thrombus formation. On the venous side, this was not so. Fibrinogen was necessary in early thrombus formation on both the arterial and venous side.

6. Metastasis Formation

Fibrinogen or fibrin around disseminated tumor cells might be important for the development of metastases. The topic has received much attention, and for this report, we shall simply make reference to one of many ways in which thrombin-like enzymes have been used to study the subject (HAGMAR, 1972).

7. Phospholipase A_2

A phospholipase A_2 with anticoagulant activity has been isolated from *Vipera berus orientale* (Eastern Europe) venom (BOFFA et al., 1976). It was separated from other phospholipase components which were not related to the anticoagulant property. Molecular weight of the 119 amino acid single polypeptide chain was 13400. Crude cephalin was hydrolyzed by the lipase (BOFFA and BOFFA, 1976). Since there was no reduction in procoagulant activity, cleavage of the β-acyl bond could not account for the inhibitory activity which was apparently due to the formation of a complex between the inhibitor and phospholipid at their clotting protein binding site.

X. Venoms and Direct Fibrinolysis

Contributions to the subject of fibrinolysis by snake venoms have a broad range, including surveys (DEUTSCH and DINIZ, 1955; OUYANG, 1957; BANERJEE et al., 1973), observations on the induction of fibrinolysis by venom (GITTER et al., 1960; KORNALÍK, 1971), or venom fractions without indications about mechanisms, lysis by the purified thromboserpentins already discussed, direct lysis of fibrinogen by isolated protein, and other observations. Lysis was recognized in some of the first studies on the defibrination syndrome produced by a Malayan pit viper bite (CHAN and REID, 1964). Lysis is associated with the appearance of fibrinogen and fibrin split products, and the best known of these can be measured quantitatively (THOMAS et al., 1970; HOQ and CASH, 1973; KOPEĆ et al., 1970a).

In the earliest papers on the clinical and experimental work already mentioned, fibrinolysis was discerned to be an important part of the overall process. By means of agarose gel filtration and other techniques, high molecular weight clottable complexes of fibrinogen, as well as degradation products, can be measured quantitatively (ASBECK et al., 1975). The infusion of purified thrombin-like enzyme is accompanied by a decrease in plasminogen and antiplasmin levels and the appearance of fibrin and fibrinogen degradation products (REGOECZI et al., 1966; PITNEY et al., 1969; EGBERG and NORDSTRÖM, 1970; STRAUB and HARDER, 1971; BARLOW et al., 1973b; KWAAN et al., 1973; COLLEN and VERMYLEN, 1973). The lysis is apparently a secondary process. It is of critical importance, for animals die if pretreated with antifibrinolytic agents (REGOECZI et al., 1966), but once the process is started, it is difficult to delay it with EACA or aprotinin (EGBERG and NORDSTRÖM, 1970). Infusion of ^{125}I fibrinogen before defibrination made it possible to detect an elevated concentration of radioactivity over the spleen (STRAUB and HARDER, 1971). Some fibrin deposits appeared in the kidneys of dogs, but apparently did not interfere appreciably with the glomerular filtration rate (EGBERG and LJUNGQVIST, 1973). Lung capillaries sometimes contained some fibrin during the first hour after injection. No organ, including lung, liver, spleen, or muscle, was damaged by infarctions. The fibrinolytic mechanisms and RES system were considered most important to account for the disappearance of the fibrin.

In an effort to obtain insight from related work, it was found that ancrod-induced soluble fibrin products display renal glomerular microclots typical of the generalized Shwartzman's reaction if rabbits are infused simultaneously with ancrod, aprotinin, and norepinephrine (MÜLLER-BERGHAUS and MANN, 1973). Blockade of the α-adrenergic receptor sites diminishes the occurrence of glomerular microclots after endotoxin injection, whereas stimulation of α-adrenergic receptor sites favors the occurrence of glomerular capillary clots. In this connection, it is sufficient only to mention that soluble fibrin monomers are precipitated by cellular basic proteins as found, for example, in polymorphonuclear leukocytes (HAWIGER et al., 1969; KOPEĆ et al., 1970b). The random thoughts of this paragraph might eventually prove to have interrelationships.

Echis carinatus venom has the unique effect of enhancing plasminogen activation by urokinase (KORNALÍK, 1963).

Purification work on the fibrinolytic principle(s) of venoms is in its beginning stages. Successful work has been completed (OUYANG and HUANG, 1976a) with *Agkistrodon acutus* (Hundred-pace snake) venom. In the isolation work, 12 fractions were first obtained from a DEAE Sephadex chromatography column. The fibrinolytic activity was mainly in one of the fractions which was repeatedly passed through a Sephadex G-75 column. It was obtained as a single component as shown by disk gel electrophoresis before and after treatment to reduce disulfide bonds and was thus most likely a single-chain compound. The molecular weight by gel filtration was 23000. The amino acid composition for an assumed molecular weight of 23000 was a follows: Lys 11, His 7, Arg 7, Asp 25, Thr 11, Ser 23, Glu 21, Pro 8, Gly 12, Ala 12, Half-Cys 8, Val 10, Met 6, Ile 15, Leu 12, Tyr 10, Phe 5, and Trp 5. In the ultracentrifuge, the preparation sedimented as a single component with $S^0_{20,w}=2.44$. The fibrinolytic protein digested mainly the Aα-chain of fibrinogen and most likely not the

Bβ- or γ-chains. The lytic agent could be considered quite potent at substrate-enzyme proportions of 1000 to 1, respectively.

In addition to the fibrinolytic, fibrinogenolytic, and caseinolytic activities, the purified fibrinolytic principle of *Agkistrodon acutus* venom possessed hemorrhagic activity (OUYANG and HUANG, 1977). Trasylol had a much higher inhibitory action on the fibrinolytic activity of the fibrinolytic principle of the venom than did EACA. Thus, the fibrinolytic action of the fibrinolytic principle was chiefly due to a direct action on fibrin. Both EDTA (5×10^{-4} M) and cysteine (5×10^{-3} M) completely inhibited the fibrinolytic, fibrinogenolytic, hemorrhagic, and caseinolytic activities of the fibrinolytic principle of the venom. Disulfide bonds might be essential for the biologic activities of the fibrinolytic principle.

The venom of *Trimeresurus mucrosquamatus* (Taiwan habu) was fractionated by using CM Sephadex C-50 (OUYANG and TENG, 1976b). Out of 20 fractions, five were found to be fibrinogenolytic, fibrinolytic, and caseinolytic. Four out of the five did not hydrolyze TAME. Four of the five additionally produced hemorrhages in the peritoneal cavity when injected there, and the protein was absorbed because there were also hemorrhages in the lungs. The fraction which did not produce hemorrhages but hydrolyzed fibrinogen was further fractionated to obtain a single component. The molecular weight was in the 20000 range. In a substrate-enzyme ratio of 500 to 1, the Bβ-chain of fibrinogen was primarily digested with the early fragments having molecular weights in the 31000, 21000, and 10000 range. Later, the Aα-chain was also degraded. One of the other fractions (TAME-negative, hemorrhagic-positive) was studied. The purified material digested primarily the Aα-chain. The enzyme was quite active in a 1 to 2000 (wt/wt) enzyme-substrate ratio. It thus appears that at least two fibrinolytic agents can be obtained from one venom. One has a preference for the Bβ-chain, while the other digests primarily the Aα-chain of fibrinogen.

XI. Snake Venoms and Thrombin Formation

One of the widely used assay procedures is the one-stage test for prothrombin activity. It simply consists of mixing oxalated plasma with a proper concentration of $CaCl_2$ solution and a strong procoagulant, such as tissue thromboplastin, the latter being commonly obtained from brain. The merits and faults of this test have been widely discussed, and some improvement in specificity for measuring prothrombin activity is achieved by using Taipan snake venom *(Oxyuranus scutellatus scutellatus)* (DENSON et al., 1971) as the procoagulant. It generates thrombin directly from prothrombin without the need of other coagulation factors except phospholipid. In patients with phenindione therapy, a more slowly reacting prothrombin than normal was detected. This excess over the normal source of prothrombin has also been demonstrated in other methods, such as by immunology (JOSSO et al., 1968; DENSON, 1971) or the use of large amounts of purified autoprothrombin C and purified Ac-globulin in the two-stage analytic procedure for the assay of prothrombin (OUYANG et al., 1971b; MÜLLER-BERGHAUS and SEEGERS, 1966). In fact, a refractory type of prothrombin, is found in normal plasma (MÜLLER-BERGHAUS and SEEGERS, 1966).

In an article written recently (KORNALÍK and BLOMBÄCK, 1975), four venoms are said to form thrombin by digestion of prothrombin; namely, *Echis coloratus*, *Echis carinatus*, *Notechis scutatus scutatus*, and *Oxyuranus scutellatus scutellatus*. In the same article, the term *ecarin* is used to designate the enzyme in *Echis carinatus* (Saw-scaled viper). Ecarin has been obtained in purified form (SCHIECK et al., 1972a). Their summary follows:

1. The procoagulant from *Echis carinatus* venom, which is known to convert prothrombin into thrombin, has been purified by chromatography on calcium hydroxylapatite and DEAE-cellulose. Final purification, when necessary, can be achieved by disc gel electrophoresis. A final concentration of 0.5 µg/ml coagulates human citrate plasma in 70 sec.

2. The bulk of hemorrhagic, caseinolytic and fibrinogenolytic activities present in the starting venom is removed during purification, but the procoagulant causes some fibrinogenolysis, gelatinolysis, caseinolysis, and hemorrhage, even when homogeneous in disc gel electrophoresis. This argues for a proteolytic nature of the procoagulant activity. It is resistant against diisopropyl fluorophosphate and is not, therefore, an esteroprotease. Other protease inhibitors (from soybean, lima bean, bovine pancreas, and bovine serum) are also without effect.

3. The molecular weight is approximately 86000 as determined by gel filtration. On isoelectric focusing in solution, its isoelectric point is pH 4.4 ± 0.1. The procoagulant is relatively unstable; for instance, its pH-stability is restricted to values between 6 and 10.

In further studies (SCHIECK et al., 1972b), ecarin was found to digest purified prothrombin directly. The fibrinolytic effect of crude venom (KORNALÍK and PUDLÁK, 1971) was removed in the purification. It was not toxic in animals pretreated with oral anticoagulants because its substrate, prothrombin, was then not in the plasma. In mice, the LD_{50} was 2.5 mg/kg when given subcutaneously, and 0.25–0.5 mg/kg when given intravenously. A report on thrombin formation from purified prothrombin with purified ecarin (KORNALÍK and BLOMBÄCK, 1975) is generally confusing, but in terms of the bovine prothrombin model (Fig. 3), the emerging fact seems to be that the venom removes profragment 1 and opens the Arg-Ile bond, which must be broken (McCOY et al., 1973a). Thus, profragment 2 remains attached to the A chain of the classic thrombin structure, with the result that the specific activity is low, but one can really not be certain, from the analytic work presented, how this activity compares with that found for thrombin by other investigators. In work by IWANAGA (1975), it was also found that there is an extended A chain consisting of the regular A chain plus profragment 2.

In other reports (MORITA et al., 1974; IWANAGA et al., 1975), purified bovine prothrombin and purified ecarin were studied. It was found that the early products of activation consist of profragment 1 and prethrombin 1. Then the Arg-Ile bond number 3 of the latter (where the A and B chains of thrombin come together in prothrombin) was split, giving profragment 2 still bound to A chain and connected to the B chain by a disulfide bond. This compound had strong esterase activity associated with weak coagulant activity and was called intermediate ECV. It is now called Δ-3 prethrombin 1. In the next step, one bond was split to produce profragment 2 and classic thrombin. In the presence of hirudin, the first step in prothrombin activation consisted of breaking the Arg-Ile bond number 3 already referred to above. This yielded Δ-3 prothrombin. In a more recent report (FRANZA et al., 1975), the activation of purified human prothrombin was studied and the pattern was the same as outlined above for bovine prothrombin. Intermediate ECV had esterase and proteolytic activity. Another presentation (KORNALÍK and BLOMBÄCK, 1975) seems to be supportive. In the nomenclature used for constructing Figure 3, the work can be summarized as follows:

Step 1: Prothrombin → profragment 1 + prethrombin 1
Step 2: Prethrombin 1 → intermediate ECV (Δ-3 prethrombin 1)
Step 3: Intermediate ECV → profragment 2 + thrombin

In presence of hirudin:

Prothrombin → Δ-3 prothrombin.

It is important to note that the sequence (without inhibitor) involved the development of predominantly esterase activity, followed by thrombin with esterase plus proteolytic activity. If they had let the thrombin undergo autolysis, coagulant activity would doubtless have disappeared. Thus, with the Auto-C-like enzyme from the venom, the sequence first described many years ago can be simulated (SEEGERS and LANDABURU, 1957), namely, the following: esterase → esterase + proteolytic → esterase. The reason for the sequence is, however, not on the same basis as the old work.

Purified ecarin was used to produce experimental thrombosis in rats (KORNALÍK and HLADOVEC, 1975). An electric current was used to produce thrombosis on the carotid artery. Injection of adequate amounts of ecarin at intervals from 1 min to 24 h before use of the electric current decreased the incidence of thrombosis. It was also found that ecarin has a weak fibrinogenolytic effect.

Echis carinatus venom was used without further purification in studies on the activation of purified prothrombin isolated from chicken plasma. Conversion of purified chicken prothrombin to thrombin with purified bovine autoprothrombin C was associated with a low yield of thrombin (WALZ, 1973). The full thrombin potential was developed with Auto-C, purified Ac-globulin, crude "cephalin," and calcium ions, but the thrombin was not stable unless glycerol was added to the activation mixture. With crude *Echis carinatus* venom, the purified chicken prothrombin was also all converted to thrombin if enough venom was used, but the thrombin rapidly lost activity. By using purified chicken prothrombin complex, a stable enzyme was generated with the venom as well as in good yield (Fig. 8). Under optimum conditions, the full thrombin yield was obtained in 60 min and was isolated from the activation mixture in purified form with a molecular weight comparable to that for mammalian thrombins, and, in like manner, it consisted of two polypeptide chains bridged by a disulfide bond.

The venom of *Echis carinatus* was found useful for the quantitative measurement of prethrombin 1 concentration in plasma during disseminated intravascular coagulation (SAKURAGAWA et al., 1975). It was possible to use the venom assay to distinguish between DIC and primary fibrinolysis.

Without further purification, the venom of the Taipan snake, *Oxyuranus s. scutellatus*, was used for the assay of prothrombin (DENSON et al., 1971; PIRKLE et al., 1972). The venom is convenient for it neither requires nor is influenced by other coagulation factors. Consequently, a one-stage assay can be used to measure prothrombin concentration in many deficient plasmas. Very likely, the venom also converts modified prothrombin to thrombin, quite as has been done with other venoms (STENFLO and GANROT, 1972; NELSESTUEN and SUTTIE, 1972) and with the prethrombin assay (OUYANG et al., 1971b). In the latter assay, large amounts of purified autoprothrombin C and purified Ac-globulin are used. The conditions and procedure for the prethrombin assay have been outlined (BAKER and SEEGERS, 1967;

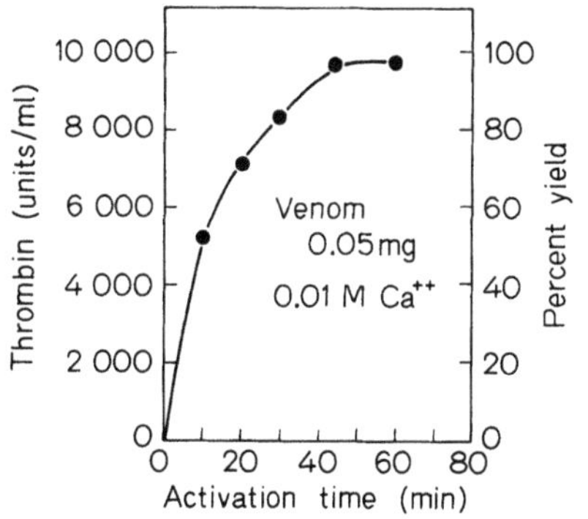

Fig. 8. Chicken prothrombin complex concentrate was incubated with 50 μg/ml of *Echis carinatus* snake venom in the presence of 0.01 M calcium ions

SEEGERS et al., 1967). The assay develops thrombin from prothrombin, as well as prethrombin 1, which means that the calcium binding sites found in profragment 1 are not *necessary* for the generation of thrombin with Auto-C + Ac-G + lipid + Ca ions because prethrombin 1 does not contain them. Prethrombin 1 only requires more procoagulant than prothrombin.

The venom of *Oxyuranus s. scutellatus* was also found to be useful as a procoagulant for a one-stage assay for prothrombin (DENSON et al., 1971) and the assay of purified prothrombin (PIRKLE et al., 1972). For a substrate of 20 μg of purified bovine prothrombin, the requirements were as follows: 5 μg crude venom, 25–250 μg of phospholipid and $CaCl_2$ 17.5 μM. This two-stage method has an advantage over the prethrombin assay because one does not need purified autoprothrombin C and purified Ac-globulin.

For one of several of the assay procedures for Ac-globulin, one makes use of the fact that Russell's viper venom can inactivate plasma Ac-globulin. The remaining plasma, like aged human oxalated plasma, is sensitive to additions of Ac-globulin (BORCHGREVINK et al., 1960). The amount of correction in the deficient plasma is proportional to the added Ac-globulin. In practice, it is necessary to take into account the fact that the venom contains a phospholipase that can inactivate crude "cephalin" in the reagents (POOL and ROBINSON, 1971).

Russell's viper venom also potentiates the activity of Ac-globulin (SCHIFFMAN et al., 1969). This activity was obtained in a separate fraction and for convenience called RVV-V. Molecular weight was in the 10000–20000 range. This factor was consumed during the potentiation of Ac-globulin activity. Adding a source of fresh Ac-globulin to a spent reaction mixture did not potentiate the activity of the newly added Ac-globulin. Once the original Ac-globulin was activated to its maximum, some thrombin did not further increase the activity. Ordinarily thrombin, up to a certain point, activates Ac-globulin, and this phenomenon is followed by inactivation of Ac-globulin (WARE et al., 1947). The balance between activation and inactivation varies from species to species so that the sera of some species, like the cow, contain Ac-globulin, while others do not. Chief examples of the latter are human and dog sera (MURPHY and SEEGERS, 1948). Although RVV-V is consumed during the potentiation of Ac-globulin, thrombin remains fully active when it potentiates Ac-globulin activity.

The RVV-V was found to be an esterase (JACKSON et al., 1971) that is inhibited by DFP and PMSF. By contrast, the Auto-III activator of the venom is not sensitive to DFP (MARKWARDT and WALSMANN, 1962). In further studies, ESMON and JACKSON (1973) compared the maximum potentiation or enhancement of Ac-globulin activity with RVV-V and found it to be the same as with thrombin. Activity of Ac-globulin in rabbit plasma was not increased by Russell's viper venom (RAPAPORT et al., 1966).

Prothrombin activation by the venom of the Tiger snake *(Notechis scutatus)* is dependent upon Ac-globulin. The venom had very little effect on fibrinogen or autoprothrombin III. Its function could be compared with the five-component system consisting of prothrombin, autoprothrombin C, Ac-globulin, phospholipid, and calcium ions (JOBIN and ESNOUF, 1966). The yield of thrombin was excellent from purified prothrombin when Ac-globulin, phospholipid, calcium ions, and venom were used. Deleting the phospholipid reduced the thrombin yield to about $^1/_{40}$th. Assuming that there is only one active principle in the venom requiring Ac-globulin, it is probably the only one known, besides autoprothrombin C, with this requirement. If and when the postulated enzyme is isolated, it most likely can be used in high concentration to generate thrombin by itself.

The generation of thrombin activity by *Oxyuranus s. scutellatus* (Taipan snake) was studied in a purified system. Partially purified Auto-C-like activity and purified bovine prothrombin were mixed. In the reaction, thrombin and degradation fragments were found to be the same whether Auto-C-like enzyme + phospholipids were used, or Auto-C + phospholipid + Ac-globulin + calcium ions (OWEN and JACKSON, 1973). The phospholipid enhanced the activity 20–30 times. The Auto-C-like activity was not inhibited by DFP (10^{-2} M), phenylmethyl-sulfonolyl fluoride (5×10^{-3} M), soybean trypsin inhibitor (1 mg/ml). It was not affected by sulfhydryl agents. It did not hydrolyze N^2-toluene-*p*-sulfonyl-L-arginine methyl ester (TAME), N^2-benzoyl-L-arginine ethyl ester (BAEE), or N-acetyl-L-tyrosine ethyl ester. From earlier work (TU et al., 1965), it was known that *Crotalidae* venoms had strong hydrolytic activity on TAME and BAEE. The *Viperidae* venoms tested were all strongly positive, but *Elapidae* venoms were all negative. No data were given for the *Hydrophidae.*

In another report, the partially purified enzyme from the Taipan snake was used for the generation of thrombin from purified *human* prothrombin (LANCHANTIN et al., 1973). The thrombin produced had the same properties as the thrombin obtained by "natural physiologic activators" with a molecular weight of about 39000 distributed to chains 32000 and 7000 respectively. Upon autolysis, the heavy chain was reduced to 19000 without change in clotting activity. This latter observation is quite different from that observed with bovine thrombin where autolysis is associated with a loss of coagulant activity but full retention and even gain in esterase activity (SEEGERS and LANDABURU, 1957; SEEGERS et al., 1974). The discrepancy is more likely due to a species difference than to the means for producing the thrombin from prothrombin.

Two interesting studies on the inhibition of thrombin formation have been completed. They are based on the original observation of OUYANG (1957). The venoms of both *Agkistrodon acutus* and *Trimeresurus gramineus* were found to be procoagulants in high concentration and anticoagulants in low concentration. The anticoagulant principle of *Agkistrodon acutus* was purified (OUYANG and TENG, 1972). Its molecular weight = 20650, $S^0_{20,w} = 2.0$ by ultracentrifugation, and isoelectric point = 4.7. It

Table 5. Amino acid composition of the anticoagulants isolated from the venoms of *T. gramineus* and *A. acutus*

Amino acid	*Anticoagulant principles of*	
	T. gramineus	*A. acutus*
Lysine	17	14
Histidine	3	5
Arginine	6	5
Aspartic acid	18	17
Threonine	7	8
Serine	6	16
Glutamic acid	12	23
Proline	7	[a]
Glycine	11	10
Alanine	7	10
Half-cystine	15	9
Valine	8	8
Methionine	3	3
Isoleucine	7	6
Leucine	8	9
Tyrosine	7	7
Phenylalanine	4	10
Tryptophan	4	
Total	150	160

[a] Small amount.

is a glycoprotein which does not possess caseinolytic, TAME esterase phospholipase A, phosphodiesterase, alkaline phosphomonoesterase, or fibrinolytic activities. Its retarding effect was only on the generation of thrombin activity. It was not due to the destruction of prothrombin but due to interference between prothrombin and its activation factors. The inhibitor, being very heat labile, was easily destroyed in activation mixtures to restore the capacity of the activation mixture to generate thrombin (OUYANG and TENG, 1973).

The anticoagulant of *Trimeresurus gramineus* venom was also purified (OUYANG and YANG, 1975). Some properties: mol wt = 19500, $S^0_{20,w} = 1.7$ and isoelectric point = 4.5. It was a glycoprotein, and, for all practical purposes, its anticoagulant function was identic with that of *Agkistrodon acutus* inhibitor. The amino acid composition of the inhibitors was somewhat similar (Table 5).

XII. Snake Venoms and Autoprothrombin C (Factor Xa) Formation

The formation of autoprothrombin C occurs under several conditions of which the main ones are mentioned. Concentrated salt solutions constitute an environment which is very favorable (ALKJAERSIG et al., 1955; SEEGERS et al., 1966). In that medium, most preparations of autoprothrombin III convert to the active enzyme by autocatalysis (KIPFER and SEEGERS, 1968). When that does not occur, the autoprothrombin III may have been modified by thrombin and/or prepared by having an enzyme inhibitor such as benzamidine hydrochloride (MARKWARDT, 1975) in the

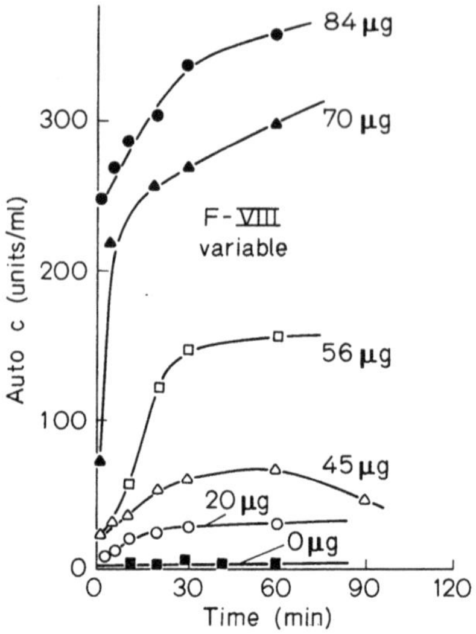

Fig. 9. With autoprothrombin III (Factor X) as substrate, enzyme activity generated in the presence of purified Factor IXa, purified Factor VIII, platelet factor 3, and calcium ions. Note that reduction of Factor VIII concentration was associated with a reduction in the rate of autoprothrombin C formation and its yield

solutions throughout the purification procedure (SEEGERS et al., 1975). Activation with tissue extract thromboplastin occurs (SEEGERS et al., 1963), and this activation is closely related to the function of Factor VII (NEMERSON, 1966). Enzymes such as trypsin, cathepsin C, and papain generate the activity. Perhaps the most interesting of all ways to obtain the enzyme is by means of the so-called intrinsic materials consisting of Factor IXa, Factor VIII, phospholipid, and calcium ions (CHUANG et al., 1972). In this system, Factor IXa is the enzyme (LUNDBLAD and DAVIE, 1964). The intrinsic materials function in much the same way as occurs in prothrombin activation (IRWIN et al., 1975). The yield of autoprothrombin C can be reduced from optimum by reducing the concentration of any one of the reactants (Fig. 9). The analogy with thrombin formation is as follows:

Auto-III	Prothrombin
↓ Ca ions	↓ Ca ions
Factor VIII	Ac-globulin
Factor IXa	Auto-C
PF-3	PF-3
Auto-C	Thrombin

Russell's viper venom is the outstanding example of a venom that generates Auto-C from its precursor. A brief historic background was written by LEE et al. (1955) and is quoted:

It has been known for many years that the venom of Russell's viper has powerful coagulant properties. Moreover, it has been suggested by several investigators that the venom can be used as a substitute for tissue thromboplastin in the determination of the prothrombin time. However, experience has shown that the results obtained with the use of the venom may not be reliable. For example, WILSON used venom for measuring the prothrombin time and found that a bleeding tendency was induced with the use of dicumarol when it was believed that the prothrombin concentration was within the therapeutic range. Apparently the venom interacted with materials in the plasma to accelerate the prothrombin time in a manner which does not occur with the use of thromboplastin. Presumably the alterations occurring in plasma in association with dicumarol therapy involved changes in the concentration of coagulant factors that do not act in conjunction with tissue thromboplastin in the same way as with the snake venom. This implies that the venom cannot simply be regarded as a powerful thromboplastin, and that it has properties which are as yet not understood in terms of our present knowledge of the blood coagulation mechanisms.

Most of the literature on the subject was written before it was realized that there are many mechanisms whereby prothrombin may become activated, and the main questions were concerned with the following: (1) is the venom like thromboplastin of tissue extracts, (2) is the venom lysing platelets or acting in conjunction with platelet products, (3) does it act directly to activate fibrinogen in a manner analogous to thrombin? Among the earlier investigators, ARTHUS described the thromboplastin-like action of the venom. HOUSSAY and SORDELLI stated that the venom has neither the activities of cytozyme nor of serozyme but enormously accelerates the formation of thrombin. In a series of toxicological studies on the venom, LEE (formerly RI) demonstrated that the Formosan daboia venom has a potent coagulant action in vivo as well as in vitro and that its action resembles that of thromboplastin but not that of thrombin. GANGULY concluded that the venom accelerates prothrombin conversion in the presence of platelets but not in their absence. He believed that the venom is a cytolytic agent enhancing the process of platelet disruption and thereby liberating what was considered to be thromboplastin. HOBSON and WITTS emphasized the dependence on calcium, and the importance of platelets. Although EDSALL considered the coagulant action of Daboia venom to be independent of the presence of formed platelets and distinctly different from that of thromboplastin, he really did not rule out the importance of materials derived from platelets because his technique included conditions favorable for platelet lysis. BIGGS cites the work of TREVAN and MACFARLANE, who showed that snake venom is most effective together with lecithin. Later LEATHES and MELLANBY observed that lecithin augments the thromboplastic activity of the venom, but that of brain extract to a lesser degree. MACFARLANE, TREVAN and ATTWOOD removed lipoidal components of horse plasma by prolonged centrifugation at high speed. When subsequently recalcified, the plasma could no longer be coagulated by addition of Daboia venom unless lecithin was also added. QUICK also showed that the prothrombin time of human plasma, normally twelve seconds, may be reduced to three seconds if lecithin and venom are used concurrently. He also remarked that tissue extracts are not affected by lecithin, and that the venom, in contrast to tissue extracts, will clot avian plasma as readily as mammalian plasma. EAGLE states that Daboia venom does not clot oxalated plasma and hence does not activate fibrinogen.

The use of Russell's viper venom (Stypven) as a substitute for thromboplastin in the one-stage prothrombin time was tried for the control of oral anticoagulant therapy (MACFARLANE, 1965). This venom converts autoprothrombin III to autoprothrombin C (X to Xa) (ESNOUF and WILLIAMS, 1962), and the activation occurs rapidly. A use for the venom was found for differentiating Factor VII from Factor X deficiency (QUICK, 1971). As QUICK states: "A prolonged prothrombin time corrected by aged serum indicates a lack of either Factor VII or Factor X, and a normal Stypven time (a prothrombin time using Russell's viper venom) makes the diagnosis of lack of Factor VII specific."

The Stypven time has been used extensively for estimating platelet Factor 3 activity. A limitation of this test is the failure to tell a difference between platelet Factor 3 as lipoprotein or the phospholipid portion of platelet Factor 3 because the procoagulant function of the two types of materials is quite different. The platelet Factor 3 material, as represented by membranes, is quite different from that which is released from platelets by adequate stimuli. The released material is not sedimented by high speed centrifugation and its chemical nature remains unknown. A modified Stypven time has been used to detect lipid procoagulant material in plasma (MACKENZIE et al., 1971). After a standard breakfast, the highest activity found in the plasma of four patients was 0.24% of that which was derived from the platelets in the blood of the same subject. This is a very minute amount of procoagulant in plasma, the significance of which is not known, and detected by a very sensitive test. In another study, no venoms were used, nor were plasmas taken after meals involved. Normal plasma was compared with delipidated plasma and no difference was found (ZOLTON and SEEGERS, 1974). The test employed purified autoprothrombin C (Factor Xa) to determine whether any lipid in plasma would enhance its capacity to generate thrombin from purified prothrombin in the presence of Ac-globulin and calcium ions. The procedure has not been applied to plasma obtained after a high fat meal.

As would be expected, the procoagulant effect of Russell's viper venom is reduced in cases of Stuart deficiency, the reduction depending upon the severity of the deficiency (HOUGIE, 1956). This is because the venom activates autoprothrombin III, and the resulting autoprothrombin C produces thrombin from prothrombin.

As an outgrowth of MACFARLANE'S interest in this venom (MACFARLANE, 1965), the current perspective has its foundations in the work of WILLIAMS and ESNOUF (1962). They isolated a protein as a physically homogeneous component with a specific activity eight times that of the crude venom. It functioned as an enzyme. At the same time, they produced the substrate (Factor X) for the venom in concentrated form (ESNOUF and WILLIAMS, 1962). The venom protein was later obtained free of esterase activity, and the activity was not destroyed by DFP or PMSF (JACKSON et al., 1971). Perhaps the simplest way to obtain the venom protein is by the procedure of SCHIFFMAN et al. (1969). This involves gel filtration on Sephadex G-200 followed by filtration through Sephadex G-100. An excellent affinity chromatography procedure has also been described (FURIE and FURIE, 1975).

The substrate, autoprothrombin III, was recently isolated as a single polypeptide chain (MATTOCK and ESNOUF, 1973). This has not been confirmed and it is usually isolated by methods that yield a product in which two polypeptide chains are bridged by a disulfide bond. The NH_2 terminal portion of the light chain is homologous with the NH_2 terminal portion of prothrombin (AGRAWAL et al., 1974; MCCOY et al., 1973b). In the activation of autoprothrombin III, calcium ions, and the venom protein are sufficient. It is essential to remove a peptide at the NH_2 terminal end of the heavy chain to generate activity. This peptide has a molecular weight near 11000 and is rich in carbohydrate (FUJIKAWA et al., 1972). Another peptide(s) can be removed to give rise to molecular variants. In the case of trypsin activation, a fragment (mol wt 3000) is removed from the COOH terminal end of the heavy chain, in addition to the peptide at the NH_2 terminal end.

In another study, autoprothrombin C was produced with various "activators" (RADCLIFFE and BARTON, 1972, 1973). Included were the viper venom protein, 25% sodium citrate solution, an insoluble form of trypsin, tissue thromboplastin, and material designed to simulate intrinsic activation conditions. In each case, the autoprothrombin C was isolated from the activation mixture and within experimental error they were similar. This contribution is very impressive and represents excellent technology. Nevertheless, at the premolecular level of observation, evidence was presented for multiple molecular forms of autoprothrombin C (DOMBROSE and SEEGERS, 1973). Differences were found in solubility, pH, and temperature stability. Further work along these lines should be productive. It will be especially interesting to see what kind of enzyme structure(s) can be derived from autoprothrombin III m because the latter is a degradation product of autoprothrombin III produced by thrombin.

The hemostatic drug marketed as Reptilase contains a Factor X-activating fraction of the venom (STOCKER and EGBERG, 1973). Apparently there are no further reports on the nature of this Factor X activator.

Echis carinatus venom has frequently been used, without further purification, to convert purified Factor X to Factor Xa (SEEGERS, 1975). Even at the most favorable concentration of the enzyme, the yield was less than 60%. Quite possibly, this activity is associated with a different molecule than the one that yields thrombin from prothrombin. It was found that purified ecarin does not activate purified Factor X (FRANZA et al., 1975), and it should be possible to obtain a specific activator for Factor X from *Echis carinatus* venom.

In one of the simple assays for Factor X, the proenzyme is first converted to maximum enzyme strength with Russell's viper venom in the presence of calcium ions. Then the amount of enzyme activity is measured by doing a partial thromboplastin time in which enzyme supplements the regular procoagulant (RENO and SEEGERS, 1967).

XIII. Snake Venoms and Platelets

1. Platelet Membrane Structural Changes Induced by Phospholipase A and Direct Lytic Factor (DLF) of Snake Venoms

There are two hemolysins in snake venoms. Phospholipase A (PhA, indirect hemolysin) lyses washed red blood cell via the formation of lysolecithin generated from extracellular or added phospholipids. DLF (direct hemolysin) lyses washed RBC of several species in the absence of lecithin (see Chapter 13 by Condrea). Both platelet and RBC are very similar in their negative-charged membranes and their responses to some factors. Phospholipid of osmotically hemolyzed RBC and intact platelet were hydrolyzed by phospholipase A of *Naja naja* and *Vipera russellii* venoms (RVV), while *Vipera palestinae* venom phospholipase A did not produce hydrolysis of phospholipid in intact platelets or intact or osmotically hemolyzed RBCs (KIRSCHMANN et al., 1964; BRADLOW and MARCUS, 1966). The striking difference between the action of RVV on RBC and platelet may be due to variation in lipid composition. Thus, the platelet lipids are readily available to the action of the enzyme. This "availability" might be determined by nonlipid components of the membrane (such as protein and polysaccharide). *Vipera palestinae* PhA does not produce hydrolysis of phospholipids in intact platelet. But lysolecithin, developed from plasma lecithin by the venom PhA both in vivo and in vitro, becomes attached to RBC and platelet (KIRSCHMANN et al., 1963). Plasma albumin is able to remove previously adsorbed lysolecithin from the platelet surface. The protective action of plasma explains the lack of platelet damage just as lack of hemolysis in vivo and in vitro (JIMÉNEZ-PORRAS, 1968; LUZZIO, 1967; CONDREA et al., 1969). However, marked decrease in platelet count can be found clinically in patients envenomated with *Vipera* or *Crotalus* venoms (RUSSELL, 1969; LYONS, 1971). This thrombocytopenia may be due mainly to intravascular clotting and minorly to platelet lysis by PhA of these venoms. Phosphotidyl ethanolamine, phosphotidyl serine, and lecithin in the human platelet are hydrolyzed by *Naja naja* venom PhA but not by *Vipera palestinae* venom PhA. The platelet phospholipids are rendered susceptible to the action of *Vipera palestinae* venom PhA by DLF of *Naja naja* venom as well as by surface active agent (KIRSCHMANN et al., 1964). Potentiation of the lytic activity of PhA by DLF is similar in the platelet as that in RBC.

The anticoagulant action of cobra venom is chiefly due to its antithromboplastin activity, but the precise mechanism has not been fully elucidated. Inactivation of Factors V, VII, VIII, IX, and other coagulation factors of platelets have also been reported (LEE, 1971). The relationship of PhA and the anticoagulant action of cobra venom has been the subject of dispute. The anticoagulant effects of PhA and DLF may be due to their action on platelets. Assaying phospholipids released from the platelet membrane by PhA of *Naja naja* and RVV, some authors (CONDREA et al., 1969; KIRSCHMANN et al., 1964) reported some similarities between lipid availability for the coagulation process and susceptibility to venom action. Cell preparations which resisted the action of venom were also inactive in in vitro coagulation systems. On the other hand, venom-sensitive cells were specifically those which were active in the coagulation system. PhA, DLF, and lysolecithin also inhibit the retracting activity of blood clot. This inhibitory effect is also due to platelet lysis or membrane structural changes (KIRSCHMANN et al., 1963).

2. Platelet Aggregation Induced by Coagulant and Noncoagulant Venoms

Platelet aggregation can be induced by snake venoms which may be coagulant or noncoagulant. Accompanying the aggregation process, nucleotides, serotonin, and other platelet factors or constituents may also be released by these venoms. DAVEY and LÜSCHER (1967) summarized the release reaction of platelet by some venoms by measuring nucleotide release as follows:

Release reaction of platelets	No release reaction of platelets
Venom factor (noncoagulative)	Venom coagulants
Crotalus terrificus	*Agkistrodon rhodostoma*
Trimeresurus okinavensis	*Crotalus adamateus*
Trimeresurus purpureomaculata	*Trimeresurus okinavensis*
	Trimeresurus purpureomaculata
	Venom esterase
	Trimeresurus okinavensis

Concerning the action of thrombin-like enzymes on platelet function, it is well established that Reptilase and ancrod do not induce platelet aggregation and do not cause clot retraction because of lack of platelet activation (DAVEY and LÜSCHER, 1967, 1968; TANGEN and BYGDEMAN, 1972; ODDVAR et al., 1973). But ADP, adrenaline, or collagen preincubated with unstirred human platelet-rich plasma induce the retraction clotted by Reptilase (DE GAETANO et al., 1973; KUBISZ, 1973, 1975; NIEWIARIOUSKI et al., 1975). Reptilase and ancrod have been extensively used to study platelet functions, such as platelet aggregation (TANGEN and BYGDEMAN, 1972; ODDVAR et al., 1973), clot retraction (DE GAETANO et al., 1973; KUBISZ, 1973), release reaction (DAVEY and LÜSCHER, 1967, 1968; DE GAETANO et al., 1973; KUBISZ, 1973), and role of platelet in generalized Schwartzman's reaction (MÜLLER-BERGHAUS and HOCKE, 1973). Recently, OUYANG and TENG (unpublished data a) studied the thrombin-like enzyme of *Agkistrodon acutus* venom on platelet aggregation using washed rabbit platelet suspension. They observed platelet aggregation using thrombin or thrombin-like enzyme (TLE). Platelet aggregation was induced by TLE only when the concentration was higher than 50 U/ml. The platelet-aggregating activity of TLE was only $^{1}/_{5000}$th of that for bovine thrombin.

The venoms of *Crotalus terrificus*, *Trimeresurus okinavensis*, and *Trimeresurus purpureomaculata* can retain their activities of releasing nucleotides from human platelet after the esterolytic and coagulant activities have been abolished by DFP (DAVEY and LÜSCHER, 1967). The exact mode of action is unknown, and the venom factor has not been purified. Recently, OUYANG and TENG (unpublished data b) isolated a strong noncoagulant inducer of platelet aggregation from the venom of *Trimeresurus mucrosquamatus*. It is effective in concentration as low as 1 μg/ml. The aggregation patterns are very similar to ADP. Its aggregating activity is dependent on Ca^{++}, decreased by adenosine, EDTA, and a SH reagent, N-ethylmaleimide, and potentiated by potassium cyanide. But the venom inducer causes platelet aggregation even when the platelet preparation is in a refractory state to ADP. This venom-aggregating agent may influence platelets in two ways: 1) affects directly on platelet membrane and 2) affects indirectly through the release of platelet constituents (especially ADP).

3. Venom Inhibitors of Platelet Aggregation

Platelet aggregation inhibitors of snake venoms have not been well-studied. Recently, BOFFA and BOFFA (1975) studied the correlation between enzymic activities and the activity of inhibiting platelet aggregation using fractions of the venom of *Vipera aspis*. They classified the inhibitors of this venom into three components: ADPase or 5'-nucleotidase, fibrinolytic enzymes, and phospholipase A. Purified ADPase from Russell's viper venom has been used to study the role of ADP in norepinephrine-induced platelet aggregation (HASLAM, 1967). The fibrinogen or fibrin degradation products (FDP) from fibrinogen or fibrin, produced by plasmin (JERUSLALNY and ZUCKER, 1966), trypsin (WILSON et al., 1968), and brinolase (fibrinolytic enzyme from *Aspergillus orizyae*) (ROSCHLAU and GAGE, 1972), can inhibit platelet aggregation. The FDP produced by α-fibrinogenase but not by β-fibrinogenase of *Trimeresurus mucrosquamatus* venom (OUYANG and TENG, 1978) inhibits the aggregation induced by ADP. In addition to hemorrhagin, the impairment of platelet aggregation is another antihemostatic effect of snake venoms (BIRAN et al., 1974).

D. Overview

We call this portion of our work an overview rather than a summary, for we feel that the preceding work is quite condensed and practically represents a summary. Our overview is an attempt to arrive at generalizations that outline the topography of the field of study. Such generalizations carry with them the hazard of oversight and overreaching. Due allowances can be made for that in return for an account that can be useful with those limitations in mind.

Blood coagulation is discussed as a cybernetic system. There are three basic chemical reactions as follows:

1. Formation of autoprothrombin C (Factor Xa)
2. Formation of thrombin
3. Formation of fibrin.

These reactions occur in the given order, and each one depends upon the previous one. Thus, formation of fibrin is due to thrombin; formation of thrombin is due to autoprothrombin C; and formation of autoprothrombin C is due to an enzymic degradation process. More than one enzyme can serve that purpose—probably Factor IXa, Factor VIIa, and autocatalysis. Each basic reaction is accelerated by accessory factors and retarded by inhibitors. The fibrin formed by thrombin is modified by fibrinoligase (Factor XIIIa). The materials required for this cybernetic system are primarily found in plasma, platelets, and fixed tissues. These materials are supplied by the bodily metabolic machinery and can be considered as being disposed of and replaced on approximately a 1-week time schedule. Many details about the three basic reactions can be described in terms of molecular biology.

The fibrin of a blood clot, as well as the fibrinogen from which the fibrin structure is made, can be digested by plasmin (fibrinolysin) to yield more or less well-defined soluble decomposition products. Plasmin is derived from its plasma precursor, plasminogen (profibrinolysin), by an activator, which itself arises from plasma proactivator. The generation of activator activity can be due to Factor XIIa. Plasminogen is also converted to plasmin by tissue activator(s), by urokinase found in urine and produced by kidney cells, and by streptokinase of bacterial origin.

The activity of plasmin is neutralized by plasma antifibrinolysins. Among these are α_1-antitrypsin and α_2-macroglobulin. Complexes of plasmin and inhibitors can dissociate and thus serve as a reservoir for plasmin activity in addition to plasminogen. Fibrinolysis is also induced by autoprothrombin II-A which functions by depressing antifibrinolysin activity.

Snake venoms contain enzymes concerned with all three basic reactions of blood coagulation. They contain fibrinolytic enzymes and inhibitors. At least eight thrombin-like enzymes have been obtained in purified form from eight different snakes. Many are single-chain glycoproteins sensitive to DFP and in the molecular weight range of 20000–40000. In the formation of fibrin, only fibrinopeptide A is removed, but in one case, primarily only fibrinopeptide B. Platelets are not aggregated by the thrombin-like enzymes unless a "cofactor" is added such as collagen, ADP, or adrenaline. Neither is there clot retraction unless the platelets are stimulated by another agent. Except for one variety, the thrombin-like enzyme from *Bothrops* venoms activates Factor XIII, whereas the enzyme from *Agkistrodon rhodostoma* does not. The thrombin-like enzymes progressively digest fibrin slowly after clot formation, and the clots are more susceptible to fibrinolysis than fibrin formed with thrombin. The thrombin-like enzymes are eliminated via urine, the RES and neutralization by inhibitors. Their activity is not reduced by heparin or hirudin.

In selected cases, the thrombin-like enzymes are useful for the management of thrombosis. In proper concentration and controlled rate of intravenous infusion, the blood becomes defibrinated, lysis is induced, and fibrinogen and fibrin degradation products appear early in high concentration and then at lower levels. Repeated infusion maintains the anticoagulation; otherwise, fibrinogen concentration builds up again. Bleeding occurs in special cases where the hemostatic mechanism is injured or inhibited. Blood viscosity drops, and blood flow is accordingly facilitated.

The maintenance of hemostasis while the coagulation mechanisms are essentially not functioning fits a three-component theory of hemostasis. This postulates that three primary mechanisms function; namely, platelets, coagulation of blood, and blood vessels. Removal of any two components results in bleeding. Defibrination removes only one.

The experimental infusion of acetylated thrombin in animals develops a pattern of responses similar to that seen with thrombin-like enzymes. The fibrinolysis induced by either agent might be due to the formation of autoprothrombin II-A which produces lysis by depressing the activity of antifibrinolysins. Whether the fibrinolysis is initiated by acetylated thrombin or thrombin-like enzymes, it is difficult to retard it with EACA or aprotinin.

Snake venoms contain enzymes that lyse fibrin(ogen) directly. The fibrinolytic principle from *Agkistrodon acutus* (Hundred-pace snake) has been obtained in purified form and has a preference for the Aα-chain of fibrinogen. Two distinct fibrinolytic principles have been obtained from *Trimeresurus mucrosquamatus* (Taiwan habu). One of these has a preference for the Bβ-chain, while the other digests primarily the Aα-chain of fibrinogen.

Several snake venoms convert prothrombin to thrombin. The principle with that property has been obtained from *Echis carinatus* venom in purified form. Early products of activation are prethrombin 1 + profragment 1 (Fig. 3). In the next step, the Arg-Ile bond between A and B chains is split, and then the profragment 2 is removed to give classic thrombin. To obtain purified chicken thrombin, the purified prothrombin was activated with the venom. The partially purified activator from the Taipan snake, *Oxyuranus s. scutellatus*, produced the same activation pattern and the same thrombin structure as physiologic activators when either purified bovine or human prothrombin served as substrate.

Like the physiologic activation of prothrombin, an Auto-C-like (Factor Xa-like) enzyme of the Tiger snake *(Notechis scutatus)* requires Ac-globulin + phospholipids + calcium ions. The partially purified Auto-C-like enzyme of the Taipan snake venom has its activity enhanced by phospholipid and calcium ions. Russell's viper venom contains an activity that destroys Ac-globulin as well as material that enhances Ac-globulin activity. The latter protein has been obtained in purified form and is inhibited by DFP.

An inhibitor has been isolated from *Agkistrodon acutus* and from *Trimeresurus gramineus* venom. Each one is a glycoprotein in the 20000 molecular weight range and reversibly inhibits the generation of thrombin in a system consisting of prothrombin + Ac-globulin + phospholipid + calcium ions.

An enzyme in Russell's viper venom converts Factor X to Xa. The enzyme has been obtained in purified form, and in the activation of Factor X removes a polypeptide (11000 daltons) from the NH_2 terminal end of the heavy chain.

Snake venoms are useful as laboratory reagents involving various tests and analytic procedures such as prothrombin analysis, autoprothrombin III analysis, fibrinogen determination, and molecular structural studies.

Acknowledgments. This work was supported by a National Science Council Research Grant of the Republic of China, Research Grant HL 03424-19 from the National Heart and Lung Institute, National Institutes of Health, U.S. Public Health Service, the McGregor Fund, and the Skillman Foundation. It is a pleasure to express our thanks to Dr. Chen-Yuan Lee, Dean, College of Medicine, National Taiwan University, for inviting us to write this review and making the arrangements that made the work possible for us.

References

Agrawal, B. B. L., McCoy, L. E., Walz, D. A., Seegers, W. H.: Some observations on the structure of autoprothrombin III (Factor X). Thrombos. Diathes. haemorrh. (Stuttg.) (Suppl.) **57**, 217—288 (1974)

Alkjaersig, N., Abe, T., Johnson, S. A., Seegers, W. H.: An accelerator of prothrombin activation derived from prothrombin. Amer. J. Physiol. **182**, 443—446 (1955)

Andersson, L.: Isolation of thrombin-like activity from the venom of *Trimeresurus okinavensis*. Haemostasis **1**, 31—43 (1972)

Asbeck, F., Lechler, E., Loo, J., Van de: Fibrinogen-Fibrin-Derivate unter Defibrasebehandlung. In: Martin, M., Schoop, W. (Eds.): Defibrinierung mit thrombin-ähnlichen Schlangengiftenzymen. Aktuelle Probleme in der Angiologie, Vol. XXVI, pp. 79—83. Bern-Stuttgart-Wien: Hans Huber 1975

Ashford, A., Bunn, D. R. G.: The effect of Arvin on reticuloendothelial activity in rabbits. Brit. J. Pharmacol. **40**, 37—44 (1970)

Ashford, A., Ross, J. W., Southgate, P.: Pharmacology and toxicology of a defibrinating substance from Malayan pit viper venom. Lancet **1968 I**, 486—489

Baker, W. J., Seegers, W. H.: The conversion of prethrombin to thrombin. Thrombos. Diathes. haemorrh. (Stuttg.) **17**, 205—213 (1967)

Baldini, M. G., Ebbe, S. (Eds.): Platelets: Production, Function, Transfusion, and Storage. New York-San Francisco-London: Grune and Stratton 1974

Ballerini, G., Seegers, W. H.: A description of clot retraction as a visual experience. Thrombos. Diathes. haemorrh. (Stuttg.) **3**, 147—164 (1959)

Banerjee, S., Devi, A., Copley, A. L.: Studies of actions of snake venoms on blood coagulation. II. Electrophoretic analysis of venoms of *Viperidae*, *Crotalidae*, *Elapidae*, and *Hydrophidae*. Thrombos. Res. **3**, 451—464 (1973)

Bang, N. U., Beller, F. K., Deutsch, E., Mammen, E. F. (Eds.): Thrombosis and Bleeding Disorders. Stuttgart: George Thieme; New York-London: Academic Press 1971

Bang, N. U., Chang, M. L.: Soluble fibrin complexes. Semin. Thromb. Hemost. **1**, 91—128 (1974)

Barlow, G. H., Devine, E. M.: A study of the relationship between ancrod and thrombin clotting units. Thrombos. Res. **5**, 695—698 (1974)

Barlow, G. H., Holleman, W. H., Lorand, L.: The action of Arvin on fibrin stabilizing factor (Factor XIII). Res. Commun. chem. Path. Pharmacol. **1**, 39—42 (1970)

Barlow, G. H., Lazer, S. L., Finley, R., Kwaan, H. C., Donahoe, J. F.: Some studies on proteins in the defibrinated state during Ancrod (A 38414) studies in normal humans. Thrombos. Res. **2**, 115—122 (1973a)

Barlow, G. H., Lewis, L. J., Finley, R., Martin, D., Stocker, K.: Immunochemical identification of Ancrod (A 38414) and Reptilase (Defibrase). Thrombos. Res. **2**, 17—22 (1973b)

Barthels, M., Seegers, W. H.: Substitution of lipids with bile salts in the formation of thrombin. Thrombos. Diathes. haemorrh. (Stuttg.) **22**, 13—27 (1969)

Bell, W. R.: Current status of therapy with Arvin. Thrombos. Diathes. haemorrh. (Stuttg.) (Suppl.) **47**, 371—378 (1971)
Bell, W. R., Bolton, G., Pitney, W. R.: The effect of Arvin on blood coagulation factors. Brit. J. Haemat. **15**, 589—601 (1968b)
Bell, W. R., Pitney, W. R.: Management of priapism by therapeutic defibrination. New Engl. J. Med. **280**, 649—650 (1969)
Bell, W. R., Pitney, W. R.: The concept of therapeutic defibrination. Thrombos. Diathes. haemorrh. (Stuttg.) (Suppl.) **39**, 285—289 (1970)
Bell, W. R., Pitney, W. R., Goodwin, J. F.: Therapeutic defibrination in the treatment of thrombotic disease. Lancet **1968a I**, 490—493
Bettex-Galland, M., Lüscher, E. F.: Thrombosthenin, the contractile protein from blood platelets and its relation to other contractile proteins. Advanc. Protein Chem. **20**, 1—35 (1965)
Biggs, R. (Ed.): Human Blood Coagulation, Haemostasis, and Thrombosis. Oxford-London-Edinburgh-Melbourne: Blackwell Scientific 1972
Biggs, R., Macfarlane, R. G. (Eds.): Treatment of Haemophilia and Other Coagulation Disorders. Philadelphia: F. A. Davis 1966
Biran, H., Dvilansky, A., Nathan, I., Live, A.: Impairement of human platelet aggregation and serotonin release caused in vitro by *Echis colorata* venom. Thrombos. Diathes. haemorrh. (Stuttg.) **30**, 191—198 (1974)
Blombäck, B.: Studies on the action of thrombic enzyme on bovine fibrinogen as measured by N-terminal analysis. Arkiv Kemi **12**, 321—335 (1958)
Blombäck, B., Blombäck, M., Nilsson, I. M.: Coagulation studies on "Reptilase", an extract of the venom from *Bothrops jararaca*. Thrombos. Diathes. haemorrh. (Stuttg.) **1**, 76—86 (1957)
Blombäck, M., Egberg, N.: Defibrase in treatment of venous thrombosis. In: Martin, M., Schoop, W. (Eds.): Defibrinierung mit thrombin-ähnlichen Schlangengiftenzymen. Aktuelle Probleme in der Angiologie, Vol. XXVI, pp. 206—213. Bern-Stuttgart-Wien: Hans Huber 1975
Blombäck, M., Egberg, N., Gruder, E., Johansson, S. A., Johnsson, H., Nilsson, S. E. G., Blombäck, B.: Treatment of thrombotic disorders with Reptilase. Thrombos. Diathes. haemorrh. (Stuttg.) (Suppl.) **45**, 51—61 (1971)
Blombäck, B., Laurent, T. C.: N-terminal and light-scattering studies on fibrinogen and its transformation to fibrin. Arkiv Kemi **12**, 137—146 (1958)
Blombäck, B., Yamashina, I.: On the N-terminal amino acids in fibrinogen and fibrin. Arkiv Kemi **12**, 299—319 (1958)
Boffa, G. A., Boffa, M. C., Winchenne, J. J.: A phospholipase A_2 with anticoagulant activity. I. Isolation from *Vipera berus* venom and properties. Biochim. biophys. Acta (Amst.) **429**, 828—838 (1976)
Boffa, M. C., Boffa, G. A.: Correlation between the enzymatic activities and the factors active on blood coagulation and platelet aggregation from the venom of *Vipera aspis*. Biochim. biophys. Acta (Amst.) **354**, 275—290 (1975)
Boffa, M. C., Boffa, G. A.: A phospholipase A_2 with anticoagulant activity II. Inhibition of the phospholipid activity in coagulation. Biochim. biophys. Acta (Amst.) **429**, 839—852 (1976)
Bonilla, C. A.: Defibrinating enzyme from Timber rattlesnake *(Crotalus h. horridus)* venom: a potential agent for therapeutic defibrination. I. Purification and properties. Thrombos. Res. **6**, 151—169 (1975)
Boquet, P.: Venins de serpents. Physio-pathologie de l'envenimation et proprieties biologiques des venins. Toxicon **2**, 5—44 (1964)
Borchgrevink, C. F., Pool, J. G., Stormorken, H.: A new assay for Factor V (proaccelerin-accelerin) using Russell's viper venom. J. Lab. clin. Med. **55**, 625—632 (1960)
Bowie, E. J. W., Thompson, Jr., J. H., Didisheim, P., Owen, Jr., C. A.: Laboratory manual of hemostasis. Philadelphia-London-Toronto: W. B. Saunders 1971
Bradlow, B. A., Marcus, A. J.: Action of snake venom phospholipase A on isolated platelet membranes. Proc. Soc. exp. Biol. (N.Y.) **123**, 889—893 (1966)
Bradshaw, R. A., Wessler, S. (Eds.): Heparin: Structure, Function, and Clinical Implications. New York-London: Plenum Press 1975
Brambel, C. E.: Proteases in the clotting mechanism. Ann. N.Y. Acad. Sci. **68**, 67—69 (1957)
Brinkhous, K. M., Shermer, R. W. (Eds.): The Platelet. Baltimore: Williams and Wilkins 1971

Broersma, R. J., McCoy, L. E., Seegers, W. H.: Production of microvascular thrombosis and lysis with acetylated thrombin. Thrombos. Diathes. haemorrh. (Stuttg.) (Suppl.) **47**, 353—360 (1971)

Brown, C. H. III., Bell, W. R., Shreiner, D. P., Jackson, D. P.: Effects of Arvin on blood platelets. In vitro and in vivo studies. J. Lab. clin. Med. **79**, 758—769 (1972)

Browse, N. L.: Vein surgery during defibrination. In: Martin, M., Schoop, W. (Eds.): Defibrinierung mit thrombin-ähnlichen Schlangengiftenzymen. Aktuelle Probleme in der Angiologie, Vol. XXVI, pp. 152—156. Bern-Stuttgart-Wien: Hans Huber 1975

Bruner-Lorand, J., Pilkington, T. R. E., Lorand, L.: Inhibitors of fibrin cross-linking: relevance for thrombolysis. Nature (Lond.) **210**, 1273—1274 (1966)

Bücherl, W., Buckley, E., Deulofeu, V. (Eds.): Venomous Animals and Their Venoms. New York-London: Academic Press 1968

Caldwell, M. J., Seegers, W. H.: Inhibition of prothrombin, thrombin, and autoprothrombin C with enzyme inhibitors. Thrombos. Diathes. haemorrh. (Stuttg.) **13**, 373—386 (1965)

Chan, K. E., Reid, H. A.: Fibrinolysis and the defibrination syndrome of Malayan viper bite. Lancet **1964 I**, 461—463

Chan, K. E., Rizza, C. R., Henderson, M. P.: A study of the coagulant properties of Malayan pit-viper venom. Brit. J. Haematol. **11**, 646—653 (1965)

Cheng, H. C., Ouyang, C.: Isolation of coagulant and anticoagulant principles from the venom of *Agkistrodon acutus*. Toxicon **4**, 235—243 (1967)

Chuang, T. F., Sargeant, R. B., Hougie, C.: The intrinsic activation of Factor X in blood coagulation. Biochim. biophys. Acta (Amst.) **273**, 287—291 (1972)

Cochrane, C. G., Revak, S. D., Wuepper, K. D.: Activation of Hageman factor in solid and fluid phases. A critical role of kallikrein. J. exp. Med. **138**, 1564—1583 (1973)

Collen, D., Vermylen, J.: Metabolism of iodine-labeled plasminogen during streptokinase and Reptilase therapy in man. Thrombos. Res. **2**, 239—249 (1973)

Colman, R. W., Bagdasarian, A., Talamo, R. C., Scott, C. F., Seavey, M., Guimaraes, J. A., Pierce, J. V., Kaplan, A. P.: Williams trait: Human kininogen deficiency with diminished levels of plasminogen proactivator and prekallikrein associated with abnormalities of the Hageman factor dependent pathways. J. clin. Invest. **56**, 1650—1662 (1975)

Condrea, E., Berzilay, M., Vries, A. de: Study of hemolysis in the lethal effect of *Naja naja* venom in the mouse and guinea-pig. Toxicon **7**, 95—98 (1969)

Copley, A. L., Banerjee, S., Devi, A.: Studies of snake venoms on blood coagulation. I. The thromboserpentin (thrombin-like) enzyme in the venoms. Thrombos. Res. **2**, 487—508 (1973)

Davey, M. G., Lüscher, E. F.: Actions of some coagulant snake venoms on blood platelets. Nature (Lond.) **207**, 730—732 (1965)

Davey, M. G., Lüscher, E. F.: Actions of thrombin and other coagulant and proteolytic enzymes on blood platelets. Nature (Lond.) **216**, 857—858 (1967)

Davey, M. G., Lüscher, E. F.: Release reaction of human platelet induced by thrombin and other agents. Biochim. biophys. Acta (Amst.) **165**, 490—506 (1968)

Davie, E. W., Fujikawa, K.: Basic mechanisms in blood coagulation. Ann. Rev. Biochem. **44**, 799—829 (1975)

Davies, J. A., Sharp, A. A., Merrick, M. V., Holt, J. M.: Controlled trial of ancrod and heparin in treatment of deep-vein thrombosis of lower limb. Lancet **1972 I**, 113—115

Denson, K. W. E.: Coagulant and anticoagulant action of snake venoms. Toxicon **7**, 5—11 (1969)

Denson, K. W. E.: The levels of Factors II, VII, IX, and X by antibody neutralization techniques in the plasma of patients receiving phenindione therapy. Brit. J. Haemat. **20**, 643—648 (1971)

Denson, K. W. E., Borrett, R., Biggs, R.: The specific assay of prothrombin using the Taipan snake venom. Brit. J. Haemat. **21**, 219—226 (1971)

Denson, K. W. E., Russell, F. E., Almagro, D., Bishop, R. C.: Characterization of the coagulant activity of some snake venoms. Toxicon **10**, 557—562 (1972)

Deutsch, E.: Blutgerinnungsfaktoren. Wien: Franz Deuticke 1955

Deutsch, H. F., Diniz, C. R.: Some proteolytic activities of snake venoms. J. biol. Chem. **216**, 17—26 (1955)

Devi, A.: Constituents of snake venoms. In: Bücherl, W., Buckley, E., Deulofeu, V. (Eds.): Venomous Animals and Their Venoms, Vol. I, pp. 119—165. New York-London: Academic Press 1968

Devi, A., Banerjee, S., Copley, A. L.: Coagulant and esterase activities of thrombin and *Bothrops atrox* venom. Toxicon **10**, 563—573 (1972)
Diener, L.: Phlebography of the lower limb in connection with Defibrase treatment of deep venous thrombosis. In: Martin, M., Schoop, W. (Eds.): Defibrinierung mit thrombin-ähnlichen Schlangengiftenzymen. Aktuelle Probleme in der Angiologie, Vol. XXVI, pp. 214—216. Bern-Stuttgart-Wien: Hans Huber 1975
Dombrose, F. A., Seegers, W. H.: Evidence for multiple molecular forms of autoprothrombin C (Factor X a). Thrombos. Res. **3**, 737—743 (1973)
Doolittle, R. F., Cassman, K. G., Chen, R., Sharp, J. J., Woodling, G. L.: Correlation of the mode of fibrin polymerization with the pattern of cross-linking. Ann. N.Y. Acad. Sci. **202**, 114—126 (1972)
Douglas, A. S.: Anticoagulant Therapy. Philadelphia: F. A. Davis 1962
Durante, L. J., Moutsos, A., Ambrose, R. B., Duncan, W. J., Fleming, W., Zinsser, H. H., Phillips, L. L.: Postprostatectomy bleeding. Ann. Surg. **156**, 781—792 (1962)
Dvilansky, A., Britten, A. F. H., Loewy, A. G.: Factor XIII assay by an isotope method. I. Factor-XIII (transamidase) in plasma, serum, leucocytes, erythrocytes, and platelets and evaluation of screening tests of clot solubility. Brit. J. Haemat. **18**, 399—410 (1970)
Eagle, H.: The coagulation of blood by snake venoms and its physiological significance. J. exp. Med. **65**, 613—639 (1937)
Edgar, W., Prentice, C. R. M.: The proteolytic action of ancrod on human fibrinogen and its polypeptide chains. Thrombos. Res. **2**, 85—95 (1973)
Egberg, N.: On interaction of serum proteins with thrombin-like enzyme from *Bothrops atrox* venom. Thrombos. Res. **1**, 637—639 (1972)
Egberg, N.: Experimental and clinical studies on the thrombin-like enzyme from the venom of *Bothrops atrox*. On the primary structure of fragment E. Acta physiol. scand. (Suppl.) **400**, 1—47 (1973)
Egberg, N.: On the metabolism of the thrombin-like enzyme from the venom of *Bothrops atrox*. Thrombos. Res. **4**, 35—53 (1974)
Egberg, N., Blombäck, M., Johnsson, H., Abildgaard, U., Blombäck, B., Diener, G., Ekeström, S., Göransson, L., Johansson, S.-A., McDonagh, J., McDonagh, R., Nilsson, S. E., Nordström, S., Olsson, P., Wiman, B.: Clinical and experimental studies on Reptilase. Thrombos. Diathes. haemorrh. (Stuttg.) (Suppl.) **47**, 379—387 (1971)
Egberg, N., Johnsson, H.: Platelet aggregation induced by ADP and thrombin in Reptilase defibrinated dogs. Thrombos. Res. **1**, 95—112 (1972)
Egberg, N., Ljungqvist, A.: On fibrin distribution in organs of dogs during defibrination with the thrombin-like enzyme from *Bothrops atrox*. Thrombos. Res. **3**, 191—207 (1973)
Egberg, N., Nordström, S.: Effects of Reptilase-induced intravascular coagulation in dogs. Acta physiol. scand. **79**, 493—505 (1970)
Ehringer, H., Dudczak, R., Lechner, K.: Rationale einer therapeutischen Defibrinierung mit Ancrod als neue Therapie bei arterieller Verschlußkrankheit. In: Martin, M., Schoop, W. (Eds.): Defibrinierung mit thrombin-ähnlichen Schlangengiftenzymen. Aktuelle Probleme in der Angiologie, Vol. XXVI, pp. 114—131. Bern-Stuttgart-Wien: Hans Huber 1975
Ehrly, A. M.: Schlangengiftenzymbehandlung (Arwin) bei der peripheren chronischen arteriellen Verschlußkrankheit. In: Martin, M., Schoop, W. (Eds.): Defibrinierung mit thrombin-ähnlichen Schlangengiftenzymen. Aktuelle Probleme in der Angiologie, Vol. XXVI, pp. 217—224. Bern-Stuttgart-Wien: Hans Huber 1975a
Ehrly, A. M.: Veränderungen der Fließeigenschaften des Blutes bei der Therapie mit Arwin. In: Martin, M., Schoop, W. (Eds.): Defibrinierung mit thrombin-ähnlichen Schlangengiftenzymen. Aktuelle Probleme in der Angiologie, Vol. XXVI, pp. 144—149. Bern-Stuttgart-Wien: Hans Huber 1975b
Esmon, C. T., Jackson, C. M.: The Factor V activating enzyme of Russell's viper venom. Thrombos. Res. **2**, 509—524 (1973)
Esmon, C. T., Jackson, C. M.: The conversion of prothrombin to thrombin. IV. The function of the fragment 2 region during activation in the presence of Factor V. J. biol. Chem. **249**, 7791—7797 (1974)
Esmon, C. T., Owen, W. G., Jackson, C. M.: A plausible mechanism for prothrombin activation by Factor X a, Factor V a, phospholipid, and calcium ions. J. biol. Chem. **249**, 8045—8047 (1974)

Esnouf, M. P., Marshall, R.: The effect of blockade of the reticuloendothelial system and of hypotension on the response of dogs to *Ancistrodon rhodostoma* venom. Clin. Sci. **35**, 261—272 (1968)
Esnouf, M. P., Tunnah, G. W.: The isolation and properties of the thrombin-like activity from *Ancistrodon rhodostoma* venom. Brit. J. Haemat. **13**, 581—590 (1967)
Esnouf, M. P., Williams, W. J.: The isolation and purification of a bovine-plasma protein which is a substrate for the coagulation fraction of Russell's viper venom. Biochem. J. **84**, 62—71 (1962)
Ewart, M. R., Hatton, M. W. C., Basford, J. M., Dodgson, K. S.: The proteolytic action of Arvin on human fibrinogen. Biochem. J. **118**, 603—609 (1970)
Fearnley, G. R.: Fibrinolysis. Baltimore: Williams and Wilkins 1965
Feddersen, C., Gormsen, J.: Plasma digestion of stabilized and nonstabilized fibrin illustrated by pH-stat titration and thromboelastography. Scand. J. clin. Lab. Invest. **27**, 175—181 (1971)
Finlayson, J. S.: Crosslinking of fibrin. Semin. Thromb. Hemost. **1**, 33—62 (1974)
Franza, Jr., B. R., Aronson, D. L., Finlayson, J. S.: Activation of human prothrombin by a procoagulant fraction from the venom of *Echis carinatus*. Identification of a high molecular weight intermediate with thrombin activity. J. biol. Chem. **250**, 7057—7068 (1975)
Fujikawa, K., Legaz, M. E., Davie, E. W.: Bovine Factor X_1 (Stuart factor). Mechanism of activation by a protein from Russell's viper venom. Biochemistry **11**, 4892—4898 (1972)
Fujikawa, K., Legaz, M. E., Kato, H., Davie, E. W.: The mechanism of activation of bovine Factor-IX (Christmas Factor) by bovine Factor XIa (activated plasma thromboplastin antecedent). Biochemistry **13**, 4508—4516 (1974)
Funk, C., Gmür, J., Herold, R., Straub, P. W.: Reptilase-R—A new reagent in blood coagulation. Brit. J. Haemat. **21**, 43—52 (1971)
Furie, B. C., Furie, B.: Interaction of lanthanide ions with bovine Factor X and their use in the affinity chromatography of the venom coagulant protein of *Vipera russelli*. J. biol. Chem. **250**, 601—608 (1975)
Gaetano, G., de, Bottecchia, D., Vermylen, J.: Retraction of reptilase-clots in the presence of agents inducing or inhibiting the platelet adhesion-aggregation reaction. Thrombos. Res. **2**, 71—84 (1973)
Gaetano, G., de, Franco, R., Donati, M. B., Bonaccorsi, A., Garattini, S.: Mechanical recording of Reptilase-clot retraction: effect of adenosine-5'-diphosphate and prostaglandin E_1. Thrombos. Res. **4**, 189—192 (1974)
Gitter, S., Levi, G., Kochwa, S., Vries, A., de, Rechnic, J., Casper, J.: Studies on the venom of *Echis coloratus*. Amer. J. trop. Med. Hyg. **9**, 391—399 (1960)
Gormsen, J., Fletcher, A. P., Alkjaersig, N., Sherry, S.: Enzymic lysis of plasma clots: The influence of fibrin stabilization on lysis rates. Arch. Biochem. **120**, 654—665 (1967)
Guest, M. M., Murphy, R. C., Bodnar, S. B., Ware, A. G., Seegers, W. H.: Physiological effects of a plasma protein: Blood pressure, leukocyte concentration, smooth and cardiac muscle activity. Amer. J. Physiol. **150**, 471—479 (1947a)
Guest, M. M., Ware, A. G., Seegers, W. H.: A quantitative study of antifibrinolysin in chick plasma: increase in antifibrinolysin activity during pteroylglutamic acid deficiency. Amer. J. Physiol. **150**, 661—669 (1947b)
Gulliver, G. (Ed.): The Works of William Hewson, F.R.S. Bartholomew Close: C. and J. Adlard 1846
Hagen, E., Wechsler, W., Zilliken, F. (Eds.): Platelets in Haemostasis. Basel-New York: S. Karger 1968
Hagmar, B.: Defibrination and metastasis formation: Effects of Arvin on experimental metastases in mice. Europ. J. Cancer **8**, 17—28 (1972)
Hall, G. H., Holman, H. M., Webster, A. D. B.: Anticoagulation by ancrod for haemodialysis. Brit. med. J. **1970 IV**, 591—593
Hardaway, R. M. III: Syndromes of disseminated intravascular coagulation. Springfield: Charles C. Thomas 1966
Harder, A. J., Stadelmann, H., Straub, P. W.: Reptilase-induced shortening of coagulation times in normal and hemophilic individuals. Thrombos. Diathes. haemorrh. (Stuttg.) **27**, 349—360 (1972)

Harder,A.J., Straub,P.W.: In vitro and in vivo induction of fibrinogen and paracoagulation by Reptilase. Thrombos. Diathes. haemorrh. (Stuttg.) **27**, 337—348 (1972)
Hardisty,R.M., Ingram,G.I.C.: Bleeding Disorders. Oxford: Blackwell Scientific 1965
Harmison,C.R., Seegers,W.H.: Some physicochemical properties of bovine autoprothrombin II. J. Biol. Chem. **237**, 3074—3076 (1962)
Haslam,R.J.: Mechanism of blood platelet aggregation. In: Johnson,S.A., Seegers,W.H. (Eds.): Physiology of Haemostasis and Thrombosis, pp. 88—112. Charles C. Thomas 1967
Hawiger,J., Collins,R.D., Horn,R.G.: Precipitation of soluble fibrin monomer complexes by lysosomal protein fraction of polymorphonuclear leukocytes. Proc. Soc. exp. Biol. (N.Y.) **131**, 349—353 (1969)
Hecht,E.R.: Lipids in Blood Clotting. Springfield: Charles C. Thomas 1965
Heilbrun,L.V.: The Dynamics of Living Protoplasm. New York: Academic Press 1956
Hemker,H.C., Loeliger,E.A., Veltkamp,J.J. (Eds.): Human Blood Coagulation. New York: Springer-Verlag; Leiden: Leiden Univ. Pr. 1969
Henriksen,R.A., Jackson,C.M.: Cooperative calcium binding by the phospholipid binding region of bovine prothrombin: a requirement for intact disulfide bridges. Arch. Biochem. **170**, 149—159 (1975)
Henriques,S.B., Henriques,O.B.: Chemical composition of snake venoms. In: Rašková,H. (Ed.): International Encyclopedia of Pharmacology and Therapeutics, Sect. 71, Vol. I, Part II, pp. 225—288. Pharmacology and Toxicology of Snake Venoms. New York: Pergamon Press 1971
Henry,R.L., Steiman,R.H.: Mechanisms of hemostasis. Microvasc. Res. **1**, 68—82 (1968)
Herzig,R.H., Ratnoff,O.D., Shainoff,J.R.: Studies on a procoagulant fraction of Southern copperhead snake venom: the preferred release of fibrinopeptide B. J. Lab. clin. Med. **76**, 451—465 (1970)
Hessel,B., Blombäck,M.: The proteolytic action of the snake venom enzymes Arvin and Reptilase on N-terminal chain-fragments of human fibrinogen. FEBS Letters **18**, 318—320 (1971)
Hewett-Emmett,D., McCoy,L.E., Hassouna,H.I., Reuterby,J., Walz,D.A., Seegers,W.H.: A partial gene duplication in the evolution of prothrombin? Thrombos. Res. **5**, 421—430 (1974)
Highsmith,R.F., Rosenberg,R.D.: The inhibition of human plasmin by human antithrombin-heparin cofactor. J. biol. Chem. **249**, 4335—4338 (1974)
Holleman,W.H., Coen,L.J.: Characterization of peptides released from human fibrinogen by Arvin. Biochim. biophys. Acta (Amst.) **200**, 587—589 (1970)
Hoq,M.S., Cash,J.D.: Studies on a direct latex agglutination technique for the semiquantitation of fibrin/fibrinogen degradation products. Thrombos. Res. **2**, 23—29 (1973)
Hougie,C.: Effect of Russell's viper venom on Stuart clotting defect. Proc. Soc. exp. Biol. (N.Y.) **93**, 570—573 (1956)
Hougie,C.: Fundamentals of Blood Coagulation in Clinical Medicine. New York-Toronto-London: McGraw-Hill 1963
Houssay,B.A., Sordella,A.: Action des venins de serpents sur la coagulation sanguine. J. Physiol. Path. Gen. **18**, 781 (1919)
Howie,P.W., Prentice,C.R.M., McNicol,G.P.: A method of antithrombin estimation using plasma defibrinated with ancrod. Brit. J. Haemat. **25**, 101—110 (1973)
Irwin,J.F.: Factor VIII in von Willebrand's disease. Semin. Thromb. Hemost. **2**, 85—104 (1975)
Irwin,J.F., Seegers,W.H., Andary,T.J., Fekete,L.F., Novoa,E.: Blood coagulation as a cybernetic system: control of autoprothrombin C (Factor Xa) formation. Thrombos. Res. **6**, 431—441 (1975)
Iwanaga,S.: Personal communication (1975)
Iwanaga,S., Morita,T., Suzuki,T.: Activation of bovine prothrombin by *Echis carinatus* venom activator. Presented at the Japan-U.S. Seminar on Hemorheology and Thrombosis, Kobe, Japan, April 28—May 2, 1975
Jackson,C.M., Gordon,J.G., Hanahan,D.J.: Separation of the tosyl arginine esterase activity from the Factor X activating enzyme of Russell's viper venom. Biochim. biophys. Acta (Amst.) **252**, 255—261 (1971)
Jeruslalny,Z., Zucker,M.B.: Some effect of fibrinogen degradation products (FDP) on blood platelet. Thrombos. Diathes. haemorrh. (Stuttg.) **15**, 413—419 (1966)

Jiménez-Porras, J. M.: Pharmacology of peptides and proteins in snake venoms. Ann. Rev. Pharmacol. **8**, 299—318 (1968)
Jiménez-Porras, J. M.: Biochemistry of snake venoms. Clin. Toxicol. **3**, 389—431 (1970)
Jobin, F., Esnouf, M. P.: Coagulant activity of Tiger snake *(Notechis scutatus scutatus)* venom. Nature (Lond.) **211**, 873—875 (1966)
Johnson, S. A. (Ed.): The Circulating Platelet. New York-London: Academic Press 1971
Johnson, S. A., Greenwalt, T. J.: Coagulation and Transfusion in Clinical Medicine. Boston: Little, Brown and Company 1965
Johnson, S. A., Guest, M. M. (Eds.): Dynamics of Thrombus Formation and Dissolution. Philadelphia: J. B. Lippincott 1969
Johnson, S. A., Monto, R. W., Rebuck, J. W., Horn, Jr. R. C. (Eds.): Blood platelets. Henry Ford Hospital International Symposium, March 17—19, 1960, Detroit, Michigan. Boston: Little, Brown and Company 1961
Jorpes, J. E.: Heparin in the Treatment of Thrombosis, 2nd Ed. London-New York-Toronto: Oxford Univ. Pr. 1946
Josso, F., Lavergne, J. M., Gouault, M., Prou-Wartelle, O., Soulier, J. P.: Différents états moléculaires du facteur II (prothrombine). Leur étude à l'aide de la staphylocoagulase et d'anticorps anti-facteur II. I. Le facteur II chez les sujets traités par les antagonistes de la vitamine K. Thrombos. Diathes. haemorrh. (Stuttg.) **20**, 88—98 (1968)
Kakkar, V. V., Flanc, C., Howe, C. T., O'Shea, M., Flute, P. T.: Treatment of deep vein thrombosis. A trial of heparin, streptokinase, and Arvin. Brit. med. J. **1969 b I**, 806—810
Kakkar, V. V., Howe, C. T., Laws, J. W., Flanc, C.: Late results of treatment of deep vein thrombosis. Brit. med. J. **1969 a I**, 810—811
Kaplan, A. P., Austen, K. F.: A pre-albumin activator of prekallikrein. J. Immunol. **105**, 802—811 (1970)
Kaplan, A. P., Austen, K. F.: The fibrinolytic pathway of human plasma. J. exp. Med. **136**, 1378—1393 (1972)
Kaplan, A. P., Meier, H. L., Mandle, Jr., R.: The Hageman factor dependent pathways of coagulation, fibrinolysis, and kinin-generation. Semin. Thromb. Hemost. **3**, 1—26 (1976)
Karpatkin, S., Karpatkin, M.: Inhibition of the enzymatic activity of thrombin by concanavalin A. Biochem. biophys. Res. Commun. **57**, 1111—1118 (1974)
Kaulla, K. N., von: Chemistry of Thrombolysis: Human Fibrinolytic Enzymes. Springfield: Charles C. Thomas 1963
Kipfer, R., Seegers, W. H.: Transformation of autoprothrombin III to autoprothrombin C in sodium citrate solution. Thrombos. Diathes. haemorrh. (Stuttg.) **19**, 204—212 (1968)
Kirschmann, C., Aloof, S., Vries, A., de: Action of lysolecithin on blood platelets. Thrombos. Diathes. haemorrh. (Stuttg.) **9**, 512—524 (1963)
Kirschmann, C., Condrea, E., Moav, N., Aloof, S., Vries, A., de: Action of snake venom on human platelet phospholipids. Arch. int. Pharmacodyn. **150**, 372—378 (1964)
Koehnlein, H. E.: Effects of various hemostyptic drugs in rats. Plast. Reconstr. Surg. **50**, 462—466 (1972)
Köhler, M.: Untersuchungen zur Wirkung einer Defibrinierung mittels Schlangengiftenzym auf den Stoffwechsel bei chronischer peripherer Arteriopathie. In: Martin, M., Schoop, W. (Eds.): Defibrinierung mit thrombin-ähnlichen Schlangengiftenzymen. Aktuelle Probleme in der Angiologie, Vol. XXVI, pp. 132—138. Bern-Stuttgart-Wien: Hans Huber 1975
Kopeć, M., Latallo, Z. S., Stahl, M., Wegrzynowicz, Z.: The effect of proteolytic enzymes on fibrin stabilizing factor. Biochim. biophys. Acta (Amst.) **181**, 437—445 (1969)
Kopeć, M., Wegrzynowicz, Z., Latallo, Z. S.: Soluble fibrin complexes and a new specific test for their detection. Thrombos. Diathes. haemorrh. (Stuttg.) (Suppl.) **39**, 219—228 (1970 a)
Kopeć, M., Wegrzynowicz, Z., Latallo, Z. S.: Precipitation of soluble fibrin monomer complexes SFMC by cellular basic proteins, and the antagonistic effect of sulfonated mucopolysaccharides. Proc. Soc. exp. Biol. (N.Y.) **135**, 675—678 (1970 b)
Kornalík, F.: Über den Einfluß von *Echis-carinata*-Toxin auf die Blutgerinnung in vitro. Folia haemat. (Lpz.) **80**, 73—78 (1963)
Kornalík, F.: Fibrinolytische Proteasen aus Schlangengiften. Folia haemat. (Lpz.) **95**, 193—208 (1971)

Kornalík, F., Blombäck, B.: Prothrombin activation induced by ecarin—a prothrombin converting enzyme from *Echis carinatus* venom. Thrombos. Res. **6**, 53—63 (1975)
Kornalík, F., Hladovec, J.: The effect of ecarin—defibrinating enzyme isolated from *Echis carinatus*—on experimental arterial thrombosis. Thrombos. Res. **7**, 611—621 (1975)
Kornalík, F., Pudlák, P.: A prolonged defibrination caused by *Echis carinatus* venom. Life Sci. **10**, 309—314 (1971)
Kowalski, E., Budzyński, A. Z., Kopeć, M., Latallo, Z. S., Lipiński, B., Wegrzynowicz, Z.: Circulating fibrinogen degradation products (FDP) in blood after intravenous thrombin infusion. Thrombos. Diathes. haemorrh. (Stuttg.) **13**, 12—24 (1965)
Kubisz, P.: Platelet release reaction and clot retraction. Thrombos. Diathes. haemorrh. (Stuttg.) **30**, 224—226 (1973)
Kubisz, P.: Retraction of reptilase clots. Thrombos. Diathes. haemorrh. (Stuttg.) **33**, 384—386 (1975)
Kwaan, H. C., Barlow, G. H.: The mechanism of action of a coagulant fraction of Malayan pit viper venom, Arvin and of Reptilase. Thrombos. Diathes. haemorrh. (Stuttg.) (Suppl.) **45**, 63—68 (1971 a)
Kwaan, H. C., Barlow, G. H.: The mechanism of action of arvin and reptilase. Thrombos. Diathes. haemorrh. (Stuttg.) (Suppl.) **47**, 361—369 (1971 b)
Kwaan, H. C., Barlow, G. H., Suwanwela, N.: Fibrinogen and its derivatives in relationship to ancrod and Reptilase. Thrombos. Res. **2**, 123—136 (1973)
Laki, K. (Ed.): Fibrinogen. New York: Marcel Dekker 1968
Laki, K., Lorand, L.: On the solubility of fibrin clots. Science **108**, 280 (1948)
Lanchantin, G. F., Friedmann, J. A., Hart, D. W.: Two forms of human thrombin. J. biol. Chem. **248**, 5956—5966 (1973)
Landaburu, R. H., Giavedoni, E., Santillan, R.: Thrombin and acetylated thrombin in the activation of fibrinolysis. Canad. J. Physiol. Pharmacol. **46**, 809—813 (1968)
Landaburu, R. H., Seegers, W. H.: The acetylation of thrombin. Canad. J. Biochem. Physiol. **37**, 1361—1366 (1959)
Latallo, Z. S., Teisseyre, E.: Evaluation of Reptilase-R and thrombin clotting time in the presence of fibrinogen degradation products and heparin. Scand. J. Haemat. (Suppl.) **13**, 261—266 (1971)
Laurent, T. C., Blombäck, B.: On the significance of the release of two different peptides from fibrinogen during clotting. Acta chem. scand. **12**, 1875—1877 (1958)
Lee, C. Y.: Mode of action of cobra venom and its purified toxins. In: Simpson, L. L. (Ed.): Neuropoisons: Their Pathophysiological Action, Vol. I, pp. 21—70. Plenum Press 1971
Lee, C.-Y., Johnson, S. A., Seegers, W. H.: Clotting of blood with Russell's viper venom. J. Mich. State med. Soc. **54**, 801—804, 824 (1955)
Liu, D. T. H., McCoy, L. E.: Tissue extract thromboplastin: Quantitation, fractionation, and characterization of protein components. Thrombos. Res. **7**, 199—211 (1975 a)
Liu, D. T. H., McCoy, L. E.: Phospholipid requirements of tissue thromboplastin in blood coagulation. Thrombos. Res. **7**, 213—221 (1975 b)
Lorand, L., Robbins, K. C.: Clotting and lysis in blood plasma. In: Kornberg, H. L., Phillips, D. C. (Eds.): MTP International Review of Science, Biochemistry, Series 1, pp. 77—100. London: Butterworth; Baltimore: Univ. Park Press 1975
Lundblad, R. L., Davie, E. W.: The activation of antihemophilic factor (Factor VIII) by activated Christmas factor (activated Factor IX). Biochemistry **3**, 1720—1725 (1964)
Luzzio, A. J.: Inhibitory properties of serum protein on the enzymatic sequence leading to lysis of red blood cells by snake venom. Toxicon **5**, 97—103 (1967)
Lyons, W. J.: Profound thrombocytopenia associated with *Crotalus ruber ruber* envenomation: a clinical case. Toxicon **9**, 337—340 (1971)
Macfarlane, R. G.: Russell's viper venom: 1934—1964. Oxford Med. School Gaz. **17**, 100—115 (1965)
Macfarlane, R. G., Barnett, B.: The haemostatic possibilities of snake-venom. Lancet **1934 II**, 985—987
MacKenzie, R. D., Blohm, T. R., Auxier, E. M.: A modified Stypven test for the determination of platelet factor 3. Amer. J. clin. Path. **55**, 551—554 (1971)

MacMillan, R. L., Mustard, J. F. (Eds.): Anticoagulants and Fibrinolysins. Philadelphia: Lea and Febiger 1961
Magnusson, S., Sottrup-Jensen, L., Petersen, T. E., Morris, H. R., Dell, A.: Primary structure of the vitamin K-dependent part of prothrombin. FEBS Letters **44**, 189—193 (1974)
Mammen, E. F., Thomas, W. R., Seegers, W. H.: Activation of purified prothrombin to autoprothrombin I or autoprothrombin II (platelet cofactor II) or autoprothrombin II-A. Thrombos. Diathes. haemorrh. (Stuttg.) **5**, 218—249 (1960)
Mann, J. R., Breeze, G. R., Beeble, T. J., Stuart, J.: Ancrod in sickle cell crisis. Lancet **1972 I**, 934—937
Marciniak, E., Murano, G., Seegers, W. H.: Inhibitor of blood clotting derived from prothrombin. Thrombos. Diathes. haemorrh. (Stuttg.) **18**, 161—166 (1967)
Marcus, A. J., Zucker, M. B.: The Physiology of Blood Platelets. New York-London: Grune and Stratton 1965
Markland, F. S., Damus, P. S.: Purification and properties of a thrombin-like enzyme from the venom of *Crotalus adamanteus* (Eastern diamondback rattlesnake). J. biol. Chem. **246**, 6460—6473 (1971)
Markwardt, F.: Inhibition of thrombin. In: Hemker, H. C., Veltkamp, J. J. (Eds.): Prothrombin and Related Coagulation Factors, pp. 116—131. Leiden: Leiden University Press 1975
Markwardt, F., Walsmann, P.: Versuche zur Klärung des Wirkungsmechanismus der thrombokinaseähnlich wirkenden Komponente des Russell-Vipern-Giftes. Thrombos. Diathes. haemorrh. (Stuttg.) 7, 86—94 (1962)
Marsh, N. A., Gaffney, P. J., Whaler, B. C.: A thrombin-like enzyme from Gaboon viper venom. I. Isolation and practical characterisation. Abstracts. Symposium on Thrombin-like Enzymes—Properties and Applications, Juli 15—17, 1975, Trier, F. R. Germany
Marsh, N. A., Whaler, B. C.: Separation and partial characterization of a coagulant enzyme from *Bitis gabonica* venom. Brit. J. Haemat. **26**, 295—306 (1974)
Marshall, R., Esnouf, M. P.: The effect of *Ancistrodon rhodostoma* venom in the dog. Clin. Sci. **35**, 251—259 (1968)
Marsten, J. L., Kok-Ewe, C., Ankeney, J. L., Botti, R. E.: Antithrombotic effect of Malayan pit viper venom on experimental thrombosis of the inferior vena cava produced by a new method. Circulat. Res. **19**, 514—519 (1966)
Martin, U., Martin, M.: Verhalten der Thrombozytenadhäsivität unter Defibrase-Therapie. In: Martin, M., Schoop, W. (Eds.): Defibrinierung mit thrombin-ähnlichen Schlangengiftenzymen. Aktuelle Probleme in der Angiologie, Vol. XXVI, pp. 102—107. Bern-Stuttgart-Wien: Hans Huber 1975
Mattock, P., Esnouf, M. P.: A form of bovine Factor X with a single polypeptide chain. Nature (Lond.) New Biol. **242**, 90—92 (1973)
Maupin, B.: Blood Platelets in Man and Animals, Vol. I. Oxford-London-Edinburgh: Pergamon Press 1969
McCoy, L. E., Griscom, H. A., Diekamp, U., Seegers, W. H.: Experimental fibrinolysis with acetylated thrombin. Thrombos. Diathes. haemorrh. (Stuttg.) (Suppl.) **47**, 339—351 (1971)
McCoy, L. E., Walz, D. A., Agrawal, B. B. L., Seegers, W. H.: Isolation of L-chain polypeptide of autoprothrombin III (Factor X): Homology with prothrombin indicated. Thrombos. Res. **2**, 293—296 (1973b)
McCoy, L. E., Walz, D. A., Seegers, W. H.: Prethrombin and the ultimate formation of thrombin. Thrombos. Res. **3**, 357—361 (1973a)
McDonagh, R. P., McDonagh, J., Duckert, F.: The influence of fibrin crosslinking on the kinetics of urokinase-induced clot lysis. Brit. J. Haemat. **21**, 323—332 (1971)
McKay, D. G.: Disseminated Intravascular Coagulation. New York: Hoeber Medical Division, Harper and Row 1965
Meaume, J.: Les venins de serpents agents modificateurs de la coagulation sanguine. Toxicon **4**, 25—28 (1966)
Mellanby, J.: The coagulation of blood. Part II. The action of snake venoms, peptone and leech extract. J. Physiol. (Lond.) **38**, 441—503 (1909)
Mitrakul, C.: Effects of Green pit viper (*Trimeresurus erythrurus* and *Trimeresurus popeorum*) venoms on blood coagulation, platelets and the fibrinolytic enzyme systems: studies in vivo and in vitro. Amer. J. Clin. Path. **60**, 654—662 (1973)

Morawitz, P.: The chemistry of blood coagulation. Springfield: Charles C. Thomas 1958
Morita, T., Nishibe, H., Iwanaga, S., Suzuki, T.: Studies on the activation of bovine prothrombin. Isolation and characterization of the fragments released from the prothrombin by activated Factor X. J. Biochem. (Tokyo) **76**, 1031—1048 (1974)
Müller-Berghaus, G., Hocke, M.: Production of the generalized Shwartzman reaction in rabbits by ancrod (Arvin) infusion and endotoxin injection. Brit. J. Haemat. **25**, 111—112 (1973)
Müller-Berghaus, G., Mann, B.: Precipitation of ancrod-induced soluble fibrin by aprotinin and norepinephrine. Thrombos. Res. **2**, 305—322 (1973)
Müller-Berghaus, G., Seegers, W.H.: Some effects of purified autoprothrombin C in blood clotting. Thrombos. Diathes. haemorrh. (Stuttg.) **16**, 707—722 (1966)
Murano, G.: The molecular structure of fibrinogen. Semin. Thromb. Hemost. **1**, 1—31 (1974)
Murano, G., Seegers, W.H., Zolton, R.P.: Autoprothrombin II-A: A competitive inhibitor of autoprothrombin C (Factor Xa). A review with additions. Thrombos. Diathes. haemorrh. (Stuttg.) (Suppl.) **57**, 305—314 (1974)
Murano, G., Wiman, B., Blombäck, B.: Human fibrinogen: some characteristics of its S-carboxymethyl derivative chains. Thromb. Res. **1**, 161—171 (1972)
Murphy, R.C., Seegers, W.H.: Concentration of prothrombin and Ac-globulin in various species. Amer. J. Physiol. **154**, 134—139 (1948)
Nahas, L., Denson, K.W.E., Macfarlane, R.G.: A study of the coagulant action of eight snake venoms. Thrombos. Diathes. haemorrh. (Stuttg.) **12**, 354—367 (1964)
Nelsestuen, G.L., Suttie, J.W.: Mode of action of vitamin K. Calcium binding properties of bovine prothrombin. Biochemistry **11**, 4961—4964 (1972)
Nelsestuen, G.L., Zytkovicz, T.H., Howard, J.B.: The mode of action of vitamin K. Identification of γ-carboxyglutamic acid as a component of prothrombin. J. biol. Chem. **249**, 6347—6350 (1974)
Nemerson, Y.: The reaction between bovine brain tissue factor and Factors VII and X. Biochemistry **5**, 601—608 (1966)
Niewiarowski, S., Regoeczi, E., Stewart, G.J., Senyi, A.F., Mustard, J.F.: Platelet interaction with polymerizing fibrin. J. clin. Invest. **51**, 685—700 (1972)
Niewiarowski, S., Stewart, J., Nath, N., Taiska, A., Lieberman, G.E.: ADP, thrombin and *B. atrox* thrombin-like enzyme in platelet dependent fibrin retraction. Amer. J. Physiol. **229**, 737—745 (1975)
Norman, P.S., Hill, B.M.: The studies of the plasmin system. III. Physical properties of the two plasmin inhibitors in plasma. J. exp. Med. **108**, 639—649 (1958)
Oddvar, T., Wik, O.K., Berman, H.J.: The effect of thrombin, reptilase, and a fibrinopeptide-B releasing enzyme from the venom of southern copperhead snake on rabbit platelet. Microvasc. Res. **6**, 342—346 (1973)
Olsen, E.J.G., Pitney, W.R.: The effect of Arvin on experimental pulmonary embolism in the rabbit. Brit. J. Haemat. **17**, 425—429 (1969)
Olson, P.S.: The contribution of platelets and fibrinogen in the early development of experimental arterial and venous thrombi. In: Martin, M., Schoop, W. (Eds.): Defibrinierung mit thrombin-ähnlichen Schlangengiftenzymen. Aktuelle Probleme in der Angiologie, Vol. XXVI, pp. 108—113. Bern-Stuttgart-Wien: Hans Huber 1975
Olsson, P., Blombäck, M., Egberg, N., Ekeström, S., Göransson, L., Johnsson, H.: Studies on the bleeding tendency and the possibility of surgery in states of Reptilase induced defibrinogenation. Thrombos. Diathes. haemorrh. (Stuttg.) (Suppl.) **47**, 389—396 (1971)
Olsson, P., Ljungqvist, A., Göransson, L.: Vein graft surgery in Defibrase-defibrinogenated dogs. Thrombos. Res. **3**, 161—172 (1973)
Olsson, P.I., Johnsson, H.: Interference of acetyl salicylic acid, heparin and fibrinogen degradation products in haemostasis of Reptilase-defibrinogenated dogs. Thrombos. Res. **1**, 135—146 (1972)
Ouyang, C.: The effects of Formosan snake venoms on blood coagulation in vitro. J. Formosan med. Ass. **56**, 435—448 (1957)
Ouyang, C., Hong, J.S.: Inhibition of the thrombin-like principle of *Agkistrodon acutus* venom by group-specific enzyme inhibitors. Toxicon **12**, 449—453 (1974)

Ouyang, C., Hong, J. S., Teng, C. M.: Purification and properties of the thrombin-like principle of *Agkistrodon acutus* venom and its comparison with bovine thrombin. Thrombos. Diathes. haemorrh. (Stuttg.) **26**, 224—234 (1971 a)

Ouyang, C., Huang, T. F.: The purification and characterization of the fibrinolytic principle of *Agkistrodon acutus* venom. Biochim. biophys. Acta (Amst.) **439**, 146—153 (1976 a)

Ouyang, C., Huang, T. F.: The properties of the purified fibrinolytic principle of *Agkistrodon acutus* snake venom. Toxicon **15**, 161—167 (1977)

Ouyang, C., Seegers, W. H., McCoy, L. E., Müller-Berghaus, G.: Metabolic formation of a prothrombin derivative. Thrombos. Diathes. haemorrh. (Stuttg.) **25**, 332—339 (1971 b)

Ouyang, C., Teng, C. M.: Comparative studies on the effects of thrombin-like enzyme of *A. acutus* venom and bovine thrombin on platelet function. (unpublished data a)

Ouyang, C., Teng, C. M.: Thrombagglutinin of *T. mucrosquamatus* venom. (unpublished data b)

Ouyang, C., Teng, C. M.: Anticoagulant effects of fibrinogen degradation products produced by α- and β-fibrinogenases of *T. mucrosquamatus* venom. Toxicon (in press) (1978)

Ouyang, C., Teng, C. M.: Purification and properties of the anticoagulant principle of *Agkistrodon acutus* venom. Biochim. biophys. Acta (Amst.) **278**, 155—162 (1972)

Ouyang, C., Teng, C. M.: The effect of the purified anticoagulant principle of *Agkistrodon acutus* venom on blood coagulation. Toxicon **11**, 287—292 (1973)

Ouyang, C., Teng, C. M.: The effects of the purified thrombin-like and anticoagulant principles of *Agkistrodon acutus* venom on blood coagulation in vivo. Toxicon **14**, 49—54 (1976 a)

Ouyang, C., Teng, C. M.: Fibrinolytic enzymes of *Trimeresurus mucrosquamatus* venom. Biochim. biophys. Acta (Amst.) **420**, 298—308 (1976 b)

Ouyang, C., Yang, F. Y.: Purification and properties of the thrombin-like enzyme from *Trimeresurus gramineus* venom. Biochim. biophys. Acta (Amst.) **351**, 354—363 (1974)

Ouyang, C., Yang, F. Y.: Purification and properties of the anticoagulant principle of *Trimeresurus gramineus* venom. Biochim. biophys. Acta (Amst.) **386**, 479—492 (1975)

Ouyang, C., Yang, F. Y.: The effects of the purified thrombin-like enzyme and anticoagulant principle of *Trimeresurus gramineus* venom on blood coagulation in vivo. Toxicon **14**, 197—201 (1976)

Owen, C. A., Bollman, J. L.: Prothrombin conversion factor of Dicumarol plasma. Proc. Soc. exp. Biol. (N.Y.) **67**, 231—234 (1948)

Owen, Jr., C. A., Bowie, E. J. W., Didisheim, P., Thompson, Jr., J. H.: The Diagnosis of Bleeding Disorders. Boston: Little, Brown and Company 1969

Owen, W. G., Jackson, C. M.: Activation of prothrombin with *Oxyuranus scutellatus scutellatus* (Taipan snake) venom. Thrombos. Res. **3**, 705—714 (1973)

Owren, P. A.: The coagulation of blood. Investigations on a new clotting factor. Acta med. scand. (Suppl.) **194** (1947)

Pechet, L., Engel, A. M., Goldstein, C., Claser, B.: The effects of infusing thrombin and its acetylated derivative. I. Studies on coagulation and fibrinolysis. Thrombos. Diathes. haemorrh. (Stuttg.) **20**, 190—201 (1968)

Pirkle, H., McIntosh, M., Theodor, I., Vernon, S.: Activation of prothrombin with Taipan snake venom. Thrombos. Res. **1**, 559—567 (1972)

Pitney, W. R.: Clinical experience with Arvin. Thrombos. Diathes. haemorrh. (Stuttg.) (Suppl.) **38**, 81—86 (1970)

Pitney, W. R., Bell, W. R., Bolton, G.: Blood fibrinolytic activity during Arvin therapy. Brit. J. Haemat. **16**, 165—171 (1969)

Pitney, W. R., Oakley, C. M., Goodwin, J. F.: Therapeutic defibrination with Arvin. Amer. Heart J. **80**, 144—146 (1970)

Pitney, W. R., Raphael, M. J., Webb-Peploe, M. M., Olsen, E. J. G.: Treatment of experimental venous thrombosis with streptokinase and ancrod (Arvin). Brit. J. Surg. **58**, 442—447 (1971)

Pitney, W. R., Regoeczi, E.: Inactivation of Arvin by plasma proteins. Brit. J. Haemat. **19**, 67—81 (1970)

Pizzo, S. V., Schwartz, M. L., Hill, R. L., McKee, P. A.: Mechanism of ancrod anticoagulation. A direct proteolytic effect on fibrin. J. clin. Invest. **51**, 2841—2850 (1972)

Poller, L. (Ed.): Recent Advances in Blood Coagulation. London: J. and A. Churchill 1969

Pool, J. G., Robinson, A. J.: A change in Russell's viper venom (Stypven): Modification of Factor V assay to compensate. J. Lab. clin. Med. **77**, 343—345 (1971)

Prentice, C. R. M., Hassanein, A. A., Turpie, A. G. G., McNicol, G. P., Douglas, A. S.: Changes in platelet behavior during Arvin therapy. Lancet **1969 I**, 644—647
Quick, A. J.: The Hemorrhagic Diseases. Springfield: Charles C. Thomas 1942
Quick, A. J.: Thromboplastin generation: Effect of the Bell-Alton reagent and Russell's viper venom on prothrombin consumption. Amer. J. clin. Path. **55**, 555—560 (1971)
Radcliffe, R. D., Barton, P. G.: The purification and properties of activated Factor X. Bovine Factor X activated with Russell's viper venom. J. biol. Chem. **247**, 7735—7742 (1972)
Radcliffe, R. D., Barton, P. G.: Comparisons of the molecular forms of activated bovine Factor X. Products of activation with Russell's viper venom, insoluble trypsin, sodium citrate, tissue factor and the intrinsic system. J. biol. Chem. **248**, 6788—6795 (1973)
Radcliffe, R., Nemerson, Y.: Activation and control of Factor VII by activated Factor X and thrombin. Isolation and characterization of a single chain form of Factor VII. J. biol. Chem. **250**, 388—395 (1975)
Rahimtoola, S. H., Raphael, M. J., Pitney, W. R., Olsen, E. J. G., Webb-Peploe, M.: Therapeutic defibrination and heparin therapy in the prevention and resolution of experimental venous thrombosis. Circulation **42**, 729—737 (1970)
Rapaport, S. I., Hjort, P. F., Patch, M. J.: Rabbit Factor V: Different effects of thrombin and venom, a source of error in assay. Amer. J. Physiol. **211**, 1477—1485 (1966)
Ratnoff, O. D.: Bleeding Syndromes. Springfield: Charles C. Thomas 1960
Regoeczi, E., Bell, W. R.: In vivo behavior of coagulant enzyme from *Agkistrodon rhodostoma* venom: Studies using ^{131}I-"Arvin." Brit. J. Haemat. **16**, 573—587 (1969)
Regoeczi, E., Gergely, J., McFarlane, A. S.: In vivo effects of *Agkistrodon rhodostoma* venom: Studies with fibrinogen ^{131}I. J. clin. Invest. **45**, 1202—1212 (1966)
Reid, H. A.: Treatment of snake-bite poisoning. Brit. med. J. **1963 I**, 1675
Reid, H. A.: A new possibility; therapeutic defibrination; afibrinogenemia due to Malayan pit viper venom. Thrombos. Diathes. haemorrh. (Stuttg.) (Suppl.) **38**, 75—79 (1970)
Reid, H. A., Chan, K. E.: The paradox in therapeutic defibrination. Lancet **1968 I**, 485—486
Reid, H. A., Chan, K. E., Thean, P. C.: Prolonged coagulation defect (defibrination syndrome) in Malayan viper bite. Lancet **1963 b I**, 621—626
Reid, H. A., Thean, P. C., Chan, K. E., Baharom, A. R.: Clinical effects of bites by Malayan viper *(Ancistrodon rhodostoma)*. Lancet **1963 a I**, 617—621
Reno, R. S., Seegers, W. H.: Two-stage procedure for the quantitative determination of autoprothrombin III concentration and some applications. Thrombos. Diathes. haemorrh. (Stuttg.) **18**, 198—210 (1967)
Riddle, J. M., Barnhart, M. I.: Eosinophil mobilization during disseminated intravascular coagulation. Thrombos. Diathes. haemorrh. (Stuttg.) (Suppl.) **36**, 99—123 (1969)
Robbins, K. C.: A study on the conversion of fibrinogen to fibrin. Amer. J. Physiol. **142**, 581—588 (1944)
Robertson Smith, D., Morag, M.: The effect of Malayan pit-viper *(Agkistrodon rhodostoma)* venom on ovine blood and the development of resistance to the anticoagulant activity of this venom. Res. Vet. Sci. **13**, 298—301 (1972)
Roschlau, W. H. E., Gage, R.: The effects of brinolase on platelet aggregation of dog and man. Thrombos. Diathes. haemorrh. (Stuttg.) **28**, 31—48 (1972)
Rosenberg, R. D., Damus, P. S.: The purification and mechanism of action of human antithrombin-heparin cofactor. J. biol. Chem. **248**, 6490—6505 (1973)
Rosenfeld, G., Nahas, L., Kelen, E. M. A.: Coagulant, proteolytic, and hemolytic properties of some snake venoms. In: Bücherl, W., Buckley, E., Deulofeu, V. (Eds.): Venomous Animals and Their Venoms, Vol. I, pp. 229—273. New York-London: Academic Press 1968
Russell, F. E.: Clinical aspects of snake venom poisoning in North America. Toxicon **7**, 33—37 (1969)
Russell, F. E., Carlson, R. W., Wainschel, J., Osborne, A. H.: Snake venom poisoning in the United States. J. Amer. med. Ass. **233**, 341—344 (1975)
Sakuragawa, N., Takahashi, K., Hoshiyama, M., Jimbo, C., Matsuoka, M., Onishi, Y.: Significance of a prothrombin assay method using *Echis carinatus* venom for diagnostic information in disseminated intravascular coagulation syndrome. Thrombos. Res. **7**, 643—653 (1975)
Sawyer, P. N. (Ed.): Biophysical Mechanisms in Vascular Homeostasis and Intravascular Thrombosis. New York: Appleton-Century-Crofts 1965

Scheraga, H. A., Laskowski, Jr., M.: The fibrinogen-fibrin conversion. Advanc. Protein Chem. **12**, 1—131 (1957)

Schieck, A., Kornalík, F., Habermann, E.: The prothrombin activating principle from *Echis carinatus* venom. I. Preparation and biochemical properties. Naunyn-Schmiedebergs Arch. Pharmacol. **272**, 402—416 (1972a)

Schieck, A., Habermann, E., Kornalík, F.: The prothrombin activating principle from *Echis carinatus* venom. II. Coagulation studies in vitro and in vivo. Naunyn-Schmiedebergs Arch. Pharmacol. **274**, 7—17 (1972b)

Schiffman, S., Theodor, I., Rapaport, S. I.: Separation from Russell's viper venom of one fraction reacting with Factor X and another reacting with Factor V. Biochemistry **8**, 1397—1405 (1969)

Seegers, W. H.: Prothrombin. Cambridge: Harvard University Press 1962

Seegers, W. H.: Prothrombin in Enzymology, Thrombosis and Hemophilia. Springfield: Charles C. Thomas 1967a

Seegers, W. H. (Ed.): Blood Clotting Enzymology. New York-London: Academic Press 1967b

Seegers, W. H.: Blood clotting mechanisms: three basic reactions. Ann. Rev. Physiol. **31**, 269—294 (1969)

Seegers, W. H.: Solving the riddle of blood clotting. Shirley A. Johnson Memorial Lecture. Thrombos. Diathes. haemorrh. (Stuttg.) (Suppl.) **54**, 9—30 (1973a)

Seegers, W. H.: Blood coagulation: a cybernetic system. Ser. Haematol. **6**, 549—578 (1973b)

Seegers, W. H.: Unpublished observations (1975)

Seegers, W. H., Andary, T. J.: Formation of prethrombin-E, thrombin, and thrombin-E and their inhibition with antithrombin and enzyme inhibitors. Thrombos. Res. **4**, 869—874 (1974)

Seegers, W. H., Cole, E. R., Harmison, C. R., Marciniak, E.: Purification and some properties of autoprothrombin C. Canad. J. Biochem. Physiol. **41**, 1047—1063 (1963)

Seegers, W. H., Diekamp, U., McCoy, L. E.: Induction of platelet aggregation with acetylated thrombin. Thrombos. Diathes. haemorrh. (Stuttg.) (Suppl.) **42**, 115—124 (1970)

Seegers, W. H., Hassouna, H. I., Hewett-Emmett, D., Walz, D. A., Andary, T. J.: Prothrombin and thrombin: Selected aspects of thrombin formation, properties, inhibition, and immunology. Sem. Thromb. Hemost. **1**, 211—283 (1975)

Seegers, W. H., Heene, D. L., Marciniak, E.: Activation of purified prothrombin in ammonium sulfate solutions: Purification of autoprothrombin C. Thrombos. Diathes. haemorrh. (Stuttg.) **15**, 1—11 (1966)

Seegers, W. H., Landaburu, R. H.: Esterase and clotting activity derived from purified prothrombin. Amer. J. Physiol. **191**, 167—173 (1957)

Seegers, W. H., Landaburu, R. H., Johnson, J. F.: Fibrinolytic properties of thrombin. Presented at the International Conference on Fibrinolysis, Princeton, New Jersey, 1960a

Seegers, W. H., Landaburu, R. H., Johnson, J. F.: Thrombin-E as a fibrinolytic enzyme. Science **131**, 726 (1960b)

Seegers, W. H., Marciniak, E., Kipfer, R. K., Yasunaga, K.: Isolation and some properties of prethrombin and autoprothrombin III. Arch. Biochem. **121**, 372—383 (1967)

Seegers, W. H., McClaughry, R. I., Fahey, J. L.: Some properties of purified prothrombin and its activation with sodium citrate. Blood **5**, 421—433 (1950)

Seegers, W. H., McCoy, L. E.: Stability conditions related to a previously unrecognized form of thrombin. Thrombos. Diathes. haemorrh. (Stuttg.) **27**, 361—362 (1972)

Seegers, W. H., McCoy, L. E., Groben, H. D., Sakuragawa, N., Agrawal, B. B. L.: Purification and some properties of autoprothrombin II-A: An anticoagulant perhaps also related to fibrinolysis. Thrombos. Res. **1**, 443—460 (1972b)

Seegers, W. H., McCoy, L., Marciniak, E.: Blood-clotting enzymology: Three basic reactions. Clin. Chem. **14**, 97—115 (1968)

Seegers, W. H., Miller, K. D., Andrews, E. B., Murphy, R. C.: Fundamental interactions and effect of storage, ether, adsorbants, and blood clotting on plasma antithrombin activity. Amer. J. Physiol. **169**, 700—711 (1952)

Seegers, W. H., Nieft, M. L., Vandenbelt, J. M.: Decomposition products of fibrinogen and fibrin. Arch. Biochem. **7**, 15—19 (1945)

Seegers, W. H., Novoa, E., Henry, R. L., Hassouna, H. I.: Relationship of "new" vitamin K-dependent Protein C and "old" autoprothrombin II-A. Thrombos. Res. **8**, 543—553 (1976)

Seegers, W. H., Sakuragawa, N., McCoy, L. E., Sedensky, J. A., Dombrose, F. A.: Prothrombin activation: Ac-globulin, lipid, platelet membrane, and autoprothrombin C (Factor Xa) requirements. Thrombos. Res. **1**, 293—310 (1972a)

Seegers, W. H., Sharp, E. A.: Hemostatic Agents. Springfield: Charles C. Thomas 1948

Seegers, W. H., Smith, H. P.: Factors which influence the activity of purified thrombin. Amer. J. Physiol. **137**, 348—354 (1942)

Seegers, W. H., Ulutin, O. N.: Autoprothrombin II-anticoagulant (autoprothrombin II-A). Thrombos. Diathes. haemorrh. (Stuttg.) **6**, 270—281 (1961)

Seegers, W. H., Walz, D. A., Reuterby, J., McCoy, L. E.: Isolation and some properties of thrombin-E and other prothrombin derivatives. Thrombos. Res. **4**, 829—859 (1974)

Seegers, W. H., Warner, E. D., Brinkhous, K. M., Smith, H. P.: The use of purified thrombin as an hemostatic agent. Science **89**, 86 (1939)

Selye, H.: Thrombohemorrhagic Phenomena. Springfield: Charles C. Thomas 1966

Sharma, G. V. R. K., Godin, P. F., Belko, J. S., Bell, W. R., Sasahara, A. A.: Arvin therapy in experimental pulmonary embolism. Amer. Heart J. **85**, 72—77 (1973)

Sharp, A. A.: Clinical use of Arvin. Thrombos. Diathes. haemorrh. (Stuttg.) (Suppl.) **45**, 69—71 (1971)

Sharp, A. A., Warren, B. A., Paxton, A. M., Allington, M. J.: Anticoagulant therapy with a purified fraction of Malayan pit viper venom. Lancet **1968 I**, 493—499

Sherry, S., Scriabine, A. (Eds.): Platelets and Thrombosis. Baltimore-London-Tokyo: University Park Press 1974

Shiau, S., Ouyang, C.: Isolation of coagulant and anticoagulant principles from the venom of *Trimeresurus gramineus*. Toxicon **2**, 213—220 (1965)

Stacher, A., Böhnel, J.: Experimentelle und klinische Untersuchungen zur hämostatischen Wirkung von Schlangengiften. Wien. klin. Wschr. **71**, 333—335 (1959)

Stachurska, J.: Inhibition of platelet aggregation by dialysable fibrinogen degradation products (FDP). Thrombos. Diathes. haemorrh. (Stuttg.) **23**, 91—98 (1970)

Stenflo, J.: A new vitamin K-dependent protein. J. biol. Chem. **251**, 355—363 (1976)

Stenflo, J., Fernlund, P., Egan, W., Roepstorff, P.: Vitamin K-dependent modifications of glutamic acid residues in prothrombin. Proc. nat. Acad. Sci. (Wash.) **71**, 2730—2733 (1974)

Stenflo, J., Ganrot, P. O.: Vitamin K and the biosynthesis of prothrombin. I. Identification and purification of a dicoumarol-induced abnormal prothrombin from bovine plasma. J. biol. Chem. **247**, 8160—8166 (1972)

Stocker, K., Barlow, G. H.: Snake venom proteases which coagulate blood: The coagulant enzyme from *Bothrops atrox* venom (batroxobin). In: Colowick, S. P., Kaplan, N. O. (Eds.): Methods in Enzymology. New York-London: Academic Press 1975b

Stocker, K., Christ, W., Leloup, P.: Characterization of the venoms of various *Bothrops* species by immunoelectrophoresis and reaction with fibrinogen agarose. Toxicon **12**, 415—417 (1974)

Stocker, K., Egberg, N.: Reptilase as a defibrinogenating agent. Thrombos. Diathes. haemorrh. (Stuttg.) (Suppl.) **54**, 361—369 (1973)

Stocker, K., Yeh, H.: A simple and sensitive test for the detection of inhibitors of Defibrase and Arwin in serum. Thrombos. Res. **6**, 189—194 (1975)

Stocker, K. F., Barlow, G. H.: Characterization of Defibrase. In: Martin, M., Schoop, W. (Eds.): Defibrinierung mit thrombin-ähnlichen Schlangengiftenzymen. Aktuelle Probleme in der Angiologie, Vol. XXVI, pp. 45—62. Bern-Stuttgart-Wien: Hans Huber 1975a

Straub, P. W., Bollinger, A., Blättler, W.: Metabolism of labelled thrombin-like snake venom enzymes. In: Martin, M., Schoop, W. (Eds.): Defibrinierung mit thrombin-ähnlichen Schlangengiftenzymen. Aktuelle Probleme in der Angiologie, Vol. XXVI, pp. 72—78. Bern-Stuttgart-Wien: Hans Huber 1975

Straub, P. W., Harder, A.: Verhalten von I^{125}-Fibrinogen bei therapeutischer Defibrinierung mit hochgereinigter Reptilase ("Defibrase"). Schweiz. med. Wschr. **101**, 1802—1804 (1971)

Tager, M., Drummond, M. C.: Implications of staphylocoagulase-thrombin and fibrinogen interaction. Thrombos. Diathes. haemorrh. (Stuttg.) (Suppl.) **39**, 291—298 (1970)

Tangen, O., Bygdeman, S.: Study of the clotting, esterase and platelet aggregating activities of thrombin, acetylated thrombin and Reptilase. Scand. J. Haematol. **9**, 333—338 (1972)

Tangen, O., Wik, O. K., Berman, H. J.: The effect of thrombin, Reptilase, and a fibrinopeptide B-releasing enzyme from the venom of the Southern copperhead snake on rabbit platelets. Microvasc. Res. **6**, 342—346 (1973)

Thomas, D. P., Niewiarowski, S., Myers, A. R., Bloch, K. J., Colman, R. W.: A comparative study of four methods of detecting fibrinogen degradation products in patients with various diseases. New Engl. J. Med. **283**, 663—668 (1970)

Tidrick, R. T., Seegers, W. H., Warner, E. D.: Clinical experience with thrombin as an hemostatic agent. Surgery **14**, 191—196 (1943)

Tocantins, L. M., Kazal, L. A. (Eds.): Blood Coagulation, Hemorrhage, and Thrombosis. New York-London: Grune and Stratton 1964

Triantaphyllopoulos, D. C., Triantaphyllopoulos, E.: Evidence of antithrombic activity of the anticoagulant fraction of incubated fibrinogen. Brit. J. Haemat. **12**, 145—151 (1966)

Tsernoglou, D., Walz, D. A., McCoy, L. E., Seegers, W. H.: A new thrombin: purification, amino acid composition and crystallization. Thrombos. Res. **1**, 533—537 (1972)

Tu, A. T., Gordon, J. P., Azucena, C.: Some biochemical evidence in support of the classification of venomous snakes. Toxicon **3**, 5—8 (1965)

Vinazzer, H.: Proteinchemische Charakterisierung und Standardisierung von Arwin. In: Martin, M., Schoop, W. (Eds.): Defibrinierung mit thrombin-ähnlichen Schlangengiftenzymen. Aktuelle Probleme in der Angiologie, Vol. XXVI, pp. 63—71. Bern-Stuttgart-Wien: Hans Huber 1975

Vries, A., de, Cohen, I.: Hemorrhagic and blood coagulation disturbing action of snake venoms. In: Poller, L. (Ed.): Recent Advances in Blood Coagulation, p. 277. London: J. and A. Churchill 1969

Walz, D. A.: Further studies on the nature and generation of thrombin. Ph.D. Dissertation, Wayne State Univ. Library, Detroit, Michigan 1973

Ware, A. G., Fahey, J. L., Seegers, W. H.: Platelet extracts, fibrin formation and interaction of purified prothrombin and thromboplastin. Amer. J. Physiol. **154**, 140—147 (1948)

Ware, A. G., Murphy, R. C., Seegers, W. H.: The function of Ac-globulin in blood clotting. Science **106**, 618 (1947)

Ware, A. G., Seegers, W. H.: Serum Ac-globulin: formation from plasma Ac-globulin; role in blood coagulation; partial purification; properties; and quantitative determination. Amer. J. Physiol. **152**, 567—576 (1948)

Warner, E. D., Brinkhous, K. M., Seegers, W. H., Smith, H. P.: Further experience with the use of thrombin as a hemostatic agent. Proc. Soc. exp. Biol. (N.Y.) **41**, 655—657 (1939)

Wetmore, R., Gurewich, V.: The role of fibrin monomer and an in vivo thrombin-induced anticoagulant in experimental venous thrombosis. Scand. J. Haematol. **12**, 204—212 (1974)

Wik, O. K., Tangen, O., McKenzie, F. N.: Blood clotting activity of Reptilase and bovine thrombin in vitro: A comparative study on seven different species. Brit. J. Haematol. **23**, 37—45 (1972)

Williams, W. J., Esnouf, M. P.: The fractionation of Russell's-viper *(Vipera russelli)* venom with special reference to the coagulant protein. Biochem. J. **84**, 52—62 (1962)

Wilson, P. A., McNicol, G. P., Douglus, A. S.: Effect of FDPs on platelet aggregation. J. clin. Pathol. **21**, 147—153 (1968)

Wintrobe, M. M.: Clinical Hematology, 7th Ed. Philadelphia: Lea and Febiger 1974

Zimmerman, T. S., Arroyave, C. M., Müller-Eberhard, H. J.: A blood coagulation abnormality in rabbits deficient in the sixth component of complement (C6) and its correction by purified C6. J. exp. Med. **134**, 1591—1600 (1971)

Zimmerman, T. S., Müller-Eberhard, H. J.: Blood coagulation initiation by a complement-mediated pathway. J. exp. Med. **134**, 1601—1607 (1971)

Zolton, R. P., Seegers, W. H.: Autoprothrombin II-A: Thrombin removal and mechanism of induction of fibrinolysis. Thrombos. Res. **3**, 23—33 (1973)

Zolton, R. P., Seegers, W. H.: Phospholipid requirements in thrombin formation. Thrombos. Res. **4**, 437—446 (1974)

Part IV

Immunological and Clinical Aspects

CHAPTER 19

Immunological Properties of Snake Venoms

P. BOQUET

A. Introduction

I. Definitions

The study of humoral immunity has been enriched in recent decades by a considerable number of observations concerning the origin, structure and specifity of antibodies.

An immunogen is a substance that generates antibody. Antigens are potential immunogens which bind specifically to antibodies. Haptens are devoid of immunogenicity but nevertheless combine to antibodies of their own, these antibodies being obtained by artificial means.

Immunogens, which are generally large molecules, possess several sites with immunological properties, called epitopes. The study of the specificity of antibodies necessitated the use of antigens with a less complex structure. By joining, through a so-called covalent bond, a very small hapten molecule of known chemical structure to an immunogen, then injecting the hapten and its vehicle into animals, LANDSTEINER (1936) achieved the synthesis of antibody specific to this hapten, thus establishing the basis of immunochemistry. Using these new investigative procedures, the immunochemists set out to locate, define, and measure the regions responsible for antigenicity on various molecules of known structure. The analytical studies of silk fibroin, ribonuclease, lysozyme, myoglobin and of synthetic polypeptides and polysaccharides are examples of this type of research. In other areas, experimenters have concentrated their attention on the problems raised in the *in vivo* recognition of antigenic structures, the memory that the animals' immune system retains from a first contact with these structures, the tolerance it sometimes shows with respect to an immunogen, the stages of synthesis of antibodies, and lastly the competition that may occur between several immunogens administered simultaneously or successively.

The literature devoted to the analysis of mechanisms of immunity shows that venoms have been used exceptionally as experimental materials. The extreme complexity of these substances is the principal reason for this. For some years, however, low-molecular-weight proteins have been extracted, in a pure state, from the venoms of *Hydrophiidae* and *Elapidae*. These antigens are carriers of a very small number of epitopes. A comparative study of their composition and their structure has recently led to the conclusion that some of them have the same protein as a common ancestor (STRYDOM, 1972a, 1973a and b). Differing from each other in their chemical nature and sometimes in their pharmacological properties, these constituents of snake venoms will provide a material of choice for future experimentation in the field of immunology.

II. Historical Data

The resistance of snake charmers to reptile venoms has been known for a very long time. This resistance, which is an expression of a state of acquired immunity, was generally obtained because of the protective nature of superficial and frequent bites by young snakes. Experimental research on resistance to snake venom did not really begin to progress until the end of the nineteenth century. Three years before the discovery by BEHRING and KITASATO (1890) of antidiphtheria and antitetanus immunity, SEWALL, an American scientist, established in 1887 that pigeons which had been injected with nonlethal doses of *Sistrurus catenatus* venom over several months withstood the injection of a dose of the same venom that was lethal for untreated animals. Later, KAUFFMAN (1893) and PHISALIX, in collaboration with BERTRAND (1894a) succeeded in conferring upon small rodents a resistance to the venom of *Vipera aspis* by vaccination with nonlethal doses of this venom. It was further demonstrated by PHISALIX and BERTRAND (1894a and b), by CALMETTE (1894a) and by FRASER (1895a and b) that the serum of these animals contained a substance that neutralized the venom. Thus the principle of serotherapy as a treatment for envenomation was established and therapeutic antivenoms were prepared in 1894 by CALMETTE and in 1895 by FRASER (a and b).

The properties of the venoms and their seric antidotes were a subject of intensive research in many countries at this time, but soon afterwards controversy arose concerning the therapeutic effects of sera obtained by immunization of horses with the venom of snakes of a single species. CALMETTE (1894a) stated that all snake venoms contained identical toxic substances and that only the relative proportions of these substances were different, depending on the species of the snakes that had produced the venom. This hypothesis was soon disproved, as it was established that the venoms of different species of snakes possess distinct properties: some coagulate the blood (LAMB, 1901; MARTIN, 1905), others inhibit coagulation (CUNNINGHAM, 1895); some disturb the functioning of the nervous centers and others that of the nerve endings (BRUNTON and FAYRER, 1874; ELLIOT, 1900). There are venoms that agglutinate and lyze mammalian erythrocytes (CALMETTE, 1902; STEPHENS, 1900; FLEXNER and NOGUCHI, 1902; NOGUCHI, 1909), while still others behave as proteolytic substances and some arrest an isolated heart in systole (ELLIOT, 1905).

A single venom may show several of these properties but, in general, a group of properties is characteristic of the venom of snakes belonging to the same zoological family. *Elapidae* and *Hydrophiidae* venoms were considered to be neurotoxic and those of *Viperidae* and *Crotalidae* to be hemotoxic and to cause necrosis. Later, however, it was observed that this was not an absolute rule.

Following the previous observations, the hypothesis of the universal nature of the neutralizing ability of the cobra antivenin, as suggested by CALMETTE, was disputed. Most experimenters acknowledged that the symptoms of venom intoxication were inhibited only by an immune serum specific to the venom responsible for the poisoning. They admitted that the effect of the same serum on poisoning produced by another venom was always weak or nonexistent (NOGUCHI, 1904; ARTHUS, 1911a, b). In connection with this, MARTIN wrote in 1904:

Some years ago, I expressed the opinion that all these constituents with the same physiological action, which have been found in different venoms, might indeed be identical ... Recent experiments by CUNNINGHAM, LAMB, TIDSWELL, FLEXNER and NOGUCHI, KYES, ROGERS and myself have, however, led me to the conclusion that many of these constituents from different venoms, even when incapable of being differentiated by their physiological action, can be so differentiated by the inability of antiserum prepared against one venom to combine with the toxin in another venom, or, expressed in terms of EHRLICH's interpretation, that although the "toxophoric" group may be similar, the "haptophor" is generally dissimilar.

B. Snake Venom is a Mosaic of Antigens

Soon, however, the experimenters had to adopt a more general view. The neutralizing power of different antivenom sera was measured on small rodents and it was established that snake venoms from the same family, and sometimes even from different families, contained toxic substances of a very similar nature, the effects of which could be attenuated or even inhibited by a specific immune serum of any of these venoms (HOUSSAY and NEGRETE, 1923).

The literature dealing with these observations is particularly abundant in the period between 1925 and 1961. Only the observations made by KRAUS (1926), MORITSCH (1926), OTTO (1927, 1928, 1929a and b, 1930), SCHLOSSBERGER et al. (1936), GRASSET (1936), TAYLOR and MALLIK (1935, 1936), VELLARD (1938), SCHÖTTLER (1955), and KEEGAN and his co-workers (1961) will be mentioned here. These were recently extended by the publications of MINTON (1967b), TIMMERMAN (1970), TU and SALAFRANCA (1974), MOHAMED et al. (1974), and BOLAÑOS et al. (1975). While on this subject, it is opportune to remember that the toxic effects of the venom of a Colubridae opistoglyphe, *Dispholidus typus*, are inhibited by immune sera specific of *Bitis arietans* (GRASSET and SCHAAFSMA, 1940), of *Echis carinatus* (CHRISTENSEN, 1968) and even of *Bothrops* (GRASSET and SCHAAFSMA, 1940) venoms.

Since experimental conditions vary from one laboratory to another it is difficult to compare all the results mentioned in the literature. It appears, however, from an overall view of the research, that snake venoms may be represented as a "mosaic of antigens," in the picturesque words of NICOLE and RAPHAEL (1925). When one considers the composition of venoms produced by ophidians belonging to the same family, and sometimes even to different families, certain fragments of this mosaic, although not strictly identical, can be seen to have very closely related characteristics (BAXTER and GALLICHIO, 1974). In the light of these observations, it appears that the venoms of *Elapidae* and *Hydrophiidae* contain antigens of similar constitution and that those of *Viperidae* and *Crotalidae* sometimes show resemblances. Venoms of these two groups can generally be distinguished from each other by the immunological properties of their components. However, even though some relationships can be established between toxins produced by snakes of different species, it is apparent that venoms derived from snakes belonging to a single species sometimes have properties, and consequently contain antigens, that vary according to the origin of the selected population. The immune serum obtained from animals immunized with the "neurotoxic" venom of *Crotalus terrificus* captured in South Brazil neutralized this venom specifically but had no effect on the strongly proteolytic venom of the same species from Venezuela (VELLARD, 1930, 1938, 1939). Similar findings have been reported by MINTON (1953, 1957), GONÇALVES (1956a and b), and PICADO (1934). REID (1963, 1964) made several observations concerning the venoms of cobras from Malaysia. While *Naja naja* venom of India was shown to be rich in toxins causing paralysis, *Naja naja* venom from Malaysia produced necrosis on which the usual anticobra serum had no effect. Finally, it was recently reported by KORNALIK and TABORSKA (1973) that individual intraspecies variability was frequent, when for example, the composition of the venoms of *Echis carinatus* and *Vipera russellii* was considered.

During the same period, the *in vivo* and *in vitro* properties of venomous secretions of ophidians had been progressively defined. KELLAWAY (1937) confirmed, by very precise experiments, the initial observations of FAYRER (1868–1869) on the curare-like effects of *Elapidae* venoms. EPSTEIN (1930) and subsequently SARKAR (1948) described the cardiac effects produced by these same venoms. ARTHUS (1919), HOUSSAY and SORDELLI (1919), MCFARLANE and BARNETT (1934), VON KLOBUSITZKY (1935) and EAGLE (1937) accumulated further observations on the presence, in the venoms of *Viperidae* and *Crotalidae*, of factors capable of accelerating or retarding blood coagulation. It was subsequently discovered that snake venoms contain many enzymes. The first experimenter to make this discovery was DELEZENNE, who, in collaboration with LEDEBT defined a phospholipid-hydrolyzing activity (DELEZENNE and LEDEBT 1911a, b).

DELEZENNE and MOREL (1919), ZELLER and MARITZ (1945), ZELLER (1948a and b, 1950), GHOSH (1936), GULLAND and JACKSON (1938a, b), BOMAN and KALETTA (1957), BOMAN (1959), YANG and CHANG (1954), YANG et al. (1959), TABORDA et al. (1952), LASKOWSKI et al. (1957), IYENGAR et al. (1938), CHAUDHURY (1946), CHANG and LEE (1955), and many others, discovered the esterase effects of various venoms: phosphatases, phosphomonoesterases, phosphodiesterases, nucleases, 5′-nucleotidases, and acetylcholinesterases. L-amino-acid-oxidase, amino-ester-hydrolase, and peptidase activities as well as a diffusion factor have been described by ZELLER (1948b), NOC (1904), HOUSSAY and NEGRETE (1918), DEUTSCH and DINIZ (1955), HAMBERG and ROCHA E SILVA (1957), HENRIQUES et al. (1958), and DURAN-REYNALS (1938). All these properties, found by *in vivo* and *in vitro* experimentation, are due to different protein components of venoms which have been disclosed by immunological techniques.

A study of these techniques leads us to consider firstly the results of experiments performed at the end of the last century. In fact, three years after the first observation of BORDET (1899) on the precipitation of the serum of an animal belonging to one species by the serum of an animal belonging to another species treated with injections of the former serum, LAMB (1902, 1904) observed that mixtures of *Naja naja* venom and its specific immune serum also became opaque and precipitated. He showed, however, that there was no relation between the precipitating ability of the immune serum and its antitoxicity. He made the important observation that the precipitating and the antitoxic agents of the serum did not develop at parallel rates during immunization. CALMETTE and MASSOL confirmed this in 1909, and indicated that an excess of antiserum suppressed the precipitation phenomena. After separating the precipitate from a mixture of venom and antivenom, CALMETTE and MASSOL found no toxicity of the insoluble material, but after heating it for one hour at 72° C in a weakly acid solution, they recovered a soluble toxic product which represented almost all the venom added to the immune serum. They concluded that the precipitate was the result of an unstable association of the venom and the antivenom.

Following this, it was shown that several precipitation zones frequently appeared in mixtures of increasing quantities of venom with a constant volume of the corresponding immune serum and *vice versa* (CESARI and BOQUETT, 1936a, b; CHRISTENSEN, 1955a). Having prepared mixtures of *Naja flava* (now called *Nava nivea*) venom and specific immune serum according to this technique, CHRISTENSEN (1953, 1955a) observed three high-precipitation zones. When heated separately at 70° C in an acidic medium (pH 2.0), each precipitate dissociated. The heat labile immune serum was destroyed and three heat stabile components, toxic for mice, were liberated. They were termed α, β, and γ toxins. By this method CHRISTENSEN demonstrated that a single venom might contain more than one toxic component. In a later series of similar experiments (CHRISTENSEN and ANDERSON, 1967), he produced evidence for the presence of a common fraction of low toxicity in the venoms of three *Dendroaspis* species: *angusticeps*, *jamesoni*, and *polylepis*. He also concluded that the dominant toxins of *Dendroaspis jamesoni* and *Dendroaspis polylepis* venoms have common antigenic structures but are not identical and differ immunologically from that of *Dendroaspis angusticeps* venom.

Knowledge of the great number of antigenic components in snake venoms and their differences and similarities depending on their origin was confirmed and widened by the use of immunological analysis involving the mutual precipitation of antigens and antibodies in a gel, as in the method developed by OUDIN (1948) and OUCHTERLONY (1948), or by the method of GRABAR and WILLIAMS (1955), and by other techniques based on the results of electrophoretic separation of proteins in a mixture, followed by precipitation of each separated protein by its specific antibody. The serum chosen for this immunochemical analysis is sometimes the specific immune serum to the venom to be studied, and sometimes a specific immune serum to another venom. In this case, antigens of very closely related composition in two different venoms are revealed by the phenomenon of crossed precipitation.

The use of one immune serum and a series of samples of venoms from different origins leads to the disclosure of components of comparable composition and sometimes to a hierarchy of these components according to their degree of immunological reactivity.

By these classic methods, numerous antigens have been described in snake venoms. It is difficult, however, to compare the results of experiments performed in widely differing conditions. Each antigen contained in a venom forms, with its specific antibodies, a precipitating system which demonstrates the presence of this antigen. Animals of different species, and even animals belonging to the same species, produce immune sera whose populations of antibodies are in proportions that vary from one immune serum to another. Incidentally, the nature and specificity of these antibodies differ according to the species they come from and the procedure of immunization. PIANTANIDA and MUIC (1954) using OUDIN's technique, defined three antigenic compounds in the venom of *Vipera ammodytes*. Precipitation of the same venom in a gel medium, by the method of OUCHTERLONY, results in definition of twelve components (AJDUKOVIC and MUIC, 1963). Lastly, immunoelectrophoresis analysis shows up eighteen components, of which eleven are positively charged and seven negatively (SKVARIL and TYKAL, 1961).

GRASSET et al. (1956), using OUCHTERLONY'S technique, established that the venoms of *Vipera aspis* and *Vipera ammodytes* contained common antigens. They also showed the existence of similar antigens in the venoms of *Vipera ammodytes*, *Vipera russellii*, *Bitis arietans*, *Bitis gabonica* (*Viperidae*), *Agkistrodon rhodostoma* and *Bothrops jararaca* (*Crotalidae*). Finally, they demonstrated the existence of a common population of antigens in the venoms of *Naja naja*, *Naja flava* (nowadays *Naja nivea*), *Bungarus fasciatus*, and *Sepedon* (actually *Hemachatus haemachatus*), all of which belong to the *Elapidae*.By contrast, the experimenters discovered that no immunological resemblance could be established between the components of venoms of *Naja naja*, *Dendroaspis angusticeps* (*Elapidae*), and *Crotalus terrificus* (*Crotalidae*).

KULKARNI and RAO (1956), studying the antigenic composition of four venoms from *Elapidae* and *Viperidae* by OUDIN'S method, determined the number of antigenic components in each venom, using four different antivenoms as precipitating reagents. They observed that several components are common to two, and sometimes even to three, of the venoms. The results of this experiment are shown in Table 1.

Thus, it is shown that two venoms of the *Elapidae* and two venoms of the *Viperidae* contain antigens of a closely related nature. But the two groups of venoms are distinguishable from each other by their immunological properties. LATIFI et al. (1973) reported, however, that an immune serum, anti-*Naja naja oxiana* venom, precipitated specifically fourteen antigens of this venom, and four to six components of venoms from *Echis carinatus*, *Vipera latifii*, *Vipera lebetina*, *Pseudocerastes persicus*, and *Agkistrodon halys*. In contrast, they observed that an immune serum against *Agkistrodon halys* venom shows up the presence of thirteen components in this venom, but only two in the venom of *Naja naja oxiana*.

TU and GANTHAVORN (1968) established that the diagrams defined by immunoelectrophoresis of the venoms from two Asian *Elapidae*, *Naja naja siamensis*, and *Naja naja atra* are very closely related when one uses an immune serum, anti *Naja naja siamensis* venom, as an agent for revealing them. This same serum, which precipitates ten components of the venom of *Naja naja siamensis*, precipitates only two in the venom of *Bungarus fasciatus* and only a single component in the venom of *Naja naja hanah* (PURANANANDA et al., 1966).

Strong cross-immunological reactions between the antigens of different South American *Micrurus* venoms were observed by COHEN et al. (1971). However, according to BARRIO and MIRANDA (1966), the composition of venoms from different subspecies of *Micrurus frontalis* differs slightly but much more considerable variations occur in venoms from representatives of the diverse subspecies of *Micrurus corallinus*.

Rattlesnake venoms have certain common characteristics. Three antigens of the same type are present in the venoms of *Crotalus atrox*, *Crotalus ruber*, *Crotalus molossus*, *Crotalus scutulatus*, and *Sistrurus miliarus*. These same venoms, and those of *Agkistrodon*, contain one, and sometimes several, similar antigenic components (MINTON, 1957). TU and ADAMS (1968) observed, however, that the composition of *Agkistrodon* venoms varies considerably according to whether the snakes are Asiatic or American in origin.

A particular observation by MINTON (1967a) warrants attention: the antigenic composition of venoms from young and adult snakes differs, and the number of antigens increases during the first year after the birth of the animals.

Table 1. Antigenic Composition of four Indian snake venoms

Venoms of:		Antivenom: (Number of rings obtained by Oudin's technique)			
		N. naja	*B. coeruleus*	*V. russellii*	*E. carinatus*
Elapidae	*N. naja*	*10*	3	1 (light)	0
	B. coeruleus	2	*9*	0	0
Viperidae	*V. russellii*	1 (light)	0	*9*	4
	E. carinatus	0	0	5	*14*

(According to KULKARNI and RAO, 1956)

In a series of very precise experiments performed according to the method of Ouchterlony, SCHENBERG (1961) demonstrated the presence of more than 30 antigens in the venoms of different populations of *Bothrops jararaca* from Brazil. More than 50 varieties of the same venom were differentiated according to the distribution of the antigens in each sample analyzed. Later, SCHENBERG (1963) studied the venoms of the subspecies of *Bothrops neuwiedi* and divided them into five main groups on the basis of their antigenic composition. He noticed that the venom extracted from snakes of the same zoological subspecies could belong to any of these antigenic groups. It thus appeared that no relationship could be established between the morphological characterization of these snakes and the composition of their venom. However, immunological techniques sometimes provide important information to zoologists. Thus, a member of the *Viperidae* from Africa, *Atractaspis microlepidota* resembles the *Elapidae* in some aspects. On this subject, MINTON (1968) has reported that the venom of this snake is precipitated by numerous immune sera specific to venoms of the *Elapidae* and by the only serum anti-*Echis* venom prepared by the Razi Institute (Iran) among all the immune sera used in this trial. The results tend to support the opinion that *Atractaspis microlepidota* is not a viperid, or not a typical viperid. However, a potent immune serum specific to *Naja* venom was unable to protect mice against the toxic effect of this venom. *Causus rhombeatus*, another of the *Viperidae* from Africa, has sometimes been compared with *Atractaspis*. MINTON (1968) has considered that the presence of more precipitin lines formed by the venom of this snake with viperid antisera than with elapid and crotalid antisera supports the keeping of the genus in the *Viperidae*. By the gel diffusion precipitation technique no antigenic relationship could be established between *Causus* and *Atractaspis* venoms. Finally, CHRISTENSEN (1955a) reported that *Causus* venom is neutralized by an antiviperid immune serum, the *Bitis* antivenom.

Taking these results as a whole, they confirm the early observations made in animal experiments on the effect of antivenoms on venoms and from the examination of anti-enzymatic properties of antivenoms *in vitro* (CESARI and BOQUET, 1935, 1936a and b, 1937). Although the application of the technique of precipitation in gel medium allowed, on a single preparation, the numbering of antigen components of the venoms and the collection of information on the existence of proteins of similar make-up in these venoms, it did not lead to the recognition of a relationship between the enumerated antigens and the physiological properties of the corresponding proteins. It is this problem we have attempted to resolve.

Our experiments consisted of extracting the principal components of *Naja nigricollis* venom (Ethiopia), of studying their physiological properties, and of defining the position of the precipitate they formed in the diagrams obtained by immunoelectrophoresis (DETRAIT and BOQUET, 1958; DETRAIT et al., 1959; BOQUET et al., 1967).

For many years, biochemists have tried to isolate the toxic components of snake venoms. The reader should refer to the chapter devoted to this subject for more detailed information. Here, however, we shall mention the works of MICHEEL and JUNG (1936), SLOTTA (1938), GHOSH and DE (1938), GONÇALVES (1956a), and SASAKI (1957), who were the original researchers in this field. In 1960–1962, CAREY and WRIGHT, using the technique of chromatography on CM cellulose, isolated a basic protein from the venom of *Enhydrina schistosa*, which was considered to be toxic to the nervous system. Only one band of precipitation was observed when this toxin was subjected to immunoelectrophoretic analysis. Shortly afterwards, CHANG and LEE (1963) described three toxins in the venom of *Bungarus multicinctus*, which they called α, β, and γ "bungarotoxins." The α bungarotoxin alters the mechanism of transmission of the nerve impulse at neuromuscular junctions in the same way as does D-tubocurarine, which competes with acetylcholine for the cholinergic receptor. The β and γ "bungarotoxins" have a presynaptic site of action. YANG (1965b) and YANG et al. (1969) later defined the biochemical characteristics of the cobrotoxin from *Naja naja atra* venom.

We owe the discovery of the two erabutoxins a and b and of the laticotoxin from *Laticauda semifasciata* and *Laticauda laticaudata* venoms to TAMIYA and ARAI (1966) and TAMIYA and SATO (1967). The molecular weights of these basic proteins are in the region of 6800 and the 62 amino acids of which they are made up are arranged in a single chain, cross-linked by four disulfide bridges. By this time the present author and his co-workers had extracted a basic protein from *Naja nigricollis* (Ethiopia) venom, by electrophoresis and by successive filtrations of the venom on dextran gels (DETRAIT et al., 1959; BOQUET et al., 1966a and b). This protein was a curare-like substance (TAZIEFF-DEPIERRE and PIERRE, 1966). Its molecular weight was low, as its sedimentation constant was 0.87. The group named it α toxin after defining its immunological characteristics. This toxin, however, contained a few impurities, detected by precipitation according to the technique of GRABAR and WILLIAMS (1955). KARLSSON et al. (1966) isolated this α toxin in a pure state, established its chemical composition, and determined its molecular weight, which was 6786. Then, EAKER and PORATH (1967) defined the sequence of its 61 amino acid residues.

Having separated the fractions containing toxins and enzymes by filtration of the venom from *Naja nigricollis* (Ethiopia) on Sephadex, the present author's group then defined the respective positions of these antigens, on the diagram obtained by immunoelectrophoresis of this venom, using the methods of HEREMANS (1960) and URIEL and coworkers (URIEL and SCHEIDEGGER, 1955; URIEL and COURCON, 1961; URIEL and AVRAMEAS, 1964) (Fig. 1). From then, it was possible to follows the progress of the operation of purification of an antigen by immunochemical analysis.

Since the α antigen of *Naja nigricollis* (Ethiopia) venom was known, the aim was to establish the presence of substances with related antigenic activity in different snake venoms (BOQUET et al., 1969). The method used was based on the principle of identification of proteins by the technique of precipitation in a gel according to the method of OUCHTERLONY, on that of HEREMANS and on the results of experiments on

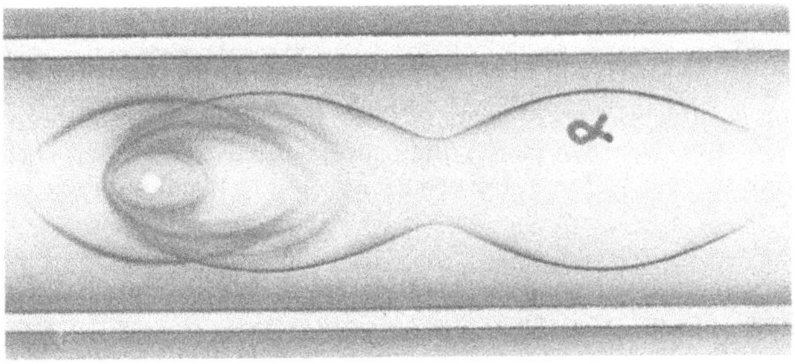

Fig. 1. Determination of α toxin by HEREMAN's technique in the immunoelectrophoretic pattern of *Naja nigricollis* (Ethiopia) venom. The precipitating serum is a reference horse immune serum anti-*Naja nigricollis* (Ethiopia) venom

exhaustion of anti-α-antibodies of a reference immune serum by samples of venoms of different origin. It was established that the venomous secretions of *Naja haje*, *Naja melanoleuca*, *Naja nivea*, *Hemachatus haemachatus* from Africa, *Naja naja oxiana* from Asia and *Naja naja philippinensis* from the Philippines islands contained an antigen which was analogous to the α protein of *Naja nigricollis* venom (Ethiopia). The presence of such a protein in *Naja haje* venom was soon confirmed by BOTES and STRYDOM (1969), who compared the composition and the primary structure of the two toxins which are chemically related. In collaboration with TAMIYA (unpubl.) it was later demonstrated that erabutoxin a was analogous to the α protein of *Naja nigricollis* (Ethiopia) venom. Finally, after the methods of separating proteins by chromatography were perfected, many constituents were extracted from snake venoms.

Owing to the relevance of these substances for the development of immunological research, although only a small number of them have been studied with regard to their antigenicity, a list of the principal ones is given in Table 2.

It seems useful to add a paragraph concerning *Echis carinatus* venom. The study made on the distribution of antigens comparable to the α toxin of *Naja nigricollis* (Ethiopia) in different venoms of the *Elapidae*, led us to a similar search for proteins of the same nature in various venoms of the *Viperidae*. None of these venoms, with exception of *Echis carinatus* from Ethiopia, contained an antigen homologous to the α toxin. The presence of a component of *Echis carinatus* venom which could be precipitated by specific anti-α-antibodies led us to propose several hypothesis. Was the component the result of an accidental mixing of *Naja* and *Echis* venoms? Was it alternatively a protein normally present in *Echis* venom? No conclusion could be drawn from the observations. The extraction, by DELORI from the same sample (unpubl., 1969) of a protein possessing the chemical characteristics of α toxin and the results of the quantitative precipitation of this protein and of the α toxin (DELORI and RONSSERAY, unpubl., 1969) by the immune serum antivenom of *Naja nigricollis* (Ethiopia) proved that the *Echis* venom had been contamined by *Naja nigricollis* (Ethiopia) venom during the course of its extraction. Subsequently, the examination of two samples of *Echis* venom, from South Africa and India, confirmed the absence of a component comparable to the curarizing α toxin. Pending more information, the *Viperidae* venoms examined were considered to contain no antigen comparable to

Table 2. Antigens isolated from snake venoms

I. Toxins reacting at the postsynaptic site of the motor endplate (curare-like toxins).

The physiopathological properties of some of these toxins have not yet been studied on nerve muscle preparations, however their paralyzing properties *in vivo* and their chemical composition and structure led to their inclusion in the group. All bind to the cholinergic receptor.

a) *Elapidae venoms:*

Toxins consisting of 60—62 amino acid residues in a single chain cross-linked by 4 disulfide bridges (Fig. 2a)

1. *Naja nivea*
   β (BOTES, 1970, 1971)
   δ (BOTES et al., 1971a and b)
2. *Naja haje (haje)*
   II (KOPEYAN et al., 1973)
   Naja haje (annulifera)
   α (BOTES and STRYDOM, 1969)
   CM 10, CM 12, CM 14 (JOUBERT, 1975c)
3. *N. melanoleuca*
   d (BOTES, 1972); F_7 (POILLEUX and BOQUET, 1972; BERGEOT-POILLEUX and BOQUET, 1975); 3.11 (SHIPOLINI et al., 1975)
4. *N. nigricollis* (Ethiopia)
   α (BOQUET et al., 1966a, b; KARLSSON et al., 1966); I, II, III (ROCHAT et al., 1974)
5. *Hemachatus haemachatus*
   II (STRYDOM and BOTES, 1971)
   IV (STRYDOM and BOTES, 1971)
6. *N. naja atra*
   Cobrotoxin (YANG et al., 1969) (Fig. 2a)
7. *N. naja philippinensis*
   I (HAUERT et al., 1974)
8. *Naja naja oxiana*
   I and II (GRISHIN et al., 1973, 1974b)
   α (ARNBERG et al., 1974)
9. *Dendroaspis viridis*
   4.11.3 (SHIPOLINI et al., 1973, 1974; BANKS et al., 1974)

Toxins consisting of 71—74 amino acid residues in a single chain cross-linked by 5 disulfide bridges (Fig. 2b)

1. *Bungarus multicinctus*
   α Bungarotoxin (CHANG and LEE, 1963; MEBS et al., 1971)
2. *N. naja siamensis*
   3 (KARLSSON et al., 1971)
3. *N. naja kaouthia* (India)
   (KARLSSON et al., 1971)
4. *N. naja naja* (India)
   T_3 (KARLSSON et al., 1971)
   N. naja naja (Pakistan)
   (KARLSSON et al., 1971)
5. *Naja naja* (India)
   A (NAKAI et al., 1971)
   B (OHTA and HAYASHI, 1974)
6. *N. naja oxiana*
   (GRISHIN et al., 1974b)
7. *Naja nivea*
   α (BOTES, 1971) (Fig. 2b)
8. *N. melanoleuca*
   b (BOTES, 1972); F_6 (POILLEUX and BOQUET, 1972); BERGEOT-POILLEUX and BOQUET, 1975); 3.9.4. (SHIPOLINI et al., 1975); F_5 (BERGEOT-POILLEUX and BOQUET, 1975)
9. *Naja haje*
   III (MIRANDA et al., 1970; KOPEYAN et al., 1973, 1975)
10. *Dendroaspis polylepis polylepis*
    γ (STRYDOM, 1972b)
11. *Dendroaspis viridis*
    4.7.3. and 4.9.3. (SHIPOLINI et al., 1973)
    I and V (BECHIS et al., 1976)
12. *Ophiophagus hannah*
    A and B (JOUBERT, 1973)
13. *Bungarus caeruleus*
    I-B-2 and I-C (MEBS et al., 1974; LEE et al., 1976)

Table 2 (continued)

b) *Hydrophiidae venoms:*

Toxins consisting of 55—62 amino acid residues in a single chain cross-linked by 4 disulfide bridges

1. *Laticauda semifasciata*
   Erabutoxins a and b (TAMIYA and ARAI, 1966); Erabutoxin c (TAMIYA and ABE, 1972)
2. *Laticauda laticaudata*
   Laticotoxins a and b (SATO et al., 1969)
3. *Enhydrina schistosa*
   (TU and TOOM, 1971) Fract. 4 and 5 (KARLSSON et al., 1972a)
4. *Lapemis hardwickii*
   (TU and HONG, 1971)
5. *Pelamis platurus*
   (TU et al., 1975) Pelamitoxin (LIU et al., 1975)
6. *Aipysurus laevis*
   a, b, c (MAEDA and TAMIYA, 1976)
7. *Hydrophis cyanocinctus*, „Hydrophitoxin" a and b (LIU et al., 1973; LIU and BLACKWELL, 1974), amino acid composition very close to that of fractions 4 and 5 of *E. schistosa*

Toxins consisting of 66 amino acid residues in a single chain cross-linked by 5 disulfide bridges

1. *Laticauda semifasciata*
   LS III (MAEDA et al., 1974). Week affinity for the cholinergic receptor

II. Toxins of which the mechanism of action is not yet entirely elucidated

Some might act like curare($^{+}$). Others have no effect on neutromuscular transmission($^{++}$). Still others act apparently like cardiotoxins but their mode of action is probably different($^{+++}$).

Elapidae venoms:

Toxins consisting of 59 amino acid residues or more in a single chain crosslinked by 4 or 5 disulfide bridges

1. *Dendroaspis polylepis*
   a^{+} (STRYDOM, 1972b) Viz (STRYDOM, 1977)
2. *Dendroaspis jamesoni*
   VN^{I}I^{+} and VN$'''$I^{+} (STRYDOM, A. J. C., 1973)
3. *Dendroaspis angusticeps*
   Ta 1 (ex VII); Ta 2 (VILJOEN and BOTES, 1973, 1974)
4. *Dendroaspis viridis*
   4.9.6. (SHIPOLINI and BANKS, 1974)
5. *Naja melanoleuca*
   3.20^{++} (SHIPOLINI et al., 1975)

A fraction $S_4 C_{II}$, extracted from *Naja melanoleuca* venom by CARLSSON (1975), consists of a single chain of 65 aminoacids cross-linked by 5 disulfide bridges. Its toxicity is very low and it is not yet known whether it reacts with the cholinergic receptor

6. *Bungarus fasciatus*
   VI A, 77 amino acid residues, mol W 9700 $^{+++}$
   VI B, 124 amino acid residues, mol W 13652 $^{+++}$
   (LIN SHIAN et al., 1975)

Table 2 (continued)

7. We shall quote here a toxin of which the chemical constitution is under study. It blocks the neuro-muscular transmission without binding to the cholinergic receptors: *Bungarus coeruleus* ceruleotoxin, acidic protein, M. W. 38000 (BON and CHANGEUX, 1975) — Has phospholipase activity.

III. Toxins acting on the cell-membranes: depolarizing agents, direct lytic factors, cardiotoxins, cytotoxins, cobramines.

Elapidae venoms:

They consist of about 60 amino acid residues in one chain crosslinked by 4 disulfide bridges:

1. *Naja naja atra* Cardiotoxin (NARITA and LEE, 1970); Cardiotoxin analog I (HAYASHI et al., 1975); Cardiotoxin analogs II and IV (KANEDA et al., 1977)
2. *Naja naja* Cytotoxin (BRAGANCA et al., 1967); Cytotoxin I (ex XI) (HAYASHI et al., 1971); Cytotoxin II (ex XII) (TAKECHI et al., 1973; IWAGUCHI et al., 1974); Cardiotoxin F_8 (FRYKLUND and EAKER, 1975a); „Cobramines“ A and B (LARSEN and WOLFF, 1968)
3. *Naja naja oxiana.* Cytotoxin (GRISHIN et al., 1974)
4. *Naja nigricollis* (Ethiopia). γ and 14 and *Naja mossambica pallida* γ (IZARD et al., 1969); (FRYKLUND and EAKER, 1975b)
5. *Naja mossambica mossambica.* Cytotoxins $V^{II}1$, $V^{II}2$, $V^{II}3$, $V^{II}4$ (LOUW, 1974a, b)
6. *Naja haje annulifera.* Cytotoxins $V^{II}1$, $V^{II}2$, $V^{II}2A$, CM_8, CM_{11}, CM_{13a}, CM 2_c, CM_{4a}, CM_7 (WEISE et al., 1973; JOUBERT, 1976a–b)
7. *Hemachatus haemachatus.* 12B (D.L.F.) (ALOOF-HIRSH et al., 1968; FRYKLUND and EAKER, 1973)
8. *Naja melanoleuca.* Cardiotoxins $V^{II}1$, $V^{II}2$, $V^{II}3$ (CARLSSON, 1974; CARLSSON and JOUBERT, 1974)
9. *Naja nivea.* Cytotoxins $V^{II}1$, $V^{II}2$, $V^{II}3$ (BOTES and VILJOEN, 1976)

IV. Toxins acting at the presynaptic site of motor nerve endings.

All are proteins of various chemical compositions and molecular weights.

a) *Elapidae venoms:*
   Bungarus multicinctus.
   β-Bungarotoxin: 180 amino acid residues, mol wt approx. 22000 has phospholipase activity) (CHANG and LEE, 1963; LEE et al., 1972; KELLY and BROWN, 1974)
   Bungarus caeruleus
   III—A and III—B more than 100 amino acid residues (MEBS et al., 1974; LEE et al., 1976)
   Notechi scutatus
   Notexin: 119 amino acid residues, 14 half-cystines; mol wt 13600 (has a phospholipase A_2 activity) (KARLSSON et al., 1972c); EAKER et al., 1974; HALPERT and EAKER, 1975); FOHLMAN et al., 1976)
   Oxyuranurus scutellatus
   Taipoxin: consisting of α, β and γ subunits (KAMENSKAYA and THESLEFF, 1974; EAKER et al., 1974)
   Naja nigricollis (Ethiopia)
   Basic phospholipase; 118 aminoacid residues, 14 half-cystines (EAKER et al., 1974; DUMAREY et al., 1975; BENOIT, unpubl.)
b) *Crotalidae venoms:*
   Crotalus durissus terrificus:
   Crotoxin (basic phospholipase A+ "Crotapotin"), (SLOTTA, 1938; FRAENKEL-CONRAT and SINGER, 1956; HABERMANN and RÜBSAMEN, 1971; Vital BRAZIL, 1972).

V. Toxic proteins whose mechanism of action is unknown
   Some act on the mechanism of muscle concentration$^+$.

a) *Viperidae venoms:*
   1. *Vipera palestinae*
      Viperotoxin, 108 amino acid residues, 6 half-cystines (MOROZ et al., 1965, 1966a and c)

Table 2 (continued)

2. *Vipera ammodytes*
Fraction F, basic (SKET et al., 1973). Fraction 4 and 5, mol wt 18600 and 22900 (SHIPOLINI et al., 1965; ALEKSIEV and SHIPOLINI, 1971)
3. *Vipera berus*
P_4: basic phospholipase (DELORI, 1971, 1973)
4. *Vipera russellii*
Toxic fraction (?) (DIMITROV and KANKONKAR, 1968)

b) *Crotalidae venoms:*
1. *Crotalus durissus terrificus*
Crotamin$^+$ amino acid residues, 6 half-cystines (GONÇALVES, 1965a and b; LAURE, 1975)
Convulxin (PRADO FRANCESCHI and VITAL BRAZIL, quoted by VITAL BRAZIL, 1972)
2. *Crotalus adamanteus*
Basic protein of Crotamin$^+$-type (BONILLA et al., 1971; LEE et al., 1973)
3. *Crotalus horridus horridus*
Basic protein of Crotamin$^+$-type (BONILLA et al., 1971; LEE et al., 1973)
4. *Crotalus viridis viridis*
Basic protein of Crotamin$^+$-type (BONILLA et al., 1971; LEE et al., 1973)
5. *Crotalus viridis helleri*
Peptide I. Peptide II (DUBNOFF and RUSSELL, 1970)

VI. Enzymes

A. *Phospholipases A_2* (phosphatidyl-acyl-hydrolases)
The amino acid sequences of a number of these phospholipases have been recently determined.

a) *Elapidae venoms:*
1. *Naja naja*
Several isoenzymes, mol wt 8500 to 20000 (SALACH et al., 1968, 1971; SHILOAH et al., 1973). One phospholipase A_2: 102 amino acid residues, II half-cystines, acidic protein (DEEMS and DENNIS, 1975)
2. *Naja naja atra*
One phospholipase A_2 mol wt 13000 (LO and CHANG, 1974). Fractions A_1 and A_2 (WAKUI and KAWAUCHI, 1961)
3. *Naja melanoleuca*
DE_I, 118 amino acid residues, 14 half-cystines, basic protein. DE_{II}, 119 amino acid residues, 14 half-cysteines, acidic protein. DE_{III}, 119 amino acid residues, 14 half-cystines, acidic protein. Mol wt of the 3 proteins 13000 (JOUBERT, 1975a)
4. *Naja nigricollis* (Ethiopia)
A_I and X, 118—121 amino acid residues, 14 half-cystines, basic protein (WAHLSTRÖM, 1971; EAKER et al., 1974; DUMAREY et al., 1975). I, Acidic protein (WAHLSTRÖM, 1971; DUMAREY and BOQUET, unpubl.)
5. *Naja mossambica mossambica*
CM_I, CM_{II}, CM_{III} (JOUBERT, 1977)
6. *Hemachatus haemachatus*
Phospholipase A (JOUBERT, 1975b)
7. *Pseudechis porphyriacus*
Fraction X_2 (DOERY and PEARSON, 1961)

b) *Hydrophiidae venoms:*
1. *Laticauda semifasciata*
Acidic phospholipase, 108 amino acid residues, 12 half-cystines, mol wt 11000 (TU et al., 1970; TU and PASSEY, 1971)
2. *Enhydrina schistosa*
Frachon VI:5, a phospholipase producing myoglobinuria (FOHLMAN and EAKER, 1977)

Table 2 (continued)

c) *Viperidae venoms:*

1. *Vipera berus*
   P_1, acidic protein mol wt 30800. P_2, acidic protein mol wt 28700. P_3, acidic protein mol wt about 11000. P_4 basic protein, 91 amino acid residues, 10 half-cysteines (toxic protein) mol wt 10300 (DELORI, 1971; 1973)
2. *Bitis arietans*
   Phospholipase A_2, 117 amino acid residues, 14 half-cystines, mol wt 14000 (HOWARD, 1975)
3. *Bitis gabonica*
   Phospholipase A_2, 118 amino acid residues, 12 half-cystines. Mol wt 14000 (BOTES and VILJOEN, 1974)
4. *Vipera palestinae*
   Several isoenzymes (SHILOAH et al., 1970)
5. *Vipera russellii*
   Several isoenzymes (SALACH et al., 1971)

d) *Crotalidae venoms:*

1. *Agkistrodon piscivorus*
   Phospholipase A_2, basic protein, mol wt 14000 (AUGUSTYN and ELLIOTT, 1970)
2. *Agkistrodon halys blomhoffii*
   A_2 II, 126 amino acid residues, 14 half-cystines, acidic protein, mol wt 13700 (KAWAUCHI et al., 1971; SAMEJIMA et al., 1974; A_2 I, 126 amino-acid residues, 14 half-cystines, basic protein, mol wt 13800 (KAWAUCHI et al., 1971)
3. *Crotalus adamanteus*
   I and II (SAITO and HANAHAN, 1962). A α and A β, mol wt 29800 (dimer) (WELLS and HANAHAN, 1969). A_2, 123 amino acid residues, 14 half-cystines, mol wt 14000 (TSAO et al., 1975), A2α, 122 amino acid residues, 14 half-cystines (HEINRIKSON et al., 1977)
4. *Crotalus atrox*
   One phospholipase A_2, 280 amino acid residues, 28 half-cystines, mol wt 29500 (dimer) (WU and TINKER, 1969; HACHIMORI et al., 1971; COLES et al., 1974)
5. *Crotalus durissus terrificus*
   Phospholipase A_2, basic protein (HORST et al., 1972). Fraction VI, 140 amino acid residues, 16 half-cystines, mol wt 16200, (toxic protein) (HABERMANN and RÜBSAMEN, 1971; OMORI-SATOH et al., 1975)
6. *Bothrops neuwiedii*
   P_1 and P_2 (VIDAL and STOPPANI, 1968, 1971a; VIDAL et al., 1972)
7. *Bothrops jararaca*
   2 phospholipases A_2 (VIDAL and STOPPANI, 1971a)
8. *Bothrops jararacussu*
   2 phospholipases A_2 (VIDAL and STOPPANI, 1971a)
9. *Bothrops atrox*
   2 phospholipases A_2 (VIDAL and STOPPANI, 1971a)

B. *Acetylcholine esterases* (acetylcholine acyl-hydrolases)

Elapidae venoms:

1. *Naja naja*
   Acetylcholine-esterase (MASSARO et al., 1971)
2. *Bungarus fasciatus*
   Acetylcholine-esterase, mol wt 130000 (probably formed by 2 subunits of 62700) (KUMAR and ELLIOT, 1973)
3. *Hemachatus haemachatus*
   Acetylcholine esterase (BJÖRK, 1961)

Table 2 (continued)

C. *Phosphatases, 5′-nucleotidases, ADPases, phosphoesterases, endonucleases, nucleosidases* (Phosphoric monoester hydrolases, diphosphonucleotide hydrolases, phosphoric-diester hydrolases, NAD glyco hydrolases). Only a very few of these enzymes have been obtained in a pure state. Their chemical composition is unknown. Some of the enzymes quoted in this table are probably still impure fractions.

a) *Elapidae venoms:*
   Hemachatus haemachatus
   5′-nucleotidase (BJÖRK, 1961)
b) *Viperidae venoms:*
   1. *Bitis arietans*
      ADPase (SCHENBERG et al., 1974)
   2. *Bitis gabonica*
      ADPase (SCHENBERG et al., 1974)
c) *Crotalidae venoms:*
   1. *Bothrops atrox*
      Alkaline phosphatase (SULKOWSKI et al., 1963). Endonuclease (GEORGATSOS and LASKOWSKI, 1962). Phosphodiesterase (exonuclease) (FELIX et al., 1960), (FRISCHAUF and ECKSTEIN, 1973). 5′-nucleotidase (SULKOWSKI et al., 1963; see also GULLAND and JACKSON, 1938a and b)
   2. *Crotalus adamanteus*
      Phosphodiesterase (exonuclease) (RICHARDS et al., 1967; SULKOWSKI and LASKOWSKI, 1974; TATSUKI et al., 1975)
   3. *Agkistrodon halys blomhoffii*
      Phosphodiesterase (exonuclease) (TATSUKI et al., 1975). Nucleotidase (TATSUKI et al., 1975)

D. *Oxidoreductases: aminoacid oxidases*
a) *Viperidae venoms:*
   Vipera palestinae
   L-amino acid oxidase, mol wt about 130000 (SHAHAM et al., 1973)
b) *Crotalidae venoms:*
   1. *Agkistrodon piscivorus*
      L-amino-acid oxidase (SINGER and KEARNEY, 1950)
   2. *Crotalus adamanteus*
      L-aminoacid oxidase, mol wt 130000—140000; protein consisting of 2 subunits of mol wt 70000 (WELLNER and MEISTER, 1960; DE KOK and RAWITCH, 1969)

E. *Aminoacid ester hydrolases*
a) *Viperidae venoms:*
   Echis coloratus
   Arginine ester hydrolase, bradykinin releasing factor (COHEN et al., 1969)
b) *Crotalidae venoms:*
   1. *Crotalus adamanteus*
      Arginine ester hydrolase, thrombin-like enzyme (MARKLAND and DAMUS, 1971)
   2. *Bothrops atrox*
      Thrombin-like enzyme (Reptilase) (STOKES, quoted by EGBERG et al., 1971)
   3. *Bothrops jararaca*
      Bradykinin releasing factor (HENRIQUES et al., 1966). Thrombin like enzyme (BLOMBÄCK et al., 1957)
   4. *Agkistrodon halys blomhoffii*
      Three arginine ester hydrolases: a) bradykinin-releasing enzyme; b) thrombin-like enzyme, and c) an arginine ester hydrolase different from the two other enzymes (SATO et al., 1965)

Table 2 (continued)

5. *Agkistrodon contortrix*
Arginine ester hydrolase, basic protein, mol wt 30000 (TOOM et al., 1970)
6. *Agkistrodon rhodostoma*
A thrombin-like enzyme (SOH and CHAN, 1974); A thrombin-like enzyme (Arvin, Ancrod) mol wt 55000 (ESNOUF and TUNNAH, 1967; COLLINS and JONES, 1972)
7. *Agkistrodon acutus*
Thrombin-like, arginine ester-hydrolase, 193 amino acid residues, 13 half-cystines, mol wt 33500 (CHENG and OUYANG, 1967; OUYANG et al., 1971)

F. *Peptidases (endopeptidases)*

a) *Viperidae venoms; Vipera russellii* Factor X converting enzyme (FURUKAWA et al., 1976)
b) *Crotalidae venoms:*
1. *Crotalus atrox*
α, β and γ proteinases (PFLEIDERER and SUMYK, 1961). α proteinase, mol wt 23000 (ZWILLING and PFLEIDERER, 1967). Two proteinases whose composition is not known were isolated by MEBS (1968). It is possible that they correspond to two of the proteinases described by PFLEIDERER and SUMYK (1961).
2. *Bothrops jararaca*
Protease A (HENRIQUES et al., 1966). HF 2 (also a hemorrhagic factor), mol wt 49700 (MANDELBAUM et al., 1974)
3. *Agkistrodon halys blomhoffii*
A, B, and C proteinases (MURATA et al., 1963). B proteinase (or HR II) (also has hemorrhagic activity (IWANAGA et al., 1965), mol wt 95000 (OSHIMA et al., 1968)
4. *Agkistrodon rhodostoma*
Caseinolytic enzyme (SOH and CHAN, 1974)
5. *Trimeresurus flavoviridis*
H_2 proteinase, mol wt 24000 (TAKAHASHI and OHSAKA, 1970a and b)

VII. Enzyme inhibitors

A. *Peptidase and proteinase inhibitors (Fig. 3)*

a) *Elapidae venoms:*
Dendroapis polylepis. Fractions I and K, 60 amino acid residues, 6 half-cystines (STRYDOM, 1973c). These fractions have low proteinase inhibitory activity but they are toxic.
b) *Viperidae venoms:*
1. *Vipera russellii*
Inhibitor I, 52 amino acid residues, 4 half-cystines, mol wt 6300. Inhibitor II, 60 amino acid residues, 6 half-cystines, mol wt 7000 (TAKAHASHI et al., 1972, 1974a—c)
2. *Hemachatus haemachatus*
Inhibitor II, 57 amino acid residues, 6 half-cystines (TAKAHASHI et al., 1974b)
c) *Crotalidae venoms:*
1. *Bothrops jararaca*
A family of low-molecular-weight bradykinin potentiators (peptidase inhibitors) (FERREIRA et al., 1970)
2. *Agkistrodon halys blomhoffii*
Bradykinin potentiators B and C (peptidase inhibitors), 11 amino acid residues, no cystine but a high proline content (KATO and SUZUKI, 1971)

B. *Phospholipase A inhibitor*
Crotalidae venom:
Bothrops neuwiedii. Phospholipase inhibitor (VIDAL and STOPPANI, 1971b)

VIII. Hemorrhagic factors

a) *Viperidae venoms:*
Vipera palestinae. Acidic protein, mol wt 44000 (GROTTO et al., 1967)
b) *Crotalidae venoms:*
1. *Agkistrodon halys blomhoffii*
HR_1, acidic protein, mol wt 80000 (OSHIMA et al., 1972)

Table 2 (continued)

2. *Trimeresurus flavoviridis*
   HR1, acidic protein, mol wt about 100000 (OMORI-SATOH and OHSAKA, 1970). HR2a and HR2b basic protein (TAKAHASHI and OHSAKA, 1970b)

IX. Anticoagulant factor.

Crotalidae venom:

Agkistrodon acutus. Fraction 6, acidic glycoprotein, mol wt 20600 (This factor does not possess caseinolytic, tosyl-arginine-methyl-ester esterase, phospholipase A, phospho-diesterase, phospho-monoesterase or fibrinolytic activities (OUYANG and TENG, 1972)

X. Nerve growth factors (NGF)

a) *Elapidae venom:*
   Naja naja. N. G. F., 117 amino acid residues, 6 half-cystines, mol wt 28000 (ANGELETTI, 1970; ANGELETTI et al., 1976)
b) *Viperidae venom:*
   Vipera russellii. N.G.F., 270 amino acid residues, 12 half-cystines, mol wt 37000 (PEARCE et al., 1972)
c) *Crotalidae venoms:*
   1. *Bothrops jararaca*
      N. G. F., mol wt 20000 to 60000 (ANGELETTI, 1968)
   2. *Crotalus adamanteus*
      N. G. F., mol wt 20000 to 60000 (ANGELETTI, 1968)
   3. *Crotalus terrificus*
      N.G.F., mol wt 20000 to 40000 (ANGELETTI, 1968)

XI. Factor reacting on the complement (C_3)
Elapidae venom:
Naja naja
Co. V. F., mol wt 144000 (NELSON, 1966; MÜLLER-EBERHARD, 1967, 1971)

---

this toxin. By the same token we recall that *Atractaspis microlepidota*, whose classification among the *Viperidae* was the object of discussion owing to some of its morphological features, produces a venom that does not contain a major toxic constituent antigenically comparable to that of the *Naja* venom (MINTON, 1968). No protein constitutionally similar to the α toxin has been found in venoms of *Crotalidae*. Finally, recent research on extracts of labial glands of three *Colubridae opisthoglyphs*: *Boiga cyanea*, *Homalopsis buccata*, and *Enhydris bocourti*, has demonstrated that these extracts were precipitable by immune sera specific to the venoms of proteroglyphs, *Elapidae* and *Viperidae*, although the glands which ensure the poisonous nature of these venoms have reached very different stages of evolution. Despite these crossed immunological reactions, the antigens contained in the glands of these three *Colubridae* did not precipitate on contact with antibody specific to α toxin of *Naja nigricollis* (Ethiopia) venom (BOQUET and SAINT GIRONS, 1972).

Progressive modifications of the structure of living molecules characterize the stages of the slow transformation of species. Researches on the hemoglobins, cytochromes, hormones, and other proteins (ACHER, 1967, 1974) are evidence of this. Similarly the results collected from studies of antigenic components of venoms will lead to the establishement of an immunological classification of these constituents, which is to be elaborated later in this chapter.

C. Stimulation of the Immune System by Venom Antigens

I. General Remarks on Antivenom Sera

Table 2 is not a systematic list of all the constituents of *Elapidae*, *Hydrophiidae*, *Viperidae*, and *Crotalidae* venoms including enzymes, toxins and other components which have been described (see Chaps. 4, 5, 8). Only the proteins extracted from these venoms in a pure, or nearly pure, state have been included. Some of them are actually the subject of comparative immunological research. However, before approaching this field, so as to follow the chronological development of experiments, we shall first briefly examine the problem of the preparation of antivenom sera.

Early this century, the main objective was to obtain, in a single immune serum, a group of antibodies capable of neutralizing toxic substances produced by snakes belonging to the most prevalent species in a defined geographical area (VITAL BRAZIL, 1911). The techniques applied to this end will not be described in detail. Generally, horse (CALMETTE, 1907), sheep (SHULOV et al., 1959), and goat (MOHAMED et al., 1966; COHEN and SELIGMAN, 1966; RUSSELL et al., 1970) have been used for obtaining. sera. CALMETTA (1894, a, b, 1907) recommended subcutaneous injection to horses of small doses of venom to which had been added an equal volume of lime hypochlorite in a one percent solution. This reagent was added to reduce the toxicity of the venom. About 16 months of immunization were necessary to obtain a good therapeutic immune serum anticobra venom. With successive improvements in immunization techniqzes, a few months, and in some cases even weeks, are adequate nowadays to ensure the production of such a serum.

Following the work of RAMON (1924) on the preparation of anatoxins and anavenoms, ARTHUS (1930), RAMON and his co-workers (1941), GRASSET and ZOUTENDYK (1932), GRASSET (1945), and CHRISTENSEN (1947) turned to the use of anavenoms, i.e. to solutions of venoms whose toxicity was depleted by the addition of formaldehyde in the proportions of 5 or 6 per 1000, the mixture being incubated at 37–40° C for several weeks.

Other procedures have been suggested for depriving snake venoms of their toxicity without altering their main immunogenic properties. Among the techniques used have been the addition of soaps (RENAUD, 1930; CESARI and BOQUET, 1937) or of thioctic acid (SAWAI et al., 1963, 1967). Glutaraldehyde (BRADE and VOGT, 1971), partial oxidation (BOQUET, 1941), photo-oxidation (KOCHOLATY, 1966; KOCHOLATY et al., 1967, 1968a and b), acetylation (DELORI et al., 1974), X-irradiation (FLOWERS, 1966), and cobalt-60 irradiation (MITTELSTAEDT et al., 1973) have also been used. LUZZIO and TREVINO (1966) injected animals with a venom-antivenom precipitate. Recently, the term toxoid has been wrongly used to include venoms treated with chelating agents, whose action is limited to the inhibition of certain enzymes (GOUCHER and FLOWERS, 1964). The various toxic factors of venoms are distinguishable by their sensitivity to these reagents; some are very labile, while others are resistant. Possible methods of depleting these toxic factors of their physiological properties are e.g., an increased dose of the reagent or prolongation of the time that the mixtures are kept at 37–40° C (CESARI and BOQUET, 1939; KONDO et al., 1970–1971).

From the experiments of BOQUET and VENDRELY (1943), GRASSET (1945) and CHRISTENSEN (1947), it appears that, all other experimental conditions being equal, the pH of the mixture of venom and formaldehyde influences the rate of the reaction. The loss of activity, which is very slow in an acid medium, is much more rapid when an alkaline medium is used. In these conditions, the venom loses its toxicity and its antigenic properties at the same time. Similar results have been reported by MOROZ-PERLMUTTER et al. (1963). In fact, these workers have observed that the fraction of *Vipera palestinae* venom responsible for the hemorrhagic phenomena seen after venom poisoning is sensitive to formaldehyde when the pH of the mixture of venom and the reagent is between 5.5 and 9.2. However, when the pH of this same mixture is less than 7.0, the neurotoxic component retains its activity. It loses this when the pH is raised to over 7, but in these conditions it also loses its antigenicity.

After being transformed into toxoids, venoms are injected subcutaneously to animals. They are often mixed with substances that are known to increase the immune response, and are called "adjuvants of immunity": aluminium hydroxide gel (CRILEY, 1956), Freund's whole adjuvant (SAWAI et al., 1961; MOROZ et al., 1966), and sodium alginate (BOLAÑOS et al, 1975).

According to CHRISTENSEN (1966 b) crude venoms adsorbed onto bentonites lose some of their toxicity and retain their immunogenicity. CHRISTENSEN'S technique consists of giving horses a first basal immunity with injections of 25–100 mg of venom adsorbed on a 2% suspension of bentonites in distilled water. As soon as traces of circulating antibodies are detected by the mouse protection test, the immunization is continued with injections of a solution of unmodified venom sterilized by filtration and preserved with 0.25% cresol. Bentonites behave not only as an adsorbant but also as an adjuvant of immunity.

Immune sera thus obtained contain populations of antibodies that combine to different antigens of venoms and consequently neutralize toxins and enzymes.

The specific effects of antivenoms, which were reported by researchers even at the end of the last century, have been studied in detail *in vivo* by ARTHUS and STAWSKA (1911), who observed the protective properties of cobra antivenom with regard to the curarizing toxin of this venom, by PRATT JOHNSON (1934), TAYLOR and MALLICK (1936), CHRISTENSEN (1955 b), and GITTER et al. (1960), who measured the neutralizing power of antivenoms with respect to factors generating hemorrhage and necrosis, and lastly by MARQUART (1951), whose work showed that viper antivenoms suppressed the effect of the diffusion factor contained in the venoms of these snakes.

As early as 1911, ARTHUS reported that addition of venom from an American *Crotalidae* to a solution of fibrinogen caused it to coagulate very rapidly. The simultaneous addition of the specific antivenom suppressed this coagulation. CESARI and BOQUET (1935, 1936) subsequently established that the sera prepared to treat European and African snake bites were also antidotes for the blood coagulation-accelerating and inhibiting factors contained in the venoms of *Vipera aspis* and *Cerastes cornutus*, whose effects they had observed in vitro. Phospholipases, phosphoesterases, certain proteases and hyaluronidase of snake venoms are inhibited by the immune sera that are specific for them (CESARI and BOQUET, 1935; CHRISTENSEN, 1955 a; ZWISSLER, 1966; ELLIOTT et al., 1973; KUMAR and ELLIOTT, 1973; NAIRN et al., 1975; BOQUET et al., 1958). The very special case of aminoacid oxidase, which precipitates on contact with corresponding antibodies, but without losing its enzymatic properties (ZELLER, 1948 b; ZWISSLER, 1966), will be considered later.

II. Immunogenic Properties of some Proteins Extracted from Snake Venoms

We have shown how a specific immune serum to a venom precipitates and inactivates not only the various toxic and enzymatic components of this venom, but also, to different degrees, homologous substances contained in other venoms. The limits of this "paraspecific" neutralization have been defined. They remain very imprecise however, because of the complexity of each of the agents involved. Study of this phenomenon requires the use of antigens in a pure state and of sera specific to these antigens. It is for this reason that we shall describe, as an example, the problem of antigenicity of some curarizing toxins recently extracted from venoms of *Elapidae* and *Hydrophiidae.*

A brief survey of the literature shows that a venom labeled with iodine, or other radioactive material, injected intravenously or intramuscularly to a rabbit or a mouse, diffuses very rapidly in the animal's system. Whatever the origin of the venom used, the radioactive material generally concentrates in the lung, liver, heart, muscle (among them the diaphragm), and, most particularly, in the renal cortex. Any urine excreted is rich in a radioactive product (SUMYK et al., 1963; LEBEZ et al., 1973; GUMAA et al., 1974). Similar results are obtained when experiments are performed with curarizing toxins such as cobrotoxin *(Naja naja atra)*, erabutoxins *(Laticauda semifasciata)*, α toxin *(Naja nigricollis, Ethiopia)* or α bungarotoxin *(Bungarus multicinctus)* (Table 2).

When these labeled toxins are injected to animals, the presence of the radioactive protein in their diaphragm is readily detected at the motor nerve endings (LEE and TSENG, 1966; SATO and TAMIYA, 1970). According to SHÜ et al. (1968), 70% of cobrotoxin labeled with ^{131}I is excreted in the urine of rabbits injected intravenously with this protein 5 h previously. Most of the radioactivity excreted in the urine 20 min after the injection was shown by gel filtration, paper electrophoresis and toxicity tests, to be in the intact cobrotoxin fraction. Four hours after the injection, half of the radioactivity in the urine appeared in the free iodine fraction.

In experiments in mouse, with tritiated α toxin from *Naja nigricollis* (Ethiopia) venom, MENEZ et al. (unpubl.) confirmed the observations of SHÜ et al. (1968). The urine contained a high proportion of radioactive products precipitable by specific antibodies to α toxin. All or part of the protein was, therefore, in the form of an antigen, but while there were always very high levels of labeled product eliminated via the kidney the proportions varied from one experiment to another. The amount of radioactive toxin detectable in the brain was always low. This fact confirmed the observation reported by LEE and TSENG (1966) and TSENG et al. (1968) working with α bungarotoxin and cobra curare like toxin, respectively.

From these experiments, it can be seen that the amounts of curarizing toxins retained in the animal's system are much reduced within a few hours of their introduction. We do not know what consequences this has on the induction of immune-mechanisms, however, the speed with which toxin molecules are eliminated is probably not without effect on antigen capture, which is the first manifestation of a series of events, the end result of which is antibody production.

To obtain an immune serum specific for the α toxin of the venom of *Naja nigricollis* (Ethiopia), rabbits were immunized with a solution of α protein, either in its original form or transformed into toxoid by the addition of formaldehyde (DUMAREY, 1971). The toxoid was prepared as follows: 0.3% formaldehyde (3.8×10^{-2} M) was added to a buffered solution (pH 7.2) of 1% toxin (1.47×10^{-4} M), and the mixture was maintained at 37° C for 7 days. Three fractions were collected when the final product was filtered on Sephadex G 50. They corresponded to several molecular populations, one of which was represented by monomers, another by dimers, and the third by several soluble small polymers among which there was a family of decamers.

The α toxin, the toxoid and its by-products were injected directly or in combination with complete Freund's adjuvant to rabbits separated into several groups (DUMAREY and BOQUET, 1972; BOQUET et al., 1974).

Because of its high toxicity the dose of α toxin administered subcutaneously in its original form during the course of immunization was very low. Neither precipitating nor antitoxic antibodies were produced.

When α toxin was mixed with Freund's complete adjuvant before injection of the same doses under the same conditions, specific antibodies for the toxin appeared in the blood of the treated animals. These, however, were in very low proportions. At higher doses, α toxoid monomers injected subcutaneously to rabbits by the usual procedure, but without the adjuvant, had a low immunogenic capacity in a preliminary experiment. A second series of experiments, performed with a toxoid sample composed exclusively of monomers, has recently demonstrated that when this soluble antigen is injected to rabbits it does not produce any precipitating, hemagglutinating or neutralizing antibodies (BOQUET et al., unpubl.).

This phenomenon is in keeping with the observation of DRESSER (1962), who demonstrated that the bovine immunoglobin G, in a solution from which all particles have been removed by centrifugation, induced a state of immunological tolerance when injected into the peritoneum of mice, while if it contained aggregates it caused the production of antibodies. The next question is whether the unresponsiveness observed when the soluble α toxoid monomer is injected to rabbit corresponds to a state of immunological tolerance. At present, no answer can be given. If, however, it is confirmed that the observed phenomenon is the consequence of an immune-paralysis, one could be led to consider it as state defined by MITCHISON (1964) and later by DRESSER and MITCHISON (1968) by the term "low zone paralysis," i.e., as a paralysis induced, after a short delay, by low quantities of antigen (NOSSAL, 1971; WEIGLE et al., 1971; DIENER and FELDMAN, 1972; LOUIS et al., 1973; COUTINHO and MOLLER, 1975; HOWARD and MITCHISON, 1975).

The polymerized toxoid, in decamer form, is only weakly immunogenic.

If Freund's complete adjuvant is added to the monomer (all other conditions being as in previous experiments), there is a production of antibodies. This production is proportional to the dose of antigen injected. Some results are shown in Tables 3 and 4 (BOQUET et al., 1974 and unpubl.).

Hyperimmunization over a long period is not, however, followed by a regular increase in serum antibodies. The animals subjected to successive injections of venom, of a pure toxin, or of toxoids prepared from these substances, produce immune sera whose specific neutralizing activity increases progressively, then very often declines. This decrease is sometimes very marked, the animal ceasing to respond to any further antigenic stimulation.

Table 3. Production of antibody specific to the α toxin of *Naja nigricollis* (Ethiopia) venom (Effect of Freund's adjuvant)

Antigen:	Bleedings: Days after priming[b]		
	52	86	114
a) *α toxoid*[a] *monomer without adjuvant*	0	0	0
b) *α toxoid*[a] *monomer + Freund's adjuvant*	35[c]	100	160

[a] α Toxin of *N. nigricollis* (Ethiopia) transformed into toxoid by addition of formaldehyde. The monomers were separated by filtration on "Sephadex" G 50.
[b] Antigen was injected subcutaneously to 5—10 rabbits of body weight 2500—3000 g. The *total* dose of antigen injected to each animal during the period of immunization was 1.9 mg.
[c] Amount (μg) of α toxin neutralized per ml of serum. The figure indicated is a mean established according to the titration of each serum. The assay in the mouse consisted of injecting the animal with a mixture of toxin and serum following the usual techniques (CHRISTENSEN, 1966a). The assay was completed by precipitation and hemagglutination tests.

Table 4. Influence of antigen dose on the production of specific antibodies to α toxin[a]

	Bleedings: Days after priming		
	52	86	114
Total dose of antigen injected mixed with Freund's adjuvant:			
α toxoid 240 μg	10[b]	10	18
α toxoid 375 μg	10	35	23
α toxoid 1900 μg	94	284	198

[a] Same conditions as in the experiments whose results are shown in Table 3.
[b] Amount (μg) of α toxin neutralized by 1 ml of serum.

The absence of detectable antibodies in the serum of rabbits injected with α toxoid in the form of soluble monomers has led to the hypothesis that this unresponsiveness might correspond to a state of immune paralysis. The question arises as to whether or not the disappearance of serum antibodies in animals subjected to long-term hyperimmunization is a phenomenon of the same nature as that defined as high zone induced paralysis by MITCHISON (1964).

The results reported in Tables 3 and 4 were obtained with methods based on those described by CHRISTENSEN (1955a, 1966b). The protocol followed by the present author consists of creating a basal immunity in animals by two subcutaneous injections of antigen with Freund's adjuvant, separated with a short interval. Animals thus treated were allowed to rest for three weeks, and then received booster injections at weekly intervals. Following this technique, priming conferred an immunological memory to immunocompetent cells (CELADA, 1971; MILLER, 1971), and the antibody level during the secondary response was much higher than that of control rabbits immunized immediately after the first injection of antigen without a break.

Experiments performed using pure toxins extracted from snake venoms and then injected to animals led to the general opinion that the use of these toxins was an

Table 5. Influence of a basal immunity on the production of antibodies by animals boostered with injections of whole venom

Dose of antigen injected for priming:	Amount of toxin (µg) neutralized by 1 ml of the serum (last bleedings 114 days after priming[a]	
α toxoid	α toxin[b]	γ toxin[b]
75 µg	114	240
whole venom of *Naja nigricollis* Formalin treated 250 µg	38	260

[a] After priming all rabbits received, by subcutaneous injections, a *total dose of 3600*µg of venom of *N. nigricollis* (Ethiopia) detoxified by formalin. The experiments were performed in the same conditions as those whose results are presented in Tables 3 and 4.
[b] The α and γ toxins are from *N. nigricollis* (Ethiopia) venom.

excellent means of obtaining therapeutic sera rich in antitoxins. DELORI et al. (1974) prepared univalent sera against various toxins of *Elapidae* venoms in the rabbit. They suggested that the mixture and final concentration of monovalent sera could be held as a multivalent antivenom of high therapeutic value. A simple method, according to BOQUET et al. (1974), consists of conferring a basal immunity on animals to be used for the production of immune sera, by injecting them subcutaneously with a purified antigen transformed into a toxoid and mixed with an adjuvant such as Freund's complete adjuvant. After the usual rest period, which follows the first immunization, the animals are injected with the whole venom which has been treated with either formaldehyde or another reagent, so as to render it nontoxic. The antitoxic power of the immune sera obtained is very much increased with respect to the toxin injected for priming. The mixture and the concentration of sera of different specificities allow to achieve a good therapeutic serum. Some experimental results are shown in Table 5.

In all the immunization experiments performed by the present author and his coworkers the response of the rabbits has varied according to the origin of the animals. Thus, rabbits of some strains synthesized large quantities of antitoxin α, while others, of different origins, produced only a little or even none at all. It is important, then, that, in future prospects, attention should be paid to these differences, which might arise from the genetic control of antibody synthesis.

An experiment by KOCHWA et al. (1959a, b) showed that repeated subcutaneous injections of *Vipera xanthina* venom to rabbits or horses produced antibodies against hemorrhagic and necrotic factors contained in the venom, but apparently not against the neurotoxin. A series of injections of this neurotoxin isolated from the same venom provoked a marked increase in the amount of antineurotoxic antibodies in these animals.

The hypothesis of antigenic competition or "antigen-induced suppression" (PROSS and EIDINGER, 1974) has often been proposed by researchers surprised to find in antivenom sera relatively low proportions of specific antibodies to certain constituents of the venoms used as immunogens. This finding does not actually rest on the results of any convincing experiment. However, it must be admitted that injection of a venom into subcutaneous tissue in an animal causes the introduction into the organism of a mixture of chemical substances of different molecular weights, electrical charges, and structures. Certain of these substances diffuse very rapidly towards deep tissues, whereas others remain *in situ* for a relatively long period.

It has been confirmed, since the observation by MICHAELIS in 1902, that when the immune mechanisms are incited by two antigens, there is a competitive effect which results in an alteration of their ability to make a response against one of the antigens (ADLER, 1957). In some cases the strongest competition occurs when one antigen is injected a few days before the other. However, antigenic competition has been observed when both are injected together.

According to BURNET'S clonal selection theory (1959), each antibody-forming cell precursor in the adult animal carries on its surface receptors capable of reacting specifically with the epitope of an antigen molecule. The specificity of the clone is genetically predetermined. Antigenic competition between apparently unrelated antigens is considered as a serious challenge.

The mechanism of antigen competition or antigen-induced suppression has been the object of numerous hypothesis. It could be the expression of an immunological specific effect such as competition for antigenic sensitive cells or a cross-reaction of the antigens and induction of tolerance. It could be also a nonspecific phenomenon such as competition for some limiting factors or some of the steps of antigen processing. The increase in the number of cells in response to the first antigen might interfere physically with the response to the second antigen (KERBEL and EIDINGER, 1971a and b; ADLER and MOLLER, 1971). Finally, it has been suggested that antigenic competition might be the consequence of the production of inhibitors of antibody synthesis (RADOVICH and TALMAGE, 1967).

The results of a recent experiment showed that the neutralizing power of serum from rabbits immunized with repeated injections of α toxoid (the total quantity administered during the entire immunization was 375 μg) was approximately equal to that of serum from animals which received, in the same conditions, formalin-treated venom of *Naja nigricollis* (Ethiopia) in a total dose of 3600 μg. If we consider that this venom contains about 10% of α toxin, we are led to the conclusion that an equal dose of α toxin injected either in a pure state or associated with various venom proteins produced an equal quantity of antibodies specific to it (see Tables 4 and 5). In the conditions of this particular experiment, the different antigens contained in the venom did not exercise any competitive effect with respect to the α protein. Although the chemical composition and the molecular weight of the factors generating hemorrhages (HR1 and HR2) (OMORI-SATOH and OHSAKA, 1970) which have been extrated from the venom of *Trimeresurus flavoviridis* and those from the toxins of *Naja nigricollis* venom (Ethiopia), which we have used, are very different, it is important to remember that factors HR1 and HR2 injected simultaneously to guinea-pigs (SADAHIRO et al., 1970) resulted in elevated levels of specific antibodies to both. However, when rabbits were primed by injections of a mixture, in Freund's adjuvant, of pure α and γ toxins of *Naja nigricollis* venom (Ethiopia) detoxified by formalin, and then given booster injections of the venom, the antitoxic level of their sera against the α toxin was lower than that of the sera of control rabbits primed with the α toxin alone. It was concluded, by hypothesis that the phenomenon could be the consequence of an antigen-induced suppression (BOQUET et al., 1974). However, other hypotheses might be put forward.

According to HANNA et al. (1968) when two antigens of different immunological specificities are injected with only a short interval, a depression of the secondary response to the second antigen is observed and the level of the immune suppression is dependent upon the dose of the first antigen (HANNA and PETERS, 1970). Does the same happen when one preimmunizes rabbits with successive injections of γ and α toxoids? Rabbits were primed with a high dose of the γ toxoid (275 µg) and received an injection of the α toxoid (75 µg) five days later. All the animals were then given booster injections of the same α toxoid. The serum of these animals possessed an antitoxic power with respect to α toxin equal to that of control animals preimmunized and then immunized by injections of α toxoid alone. It appears, then, that the problem of antigenic competition between components of the same venom will have to be the subject of fresh research in order that practical conclusions may be drawn.

Before bringing to an end this section, it seems worthwhile to recall the results of an experiment by WU and CINADER (1971), who injected, by the same route, a strong immunogen followed by a weak one. They observed an augmentation of the immune response to the latter, which did not occur when the weak immunogen was injected first. Similarly, RUBIN and COONS (1972a and b) observed that the addition *in vitro* of an antigen to a population of cells formerly primed to this antigen resulted in the enhancement of the response to another unrelated antigen. The venoms contain both proteins of high molecular weight, which might behave as strong antigens, and small molecules, which may be considered as so many weak antigens. The problem is to know whether the former, in certain circumstances, favors the production of antibodies specific to the latter. Are other substances able to transform a weak antigen into an immunogen? This question opens the discussion in the following section.

III. Role of Adjuvant Substances

If we consider the results reported in Table 3, the role of adjuvant substances appears to be an essential one if an animal is immunized with injections of the monomeric form of α toxoid. It is probable that adjuvants are equally important in setting in motion the mechanisms for production of specific antibodies to numerous other weakly immunogenic proteins contained in snake venoms.

The effects of adjuvants are multiple, and each adjuvant possesses its individual properties. However, oily adjuvants, such as Freund's adjuvant, produce characteristic reactions in the tissues. Granulomas that develop there contain numerous active cells, macrophages, lymphocytes, and plasma cells.

The antigen incorporated in the adjuvant is slowly liberated into a medium rich in migratory cells. However, this depot effect might be no more than a contributory factor to the mode of action of the adjuvant. In the lymph node, which drains the site of the injection, adjuvants may facilitate the contact between macrophages and lymphocytes. It has been established that some adjuvants are potent mediators of the sequestration of lymphocytes in the node and that a "trapping" mechanism is mediated mainly through macrophages (FROST and LANCE, 1973). By that time, the antigen could have been chemically modified, aggregated, adsorbed onto particles, or even denatured. Particulate antigen associates easily with the membrane of macrophages, which is thought to facilitate its "presentation" to immunocompetent cells. It is now generally accepted that these cells are lymphocytes bearing on their surfaces receptors capable of interacting with antigenic substances.

The response to many antigens requires three categories of cells: thymus-derived (T) and bone marrow-derived (B) cells, lymphocytes, and accessory cells (TALMAGE, 1974) of the macrophage type (FELDMAN and UNANUE, 1971). The bone marrow-derived (B) cells produce the antibodies. They are triggered by the thymus-derived (T) cells called helper lymphocytes (MILLER and MITCHELL, 1968; MITCHELL and MILLER, 1968; MILLER, 1971; MILLER et al., 1971; MITCHISON et al., 1970; SCHIRRMACHER and WIGZELL, 1972). Some antigens, which have a structure of a large number of repeating determinants, act directly on B lymphocytes.

The macrophage is considered to process the antigen or to "present" it to immunocompetent cells (ASKONAS and JAROSKOVA, 1970; FELDMAN, 1972), and to exert a stimulus on these cells to divide and differentiate (DRESSER and PHILLIPS, 1973). In one series of experiments, UNANUE and co-workers (1969) showed that the adjuvant exerts its enhancing effect on antibody-producing cells only after uptake by macrophages. There is now much evidence that the cells initially involved in the action of adjuvants are, at least partly, macrophages (SPITZNAGEL and ALLISON, 1970a) and that, in some circumstances, adjuvants increase the efficiency of the interaction of these macrophages with bone marrow-derived cells, by-passing the requirement of thymus-derived helpers. Adjuvants may also enhance the macrophage-stimulating effect on T helpers so that their effect on B cells is augmented.

There is some evidence to suggest that macrophages concentrate antigen that is presented to the thymus-derived lymphocytes in a highly immunogenic form. However, it has recently been proposed that T cells might concentrate antigen on macrophages, which, in turn, stimulate the response of B cells; and some experimenters have suggested that T cells cooperate with B cells via a nonantigen specific factor which constitutes a second signal (DUTTON et al., 1971; MARRACK-HUNTER and KAPPLER, 1975).

An important observation is that antibody formed against an antigen is probably dependent on a switch mechanism and that adjuvants increase the probability that immunocompetent cells, especially T cells, are turned on. Consequently, adjuvants should be more effective in increasing antibody synthesis against antigens that are T-dependent (ALLISON, 1973). As adjuvants are necessary to set in motion the mechanism of antibody production against the α toxin (Table 2) this small protein may be considered to be T-dependent.

One of the effects of adjuvants may be to bring about the release from macrophages of a factor that stimulates proliferation of immunocompetent cells (ALLISON and DAVIES, 1971). Several adjuvants are active surface agents (GALL, 1966). They affect the structure of plasma and lysosomal membranes (SPITZNAGEL and ALLISON, 1970b; HOWARD et al., 1973). This property might facilitate contacts and eventually the formation of temporary bridges between cells such as macrophages, dendritic cells, and lymphocytes. In addition, multiplication of immunocompetent cells is often associated with labilization of lysosomes (MAILLARD and BLOOM, 1972). In relation to this it should be remembered that the direct lytic factor of *Naja naja* venom (cf. Table 2) associated with the phospholipase A_2 of the same venom has the property of impairing lysosomal membranes (KRAMAR et al., 1971).

Table 6. Comparative study of the action of three adjuvants on the productions of specific anti-α-toxin antibodies[a]

Nature of the adjuvant	Total dose of antigen injected	Bleedings: Days after priming		
		52	86	114
Sodium alginate	1900 μg of α toxoid	10[b]	24	28
Bentonites	934 μg of α toxin	9	13	—
Bentonites	5910 μg of α toxoid	10	10	—
Freund's adjuvant	1900 μg of α toxoid	94	284	198

[a] Same experimental conditions as those reported in Table 3.
[b] Amount (μg) of α toxin neutralized by 1 ml of immune serum (see Table 3).

By inducing cell destruction, adjuvants also liberate nucleic acids, which, in turn, enhance the immune response (BRAUN and NAKATO, 1967; JOHNSON et al., 1968). Another consequence of their surface activity is that they stimulate adenyl cyclase, which increases the level of cyclic AMP in cells. This can have the effect, for example, of restoring the ability to synthesize antibodies in neonatally thymectomized mice (KOOK and TRAININ, 1974, 1975).

Finally, adjuvants could influence the synthesis of various hormones, which would modify protein synthesis and consequently antibody synthesis (JOLLES and PARAF, 1973).

It seemed important to compare the effects of different adjuvants on the production of antibodies by a pure protein extracted from venoms, for example, α protein from the venom of *Naja nigricollis* (Ethiopia), which has already been used in many experiments. For this purpose, three adjuvants of different types and with different properties were chosen: the bentonites, which are particles and are considered to act on lysosomal membranes (ALLISON et al., 1966), sodium alginate, known for its depot effect (AMIES, 1959), and lastly Freund's adjuvant, which is responsible for granuloma formation and cellular multiplication, particularly of macrophages, in situ. The results shown in Table 6 demonstrate the particularly favorable effect of Freund's adjuvant. In the same experimental conditions, alginate only exercised a weak adjuvant effect. As for the bentonites, their effect was practically nonexistent. Adsorbed onto this substance and then injected subcutaneously into rabbits in nonlethal doses, α toxin elicited the production of only small amounts of antibody. It did not have any greater effect after being transformed into toxoid by the addition of formaldehyde and then adsorbed onto bentonites and injected to rabbits in very high doses. However, the results were different when instead of α toxoid, a venom from any of the African *Elapidae* was injected to horses in the same conditions (CHRISTENSEN, 1955a; 1966b; BOQUET, unpubl.). Using this technique, therapeutic antivenoms have been prepared. The poor response to injections of α toxin adsorbed on bentonites in the rabbit poses a problem as to the mechanism of action of this adjuvant: is its effect different in different species? Do strong immunogens associated with weak immunogens of the venom adsorbed on bentonites promote the synthesis of antibodies specific to the latter? At the current stage of our knowledge, no answer can be given. Freund's adjuvant is incontestably the most effective. Certainly, it is not completely without drawbacks, such as the causation of a particular type of abscess and of allergic sensitivity. However, the development of research on various extracts of the tuberculosis bacillus and of various other bacteria should soon allow experimenters to use substances whose effects are limited to an adjuvant action (SCHENCK et al., 1969; TANAKA et al., 1971; JOLLES and PARAFF, 1973; CHEDID et al., 1975).

Other procedures have been used to augment the immunogenic power of weak antigens from venoms. For this purpose, MOROZ et al. (1963, 1966a and c) injected rabbits and horses with a neurotoxic fraction from *Vipera palestinae* venom bound to a soluble carboxymethyl-cellulose. They obtained a good antitoxic immune serum. AHARONOV et al. (1974) reported that the immunological response of animals injected with a polyalanylated long toxin of *Naja naja siamensis* venom was less than that obtained in the control test with the unmodified toxin.

IV. Other Examples of Immunogenicity of Proteins Extracted in a Pure Form from Snake Venoms

Some aspects of the problem concerning the antigenic properties of α toxin of *Naja nigricollis* (Ethiopia) have been mentioned in this chapter, and the optimal conditions for production of anti-α-antibodies have also been described. Other proteins extracted from the venoms of various species of snakes have been used with the aim of preparing specific immune sera for each one. Thus, SATO et al. (1972), using rabbits, injected the toxoids (mixed with Freund's adjuvant) obtained from two "short" curare-like toxins from the venom of *Laticauda semifasciata*, the erabutoxins a and b, which differ from each other by a single amino acid. To solutions of these two erabutoxins, in the concentration of 5% (weight), buffered at pH 7,0, 2% of formaldehyde (volume) was added. These mixtures were maintained at 37° C for five days. The amino and guanidino groups of the native toxins were 5 and 3 respectively. These groups were not effectively detectable after formalin treatment. The two toxoids were aggregates of 10 molecules. The sera obtained by SATO and his colleagues cross-precipitated and neutralized erabutoxins a and b.

Using a similar procedure, CHANG and YANG (1969) prepared an immune serum specific for the short neurotoxin of *Naja naja atra*. Applying KABAT'S technique (1961), they established that the ratio of antibody to antigen in the mixtures where the precipitation was optimal, i.e., in the so-called equivalence zone, was 1.7 to 1.5, and they estimated that there are three antigenic determinants on the surface of the toxin molecule. CLARK et al. (1972) described a method that resulted in production of a serum specific for α bungarotoxin. DUMAREY and BOQUET (unpubl., 1974) used a rabbit immune serum against the γ toxin of the venom from *Naja nigricollis* (Ethiopia) in various experiments.

By immunizing guinea-pigs by means of toxoids derived from hemorrhage generating factors HR1 and HR2 (cf. Table 2) from the venom of *Trimeresurus flavoviridis*, KONDO et al. (1971b, 1973) obtained specific immune sera to these antigens. The adjuvant chosen for these experiments was aluminium phosphate. DELORI (1973) injected rabbits with a mixture of Freund's adjuvant and a phospholipase known as P_4 (cf. Table 2), which he extracted from the venom of *Vipera berus*. The resulting immune serum precipitated phospholipase P_4 and inhibited its in vivo toxic effects. However its action on the enzymic activity of the protein was not studied. The two other phospholipases of the same venom did not precipitate on contact with this immune serum. Antisera were recently raised against nerve growth factors isolated from the venoms of *Vipera ammodytes*, *Dendroaspis viridis* and *Agkistrodon rhodostoma* (BAILEY et al., 1976).

SHAHAM et al. (1973), using a fraction of *Vipera palestinae* venom containing L-amino acid oxidase as antigen (cf. Table 2), obtained an immune serum that specifically precipitated the enzyme. According to ZWISSLER (1966) and other workers whose findings have already been mentioned, the specific antibodies to L-amino acid oxidase do not inhibit the catalytic action of this enzyme. A certain number of other enzymes behave in this way but L-amino-acid-oxidase is particularly interesting. ZIMMERMAN et al. (1971) have prepared an immune serum specific to the enzyme they obtained by chromatography of *Crotalus adamanteus* venom. This L-amino-acid-oxidase undergoes reversible inactivation when subjected to different conditions. The active, inactive, and reactive enzyme, and particularly the "warm" and "frozen" inactive forms, have been the subject of a number of studies which demonstrated that active and inactive forms corresponded to identical proteins. The only difference observed suggested that the inactivation affected the environment of the flavin, which is the prosthetic group of the enzyme. Immunological studies of this L-amino-acid-oxidase led researchers to assume that inactivation and reactivation are the consequence of some conformational change in the enzyme. Since reactivated enzyme appeared to be immunologically identical to the native enzyme, it was likely that its conformation had been restored to the native form. Antibodies specific to the active form did not inhibit the enzyme but protected it against inactivation. Following the rate of reactivation of either warm or frozen inactivated enzyme in the presence of antibodies, a faster initial rate of reactivation than that of a control preparation was observed. The reaction of the antibodies with the corresponding epitopes must be such as to maintain or promote the molecule in a configuration favorable for enzymic activity. Thus, the antibodies do not appear to bind or to block the active site of the enzyme.

V. Relationships Between Chemical Composition, Structure and Immunological Properties of Some Antigens of Snake Venoms

The observations reported in the preceding paragraph lead to the problem of relationships existing between the structures of the best known proteins of snake venoms, their functions and their antigenic properties. Among all the proteins listed in Table 2, the short and long toxins, in particular, lend themselves to such a study. Comparing the composition of these proteins, STRYDOM (1973a and b) established phylogenic relationships between them, and considered that the second constitued a branch detached during the evolution of the ophidian species from the main group represented by the first.

Using the small curare-like proteins, whose chemical composition is given in Table 2, researchers have undertaken experiments of two types. Firstly, chemical modifications of these proteins have shown the importance of certain amino acid residues and have yielded antigens deprived of their toxic properties but whose immunological specificity is not at all, or only slightly modified. Secondly, analogous toxins have been compared and then classified according to the usual immunological techniques. The immunological distances that separate them from each other was then estimated. The final objective of these experiments was to define immunological active regions of these proteins.

At the beginning of this article, experiments performed on ribonuclease, lysozyme and myoglobin were quoted. For more information on this subject the reader is referred to the excellent general reviews by BENJAMINI et al. (1972) and REICHLIN (1975).

Before the study of venom toxins is described, it seems important to mention some observations made by ATASSI (1975) whose research on myoglobin led him to the following conclusions, which we summarize:

The site of the antigenic reactive region on a natural protein is small: 6–7 amino acid residues. (According to RUDE (1971), however, there may be as many as 15, or even 20.)

Interactions of the reactive regions of myoglobin with corresponding antibody sites are predominantly polar.

Two or more reactive regions, which may be distant in sequence but close if we consider the three-dimensional structure, may form an epitope.

At any rate the region considered as a determinant is invariably a reactive one with every immune serum. However, when it reacts with specific immune sera, an antigenic region has well-defined boundaries and the variability of these boundaries is small.

Antigenic reactive regions should be expected to occupy surface areas in highly accessible locations. However, the opinion that every bend may contain a reactive region is erroneous.

The immunological reactivity of antigenic proteins is highly influenced by changes in their conformation.

The environment of an amino acid type determines its involvement in the antigenic structure of a globular protein.

Finally, the immunochemical cross-reactions of two proteins are not necessarily effected through all equivalent antigenic reactive regions on the surface of the two proteins. If equivalent reactive regions on the two proteins contribute to the parallel cross-reactions, they may not do so with equal affinity. Their behavior may be complicated by any differences in conformation between the two proteins that may take place as a result of evolutionary amino acid replacement.

We shall now expound a few observations concerning the relationships between the structure, the toxic properties and the antigenic activities of some curare-like toxins in snake venoms.

1. Chemical Modifications

a) Influence of S-S Bridges

YANG (1967) found that splitting of the disulfide bridges of cobrotoxin from *Naja naja atra* venom (cf. Table 2 and Fig. 2a) deprived this protein of its biological activities. A progressive reoxidation restored the structure of the molecule which also recovered its antigenicity. The observation of BOTES (1974) gave more precise information about the role of the disulfide bridges in the maintenance of biological properties of long α toxin of *Naja nivea* venom (cf. Table 2). At an equimolar concentration of dithio-erythritol to toxin, one disulfide bridge is cleaved selectively be-

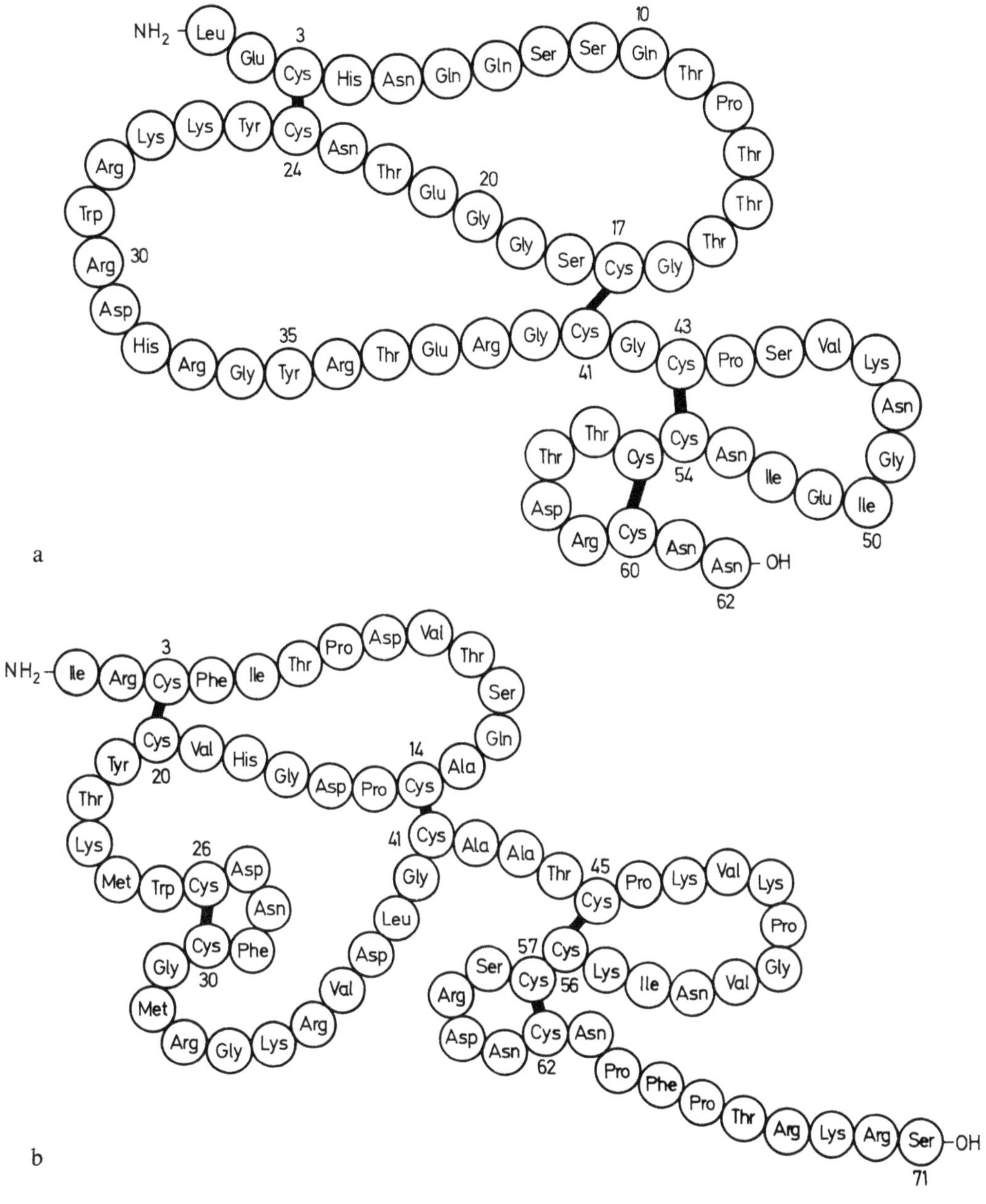

Fig. 2. (a) Cobrotoxin of *Naja naja atra* venom (YANG, 1969, by permission); (b) α toxin of *Naja nivea* venom (BOTES, by permission)

tween half-cystines 26 and 30 (Fig. 2b), which comprise the additional loop of long toxins. This conformational change is small and the modified toxin still binds to the cholinergic receptor. However, it binds with less affinity than the native toxin. It also reacts with antibodies specific for the unmodified protein. The conclusion is that the rupture of one disulfide bond has no drastic effect on the conformation of the molecule and the modified region does not seem to contribute toward the antigenic make-up of the toxin. Increasing the concentration of dithio-erythritol leads to random cleavage of the other disulfide bridges and the molecule loses its biological activities.

b) *Modification of Amino-Groups*

Modification of one arginine residue of the three that erabutoxin a possesses does not modify its antigenicity (TU et al., 1971). In order to differentiate the functionally important arginine residues of cobrotoxin, YANG et al. (1974) treated this toxin with phenylglyoxal at various pH. The arginine (Arg) residues modified at pH 6.0, 6.7, 7.5, and 8.0 were respectively: Arg 28; Arg 28 and 33; Arg 28, 30 and 33, and Arg 28, 30, 33 and 36 (cf. Fig. 2a). Arg 28-modified cobrotoxin retained its full lethality and its antigenic properties. The lethal activity of Arg 28 and 33-modified toxin dropped suddenly but the antigenic activity of the molecule was not altered significantly. When an additional Arg 30 was modified, the toxicity of the protein was destroyed almost completely and its antigenic activity decreased by about 30%. Cobrotoxin lost its biological activities when Arg 28, 30, 33, and 36 were modified. The experimenters suggested that Arg 30 and 36 might be related to the antigenic specificity of this toxin (YANG et al., 1977).

Recent observations by CHANGEUX et al. (1970), by BOURGEOIS et al. (1971), and by MILEDI et al. (1971) indicate that some of the short and long neurotoxins bind firmly to nicotinic acetylcholine receptors. Although the mechanism of binding is not known exactly, the hypothesis has been proposed that this mechanism might involve an interaction between the receptor and at least one of the cationic groups of these toxins. Acetylation, carbamylation and guanidination of cationic groups of long toxins of *Naja naja siamensis* and *Naja naja naja* (cf. Table 2) have been performed by KARLSSON et al. (1972b), who demonstrated the importance of certain of these groups in the preservation of toxicity of the molecule. When acetylated, the curarizing proteins lose their toxicity, but maintain their antigenicity (DELORI et al., 1974).

The reagent generally used to transform the toxins into toxoids is formaldehyde. The action of formaldehyde on proteins is mainly due to its affinity for the free amino groups of the lysine residues. The mechanism of the reaction has been studied thoroughly by FRAENKEL-CONRAT and OLCOTT (1948) and by BLASS (1961). BLASS et al. (1969) described the mechanism of transformation of diphtheria toxin into anatoxin by the use of formalin. Part of the reagent becomes fixed to the protein in the form of methylene bridges between the amino-groups of the lysine residues and other functional groups of the amino acids, including those of tyrosine. BLASS and coworkers demonstrated that four molecules of formalin take part in the formation of methylene bridges between neighboring residue of lysine and tyrosine during the transformation of the diphtheria toxin into an anatoxin. This observation led DUMAREY (1971) to investigate to what extent the single tyrosine (No. 24) of the α toxin of *Naja nigricollis* (Ethiopia) venom reacts with formalin during the transformation of this toxin into a toxoid.

After determination of the optimum conditions under which the toxin was deprived of its lethal properties by formalin, it was established that destruction of toxicity was always accompanied by a slight modification of antigenic properties as

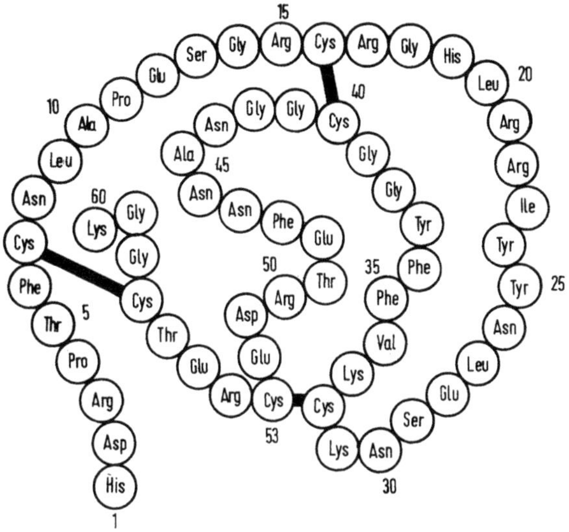

Fig. 3. Proteinase inhibitor of *Vipera russellii* venom. (TAKAHASHI et al., 1972, 1974, by permission)

measured by quantitative precipitation and passive hemagglutination. The acid-labile formalin was eliminated from the toxoid, which was submitted to hydrolysis and then to chromatoelectrophoresis. By this procedure it was shown that Tyr 24 does not take part in the formation of a methylene bridge. It was concluded that the change in biological properties of the molecule resulted from the fixation of formalin onto active groups other than those of Tyr 24, and that this amino acid residue is buried in the molecule. In addition, it has already been mentioned that the toxoid is in the form of a mixture of molecular populations composed of monomers, dimers, and small aggregates composed of 10 units. In relation to this, it should be noted that glutaraldehyde in high and low doses provokes a high degree of polymerization of α toxin. The aggregates are formed as large insoluble particles, which do not cause appearance of antibodies when they are injected, associated with an adjuvant, into the animal. Mixed with an anti-α-toxin immune serum, these aggregates do not modify the precipitating power of this serum with respect to native toxin. Animals subjected to injections of antigen treated with glutaraldehyde are not rendered tolerant to this antigen. They respond normally by production of antitoxin when they are immunized, in usual conditions, by injections of the α toxoid prepared with formaldehyde. Reducing the dose of glutaraldehyde, shortening the contact time between the reagents, and stopping the action of glutaraldehyde by the addition of lysine, resulted in the formation of a weakly polymerized toxoid, which remains immunogenic. Its activity, however, is inferior to that of the toxoid obtained by treating α toxin with formaldehyde (DUMAREY and BOQUET, unpubl.).

Since the experimental conditions of BRADE and VOGT (1971) were different, the results of these authors cannot be compared with those described here. In fact, BRADE and VOGT treated cobra venom with glutaraldehyde. Serum of rabbits injected with high doses of the product contained antibodies which precipitated various antigens of the venom and neutralized its toxic constituents. In these conditions, the binding between molecules of identical constitution is not effected by glutaraldehyde, but links are created at random between the molecules of different constitution and different molecular weights which constitute the cobra venom. Some of them probably behave as carriers.

Another procedure consists of blocking cationic groups of the protein by thioisocyanates. YANG et al. (1967), then CHANG (1970), thiocarbamylated cobrotoxin (Table 2 and Fig. 2a). Three residues of lysine and N-terminal leucine were carbamylated. The protein lost its toxicity and was transformed into a toxoid. When injected to rabbits, this toxoid, mixed with Freund's adjuvant, produced an immune serum that precipitated and neutralized the native toxin. Immunodiffusion showed that the precipitin lines corresponding to the toxin and to the toxoid fused. In addition, the graphs corresponding to the results of quantitative precipitin reactions showed no significant differences between homologous and heterologous reactions.

By the same technique, the α toxin of *Naja nigricollis* (Ethiopia) venom was depleted of its toxicity and a specific rabbit immune serum was prepared. This serum precipitated and neutralized the α toxin. However, a comparison of the quantitative precipitin curves, drawn from the results of experiments with the toxin and the toxoid (Fig. 4), led BOQUET and RONSSERAY (unpubl., 1972) to conclude that carbamylation has slightly modified the antigenic specificity of the protein. Were some of

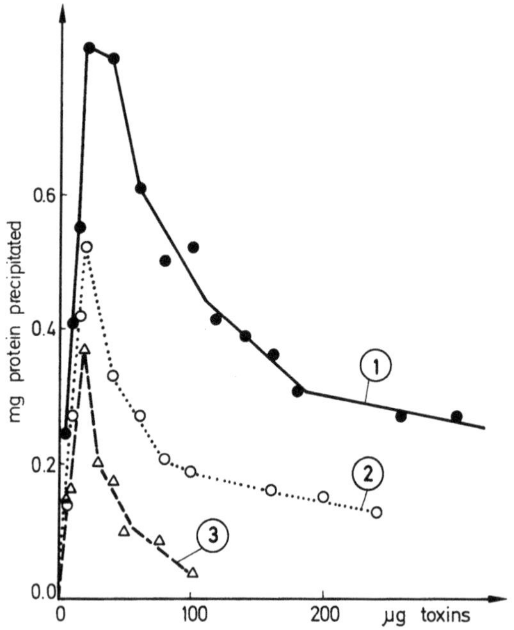

Fig. 4. Quantitative precipitation curves. (1) α toxin of *N. nigricollis* (Ethiopia) venom treated with F.i.t.c.* + rabbit serum anti-α toxin of *N. nigricollis* (Ethiopia) venom treated with F.i.t.c. (2) Native α toxin of *N. nigricollis* (Ethiopia) venom + rabbit serum anti-α toxin of *N. nigricollis* (Ethiopia) venom treated with F.i.t.c. (3) α toxin of *N. nigricollis* (Ethiopia) venom treated with F.i.t.c. + rabbit serum anti-α toxin of *N. nigricollis* (Ethiopia) venom treated with F.i.t.c. absorbed by native α toxin

* F.i.t.c. = fluoresceine isothiocyanate

the carbamylated groups responsible for this alteration? To answer this question, the γ toxin of the same venom which is chemically but not immunologically related to the α toxin, was treated with the same reagent and mixed with the rabbit immune serum. No precipitation occurred.

c) Modification of Histidyl Residues

Erabutoxins a and b of *Laticauda semifasciata* have the same antigenic specificity (cf. Table 2). The only difference between them concerns amino acid residue 26, where Asn in erabutoxin a is substituted for His in erabutoxin b. The two toxins contain a common histidyl residue No. 7 and a common tyrosyl residue No. 25. Iodination of erabutoxin b involves His 26, while in the same conditions erabutoxin a does not fix iodine. The tyrosine at 25 is not accessible to iodine in the two toxins. Fixation of iodine by His 26 of erabutoxin b does not diminish the intensity of the precipitation of this antigen by a specific immune serum to the native toxin (SATO and TAMIYA, 1970). The two histidyl residues of cobrotoxin of *Naja naja atra* venom (Table 2 and Fig. 2a), which is chemically related to erabutoxin b, do not react with iodine (HUANG et al., 1973). It is His 4 that is iodinated in α toxin of *Naja nigricollis* venom (MENEZ, pers. comm.). Precipitation tests demonstrate that the iodinated α toxin reacts like native toxin in the presence of antibodies specific to this native toxin. It thus appears that the two histidyl residues, 26 of erabutoxin b and 4 of α toxin, are not essential for the maintenance of the antigenic properties of the two molecules.

d) Modification of Tryptophanyl Residues

The sequence of amino acids Cys-Tyr-X-(Lys or Glu)-Y-Trp occupies approximately the same position in molecules of different short curare-like toxins of *Elapidae* and *Hydrophiidae* venoms generally containing only one tryptophan residue. Some toxins, however, have a second tryptophan residue. It has been considered that the first of these has an essential role in the maintenance of the toxins' ability to fix to the cholinergic receptor.

Modification of this residue should provide important information on the structure of the molecule. The tryptophan residue No. 29 of erabutoxin a, one of the short toxins from *Laticauda semifasciata* venom, was modified by SETO et al. (1970) with N-bromosuccinimide or 2-hydroxy-5-nitro-benzyl bromide (Koshland's reagent). This treatment deprived the protein of its toxicity. The modified toxin was still antigenic and the corresponding precipitin line, observed by the immunodiffusion test, fused with that of the native protein. These results were confirmed by TU et al. (1971). According to CHANG and HAYASHI (1969), the only tryptophan residue of cobrotoxin, the short toxin of *Naja naja atra*, could be converted into formyl kynurenine by ozonization in formic acid. The residual activity of the cobrotoxin was low. Later, CHANG and YANG (1973), with the same object in mind, used different procedures for selectively altering the tryptophan residue in the same toxin: ozonization in the presence of formic acid, oxidation by N-bromo-succinimide, or treatment with 2-hydroxy-5-nitrobenzyl bromide or 2-nitrophenyl sulphenyl chloride. The modified protein was deprived of its toxicity and was used for immunizing rabbits. In comparing results of experiments performed with the four different reagents, CHANG and YANG have shown that 2-hydroxy-5-nitrobenzyl cobrotoxin was the best immuno-

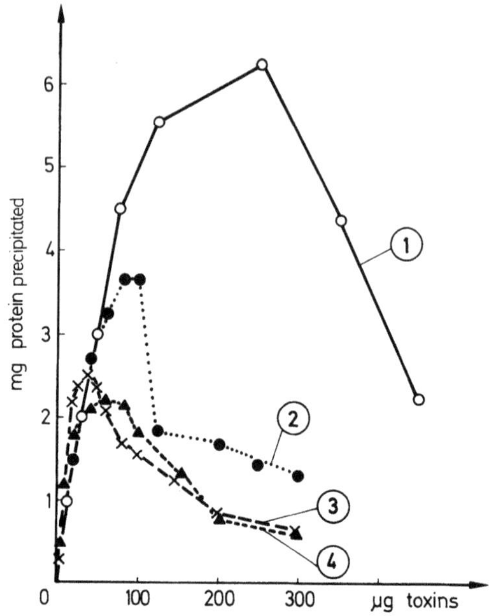

Fig. 5. (1) α toxin of *N. nigricollis* (Ethiopia) venom + rabbit serum anti-α toxoid (formalin-treated) of *N. nigricollis* (Ethiopia) venom. (2) α toxin of *N. nigricollis* (Ethiopia) venom treated with Koshland's reagent + rabbit serum anti-α toxin of *N. nigricollis* (Ethiopia) venom treated with Koshland's reagent. (3) Native α toxin of *N. nigricollis* (Ethiopia) venom + rabbit serum anti-α toxin treated with Koshland's reagent. (4) α toxin treated with Koshland's reagent + rabbit serum anti-α toxoid (formalin-treated)

gen. The patterns of immunodiffusion were the same for both native and modified toxins.

At the same time, KARLSSON et al. (1973) treated a short curare-like toxin of *Naja naja siamensis* venom (cf. Table 2) with 2-hydroxy-5-nitrobenzyl bromide and a long toxin of the same venom (cf. Table 2) by ozonization. With Koshland's reagent, polymerization occurred. Monomers and dimers were slightly toxic and the polymers were not. Ozonization gave a derivative with a residual activity. The experimenters stated that the invariant tryptophan of neither short and long toxins appears to be a functionally essential group directly involved in the toxic action. The recent observation of MENEZ et al. (1976) has led to the opinion that short toxin molecules, which were the subject of their study, possess a narrow region limited to certain amino acids, including Tyr and Trp, whose conformation underwent modifications following experimental procedures. MENEZ and his co-workers consider that, in the current state of our knowledge, no relationship could be definitely established between this property and the mechanism by which toxin molecules fix themselves to the cholinergic receptor. In addition, CHICHEPORTICHE et al. (1972) demonstrated that formylation of a short toxin, the toxin I of *Naja haje* venom (cf. Table 2), has no effect on the toxin activity of the molecule, and they concluded that it did not seem likely that the tryptophan located after the third half-cystine took part in the non-covalent interaction that stabilizes the association of the molecule with the cholinergic receptor. They suggest that the indole side chain of the tryptophan, like the phenol part of the tyrosyl residue, "is involved in the stabilization of an adequate geometry for the active site." Similar results were reported by OHTA and HAYASHI (1974) during research on the role of tryptophan in a long toxin from *Naja naja* venom (cf. Table 2).

Modifications of its sole tryptophan residue do not seem to deprive the α toxin molecule of *Naja nigricollis* (Ethiopia) venom of its antigenicity. Following the technique of KARLSSON et al. (1973), this toxin was treated with Koshland's reagent. The residual toxicity of the monomer was low. When mixed with Freund's adjuvant and then injected to rabbits, it caused the appearance of precipitating antibodies and antitoxins specific to α protein in the animal's serum. In this respect, it behaved as a toxoid. However, the curves determined by quantitative precipitation of the native and modified toxins showed that the antigenic specificity of the toxoid is not identical to that of the original toxin. A limited modification of the conformation of the molecule could perhaps be one of the determining causes of this phenomenon (BOQUET and RONSSERAY, unpubl.) (Fig. 5).

e) *Modification of Tyrosyl Residues*

The first experiments of SATO and TAMIYA (1970) showed that the only tyrosyl residue of erabutoxin b was "buried." The same is true for the single tyrosyl residue of short toxins of *Lapemis hardwickii* (cf. Table 2) (RAYMOND and TU, 1972) and of *Naja nigricollis* (Ethiopia) (DUMAREY, 1971). Cobrotoxin (Fig. 2a) (YANG et al., 1969) contains two tyrosyl residues. Residue 25, whose presence is well-established in other toxins, is also buried. When this residue is modified with an appropriate reagent, the molecule loses its biological properties. The second tyrosyl residue (No. 35) of cobrotoxin can be nitrated without altering the properties of the molecule (CHANG et al., 1971). However, under conditions of submaximal iodination in the presence of guanidine HCl, both tyrosyl residues were modified. Surprisingly, the toxicity and antigenicity remained unchanged (HUANG et al., 1973).

When the amino acid sequences of curare-like toxins are examined, it can be observed that they contain a very low proportion of aromatic amino acids. According to SELA and ARNON (1960), ARNON and SELA (1960), SELA et al. (1962), aromatic amino acids such as tyrosine consistently enhanced the immunogenicity of gelatin and synthetic polypeptide-antigens. However, this is not necessarily due to the aromatic character of these amino acids, as the attachment of cyclohexylalanine also enhances immunogenicity. The question arose as to whether the fixation of tyrosine to the α toxin of *Naja nigricollis* (Ethiopia) venom would increase its immunogenic power. Tyrosine (2.6×10^{-3} M) was incorporated into a mixture of the toxin and formaldehyde prepared according to the method of DUMAREY (1971). Chromatoelectrophoresis of the hydrochloric acid hydrolysate of the protein, free from acid-labile formaldehyde and excess polymerized tyrosine, demonstrated a compound "lysine-methylene tyrosine" (BLASS, 1961), which did not appear in the chromatoelectrophoregram of toxin treated by formaldehyde alone (DUMAREY, 1971), because of the buried position of the only tyrosyl residue of this molecule. The presence of such a compound demonstrated that tyrosine molecules were attached to the protein. When injected in low doses into 16 rabbits the average titer of the sera collected was much higher than that from control rabbits immunized by injections of the toxoid

Table 7. Antitoxic activity of sera obtained by immunization of rabbits with α toxoid obtained in different conditions

Reagent used to prepare the toxoid and total dose of toxoid injected (μg)		Dose of α toxin neutralized by 1 ml of serum (μg). Bleedings: Days after the 1st immunization	
		86	122
1 – formic aldehyde	(240)	10	18
2 – formic aldehyde	(375)	10	35
3 – formic aldehyde	(1900)	94	284
4 – formic aldehyde + tyrosine	(240)	86	70
5 – Koshland's reagent	(1900)	80	162
6 – acetic anhydride[a]	(1900)	112	138
7 – glutaraldehyde	(1900)	38	68
8 – fluoresceine isothiocyanate	(1900)	41	52

(For technical information, see Table 3.)
[a] The toxoid was treated with hydroxylamine.

without tyrosine. However, when high doses of antigen were administered, no differences were observed between the antitoxic activity of the sera of animals that received the tyrosyl antigen, and that of the controls, as if there was a ceiling of synthesis of antibodies in the conditions of the experiment (DUMAREY and BOQUET, 1974, and unpubl.).

Table 7 summarizes the results of a comparative study of the neutralizing ability of antisera from rabbits injected with α toxin transformed into toxoid by different reagents.

f) The Problem of Aminoacid Residue Modifications

The observations reported led us to conclude that the use of chemical reagents reacting selectively on certain amino acid residues provides information about the antigenic properties of some short and long toxins extracted from snake venoms. With the exception of the 5th disulfide bridge of long toxins, the rupture of which does not seem to influence the antigenicity of the molecule profoundly (BOTES, 1974), the other bonds of this type are essential for the maintenance of these properties. Modification of the tyrosyl residue near the third half-cystine generally causes the molecule to lose its biological properties. In contrast, a modification of the only tryptophan residue of most curare-like toxins or of some of the cationic groups, which results in a modification of the total charge of the molecule, transforms it into a toxoid. Lys 27 and 47 of erabutoxin b seem to be (HOZI and TAMIYA, personal communication) essential in this transformation. Whatever the mechanism of this phenomenon may be the immunologically active areas distributed on the surface of the toxin molecule do not seem to undergo a profound alteration. Since the entire molecule has only a low molecular weight, its surface cannot be extensive. Consequently, the number of active superficial areas is probably reduced. Immunological studies demonstrated that there are at least three antigenic sites on cobrotoxin (CHANG and YANG, 1969). In these conditions, molecular alteration resulting in loss of toxicity and conservation of antigenicity may be the consequence of only a minimal structural modification.

Another procedure used for defining immunologically active regions of a protein consists in fragmenting it by partial enzyme digestion and examining the properties of separately collected fragments. This procedure has been applied to the study of myoglobin, lysozyme and some other proteins whose structure is known (CRUMPTON and WILKINSON, 1965; ATASSI and SAPLIN, 1968; MARON et al., 1972). No results have so far been obtained by submitting α toxin of *Naja nigricollis* (Ethiopia) venom, either in its original form, or in a reduced form, to a trypsic digestion. We must hope, however, that this method will provide useful information in the near future.

2. Immunological Analysis

Study of the antigenic regions of these curare-like toxins can be undertaken in a very different way. By comparing the immunological properties of the cytochromes C, of known chemical structure, MARGOLIASH et al. (1967, 1970) and NISONOFF et al. (1970) have defined some of their antigenic determinants. The curare-like toxins of *Elapidae* and *Hydrophiidae* lend themselves to a study based on the same principles. It is for this reason that we performed a series of experiments designed to establish an immunological classification of the principal toxins of known composition which had been isolated from venoms of these snakes (Table 8) (BOQUET et al., 1970, 1973b).

Nineteen toxins behaving either as curarizing proteins or as agents modifying the permeability of cell membranes (cardiotoxins, cytotoxins) were compared following the usual techniques of precipitation, double diffusion in gel, inhibition of precipitation, and quantitative precipitation. A certain number of antivenoms of *Naja nigricollis* (Ethiopia), *Naja haje*, *Naja naja*, *N. naja philippinensis*, and *Hemachatus haemachatus* were used as reference sera. These 19 different basic toxins fall into three immunological groups. Group I is represented by proteins consisting of a single chain of 61 to 62 amino acid residues containing four disulfide bonds (short toxins). Group II includes proteins related to *Naja nigricollis* (Ethiopia) γ toxin, which is a 60-amino acid residue molecule containing eight half-cystines. Proteins belonging to group III are made up of 71–74 amino acid residues in a single chain cross-linked by five disulfide bonds (long toxins).

Toxins belonging to the immunological groups I and III behave as curare-like substances.

Proteins of group II act as cardiotoxins and cytotoxins and alter the permeability of the cell membrane.

This attempt to classify toxic proteins of *Elapidae* and *Hydrophiidae* venoms will need to be extended in the future. New toxins recently extracted from snake venoms will probably necessitate the inclusion of several new groups or subgroups. This might be the case for fractions LS III from *Laticauda semifasciata* venom (MAEDA and TAMIYA, 1974), S_4C_{11} from *Naja melanoleuca* venom (CARLSSON, 1975), and TA_2 from *Dendroaspis angusticeps* venom (VILJOEN and BOTES, 1974). In fact, immune sera used to characterize these proteins have not permitted their classification into one of the three proposed groups.

The primary structures of the proteins belonging to groups I and II have resemblances in both amino acid sequence and location of disulfide bridges. STRYDOM

Table 8. Immunological classification of some toxic proteins isolated from the venoms of *Elapidae* and *Hydrophiidae*

Immuno-logical group	Name of the toxin:	Species	Chemical constitution	Pharmacological properties
I	α1 (KARLSSON et al., 1966) (BOQUET et al., 1966a and b) (EAKER and PORATH, 1967)	*N. nigricollis* (Ethiopia) (c)	61 A.A., 8 H.C.	Curare-like
	α2 (a)	*N. nigricollis* (Ethiopia) (c)	60—61 A.A.	Curare-like
	α3 (b)	*N. nigricollis* (Ethiopia) (c)		
	α (BOTES and STRYDOM, 1969) (d)	*N. haje*	61 A.A., 8 H.C.	Curare-like
	II (MIRANDA et al., 1970) (KOPEYAN et al., 1973)	*N. haje*	61 A.A., 8 H.C.	
	Cobrotoxin (YANG et al., 1969)	*N. naja atra*	62 A.A., 8 H.C.	Curare-like
	d (BOTES, 1972) (e)	*N. melanoleuca*	61 A.A., 8 H.C.	Curare-like
	I (HAUERT et al., 1974)	*N. naja philippinensis*	61 A.A., 8 H.C.	
	Erabutoxin a (TAMIYA et al., 1966)	*Laticauda semifasciata*	62 A.A., 8 H.C.	Curare-like
	Erabutoxin b (TAMIYA et al., 1966)	*Laticauda semifasciata*	62 A.A., 8 H.C.	
	Laticotoxin a (SATO et al., 1969)	*Laticauda laticaudata*	62 A.A., 8 H.C.	
II	γ (IZARD et al., 1969) (f)	*N. nigricollis* (Ethiopia)	60 A.A., 8 H.C.	Cardiotoxin, Cytotoxin
	F_7 (IZARD et al., 1970) (g)	*N. naja philippinensis*	60 A.A., 8 H.C.	
	γ (IZARD et al., 1970) (g)	*Naja haje*	N.D.	
III	F_3 (KARLSSON et al., 1971)	*Naja naja*	71 A.A., 10 H.C.	Curare-like
	III (MIRANDA et al., 1970)	*Naja haje*	71 A.A., 10 H.C.	
	b (BOTES, 1972) (h)	*N. melanoleuca*	71 A.A., 10 H.C.	
	3.9.4. (SHIPOLINI et al., 1974) (i)	*N. melanoleuca*	71 A.A., 10 H.C.	
	α Bungarotoxin (CHANG and LEE, 1963; MEBS et al., 1971)	*Bungarus multicinctus*	74 A.A., 10 H.C.	

Key:
A.A. Amino acid
H.C. = Half-cystine.
N.D. = Not determined.
(a) = Unpublished experiments by DUMAREY et al. (1972). This toxin may be the same as that described by KOPEYAN et al. (1973).
(b) = Unpublished experiments by DUMAREY et al. (1972).
(c) = This variety is now called *N. mossambica.*
(d) = This toxin is identical to that described by MIRANDA et al. (1970).
(e) = This toxin is identical to that described by POILLEUX and BOQUET (1972) and BERGEOT-POILLEUX and BOQUET (1975), which was used in these experiments.
(f) = This toxin is identical to that described by FRYKLUND and EAKER (1975a and b).
(g) = Unpublished experiments by IZARD (1970). Amino acid analysis by MAIRE and HAUERT.
(h) = This toxin is identical to fraction F_6 isolated by POILLEUX and BOQUET (1972), which was used in these experiments.
(i) = This toxin is identical to fraction F_5 isolated by POILLEUX and BOQUET (1972), which was used in these experiments.

(1973a and b) has demonstrated that phylogenic relationships exist between them. There are, however, significant differences between their amino acid composition. The content of evenly distributed lysine residues is higher in the molecules of proteins of group II than in those of proteins of group I. Besides, the amino acids of the N-terminal half of toxins of group II are predominantly hydrophobic, whereas they are hydrophilic in those of group I. Apparently, no antigenic relationship exists between the two groups. This was to be expected. Thus BREW et al. (1967) have made a comparative study of lysozyme and bovine lactalbumin. The molecular weight of the two proteins is of the same order of magnitude and their internal bonds are in the form of disulfide bridges whose arrangement is similar. Both have their origin in a protein diversified by successive mutations. Despite these resemblances, the two proteins differ immunologically (ATASSI et al., 1970). However, a weak but quite definite reciprocal cross-reaction has been demonstrated by passive cutaneous anaphylaxis and passive hemagglutination (STROSBERG et al., 1970; MARON et al., 1972). Will such sensitive immunological methods allow the establishment of antigenic relationships between toxins of group I and II? If this should happen, the limits between the two groups will be obliterated, and group II will become merely a subdivision of group I.

In comparative studies of the immunological properties of three phospholipases extracted from *Naja melanoleuca* venom by JOUBERT (1975a and b) (cf. Table 2) and those of two toxic phospholipases A_2 isolated from *Naja nigricollis* (Ethiopia) venom (cf. Table 2), it has been found that all these enzymes contain common antigenic determinants, this being demonstrated by precipitation in gel by means of two immune sera specific to *Naja nigricollis* (Ethiopia) and *Naja melanoleuca* venoms (DUMAREY and BOQUET, 1975, unpubl.). NAIRN et al. (1975) observed that specific antisera to *Naja naja* and *Naja nigricolis* venoms inhibited *in vitro* phospholipase A_2 activities of the venoms of only closely related species *(Naja melanoleuca)*. It was also reported that acetylcholinesterase of different venoms of *Elapidae* have common antigenic sites (ELLIOTTet al., 1973; KUMAR and ELLIOTT, 1973).

In the same order of facts, BAILEY et al. (1976) reported that the nerve growth factors from five different snake venoms were immunologically related.

The evolutionary changes that occur in the composition and structure of a protein may be very extensive even though its catalytic or toxic activities are not affected. Immunochemical analysis of cytochromes C from various origins (MARGOLIASH et al., 1967; NISONOFF et al., 1970) led to the conclusion that there is a rough correlation between the differences in the amino acid composition of these proteins and their capacity to cross-react immunologically. Following the results of such experiments we have been led to consider the immunological distance separating snake toxins belonging to a group of homologous proteins. Comparative studies of the primary structure of these toxins encouraged the present author and his co-workers to try to establish a hierarchy based on their structural characteristics and their antigenic properties. To this end, a certain number of short curare-like toxins belonging to the immunological group I have been subjected to the test of quantitative precipitation, using reference immune sera (Fig. 6).

A comparison of the antibody-antigen ratio in the so-called equivalence zone allowed us to distribute into three subgroups the following seven short curare-like toxins: α toxin of *Naja nigricollis* (Ethiopia) venom (BOQUET et al., 1966a and b;

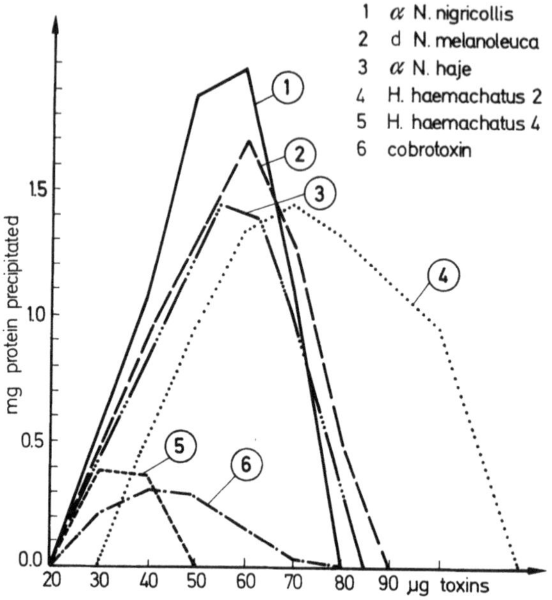

Fig. 6. Quantitative precipitation curves of different toxins (curare-like) of Elapidae venoms, all belonging to immunological group I. The precipitating immune serum is a reference horse anti-venom of *Naja nigricollis* (Ethiopia)

KARLSSON et al., 1966), D toxin of *Naja melanoleuca* venom (BOTES, 1972), α toxin of *Naja haje* venom (BOTES and STRYDOM, 1969), toxins 2 and 4 of *Hemachatus haemachatus* venom (STRYDOM and BOTES, 1971), cobrotoxin of *Naja Naja atra* (YANG et al., 1969) and erabutoxin b of *Laticauda semifasciata* venom (TAMIYA and ARAI, 1966) (cf. Table 2).

Subgroup a includes α toxins [*N. nigricollis* (Ethiopia) and *N. haje*)], D toxin *(N. melanoleuca)*, and toxin 2 *(H. haemachatus)*.

Subgroup b includes cobrotoxin *(N. n. atra)* and toxin 4 *(H. haemachatus)*. No precipitation occurred in the mixtures of erabutoxin b and the reference immune serum anti-*Naja nigricollis* (Ethiopia) venom. However, by affinity chromatography, DETRAIT and BOQUET (unpublished experiments, 1973, 1974), using erabutoxin b covalently linked to Sepharose 4 B, extracted from the same reference immune serum antibodies reacting with the α toxin of *Naja nigricollis* (Ethiopia) venom[1]. No precipitation occurred when these antibodies were mixed with erabutoxin b, but surprisingly they precipitated when in contact with the α toxin. No definite explanation has yet been given for this phenomenon; however, it was concluded that erabutoxin b of *Laticauda semifasciata* venom should be classified in a third *subgroup c*.

If, starting from the N-terminal amino acid, we consider the loops I, II, III, and IV formed by the α toxin molecule of *Naja nigricollis* (Ethiopia) venom (Fig. 7), we find that the three other toxins of subgroup "a" are distinguishable from this last by subtitution at certain residues. As the antibody-antigen ratios in the zone of equiva-

---

[1] Among many immune sera anti-*Naja nigricollis* (Ethiopia) venom tested, only a few precipitated when in contact with the erabutoxins.

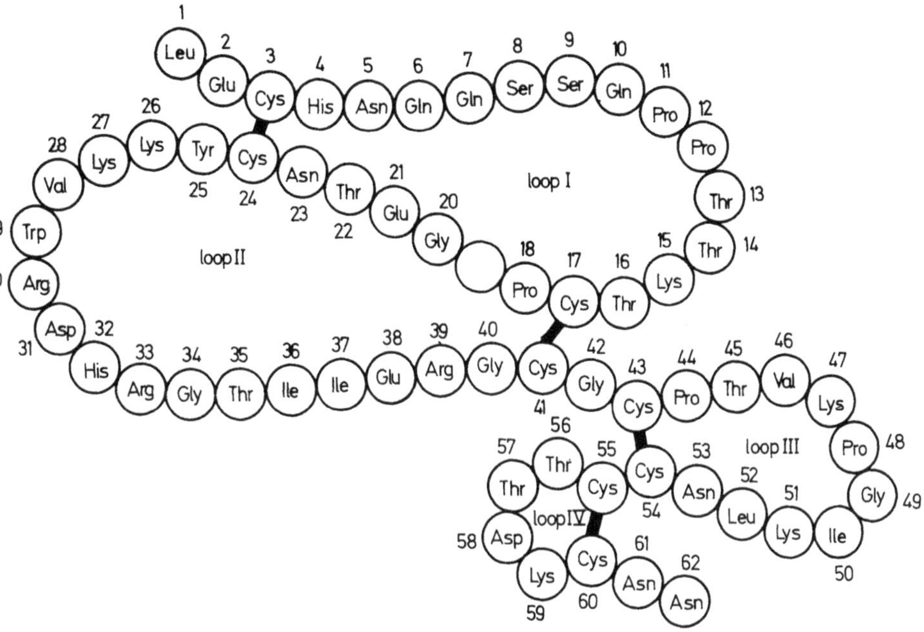

a

TOXINS \ A.A.	1	2	4	7	11	12	15	16	18	19	21	22	23	26	28	30	32	35	36	37	45	48	50	51	52	53	56	57	58	59	61
			LOOP 1											LOOP 2							LOOP 3						LOOP 4				
α N. nigricollis	Leu	Glu	His	Gln	Pro	Pro	Lys	Thr	Pro		Glu	Thr	Asn	Lys	Val	Arg	His	Thr	Ile	Ile	Thr	Pro	Ile	Lys	Leu	Asn	Thr	Thr	Asp	Lys	Asn
d. N. melanoleuca	Met														Gln	Ser					Ser	Lys	Val		Ile					Arg	
α N. haje		Gln													Arg			Ser	Ser	Thr	Ser	Lys		Glu	Ile						
H. haemachatus 2								Ser			Asp			Asn	Arg									Asn		Lys				Arg	
H. haemachatus 4					Thr		Gln								Gln			Ser	Arg	Thr						Lys				Arg	Lys
cobrotoxin					Thr		Thr	Gly	Ser	Gly					Arg			Tyr	Arg	Thr	Ser	Asn		Glu	Ile					Arg	
erabutoxin b	Arg	Ile	Phe	His		Glu				Ser	Ser	Glu	Ser	His	Gln	Ser	Phe									Ser	Glu	Ser	Glu	Val	
TOXINS \ A.A.	1	2	4	7	11	12	15	16	18	19	21	22	23	26	28	30	32	35	36	37	45	48	50	51	52	53	56	57	58	59	61

b

Fig. 7. (a) *Naja nigricollis* (Ethiopia) α toxin. Loops I, II, III, IV. (b) Comparison of amino acid sequences of short curare-like toxins of *Elapidae* venoms, all belonging to immunological group I

lence determined by quantitative precipitation of the four toxins by the same immune serum are closely related, we may consider that the difference of composition of the corresponding chains of amino acids has only little effect on the result of the experiment, and that the antibodies reacting specifically with α toxin of *Naja nigricollis* (Ethiopia) venom react also with the corresponding epitopes of the other toxins but with less affinity.

The differences of composition between α toxin of this venom and the cobrotoxin of *Naja naja atra* venom are much more important and involve 14 amino acid residues. If the substitutions in loop III are comparable with those stated for the α toxin of *Naja haje*, with the exception of amino-acid 48, which is altered from a proline to an asparagine, the main changes occur in the composition of loops I and II. Thus proline-11, lysine-15, and threonine-16 in loop I are replaced by two threonines and one glycine. In the common region of loops I and II, a serine substitutes for a proline 18, and a supplementary amino acid, a glycine, is inserted between this serine and the following glycine, which is common to the three other toxins. Finally, if the only modification of the following 14 amino acid residues of loop II is limited to the substitution of an arginine at the valine 28 as in the α toxin of *Naja haje* venom, the most important changes are located in the distant sequence, Thr 35-Ile 36-Ile 37, which becomes Tyr 35-Arg 36-Thr 37.

The number of substitutions of amino acid residues in toxin 4 of *Hemachatus haemachatus* venom is reduced to nine. As in cobrotoxin, proline 11 is replaced by a threonine. A glutamine substitutes for lysine 15. Amino acid residues 16, 18, 19 are identical in α toxin of *Naja nigricollis* (Ethiopia) venom and in toxin 4 of *Hemachatus haemachatus* venom. The main change is located, as in cobrotoxin, in the sequence Thr 35-Ile 36-Ile 37, which becomes Ser 35-Arg 36-Thr 37.

On the basis of these facts and of the work of RYDEN et al. (1973), who proposed the hypothesis that loop III constitutes a hydrophobic nucleus covered by the other three loops, one is led to suppose that an immunologically active zone could occupy part of loop II. As the modification of tryptophan 29 by Koshland's reagent does not greatly alter the antigenicity of the short curare-like toxins, attention is drawn to the major variation which the composition of the short sequence of amino acid residues 35, 36, and 37 undergoes. Despite the absence of an alteration of the antigenicity of the cobrotoxin molecule following modification of tyrosine 35 noted by HUANG et al. (1973), one is led to the hypothesis that the variation reported influences the composition and in consequence the immunological affinity or specificity of an antigenic site. Such an hypothesis does not imply, in any way, that an epitope could be limited to a short fragment of this second loop, whose largest part, according to the recent observations of LOW et al. (1976) and TSERNOGLOU and PETSKO (1976) is at the surface of the molecule. The participation of other amino acids, which, may be nearby, due to the folding of the chain, cannot be excluded (GABEL et al., 1976).

Still more important alterations of specific antigenicity have been observed in the course of similar experiments performed with erabutoxin b of *Laticauda semifasciata* venom. Eighteen aminoacid residues distinguish this toxin from the α protein of *Naja nigricollis* (Ethiopia) venom. If these are mostly spread along the length of the chain with the exception of an important part of the second loop including the sequence from aminoacid residues 33 to 41, which may include a common antigenic site to both toxins, four of them form the fourth loop. The composition of this is: Thr-Thr-Asp-Lys in α toxin and Glu-Ser-Glu-Val in erabutoxin b, this last loop occupying an exposed region of the molecule (LOW et al., 1976; TSERNOGLOU and PERSKO, 1976). The question remains as to whether or not it is involved as part of an antigenic site. Experiments with synthetic peptides (IVANOV, 1974) should doubtless solve this problem.

In our present state of knowledge, we can draw the following conclusions: the toxins extracted from venoms of *Hydrophiidae* and *Elapidae* can temporarily be divided into three serological groups, and at least three subgroups constitute the serological group I. Two regions of the molecules of the curare-like short toxins may be considered as eventual antigenic sites. There is no evidence that all or part of the active site of short curare-like toxins, i.e., of the regions still undetermined which have a specific affinity for cholinergic receptors, can correspond to an epitope or a part of an epitope. On the other hand, we do not know the mechanism by which the antibodies inhibit the fixation of these toxins onto their specific receptor. If the physiologically active region of the curare-like protein constitutes neither an epitope nor part of an epitope, its inactivation may be considered as the result of steric hindrance by one or several molecules of antibody. It might also be the consequence of a slight modification of the conformation of the toxic molecule produced by antibody fixation, or, lastly the maintenance of a conformation unsuitable to fit on the cholinergic receptor.

D. Nature of Antivenom Antibodies, and Measurement of the Activity of Immune Sera

Our knowledge of the nature of antivenom antibodies is very limited. GRAFIUS and EDWARDS (1958) established that the antibodies specific to the venom of *Crotalus adamanteus*, produced in rabbits, are IgG immunoglobulins. Antibodies of rabbit serum rendered immune by injection of α bungarotoxin belong to the IgG category (CLARK et al., 1972). DETRAIT and BOQUET (1972), having fixed the α toxin from *Naja nigricollis* (Ethiopia) venom onto Sepharose, according to the method of AXEN et al. (1967), extracted specific antibodies to this toxin from a horse serum anti-*Naja nigricollis* venom. These antibodies had all the characteristics of IgT. By the same technique AHARONOV et al. (1974) have separated antibodies to a curare-like toxin of *Naja naja siamensis* venom (cf. Table 2) from the serum of rabbits previously immunized by injections of this toxin. By gel filtration on Sephadex G 100 of a dissociated cobrotoxin—antibody complex with formic acid (0.53 M, pH 2.05), CHANG and YANG (1969) obtained purified rabbit IgG which precipitated specifically cobrotoxin. The purified antibody was digested with papain and the univalent fragments formed soluble antigen-antibody complexes with the toxin. Later on, YANG et al. (1977) obtained non-precipitating antibodies and precipitating antibodies by hyperimmunization of rabbits with cobrotoxin.

No definitive results concerning the problem of the affinity of antibodies reacting with the toxic components of snake venoms have yet been published. Recently, YANG et al. (1977) reported that nonprecipitating antibodies from rabbits immune sera specific to cobrotoxin neutralized this toxin.

One important question was raised years ago, following observations showing that snakes were resistant to their own venoms and sometimes to the injection of venoms of snakes belonging to other species. Soon after, it was demonstrated that the blood of these reptiles contains proteins inhibiting the activity of venoms. Recent studies have shown that the mechanism of the resistance is a complex phenomenon and that the neutralizing proteins might be different from antibodies (OVADIA et al., 1977). These facts will be discussed in the course of another chapter.

For more information about the measurement of activity of antivenom sera for therapeutic use, the reader should turn to the chapter devoted to this problem. We think, however, that it is necessary to remember the opinion expressed on this subject by JERNE and WOOD (1949). According to these authors, the measurement of biological effects of a substance requires that its characteristic action should not be altered by the presence of associated factors. Considering the problem of antivenom titration, JERNE and WOOD came to the conclusion that the main toxins of snake venoms should be separated and each one be used as the test toxin.

These arguments encouraged the author to establish an *in vitro* method for titrating antitoxic antibodies in sera prepared against *Elapidae* venoms. The inhibition *in vivo* of a toxin by its specific antibodies is a complex phenomenon. Our object was to try to find out whether a connection could be established between this phenomenon and the precipitation that occurs *in vitro* when both reagents are mixed. The method of precipitation of antigens by their specific antibodies in a gel seemed suitable for this test. We turned to two classic procedures: radial immunodiffusion according to MANCINI (1965), and immunoelectrophoresis after LAURELL (1965). In both cases, the gel in which the antigen is to diffuse contains a certain proportion of a reference immune serum. The area of the circular zone of precipitation (in MANCINI's method) and the height or the area of the opaque "rocket" defined by electrophoresis, according to LAURELL's technique, are proportional to the quantity of antigen added in the assay. Our technique consisted of pouring a mixture of a constant dose of toxin and increasing quantities of a horse immune serum of unknown activity into the wells in two preparations, one of which was used for immunodiffusion assay and the other for electrophoresis. The toxin that remains uncombined with the antibody diffuses in the gel (in the first preparation) or emigrates under the influence of an electric current (in the second). Thus it is possible to define by difference the quantity of toxin combined to unit volume of immune serum added. Compared to the results of the usual procedure of titration *in vivo*, the results of the two methods were not identical, but there was a constant ratio of about 2 between them. Quantities of *Naja nigricollis* (Ethiopia) α toxin fixed per ml of serum, as defined by the results of immunodiffusion according to MANCINI, and by those of in vivo tests according to CHRISTENSEN (1966a), were of the same order (MANGALO et al., 1977).

The use of special methods is sometimes necessary when a measure of the inhibitory power of specific antibody to a particular component of a venom is required. To our knowledge there are no reference methods in this situation. A mention may be given, however, to the procedure of KONDO et al. (1971a), for measuring the *in vivo* inactivation of hemorrhage-generating factors, and to the *in vitro* assay of antiphospholipases proposed by STANIC (1960).

Generally, immunological procedures can be usefully applied when one wishes to observe the intensity of a reaction between an antigen and corresponding antibodies: quantitative precipitation, hemagglutination, complement fixation, or even the particularly sensitive technique recently proposed by HAIMOVICH et al. (1970), which consists in conjugating a protein and a bacteriophage, and then measuring the degree of inhibition of this bacteriophage by specific immune sera to the protein (AHARONOV et al., 1974). The use of these different procedures sometimes presents difficulties which should be recognized. All immune responses are heterogeneous. The mode of expression depends on the nature of the antigen employed, on the method of immunization, and on other factors. The phenomenon of immune deviation (ASHERSON and STONE, 1965) provides an example of this heterogeneity. According to WHITE et al. (1963) guinea-pigs immunized by injections of a simple water-in-oil emulsion of ovalbumin produced, three weeks later, an antibody response entirely confined to the γ_1 globulins, However, when mycobacteria were added to the emulsion, γ_2 immunoglobins appeared. It is well known that these γ_2 immunoglobins are much more active in complement fixation than the γ_1.

E. Hypersensitivity to Snake Venoms

In 1912, ARTHUS reported that repeated subcutaneous injections of cobra venom, given in nonlethal doses to rabbits, induced a state of anaphylactic sensitivity. SHKENDEROV (1974), studying the anaphylactogenic properties of bee venom, established that the high-molecular-weight proteins such as phospholipase A and hyaluronidase caused sensitization, while the peptides apamin and melittin had no sensitizing action. Our knowledge is still very poor regarding the mechanisms of hypersensitivity to snake venoms and the nature of sensitizing factors.

Researchers who work with venoms in a powder form often become allergic (PARRISH et al., 1957). Spasmodic coryza, asthma, and various edemas are the most frequent symptoms of this allergy (BARRIO, 1954). Sensitization and triggering of clinical symptoms are, sometimes, produced by different venoms (PARRISH et al., 1957). Hypersensitivity states are detected by the usual cutaneous reactions. The Prausnitz-Kustner test provides a diagnosis. Guinea-pigs previously sensitized by subcutaneous injections of 200 µg of *Vipera ammodytes* venom, or by inhalation of this venom, become shocked by the intracardiac administration of a very low dose of the same venom. Isolated uterus from animals sensitized by inhalation contracted not only in response to a very dilute solution of *Vipera ammodytes* venom but also to solutions of *Naja naja* and *Bungarus caeruleus* venoms (STANIC, 1956). This relates to an old observation by HEYMANS (1921): the isolated heart of a rabbit rendered hypersensitive to *Crotalus adamanteus* venom stops in systole, more rapidly than that of an untreated rabbit, when both are perfused with a solution containing a small quantity of the same venom.

F. Action of Snake Venoms on Cellular and Humoral Factors of Immunity

We have described the importance of the role of macrophages and lymphocytes in the production of humoral immunity. Only a few observations suggest that the venoms have a direct action on these cells. Some experiments, however, encourage us to consider possible relationships.

Injection of *Crotalus* venom into a dog does not modify the number of white cells, nor the relative proportions of polymorphonuclear leucocytes, lymphocytes and large monocytes in its blood (ESSEX and MARKOWITZ, 1930). According to REID et al. (1963), the number of blood leucocytes in victims of *Agkistrodom rhodostoma* bites is normal, but intoxication by certain of the *Hydrophiidae* and *Viperidae* venoms is characterized by leucocytosis (REID et al., 1963; EFRATI and REID, 1953). Injection of *Crotalus adamanteus* venom in dogs produced an increase in the proportion of circulating polymorphonuclear leucocytes (RADOMSKI, et al., 1959), but in dogs experimentally injected with *Crotalus atrox* venom the number of basophils in the blood decreases rapidly (OBERER, 1962).

We do not know the effects of venom intoxication on macrophages and lymphocytes. Phospholipase and proteolytic enzymes doubtless contribute to their destruction in envenomated tissues. It appears that the membrane permeability of lymphocytes may be modified in guinea-pigs injected with *Echis carinatus* venom: lymphocytes of the intoxicated animals absorb fluorescein *in vivo* and *in vitro*, and the venom fraction which provokes this alteration is that containing a protease (COHEN et al., 1966). One must consider that proteins of *Elapidae* venoms, known as cardiotoxins, direct lytic factors, cytotoxins, etc., exercise on all cells a very marked effect. Thus, BRAGANCA et al. (1967) extracted from the venom of *Naja naja* a basic protein which had strong cytotoxic effect on Yoshida sarcoma cells. However, human leucocytes, rat lymphocytes and bone marrow cells were less sensitive. This toxin attached to the membrane of the cells (PATEL et al., 1969). Rat monocytes appear to be resistant to cobra venom (SATO et al., 1964). Toxicity of γ toxin of *Naja nigricollis* (Ethiopia) venom for KB cells was demonstrated in vitro by diminution of amino acid transport, nucleotide triphosphate content and oxygen consumption (BOQUET JR, 1970). Finally LEE et al. (1971) extracted three fractions from *Naja naja atra* venom which also exerted cytopathic effects on different types of cultured cells.

The mechanism by which these cytotoxins alter the permeability of the cell membrane has been the subject of many hypotheses (CONDREA, 1974; VOGT et al., 1970; KEUNG et al., 1975). The problem is still to be elucidated and the question remains as to whether or not these proteins, which are contained in relatively high proportion in *Elapidae* venoms, exercise an effect on the behavior of immunologically competent cells.

According to long-established observations by MORGENROTH and KAYA (1908), by COCA (1914) and by HIRSCHFELD and KLINGER (1915), cobra venom deprives guinea-pig serum of its complementary power. At the time of these observations, complement was considered to be a chain formed from four components, two of which were resistant to heating to 56° C. As long ago as 1912, RITZ demonstrated that complement inhibited by cobra venom was reactivated by the addition of serum heated to 56° C. In a careful study of *Bothrops* venom, also an inhibitor of complement, BIER (1932), then TODA and MITSUE (1933), attributed this inhibitory effect to the destruction of one of the late-acting components. The attention of most workers was soon concentrated on the mechanisms of activation of the third component (MUTSAARS and BARTELS-VIROUX, 1947). It is now considered that the activation of the complement system (C) results in the participation of nine different proteins designated by the symbols C_1, C_2, ..., C_9. A chain reaction confers, successively and temporarily, enzymic activities on these proteins. The ultimate manifestations of these activities are defined lesions of cell membranes. Degradation products liberated in the course of these reactions intervene in a number of immunological events, in the development of inflammatory phenomena, and in blood coagulation.

Activation of the third (C_3) component of complement can be considered as an essential step in the series of events whose end result is cytolysis. This activation is the consequence of mechanisms summarized briefly here. Usually the first component, C_1, which is itself composed of three subunits, is fixed by the linking of one of these subunits (C_1q) to a molecule of immunoglobulin M, or to two molecules of immunoglobulin G associated with an antigen, for example an erythrocyte membrane. The adjacent subunit (C_1s) then acquires esterase properties. It activates next C_4, and subsquently C_2. In this way the complex, C_3 convertase, is formed. In its turn it activates C_3. This is the so-called classical pathway, and the reactions continue, resulting in cell lysis. However, other mechanisms, which, by-passing the first step of activation, activate C_3 directly. These alternative activating mechanisms lead to lysis of unsensitized erythrocytes, i.e., to lysis in the absence of antibodies.

According to NELSON (1966), MÜLLER-EBERHARD (1967), COCHRANE et al. (1968), BALLOW and COCHRANE (1969), PICKERING et al. (1969), MÜLLER-EBERHARD (1971), BITTER-SUERMAN et al. (1972), HUNSICKER et al. (1973), a purified anti-complementary protein (mol wt 144000) of *Naja naja* venom (C.V.F.) when complexed with a pro-inactivator, which is a thermolabile 5.55 S globulin, causes inactivation of C_3. However, evidence was presented that constitution of the complex, requires the participation of two seric factors called factor B and D for its full activity. The complex consists of cobra venom factor (C.V.F.) and activated factor B which is a fragment of B cleaved by activated factor D when B is bound to cobra venom factor (C.V.F.). This complex acts like an enzyme and activates C_3. Research workers, then, were led to consider the action of cobra venom not any longer as an inactivator of C_3, but, on the contrary, as an activator (GÖTZE et al., 1970, 1971). The serum "proinactivator" was designed as a "pro-activator" and its action was compared to that of activated C_4C_2 complex (C_4b 2a), the C_3 convertase. The activation of C_3 is then followed by a secondary decay of C_3 fragments (BITTER-SUERMAN et al. 1972).

A second anti-complement factor (mol wt 800000) has been extracted from *Naja naja* venom. However, the site of action of this heavy factor seems to be upon one of the early components of the complement system (BALLOW and COCHRANE, 1969).

The principal effect noted after treatment of animals with the cobra venom factor (C.V.F.) isolated by MÜLLER-EBERHARD (1967) was an inhibition of the accumulation of neutrophil phagocytes at the site of an antigen antibody reaction. The development of the Arthus phenomenon was also prevented (COCHRANE et al., 1970).

It has been suggested that C_3 may play an important part in the induction of antibody response (DUKOR et al., 1974). Activated C_3 was supposed to act as a second signal for B cells inducing the secretion of antibodies, or, when bound to macrophage surfaces, to assist T and B cells cooperation in thymus-dependent response. Experiments by PRYJMA and HUMPHREY (1975) on the response of mice injected with different immunogens after prolonged C_3 depletion by cobra venom factor (C.V.F.) dó not support the hypothesis that C_3 activation is a necessary condition for stimulation of B cells by the T cell-independent immunogens or a sufficient one to enable a T cell-dependent immunogen to escape the need for T-cell help. However, they do not provide arguments to allow one to reject the hypothesis that C_3 activation plays a role in the T-B lymphocyte cooperation.

Having attempted to bring to the fore some of the problems posed by the results of still fragmentary research on the immunology of venoms, the reader is left, by way of a conclusion, with a few lines from a publication of ZIMMERMAN et al. (1971):

> "The highly sensitive methods of immunology are often helpful where other methods fail in demonstrating conformational or structural changes or differences in substances which can evoke and react with antibodies."

Acknowledgements. I am grateful to C. DUMAREY, F. FOUQUE, D. JOSEPH, C. PHILIBERT and A. M. RONSSERAY for their collaboration in the experimental work, to C. DUMAREY for her help to revise the bibliography, and E. MAC CALL for her translation of both chapters:

— "History of snake venom research",
— "Immunological properties of snake venoms".

I also thank Professors D. P. BOTES, C. Y. LEE, N. TAMIYA, and C. C. YANG for their generous gifts of snake toxins.

References

Acher, R.: Evolution de la structure des protéines. Bull. Soc. chim. Biol. (Paris) **49**, 609—611 (1967)

Acher, R.: L'évolution moléculaire au niveau des protéines. Biochimie **56**, 1—19 (1974)

Adler, F. L.: Antibody formation after injection of heterologous immunoglobulin — II. Competition of antigens. J. Immunol. **78**, 201—210 (1957)

Adler, F. L., Moller, G.: Antigenic competition. 1st International Congress of Immunology, Washington. In: Amos, B. (Ed.): Progress in Immunology, pp. 1511—1514. New York: Academic 1971

Aharonov, A., Gurari, D., Fuchs, S.: Immunochemical characterization of *Naja siamensis* toxin and of a chemically modified toxin. Europ. J. Biochem. **45**, 297—303 (1974)

Ajdukovic, A. D., Muic, N.: Double diffusion analysis of the *Vipera ammodytes* venom. Arch. Hig. Rada. Toksikol. **14**, 107—110 (1963)

Akatsuka, K.: Immunological studies of snake venoms. Jap. J. exp. Med. **14**, 147—183 (1936)

Aleksiev, B., Shipolini, R.: Further investigations on the fractionation and purification of the toxic components from the venom of the Bulgarian viper *(Vipera ammodytes ammodytes)*. Hoppe-Seylers Z. physiol. Chem. **352**, 1183—1188 (1971)

Allison, A. C.: The effect of adjuvants on different cell types and their interaction in immune responses. In: Immunopotentation (Ciba Foundation Symposium No. 18), pp. 73—79. Amsterdam: North-Holland 1973

Allison, A. C., Davies, A. J. S.: Requirement of thymus-dependent lymphocytes for potentiation by adjuvants of antibody formation. Nature (Lond.) **233**, 330—332 (1971)

Allison, A. C., Harington, J. S., Birbeck, M.: An examination of cytotoxic effects of silica on macrophages. J. exp. Med. **124**, 141—153 (1966)

Aloof-Hirsch, S., de Vries, A., Berger, A.: The direct lytic factor of cobra venom; purification and chemical characterization. Biochim. biophys. Acta (Amst.) **154**, 53—60 (1968)

Amies, C. R.: The use of topically formed calcium alginate as a depot substance in active immunization. J. Path. Bact. **77**, 435—442 (1959)

Angeletti, R. H.: Studies of the nerve growth factor (NGF) from snake venoms. Gel filtration patterns of crude venoms. J. Chromatogr. **36**, 535—537 (1968)

Angeletti, R. H.: Nerve growth factor from cobra venom. Proc. nat. Acad. Sci. (Wash.) **65**, 668—674 (1970)

Angeletti, R. H., Frazier, W. A., Jacobs, J. W., Niall, H. D., Bradshaw, R. A.: Purification, characterization and partial amino acid sequence of nerve growth factor from cobra venom. Biochemistry **15**, 26—34 (1976)

Arnberg, H., Eaker, D., Fryklund, L., Karlsson, E.: Amino acid sequence of oxiana α, the main neurotoxin of the venom of *Naja naja oxiana*. Biochim. biophys. Acta (Amst.) **359**, 222—232 (1974)

Arnon, R., Sela, M.: Studies on the chemical basis of the antigenicity of proteins. II. Antigenic specificity of polytyrosyl gelatin. Biochem. J. **75**, 103—109 (1960)

Arthus, M.: De la spécificité des sérums antivenimeux. Sérum anticobraïque et venins d'Hamadryas *(Naja bungarus)* et de Krait *(Bungarus coeruleus)*. C.R. Acad. Sci. [D] (Paris) **153**, 394—397 (1911 a)

Arthus, M.: De la spécificité des sérums antivenimeux. Sérum anticobraïque, antibothropique et anticrotalique. Venins de *Lachesis lanceolatus*, de *Crotalus terrificus* et *de Crotalus adamanteus*. C.R. Acad. Sci. [D] (Paris) **153**, 1504—1507 (1911 b)

Arthus, M.: Etudes sur le venin de serpents. III. Envenimation et anaphylaxie. Int. Arch. Physiol. **12**, 271—288 (1912)
Arthus, M.: Venin de Daboïa et extraits d'organes. C.R. Soc. Biol. (Paris) **82**, 1156—1158 (1919)
Arthus, M.: Les anavenins. II. Immunisation par les anavenins. J. Physiol. Path. Gén. **28**, 773—788 (1930a)
Arthus, M.: Les anavenins. III. Anaphylaxie engendrée par les anavenins. J. Physiol. Pathol. Gén. **28**, 800—815 (1930b)
Arthus, M., Stawska, B.: Venins et antivenins. C.R. Acad. Sci. (Paris) **153**, 355—357 (1911)
Asherson, G.L., Stone, S.H.: Selective and specific inhibition of 24 hours skin reactions in the guinea pig. I. Immune deviation: description of the phenomenon and the effect of splenectomy. Immunology **9**, 205—217 (1965)
Askonas, B.A., Jaroskova, L.: Macrophages as helper cells in antibody induction. In: Sterzl, J., Riha, I. (Eds.): Developmental Aspect of Antibody Formation and Structure, Vol. II, pp. 531—546. New York: Academic 1970
Atassi, M.Z.: Antigenic structure of myoglobin: the complete immunochemical anatomy of a protein and conclusions relating to antigenic structure of proteins. Immunochemistry **12**, 423—438 (1975)
Atassi, M.Z., Habeeb, A.F.S.A., Rydstedt, L.: Lack of immunochemical cross-reaction between lysozyme and α lactalbumin and comparison of their conformations. Biochim. biophys. Acta (Amst.) **200**, 184—187 (1970)
Atassi, M.Z., Saplin, B.J.: Immunochemistry of sperm-whale myoglobin. I. The specific interaction of some tryptic peptides and of peptides containing all the reactive region of the antigen. Biochemistry **7**, 688—698 (1968)
Augustyn, J.M., Elliott, W.B.: Isolation of a phospholipase A from *Agkistrodon piscivorus* venom. Biochim. biophys. Acta (Amst.) **206**, 98—108 (1970)
Axen, R., Porath, J., Ernback, S.: Chemical coupling of peptides and proteins to polysaccharides by means of cyanogen halides. Nature (Lond.) **214**, 1302—1304 (1967).
Bailey, G.S., Banks, B.E.C., Carstairs, J.R., Edwards, D.C., Pearce, F.L., Vernon, C.A.: Immunological properties of nerve growth factors. Biochim. biophys. Acta (Amst.) **437**, 259—263 (1976)
Ballow, M., Cochrane, C.G.: Two anticomplementary factors in cobra venom: Hemolysis of guinea pig erythrocytes by one of them. J. Immunol. **103**, 944—952 (1969)
Balozet, L.: Les antigènes des venins de Cerastes et de Lebetine étudiés par la précipitation en milieu gélifié. Arch. Inst. Pasteur Algér. **37**, 292—296 (1959)
Banks, B.E.C., Miledi, R., Shipolini, R.A.: The primary sequences and neuromuscular effects of three neurotoxic polypeptides from the venom of *Dendroaspis viridis*. Europ. J. Biochem. **45**, 457—468 (1974)
Barrio, A.: Alergia al veneno de serpiente cascabel *(Crotalus terrificus terrificus)*. Rev. Inst. Malbran **16**, 219—223 (1954)
Barrio, A., Miranda, M.E.: Estudio comparativo morfologico e immunologico entre las differentes entidades del genero *Micrurus* wagler (Ophidia Elapidae) de la Argentina. Mem. Inst. Butantan **33**, 869—879 (1966)
Baxter, E.H., Gallichio, H.A.: Cross-neutralization by tiger snake *(Notechis scutatus)* antivenene and sea snake *(Enhydrina schistosa)* antivenene against several sea snake venoms. Toxicon **12**, 273—278 (1974)
Bechis, G., Granier, C., Van Reitschoten, J., Jover, E., Rochat, H., Miranda, F.: Purification of six neurotoxins from the venom of *Dendroaspis viridis*. Primary structure of two long toxins. Europ. J. Biochem. **68**, 445—456 (1976)
Behring, E., von, Kitasato, S.: Über das Zustandekommen der Diphtherie-Immunität und der Tetanus-Immunität bei Tieren. Deutsch. med. Wschr. **16**, 1113—1114 (1890)
Benjamini, E., Michaeli, D., Young, J.D.: Antigenic determinants of proteins of defined sequences. In: Current Topics in Microbiology and Immunology, No. 58, pp. 85—134. Berlin: Springer 1972
Bergeot-Poilleux, G., Boquet, P.: Remarques à propos de trois neurotoxines du venin de *Naja melanoleuca*. C.R. Acad. Sci. [D] (Paris) **280**, 1757—1759 (1975)
Bier, O.: Inactivation de l'alexine par le venin de *Bothrops*. Z. Immun.-Forsch. **77**, 187—194 (1932)

Bitter-Suermann, D., Dietrich, M., König, W., Hadding, U.: By pass-activation of the complement system starting with C_3. I. Generation and function of an enzyme from a factor of guinea pig serum and cobra venom. Immunology **23**, 267—281 (1972)

Björk, W.: Partial purification of phosphodiesterase, 5'-nucleotidase, lecithinase A, and acetylcholine esterase from Ringhals cobra venom. Biochim. biophys. Acta (Amst.) **49**, 195—204 (1961)

Blass, J.: A propos de l'absence des taches de tyrosine sur les chromatogrammes des hydrolysats acides des anatoxines. Ann. Inst. Pasteur **101**, 687—702 (1961)

Blass, J., Bizzini, B., Raynaud, M.: Etude sur le mécanisme de la détoxification des toxines protéiques par le formol. II. Fixation quantitative du formol. Ann. Inst. Pasteur **116**, 501—521 (1969)

Blombäck, B., Blombäck, M., Nilsson, I. M.: Coagulation studies on "reptilase", an extract of the venom of *Bothrops jararaca*. Thrombos. Diathes. haemorrh. (Stuttg.) **1**, 76 (1957)

Boche, R. D., Russell, F. E.: Passive hemagglutination studies with snake venom and antivenin. Toxicon **6**, 125—130 (1968)

Bolaños, R., Cerdas, L., Taylor, R.: The production and characteristics of a coral snake *(Micrurus mipartitus hertwigi)* antivenin. Toxicon **13**, 139—142 (1975)

Boman, H. G.: On the specificity of the snake venom phosphodiesterase. Ann. N.Y. Acad. Sci. **81**, 800—803 (1959)

Boman, H. G., Kaletta, U.: Chromatography of rattle snake venom. A separation of three phosphodiesterases. Biochim. biophys. Acta (Amst.) **24**, 619—631 (1957)

Bon, C., Changeux, J. P.: Ceruleotoxin: an acidic neorotoxin from the venom of *Bungarus caerulus* which blocks the response to a cholinergic agonist without binding to the cholinergic receptor site. FEBS Letters **52**, 212—216 (1975)

Bonilla, C. A., Fiero, M. K., Frank, L. P.: Isolation of a basic protein neurotoxin from *Crotalus adamanteus* venom. In: deVries, A., Kochva, E. (Eds.): Toxin of Animal and Plant Origin, Vol. I, pp. 343—359. London: Gordon and Breach 1971

Boquet, P.: Rôle du cuivre en quantités infinitésimales dans l'atténuation des venins de *Vipera aspis* et de *Naja tripudians* et d'une toxine végétale, la ricine, par le peroxyde d'hydrogène. Ann. Inst. Pasteur **66**, 379—396 (1941)

Boquet, P., Detrait, J., Farzanpay, R.: Recherches biochimiques et immunologiques sur le venin des serpents. III. Etude des analogues de l'antigène α du venin de *Naja nigricollis*. Ann. Inst. Pasteur **116**, 522—542 (1969)

Boquet, P., Dumarey, C., Bergeot, G., Ronsseray, A. M.: Immunological properties of some proteins of snake venoms. 4th International Symposium on Animal, Plant, and Microbial toxins. Tokyo 1974

Boquet, P., Dumarey, C., Izard, Y.: Studies on the immunogenic activity of toxin α of *Naja nigricollis* venom. In: Kaiser, E. (Ed.): Animal and Plant Toxins, pp. 211—217. Munich: Goldmann 1973a

Boquet, P., Izard, Y., Detrait, J.: Recherche sur le facteur de diffusion des venins de serpents. C.R. Soc. Biol. (Paris) **152**, 1363–1365 (1958)

Boquet, P., Izard, Y., Jouannet, M., Meaume, J.: Recherches biochimiques et immunologiques sur les venins de serpents. I. Essais de séparation des antigènes du venin de *Naja nigricollis* par filtration sur Sephadex. Ann. Inst. Pasteur **111**, 719—732 (1966a)

Boquet, P., Izard, Y., Jouannet, M., Meaume, J.: Etude de deux antigènes toxiques du venin de *Naja nigricollis*. C.R. Acad. Sci. [D] (Paris) **262**, 1134—1137 (1966b)

Boquet, P., Izard, Y., Meaume, J., Jouannet, M.: Recherches biochimiques et immunologiques sur le venin de serpents. II. Etude des propriétés enzymatiques et toxiques des fractions obtenues par filtration du venin de *Naja nigricollis* sur Sephadex. Ann. Inst. Pasteur **112**, 213—235 (1967)

Boquet, P., Izard, Y., Ronsseray, A. M.: Essai de classification des protéines toxiques extraites des venins de serpents. C.R. Acad. Sci. [D] (Paris) **271**, 1456—1459 (1970)

Boquet, P., Poilleux, G., Dumarey, C., Izard, Y., Ronsseray, A. M.: An attempt to classify the toxic proteins of Elapidae and Hydrophiidae venoms. Toxicon **11**, 333—340 (1973b)

Boquet, P., Saint Girons, H.: Étude immunologique des glandes salivaires du vestibule buccal de quelques *Colubridae opistoglyphes*. Toxicon **10**, 635—644 (1972)

Boquet, P., Vendrely, R.: Influence du pH sur la transformation du venin de cobra en anavenin par l'aldehyde formique; préparation d'un anavenin. solide. C.R. Soc. Biol. (Paris) **137**, 179—180 (1943)
Boquet, P., Jr.: Action de la toxine γ du venin de *Naja nigricollis* sur les cellules KB cultivées "in vitro". C.R. Acad. Sci. (Paris) **271**, 2422—2425 (1970)
Bordet, J. (1899): Quoted in: Bordet, J.: Traité de l'Immunité. Paris: Masson 1920
Botes, D. P.: Purification and amino acid sequence of three neurotoxins from the Cape Cobra *(Naja nivea)*. Toxicon **8**, 125—126 (1970)
Botes, D. P.: The amino acid sequences of toxin α and β from *Naja nivea* venom and the disulfide bonds of toxin α. J. biol. Chem. **246**, 7383—7391 (1971)
Botes, D. P.: Snake venom toxins. The amino acid sequences of toxins b and d from *Naja melanoleuca* venom. J. biol. Chem. **247**, 2866—2871 (1972)
Botes, D. P.: Snake venom toxins. The reactivity of the disulphide bonds of *Naja nivea* toxins. Biochim. biophys. Acta (Amst.) **359**, 242—247 (1974)
Botes, D. P., Strydom, D. J.: A neurotoxin, toxin α, from Egyptian cobra *(Naja haje haje)* venom. J. biol. Chem. **244**, 4147—4157 (1969)
Botes, D. P., Strydom, D. J., Anderson, C. G., Christensen, P. A.: Snake venom toxins. Purification and properties of three toxins from *Naja nivea* (Linneus) (Cape cobra) venom and the amino acid sequence of toxin δ. J. biol. Chem. **246**, 3132—3139 (1971 a)
Botes, D. P., Strydom, D. J., Strydom, A. J. C., Joubert, F. J., Christensen, P. A., Anderson, C. G.: The purification and amino acid sequence of three neurotoxins from the Cape cobra *(Naja nivea)* venom. In: deVries, A., Kochva, E. (Eds.): Toxins of Animal and Plant Origin, Vol. I, pp. 281—292. London: Gordon and Breach 1971 b
Botes, D. P., Viljoen, C. C.: Purification of phospholipase A from *Bitis gabonica* venom. Toxicon **12**, 611—619 (1974)
Botes, D. P., Viljoen, C. C.: The amino acid sequences of three noncurarimimetic toxins from *Naja nivea* venom. Biochim. biophys. Acta (Amst.) **446**, 1—9 (1976)
Bourgeois, J. P., Tsuji, S., Boquet, P., Pillot, J., Ryter, A., Changeux, J. P.: Localization of the cholinergic receptor protein by immunofluorescence in cell electroplax. FEBS Letters **16**, 92—94 (1971)
Brade, V., Vogt, W.: Immunization against cobra venom. Experientia (Basel) **27**, 1338 (1971)
Braganca, B. M., Patel, N. T., Badrinath, P. G.: Isolation and properties of a cobra venom factor selectively cytotoxic to Yoshida sarcoma cells. Biochim. biophys. Acta (Amst.) **136**, 508—520 (1967)
Braun, W., Nakano, M.: Antibody formation: stimulation by polyadenylic and polycitidylic acids. Science **157**, 819—821 (1967)
Brew, K., Vanaman, T. C., Hill, R. L.: Comparison of the amino acid sequence of bovine lactalbumin and hen egg white lysozyme. J. biol. Chem. **242**, 3747—3749 (1967)
Brunton, T. L., Fayrer, J.: On the nature and physiological action of the poison of *Naja tripudians* and other Indian venomous snakes. Proc. roy. Soc. Lond. [Biol.] **22**, 68—133 (1874)
Burnet, F. N.: The Clonal Selection Theory of Acquired Immunity. Nashville,, Ten.: Vanderbilt University Press 1959
Calmette, A.: L'immunisation artificielle des animaux contre le venin des serpents et la thérapeutique expérimentale des morsures venimeuses. C.R. Acad. Sci. [D] (Paris) **118**, 720 (1894 a)
Calmette, A.: Contribution á l'étude du venin des serpents. Immunisation des animaux et traitements de l'envenimation. Ann. Inst. Pasteur **8**, 275—291 (1894 b)
Calmette, A.: Sur l'action hémolytique de venin de cobra. C.R. Acad. Sci. [D] (Paris) **134**, 1446—1447 (1902)
Calmette, A.: Les Venins, les Animaux Venimeux et la Sérothéraphie Antivenimeuse. Paris: Masson 1907
Calmette, A., Massol, L.: Les précipitines du sérum antivenimeux vis à vis-du-venin de cobra. Ann. Inst. Pasteur **23**, 155—165 (1909)
Carey, J. E., Wright, E. A.: Isolation of the neurotoxic component of the venom of the sea snake "*Enhydrina schistosa*". Nature (Lond.) **185**, 103—104 (1960)
Carey, J. E., Wright, E. A.: Studies on the fractions of the venom of the sea snake "*Enhydrina schistosa*". Aust. J. exp. Biol. med. Sci. **40**, 427—435 (1962)

Carlsson, F. H.: Snake venom toxins. The primary structure of protein S_4C_{11}. A neurotoxin homologue from the venom of forest cobra *(Naja melanoleuca)*. Biochim. biophys. Acta (Amst.) **400**, 310—321 (1975)

Carlsson, F. H.: Snake venom toxins. The primary structures of two novel cytotoxin homologues from the venom of forest cobra *(Naja melanoleuca)*. Biochem. biophys. Res. Commun. **59**, 269—275 (1974)

Carlsson, F. H., Joubert, F. J.: The isolation and purification of three cytotoxin homologues from the venom of forest *(Naja melanoleuca)* and the complete amino acid sequence of toxin V^{11} 1. Biochim. biophys. Acta (Amst.) **336**, 453—469 (1974)

Celada, F.: The cellular basis of immunologic memory. Prog. Allergy (Basel) **15**, 223—267 (1971)

Cesari, E., Boquet, P.: Recherches sur les antigènes des venins et les anticorps des sérums antivenimeux. I. Venin de *Vipera aspis* et sérums antivipérins *(V. aspis)*. Ann. Inst. Pasteur **55**, 307—330 (1935)

Cesari, E., Boquet, P.: Recherches sur les antigènes des venins et les anticorps des sérumss antivenimeux. II. Venin de *Cerastes cornutus* et sérums antiviperins *(C. cornutus)*. Ann. Inst. Pasteur **56**, 171—196 (1936a)

Cesari, E., Boquet, P.: Recherches sur les antigènes des venins et les anticorps des sérums antivenimeux. III. Venin de *Naja tripudians* et sérum anti-cobraique. Ann. Inst. Pasteur **56**, 511—535 (1936b)

Cesari, E., Boquet, P.: Détoxication du venin de *Vipera aspis* par le ricinoléate de soude; vaccination du lapin par le venin détoxiqué. C.R. Soc. Biol. **125**, 231—234 (1937)

Cesari, E., Boquet, P.: Sur le mécanisme de la détoxication du venin de *Vipera aspis* par l'aldéhyde formique. C.R. Soc. Biol. (Paris) **130**, 19—22 (1939)

Chang, C. C.: Immunological studies on fluorescein-thiocarbamylated and reduced S-carboxymethylated cobrotoxin. J. Biochem. (Tokyo) **67**, 343—352 (1970)

Chang, C. C., Hayashi, K.: Chemical modification of the tryptophan residue in "Cobrotoxin". Biochem. biophys. Res. Commun. **37**, 841—846 (1969)

Chang, C. C., Lee, C. Y.: Cholinesterase and anticholinesterase activities in snake venoms. J. Formosan med. Ass. **54**, 103—112 (1955)

Chang, C. C., Lee, C. Y.: Isolation of neurotoxins from the venom of *Bungarus multicinctus* and their mode of neuromuscular blocking action. Arch. int. Pharmacodyn. **144**, 241—257 (1963)

Chang, C. C., Yang, C. C.: Immunochemical studies on "Cobrotoxin". J. Immunol. **102**, 1437—1444 (1969)

Chang, C. C., Yang, C. C.: Immunochemical studies on the tryptophan-modified cobrotoxin. Biochim. biophys. Acta (Amst.) **295**, 595—604 (1973)

Chang, C. C., Yang, C. C., Hamaguchi, K., Nakai, K., Hayashi, K.: Studies on the status of tyrosyl residues in cobrotoxin. Biochim. biophys. Acta (Amst.) **236**, 164—173 (1971)

Changeux, J. P., Kasai, M., Lee, C. Y.: Use of a snake venom toxin to characterize the cholinergic receptor protein. Proc. nat. Acad. Sci. (Wash.) **67**, 1241—1247 (1970)

Chaudhury, D. K.: Studies on cholinesterase. Ann. Biochem. exp. Med. **6**, 91 (1946)

Chedid, L., Audibert, F., Bona, C.: Activités adjuvantes et mitogènes de lipopolysaccharides détoxifiées. C.R. Acad. Sci. [D] (Paris) **280**, 1197—1200 (1975)

Cheng, H. C., Ouyang, C.: Isolation of coagulant and anticoagulant principles from the venom of *Agkistrodon acutus*. Toxicon **4**, 235—243 (1967)

Chicheportiche, R., Rochat, C., Sampieri, F., Lazdunski, M.: Structure—function relationships of neurotoxins isolated from *Naja haje* venom. Physico-chemical properties and identification of the active site. Biochemistry **11**, 1681—1691 (1972)

Chicheportiche, R., Vincent, J. P., Kopeyan, C., Schweitz, H., Lazdunski, M.: Structure-function relationship in the binding of snake neurotoxins to the Torpedo membrane receptor. Biochemistry **14**, 2081—2091 (1975)

Christensen, P. A.: Formol detoxication of Cape cobra *(Naja flava)* venom. S. Afr. J. med. Sci. **12**, 71—75 (1947)

Christensen, P. A.: Problems of antivenene standardization revealed by the flocculation reaction. Bull. Wld Hlth Org. **9**, 353—370 (1953)

Christensen, P. A.: South African Snake Venoms and Antivenoms. Johannesburg: S. Afr. Inst. med. Res. 1955a

Christensen, P. A.: The ability of antivenom to inhibit the skin reaction and various "in vitro" reactions caused by venom. In: S. Afr. Snake Venoms and Antivenoms. Johannesburg: S. Afr. Inst. Med. Res. 1955 b
Christensen, P. A.: Venom and antivenom potency estimation. Mem. Inst. Butantan **33** (I), 305—326 (1966 a)
Christensen, P. A.: The preparation and purification of antivenoms. Mem. Inst. Butantan **33** (I), 245—250 (1966 b)
Christensen, P. A.: Venoms of central and south African snakes. In: Bücherl, W., Buckley, E., Delofeu, V. (Eds.): Venomous Animals and their Venoms, Vol. I, pp. 437—461. New York: Academic 1968
Christensen, P. A., Anderson, C. G.: Observations on *Dendroaspis* venoms. In: Russell, F. E., Saunders, P. R. (Eds.): Animals' Toxins, pp. 223—234. New York: Pergamon 1967
Clark, D. G., MacMurchie, D. D., Elliott, E., Wolcott, R. G., Landel, A. M., Raftery, M. A.: Elapid neurotoxins. Purification, characterization, and immunochemical studies of α bungarotoxin. Biochemistry **11**, 1663—1668 (1972)
Coca, A. F.: A study of anticomplementary action of yeast of certain bacteria and of cobra-venom. Z. Immun.-Forsch. **21**, 604—622 (1914)
Cochrane, C. G., Müller-Eberhard, H. J., Aikin, B. S.: Depletion of plasma complement "in vivo" by a protein of cobra venom: its effect on various immunologic reactions. J. Immunol. **105**, 55—69 (1970)
Cochrane, C. G., Müller-Eberhard, H. J., Fjellstrom, K. E.: Capacity of a cobra venom protein to inactivate the third component (C'3) and to inhibit immunologic reactions. J. clin. Invest. **47**, 21 a (1968)
Cohen, I., Djaldetti, M., Sanbank, U., Klibansky, C., de Vries, A.: Fluorescein staining of guinea pig lymphocytes induced by *Echis colorata* venom. Experientia (Basel) **22**, 662 (1966)
Cohen, I., Zur, M., Kaminsky, E., de Vries, A.: Isolation and characterization of kinin releasing enzyme of *Echis coloratus* venom. Toxicon **7**, 3—4 (1969)
Cohen, P., Berkeley, W. H., Seligmann, E. B., Jr.: Coral snake venoms: "in vitro" relation of neutralizing and precipitating antibodies. Amer. J. trop. Med. Hyg. **20**, 646—649 (1971)
Cohen, P., Seligmann, E. B., Jr.: Immunologic studies of coral snake venom. Mem. Inst. Butantan **33**, (1) 339—347 (1966)
Coles, E., McIlwain, D. L., Rapport, M. M.: The activity of pure phospholipase A_2 from *Crotalus atrox* venom on myelin and pure phospholipids. Biochim. biophys. Acta (Amst.) **337**, 68—78 (1974)
Collins, J. P., Jones, J. G.: Studies on the active site of IRC-50 Arvin, the purified coagulant enzyme from *Agkistrodon rhodostoma* venom. Europ. J. Biochem. **26**, 510—517 (1972)
Condrea, E.: Membrane-active polypeptides from snake venoms; cardiotoxins and haemocytotoxins. Experientia (Basel) **30**, 121—129 (1974)
Coutinho, A., Moller, G.: Thymus-independent B-cell induction and paralysis. Advance Immunol. **21**, 133—236 (1975)
Criley, B. R.: Development of a multivalent antivenin for the family of Crotalidae venoms. In: Buckley, E., Porges, N. (Eds.): Venoms, pp. 373—380. Amer. Ass. Adv. Sci., pub. No. 44. Washington 1956
Crumpton, M. J., Wilkinson, J. M.: The immunological activity of some of the chymotryptic peptides of sperm-whale myoglobin. Biochem. J. **94**, 545—556 (1965)
Cunningham, D. D.: The physiological action of snake venoms. Sci. Mem. med. Offs. India, **9**, (1895) (quoted by Phisalix, M.: Les Animaux Venimaux et les Venins. Paris: Masson (1922)
Deems, R. A., Dennis, E. A.: Characterization and physical properties of the major form of phospholipase A_2 from cobra venom *(Naja naja naja)* that has a molekular weight of 11000. J. biol. Chem. **250**, 9008—9012 (1975)
De Garilhe, M. P., Laskowski, M.: Chromatographic purification of phosphodiesterase from rattle snake venom. Fed. Proc. **14**, 200 (1955 a)
De Garilhe, M. P., Laskowski, M.: Studies of the phosphodiesterase from rattlesnake venom. Biochim. biophys. Acta (Amst.) **18**, 370—378 (1955 b)
De Kok, A., Rawitch, A. B.: Studies on L-amino acid oxidase. II. Dissociation and characterization of its subunits. Biochemistry **8**, 1405—1411 (1969)

Delezenne, C., Ledebt, S.: Action du venin de cobra sur le sérum de cheval. Ses rapports avec l'hémolyse. C.R. Acad. Sci. [D] (Paris) **152**, 790—792 (1911a)
Delezenne, C., Ledebt, S.: Formation de substances hémolytiques et toxiques aux dépens du vitellus de l'oeuf soumis à l'action du venin de cobra. C.R. Acad. Sci. [D] (Paris) **153**, 81—84 (1911b)
Delezenne, C., Morel, H.: Action catalytique des venins de serpents sur les acides nucléiques. C.R. Acad. Sci. [D] (Paris) **168**, 244—246 (1919)
Delori, P.: Isolement, purification et étude d'une phospholipase A_2 toxique du venin de *Vipera berus*. Biochimie **53**, 941—942 (1971)
Delori, P.: Purification et propriétés physicochimiques, chimiques et biologiques d'une phospholipase A_2 toxique isolée du venin de serpent Viperidae: *Vipera berus*. Biochimie **55**, 1031—1045 (1973)
Delori, P., Miranda, F., Rochat, H.: Recent progress in immunological study of scorpions and snakes venoms and toxins (Abstract). 4th International Symposium on Animal, Plant and Microbial Toxins. Tokyo 1974
Detrait, J., Boquet, P.: Séparation des constituants du venin de *Naja naja* par électrophorèse. C.R. Acad. Sci. [D] (Paris) **246**, 1107—1109 (1958)
Detrait, J., Boquet, P.: Isolement des anticorps antitoxine α_1 du venin de *Naja nigricollis* au moyen du Sépharose. C.R. Acad. Sci. [D] (Paris) **274**, 1765—1767 (1972)
Detrait, J., Izard, Y., Boquet, P.: Séparation par électrophorèse des constituants toxiques des venins de *Naja naja* et de *Naja nigricollis*. C.R. Soc. Biol. (Paris) **153**, 1722—1724 (1959)
Deutsch, H.F., Diniz, C.R.: Some proteolytic activities of snake venoms. J. biol. Chem. **216**, 17—26 (1955)
Diener, E., Feldman, M.: Relationships between antigen and antibody induced suppression of immunity. Transplant Rev. **8**, 76—102 (1972)
Dimitrov, G., Kankonkar, R.C.: Fractionation of *Vipera russellii* venom by gel filtration. Toxicon **5**, 213—221 (1968)
Doery, H.M., Pearson, J.E.: Haemolysins in venoms of Australian snakes. Observations on the haemolysins of the venoms of some Australian snakes and the separation of phospholipase A from the venom of *Pseudechis porphyriacus*. Biochem. J. **78**, 820—827 (1961)
Dresser, D.W.: Specific inhibition of antibody production. III. Paralysis induced in adult mice by small quantities of protein antigen. Immunology **5**, 378—388 (1962)
Dresser, D.W., Mitchison, N.A.: The mechanism of immunological paralysis. Advanc. Immunol. **8**, 129—181 (1968)
Dresser, D.W., Phillips, J.M.: The cellular target for the action of adjuvants: T adjuvant. In: Immunopotentation (Ciba Foundation Symposium no. 18). pp. 2—28. Amsterdam: North-Holland 1973
Dubnoff, J.W., Russell, F.E.: Isolation of a lethal protein and peptide from *Crotalus viridis helleri* venom. Proc. West Pharmacol. Soc. **13**, 98 (1970)
Dukor, P., Schumann, G., Gisles, R.H., Dierich, M., König, W., Hadding, U., Bitter-Suermann, D.: Complement-dependent B-cell activation by cobra factor and other mitogens. J. exp. Med. **139**, 337—354 (1974)
Dumarey, C.: Recherches biochimiques et immunologiques sur le venin des serpents. IV. Action de l'aldéhyde formique sur la toxine alpha du venin de *Naja nigricollis*. Ann. Inst. Pasteur **121**, 675—688 (1971)
Dumarey, C., Boquet, P.: Pouvoir immunogène de la toxine α du venin de *Naja nigricollis* polymérisée par l'aldéhyde formique. C.R. Acad. Sci. [D] (Paris) **275**, 3053—3055 (1972)
Dumarey, C., Sket, D., Joseph, D., Boquet, P.: Étude d'une phospholipase basique du venin de *Naja nigricollis*. C.R. Acad. Sci. [D] (Paris) **280**, 1633—1635 (1975)
Duran-Reynals, F.: Content in spreading factor and toxins in organs and poisonous secretions of snakes. Proc. Soc. exp. Biol. (N.Y.) **38**, 763—766 (1938)
Dutton, W., Falkoff, R., Hirst, J.A., Hoffmann, M., Kappler, J.W., Kettman, J.R., Lesley, J.F., Vann, D.: Is there evidence for a non-antigen specific diffusable chemical mediator from the thymus-derived cell in the initiation of the immune response? (1st International Congress of Immunology). In: Amos, B. (Ed.): Progress in Immunology, pp. 355—368. New York: Academic 1971

Eagle, H.: The coagulation of blood by snake venoms and its physiologic significance. J. exp. Med **65**, 613—639 (1937)
Eaker, D.: Snake venom toxins reacting post and pre-synaptically at the neuromuscular junction. Bull. Inst. Pasteur **74**, Abstr. 9 (1976)
Eaker, D., Halpert, J., Fohlman, J., Karlsson, E.: Structural nature of presynaptic neurotoxins from the venoms of the Australian tiger snake *(Notechis scutatus scutatus)* and Taipan *(Oxyuranus scutellatus scutellatus)*. 4th International Symposium an Animal, Plant, and Microbial Toxins, Tokyo 1974
Eaker, D., Porath, J.: The amino acid sequence of a neurotoxin from *Naja nigricollis* venom. (Abstract) Jap. J. Microbiol. **11**, 353—355 (1967)
Efrati, P., Reif, L.: Clinical and pathological observations on sixtyfive cases of viper bites in Israel. Am. J. trop. Med. Hyg. **2**, 1085—1108 (1953)
Egberg, N., Blombäck, M., Johnsson, H.: Clinical and experimental studies on reptilase. Thrombosis (Suppl.) **47**, 379—387 (1971)
Elliot, R. H.: An account of some researches into the nature and action of snake venoms. Brit. med. J. **1900 I**, 309—313
Elliot, R. H.: A contribution to the study of the action of India cobra. Phil. Trans. B **197**, 361—406 (1905)
Elliott, W. B., McLean, R. L., Massaro, E. J.: Immunological identity of esterases present in elapid venoms. In: Kaiser, E. (Ed.): Animal and Plant Toxins, pp. 104—110. Munich: Goldmann 1973
Epstein, D.: The pharmacology of the venom of the Cape cobra *(Naja flava)*. Q.J. exp. Physiol. **20**, 7—19 (1930)
Esnouf, M. P., Tunnah, G. W.: The isolation and properties of the thrombin-like activity from *Agkistrodon rhodostoma* venom. Brit. J. Haematol. **13**, 581—590 (1967)
Essex, H. E., Markowitz, J.: The physiologic action of rattlesnake venom (Crotalin) III. The influence of crotalin on blood, "in vitro" and "in vivo". Amer. J. Physiol. **92**, 335—341 (1930)
Fayrer, J.: On the action of cobra poison, Edinb. med. J. **14**, 522—529, 915—923, 966—1011 (1868—1869)
Feldman, M.: Cell interaction in the immune response "in vitro". II. The requirement for macrophages in lymphoid cell collaboration. J. exp. Med. **135**, 1049—1058 (1972)
Feldman, M., Unanue, E. R.: Macrophages: Their role in the induction of immunity. In: Amos, B. (Ed.): Progress in Immunology, pp. 1379—1382. New York: Academic 1971
Felix, F., Potter, J. L., Laskowski, M.: Action of venom phosphodiesterase on deoxyribonucleotides carrying a mono-esterified phosphate on carbon 3'. J. biol. Chem. **235**, 1150 (1960)
Ferreira, S. H., Bartelt, D. C., Greene, L. J.: Isolation of bradykinin-potentiating peptides from *Bothrops jararaca* venom. Biochemistry **9**, 2583—2593 (1970)
Flexner, S., Noguchi, H.: Snake venom in relation to haemolysis, bacteriolysis and toxicity. J. exp. Med. **6**, 277—301 (1902)
Flowers, H. H.: Effects of X-irradiation on the antigenic character of *Agkistrodon piscivorus* (cotton mouth moccassin) venom. Toxicon **3**, 301—304 (1966)
Fohlman, J., Eaker, D.: Isolation and characterization of a lethal myotoxic phospholipase A from the venom of the common sea snake *Erhydrina schistosa* causing myoglobinuria. Toxicon **15**, 385—394 (1977)
Fohlmann, J., Eaker, D., Karlsson, E., Thesleff, S.: Taipoxin, an extremely potent presynaptic neurotoxin from the venom of the Australian snake Taipan *(Oxyuranus scutellatus)*. Isolation, characterization, quaternary structure and pharmacological properties. Europ. J. Biochem. **68**, 457—469 (1976)
Fraenkel-Conrat, H., Olcott, H. S.: Reaction of formaldehyde with protein. VI. Cross-linking of amino groups with phenol, imidazole, or indole groups. J. biol. Chem. **174**, 827—843 (1948)
Fraenkel-Conrat, H., Singer, B.: Fractionation and composition of "Crotoxin". Arch. biochem. Biophys. **60**, 64—73 (1956)
Fraser, T. R.: The rendering of animals immune against the venom of the Cobra and other serpents and on the antidotal properties of the blood serum of the immunized animals. Brit. med. J. **1895a I**, 1309—1312
Fraser, T. R.: The treatment of snake poisoning with antivenin derived from animals protected against serpent's venom. Brit. med. J. **1895b II**, 416

Frischauf, A. M., Eckstein, F.: Purification of a phosphodiesterase from *Bothrops atrox* venom by affinity chromatography. Europ. J. Biochem. **32**, 479—485 (1973)

Frost, P., Lance, E. M.: The relation of lymphocyte trapping to the mode of action of adjuvants. In: Immunopotentation (Ciba Foundation Symposium No. 18), pp. 29—45. Amsterdam: North-Holland 1973

Fryklund, L., Eaker, D.: Complete amino acid sequence of the non neurotoxic hemolytic protein from the venom of *Hemachatus haemachatus* (African ringhals cobra). Biochemistry **12**, 661—667 (1973)

Fryklund, L., Eaker, D.: The complete amino acid sequence of cardiotoxin from the venom of *Naja naja* (Cambodian cobra). Biochemistry **14**, 2860—2865 (1975a)

Fryklund, L., Eaker, D.: The complete covalent structure of a cardiotoxin from the venom of *Naja nigricollis* (African black-necked spitting cobra). Biochemistry **14**, 2865—2871 (1975b)

Fryklund, L., Eaker, D., Karlsson, E.: The amino acid sequences of the two principal neurotoxins of *Enhydrina schistosa* venom. Biochemistry **11**, 4633—4640 (1972)

Furukawa, Y., Matsunaga, Y., Hayashi, K.: Purification and characterization of a coagulant protein from the venom of Russell's viper. Biochem. biophys. Acta **453**, 48—61 (1976)

Gabel, D., Rasse, D., Scheraga, H. A.: Search for low-energy conformations of a neurotoxic protein by means of predicative rules, test for hard sphere overlaps and energy minimization. Int. J. Pept. Prot. Res. **8**, 237—252 (1976)

Gall, D.: The adjuvant activity of aliphatic nitrogenous bases. Immunology **11**, 369—386 (1966)

Georgatsos, J. G., Laskowski, M.: Purification of an endonuclease from the venom of *Bothrops atrox*. Biochemistry **1**, 288—295 (1962)

Gerson, R. K., Kondo, K.: Antigenic competition between heterologous lymphocytes. J. Immunol. **106**, 1524—1531; 1532—1539 (1971)

Ghosh, B. N.: Enzymes in snake venom. I. Action on hemoglobin and on protein solutions of different pH. J. Indian chem. Soc. **13**, 450—455 (1936)

Ghosh, B. N., De, S. S.: Investigation on the isolation of the neurotoxin and haemolysin of cobra (*Naja naja*) venom. Indian J. med. Res. **25**, 779—786 (1938)

Githens, T. S., Wolff, N. O'C.: The polyvalency of crotalidic antivenins. II. Comparison of polyvalent crotalidic antivenin with monovalent *Crotalus d. durissus* antivenin. J. Immunol. **37**, 41—45 (1939)

Gitter, S., Levi, G., Kochwa, S., de Vries, A., Rechnic, J., Casper, J.: Studies on the venom of "*Echis colorata*". Amer. J. trop. Med. Hyg. **9**, 391—399 (1960)

Götze, O., Müller-Eberhard, H. J.: Lysis of erythrocytes by complement in the absence of antibody. J. exp. Med. **132**, 898—915 (1970)

Götze, O., Müller-Eberhard, H. J.: The C3 activation system; an alternate pathway of complement activation. J. exp. Med. **134**, 90—108 (1971)

Gonçalves, J. M.: Purification and properties of Crotamine. In: Buckley, E., Porges, N. (Eds.): Venoms, pp. 261—274. Amer. Ass. Adv. Sci., pub. No. 44. Washington 1956a

Gonçalves, J. M.: Estudos sobre venenos de serpentes brasileiras. II. *Crotalus terrificus crotaminicus* subspecie biologica. Ann. Acad. Brasil. Cienc.(Buenos Aires) **28**, 365—367 (1956b)

Goucher, C. R., Flowers, H. H.: The chemical modification of necrogenic and proteolytic activities of *Agkistrodon piscivorus* venom and the use of EDTA to produce a venom toxoid. Toxicon **2**, 139—147 (1964)

Grabar, P., Williams, C. A.: Methode immuno-électrophorétique d'analyse de mélanges de substances antigéniques. Biochim. biophys. Acta (Amst.) **17**, 67—74 (1955)

Grafius, M. A., Edwards, H. N.: An electrophoretic study of the antibody production in rabbits immunized against rattlesnake venom. Naval. Med. Field Res. Lab. **8**, 133—154 (1958)

Grasset, E.: Sur les rapports de spécificité des antigènes venimeux dans la polyvalence et le titrage des sérums antivenimeux. Bull. Org. Hyg., S.D.N. **5**, 407—431 (1936)

Grasset, E.: Anavenoms and their use in the preparation of antivenomous sera. Polyvalent anti-*Bitis arietans*—*Naja flava* serum and specific antivenenes against African viperine and colubrine venoms. Trans. roy. Soc. trop. Med. Hyg. **38**, 463—468 (1945)

Grasset, E., Pongratz, E., Brechbuhler, T.: Analyse immunochimique des constituants des venins de serpents par la méthode de précipitation en milieu gélifié. Ann. Inst. Pasteur **91**, 162—186 (1956)

Grasset, E., Schaafsma, A.: Recherches sur les venins des Colubridés opisthoglyphes africains. I. *Dispholidus typus*. Bull. Soc. Path. Exot. **33**, 114—131 (1940)
Grasset, E., Zoutendyk, A.: Méthode rapide de préparation de sérums antivenimeux polyvalents-antivipéridés et cobras au moyen des anavenins formolés. C.R. Soc. Biol. (Paris) **111**, 432—444 (1932)
Grishin, E. V., Sukhikh, A. P., Adamovich, T. B., Ovchinnikov, Yu. A., Yukelson, L. Ya.: The isolation and sequence determination of a cyotoxin from the venom of the middle Asian cobra *Naja naja oxiana*. FEBS Letters **48**, 179—183 (1974a)
Grishin, E. V., Sukhikh, A. P., Ovchinnikov, Yu. A.: Structural studies of the toxic components of the cobra *Naja naja oxiana* venom. (Abstract). 4th International Symposium on Animal, Plant, and Microbial Toxins, Tokyo, 1974b
Grishin, E. V., Sukhikh, A. P., Lukyanchud, N. N., Slobodyan, L. N., Lipkin, V. M., Ovchinnikov, Yu. A.: Amino acid sequence of neurotoxin II from *Naja naja oxiana* venom. FEBS Letters **36**, 77—78 (1973)
Grotto, L., Moroz, C., de Vries, A., Goldblum, N.: Isolation of *Vipera palestinae* hemorrhagin and distinction between its hemorrhagic and proteolytic activities. Biochim. biophys. Acta (Amst.) **133**, 356—362 (1967)
Gulland, J. M., Jackson, E. M.: Phosphoesterases of bone and snake venoms. Biochem. J. **32**, 590—596 (1938a)
Gulland, J. M., Jackson, E. M.: 5-Nucléotidase. Biochem. J. **32**, 597—601 (1938b)
Gumaa, K. A., Osman, O. H., Kertesz, G.: Distribution of I^{125}-labelled *Bitis arietans* venom in the rat. Toxicon **12**, 565—568 (1974)
Habermann, E., Rübsamen, K.: Biochemical and pharmacological analysis of the so-called crotoxin. In: De Vries, A., Kochva, E. (Eds.): Toxins of Animal and Plant Origin, Vol. I, pp. 333—341. London: Gordon and Breach 1971
Hachimori, Y., Wells, M. A., Hanahan, D. J.: Observations on the phospholipase A_2 of *Crotalus atrox*. Molecular weight and other properties. Biochemistry **10**, 4084—4089 (1971)
Haimovich, J., Hurwitz, E., Novik, N., Sela, M.: Preparation of protein bacteriophage conjugates and their use in detection of anti-protein antibodies. Biochim. biophys. Acta (Amst.) **207**, 115—124 (1970)
Halpert, J., Eaker, D.: Amino acid sequence of a presynaptic neurotoxin from the venom of *Notechis scutatus scutatus* (Australian tiger snake). J. biol. Chem. **250**, 6990—6997 (1975)
Hamberg, U., Rocha e Silva, M.: Release of bradykinin as related to the esterase activity of trypsin and of the venom of *Bothrops jararaca*. Experientia (Basel) **13**, 489—490 (1957)
Hanna, M. G., Jr., Francis, M. W., Peters, L. C.: Localization of ^{125}I-labelled antigen in germinal centres of mouse spleen: effects of competitive injection of specific or non-cross-reacting antigen. Immunology **15**, 75—91 (1968)
Hanna, M. G., Peters, L. C.: The effect of antigen competition on both the primary and secondary immune capacity in mice. J. Immunol. **104**, 166—177 (1970)
Hauert, J., Maire, M., Sussmann, A., Bargetzi, J. P.: The major lethal neurotoxin of the venom of *Naja naja philippinensis*. Int. J. Pept. Prot. Res. **6**, 201—222 (1974)
Hayashi, K., Takechi, M., Sasaki, T.: Amino acid sequence of cytotoxin I from the venom of the Indian cobra *(Naja naja)*. Biochem. biophys. Res. Commun. **45**, 1357—1362 (1971)
Hayashi, K., Takechi, M., Sasaki, T., Lee, C. Y.: Amino acid sequence of cardiotoxin-analogue I from the venom of *Naja naja atra*. Biochem. biophys. Res. Commun. **64**, 360—366 (1975)
Heinrikson, L. H., Krueger, E. E., Keim, F. S.: Amino acid sequence of phospholipase A_2 from the venom of *Crotalus adamanteus*. A new classification of phospholipases A_2 based upon structural determinants. J. biol. Chem. **252**, 4913—4921 (1977)
Henriques, O. B., Lavras, A. A. C., Fichman, M., Mandelbaum, F. R., Henriques, S. B.: The proteolytic activity of the venom of "*Bothrops jararaca*". Biochem. J. **68**, 597—605 (1958)
Henriques, O. B., Mandelbaum, F. R., Henriques, S. B.: Proteolytic enzymes of *Bothrops* venom. Mem. Inst. Butantan **33**, 359—369 (1966)
Heremans, J. F.: Les Globulines Sériques du Système γ. Brussels: Arscia; Paris: Masson 1960
Heymans, C.: Sur l'anaphylaxie du coeur isolé du lapin. C.R. Soc. Biol. (Paris) **85**, 419—420 (1921)
Hirschfeld, L., Klinger, R.: The inactivation of the serum by cobra poison. Biochem. Z. **70**, 398 (1915)

Horst, J., Hendon, R. A., Fraenkel-Conrat, H.: The active components of Crotoxin. Biochem. biophys. Res. Commun. **46**, 1042—1045 (1972)
Houssay, B. A., Negrete, J.: Propriedades precipitantes espicificas de los sueros antiofidicos. Rev. Inst. Bact. (Buenos Aires) **1**, 15—31 (1917)
Houssay, B. A., Negrete, J.: Esdutios sobre venenos de serpientes. III. Accion de los venenos de serpientes sobre las substancias proteicas. Rev. Inst. Bact. (Buenos Aires) **1**, 335—370 (1918)
Houssay, B. A., Negrete, J.: Spécificité de l'action antitoxique des sérums antivenimeux. C.R. Soc. Biol. (Paris) **89**, 454—455 (1923)
Houssay, B. A., Sordelli, A.: Action des venins sur la coagulation sanguine. J. Physiol. Path. Gén. **18**, 781—811 (1919)
Howard, J. C., Mitchison, N. A.: Immunological tolerance. Prog. Allergy **18**, 43—96 (1975)
Howard, J. C., Scott, M. T., Christie, G. H.: Cellular mechanism underlying the adjuvant activity of *Corynebacterium parvum;* interaction of activated macrophages with T and B lymphocytes. In: Immunopotentiation, G. E. Wolstenholme, J. Knight (Eds.), (Ciba Foundation Symposium N. 28), pp. 101—120. Amsterdam: North-Holland 1973
Howard, N. L.: Phospholipase A_2 from puff adder *(Bitis arietans)* venom. Toxicon **13**, 21—30 (1975)
Huang, J. S., Liu, S. S., Ling, K. H., Chang, C. C., Yang, C. C.: Iodination of "Cobrotoxin". Toxicon **11**, 39—45 (1973)
Hunsicker, L. G., Ruddy, S., Austen, K. F.: Alternate complement pathway: factors involved in cobra venom factor (Co VF) activation of the third component of complement (C'3). J. Immunol. **110**, 128—138 (1973)
Iizuka, K., Murata, Y., Satake, M.: Studies on snake venom. X. On the antigen-antibody reaction of Formosan and Japanese snake venoms with commercial antiserum. J. Pharm. Soc. Jap. **80**, 1035—1039 (1960)
Ivanov, V. T.: Synthetic studies of α "Bungarotoxin" (Abstract). 4th International Symposium on Animal, Plant, and Microbial Toxins, Tokyo, 1974
Iwaguchi, I., Takechi, M., Hayashi, K.: Cytocidal activity of cytotoxin from Indian cobra venom and its derivatives against experimental tumors (Abstract). 4th International Symposium on Animal, Plant, and Microbial Toxins, Tokyo, 1974
Iwanaga, S., Omori, I., Oshima, G., Suzuki, T.: Studies on snake venoms XVI. Demonstration of a proteinase with hemorrhagic activity in the venom of *Agkistrodon halys blomhoffii.* J. Biochem. (Tokyo) **57**, 392—401 (1965)
Iyengar, N. K., Sehra, H. B., Mukergi, B., Chopra, R. N.: Choline esterase in cobra venom. Curr. Sci. Ind. **7**, 51—53 (1938)
Izard, Y., Boquet, M., Ronsseray, A. M., Boquet, P.: Isolement d'une protéine toxique du venin de *Naja nigricollis:* la toxine gamma. C.R. Acad. Sci. [D] (Paris) **269**, 96—97 (1969)
Jerne, N. K., Wood, E. C.: The validity and meaning of the results of biological assays. Biometrics **5**, 273—299 (1949)
Johnson, A. G., Schmidtke, J., Meritt, K., Han, I.: Enhancement of antibody formation by nucleic acids and their derivatives. In: Plescia, O. J., Braun, W. (Eds.): Nucleic Acids in Immunology, pp. 379—385. Berlin-New York: Springer 1968
Jolles, P., Paraf, A.: Chemical and Biological Basis of Adjuvants. Berlin-Heidelberg-New York: Springer 1973
Joubert, F. J.: Snake venom toxins from *Ophiophagus hannah* (king cobra venom.) Biochim. biophys. Acta (Amst.) **317**, 85—98 (1973)
Joubert, F. J.: *Naja melanoleuca* (forest cobra) venom. The amino acid sequence of phospholipase A fractions DEI, DEII, DEIII. Biochim. biophys. Acta (Amst.) **379**, 229—359 (1975a)
Joubert, F. J.: *Hemachatus haemachatus* venom. The amino acid sequence of phospholipase A. Europ. J. Biochem. **52**, 539—544 (1975b)
Joubert, F. J.: The amino acid sequence of three toxins (CM 10, CM 12, CM 14) from *Naja haje annulifera.* Hoppe Seylers Z. physiol. Chem. **356**, 52—72 (1975c)
Joubert, F. J.: The amino acid sequence of three toxins (CM 8, CM 11, and CM 13a) from *Naja haje annulifera* (Egyptian cobra). Europ. J. Biochem. **64**, 219—232 (1976a)
Joubert, F. J.: The amino acid sequences of three toxins (CM 2c, CM 4a, and CM 7) from the venom of *Naja haje annulifera* (Egyptian cobra) venom. Hoppe-Seylers Z. physiol. Chem. **357**, 1735—1750 (1976b)

Joubert, F. J.: *Naja mossambica mossambica* venom. Purification, some properties and amino acid sequences of three phospholipases A (CM I, CM II, CM III). Biochim. biophys. Acta (Amst.) **477**, 216—227 (1977)

Joubert, F. J., Van der Walt, S. J.: *Naja melanoleuca* (Forest Cobra) venom. Purification and some properties of phospholipases A. Biochim. biophys. Acta (Amst.) **379**, 317—328 (1975)

Kabat, E. A.: Precipitin reaction. In: Kabat, E. A., Mayer, M. (Eds.): Experimental Immuno-chemistry, 2nd Ed., pp. 22—96. Springfield, Ill.: Thomas 1961

Kamenskaya, M., Thesleff, S.: The neuromuscular blocking action of an isolated toxin from the Elapidae *Oxyuranus scutellatus*. Acta physiol. scand. **90**, 716—724 (1974)

Kaneda, N., Sasaki, T., Hayashi, K.: Primary structure of cardiotoxin analogs II and IV from the venom of *Naja naja atra*. Biochim. biophys. Acta (Amst.) **491**, 53—66 (1977)

Karlsson, E., Arnberg, H., Eaker, D.: Isolation of the principal neurotoxins of two *Naja naja* subspecies. Europ. J. Biochem. **21**, 1—16 (1971)

Karlsson, E., Eaker, D., Drevin, H.: Modification of the invariant tryptophan residue of two *Naja naja* neurotoxins. Biochim. biophys. Acta (Amst.) **328**, 510—519 (1973)

Karlsson, E., Eaker, D., Fryklund, L., Kadin, S.: Chromatographic separation of *Enhydrina schistosa* common sea snake) venom and the characterization of two principal neurotoxins. Biochemistry **11**, 4628—4633 (1972a)

Karlsson, E., Eaker, D., Ponterius, G.: Modification of amino groups in *Naja naja* neurotoxins and the preparation of radioactive derivatives. Biochim. biophys. Acta (Amst.) **257**, 235—248 (1972b)

Karlsson, E., Eaker, D., Porath, J.: Purification of a neurotoxin from venom of *Naja nigricollis*. Biochim. biophys. Acta (Amst.) **127**, 505—520 (1966)

Karlsson, E., Eaker, D., Rydén, L.: Purification of a presynaptic neurotoxin from the venom of the Australian tiger snake *(Notechis scutatus scutatus)*. Toxicon **10**, 405—413 (1972c)

Kato, H., Suzuki, T.: Bradykinin-potentiating peptides from the venom of *Agkistrodon halys blomhoffii*. Isolation of five bradykinin potentiators and the amino acid sequence of two of them, potentiators B and C. Biochemistry **10**, 972—980 (1971)

Katz, D. H., Paul, W. E., Benacerraf, B.: Carrier function in anti-hapten antibody responses. VI. Establishment of experimental conditions for either inhibitory or enhancing influences of carried-specific cells on antibody production. J. Immunol. **110**, 107—117 (1973)

Kauffman, M.: Les Vipères de France. Paris: Asselin & Houzeau 1893

Kawauchi, S., Samejima, Y., Iwanaga, S., Suzuki, T.: Amino acid compositions of snake venom phospholipase A_2. J. Biochem. (Tokyo) **69**, 433—437 (1971)

Keegan, H. L., Whittemore, F. W., Flanigan, J. F.: Heterologous antivenin in neutralization of north American coral snake venom. Public. Hlth Rep. (Wash.) **76**, 540—542 (1961)

Kellaway, C. H.: Snake venoms. I. Their constitution and therapeutic applications. II. Their peripheral action. III. Immunity. Bull. Johns Hopkins Hosp. **60**, 1—17; 18—39; 159—177 (1937)

Kelly, R. B., Brown, F. R.: Biochemical and physiological properties of a purified snake venom neurotoxin which acts presynaptically. J. Neurobiol. **5**, 135—150 (1974)

Kerbel, R. S., Eidinger, D.: New hypothesis on antigenic competition based on cell interactions in the immune response. Nature (Lond.) **232**, 26—28 (1971a)

Kerbel, R. S., Eidinger, D.: Further studies on antigenic competition. III. A model to account for the phenomenon based on a deficiency of cell to cell interaction in immune lymphoid cell populations. J. exp. Med. **133**, 1043—1073 (1971b)

Ketusinh, O., Puranamanda, C.: A preliminary electrophoretic study of unimmunized and immunized horse sera using haemotoxic and neurotoxic antigens. Proc. Symp. Diamon. Jubilée, Haffkine Inst. **14**, 131—134 (1959)

Keung, W. M., Yip, T. T., Kong, Y. C.: The chemistry and biological effects of cardiotoxin from the chinese cobra *(Naja naja Linn.)* on hormonal responses in isolated cell system. Toxicon **13**, 239—251 (1975)

Klobusitzky, D. von: Biochemische Studien über die Gifte der Schlangengattung *Bothrops*. I. Die blutgerinnungsfördernde Wirkung und die Reinigung der Giftdrüsensekrete der *Bothrops jararaca*. Arch. exp. Path. Pharmak. **179**, 205—216 (1935)

Kocholaty, W. F.: Detoxification of *Crotalus atrox* venom by photooxidation in the presence of methylene blue. Toxicon **3**, 175—186 (1966)

Kocholaty, W. F., Ashley, B. D., Billings, T. A.: An immune-serum against the North american coral snake *(Micrurus fulvius fulvius)* venom obtained by photooxidative detoxification. Toxicon **5**, 43—46 (1967)

Kocholaty, W. F., Goetz, J. C., Ashley, B. D., Billings, T. A., Ledford, E. B.: Immunogenic response of the venoms of fer-de-lance, *Bothrops atrox asper*, and la cascabella, *Crotalus durissus durissus*, following photooxidative detoxification. Toxicon **5**, 153—158 (1968 a)

Kocholaty, W. F., Ledford, E. B., Billings, T. A., Goetz, J. C., Ashley, B. D.: Immunization studies with *Naja naja* venom detoxified by photooxidation. Toxicon **5**, 159—163 (1968 b)

Kochwa, S., Gitter, S., Strauss, A., de Vries, A., Leffkowitz, M.: Immunologic study of *Vipera xanthina palestinae* venom and preparation of potent antivenin in rabbits. J. Immunol. **82**, 107—115 (1959 a)

Kochwa, S., Izard, Y., Boquet, P., Gitter, S.: Sur la préparation d'un immun-sérum équin antivenimeux au moyen des fractions neurotoxiques isolées du venin de *Vipera xanthina palestinae*. Ann. Inst. Pasteur **97**, 370—376 (1959 b)

Kondo, H., Kondo, S., Sadahiro, S., Yamauchi, K., Murata, R.: Standardization of *Trimeresurus flavoviridis* (Habu) antivenin. Jap. J. med. Sci. Biol. **24**, 323—327 (1971 a)

Kondo, H., Kondo, S., Sadahiro, S., Yamauchi, K., Ohsaka, A., Murata, R.: Preparation and immunogenicity of Habu *(Trimeresurus flavoviridis)* toxoid. In: de Vries, A., Kochra, E. (Eds.): Toxins of Animal and Plant Origin, Vol. III, pp. 845—862. London: Gordon and Breach 1973

Kondo, S., Sadahiro, S., Yamauchi, K., Kondo, H., Murata, R.: Preparation and standardization of toxoid from the venom of *Trimeresurus flavoviridis* (Habu). Jap. J. med. Sci. Biol. **24**, 281—294 (1971 b)

Kook, A. I., Trainin, N.: Hormone like activity of a thymus humoral factor on the induction of immune competence in lymphoid cells. J. exp. Med. **139**, 193—207 (1974)

Kook, A. I., Trainin, N.: The control exerted by thymic hormone (THF) on cellular cAMP levels and immune reactivity of spleen cells in the MLC assay. J. Immunol. **115**, 8—14 (1975)

Kopeyan, C., Miranda, F., Rochat, H.: Amino acid sequence of toxin III of *Naja haje*: Europ. J. Biochem. **58**, 117—122 (1975)

Kopeyan, C., Van Rietschofen, J., Martinez, G., Rochat, H., Miranda, F.: Characterization of five neurotoxins isolated from the venom of two Elapidae snakes *Naja haje* and *Naja nigricollis*. Europ. J. Biochem. **35**, 244—250 (1973)

Kornalik, F., Taborska, E.: Individual interspecies variability in the composition of some Viperidae venoms. In: Kaiser, E. (Ed.): Symposium on Animal and Plant Toxins, pp. 98—103. Munich: Goldman 1973

Kramar, R., Lambrechter, R., Kaiser, E.: The release of acid hydrolase from lysosomes by animal venoms. Toxicon **9**, 125—129 (1971)

Kraus, R.: Zur Serumtherapie der Bisse durch europäische Vipern. Wien. klin. Wschr. **39**, 744—745 (1926)

Kulkarni, M. E., Rao, S. S.: Antigenic composition of the venoms of poisonous snakes of India. In: Buckley, E., Porges, N. (Eds.): Venoms, pp. 175—180. Amer. Ass. Adv. Sci., pub. No. 44. Washington 1956

Kumar, V., Elliott, W. B.: The acetylcholinesterase of *Bungarus fasciatus* venom. Europ. J. Biochem. **34**, 586—592 (1973)

Lamb, G.: On the action of snake venom on the coagulability of the blood. Indian. med. Gaz. **36**, 443—455 (1901)

Lamb, G.: On the precipitin of cobra venom. A means of distinguishing between the proteins of different snake poisons. Lancet **1902 II**, 431

Lamb, G.: On the precipitin of cobra venom. Lancet **1904 I**, 916

Landsteiner, K.: The Specificity of Serological Reactions. Springfield, Ill.: Thomas 1936

Larsen, P. R., Wolf, J.: The basic proteins of cobra venom. I. Isolation and characterization of Cobramines A and B. J. biol. Chem. **243**, 1283—1289 (1968)

Laskowski, M., Hagerty, G., Laurila, U. R.: Phosphodiesterase from rattlesnake venom. Nature (Lond.) **180**, 1181—1182 (1957)

Lafiti, M., Farzanpay, R., Tabatabai, M.: Comparative studies of Iranian snake venoms by gel diffusion and neutralization tests. In: Kaiser, E. (Ed.): Symposium on Animal and Plant Toxins. Munich: Goldmann 1973

Laure, C. J.: The primary structure of Crotamine. Hoppe Seylers Z. physiol. Chem. **356**, 213—215 (1975)

Laurell, C. B.: Antigen-antibody crossed electrophoresis. Ann. Biochem. **10**, 358—361 (1965)

Lebez, D., Gubensek, F., Turk, V.: Distribution of some toxic fractions 75Se labeled *Vipera ammodytes* venom in experimental animals. In: De Vries, A., Kochwa, E. (Eds.): Toxins of Animal and Plant Origin, Vol. III, pp. 1067—1074. London: Gordon and Breach 1973

Lee, C. Y.: Chemistry and pharmacology of polypeptide toxins in snake venoms. Ann. Rev. Pharmacol. **12**, 265—286 (1972)

Lee, C. Y., Chang, C. C., Chiu, T. H., Chiu, P. J. S., Tseng, T. C., Lee, S. Y.: Pharmacological properties of cardiotoxin isolated from Formosan cobra venom. Arch. Pharmakol. exp. Path. **259**, 360—374 (1968)

Lee, C. Y., Chang, S. L., Kau, S. T., Luh, S. H.: Chromatographic separation of the venom of *Bungarus multicinctus* and characterization of its components. J. Chromatogr. **72**, 71—82 (1972)

Lee, C. Y., Chen, Y. M., Mebs, D.: Chromatographic separation of the venom of *Bungarus caeruleus* and pharmacological characterization of its components. Toxicon **14**, 451—457 (1976)

Lee, C. Y., Huang, M. C., Bonilla, C. A.: Mode of action of purified basic proteins from three rattle snake venoms on neuromuscular junctions of the chick biventer cervicis muscle. In: Kaiser, E. (Ed.): Symposium On Animal and Plant Toxins, pp. 173—178. Munich: Goldmann 1973

Lee, C. Y., Lin, J. S., Wei, J. W.: Indentification of cardiotoxin with cobramine B, DLF, toxin γ, and cobra venom cytotoxin. In: de Vries, A., Kochva, E. (Eds.): Toxins of Animal and Plant Origin, pp. 307—318. London: Gordon and Breach 1971

Lee, C. Y., Tseng, L. F.: Distribution of *Bungarus multicintus* venom following envenomation. Toxicon **3**, 281—290 (1966)

Lin Shian, S. Y., Huang, M. C., Lee, C. Y.: A study of cardiotoxic principles from the venom of *Bungarus fasciatus* (Schneider). Toxicon **13**, 189—196 (1975)

Liu, C. S., Blackwelf, R. Q.: Hydrophitoxin b from *Hydrophis cyanocinctus* venom. Toxicon **12**, 542—546 (1974)

Liu, C. S., Huber, G. S., Lin, C. S., Blackwell, R. Q.: Fractionation of toxins from *Hydrophis cyanocinctus* venom and determination of amino acid composition and end groups of hydrophitoxin a. Toxicon **11**, 73—79 (1973)

Liu, C. S., Wang, C. L., Blackwell, R. Q.: Isolation and partial characterization of "Pelamitoxin" A from *Pelamis platurus* venom. Toxicon **13**, 31—36 (1975)

Lo, T. B., Chang, W. C.: Studies on phospholipase A from Formosan *(Naja naja atra)* venom (Abstract). 4th Symposium on Animal, Plant, and Microbial toxins. Tokyo, 1974

Louis, J., Chiller, M., Weigle, W. O.: Fate of antigen binding cells in unresponsive and immune mice. J. exp. Med. **137**, 461—470 (1973)

Louw, A. I.: Snake venom toxins. The complete amino acid sequence of cytotoxin $V^{11}4$ from the venom of *Naja mossambica mossambica*. Biochem. biophys. Res. Commun. **58**, 1022—1029 (1974a)

Louw, A. I.: Snake venom toxins. The amino acid sequences of three cytotoxin homologues from *Naja mossambica mossambica* venom. Biochim. biophys. Acta (Amst.) **336**, 481—495 (1974b)

Low, B. W., Potter, R., Jackson, R. B., Tamiya, N., Sato, S.: X-ray crystallographic study of the "Erabutoxins" and of a diiodo derivative. J. biol. Chem. **246**, 4366—4368 (1971)

Low, B. W., Preston, H. S., Sato, A., Rosen, L. S., Searl, J. E., Rudko, A. D., Richardson, J. S.: Three dimensional structure of erabutoxin b neurotoxic protein; inhibitor of acetyl choline receptor. Proc. nat. Acad. Sci. (Wash.) **73**, 2991—2994 (1976)

Luzzio, A. J., Trevino, G. S.: Precipitin and neutralizing antibody response elicited by "*Crotalus atrox*" antivenom precipitate. Proc. Soc. exp. Biol. (N.Y.) **122**, 295—299 (1966)

Macfarlane, R. G., Barnett, B.: Haemostatic possibilities of snake-venom. Lancet **1934 II**, 985—987

Maeda, N., Tamiya, N.: Isolation, properties and amino acid sequences of three neurotoxins from the venom of sea snake *Aepisurus laevis*. Biochem. J. **153**, 79—87 (1976)

Maeda, N. N., Chen, Y., Tamiya, M., Lee, C. Y.: The isolation, properties and amino acid sequence of *Laticauda semifasciata* III, a weak and reversible neurotoxin from the sea snake *Laticauda semifasciata* (Abstract). 4th International Symposium on Animal, Plant, and Microbial Toxins. Tokyo, 1974

Maillard, J., Bloom, B. P.: Immunological adjuvants and the mechanism of cell cooperation. J. exp. Med. **136**, 185—190 (1972)
Mallick, S. M. K.: The applicability of floculation tests to the standardization of antivenin. Indian J. med. Res. **23**, 525—529 (1935)
Mancini, G., Carbonara, A. O., Heremans, J. F.: Immunochemical quantitation of antigens by single radial immunodiffusion. Immunochemistry **2**, 235—254 (1965)
Mandelbaum, F. R., Reichl, A. P., Assakura, M. T.: Some physical and biochemical characteristics of HF_1, the haemorrhagic factor in the venom of *Bothrops jararaca* (Abstract). 4th International Symposium on Animal, Plant, and Microbial Toxins. Tokyo, 1974
Mangalo, R., Fouque, F., Boquet, P.: Recherches biochimiques et immunologiques sur le venin des serpents. V. Application des techniques immunochimiques au titrage des anticorps spécifiques de la toxine α du venin de *Naja nigricollis*. Ann. Immunol. (Inst. Pasteur) **128** C, 841—850 (1977)
Margoliash, E., Nisonoff, A., Reichlin, M.: Immunological activity of cytochrome C. I Precipitating antibodies to monomeric vertebrate cytochrome C. J. biol. Chem. **245**, 931—939 (1970)
Margoliash, E., Reichlin, M., Nisonoff, A.: The relation of immunological activity and primary structure in cytochrome C. In: Kamachandran, G. N. (Ed.): Conformation of Biopolymers. New York: Academic 1967
Markland, F. S., Damus, P. S.: Purification and properties of a thrombin-like enzyme from the venom of *Crotalus adamanteus* (Eastern diamon back rattlesnake). J. biol. Chem. **246**, 6460—6473 (1971)
Maron, E., Shiozawa, C., Arnon, R., Sela, M.: Chemical and immunological characterization of a unique antigenic region in lysozyme. Biochemistry **10**, 763—771 (1971)
Maron, E., Webb, C., Teitelbaum, D., Arnon, R.: Cell-mediated vs humoral response in the cross-reaction between hen egg-white lysozyme and bovine α lactalbumin. Europ. J. Immunol. **2**, 294—297 (1972)
Marquart, H.: La sérothérapie antivenimeuse. Recherches sur la neutralisation des facteurs de diffusion des venins. Rev. Immunol. (Paris) **15**, 262—270 (1951)
Marrack-Hunter, P. C., Kappler, J. W.: Antigen-specific and non-specific mediators of T cell/B cell cooperation. J. Immunol. **114**, 1116—1125 (1975)
Martin, C. J.: The contribution of experiments with snake venom to the development of our knowledge of immunity. Brit. med. J. **1904 II**, 574—577
Martin, C. J.: Observations upon fibrin-ferments in the venoms of snakes and the time relation of their action. J. Physiol. (Lond.) **32**, 207—215 (1905)
Massaro, E. J., McLean, R. L., Elliott, W. B.: A fractionation procedure for *Naja naja* venom. In: deVries, A., Kochva, E. (Eds.): Toxins of Animal and Plant Origin, Vol. I, pp. 259—279. London: Gordon and Breach 1971
Mebs, D.: Vergleichende Enzymuntersuchungen an Schlangengiften unter besonderer Berücksichtigung ihrer Casein-spaltenden Proteasen. Hoppe-Seylers Z. physiol. Chem. **349**, 1115—1125 (1968)
Mebs, D., Lee, C. Y., Chen, Y. M., Iwanaga, S.: Chemical and pharmacological characterization of toxic polypeptides from four *Elapidae* venoms. 4th International Symposium on Animal, Plant, and Microbial Toxins. Tokyo, Japan, 1974
Mebs, D., Narita, K., Iwanaga, S., Samejima, Y., Lee, C. Y.: Amino acid sequence of α Bungarotoxin from the venom of *Bungarus multicinctus*. Biochem. biophys. Res. Commun. **44**, 711—716 (1971)
Menez, A., Bouet, F., Fromageot, P., Tamiya, N.: On the role of tyrosyl and tryptophanyl residues in the conformation of two snake neurotoxins. Bull. Inst. Pasteur **74**, 57—64 (1976)
Michaelis, L.: Untersuchungen über Eiweißpräzipitine, zugleich ein Beitrag zur Lehre von der Eiweißverdauung. Dtsch. med. Wschr. **2**, 733—736 (1902)
Micheel, F., Jung, F.: Zur Kenntnis der Schlangengifte. Hoppe-Seylers Z. physiol. Chem. **239**, 217—230 (1936)
Miledi, R., Molinoff, P., Potter, L. T.: Isolation of the cholinergic receptor of torpedo electric tissue. Nature (Lond.) **229**, 354—357 (1971)
Miller, J. F. A. P.: Interaction between thymus dependent (T) cells and bone marrow derived (B) cells in antibody response. In: Makela, O., Cross, A., Kosunen, T. U. (Eds.): Cell Interactions and Receptor Antibodies in Immune Response, pp. 293—309. New York: Academic 1971

Miller, J. F. A. P., Basten, A., Sprent, J., Cheers, C.: Interaction between lymphocytes in immune responses. Cell. Immunol. **2**, 469—495 (1971)

Miller, J. F. A. P., Mitchell, G. F.: Cell to cell interaction in the immune response. I. Hemolysin—forming cells in neonatally thymectomized mice reconstitued with thymus or thoracic duct lymphocytes. J. exp. Med. **128**, 801—820 (1968)

Minton, S.: Antigenic relationships of the venom of *Atractaspis microlepidota* to that of other snakes. Toxicon **6**, 59—64 (1968)

Minton, S. A.: Variation in venom samples from Copperheads *(Agkistrodon contortrix mokeson)* and timber rattlesnakes *(Crotalus horridus horridus)*. Copeia **4**, 212—215 (1953)

Minton, S. A.: An immunological investigation of rattlesnake venoms by the agar diffusion method. Amer. J. trop. Med. Hyg. **6**, 1097—1107 (1957)

Minton, S. A.: Observations on toxicity and antigenic makeup of venoms from juvenile snakes. In: Russell, F. E., Saunders, P. D. (Eds.): International Symposium on Animal Toxins, pp. 211—222. Oxford: Pergamon 1967a

Minton, S. A.: Paraspecific protection by Elapidae and sea snake antivenins. Toxicon **5**, 47—55 (1967b)

Miranda, F., Kupeyan, C., Rochat, H., Rochat, C., Lissitzky, S.: Purification of animal neurotoxins. Isolation and characterization of four neurotoxins from two different sources of *Naja haje* venom. Europ. J. Biochem. **17**, 477—484 (1970)

Mitchell, G. F., Miller, J. F. A. P.: Cell to cell interaction in the immune response. II. The source of hemolysin-forming cells in irradiated mice given bone lymphocytes. J. exp. Med. **128**, 821—837 (1968)

Mitchison, N. A.: Induction of immunological paralysis in two zones of dosage. Proc. R. Soc. Lond. [Biol.] **161**, 275—292 (1964)

Mitchison, N. A.: The relative ability of T and B lymphocytes to see protein antigen. In: Makela, O., Cross, A., Kosunen, T. U. (Eds.): Cell Interaction and Receptor Antibodies in Immune Response, pp. 249—260. New York: Academic 1971

Mitchison, N. A., Rajensky, K., Taylor, R. S.: Cooperation of antigenic determinants and of cells in the induction of antibodies. In: Sterzl, J., Riha, I. (Eds.): Developmental Aspects of Antibody Formation and Structure, Vol. II, pp. 547—561. New York: Academic 1970

Mittelstaedt, J. S., Shaw, S. M., Tiffany, L. W.: The detoxifying effect of cobalt-60 radiations of the venom of the hooded cobra, *Naja naja*. In: De Vries, A., Kochva, E. (Eds.): Toxins of Animal and Plant Origin, Vol. III, pp. 887—896. London: Gordon and Breach 1973

Mohamed, A. H., Bakr, I. A., Kamel, A.: Egyptian polyvalent anti-snake bite serum; technic of preparation. Toxicon **4**, 69—72 (1966)

Mohamed, A. H., Darwish, M. A., Hani-Ayobe, M.: Immunological studies on an Egyptian bivalent *Naja* antivenin. Toxicon **12**, 321—323 (1974)

Moller, G., Sjoberg, O.: Studies on the mechanism of antigenic competition. In: Makela, O., Cross, A., Kosunen, T. U. (Eds.): Cell Intraction and Receptor Antibodies in Immune Responses, pp. 419—432. New York: Academic 1971

Morgenroth, J., Kaya, R.: Über eine komplementzerstörende Wirkung des Kobragiftes. Biochem. Z. **8**, 378—382 (1908)

Moritsch, P.: Zur Serumtherapie der Bisse durch europäische Vipern. Wien. klin. Wschr. **39**, 1514—1515 (1926)

Moroz, C., de Vries, A., Goldblum, N.: Preparation of an antivenin against *Vipera palestinae* venom with high antineurotoxic potency. Toxicon **4**, 205—208 (1966a)

Moroz, C., de Vries, A., Goldblum, N.: Preparation of horse antiserum against *Echis colorata* (Gunther) venom and determination of its capacity to neutralize the toxic afibrinogenemic and thrombocytopenic actions of *Echis colorata* and *Echis carinata* venoms. Ann. Inst. Pasteur **110**, 276—282 (1966b)

Moroz, C., de Vries, A., Sela, M.: Isolation and characterization of a neurotoxin from *Vipera palestinae* venom. Biochim. biophys. Acta (Amst.) **124**, 136—146 (1966c)

Moroz, C., Goldblum, N., de Vries, A.: Preparation of *Vipera palestinae* antineurotoxin using carboxymethyl-cellulose-bound neurotoxin as antigen. Nature (Lond.) **200**, 697—698 (1963)

Moroz-Perlmutter, C., Goldblum, N., de Vries, A., Gitter, S.: Detoxification of snake venoms and venom fractions by formaldehyde. Proc. Soc. exp. Biol. (N.Y.) **112**, 595—598 (1963)

Moroz, C., de Vries, A., Sela, M.: Chemical characterization of viperotoxin. Israel J. Chem. **3**, 108 (1965)
Müller-Eberhard, H. J.: Mechanism of inactivation of the third component of human complement (C'3) by cobra venom (Abstr.) Fed. Proc. **26**, 744 (1967)
Müller-Eberhard, H. J.: Biochemistry of complement. In: Amos, B. (Ed.): Progress in Immunology, pp. 553—565. New York: Academic 1971
Munjal, D., Elliott, W. B.: Further studies on the properties of phospholipase A from honeybee *(Apis mellifera)* venom. Toxicon **10**, 367—375 (1972)
Murata, Y., Satake, M., Suzuki, T.: Studies on snake venom. XII. Distribution of proteinase activities among Japanese and Formosan snake venoms. J. Biochem. (Tokyo) **53**, 431—436 (1963)
Mutsaars, W., Bartels-Viroux, J.: Recherches sur un facteur favorisant la destruction du troisième composant du sérum chauffé de cobaye par le venin de cobra. Ann. Inst. Pasteur **73**, 451—471 (1947)
Nair, B. C., Nair, C., Elliott, W. B.: Action of antisera against homologous and heterologous snake venom phospholipases A_2. Toxicon **13**, 453—456 (1975)
Nakai, K., Sasaki, T., Hayashi, K.: Amino acid sequence of toxin A from the venom of the Indian cobra *(Naja naja)*. Biochem. biophys. Res. Commun. **44**, 893—897 (1971)
Narita, K., Lee, C. Y.: The amino acid sequence of cardiotoxin from Formosan cobra *(Naja naja atra)* venom. Biochem. biophys. Res. Commun. **41**, 339—343 (1970)
Nelson, R. A.: Survey Ophtal. **11**, 498 (1966) (quoted by Hunsicker, L. G., Ruddy, S., Austen, K. F. In: Alternative Complement Pathway. J. Immunol. **110**, 128—138 (1973)
Nicolle, M., Raphael, A.: (quoted by: Nicolle, M., Boquet, A.: Elements de Microbiologie Générale et d'Immunologie, p. 268. Paris: Doin 1925)
Nisonoff, A., Reichlin, M., Margoliash, E.: Immunological activity of cytochrome C. II. Localization of a major antigenic determinant of human cytochrome C. J. biol. Chem. **245**, 940—946 (1970)
Noc, F.: Sur quelques propriétés physiologiques des différents venins de serpents. Ann. Inst. Pasteur **18**, 387—406 (1904)
Noguchi, H.: Paraspecific properties of antivenins. Brit. med. J. **1904 II**, 580—581
Noguchi, H.: Snake Venoms. Washington: Carnegie Institution 1909
Nossal, G. J. V.: Recent advances in immunological tolerance. In: Amos, B. (Ed.): Progress in Immunology, pp. 665—677. New York: Academic 1971
Oberer, D.: Effect of snake venoms on rabbit basophil leucocytes. Biochem. Pharmacol. **11**, 9—15 (1962)
Ohta, M., Hayashi, K.: Chemical modification of the tryptophan residue in toxin B from the venom of the Indian cobra. Biochem. biophys. Res. Commun. **57**, 973—979 (1974)
Omori-Satoh, T., Lang, J., Breithaupt, H., Habermann, E.: Partial amino acid sequence of the basic *Crotalus* phospholipase A. Toxicon **13**, 69—71 (1975)
Omori-Satoh, T., Ohsaka, A.: Purification and some properties of hemorrhagic principle in the venom of *Trimeresurus flavoviridis*. Biochim. biophys. Acta (Amst.) **207**, 432—444 (1970)
Oshima, G., Matsuo, Y., Iwanaga, S., Suzuki, T.: Studies on snake venoms. XIX. Purification and some physico-chemical properties of proteinases a and c from the venom of *Agkistrodon halys blomhoffii*. J. Biochem. (Tokyo) **64**, 227—238 (1968)
Oshima, G., Omori-Satoh, T., Iwanaga, S., Suzuki, T.: Studies on snake venom hemorrhagic factor I (HR-I) in the venoms of *Agkistrodon halys blomhoffii*. Its purification and biological properties. J. Biochem. (Tokyo) **72**, 1483—1494 (1972)
Otto, R.: Zur Serumtherapie bei Bissen durch europäische Vipern. Klin. Wschr. **6**, 1948—1950 (1927)
Otto, R.: Vergleichende Untersuchungen mit Schlangengiftserum und Viperngiften verschiedener Herkunft. Z. Hyg. Infekt. **109**, 272—285 (1928)
Otto, R.: Untersuchungen über die Toxine europäischer Viperinen. Z. Hyg. Infekt. **110**, 82—92 (1929a)
Otto, R.: Untersuchungen über die Wirkung verschiedener Schlangen-Gift-Antisera auf das Berne-Kreuzottern Toxin. Z. Hyg. Infekt. **110**, 513—515 (1929b)
Otto, R.: Zur Wirkung der Schlangengiftantisera auf die Gifte europäischer Ottern. Z. Hyg. Infekt. **111**, 503—510 (1930)

Ouchterlony, O.: "In vitro" method for testing the toxin producing capacity of diphtheria bacteria. Acta path. microbiol. scand. **25**, 186—191 (1948)

Oudin, J.: L'analyse immunochimique qualitative, méthode par diffusion des antigènes au sein de l'immunsérum précipitant gélosé. Ann. Inst. Pasteur **75**, 30—51 (1948)

Ouyang, C., Hong, J.S., Teng, C.M.: Purification and properties of the thrombin-like principle of *Agkistrodon acutus* venom and its comparison with the bovine thrombin. Thrombos. Diathes. haemorrh. (Stuttg.) **26**, 224—234 (1971)

Ouyang, C., Teng, C.M.: Purification and properties of the anticoagulant principle of *Agkistrodon acutus* venom. Biochim. biophys. Acta (Amst.) **278**, 155—162 (1972)

Ovadia, M., Kochva, E., Moav, B.: Neutralization mechanism of *Vipera palestinae* neurotoxin by a purified factor from homologous serum. Biochim. biophys. Acta (Amst.) **491**, 370—386 (1977)

Parrish, H.M., Watt, H.F., Arnold, J.D.: Human allergy resulting from North American snake venoms. J. Florida med. Ass. **43**, 1116—1119 (1957)

Patel, T.N., Braganca, B.M., Bellare, R.A.: Changes produced by cobra venom cytotoxin on the morphology of Yoshida sarcoma cells. Exp. Cell Res. **57**, 289—297 (1969)

Pearce, F.L., Banks, B.E.C., Banthorpe, D.V., Berry, A.R., Davies, H.S., Vernon, C.A.: The isolation and characterization of nerve-growth factor from the venom of *Vipera russellii*. Europ. J. Biochem. **29**, 417—425 (1972)

Pfleiderer, G., Sumyk, G.: Investigation of snake venom enzymes. I. Separation of rattlesnake venom proteinases by cellulose ion-exchange chromatography. Biochim. biophys. Acta (Amst.) **51**, 482—493 (1961)

Phisalix, C., Bertrand, G.: Atténuation du venin de vipère par la chaleur et vaccination du cobaye contre ce venin. Le sérum sanguin des animaux vaccinés. C.R. Soc. Biol. (Paris) **46**, 148—150 (1894a)

Phisalix, C., Bertrand, G.: Sur la propriété antitoxique du sang des animaux vaccinés contre le venin de vipère. C.R. Acad. Sci. [D] (Paris) **118**, 356—358 (1894b)

Piantanida, M., Muic, N.: The antigenic composition of *Ammodytes* viper venom. J. Immunol. **73**, 115—119 (1954)

Picado, C.: Immunité hétérologue des animaux immunisés contre le venin bothropique. C.R. Soc. Biol. (Paris) **116**, 419 (1934)

Pickering, R.J., Wolfson, M.R., Good, R.A., Gewurz, H.: Passive hemolysis by serum and cobra venom factor: a new mechanism inducing membrane damage by complement. Proc. nat. Acad. Sci. (Wash.) **62**, 521—527 (1969)

Poilleux, G., Boquet, P.: Propriétés de trois toxines isolées du venin d'un Elapidae: *Naja melanoleuca*. C.R. Acad. Sci. [D] (Paris) **274**, 1953—1956 (1972)

Pratt Johnson, J.: The estimation of haemorrhagin in venom by an intra-dermal method and a potency test of antivenom sera for antihaemorrhagin. J. Path. Bact. **39**, 704—706 (1934)

Pross, H.F., Eidinger, D.: Antigenic competition: a review of nonspecific antigen-induced suppression. Advanc. Immunol. **18**, 133—168 (1974)

Pross, H.F., Novak, T., Eidinger, D.: "In vitro" studies of "antigenic competition". I. The comparative responses of normal and "immune" lymphoid cell populations. Cell. Immunol. **2**, 445—457 (1971)

Pryjma, J., Humphrey, J.H.: Prolonged C3 depletion by cobra venom factor in thymus-deprived mice and its implication for the role of C3 as an essential second signal for B-cell triggering. Immunology **28**, 569—576 (1975)

Purananda, C., Lauhatirananda, P., Ganthavorn, S.: Cross immunological reactions in snake venoms. Mem. Inst. Butantan **33**, 1, 327—330 (1966)

Radomski, J.L., Miale, J.B., Deichmann, W.B., Fisher, J.A.: Hematologic effects of *Crotalus adamanteus* (rattlesnake) venom. Arch. Toxikol. **17**, 365—372 (1959)

Radovich, J., Talmage, D.W.: Antigenic competition: cellular or humoral? Science **158**, 512—514 (1967)

Ramon, G.: Des anatoxines. C.R. Acad. Sci. [D] (Paris) **178**, 1436—1439 (1924)

Ramon, G., Boquet, P., Richou, R., Nicol, L.: Les anavenins spécifiques et les substances adjuvantes et stimulantes de l'immunité dans la production des sérums antivenimeux respectivement dirigés contre les venins de *Cerastes cornutus* et de *Naja haje*. Ann. Inst. Pasteur **67**, 355—358 (1941)

Raudonat, H. W., Holler, B.: Über die herzwirksame Komponente des Kobragiftes "Cardiotoxin". Arch. exp. Path. Pharmak. **233**, 431—437 (1958)

Raymond, M. L., Tu, A. T.: Role of tyrosine in sea snake neurotoxin. Biochim. biophys. Acta (Amst.) **285**, 498—502 (1972)

Reichlin, M.: Amino acid substitution and antigenicity of globular proteins. Advanc. Immunol. **20**, 71—123 (1975)

Reid, H. A.: Snake bites in Malaya. In: Keegan, H. L., Macfarlane, W. V. (Eds.): Venomous and Poisonous Animals and Noxious Plants of the Pacific Region, pp. 355—362. Oxford: Pergamon 1963

Reid, H. A.: Cobra-bites. Brit. med. J. **1964 II**, 540—545

Reid, H. A., Thean, P. C., Chang, K. E., Baharom, A. R.: Clinical effects of bites by Malayan viper (*Agkistrodon rhodostoma*). Lancet **1963 I**, 617—621

Renaud, M.: Immunisation contre le venin de cobra par les complexes venins-savons. C.R. Soc. Biol. (Paris) **103**, 143—144 (1930)

Richards, G. M., Tutas, D. J., Wechter, W. J., Laskowski, M.: Hydrolysis of dinucleoside monophosphates containing arabinose in various internucleotide linkages by exonuclease from the venom of *Crotalus adamanteus*. Biochemistry **6**, 2908—2914 (1967)

Ritz, H.: Über die Wirkung des Cobragiftes auf die Komplemente. Z. Immun.-Forsch. **13**, 62—63 (1912)

Rochat, H., Gregoire, J., Martin-Moutot, N., Menashe, M., Kopeyan, C., Miranda, F.: Purification of animal neurotoxins: isolation and characterization of three neurotoxins from the venom of *Naja nigricollis* (mossambica) Peters. FEBS Letters **42**, 335—339 (1974)

Rubin, A. S., Coons, A. H.: Specific heterologous enhancement of immune responses. II. Immunological memory cells of thymic origin. J. exp. Med. **135**, 437—441 (1972a)

Rubin, A. S., Coons, A. H.: Specific heterologous enhancement of immune responses. IV. Specific generation of a thymus-derived enhancing factor. J. exp. Med. **136**, 1501—1517 (1972b)

Rude, E.: Antigens and immunogenicity. FEBS Letters **17**, 6—10 (1971)

Russel, F. E., Timmerman, W. F., Meadows, P. E.: Clinical use of antivenin prepared from goat serum. Toxicon **8**, 63—65 (1970)

Rydén, L., Gabel, D., Eaker, D.: A model of the three-dimensional structure of snake venom neurotoxins based on chemical evidence. Int. J. Pept. Prot. Res. **5**, 261—273 (1973)

Sadahiro, S., Kondo, S., Yamauchi, K., Kondo, H., Murata, R.: Studies on immunogenicity of toxoids from Habu (*Trimeresurus flavoviridis*) venom. Jap. J. med. Sci. Biol. **23**, 285—289 (1970)

Saito, K., Hanahan, D. J.: A study of the purification and properties of the phospholipase A of *Crotalus adamanteus* venom. Biochemistry **1**, 521—532 (1962)

Salach, J. I., Turini, P., Hauber, J., Seng, R., Tisdale, H., Singer, T. P.: Isolation of phospholipase A isoenzymes from *Naja naja* venom and their action on membrane bound enzymes. Biochem. biophys. Res. Commun. **33**, 936—941 (1968)

Salach, J. I., Turini, P., Seng, R., Hauber, J., Singer, T. P.: Phospholipase A of snake venoms. I. Isolation and molecular properties of isoenzymes from *Naja naja* and *Vipera russellii* venoms. J. biol. Chem. **246**, 331—339 (1971)

Samejima, Y., Iwanaga, S., Suzuki, T.: Complete amino acid sequence of phospholipase A_2 isolated from *Agkistrodon halys blomhoffii* venom. FEBS Letters **47**, 348—351 (1974)

Sarkar, N. K.: Existence of cardiotoxic principle in cobra venom. Ann. Biochem. exp. Med. **8**, 11—22 (1948)

Sasaki, T.: Chemical studies on the poison of Formosan cobra. II. The terminal amino acid residues of purified poison (neurotoxin). J. Pharm. Soc. Jap. **77**, 845—847 (1957)

Satake, M., Murata, Y., Suzuki, T.: Studies on snake venom. XIII. Chromatographic separation and properties of three proteinases from *Agkistrodon halys blomhoffii* venom. J. Biochem. (Tokyo) **53**, 438—447 (1963)

Sato, T., Iwanaga, S., Mizushima, Y., Suzuki, T.: Studies on snake venoms. XV. Separation of arginine esterhydrolase of *Agkistrodon halys blomhoffii* venom into three enzymatic entities: "bradykinin releasing", "clotting", and "permeability increasing". J. Biochem. (Tokyo) **57**, 380—391 (1965)

Sato, I., Ryan, K. W., Mitsuhashi, S.: Studies on habu snake venom. VI. Cytotoxic effect of Habu *(Trimeresurus flavoviridis Hallowell)* and cobra *(Naja naja)* venoms on the cells "in vitro". Jap. J. exp. Med. **34**, 119—124 (1964)

Sato, S., Abe, T., Tamiya, N.: Binding of iodinated "Erabutoxin b" a sea snake toxin to the end-plates of the mouse diaphragm. Toxicon **8**, 313—315 (1970)

Sato, S., Ogahara, H., Tamiya, N.: Immunochemistry of "Erabutoxins". Toxicon **10**, 239—243 (1972)

Sato, S., Tamiya, N.: Iodination of Erabutoxin b: Diiodohistidine formation. J. Biochem. (Tokyo) **68**, 867—872 (1970)

Sato, S., Yoshida, H., Abe, H., Tamiya, N.: Properties and biosynthesis of a neurotoxic protein of the venom of sea snakes *Laticauda laticaudata* and *Laticauda colubrina*. Biochem. J. **115**, 85—90 (1969)

Sawai, Y., Kawamura, Y., Fukuyama, T., Keegan, H. L.: Studies on the inactivation of snake venoms by dihydrothioctic acid. Jap. J. exp. Med. **37**, 121—128 (1967)

Sawai, Y., Makino, M., Kawamura, Y.: Studies on the antitoxic action of dihydrolypoic acid (dihydrothioctic acid), and tetracycline against Habu snake *(Trimeresurus flavoviridis Hallowell)* venom. In: Keegan, H. L., Macfarlane, W. V. (Eds.): Venomous and Poisonous Animals and Noxious Plants of the Pacific Area, pp. 327—335. Oxford: Pergamon 1963

Sawai, Y., Makino, M., Miyasaki, S., Kato, K., Adachi, H., Mitsuhashi, S., Okonogi, T.: Studies on the improvement of treatment of Habu snake bite. I. Studies on the improvement of habu snake antivenin. Jap. J. exp. Med. **31**, 137—150 (1961)

Schenberg, S.: Analise imunologica (micro-difusao em gel) de venenos individuals de *Bothrops jararaca*. Cienca Cultura **13**, 225—230 (1961)

Schenberg, S.: Immunological (Ouchterlony method) indentification of intrasubspecies qualitative differences in snake venom composition. Toxicon **1**, 67—75 (1963)

Schenberg, S., Pereira Lima, F. A., Schiripa, L. N., Nagamori, A.: A snake venom ADPase (Abstract). 4th International Symposium on Animal, Plant, and Microbial Toxins. Tokyo, 1974

Schenck, J. R., Hargie, M. P., Brown, M. S., Erbert, D. S., Yoo, A. L., McIntire, C.: The enhancement of antibody formation by *Escherichia coli* lipopolysaccharid acid-detoxified derivatives. J. Immunol. **102**, 1411—1422 (1969)

Schirrmacher, V., Wigzell, H.: Immune response against native and chemically modified albumin in mice. I. Analysis of non-thymus processed (B) and thymus processed (T) cell response against methylated bovine serum albumin. J. exp. Med. **136**, 1617—1630 (1972)

Schlossberger, H., Bieling, R., Demnitz, H.: Untersuchungen über Antitoxine gegen Schlangengifte und die Herstellung eines Heil-Serums gegen die Gifte der europäischen und mediterranen Ottern. In: Die europäischen und mediterranen Ottern und ihre Gifte, pp. 111—158. Marburg-Lahn: Behring 1936

Schöttler, W. H. A.: Serological analysis of venoms and antivenins. Bull. Org. Mond. Sante **12**, 877—903 (1955)

Sela, M., Arnon, R.: Studies on the chemical basis of the antigenicity of proteins. I. Antigenicity of polypeptidyl gelatins. Biochem. J. **75**, 91—102 (1960)

Sela, M., Fuchs, S., Arnon, R.: Studies on the chemical basis of the antigenicity of proteins 5 Synthesis, characterization and immunogenicity of some multi-chain and linear polypeptides containing tyrosine. Biochem. J. **85**, 223—235 (1962)

Seto, A., Sato, S., Tamiya, N.: The properties and modification of tryptophan in a sea snake toxin, "Erabutoxin". Biochim. biophys. Acta (Amst.) **214**, 483—489 (1970)

Sewall, H.: Experiments on the preventive inoculations of rattlesnake venom. J. Physiol. (Lond.) **8**, 203—210 (1887)

Shaham, N., Bdolah, A., Kochva, E.: Isolation of L-amino acid oxidase from *Vipera palestinae* venom and preparation of a monospecific antiserum in rabbits. In: deVries, A., Kochva, E. (Eds.): Toxins of Animal and Plant Origin, Vol. III, pp. 919—925. London: Gordon and Breach 1973

Shands, J. W.: The immunological role of the macrophage. In: Cruickshank, R., Weir, D. M. (Eds.): Modern Trends in Immunology, pp. 86—118. London: Butterworths 1967

Shiloah, J., Berger, A., Klibansky, C.: Purification of isoenzymes from cobra *Naja naja* and *Vipera palestinae* venoms Toxicon **8**, 153—154 (1970)

Shiloah, J., Klibansky, C., de Vries, A.: Phospholipase isoencymes from *Naja naja* venom. I. Purification and partial characterization. Toxicon **11**, 481—490 (1973)
Shipolini, R. A., Bailey, G. S., Banks, B. E. C.: The preparation of neurotoxin from the venom of *Naja melanoleuca* and the primary sequence determination. Europ. J. Biochem. **42**, 203—211 (1974)
Shipolini, R. A., Bailey, G. S., Edwardson, J. A., Banks, B. E. C.: Separation and characterization of polypeptides from the venom of *Dendroaspis viridis*. Europ. J. Biochem. **40**, 337—344 (1973)
Shipolini, R. A., Banks, B. E. C.: The amino acid sequence of a polypeptide from the venom of *Dendroaspis viridis*. Europ. J. Biochem. **49**, 399—405 (1974b)
Shipolini, R. A., Ivanov, C. P., Dimitrov, G.: Composition of the low molecular fraction of the Bulgarian viper venom. Biochim. biophys. Acta (Amst.) **104**, 292—295 (1965)
Shipolini, R. A., Kissonnerghis, M., Banks, B. E. C.: The primary structure of a major polypeptide component from the venom of *Naja melanoleuca*. Europ. J. Biochem. **56**, 449—454 (1975)
Shkenderov, S.: Anaphylactogenic properties of bee venom and its fractions. Toxicon **12**, 529—534 (1974)
Shü, I. C., Ling, K. H., Yang, C. C.: Study on I^{131} cobrotoxin. Toxicon **5**, 295—301 (1968)
Shulov, A., Ginsburg, H., Weissmann, A., Flesh, Y., Dishon, T.: La préparation d'un antivenin contre la vipère palestinienne par l'emploi d'un venin frais. Harefuah. J. med. Ass. Israel **56**, 55—58 (1959)
Shulov, A., Nelken, D., Schillinger, G.: Méthode sérologique pour le titrage des serums antiveni-meux. Ann. Inst. Pasteur **102**, 117—122 (1962)
Singer, T. P., Kearney, E. B.: The L-amino-acid-oxidases of snakes venoms. II. Isolation and characterization of homogeneous L-amino-acid-oxidase. Arch. Biochem. **29**, 190—209 (1950)
Sket, D., Gubensek, F., Adamic, S., Lebez, D.: Action of a partially purified basic protein fraction from *Vipera ammodytes* venom. Toxicon **11**, 47—53 (1973)
Skvaril, P., Tykal, P.: Investigation of antigen composition of the venom of *Vipera ammodytes*. Coll. Czechosl. Chem. Commun. **26**, 1479—1482 (1961)
Slotta, K. H.: A crotoxina primeru substancia pura dos venenos ofidicios. Ann. Acad. Brasil. Sci. **10**, 195 (1938)
Soh, K. S., Chan, K. E.: Caseinolytic and esteratic activities of Malayan pit viper venom and its proteolytic and thrombin-like fractions. Toxicon **12**, 151—158 (1974)
Spitznagel, J. K., Allison, A. C.: Mode of action of adjuvant effects on antibody response to macrophages associated bovine serum albumin. J. Immunol. **104**, 128—139 (1970a)
Spitznagel, J. K., Allison, A. C.: Mode of action of adjuvants: retinol and other lysosome-labilizing agents as adjuvants. J. Immunol. **104**, 119—127 (1970b)
Stanic, M.: Allergenic properties of venom hypersensitiveness in man and animals. In: Buckley, E., Porges, N. (Eds.): Venoms, pp. 181—188. Amer. Ass. Adv. Sci., pub. No. 44, Washington 1956
Stanic, M.: A modified Calmette's "in vitro" method for the titration of the antiphosphatidase a antibodies in the antivenin against the *Vipera ammodytes* venom. Path. Microbiol. (Basel) **23**, 30—35 (1960)
Stephens, J. W. W.: On the hemolytic action of snake toxins and toxin sera. J. Path. Bact. **6**, 273 (1900)
Strosberg, A. D., Nihoul-Deconink, C., Kanarek, L.: Weak immunological cross-reaction between bovine α lactalbumin and hen's egg white lysozyme. Nature (Lond.) **207**, 1241—1242 (1970)
Strydom, A. J. C.: Snake venom toxins. The amino acid sequences of two toxins from *Dendroaspis jamesoni kaimosea* (jameson's mamba) venom. Biochim. biophys. Acta (Amst.) **328**, 491—509 (1973)
Strydom, A. J. C., Botes, D. P.: Snake venom toxins. Purification, properties, and complete amino acid sequence of two toxins from ringhals *(Hemachatus haemachatus)* venom. J. biol. Chem. **246**, 1341—1349 (1971)
Strydom, D. J.: Phylogenetic relationships of proteroglyphae toxins. Toxicon **10**, 39—45 (1972a)
Strydom, D. J.: Snake venom toxins: the amino acid sequences of two toxins from *Dendroaspis polylepis polylepis*. J. biol. Chem. **247**, 4029—4042 (1972b)
Strydom, D. J.: Snake venom toxins: the evolution of some of the toxins found in snake venoms. Syst. Zool. **22**, 596—608 (1973a)

Strydom, D. J.: Snake venom toxins. Structure-function relationships and phylogenetics. Comp. Biochem. Physiol. [B] **44**, 269—281 (1973b)
Strydom, D. J.: Protease inhibitors as snake toxins. Nature (Lond.) **243**, 88—89 (1973c)
Strydom, D. J.: The amino acid sequence of toxin Vi2, a homologue of pancreatic trypsin inhibitor from *Dendroaspis polylepis polylepis* (black mamba) venom. Biochim. biophys. Acta (Anst.) **491**, 361—369 (1977)
Sulkowski, E., Björk, W., Laskowski, M.: A specific and nonspecific alkaline monophosphatase in the venom of *Bothrops atrox* and their occurence in a purified venom phosphodiesterase. J. biol. Chem. **238**, 2477—2486 (1963)
Sulkowski, E., Laskowski, M.: Venom exonuclease (phosphodiesterase) immobilized on concanavalin-A-sepharose. Biochem. biophys. Res. Commun. **57**, 463—468 (1974)
Sumyk, G., Lal, H., Hawrylewicz, E. J.: Whole animal autoradiographic localization of radioiodine labeled cobra venom in mice. Fed. Proc. **22**, 668 (1963)
Taborda, A. R., Taborda, L. C., Williams, J. N., Jr., Elvehjem, C. A.: A study of the desoxyribonucleases activity of snake venoms. J. biol. Chem. **195**, 207—213 (1952)
Takahashi, H., Iwanaga, S., Suzuki, T.: Isolation of a novel inhibitor of kallikrein, plasmin, and trypsin from the venom of Russell's viper *(Vipera russellii)*. FEBS Letters **27**, 207—210 (1972)
Takahashi, H., Iwanaga, S., Kitagawa, T., Hokama, Y., Suzuki, T.: Snake venom proteinase inhibitors. II. Chemical structure of inhibitor II isolated from the venom of Russell's viper *(Vipera russellii)*. J. Biochem. (Tokyo) **76**, 721—733 (1974a)
Takahashi, H., Iwanaga, S., Kitagawa, T., Hokama, Y., Suzuki, T.: Novel proteinase inhibitors in snake venoms: Distribution, isolation and amino acid sequence. In: Fritz, H., Tschesche, H., Greene, L. J., Eruscheit, E. (Eds.): Bayer Symposium V: Proteinase Inhibitors, pp. 265—276. Berlin-Heidelberg-New York: Springer 1974b
Takahashi, H., Iwanaga, S., Hokama, Y., Suzuki, T., Kitagawa, T.: Primary structure of proteinase inhibitor II isolated from the venom of Russell's viper *(Vipera russellii)*. FEBS Letters **38**, 217—221 (1974c)
Takahashi, T., Ohsaka, A.: Purification and characterization of a proteinase in the venom of *Trimeresurus flavoviridis*. Complete separation of the enzyme from hemorrhagic activity. Biochim. biophys. Acta (Amst.) **198**, 293—307 (1970a)
Takahashi, T., Ohsaka, A.: Purification and some properties of two hemorrhagic principles (HR_2a and HR_2b) in the venom of *Trimeresurus flavoviridis;* complete separation of the principles from proteolytic activity. Biochim. biophys. Acta (Amst.) **207**, 65—75 (1970b)
Takechi, M., Hayashi, K., Sasaki, T.: The amino acid sequence of cytotoxin II from the venom of Indian cobra *(Naja naja)*. Molec. Pharmacol. **8**, 446—451 (1973)
Takechi, M., Sasaki, T., Hayashi, K.: The N-terminal amino acid sequences of two basic cytotoxic proteins from the venom of the Indian cobra. Naturwissenschaften **6**, 323—324 (1971)
Talmage, D.: The role of auxiliary cells in antigen induced response (Summary). Immunochemistry **11**, 102 (1974)
Tamiya, N., Abe, H.: The isolation, properties and amino acid sequence of "Erabutoxin" c, a minor neurotoxic component of the venom of a sea snake *Laticauda semifasciata*. Biochem. J. **130**, 547—555 (1972)
Tamiya, N., Arai, H.: Studies on sea snake venoms. Crystallization of "Erabutoxins" a and b from *Laticauda semifasciata* venom. Biochem. J. **99**, 624—630 (1966)
Tamiya, N., Arai, H., Sato, S.: Studies on sea snake venoms: crystallization of "Erabutoxins" a and b from *Laticauda semifasiata* venom, and of "Laticotoxin", a from *Laticauda laticaudata* venom. In: Russell, F. E., Saunders, P. R. (Eds.): Animal Toxins, pp. 249—258. Oxford: Pergamon 1966
Tamiya, N., Sato, S.: Studies on snake venom: Structure and function of crystalline toxins of sea venom *Laticaudinae*. 7th Inter. Congress. Biochem., Hakone Symp., Tokyo, Abstr. 497 (1967)
Tanaka, A., Ishibashi, T., Sugugima, K., Takamoto, M.: Immunological adjuvants. VI. An acetylated mycobacterial adjuvant lacking competing antigenicity. Z. Immun.-Forsch. **142**, 303—317 (1971)
Tatsuki, T., Iwanaga, S., Oshima, G., Suzuki, T.: Snake venom NAD nucleotidase: its occurence in the venom from the genus *Agkistrodon* and purification and properties of the enzyme from the venom of *Agkistrodon halys blomhoffii*. Toxicon **13**, 211—220 (1975)

Tatsuki, T., Iwanaga, S., Suzuki, T.: A simple method for preparation of snake venom phosphodiesterase almost free from 5'-nucleotidase. J. Biochem. (Tokyo) **77**, 831—836 (1975)
Taylor, J., Mallik, S. M. K.: Observation on the neutralization of the "hemorrhagin" of certain viper venoms by antivenin. Indian J. med. Res. **23**, 121—130 (1935)
Taylor, J., Mallick, S. M. K.: The action of rattlesnake and moccasin venoms as compared with Indian viper venoms. Indian J. med. Res. **24**, 273—279 (1936)
Taylor, J., Mallick, S. M. K., Ahuja, M. L.: The coagulant action of blood of Daboia and *Echis* venoms and its neutralization. Indian J. med. Res. **23**, 131—140 (1935)
Tazieff-Depierre, F., Pierre, J.: Action curarisante de la toxine α de *Naja nigricollis*. C.R. Acad. Sci. [D] (Paris) **263**, 1785—1788 (1966)
Timmerman, W. F.: Immunological studies with *Crotalus* venom. Proc. west. Pharmacol. Soc. **13**, 105—110 (1970)
Toda, T., Mitsuse, B.: Studien über die Komponenten des hämolytischen Komplements. Z. Immun.-Forsch. **78**, 62—81 (1933)
Toom, P. M., Solie, T. N., Tu, A. T.: Characterization of a nonproteolytic arginine ester-hydrolysing enzyme from snake venom. J. biol. Chem. **245**, 2549—2555 (1970)
Tsao, F. H. C., Keim, P. S., Heinrikson, R. L.: *Crotalus adamanteus* phospholipase A2α: subunit structure, NH_2-terminal sequence, and homology with other phospholipase. Arch. Biochem. Biophys. **167**, 706—717 (1975)
Tseng, L. F., Chiu, T. H., Lee, C. Y.: Absorption and distribution of 131 abeled Cobra venom and its purified toxins. Toxicol. appl. Pharmacol. **12**, 526—535 (1968)
Tsernoglou, D., Petsko, G. A.: The crystal structure of a postsynaptic neurotoxin in from sea snake at 2.2 Å resolution. FEBS Letters **68**, 1—14 (1976)
Tu, A. T., Adams, B. L.: Phylogenetic relationships among venomous snakes of the genus *Agkistrodon* from Asia and the North American continent. Nature (Lond.) **217**, 760—762 (1968)
Tu, A. T., Ganthavorn, S.: Comparison of *Naja naja siamensis* and *Naja naja atra* venoms. Toxicon **5**, 207—212 (1968)
Tu, A. T., Hong, B. S.: Purification and chemical studies of a toxin from the venom of *Lapemis hardwickii*. J. biol. Chem. **246**, 2772—2779 (1971)
Tu, A. T., Hong, B. S., Solie, T. N.: Characterization and chemical modification of toxins isolated from the venom of sea snake, *Laticauda semifasciata*, from Philippines. Biochemistry **10**, 1295—1304 (1971)
Tu, A. T., Passey, R. B.: Phospholipase A from sea snake venom and its biological properties. In: deVries, A., Kochva, E. (Eds.): Toxins of Animal and Plant Origin, Vol. I, pp. 419—436. London: Gordon and Breach 1971
Tu, A. T., Passey, R. B., Toom, P. M.: Isolation and characterization of phospholipase A from sea snake *Lacticauda semifasciata* venom. Arch. Biochem. Biophys. **140**, 96—106 (1970)
Tu, A. T., Salafranca, E. S.: Immunological properties and neutralization of sea snake venoms (II). Amer. J. trop. Med. Hyg. **23**, 135—138 (1974)
Tu, A. T., Shen, T., Bieber, A. L.: Purification and chemical characterization of the major neurotoxin from the venom of *Pelamis platurus*. Biochemistry **14**, 3408—3413 (1975)
Tu, A. T., Toom, P. M.: Isolation and characterization of the toxic component of *Enhydrina schistosa* (common sea snake) venom. J. biol. Chem. **246**, 1012—1016 (1971)
Unanue, E. R., Askonas, B. A., Allison, A. C.: A role of macrophages in the stimulation of immune responses by adjuvants. J. Immunol. **103**, 71—78 (1969)
Uriel, J., Avrameas, S.: Mise en évidence d'hydrolases pancréatiques après électrophorèse et immuno-électrophorèse en agarose. Ann. Inst. Pasteur **106**, 396—407 (1964)
Uriel, J., Courcon, J.: Caractérisation des ribonucléases après électrophorèse en gélose. C.R. Acad. Sci. [D] (Paris) **253**, 1876—1877 (1961)
Uriel, J., Scheidegger, J. J.: Electrophorèse en gélose et coloration des constituants. Bull. Soc. chim. Biol. **37**, 165—168 (1955)
Vellard, J.: Spécificité des sérums anti-ophidiques. Ann. Inst. Pasteur **44**, 148—170 (1930)
Vellard, J.: Propriétés du venin des principales espèces de serpents du Vénézuala. Ann. Inst. Pasteur **60**, 511—548 (1938)
Vellard, J.: Variations géographiques du venin de *Crotalus terrificus*. C.R. Soc. Biol. [D] (Paris) **130**, 463—464 (1939)

Vidal, J. C., Cattaneo, P., Stoppani, A. O. M.: Some characteristic properties of phospholipases A_2 from *Bothrops neuwiedii* venom. Arch. Biochem. Biophys. **151**, 168—179 (1972)
Vidal, J. C., Stoppani, A. O. M.: Purification de la phospholipase A du venin de *Bothrops neuwiedii*. C.R. Soc. Biol. (Paris) **162**, 1615—1616 (1968)
Vidal, J. C., Stoppani, A. O. M.: Isolation and purification of two phospholipases A from *Bothrops* venom. Arch. Biochem. Biophys. **145**, 543—556 (1971 a)
Vidal, J. C., Stoppani, A. O. M.: Isolation and properties of an inhibitor of phospholipase A from *Bothrops neuwiedii* venom. Arch. Biochim. Biophys. **147**, 66—76 (1971 b)
Viljoen, C. C., Botes, D. P.: Snake venom toxins. The purification and amino acid sequence of toxin F. VII. From *Dendroaspis angusticeps* venom. J. biol. Chem. **248**, 4915—4919 (1973)
Viljoen, C. C., Botes, D. P.: Snake venom toxins. The purification and amino acid sequence of toxin T A_2 from *Dendroaspis*. J. biol. Chem. **249**, 366—372 (1974)
Vital Brazil, O.: La défense contre l'Ophidisme. Sao Paulo: Pocai & Weiss 1911
Vital Brazil, O.: Neurotoxins from the South American rattle-snake venom. J. Formosan med. Ass. **71**, 394—400 (1972)
Vogt, W., Patzer, P., Lege, L., Oldigs, H. D., Wille, G.: Synergism between phospholipase A and various peptides and SH-reagents in causing haemolysis. Arch. Pharmakol. **265**, 442—454 (1970)
Wahlström, A.: Purification and characterization of phospholipase A from the venom of *Naja nigricollis*. Toxicon **9**, 45—56 (1971)
Wakui, K., Kawauchi, S.: Properties of the two lecithinases A in snake venom. J. pharm. Soc. Jap. **81**, 1394—1400 (1961)
Weigle, W. O., Chiller, J. M., Habitch, G. S.: Immunological unresponsiveness: cellular kinetics and interactions. In: Amos, B. (Ed.): Progress in Immunology, pp. 311—322. New York: Academic 1971
Weise, K. H. K., Carlsson, F. H. H., Joubert, F. J., Strydom, D. J.: The purification of toxins $V^{11}I$ and $V^{11}2$, two cytotoxin homologues from banded Egyptian cobra *(Naja haje annulifera)* venom, and the complete amino acid sequence of toxin $V^{11}I$. Hoppe-Seylers Z. physiol. Chem. **354**, 1317—1326 (1973)
Wellner, D., Meister, A.: Crystalline L-amino acid oxidase of *Crotalus adamanteus*. J. biol. Chem. **235**, 2013—2018 (1960)
Wells, M. A., Hanahan, D. J.: Studies on phospholipase A. I. Isolation and characterization of two enzymes from *Crotalus adamanteus* venom. Biochemistry **8**, 414—424 (1969)
White, R. G.: Concepts of mechanism of action of adjuvants. In: Boreck, F. (Ed.): Immunogenicity, pp. 112—130. Amsterdam: North-Holland 1972
White, R. G., Jenkins, G. C., Wilkinson, P. C.: The reproduction of skin sensitizing antibody in the guinea-pig. Int. Arch. Allergy **22**, 156—165 (1963)
Wu, C. Y., Cinader, B.: Antigenic promotion. Increase in hapten specific plaque-forming cells after pre-injection with structurally unrelated macromolecules. J. exp. Med. **134**, 693—712 (1971)
Wu, T. W., Tinker, D. O.: Phospholipase A_2 from *Crotalus atrox* venom. I. Purification and some properties. J. Biochem. (Tokyo) **8**, 1558—1568 (1969)
Yang, C. C.: Enzymic hydrolysis and chemical modification of cobrotoxin. Toxicon **3**, 19—23 (1965 a)
Yang, C. C.: Crystallization and properties of cobrotoxin from Formosan cobra venom. J. biol. Chem. **240**, 1616—1618 (1965 b)
Yang, C. C.: The disulfide bonds of cobrotoxin and their relationship to lethality. Biochim. biophys. Acta (Amst.) **133**, 346—355 (1967)
Yang, C. C., Chang, L. T.: Studies on the phosphatase activities of Formosan snake venoms. J. Formosan med. Ass. **53**, 609—616 (1954)
Yang, C. C., Chang, C. C., Liou, I. F.: Studies on the status of arginine residues in Cobrotoxin. Biochim. biophys. Acta (Amst.) **365**, 1—14 (1974)
Yang, C. C., Chang, C. C., Wei, H. C.: Studies on fluorescent cobrotoxin. Biochim. biophys. Acta (Amst.) **147**, 600—602 (1967)
Yang, C. C., Chen, C. J., Su, C. C.: Biochemical studies on the Formosan snakes venoms. IV. The toxicity of Formosan cobra venom and enzyme activities. J. Biochem. (Tokyo) **46**, 1201—1209 (1959)

Yang, C. C., Chiu, W. C., Kao, K. C.: Biochemical studies on the snake venoms. VII. Isolation of venom cholinesterase by zone electrophoresis. J. Biochem. (Tokyo) **48**, 706—713 (1960)
Yang, C. C., Lin, M. F., Chang, C. C.: Purification of anticobrotoxin antibody by affinity chromatography. Toxicon **15**, 51—62 (1977)
Yang, C. C., Yang, H. J., Huang, J. S.: The amino acid sequence of cobrotoxin. Biochim. biophys. Acta (Amst.) **188**, 65—77 (1969)
Zeller, E. A.: Über eine Adenosintriphosphorsäure (ATP) spaltendes Enzym der Schlangengifte. Experientia (Basel) **4**, 194—197 (1948 a)
Zeller, E. A.: Enzymes of snakes venoms and their biological significance. Advanc. Enzymol. **8**, 459—495 (1948 b)
Zeller, E. A.: The formation of pyrophosphate from adenosine triphosphate in the presence of a snake venom. Arch. Biochem. **28**, 138—139 (1950)
Zeller, E. A., Maritz, A.: Über eine neue L-aminosäure-oxidase (ophio-L-aminosäure-oxidase). Helv. chim. Acta **28**, 365—379 (1945)
Zimmerman, S. E., Brown, R. K., Curti, B., Massey, V.: Immunochemical studies of L-amino acid oxidase. Biochim. biophys. Acta (Amst.) **229**, 260—270 (1971)
Zwilling, R., von, Pfleiderer, G.: Eigenschaften der α-Protease aus dem Gift von *Crotalus atrox*. Hoppe-Seylers Z. physiol. Chem. **348**, 519—524 (1967)
Zwissler, O.: The role of enzymes in the process responsible for the toxicity of snake venoms (an immunological study). Mem. Inst. Butantan **33**, 281—291 (1966)

CHAPTER 20

Production and Standardization of Antivenin

P. A. CHRISTENSEN

A. Introduction

The international name for antisera prepared for the treatment of snake bite poisoning is *antivenenum*, followed by the zoologic name or names of the species of snake from which the antigens were derived and the name of the species of animal in which the antiserum was made (WHO Expert Committee on Biological Standardization, 1971). The proper name in English, *antivenene*, suggested by FRASER (1895) has lost ground to antivenin, adopted from the French via America. The expression antivenine, occasionally seen, is of doubtful merit, and the plain name antivenom is somehow seldom used.

The experimental preparation of antivenin for the first time just before the turn of the century (PHISALIX and BERTRAND, 1894; CALMETTE, 1894) was a natural sequence to the discovery of bacterial antitoxins (BEHRING and KITASATO, 1890), and the study and development of antivenins ever since have closely followed the lines adopted for bacterial antitoxins, though not always with the same measure of success. Any procedure described for hyperimmunization with bacterial toxins, including attempted detoxicification of the antigens with retention of antigenicity and the use of adsorbants and adjuvants to enhance the immune response, has also been tried in antivenin production. The technique for potency assay is essentially the same for antitoxins and antivenins, and methods of purifying and concentrating antivenins by salt fractionation (GRASSET, 1932; GREVAL, 1934) were originally described for bacterial antitoxins and so were the current methods which involve digestion with pepsin.

Details of the preparation of antivenin for experimental purposes may be found in numerous publications, but little has been written about the production of therapeutic antivenins, and the account presented here is of necessity, but without prejudice, based on procedures in this laboratory. Conditions in other laboratories working with different venoms may favor other procedures (ARANTES and BRANDÃO, 1948a; CRILEY, 1956; LEON and SALAFRANCA, 1956; SAWAI et al., 1961; MOHAMED et al., 1966, 1973a, b, c; LATIFI and MANHOURI, 1966; CHATTERJEE et al., 1968; BOLAÑOS et al., 1975) and the immunization schedules in particular may vary in detail. The paucity of information is undoubtedly not due to any reluctance to share information, but rather because there has been nothing startling to report. The number of different antivenins has increased and their purity has been improved, but the methods of immunization have hardly altered, and the potency of antivenins still bears no comparison with that of bacterial antitoxins. Tested in mice, the number of lethal venom doses neutralized per ml of a good antivenin may be counted in hundreds, whereas for tetanus toxin and antitoxin of comparable protein concentration, the corresponding figure would amount to hundreds of thousands.

B. Antivenin Production

I. The Animal

Sera against snake venoms intended for therapeutic use have occasionally been raised in goats (COHEN and SELIGMANN, 1966; MOHAMED et al., 1966; RUSSELL et al., 1970; KOCHOLATY et al., 1971), and a *Chironex fleckeri* antivenin derived from sheep is available in Australia for the treatment of stings by this jelly fish (BAXTER and MARR, 1974), but all commercial snake antivenins are prepared in horses (MINTON, 1974).

The use of horses for the production of therapeutic sera was first described by ROUX and MARTIN (1894). It is the natural animal to choose. Horses are easy to handle, thrive in most climates, yield large volumes of serum, and methods of purifying horse serum are well-developed. Big horses are obviously preferable because of their larger blood volume, but breed and age are not important. Penicillin must not be given during immunization (European Pharmacopoeia, 1971) and streptomycin should possibly also be avoided (WHO Expert Committee on Biological Standardization, 1969). Blood should be drawn only from healthy animals; minor defects such as poor vision or lameness do not preclude their use. Tetanus is a common disease among horses, and they should be immunized prophylactically. Not only is this in the manufacturer's own interest, but it would prevent a repetition of the St. Louis tragedy, in which 14 fatalities were caused by tetanus toxin contained in injected diphtheria antitoxin drawn from a horse 2 days before it showed obvious signs of tetanus (FUNKHOUSER, 1901).

A risk of some untoward reaction is attached to the injection of serum from any animal, and horse serum has gained a particularly bad reputation in this respect, undoubtedly because it has been more widely used than sera from other animals. The incidence of the delayed type of reaction, serum sickness, has been drastically reduced by the introduction of pepsin-digested sera, but is still to be expected in 5–8% of persons treated. More dreaded is the acute anaphylactic reaction that can be elicited in persons hypersensitive to horse protein. Hypersensitivity may be naturally acquired, but some individuals in any population have become sensitized as the result of serum injections, commonly prophylactic injections of tetanus antitoxin. The number is diminishing due to several factors, namely the increasing use of toxoid for active immunization and the appreciation of the long duration of the immunity induced, the replacement of serum by chemotherapeutics and antibiotics in the treatment of some diseases, and to a lesser extent the availability of human antitoxic immunoglobulins.

Fatal anaphylaxis is undoubtedly a rare occurrence, but how rare remains unknown. Antivenin and bacterial antitoxins are alike, and PARK (1928), who had much experience in the treatment of diphtheria, stated that one death had occurred for every 50000 persons injected with antitoxin. Many clinicians suspect that the risk may be somewhat greater than this, but acceptable statistics are not available. The five deaths recorded by KOJIS (1942) in 6211 personally observed patients all resulted from second injections of antitoxin given 2–3 weeks after the first and, therefore, do not reflect the risk to a population at large. A questionnaire has for many years been enclosed with every ampoule of antivenin issued by this laboratory. Of the 3500 completed and returned questionnaires, 76 described the death of the patient. Anaphylaxis was the obvious cause of death in one case and could not be absolutely excluded in two others. Mortality rates based on such data would be high because uneventful snakebites are less likely to be reported, but they are not in conflict with the view that the risk of death from serious snakebite poisoning is greater than the risk attached to the injection of antivenin.

Considering the underlying immune mechanism, there is no reason to believe that serum sickness would be less common if serum from an animal other than the horse were used. Anaphylactic shock is said to be observed more often after first than after subsequent injections of horse serum (PARK, 1928; PARISH and CANNON, 1961). This would incriminate naturally acquired hypersensitivity, and naturally acquired sensitivity to other animal proteins, bovine proteins in particular, is probably just as widespread among human beings. The availability of nonequine antivenin would, of course, be a comfort to those specifically sensitive to horse protein and unavoidably exposed to snakebite, but no manufacturer is likely for this reason to abandon the use of horses for mass production.

II. The Antigens

Which venoms to use as antigens must obviously be determined by the frequency of bites by different snakes, the severity of the effects, and the availability of venom. Availability is essential for continued large scale serum production but goes usually hand in hand with the frequency of bites by the different species, and to some extent, with the severity of the effects, because larger snakes delivering much venom tend to do most damage. Shortage of venom may force a manufacturer to rely on cross-neutralization in areas where a dangerous genus is represented by numerous species. The genus *Crotalus* is a case in point; careful selection of antigens among the available venoms enables preparation of antivenins with wide cross-neutralizing powers (CRILEY, 1956; GINGRICH and HOHENADEL, 1956).

Some manufacturers maintain and milk snakes in their laboratories. Others, including this Institute, purchase the venom from reputable dealers. Whichever the case, research workers requiring antivenins of strict specificity should use commercial preparations with caution; the horses from which they were derived could unwittingly or on purpose have been injected with venoms other than those against which potency is claimed on the label.

In the majority of snakebites, the culprit is not seen or not identified, and this is one of the reasons why polyvalent sera are preferable to monovalent, except in areas where dangerous bites are almost exclusively due to a single species. The WHO Expert Committee on Biological Standardization (1971) does not favor the use of polyvalent preparations, possibly due to a misconception. Specific neutralization is obviously preferable to cross-neutralization, but polyvalent sera are specific. They should not be prepared by blending several monovalent sera, which would amount to a dilution of the different sera with lowering of the specific potencies. The horses should be immunized with all the antigens, and the specific potencies of their sera should not be lower than those of corresponding monovalent sera.

Horses given only one venom soon reach a state of immunity which does not improve unless the venom dose is increased quite out of proportion to the rise in antibody titer, and such monovalent horses usually maintain their serum titer to this particular venom after they have been transferred to the production of polyvalent serum (MOHAMED et al., 1973c). This Institute prepared some years ago two polyvalent sera for general use, a polyvalent *Bitis*, *Hemachatus*, *Naja* antivenin and a polyvalent *Dendroaspis* (mamba) antivenin. Large areas of the part of Africa for which these sera were intended are shared by vipers, cobras, and mambas, and both sera had, therefore, to be available in quantity. During 1970, the production of antivenin was stopped for some time while the *Bitis*, *Hemachatus*, *Naja* horses were immunized basically with *Dendroaspis* venoms, and the *Dendroaspis* horses with *Bitis*, *Hemachatus*, and *Naja* venoms. Both groups were thereafter immunized with all the venoms. The original specific potencies of the resulting sera remained unaltered for both groups, and the "new" potencies increased steadily. The two preparations were replaced by a single *Bitis*, *Dendroaspis*, *Hemachatus*, *Naja* antivenin at the end of 1971 when full polyvalent potency could be assured.

Competition among antigens discussed in Chapter 19 may be a rare phenomenon (BOYD, 1966) and does not seem to be a problem in the production of polyvalent antivenin, but the number of antigens in each venom is in any case large, and the antibody response in general too poor for this effect to be discernible. Rather than competing with each other, it is very probable that some venoms in a mixture may exert an adjuvant action on others, which could be one of the reasons why monovalent horses sometimes show disappointing serum titers (ARANTES and BRANDÃO, 1948b).

Polyvalent antivenin is easier to carry and store than a selection of different monovalent sera, and it is relatively cheaper to produce. As is the case for most therapeutic substances, the materials required, and the salaries paid to the technical staff engaged in production add comparatively little to the cost of antivenin. The administrative expenses, ampouling, packing, and maintenance of the horses are important items, the cost of which should remain the same per vial irrespective of the valency of its contents.

Once immunized, a horse will tolerate large single venom doses, but new horses are easily killed or injured, and to give them their first, basic, immunity with unmodified venom may be tedious although it can be done.

An atoxic, yet antigenic, preparation would offer obvious advantages over unmodified venom in the immunization of new horses. PHISALIX and BERTRAND (1894) used heat-treated venom in their experiments, and CALMETTE (1894), who tried various substances, recommended hypochlorite-treated venom. Mixtures of lipids and venom (VELLARD, 1930; MAITRA and MALLICK, 1932; RICHOU and NICOL, 1935; NICOL and MUSTAFA, 1936) and mixtures of soap and venom (RENAUD, 1930; CESARI and BOQUET, 1937) have been used as antigens; the comparative innocuity of such mixtures presumably being due to a decreased rate of absorption. SHORTT and MALLICK (1935) detoxified *Vipera russellii* venom solutions by photo-oxidation in the presence of methylene blue, but found the antigenic properties to be destroyed. More recent and detailed experimentation has shown that not only this venom but also those of *Crotalus atrox* and *Agkistrodon piscivorus* treated in this way can be used with reasonable safety as antigens in rabbits (KOCHOLATY, 1966; KOCHOLATY and ASHLEY, 1966). BOQUET (1941) detoxified venoms by the action of hydrogen peroxide in the presence of traces of copper, and GRASSET and ZOUTENDYK (1933) tried bile-detoxified venom and venom treated with an organic gold preparation. Neither method was of practical value because of the untoward effects produced by such inactivated venoms. To use underneutralized venom-antivenom mixtures can be risky, and fully neutralized mixtures are poor antigens. Treatment with formalin (RAMON, 1924, 1925; BÄCHER et al., 1925; MARTIN, 1925; ARTHUS, 1930; GRASSET and ZOUTENDYK, 1932) will certainly render venoms atoxic, at a rate which increases rapidly with increasing pH (BOQUET and VENDRELY, 1943; GRASSET, 1945), but this change is accompanied by a large loss in antigenicity (CHRISTENSEN, 1947; MOROZ-PERLMUTTER et al., 1963; SALAFRANCA, 1972). The use of formol-toxoided venoms (anavenom) is, therefore, wasteful of venom and can in the large doses required for hyperimmunization be the cause of unnecessary suffering of the horses. It was, however, for many years, the antigen most commonly used in antivenin-producing establishments.

Actually no detoxification is necessary if the venom is adsorbed on some inert carrier. The comparative harmlessness of adsorbed venom is presumably due to a decreased rate of absorption from the site of injection and the good response due to a prolonged stimulation by antigen held subcutis, apart from any possible adjuvant effect of the adsorbant (see Chapter 19).

In principle, this method originated with CALMETTE (1894) who recorded that a small piece of chalk impregnated with venom and coated with collodion and inserted under the skin of a rabbit would serve as a continued stimulation from an artificial gland, a suggestion he credited to Dr. ROUX, in whose laboratory he was working.

A number of adsorbants have been studied by several workers, mostly for the purpose of venom purification rather than immunization. Of the substances tested, aluminium phosphate and aluminium hydroxide are today widely used as adjuvants in vaccination of human beings with bacterial toxoids and some other vaccines. CRILEY (1956) has successfully used 1% venom solutions containing 10% aluminium hydroxide gel (Amphojel) in the preparation of pit viper antivenin. Aluminium hydroxide gels with constant adsorbant properties are notoriously difficult to prepare, and those made in this laboratory failed to adsorb *Naja* venom. Aluminium phosphate adsorbed too little to be used with safety, but the adsorption by bentonite was found to be complete and nonselective (CHRISTENSEN, 1955), an admirable property for the purpose of immunization. The original source of this particular bentonite, which is still in use, is unfortunately obscure. Unfortunately, because not all preparations appear to be satisfactory.

Venom adsorbed to a suitable bentonite may safely be used for primary immunization (CHRISTENSEN, 1955, 1966a; CHATTERJEE et al., 1968; MOHAMED et al., 1973a, b; LATIFI, 1975). Its use is discontinued as soon as traces of circulating antibody are detectable by a mouse protection test, and immunization is thereafter continued with nonadsorbed venom solutions, as detailed below.

The injection of bentonite suspensions can cause the formation of a small sterile abscess that requires incision, but the lesion heals in a few days and does not upset the horses; the loss of some antigenic material through the incision does not affect

Table 1. The intravenous and subcutaneous LD_{50} in μg of different snake venoms for mice weighing 16–18 g

Venom	Intravenous		Subcutaneous	
	LD_{50}	5% fiducial limits	LD_{50}	5% fiducial limits
Naja nivea	9.7	10.8– 9.1	12.3	13.0– 11.6
Naja melanoleuca	16	18.5–14.9	25	28.5– 22.0
Naja haje	21	23.5–19.2	29	33.8– 25.6
Naja nigricollis	23	28.9–19.9	48	51.4– 43.5
Hemachatus haemachatus	29	35.1–26.1	30	34.4– 26.0
Dendroaspis polylepis	8.3	8.9– 7.7	9.3	10.7– 8.3
Dendroaspis viridis	12.0	13.3–10.9	13.5	15.2– 12.2
Dendroaspis jamesoni	16	18.6–14.4	17	19.3– 15.6
Dendroaspis angusticeps	44	57.5–37.8	57	64.9– 49.1
Bitis arietans	9.7	10.6– 8.8	74	107.5– 59.4
Bitis gabonica	11.5	12.9–10.4	100	117.0– 85.5
Echis carinatus	22	30.9–16.3	151	177.4–134.3

the antibody response noticeably. The purpose of using bentonite or similarly acting adjuvants is to shorten the time taken to produce significant immunity with safety. Any benefit derived from their use for hyperimmunization is at most slight, and far outweighed by disadvantages when commercial antivenin production is considered. Immune horses are valuable and normally have a long productive life, 15 years or more is not unusual. They should not be exposed to the perpetual discomfort and irreversible tissue injury that may result from the use of some adjuvants.

Freund's adjuvant (FREUND, 1947) has been used in the preparation of *Trimeresurus* antivenin (SAWAI et al., 1961), but no difference was observed in the responses of comparable groups of already immune horses immunized in this laboratory with or without Freund's complete adjuvant. This was not an altogether displeasing finding because the local lesion it causes can be a pitiful sight, and the excessive formation of scar tissue after repeated injections can make further immunization impracticable. LATIFI (1975) also rejected Freund's adjuvant because of undesirable effects and uses a harmless adjuvant containing olive oil and gum arabic to stimulate the response to the otherwise plain venom solutions employed in the preparation of Iranian antivenins. Undesirable effects would undoubtedly be slight with an adjuvant such as aluminium hydroxide (CRILEY, 1956), and probably minimal with sodium alginate (BOLAÑOS et al., 1975), when the separate injection of calcium chloride into the same site, as originally suggested (SLAVIN, 1950), is omitted.

Freeze-dried venoms may be preferable, but neither the hardy elapid venoms nor the more labile viper venoms alter significantly for the purpose of immunization if they are dried with care by evaporation in a vacuum over a desiccant. This cannot, of course, be assured if the venoms are bought, but purchased venom should be tested for potency and specific antibody-binding power by immunodiffusion and mouse protection tests. This should in any case be done for the sake of identification; serious complications can arise if mislabeled venoms are injected.

The venoms used as antigens in this laboratory are listed in Table 1. The LD_{50} values shown in the table were determined for laboratory reference preparations.

Echis carinatus venom is used in the preparation of a monovalent serum but not in the production of polyvalent antivenin.

Separate solutions of individual venoms are preferred to stock solutions of ready mixed venoms, firstly because they allow for flexibility of dosage and secondly, because of the possible enzymic-degrading effect one venom could have on another in mixed solutions.

10 g of venom are dissolved per liter of distilled water containing 0.9% (wt/vol) sodium chloride and 0.25% (vol/vol) cresol; a month's requirement is prepared at a time. The solutions are clarified by filtration through a paper pad or a gamma filter (Whatman) and sterilized by filtration through an asbestos (Seitz) pad. Seitz filtration may cause some loss by adsorption of certain venom components such as phospholipase (CHOPRA et al., 1942) and phosphatases (HURST and BUTLER, 1951), but this is unimportant and reliable sterilization is essential. The solutions are kept in the cold room in dispensing flasks with rubber tubing and hooded nozzles attached, and the volumes needed for a group of horses are measured in sterile measuring cylinders and mixed. The solutions should be tested for sterility before use. Meat particle broth is not always suitable in tests for freedom from anaerobic contaminants because some venoms, even elapid venoms, may digest the meat and cause turbidity, in which case a thioglycollate medium is preferable.

The adsorbant consists of a 2% suspension of bentonite prepared in distilled water under stirring. The suspension is left overnight in a glass cylinder in the cold room. Rejecting the bottom portion with coarser particles, it is thereafter decanted and 5-ml, 7.5-ml, and 10-ml volumes are dispensed into 25-ml rubber-stoppered bottles. The bottles are sterilized at 120° C for 30 min in the autoclave and stored until required for use.

In preparing a dose for injection, the venom solution, or the mixture of several solutions if the dose is to contain more than one venom, is mixed with an equal volume of the bentonite suspension. After thorough shaking, the mixture may be injected immediately or left until later, whichever is convenient.

III. Immunization

1. New Horses

If only one venom is given, a horse will usually have demonstrable circulating antivenom 1 or 2 weeks after two doses containing 50 mg and 100 mg, respectively, given with an interval of 3 weeks between the doses. Three spaced doses of 25 mg, 50 mg, and 50 mg have also been used.

A number of monovalent sera have been prepared for experimental use, but new horses are otherwise always given bentonite mixtures containing all the venoms. Eight doses are given at weekly intervals. The first four contain a mixture of 5 mg of each venom and are followed by two doses of 10 mg, one of 15 mg and one of 20 mg of each venom. Additional doses of one or other of the venoms may be required if a serum sample taken at this stage fails to pass the following neutralization test.

The serum is mixed with solutions of laboratory reference venoms, one mixture for each venom, so that a dose of 0.6 ml will contain 0.5 ml of serum and 0.1 ml of venom solution. The concentration of the venom solution is such that 0.1 ml will contain from two to three times the LD_{99} calculated from the dose-response regression. Four mice are tested intravenously for each venom and all should survive.

When this requirement has been satisfied, the horses are given increasing but cautious doses of plain venom solutions three times per week for 2 weeks. They are thereafter bled and rested for 5 weeks before they receive a second course of slightly larger doses. From the third course onward, they are considered fully immune and treated accordingly.

2. Immune Horses

The immunization cycle for already immune horses is made up of 2 weeks for injections, 1 week for blood collection, and 5 weeks of rest. The available horses are divided into eight groups. On the 1 st day of any week one group will have completed a rest period and be ready for immunization, and two groups will be under immunization at any time throughout the year.

A standard dosage scheme is used for all horses in order to further simplify the work in stables and laboratory. During the 14 days of immunization, the horses are given six injections. The individual doses are not of the same volume or venom composition, but the volume injected is never in excess of 40 ml, and the amount of any one venom not larger than 100 mg, under normal circumstances.

All injections are given intramuscularly or subcutaneously in the tissues of the neck.

IV. Collection and Processing of Plasma

The horses are bled from the jugular vein into a sodium citrate solution. Depending on the size of the horse, from 8–10 liters of blood are removed on each of two occasions, separated by 3 days. The plasma is separated from the corpuscles by continuous centrifugation and sufficient cresol is added to give a concentration of 0.3%. The cresol prevents bacterial growth while the plasma awaits treatment and is also essential for a satisfactory result of the purification process. In order to prevent undue protein denaturation, it is convenient to add the cresol under agitation as a spray mixed with ether.

About five such blood lettings annually do not make the horses anemic or otherwise impair their health. To carry out the blood separation aseptically and return the red cells to the horses could probably increase the overall plasma yield by allowing more frequent bleeding but would be cumbersome and costly where many horses are handled. BAXTER et al. (1972) who used the technique for the preparation of *Chironex fleckeri* antivenin in a sheep concluded that plasmapheresis is useful when a valuable antigen is used and maximum yields are required over a short period.

Pope's method of purifying bacterial antitoxins (POPE, 1939a, b) is equally well applied to antivenins (PIROSKY et al., 1942; GRASSET and CHRISTENSEN, 1947; HÖXTER and DECOUSSAU, 1948; LATIFI and MANHOURI, 1966). A short digestion of the plasma yields two fractions from the antitoxic globulin; a relatively heat-stable fraction which possesses the antigen-binding sites, and another, in this respect inert fraction which is heat labile and removed by controlled heat denaturation. The discarded fraction is the main carrier of the globulin's species-specific antigenic sites, and the advantages of the method over simple salt fractionation methods are, therefore, twofold: less protein per unit dose and a reduced risk of reaction to the same amount of injected protein. Sera treated in this way are usually termed refined antisera (British Pharmaceutical Codex, 1968), to distinguish them from preparations purified by other means. The details of the purification process used here are essentially as described by HARMS (1948).

Other methods of pepsin purification (PARFENTJEV, 1934, 1936; HANSEN, 1941) require longer digestion and the removal of inactive material by adsorption. They are laborious and have not been used in the production of antivenins. However, adsorption with aluminium hydroxide (HANSEN, 1941) has been used to give a final polish to globulins obtained by Pope's process (LATIFI, 1975). Treatment of purified antitoxin with DEAE Sephadex A-50 has been used for the same purpose by HRISTOVA (1968) whose good results were confirmed here with bacterial antitoxins (ANDERSON, 1968), but antivenins were not improved under the conditions described nor by modification in the adsorbing and eluting conditions.

Taking both potency and turbidity into consideration, the results of accelerated degradation tests carried out on antivenin prepared here indicate that the maximum stability is at about pH 7 and not at pH 6 (European Pharmacopoeia, 1971).

C. Antivenin Standardization

The standardization of antivenin does not differ in principle from the standardization of other antitoxins which JERNE (1951) in his study of avidity has shown to be based on wrong assumptions. The troublesome deviations from assumed behavior of sera are fortunately minimal for hyperimmune sera, and all antivenins fall into this category. Some irregularities ascribable to lack of avidity are occasionally observed when sera are assayed with heterologous venoms, but the commonest and most striking irregularity which foils the standardization of antivenin has nothing to do with this problem.

When antivenin potency is assayed, it is customary to mix venom and serum in different proportions keeping the concentration of either the one or the other reagent constant, and to test the mixtures for free venom by injecting them into laboratory animals; the expression of potency is based on the composition of the particular harmless mixture in which the venom-serum ratio is at a maximum. Rather than to mix the reagents before they are injected, some workers have preferred to simulate the sequence in naturally occurring snakebite and inject the venom under the skin of the mice followed by serum into a vein (SCHÖTTLER, 1952; BALOZET, 1959). It could reasonably be expected that the latter way of testing would require more serum to neutralize a given amount of venom, but this would not matter if the estimates of relative potencies obtained by the two methods for different sera were concordant. This was the case when three sera were tested simultaneously by the two methods against two African cobra (*Naja nivea* and *N. haje*) and two African viper (*Bitis arietans* and *B. gabonica*) venoms (CHRISTENSEN, 1967). The three sera could be placed in the same order of potency with good agreement between pairs of relative potency estimates. For the *Naja* venoms, the ED_{50} values of the sera were persistently but not significantly higher when serum and venom were injected separately. The converse was the surprising finding for the *Bitis* venom. The explanation offered was that the mice did not die from the local venom effect but from the action of lethal components, constituting only part of the venoms injected, passing into the circulation; local tissue damage would tend to hinder the already slow absorption of toxins of comparatively large molecular size. Injected in a mixture, the serum would have to neutralize all the lethal toxin in order to protect, but injected separately into the blood stream it would only have to cope with the smaller amount of absorbed lethal toxin, and less serum would suffice.

In these experiments, the subcutaneous venom dose was immediately followed by serum intravenously. Any pause between the two injections would alter the result. The longer the delay, the larger the ED_{50} and the flatter the dose-response curve (CHRISTENSEN, 1969). Precise timing is possible in special experiments but is hardly a practical proposition in routine assays, and the separate injection of venom and serum does not seem to offer any advantages over the more convenient method of premixing the reagents.

It should be stressed that the mixtures were injected subcutaneously and not intravenously, because some venoms contain toxins that are lethal intravenously but comparatively harmless injected under the skin, and discrepancies between the titers could be expected if the mixtures had been injected intravenously; even the results of the premixing method may for this reason depend on the route of injection, as discussed below.

These observations were made with refined and specific antivenins; nonavid sera might have behaved differently, but this was not examined. The seemingly paradoxic findings in experiments of a similar nature (KOCHOLATY et al., 1968) are not necessarily in conflict with the findings recorded here, but may possibly be explained by nonavidity of the experimental sera and paraspecificity against *Crotalus d. durissus* venom of the commercial antivenin employed in the tests.

CAREY and WRIGHT (1960) examined an experimental *Enhydrina schistosa* antivenin prepared in a rabbit by the two methods. The limited data recorded in Tables IV and V of their publication show agreement between the results, but the serum was clearly less effective when tested by a method referred to as the in vivo method (Table V). By this method, the mice received 0.1 ml of antiserum intraperitoneally or intravenously and were challenged with venom 30 or 60 min later. Obviously, only part of the injected antitoxin would be circulating at this time and much of the venom would have free access to its target. This technique would hardly be considered for the purpose of standardization.

Having established the amount of venom neutralized by a certain amount of serum, it is common practice to express the potency of commercial antivenins as the calculated amount of venom expected to be neutralized by 1 ml of serum and to state this amount in mg or in number of mouse lethal doses, sometimes referred to as units, to lend an air of respectability to the statement. In such calculations, it is taken for granted that any multiple of the amount of venom neutralized in the test would require the same multiple amount of serum for its neutralization, i.e., that the "law" of combination in multiple proportions would apply, which is seldom the case. Others may have realized it, but it was left for BANIĆ and LJUBETIĆ (1938) to stress that the amount of serum required to protect an animal from the effect of two lethal venom doses is larger than twice the amount required for protection against one lethal dose, and to suggest an assay method which takes care of this.

The law of multiple proportions implies that the "neutral points" obtained by testing serum with venom at many concentration levels will fall on a straight line if recorded graphically in a system of coordinates in which the axes express the concentrations of serum and venom in the injected mixtures. The method of BANIĆ and LJUBETIĆ was modified later the same year by IPSEN (1938) who proposed the slope of the neutralization curve as the expression for the titer of a serum. This would have solved the problem if the curves were linear, as they appeared to be in the standardization experiments with IPSEN'S method presented by GRASSET (1940/41, 1949), TAYLOR (1940), and HAZRA et al. (1945/46), but other workers observed marked deviations from linearity in similar experiments (GOYAL, 1949; SCHÖTTLER, 1952). Linearity is in fact the exception not the rule. The usual finding is that neutralization curves examined over a sufficiently wide range of doses will show a change of slope, sometimes abrupt, but often gradual with curvature convex toward the venom axis, not toward the serum axis as could be expected with sera lacking in avidity, and attempts have been made to describe this seemingly complex relationship in mathematic terms (EICHBAUM, 1947; KRAG and BENTZON, 1966). No attention had been paid to the observation by SCHLOSSBERGER et al. (1936) who noted that the amount of a venom neutralized by some sera would increase with increasing serum dose up to a point beyond which further serum additions were without effect because the sera lacked antibody to some venom component. The authors did not elaborate, but it is an obvious conclusion that further additions of other sera which possessed some antibody to this component would have had some effect, though may be not of the same magnitude as the earlier serum additions, i.e., the neutralization curve would change slope. The degree of the change would vary from one serum to another depending on the concentration of antibody to this less dominant component; the lower the concentration, the larger would be the change of slope until, in the absence of any antibody, the curve would become parallel to the serum axis.

This interpretation deals adequately with the anomalies encountered when antivenoms are tested with crude venoms, and it was substantiated by results obtained in experiments with *Naja nivea* venom which was shown to contain three antigenically distinct toxins, called α-, β-, and γ-toxin in order of decreasing lethal importance (CHRISTENSEN, 1953). Tested with specific serum, this venom gave the usual type of neutralization curve showing a change of slope, quite abrupt as often is the case in tests with elapid venoms, and dividing the curve into two linear portions. Assaying the serum separately with preparations of the three toxins obtained by heat and acid treatment of specific antigen-antibody floccules, the first part of the curve obtained with whole venom could be shown to represent the neutralization of α-toxin by α-antitoxin, and the second part the neutralization of γ-toxin by γ-antitoxin. The concentration of β-antitoxin was in this serum, as in all other specific sera tested later, too high to interfere in the assay. A fourth distinct component, δ-toxin, has since been described (BOTES et al., 1971). It is immunochemically related to β-toxin, and the two would probably coflocculate and, therefore, not be separable by the earlier immunologic technique.

The upper curve shown in Figure 1 illustrates the result obtained when the international standard preparation of *Naja* antivenin was assayed with *N. nivea*

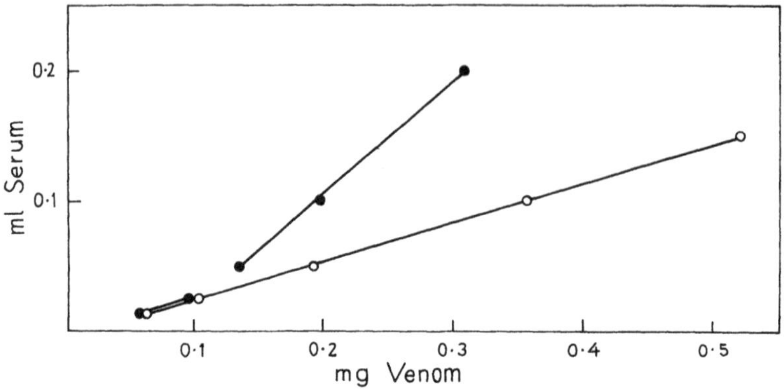

Fig. 1. Neutralization curves for *Naja nivea* venom and a polyvalent *Naja* antivenin determined in mice. ● Intravenous test. ○ Subcutaneous test

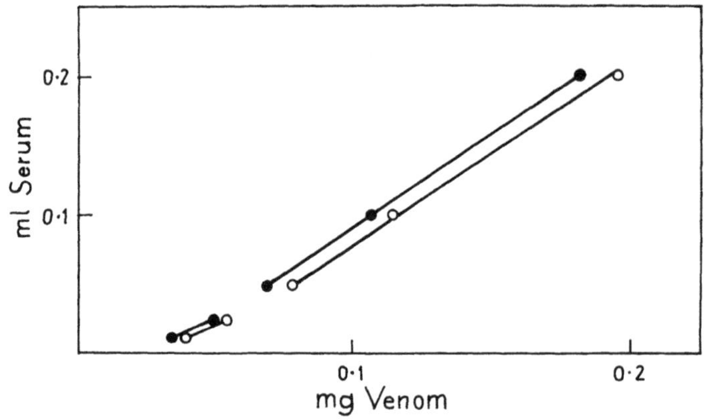

Fig. 2. Neutralization curves for *Naja haje* venom and a monovalent *N. haje* antivenin determined in mice. ● Intravenous test. ○ Subcutaneous test

venom intravenously in mice. It consists of the usual two linear components, the lower left part representing the α-toxin-antitoxin system, the other the γ-toxin-antitoxin system. A curve of similar shape would have been obtained if another serum had been included in the test, and by comparing the slopes of the corresponding parts of two such curves, it would be possible to express the relative anti-α and anti-γ potencies of the two sera. The anti-β and anti-δ potencies would remain obscure because these toxins would be fully neutralized by their common antibody in all the mixtures tested. The anti-α and anti-γ potency estimates obtained would be valid in this case, but if unknown sera were assayed at only one or two arbitrary test levels, it might be uncertain which antitoxin was operating and one might even be comparing the anti-α potency of one serum with the anti-γ potency of the other.

Having determined the neutralization curve for a serum intravenously in mice, one would expect to get a curve of similar shape if the test were repeated subcutaneously and the relative importance of the different toxic components were the same by either route, but this is not always so. The different *Bothrops* venoms examined by

SCHÖTTLER (1955/56) could, for instance, be placed in one order of potency when mice were injected intravenously and in a different order when the test was carried out subcutaneously. This, as he pointed out, would indicate that the main lethal factor differed for the two routes of injection. The predominant toxin in African venoms so far examined appears to be the same by either route, but the subcutaneous and intravenous neutralization curves can sometimes differ in shape because minor components may be comparatively harmless when injected under the skin.

The curves in Figure 1 serve as an example. The result obtained subcutaneously is represented by the lower, linear curve which is determined by α-toxin and antitoxin throughout the tested range with no signs of interference by γ-toxin. The subcutaneous LD_{50} of γ-toxin, which is probably a cardiotoxin, is from eight to ten times larger than the intravenous LD_{50}. Extrapolation to the abscissa in Figure 1 will indicate that one intravenous LD_{50} of γ-toxin was contained in about 0.08 mg of the test venom, and mixtures containing venom well in excess of 0.5 mg would have had to be injected if the effect of free γ-toxin were to have been demonstrated subcutaneously.

A similar situation has been observed with the venom of *Hemachatus haemachatus* and the two vipers *Bitis arietans* and *B. gabonica*, whereas the neutralization curves for venoms of the cobras *Naja haje*, *N. melanoleuca*, and *N. nigricollis* are determined by at least two toxins in the subcutaneous as well as the intravenous tests (CHRISTENSEN, 1966b).

The intravenous route is most convenient to use; an unaided worker can handle many mice in a short time and faulty injections can be spotted at once. The subcutaneous route could be considered preferable in situations such as that illustrated by Figure 1. The performance of assays by both routes would be advisable with venoms containing lethal toxins of route-dependent predominance. When this is not the case, the intravenous and subcutaneous neutralization curves for an antivenin will differ in position, but corresponding parts of the curves will be parallel (Figs. 1 and 2). The difference in position will about equal the difference between the intravenous and the subcutaneous LD_{50} of the active lethal component in terms of whole venom (Table 1).

This is true in tests with specific antivenins which, therefore, could be tested by either route with such venoms. The curves obtained with a related (paraspecific) venom are usually not parallel, and the subcutaneous test will yield the higher potency estimate. This is probably an avidity phenomenon. The paraspecific venom-antivenom complex would tend to dissociate when injected intravenously, whereas its stability would rather increase under the skin because of the concentration resulting from water absorption.

Points on a neutralization curve are determined either as the ED_{50} of the serum for a fixed dose of venom or the LD_{50} of venom injected with a fixed dose of serum. The two methods of preparing mixtures lead to closely the same result at comparable concentration levels. The mixture may be injected at once or may be left for some time, possibly in a warm spot, to allow antigen and antibody to combine firmly before they are injected. This is immaterial in tests with the specific venoms used in the preparation of the antisera but may affect the results when sera are tested for paraspecific potency. The same applies to the speed with which the mixtures are injected intravenously (CHRISTENSEN, 1966b).

The position with regard to the neutralization of venoms by antivenins may be summarized as follows.

All venoms contain more than one and often several antigenically different lethal toxins, each of which combines with its antitoxin according to the law of multiple proportions.

The neutralization curve will have its origin at a point on the venom dose axis corresponding to the LD_{50} of the predominant toxin, which will be in agreement with the LD_{50} of whole venom unless antigenically distinct toxins have joint action and contribute to the effect produced by the LD_{50} of whole venom.

The neutralization curve is only truly linear if the serum under test contains the relatively least amount of antibody to the dominant toxin. A valid estimate of the relative potency of different sera against this particular toxin component will be obtained if they all give this type of curve.

The curve will not be linear but show a change of slope if a serum contains relatively less antibody to a component of minor lethal importance, and if the potency of the serum allows the use of sufficiently high venom doses. Valid potency estimates against known venom toxins could be obtained from corresponding linear parts of the curve.

The point at which the curve begins to change direction and the steepness of the changed slope depend on the magnitude of the LD_{50} of the minor component in terms of whole venom and on the concentration of antitoxin to this component. Extrapolation to the venom axis will give an estimate of the amount of venom which contains an LD_{50} of the component.

Further changes in direction, sometimes resulting in gentle curvature, may occur if the serum's concentration of antitoxin to even less lethal components is still lower.

The outcome of a neutralization test may depend on the route of injection, subcutaneous or intravenous, if different lethal toxins predominate. The route is otherwise unimportant in tests with specific sera, whereas paraspecific sera may give discrepant results.

These considerations would apply whichever kind of animal was used in the tests, and they would confound comparison of antivenin potencies determined in different species.

It is well-known that the resistance to different venoms may vary from one kind of animal to another, and a highly resistant species would obviously not be chosen for antivenin standardization. Slight variations in susceptibility might feasibly affect the precision of a potency estimate, but the relative potencies of different sera should be in agreement irrespective of the animal used if the same toxin-antitoxin system is known to operate in all cases. This would usually be a moot point with whole venom as the test toxin.

No systematic studies are available comparing the use of different animals in antivenin standardization, but some observations made by GOYAL (1949) are interesting in retrospect. Working with mice, rats, guinea-pigs, rabbits, and monkeys and using a fixed serum dose, the assay results were reasonably acceptable in tests with cobra venom. But for *Vipera russellii* venom, he recorded that widely divergent amounts of venom were neutralized in different species by different routes. There is, however, a strikingly high correlation, almost a linear relationship, between the amounts of venom shown to be neutralized intravenously and the weight of the mammals used, irrespective of their kind; the value recorded for pigeons does not fit this picture. This could indicate that the serum contained little or no antibody to a minor toxic component to which the animals were about equally susceptible, and that the titers recorded in Table 1 in GOYAL's publication in reality were lethal doses of this component for animals of different body mass. Table II in the same publication shows details of antivenin assays with daboia venom in pigeons and guinea-pigs of comparable weights. Graphic recording of the results reveals a fair agreement for the three lowest test levels, but the curve for pigeons becomes thereafter extremely steep, though linear. LEE and TSENG (1969) have shown that the high lethality to *Bungarus* venom in pigeons and other birds is chiefly due to their high susceptibility to β-bungarotoxin, and GOYAL's experiment undoubtedly demonstrates the presence in *V. russellii* venom of a component to which pigeons are highly susceptible.

Sex-dependent susceptibility differences have never been observed in this laboratory, but DOSSENA (1949) recorded that female mice, rats, and guinea-pigs were more resistant than males to *Naja nivea* venom, and according to SCHÖTTLER (1952), there is an indication that this applies to *Crotalus* and *Bothrops* venoms as well. Yet, HENRIQUES and her co-workers (1959) noted a larger LD_{50} for male mice, but stressed, as did SCHÖTTLER, that the results were inconclusive. It is probably fair to conclude that the sex of the mice used in venom work is not important.

Whenever it is possible, it is always desirable to replace methods which demand the use of animals by tests carried out in glassware, and similarly, tests carried out, for instance, in the skin of animals are preferable to tests which necessitate their death, as long as these ways of testing measure the same thing with comparable precision. Many examples of such substitution tests could be drawn from the field of bacteriology, but the therapeutic value of antivenins still has to be assessed on their life-saving properties in animals.

Precipitation in mixtures of venom and antiserum from rabbits was originally observed by LAMB (1902, 1904) and has since been amply confirmed. It is especially interesting to note that CALMETTE and MASSOL, who worked with cobra venom and horse serum as early as 1909, described all the essential features of the particular antigen-antibody precipitation which, as the Ramon flocculation reaction (RAMON, 1922), is universally used in the standardization of bacterial toxoids and antitoxins. RAMON's observation sparked off interest in the possibility of also standardizing antivenins by flocculation and much has been published to little avail, because the multitude of individual antigen-antibody flocculations which take place with crude venom makes attempts at interpretation in terms of titer futile.

Many of the antienzymes contained in antivenins could undoubtedly be assayed with ease and precision unless antigenically distinct enzymes happened to act on the same substrate. But the results of such assays would not express the therapeutic value of a serum because most neurotoxins are devoid of any known enzymic activities (LEE, 1970, 1972), and the part played by enzymes in the lethal effect of cytotoxic venoms has still to be unraveled (OUYANG and SHIAU, 1970). Even the blood clotting caused by some venoms is rarely in itself the cause of death, and a serum's ability to prevent clotting in vitro is not related to its protective titer, as illustrated by experiments with *Bothrops* venom (EICHBAUM, 1947).

Some venoms are more likely to lead to permanent damage due to tissue destruction than to the loss of human life, and it cannot be excluded that properties such as, for instance, the antihemorrhagic potency of a serum would be a better indicator of its therapeutic value than its ability to save the lives of mice. Activity in this respect is conveniently tested in the skin of laboratory animals (PRATT-JOHNSON, 1934), but again, the interpretation of the tests is complicated because similar effects may be caused by more than one venom component (CHRISTENSEN, 1955). Effective standardization of antivenin is, however, possible with isolated single hemorrhagic factors (OHSAKA et al., 1966; KONDO et al., 1971).

D. Conclusions

Antivenins can sometimes be very effective in comparatively small doses (WARRELL et al., 1974), but unreasonably large volumes are commonly required in the treatment of grave poisoning (MINTON, 1974). Ease of handling and regulations put a limit to the solid contents of therapeutic sera, leaving no room for a reduction of the dose volume by concentration, and further fragmentation of the antitoxic globulins, even if feasible, would contribute comparatively little toward a dose reduction. The obvious solution would be to improve the raw material, the immune plasma, by the use of better antigens. Immunization with purified venom fractions (KOCHWA et al., 1959) coupled to a suitable carrier in order to enhance their antigenicity (MOROZ et al., 1963) has undoubtedly been considered in many production centers. The selection and isolation of appropriate antigens from viper and pit viper venoms may still present problems, but the essential elapid antigens, the neurotoxins, could be made available in quantity from the venoms of many snakes. The use of venom fractions for immunization would be costly and the immune response would have to be increased many-fold to offset the cost and make it a practical proposition.

Valid potency estimates should be independent of experimental conditions (JERNE and WOOD, 1949). The results of antivenin potency assays with whole venom as test toxin depend on the venom preparation, the test animal, the route of injection, and the serum-venom concentration in a given volume of the injected mixtures. True standardization is obviously impossible by the assay methods currently used. Yet some form of potency control is necessary in the laboratory and sometimes required by licensing authorities and, within their limitations, simple tests with whole venom can serve this purpose. The results can be reasonably reproducible provided that all the conditions of the test are kept constant and that the same reference preparation of venom is used. A fair quantity of venom should be put aside for use as reference preparation because, as pointed out by SCHÖTTLER (1958), once nearing exhaustion it would be impossible to replace it by another preparation with identic quality. Judged by the lethal toxicity, most venoms are very stable in the dry form, but constancy of the LD_{50} during storage reflects the stability of the lethal powers of the predominant toxin and tells nothing about minor toxins or about possible changes in antigenic character, which TRETHEWIE and KHALED (1973) have shown can occur. It is, therefore, advisable to establish not only a reference venom preparation, but also a reference antivenin, and to examine from time to time the position and shape of the neutralization curve for the two preparations, in order to ensure against undetected alterations in the antibody-binding powers of the toxins. The serum chosen would obviously be freeze-dried, even if refined sera for practical purposes may remain unchanged indefinitely in the cold room (CHRISTENSEN, 1975).

All obstacles in the way of antivenin standardization would be removed if single toxins could be used in the assays. A complete statement of antitoxin potencies of an antivenin could be made if all the components contributing toward a venom's total toxicity were available as isolates, but even a valid statement of potency against the predominant toxin would be preferable to often meaningless statements based on assays with whole venom. Sera containing antitoxin only against the predominant toxin would not prevent death from lethal amounts of other components injected in a bite, but it could with reason be assumed that a serum prepared with crude venom as the antigen and showing high titer against the predominant toxin would be effective against lesser toxins also, and this could be verified in tests with crude venom. The amounts of such fractions needed for potency testing would be moderate, particularly if their use was restricted to the final standardization of batches of antivenin.

E. List of Antivenin Producers[1]

Algeria	Institut Pasteur d'Algerie, Rue Docteur Laveran, Algiers
Argentina	Instituto Nacional de Microbiologia, Vélez Sarsfield 563, Buenos Aires
Australia	Commonwealth Serum Laboratories, 45 Poplar Road, Parkville, Victoria 3052
Brazil	Instituto Butantan, Caixa Postal 65, São Paulo
Colombia	Instituto Nacional de Salud, Calle 57, Numero 8—35, Bogotá, D. E.
Costa Rica	Instituto Clodomiro Picado, Universidad de Costa Rica, Ciudad Universitaria
Egypt	Ain Shams University, Cairo
France	Institute Pasteur Production, Rue du Docteur Roux, 75725 Paris, Cedex 15
Germany	Behringwerke AG, Postfach 167, D-355 Marburg-Lahn
India	Central Research Institute, Kasauli, Punjab
	Haffkine Institute, Bombay
Indonesia	Pasteur Institute, Postbox 47, Bandung
Iran	Institut d'Etat des Serums et Vaccins Razi, Boîte postale 656, Téhéran
Israel	Rogoff Wellcome Research Laboratories, Beilinson Hospital, P.O.B. 85, Petah Tikva
Italy	Instituto Sieroterapico e Vaccinogeno "SCLAVO" Via Fiorentina, Siena
Japan	Institute for Medical Science, University of Tokyo, Shiba Shirokane-daimachi Minato-ku, Tokyo
	Laboratory of Chemotherapy and Serum Therapy, Kumamoto City, Kyushu
	The Takeda Pharmaceutical Co., Osaka
Mexico	Instituto Nacional de Higiene, Czda. M. Escobedo No. 20, Mexico 13, D.F.
	Laboratorios MYN, S.A., Av. Coyoacan 1707, Mexico 12, D.F.
Philippines	Bureau of Research and Laboratories, P.O. Box 911, Manila
Republic of South Africa	South African Institute for Medical Research, Hospital Street, P.O. Box 1038, Johannesburg 2000
Russia	Tashkent Institute, Ministry of Health, Moscow
Taiwan	National Institute of Preventive Medicine, Nang Kang, Taipei
Thailand	Queen Saovabha Memorial Institute, Rama IV Street, Bangkok
Venezuela	Laboratorio Behrens, Calle Real de Chapellin, Apartado 62, Caracas, D.F.
Viet Nam	Institut Pasteur, Nha Trang
Yugoslavia	Institute of Immunology, Rockefellerova 2, Zagreb

[1] Some information about the different products may be found in publications by TAUB (1964) and the Department of the Navy, Bureau of Medicine and Surgery (1968). The manuscript for the latter publication was submitted for publication in November, 1965.

References

Anderson, C. G.: Annual Report, p. 91. Johannesburg: S. Afr. Inst. Med. Res. 1968

Arantes, J. B., Brandão, C. H.: Antigenos e anticorpos botrópicos. I. Contribuição ao estudo da dosagem dos soros a antibotrópicos polivalentes. Mem. Inst. Butantan **21**, 153—178 (1948a)

Arantes, J. B., Brandão, C. H.: Antigenos e anticorpos botrópicos. II. Contribuiçao ao estudo da produção de soros antibotrópicos monovalentes. Mem. Inst. Butantan **21**, 255—260 (1948b)

Arthus, M.: Les anavenins. I. Mem. Destruction de la toxicité des venins par le formol. J. Physiol. Path. gén. **28**, 529—543 (1930)

Bächer, S., Kraus, R., Loewenstein, E.: Über Toxoide. III. Mitteilung. Zur Frage der aktiven Schutzimpfung gegen Schlangengifte. Z. Immun.-Forsch. **45**, 93—96 (1925)

Balozet, L.: La mesure de l'efficacité thérapeutique des sérums antivenimeux. Arch. Inst. Pasteur Algér. **37**, 387—400 (1959)

Banić, M., Ljubetić, T.: Die Titration eines Serums gegen Schlangengift an Mäusen (Serum anti-*Vipera ammodytes*). Z. Hyg. Infekt.-Kr. **120**, 390—407 (1938)

Baxter, E. H., Marr, A. G. M.: Sea wasp *(Chironex fleckeri)* antivenene: neutralizing potency against the venom of three other jelly fish species. Toxicon **12**, 223—229 (1974)

Baxter, E. H., Walden, N. B., Marr, A. G.: Intensive repeated plasmapheresis for maximum yields of antibodies from a sheep immunized with a valuable antigen. Lab. Anim. Sci. **22**, 109—111 (1972)

Behring, E. von, Kitasato, S.: Über das Zustandekommen der Diphtherie-Immunität und der Tetanus-Immunität bei Tieren. Dtsch. med. Wschr. **16**, 1113—1114 (1890)

Bolaños, R., Cerdas, L., Taylor, R.: The production and characteristics of coral snake *(Micrurus mipartitus hertwigi)* antivenin. Toxicon **13**, 139—142 (1975)

Boquet, P.: Rôle du cuivre en quantités infinitésimal dans l'atténuation des venins de *Vipera aspis* et de *Naja tripudians* et d'une toxine végétale, la ricine, par le peroxyde d'hydrogène. Ann. Inst. Pasteur Lille **66**, 379—396 (1941)

Boquet, P., Vendrely, R.: Influence du pH sur la transformation de venin de cobra en anavenin par l'aldéhyde formique; préparation d'un anavenin solide. C.R. Soc. Biol. (Paris) **137**, 179—180 (1943)

Botes, D. P., Strydom, D. J., Anderson, C. G., Christensen, P. A.: Purification and properties of three toxins from *Naja nivea* (Linnaeus) (Cape cobra) venom and the amino acid sequence of toxin δ. J. biol. Chem. **246**, 3132—3139 (1971)

Boyd, W. C.: Fundamentals of Immunology, 4th Ed., p. 126. New York: Interscience Publishers 1966

British Pharmaceutical Codex 1968, p. 899. London: Pharmaceutical Press 1968

Calmette, A.: Contribution à l'étude du venin des serpents. Immunization des animaux et traitement de l'envenimation. Ann. Inst. Pasteur Lille **8**, 275—971 (1894)

Calmette, A., Massol, L.: Les précipitines du sérum antivenimeux vis-à-vis du venin de cobra. Ann. Inst. Pasteur Lille **23**, 155—165 (1909)

Carey, J. E., Wright, E. A.: The toxicity and immunological properties of some sea-snake venoms with particular reference to that of *Enhydrina schistosa*. Trans. roy. Soc. trop. Med. Hyg. **54**, 50—67 (1960)

Cesari, E., Boquet, P.: Détoxication du venin de *Vipera aspis* par le ricinoleate de soude; vaccination du lapin par le venin detoxiqué. C.R. Soc. Biol. (Paris) **125**, 231—234 (1937)

Chatterjee, S. C., Dass, B., Devi, P.: A comparative study of different methods of hyperimmunization of horses for the preparation of polyvalent anti-snake venom serum. Indian J. med. Res. **56**, 678—685 (1968)

Chopra, R. N., Chowhan, J. S., Chopra, I. C.: Sterilization of snake venom preparations. Indian med. Gaz. **77**, 23—26 (1942)

Christensen, P. A.: Formol detoxication of Cape cobra *(Naja flava)* venom. S. Afr. J. med. Sci. **12**, 71—75 (1947)

Christensen, P. A.: Problems of antivenene standardization revealed by the flocculation reaction. Bull. Wld. Hlth. Org. **9**, 353—370 (1953)

Christensen, P. A.: South African Snake Venoms and Antivenoms, pp. 40, 56. Johannesburg: S. Afr. Inst. Med. Res. 1955

Christensen, P. A.: The preparation and purification of antivenoms. Mem. Inst. Butantan **33**, 245—250 (1966a)

Christensen, P. A.: Venom and antivenom potency estimation. Mem. Inst. Butantan **33**, 305—325 (1966b)
Christensen, P. A.: Remarks on antivenin potency estimation. Toxicon **5**, 143—145 (1967)
Christensen, P. A.: The treatment of snakebite. S. Afr. med. J. **43**, 1253—1258 (1969)
Christensen, P. A.: The stability of refined antivenin. Toxicon **13**, 75—77 (1975)
Cohen, P., Seligmann, Jr., E. B.: Immunological studies of coral snake venom. Mem. Inst. Butantan **33**, 339—347 (1966)
Criley, B. R.: Development of a multivalent antivenin for the family *Crotalidae*. In: Venoms. Washington, D.C.: A.A.A.S. 1956
Department of the Navy, Bureau of Medicine and Surgery: Poisonous snakes of the world. Washington, D.C.: U.S. Government Printing Office 1968
Dossena, P.: Recherches sur l'influence des hormones sexuelles dans l'intoxication expérimentale par le venin de *Naja flava* (Cape cobra). Acta Trop. (Basel) **6**, 251—267 (1949)
Eichbaum, F. W.: A dilution phenomenon in the titration of antivenins (anti-bothropic sera). J. Immunol. **57**, 101—114 (1947)
European Pharmacopoeia, Vol. II, pp. 151, 152. Sainte-Ruffine: Maisonneuve S.A. 1971
Fraser, T. R.: The rendering of animals immune against the venom of the cobra and other serpents; and on the antidotal properties of the blood serum of the immunized animals. Brit. med. J. **1**, 1309—1312 (1895)
Freund, J.: Some aspects of active immunization. Ann. Rev. Microbiol. **1**, 291—308 (1947)
Funkhouser, R. M.: The coroner's verdict in the St. Louis tetanus cases. N.Y. med. J. **74**, 977 (1901)
Gingrich, W. C., Hohenadel, J. C.: Standardization of polyvalent antivenin. In: Venoms. Washington, D.C.: A.A.A.S. 1956
Goyal, R. K.: Standardization of daboia and cobra antivenines. Trans. roy. Soc. trop. Med. Hyg. **42**, 381—392 (1949)
Grasset, E.: Concentration of polyvalent African antivenom serum. Trans. roy. Soc. trop. Med. Hyg. **26**, 267—272 (1932)
Grasset, E.: On the standardization of African viper *(Bitis arietans)* and Cape cobra *(Naja flava)* antivenenes. Bull. Hlth. Org. L. o. N. **9**, 476—491 (1940/41)
Grasset, E.: Anavenoms and their use in the preparation of antivenomous sera. Trans. roy. Soc. trop. Med. Hyg. **38**, 463—488 (1945)
Grasset, E.: Standardization of the cobra *(Naja flava)* antibody. Bull. Wld. Hlth. Org. **2**, 69—83 (1949)
Grasset, E., Christensen, P. A.: Enzyme-purification of polyvalent antivenene against Southern and Equatorial African colubrine and viperine venoms. Trans. roy. Soc. trop. Med. Hyg. **41**, 207—211 (1947)
Grasset, E., Zoutendyk, A.: Méthode rapide de préparation de sérums antivenimeux polyvalents—antivipéridés et cobras—au moyen des anavenins formolés. C.R. Soc. Biol. (Paris) **111**, 432—444 (1932)
Grasset, E., Zoutendyk, A.: Detoxication of snake venoms, and the application of the resulting antigens to rapid methods of antivenomous vaccination and serum production. Brit. J. exp. Path. **14**, 308—317 (1933)
Greval, S. D. S.: Concentration of antivenene by the ammonium sulphate method. Indian J. med. Res. **22**, 365—371 (1934)
Hansen, A.: Studier over Isolering af det antitoxinbaerende Protein fra andre Serumbestanddele. Copenhagen: Ejnar Munksgaard 1941
Harms, A. J.: The purification of antitoxic plasmas by enzyme treatment and heat denaturation. Biochem. J. **42**, 390—397 (1948)
Hazra, A. K., Lahiri, D. C., Sokhey, S. S.: On the standardization of Haffkine Institute polyvalent anti-snake-venom serum against the venoms of the four common Indian snakes (cobra, common krait, Russell's viper and saw-scaled-viper). Bull. Hlth. Org. L. o. N. **12**, 384—393 (1945/46)
Henriques, O. B., Fichman, M., Henriques, S. B., Ferraz de Oliveira, M. C.: Fractionation of the venom of *Bothrops jararaca* by ammonium sulphate. Purification of some of the fractions obtained. Mem. Inst. Butantan **29**, 181—195 (1959)
Höxter, G., Decoussau, D.: Concentraçao, purifiçao e controle físico-químico dos soros antitóxicos e antipeçonhentos. Mem. Inst. Butantan **21**, 187—202 (1948)

Hristova, G.: Application of DEAE-Sephadex A-50 for additional purification of antitoxic sera. Z. Immun.-Forsch. **135**, 439—488 (1968)
Hurst, R. O., Butler, G. C.: The chromatographic separation of phosphatases in snake venoms. J. biol. Chem. **193**, 91—96 (1951)
Ipsen, J.: Progress report on the possibility of standardizing anti-snake venom sera. Bull. Hlth. Org. L. o. N. **7**, 785—801 (1938)
Jerne, N. K.: A study of avidity based on rabbit skin responses to diphtheria toxin-antitoxin mixtures. Acta path. microbiol. scand. Suppl. **87**, 1—183 (1951)
Jerne, N. K., Wood, E. C.: The validity and meaning of the results of biological assays. Biometrics **5**, 273—299 (1949)
Kocholaty, W.: Detoxification of *Crotalus atrox* venom by photooxidation in the presence of methylene blue. Toxicon **3**, 175—186 (1966)
Kocholaty, W., Ashley, B. D.: Detoxification of Russell's viper (*Vipera russellii*) and water moccasin (*Agkistrodon piscivorus*) venoms by photooxidation. Toxicon **3**, 187—194 (1966)
Kocholaty, W. F., Billings, T. A., Ashley, B. D., Ledford, E. B., Goetz, J. C.: Effect of the route of administration on the neutralizing potency of antivenins. Toxicon **5**, 165—170 (1968)
Kocholaty, W. F., Bowles-Ledford, E., Daly, J. G., Billings, T. A.: Preparation of coral snake antivenin from goat serum. Toxicon **9**, 297—298 (1971)
Kochwa, S., Izard, Y., Boquet, P., Gitter, S.: Sur la préparation d'un immunsérum équin antivenimeux au moyen des fractions neurotoxiques isolées du venin de *Vipera xanthina palestinae*. Ann. Inst. Pasteur Lille **97**, 370—376 (1959)
Kojis, F. G.: Serum sickness and anaphylaxis. Analysis of 6211 patients treated with horse serum for various infections. Amer. J. Dis. Child. **64**, 93—143, 313—350 (1942)
Kondo, H., Kondo, S., Sadahiro, S., Yamauchi, K., Ohsaka, A., Murata, R.: Standardization of antivenine. II. A method for determination of antihemorrhagic potency of Habu antivenine in the presence of two hemorrhagic principles and their antibodies. Jap. J. med. Sci. Biol. **18**, 127—141 (1971)
Krag, P., Bentzon, M. W.: Antivenin testing at different venom levels. Mem. Inst. Butantan **33**, 251—280 (1966)
Lamb, G.: On the precipitin of cobra venom: a means of distinguishing between the proteins of different snake poisons. Lancet **1902 II**, 431—435
Lamb, G.: On the precipitin of cobra venom. Lancet **1904 I**, 916—921
Latifi, M.: Personal communication, 1975
Latifi, M., Manhouri, H.: Antivenin production. Mem. Inst. Butantan **33**, 893—898 (1966)
Lee, C. Y.: Elapid neurotoxins and their mode of action. Clin. Toxicol. **3**, 457—472 (1970)
Lee, C. Y.: Chemistry and pharmacology of polypeptide toxins in snake venoms. Ann. Rev. Pharmacol. **12**, 265—286 (1972)
Lee, C. Y., Tseng, L. F.: Species differences in susceptibility to elapid venoms. Toxicon **7**, 89—93 (1969)
Leon, W. de, Salafranca, E.: Cobra-anti-venom serum production at the Alabang Serum and Vaccine Laboratories. Philipp. J. Sci. **84**, 477—486 (1956)
Maitra, G. O., Mallick, S. M. K.: Observations on the detoxication of daboia venom by hepatic lipoids with a note on the anti-viperine potency of Kasauli antivenene. Indian J. med. Res. **20**, 327—334 (1932)
Martin, C. de C.: The effect of formalin on snake venoms. I. Diminution of toxicity of cobra venom. Indian J. med. Res. **12**, 807—810 (1925)
Minton, S. A., Jr.: Venom diseases, p. 171. Springfield (Illinois): Charles C. Thomas 1974
Mohamed, A. H., Bakr, I. A., Kamel, A.: Egyptian polyvalent anti-snakebite serum; technic of preparation. Toxicon **4**, 69—72 (1966)
Mohamed, A. H., Darwish, M. A., Hani-Ayobe, M.: Immunological studies on Egyptian cobra antivenin. Toxicon **11**, 31—34 (1973a)
Mohamed, A. H., Darwish, M. A., Hani-Ayobe, M.: Immunological studies on *Naja nigricollis* antivenin. Toxicon **11**, 35—38 (1973b)
Mohamed, A. H., Darwish, M. A., Hani-Ayobe, M.: Immunological studies on Egyptian polyvalent antivenins. Toxicon **11**, 457—460 (1973c)
Moroz, C., Goldblum, N., de Vries, A.: Preparation of *Vipera palestinae* antineurotoxin using carboxymethyl-cellulose-bound neurotoxin as antigen. Nature (Lond.) **200**, 697—698 (1963)

Moroz-Perlmutter, C., Goldblum, N., de Vries, A., Gitter, S.: Detoxification of snake venoms and venom fractions by formaldehyde. Proc. Soc. exp. Biol. (N.Y.) **112**, 595—598 (1963)
Nicol, L., Mustafa, A.: Le cholestérol est-il capable de protéger le cobaye contre l'intoxication due aux venins? C.R. Soc. Biol. (Paris) **121**, 496—498 (1936)
Ohsaka, A., Kondo, H., Kondo, S., Kurokawa, M., Murata, R.: Problems in determination of antihemorrhagic potency of Habu (*Trimeresurus flavoviridis*) antivenine in the presence of multiple hemorrhagic principles and their antibodies. Mem. Inst. Butantan **33**, 331—337 (1966)
Ouyang, C., Shiau, S. Y.: Relationship between pharmacological actions and enzymatic activities of the venom of *Trimeresurus gramineus*. Toxicon **8**, 183—191 (1970)
Parfentjev, I.: U.S. Patent 2065196 (1934)
Parfentjev, I.: U.S. Patent 2123198 (1936)
Parish, H. J., Cannon, D. A.: Antisera, Toxoids, Vaccines, and Tuberculins in Prophylaxis and Treatment, 5th Ed., p. 23. Edinburgh-London: Livingstone 1961
Park, W. H.: Deleterious effects from serum injections. Amer. J. publ. Hlth. **18**, 354—359 (1928)
Phisalix, C., Bertrand, G.: Sur la propriété antitoxique du sang des animaux vaccinés contre le venin de vipère. C.R. Acad. Sci. (Paris) **118**, 356—358 (1894)
Pirosky, I., Sampayo, R., Franceschi, C.: Obtención y purificación de suero anti *Latrodectus*. Rev. Soc. argent. Biol. **18**, 169—175 (1942)
Pope, C. G.: The action of proteolytic enzymes on the antitoxins and proteins of immune sera. I. True digestion of the proteins. Brit. J. exp. Path. **20**, 132—149 (1939a)
Pope, C. G.: The action of proteolytic enzymes on the antitoxins and proteins of immune sera. II. Heat denaturation after partial enzyme action. Brit. J. exp. Path. **20**, 201—212 (1939b)
Pratt-Johnson, J.: The estimation of haemorrhagin in venom by an intradermal method and a potency test of antivenomous sera for antihaemorrhagin. J. Path. Bact. **39**, 704—706 (1934)
Ramon, G.: Floculation dans un mélange neutre de toxine-antitoxine diphtériques. C.R. Soc. Biol. (Paris) **86**, 661—663 (1922)
Ramon, G.: Des anatoxines. C.R. Acad. Sci. (Paris) **178**, 1436—1439 (1924)
Ramon, G.: Sur l'anatoxine diphtérique et sur les anatoxines en général. Ann. Inst. Pasteur Lille **39**, 1—21 (1925)
Renaud, M.: Immunization contre le venin de cobra par les complexes venins-savons. C.R. Soc. Biol. (Paris) **103**, 143—144 (1930)
Richou, R., Nicol, L.: Sur l'injection à l'animal d'expérience du venin de cobra incorporé à la lanoline. C.R. Soc. Biol. (Paris) **118**, 939—941 (1935)
Roux, M. E., Martin, M. L.: Contribution à l'étude de la diphtérique. Ann. Inst. Pasteur Lille **8**, 639—661 (1894)
Russell, F. E., Timmerman, W. F., Meadows, P. E.: Clinical use of antivenin prepared from goat serum. Toxicon **8**, 63—65 (1970)
Salafranca, E. S.: Irradiated cobra (*Naja naja philippinenses*) venom. Jap. J. med. Sci. Biol. **25**, 206 (1972)
Sawai, Y., Makino, M., Miyasaki, S., Kato, K., Adachi, H., Mitsuhashi, S., Okonogi, T.: Studies on the improvement of treatment of Habu snake bite. I. Studies on the improvement of Habu snake antivenin. Jap. J. exp. Med. **31**, 137—150 (1961)
Schlossberger, H., Bieling, R., Demnitz, A.: Untersuchungen über Antitoxine gegen Schlangengifte und die Herstellung eines Heilserums gegen die Gifte der europäischen und mediterranen Ottern. Behringwerke-Mitt. **7**, 111—158 (1936)
Schöttler, W. H. A.: Problems of antivenin standardization. Bull. Wld. Hlth. Org. **5**, 293—320 (1952)
Schöttler, W. H. A.: Miscellaneous observations on snake venoms and antivenins. Mem. Inst. Butantan **27**, 85—105 (1955/56)
Schöttler, W. H. A.: Reference toxins for antivenin standardization. Bull. Wld. Hlth. Org. **19**, 341—361 (1958)
Shortt, H. E., Mallick, S. M. K.: Detoxication of snake venoms by the photodynamic action of methylene blue. Indian J. med. Res. **22**, 529—536 (1935)
Slavin, D.: Production of antisera in rabbits using calcium alginate as an antigen depot. Nature (Lond.) **165**, 115—116 (1950)
Taub, A. M.: Antivenins available for the treatment of snake bite. Toxicon **2**, 71—77 (1964)

Taylor, J.: Observations relative to the standardization of cobra antivenine. Indian J. med. Res. **28**, 279—290 (1940)

Trethewie, E. R., Khaled, L.: Changes in antigenic character of fresh Australian snake venom upon aging. Toxicon **11**, 55—58 (1973)

Vellard, J.: Vaccination antivenimeuse. C.R. Acad. Sci. (Paris) **190**, 826—828 (1930)

Warrell, D. A., Davidson, N. McD., Ormerod, L. D., Pope, H. M., Watkins, B. J., Greenwood, B. M., Reid, H. A.: Bites by the saw-scaled or carpet viper *(Echis carinatus)*: Trial of two specific antivenoms. Brit. med. J. **4**, 437—440 (1974)

WHO Expert Committee on Biological Standardization: Requirement for immune sera of animal origin (Requirement for Biological Substances No. 18). Wld. Hlth. Org. techn. Rep. Ser. No. **413**, 45—59 (1969)

WHO Expert Committee on Biological Standardization: Requirements for snake antivenins (Requirement for Biological Substances No. 21). Wld. Hlth. Org. techn. Rep. Ser. No. **463**, 27—44 (1971)

CHAPTER 21

Common Antigens in Snake Venoms

S. A. MINTON, JR.

A. Introduction

Differences among venoms of snake species geographically and phylogenetically remote from each other were observed by pioneer workers on snake venoms. FAYRER (1872) noted differences in the effects of various Indian snake venoms on animals. MITCHELL and REICHERT (1886) found significant differences in the concentrations of globulins and peptones in venoms of the rattlesnake *(Crotalus adamanteus)*, water moccasin *(Agkistrodon piscivorus)*, and cobra *(Naja naja)*. They also found these venoms differed in their pharmacologic effects and in the tissue changes produced. WOLFENDEN (1886) reported on chemical differences between venoms of the cobra and Russell's viper *(Vipera russellii)*, concluding that they depended on modifications of the protein molecule. It soon became apparent that the composition of snake venoms could not be adequately defined by the biochemical techniques of the day, and the venom components were generally classified by their pharmacologic effects as neurotoxins, hemorrhagins, cytolysins, etc. Soon after SEWALL'S (1887) demonstration of the immunogenic properties of snake venom and the development of bacterial antitoxins, therapeutic antisera to snake venoms were developed on a more or less empiric basis with imperfect understanding of the nature and complexity of the venoms.

The first attempt at antigenic comparison of snake venoms was that of LAMB (1902) who used an antiserum prepared in rabbits against cobra *(Naja naja)* venom in precipitin reactions against homologous venom and venoms of Russell's viper, saw-scaled viper *(Echis carinatus)*, banded krait *(Bungarus fasciatus)*, and tiger snake *(Notechis scutatus)*. A cross-reaction was observed only with Russell's viper venom. Later (LAMB, 1904), he extended observations to venoms of the king cobra *(Ophiophagus hannah)*, Indian krait *(Bungarus caeruleus)*, a sea snake *(Enhydrina schistosa)*, green tree viper *(Trimeresurus gramineus)*, and a rattlesnake *(Crotalus adamanteus)*. Weak cross-reactions were observed with venoms of the green tree viper and sea snake. LAMB commented on the apparent absence of correlation between the precipitin reactions and the phylogenetic relationships of the snakes. He observed no reaction between the serum of the cobra and its own venom or between his cobra venom antiserum and cobra serum. However, he did obtain a precipitin reaction between serum of a rabbit immunized against cobra serum and a solution of cobra venom. HUNTER (1905) also observed a precipitin reaction between antiserum to cobra venom and Russell's viper venom as well as a reaction between antiserum to Russell's viper venom and cobra venom. He likewise confirmed the presence of common antigens in serum and venom of both these snakes. FLEXNER and NOGU-

CHI (1904) prepared antisera to rattlesnake venom in both rabbits and dogs and noted precipitin reactions with homologous venom but not with venoms of cobra or Russell's viper. All of these investigators failed to find any correlation between the precipitin titer of their antisera and the ability of the antiserum to neutralize the lethal effects of venom in animals. They believed the substances responsible for the precipitin reactions were unrelated to the substances responsible for toxicity. This view was challenged by CALMETTE and MASSOL (1909). For almost half a century, there was little interest in precipitin reactions of snake venoms, although AKATSUKA (1936) reported that antiserum against venom of the habu *(Trimeresurus flavoviridis)* gave weak reactions with venoms of *Naja naja* and *Bothrops jararaca*. AMARAL (1928) recognized 12 "antigenic principles" in snake venoms; however, true antigenicity was demonstrated only for lecithinase (=phospholipase A of current workers).

B. Paraspecific Neutralization in Animals

In the meantime, considerable interest focused on the immunologic relationships of venoms as measured by animal protection tests. GITHENS and BUTZ (1929) found serum of an animal immunized against venom of *Crotalus atrox* effectively neutralized venoms of five other species of North American rattlesnakes and was less effective against two North American *Agkistrodon*. It had little capacity to neutralize venoms of the neotropical pit vipers, *Crotalus durissus terrificus* and *Bothrops atrox*. All rattlesnake venoms contained components which bound antibodies but were not acutely toxic. In later studies, GITHENS and WOLFF (1939) divided North American pit viper venoms into three antigenic groups: rattlesnake venoms producing delayed paralytic symptoms (e.g., *Crotalus scutulatus*, *C. tigris*, *Sistrurus catenatus*), all other rattlesnake venoms, and *Agkistrodon* venoms. Antiserum against venom of the Central American *Crotalus d. durissus* was more effective than a polyvalent North American antivenin against venoms of the first group. When mice rather than pigeons were used as test animals, polyvalent *Crotalus* antivenin gave some protection against venoms of three species of *Bothrops* but little or none against three species of *Vipera* and *Bitis arietans*. PICADO (1930) recognized two "neurotoxins" in the venoms of Costa Rican arboreal vipers, one of which was shared with *Crotalus durrissus* and the other with terrestrial *Bothrops* species.

Antigenic diversity among venoms of Australian elapid snakes was shown by KELLAWAY (1930) who found that guinea-pigs immunized to tiger snake venom were not protected against venoms of the brown snake *(Demansia textilis)*, black snake *(Pseudechis porphyriacus)*, and death adder *(Acanthophis antarcticus)*, although they were protected against those of the Australian copperhead *(Denisonia superba)* and taipan *(Oxyuranus scutellatus)*. Immunization against *Acanthophis* protected against tiger snake and copperhead. Guinea-pigs immunized against Russell's viper venom showed no immunity to Australian elapid venoms; experiments with cobra venom-immunized guinea pigs were inconclusive.

TAYLOR and MALLICK (1935) found antivenin produced against venoms of the Indian cobra and Russell's viper partially neutralized the hemorrhagic activity of saw-scaled viper *(Echis carinatus)* and European viper *(Vipera berus)* venoms. African puff adder *(Bitis arietans)* antivenin neutralized the hemorrhagic activity of Russell's viper, European viper, and saw-scaled viper venoms. There was no cross-neutralization of lethal activity with any of these viper venoms. Cross-protection between the venoms of two cobra species, *Naja naja* of India and *N. nivea* of South Africa, was found to be almost complete; neither cobra antivenin neutralized venom of the banded krait (AHUJA, 1935).

Venom of one of the few dangerous colubrids, *Dispholidus typus*, was not neutralized by five elapid antivenins despite the presumed affinity between elapids and colubrids. Antivenins against an African viper, *Bitis arietans*, and a South American pit viper, *Bothrops* sp., showed slight protection (GRASSET and SCHAFFSMA, 1940).

Despite the close interrelationship of the European vipers, mouse protection tests showed comparatively little cross-neutralization of venoms of *Vipera ammodytes*, *V. aspis*, and *V. berus*. *V. aspis* antivenin showed the greatest degree of paraspecific action (KOIVASTIK, 1949).

Evidence for sharing of antigens in venoms of remotely related snakes has come from studies on the paraspecific action of commercially produced antivenins. SCHÖTTLER (1951) found *Bothrops* and *Crotalus* antivenins of South American origin neutralized venoms of European vipers of three species but were ineffective against venoms of one Asian and two North American species of the pit viper genus *Agkistrodon*. MINTON (1976) found a polyvalent American pit viper antivenin showed slight to moderate neutralizing ability against venoms of several Old World vipers but not against *Echis* sp. or *Vipera russellii*. KEEGAN et al. (1962) carried out neutralization tests with 15 monovalent and polyvalent antivenins and venoms of ten species of snakes and found no marked correlation of paraspecific action with relationship of the snake species involved. Unexpected results included neutralization of *Notechis scutatus* venom by a South American coral snake antivenin and neutralization of *Naja naja* and *Ophiophagus hannah* venoms by *Echis carinatus* antivenin. Venoms of *Vipera ammodytes* and *V. xanthina palaestinae* were neutralized fairly well by heterologous antivenins of American and African origin, while venoms of *V. russellii*, *Echis carinatus*, and *Bitis nasicornis* were, for the most part, neutralized only by specific antivenins. Similar results were found in an evaluation of antivenins for use against snakes of southeast Asia. Only five of nine cobra antivenins tested were effective against venoms of mainland *Naja naja*, *N. n. atra* of Taiwan, and, *N. n. philippinensis* of the Philippines, while no antivenin tested satisfactorily neutralized venoms of *Agkistrodon rhodostoma* and *Bungarus fasciatus*. Only specific antivenins neutralized venoms of *Agkistrodon acutus* and *Trimeresurus stejnergeri* (KEEGAN et al., 1964). Antivenins produced against venoms of certain Australian elapid snakes, particularly *Notechis scutatus*, *Acanthophis antarcticus*, and *Oxyuranus scutellatus*, neutralized nine *Naja* venom samples from both Asian and African sources, as well as venoms of six other species of elapids and one sea snake. Only *Notechis* antivenin neutralized venom of the coral snake *Micrurus fulvius*. Cobra, krait, mamba, and coral snake antivenins showed less paraspecific effect against other elapid venoms (MINTON, 1967b).

C. Demonstration of Common Antigens by Immunodiffusion

The development of immunodiffusion techniques by OUDIN (1946) and OUCHTERLONY (1949) permitted a much better immunologic analysis of complex mixtures of antigens such as snake venoms. KULKARNI and RAO (1956) used the Oudin technique

Table 1. Results of OUCHTERLONY immunodiffusion reactions between 18 representative snake venoms (10 mg/ml) and six commercial monovalent antisera. Numbers in boldface indicate distinct precipitin bands, those in parentheses faint bands. Observations made after 6 days at room temperature (ca. 25° C)

Venom	Antiserum					
	Naja naja	*Notechis scutatus*	*Vipera x. palaestinae*	*Echis carinatus*	*Trimeresurus flavoviridis*	*Agkistrodon halys*
Naja n. naja	5	2	(1)	0	0	0
Naja nigricollis	4	2	0	0	0	0
Notechis scutatus	0	5 (1)	0	0	0	0
Bungarus fasciatus	(1)	(1)	2	2	2	(2)
Micrurus fulvius	0	2	(1)	0	0	0
Dendroaspis angusticeps	(1)	0	0	0	0	0
Crotalus adamanteus	0	(1)	3	2	1	(2)
Crotalus d. terrificus	(1)	1	2 (1)	1	2	1 (1)
Trimeresurus flavoviridis	0	0	2 (1)	1	4 (1)	1 (2)
Agkistrodon piscivorus	0	(1)	2 (1)	1	2 (1)	1 (3)
Agkistrodon rhodostoma	(1)	1	2	1	1 (1)	2 (2)
Bothrops asper	2	(2)	2	2	2	1 (2)
Vipera x. palaestinae	0	0	7	1	0	1 (1)
Echis carinatus	(2)	0	3 (1)	3 (1)	0	1 (1)
Cerastes cerastes	0	1	3	4	1	1 (1)
Pseudocerastes persicus fieldi	0	0	3	0	(2)	2
Bitis arietans	0	0	3	2	0	0
Causus rhombeatus	(1)	0	3	2	0	1 (2)

to analyze venoms of four Indian Snakes, while GRASSET et al. (1956) used the OUCHTERLONY technique in an extensive antigenic analysis involving venoms of vipers, pit vipers, and elapids from Europe, Asia, Africa, and the Americas. MINTON (1957) investigated venoms of 14 species of rattlesnakes and a few other pit vipers, and BALOZET (1959) reported on venoms of several African vipers. Sea snake venoms were studied by CAREY and WRIGHT (1960) and BARME (1963). An extensive study of in vitro reactions between venoms and antivenom sera was published by SCHWICK and DICKGIESSER (1963). From all these studies, certain generalizations emerged. Venoms of closely related snakes such as rattlesnakes tended to have most of their antigens in common, although there were certain exceptions, e.g., marked antigenic differences between venoms of subspecies of *Vipera ammodytes* were demonstrated by SCHWICK and DICKGIESSER (1963). Venoms of Asian and African cobras showed a close antigenic relationship, and the early observation of common antigens in Indian cobra and Russell's viper venoms was confirmed. Despite certain similarities in their neuroparalytic activity, no common antigens were detected in venoms of the Asian cobra and the tropical rattlesnakes. In general, viper venoms showed a greater total number of antigens than those of elapids which, in turn, had more venom antigens than sea snakes.

Expansion of the scope of immunologic investigations of snake venoms showed increasing numbers of common antigens in venoms of snakes phylogenetically and geographically remote. Common antigens in the venoms of Russell's viper and two pit vipers of southeast Asia, *Agkistrodon rhodostoma* and *Trimeresurus popeorum*, were demonstrated by PURANANANDA et al. (1966), although there was no cross-neutralization of toxicity. *Vipera lebetina* antivenin produced at the Razi Serum and Vaccine Institute, Tehran, Iran gave precipitin reactions with 15 pit viper venoms (five *Agkistrodon*, five *Bothrops*, and five *Crotalus*). Most of the venoms showed two precipitin lines; however, four were seen with venom of *Bothrops ophryomegas* and three each with *B. schlegeli* and *Agkistrodon piscivorus* (MINTON, unpublished). In a comparison of venoms of adult and juvenile rattlesnakes (*Crotalus horridus atricaudatus*), common antigens were found in the venom of this species and various Old World vipers, notably *Vipera russellii*, *V. xanthina*, *Echis carinatus*, and *Trimeresurus flavoviridis*. Some were present in all rattlesnake venom samples, others only in juveniles 28–29 days old (MINTON, 1967a). Table 1 and Figures 1 and 2 illustrate the widespread sharing of venom antigens by vipers of different groups.

The pit viper genus *Agkistrodon* is the only poisonous snake genus with representatives in both Eurasia and America. Venoms of three American and two Asian species were studied by TU and ADAMS (1968) who found immunologic differences roughly proportional to geographic distance between species, although venom of *A. halys blomhoffii* of Japan was antigenically as close to *A. contortrix* and *A. piscivorus* of North America as to *A. rhodostoma* of southeast Asia. Among six Asian *Agkistrodon*, venoms of *A. h. blomhoffii*, *A. h. brevicaudus*, *A. caliginosus*, and *A. halys caucasicus* gave quite similar immunodiffusion patterns, while those of *A. acutus* and *A. rhodostoma* differed markedly from this group and from each other. The differences were also reflected in cross-neutralization of lethal and hemorrhagic effects. Finally, there was a good correlation with conventional taxonomy, the first four forms being considered closely related and probably conspecific, while *A. rhodostoma* is highly divergent and sometimes assigned to a separate monotypic genus. *A. acutus* may be closer to American members of the genus than to other Asian species (KAWAMURA, 1974).

DETRAIT et al. (1960) described a neurotoxic component common to the venoms of the cobras, *Naja naja* and *N. nigricollis* and the saw-scaled viper, *Echis carinatus*. In immunoelectrophoresis preparations of venom of *N. nigricollis*, BOQUET et al. (1966) associated biologic activities with six of ten precipitin arcs. One antigen, "toxin-α," was identified as the component present in *Echis* venom. Subsequently (BOQUET et al., 1969), an antigen of this type was identified in venoms of eight kinds of snakes, seven of which were cobras (*Naja* or *Hemachatus*). It was detected in

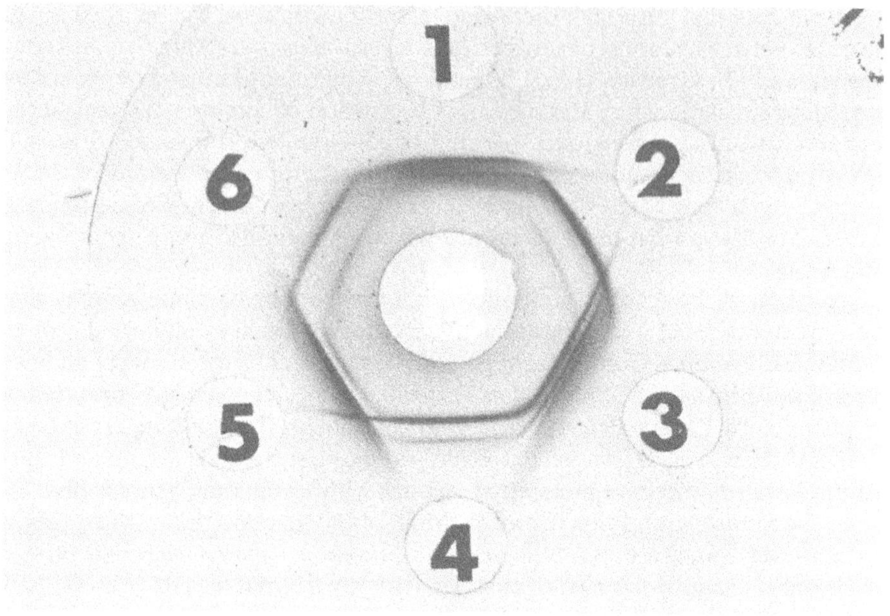

Fig. 1. Immunodiffusion reactions of six pit viper venoms against *Vipera xanthina palaestinae* commercial antiserum. 1) *Agkistrodon piscivorus*, 2) *Trimeresurus flavoviridis*, 3) *Crotalus adamanteus*, 4) *Crotalus durissus terrificus*, 5) *Bothrops atrox asper*, 6) *Agkistrodon rhodostoma*

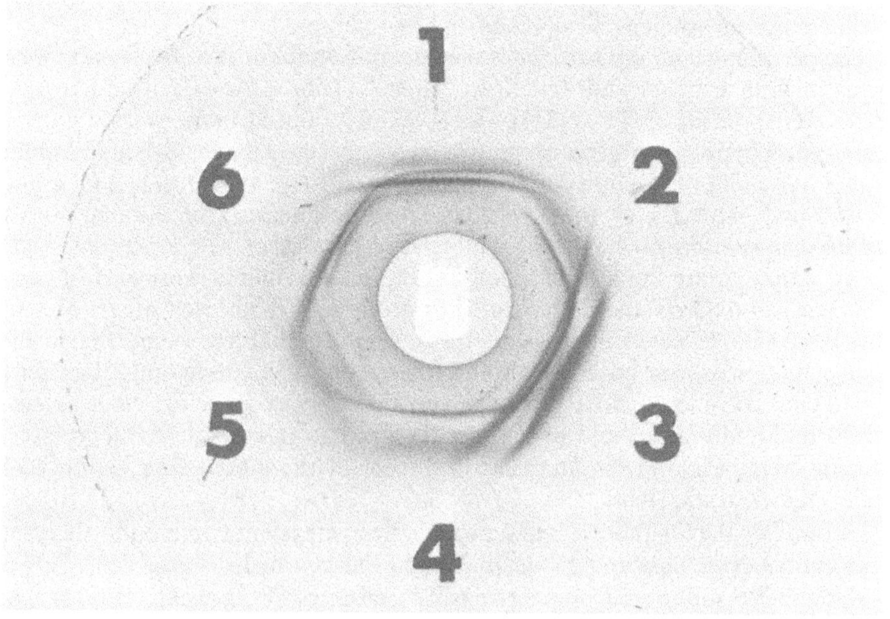

Fig. 2. Immunodiffusion reactions of six Old World viper venoms against polyvalent antiserum (Wyeth Inc.) produced against venoms of four American pit vipers. 1) *Vipera xanthina palaestinae*, 2) *Echis carinatus*, 3) *Cerastes cerastes*, 4) *Bitis arietans*, 5) *Causus rhombeatus*, 6) *Pseudocerastes persicus fieldi*

venom of *Echis* from Ethiopia but not in venom samples from *Echis* of other geographic areas. The authors suggested that this antigen was produced only by certain geographic races or individuals of *Echis* or that some batches of *Echis* venom were contaminated with cobra venom. Recent work indicates the latter hypothesis most likely (BOQUET, personal communication). MOHAMED et al. (1973a, b) found antisera to the cobras *Naja haje* and *N. nigricollis* gave cross precipitin reactions with venoms of two species of *Echis*, two species of *Cerastes*, two species of *Bitis*, and *Trimeresurus flavoviridis*, all vipers or pit vipers. Reactions were strongest with *Cerastes* and *Echis* venoms and also involved some degree of neutralization of these venoms. Immunodiffusion and immunoelectrophoresis studies of a bivalent *Cerastes* antiserum showed the presence of antigens common to this genus and other genera of Middle Eastern vipers, as well as weak reactions with cobra venoms (HASSAN and EL-HAWARY, 1975).

Immunodiffusion experiments with venoms of four widely distributed sea snake species showed a somewhat closer affinity between *Enhydrina schistosa* and *Lapemis hardwickii* than between *Enhydrina* and *Hydrophis cyanocinctus* and *Pelamis platurus* (TU and GANTHAVORN, 1969). *Enhydrina* antiserum showed strong precipitin arcs when reacted with *Praescutata viperina* venom but only a very faint arc with two species of *Laticauda* (TU and SALAFRANCA, 1974). Antiserum against venom of the terrestrial tiger snake *(Notechis scutatus)* was more effective than sea snake *(Enhydrina)* antiserum in neutralizing venoms of eight of nine sea snakes, the exception being *Enhydrina* itself. Immunodiffusion reations showed *Notechis* venom shared one or two antigens with all sea snake venoms tested, while *Enhydrina* venom had no antigens in common with venoms of *Hydrophis spiralis* and *Aipysurus laevis* (BAXTER and GALLICHIO, 1974). Although the polypeptide neurotoxins of sea snakes are similar to those of elapids, few venom antigens are shared with Asian and African elapids (Fig. 3).

MUNJAL and ELLIOTT (1972) succeeded in correlating histochemical and immunodiffusion data for a number of elapid venoms. An esterase hydrolyzing β-napthyl acetate was found immunologically identic in venoms of four out five species of *Naja*, *Ophiophagus hannah*, and *Micrurus fulvius*. Another esterase with this activity was found in the venom of *Bungarus fasciatus* and showed partial identity with antigens in venoms of four species of *Naja* and *M. fulvius*. The esterase hydrolyzing β-carbonaphthoxycholine was immunologically identic in venoms of four species of *Naja*, two species of *Bungarus*, *O. hannah*, and *M. fulvius*. Indoxyl acetate esterase was identic in venoms of *Naja*, *O. hannah*, and *M. fulvius*. This enzyme was present in venoms of mambas *(Dendroaspis)* but was immunologically distinct from that of the other elapids studied. No common antigens were detected in the venoms of these elapids and venoms of an African viper, *Bitis nasicornis*, and North American pit viper, *Agkistrodon piscivorus*. Venom of *Bitis arietans* showed a single precipitin line when reacted with *Bungarus fasciatus* antiserum.

Thrombin-like enzymes of nine pit vipers of the genus *Bothrops* showed distinctive differences in mobility on immunoelectrophoresis, although those between *B. moojeni* and *B. marajoensis* were slight. All showed multiple precipitin arcs with polyvalent *Bothrops* antivenin (STOCKER et al., 1974).

Inhibition of venom phospholipase activity of seven venoms by antisera showed probable immunologic identity of the enzymes of *Naja naja* and *N. melanoleuca*

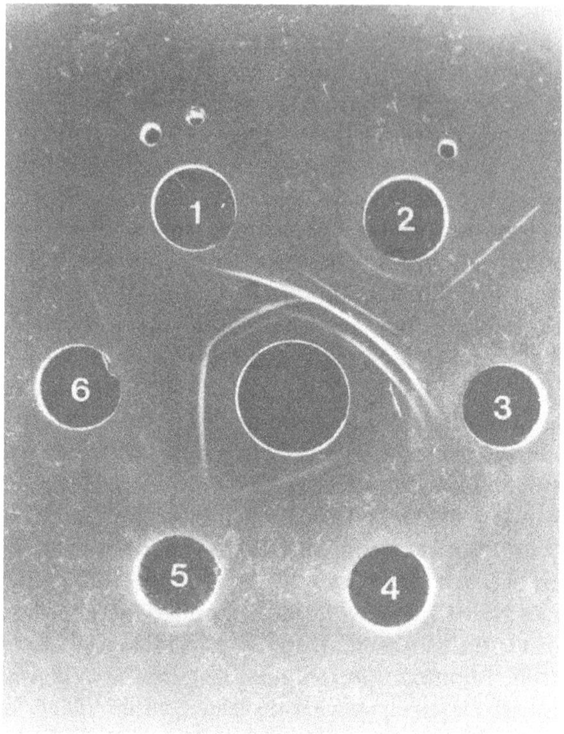

Fig. 3. Immunodiffusion reactions of six elapid venoms against sea snake *(Enhydrina schistosa)* antiserum. 1) *Naja n. naja*, 2) *Notechis scutatus*, 3) *Bungarus fasciatus*, 4) *Micrurus fulvius*, 5) *Dendroaspis angusticeps*, 6) *Naja nigricollis*

while that of *N. nigricollis* was partially identic requiring about eight times as much antiserum for neutralization. *N. nigricollis* phospholipase A was quite effectively neutralized by *Echis carinatus* antiserum, however. *Bungarus fasciatus* phospholipase A was inhibited only by homologous antiserum, but *B. fasciatus* antiserum to some degree inhibited phospholipase A activity of *Naja* venoms and *Crotalus scutulatus* venom. Polyvalent crotalid antivenin inhibited *Echis carinatus* and *Bitis gabonica* enzymes although to a lesser degree than it inhibited *Crotalus* (NAIR et al., 1975).

Antigenic relationships among venoms have occasionally been used in attempts to clarify the taxonomic status of certain venomous snakes. Venom of *Atractaspis microlepidota*, a member of a genus traditionally classified with the Viperidae, reacted with ten of 16 elapid antisera but with only 3 of 13 viperid antisera. This supports morphologic evidence that *Atractaspis* is not a member of the Viperidae or the Elapidae although possibly closer to the latter family. Venom of *Causus rhombeatus*, representing a group of primitive African vipers sometimes considered related to *Atractaspis*, reacted with 12 of 13 viperid antisera and with 8 of 16 elapid antisera. This supports retention of *Causus* in the Viperidae. The wide cross-reactivity of its venom may reflect its primitive status (MINTON, 1968a). Antiserum against venom of the African colubrid, *Dispholidus typus*, reacted with 26 of 33 viperid venoms showing double-line reactions with several pit vipers (*Agkistrodon piscivorus*, *A. halys caucasicus*, *Crotalus ruber*, and *Trimeresurus okinavensis*). A weak reaction was seen with one of ten elapid venoms, that of *Naja nigricollis*. Most of the precipitin lines were faint, and there did not seem to be more than three antigens involved in the cross-reactions. Similarly, *Dispholidus* venom reacted with several pit viper antisera; however, reactions were also seen with antisera against venoms of certain Australian elapids, notably *Pseudechis papuanus* (MINTON, unpublished). The significance of these observations is unclear, although they confirm earlier work based on venom neutralization. It is possible that colubrid venoms represent a primitive type from which viperid venoms evolved; however, they also share antigens with certain elapids.

D. Common Antigens in Venom and Snake Serum

The presence of common antigens in Asian cobra serum and venom first reported by LAMB in 1902 was confirmed by TU and GANTHAVORN (1968). MINTON (1973) observed numerous reactions between antivenins and snake sera, as well as between snake venoms and antisera to snake sera. Reactions between snake sera and antivenins were stronger and usually showed the presence of more antigens than reactions between venoms and antisera to snake sera. Moreover, antivenins of the same type from different producers varied considerably. Despite the variation observed, the evidence is very strong that several common antigens occur in the serum and venom of snakes. Some of these antigens have also been demonstrated in the serum of a variety of nonvenomous snakes. Primitive species such as *Boa constrictor* and *Eryx conicus* showed weaker reactions than the more advanced ones such as *Natrix sipedon* and *Elaphe obsoleta*. The chemical nature of the cross-reacting antigens in serum and venom is little known. In immunoelectrophoresis preparations, most of the arcs lie in the approximate position of β-globulin arcs of snake serum. A fraction of cobra venom with high phospholipase A activity has been identified in cobra serum, in serum of an Australian elapid, *Denisonia superba*, and serum of a sea snake, *Hydrophis melanocephalus*. It was not detected in serum of another sea snake, *Lapemis hardwickii*, nor in serum from four nonvenomous snakes (MINTON, unpublished). The anticomplementary protein in *Naja naja* venon is reported to be an altered form of the third component of complement (C3) of cobra serum (ALPER and BALAVITCH, 1976).

E. Discussion and Summary

Immunologic investigations of snake venoms are still confined to a relatively small number of species of medical importance whose venoms are readily available, and the chief criterion of immunologic relationship has been the cross-neutralization of toxicity. In only a few studies, e.g., MUNJAL and ELLIOTT (1972); NAIR et al. (1975) have investigators traced well-defined enzyme activities in the venoms of various snakes. In other instances, immunodiffusion patterns of whole venoms have been compared. Table 1 shows the reactions of 18 representative snake venoms in OUCHTERLONY immunodiffusion reactions against six commercial monovalent antisera. Whatever method is used, there is only a rough correlation between antigenic relationships of venoms and the phylogenetic relationships of the snakes that produce them. One of the best correlations is in the pit viper genus *Agkistrodon* where antigenic differences in venoms reflect morphologic differences and degree of geographic separation. The rattlesnakes (*Crotalus* and *Sistrurus*) are a closely related species group whose venoms diverge little antigenically, the most striking difference being the evolution of a predominantly neuroparalytic venom in the *C. durissus* complex and in *C. scutulatus* and possibly *C. tigris*. The large neotropical pit viper genus *Bothrops* has been little studied from the standpoint of venom antigens. On the basis of toxicity and pharmacologic activity, venoms of *B. cotiara*, *B. erythromelas*, and *B. insularis* appear to differ significantly from the generic mode (AMARAL, 1925; KAISER and MICHL, 1971). The equally large tropical Asian pit viper genus *Trimeresurus* which seems to have evolved in parallel with *Bothrops* also has not been extensively investigated immunologically. Venom of *T. wagleri* contains an apparently unique toxin and shows considerable antigenic difference from venom of *T. flavoviridis*, but venoms of *T. albolabris* and *T. okinavensis* are equally divergent (MINTON, 1968b). Available evidence suggests venoms of *Trimeresurus* are no closer antigenically to those of *Bothrops* than they are to those of *Agkistrodon* or *Crotalus*.

Venoms of the Old World vipers without heat-sensing pits (Viperinae) show no particular relationship at the subfamily level. Considerable antigenic differences are documented for venoms in the genus *Vipera*. This also seems to be true of the species of *Bitis*. Considerable sharing of venom antigens occurs among *Echis*, *Cerastes*, and *Eristicophis*, suggesting that these three genera may be the result of an adaptive radiation into the Afro-Asian desert zone. Another desert genus, *Pseudocerastes*, shows a remarkable antigenic difference between venoms of the Middle Eastern form, *fieldi*, and the Iran-Pakistan form, *persicus*, (Fig. 4). Antisera to venoms of *Echis carinatus*, *Vipera lebetina*, and *V. xanthina palaestinae* react with pit viper venoms extensively, while *Bitis* antiserum is more specific. Venoms of *Causus*, *Echis*, and *Cerastes* are remarkable for their sharing of antigens with pit vipers and elapids. *Causus* is generally accepted as a genus of primitive vipers from which other viperine stocks may have evolved. Its venom may be intermediate between colubrid venoms and those of the more advanced vipers (see Table 1 and Figs. 1 and 2).

Elapid venoms are better known biochemically than those of other snakes with some 50 polypeptide toxins now isolated and characterized along with a number of venom enzymes. The chemistry and evolution of these toxins has recently been reviewed by YANG (1974). Cobras of the genus *Naja* are widely distributed in Africa and southern Asia. It should be mentioned that the taxonomy of Asian cobras is in a state of confusion, especially with regard to the mainland races. Some subspecies, e.g., *N. n. siamensis* and *N. n. kaouthia*, are inadequately defined and their ranges poorly known. Antigenically, venoms of African *N. nivea* and *N. melanoleuca* are closer to Indian *N. naja* than to African *N. nigricollis*. Similarly venoms of cobras from Iran and Russian Asia (*N. naja oxiana*) and from Taiwan (*N. n. atra*) differ from southeast Asian cobra venoms to a greater degree than the latter differ from most African cobra venoms. Cobra-like snakes of other genera, e.g., *Ophiophagus*, *Hemachatus*, appear to have venoms that share many antigens with *Naja*.

The mambas (*Dendroaspis*) share few venom antigens with other snakes, and venoms of the four species differ considerably among themselves. The toxins of krait (*Bungarus*) venoms are antigenically distinct from those of most other elapid ven-

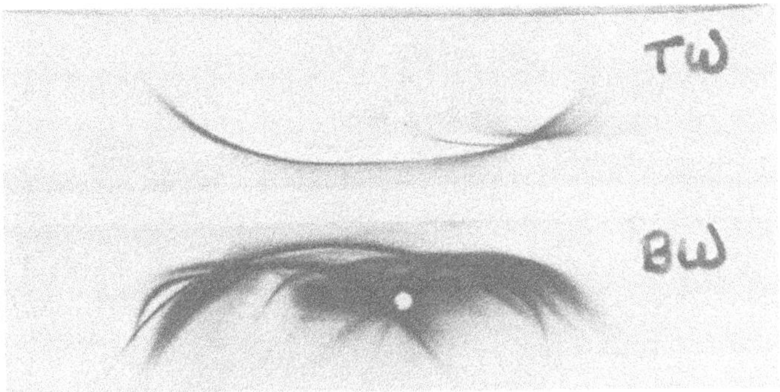

Fig. 4. Immunoelectrophoresis preparation of venoms of *Pseudocerastes persicus fieldi* (Israel) in upper well and *P. p. persicus* (Iran) in lower well. Preparation run 60 min at 7.4 v/cm and developed with *P. p. persicus* antiserum

oms; however, their neutralization by tiger snake, death adder, and taipan antivenins shows they are shared with at least some Australian snakes. Venom of *B. fasciatus* has two antigens in common with several viperid venoms (Table 1); one of these is also present in *B. caeruleus* and *B. multicinctus* venoms. Venoms of only a few of Australia's numerous species of elapids have been carefully studied. Evidence from animal protection tests indicates widespread sharing of toxin antigens among *Notechis*, *Acanthophis*, *Oxyuranus*, *Pseudechis*, and *Denisonia* with many of these antigens being shared with other elapid genera. On the other hand, *Demansia textilis* and probably some of its near relatives form another group on the basis of toxin antigens (COULTER et al., 1974). Except for a few species, venoms of the American coral snakes are poorly known. Venoms of such species as *Micrurus fulvius*, *M. frontalis*, *M. caricauda*, and *M. nigrocinctus* appear to have many common antigens, while those of *M. mipartatus* and *Micruroides euryxanthus* belong to other antigenic groups (COHEN et al., 1966, 1968, 1971).

Sea snakes have few venom antigens in common with Asian and African elapids. However, there is considerable sharing of antigens with some Australian elapids, a circumstance that tends to support the derivation of most sea snakes from Australian elapid stock (MCDOWELL, 1969). Among the sea snakes themselves, there seems to be considerable variation in antigenic composition of the venoms, although only a few species have been evaluated. NARITA et al. (1972) consider the antigenic simplicity of sea snake venoms evidence for their primitive nature; however, nearly all anatomic and physiologic evidence points to the sea snakes being a comparatively recent product of ophidian evolution (MINTON and DACOSTA, 1975).

The only colubrid venom to have been studied from the viewpoint of antigenic makeup is that of the boomslang, *Dispholidus typus*. Its affinity with viperids rather than elapids has already been mentioned. The antigenic nature of other colubrid venoms as well as that of the oral secretions of aglyphous colubrids is an interesting field for future investigation, particularly since there are several reports of envenomation by presumably "nonvenomous" snakes (MEBS, 1977).

Research on the antigenic relationships of snake venoms has often been done using commercially produced therapeutic antisera. Workers using such antisera

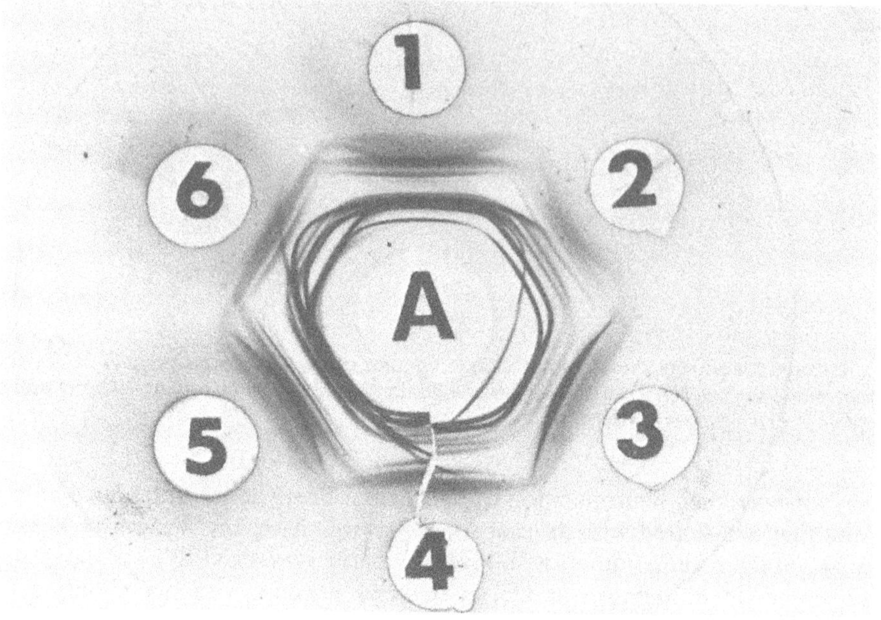

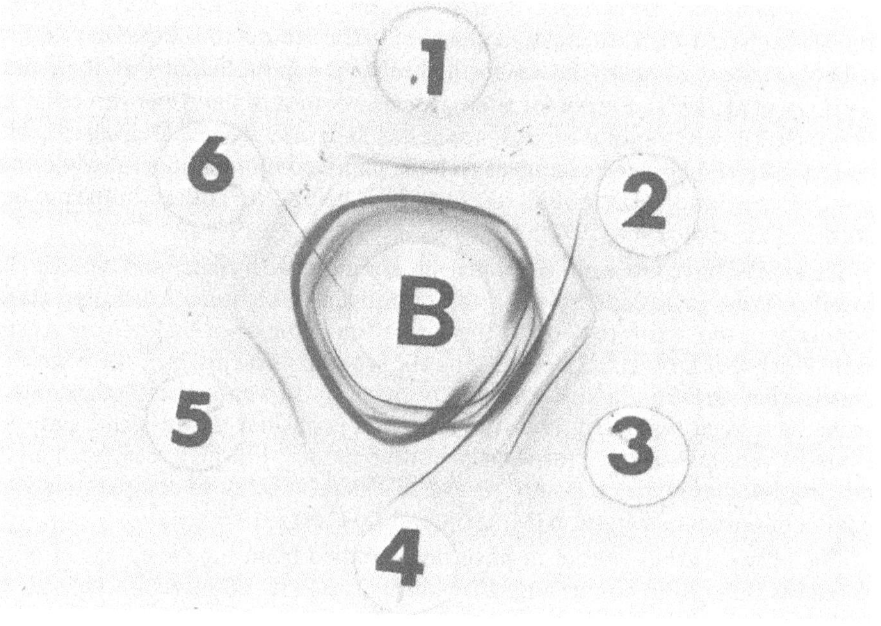

Fig. 5A–D. Immunodiffusion reactions of six Asian cobra venoms against four commercial antisera. Venoms are: 1) *Naja n. naja* (Karachi), 2) *Naja n. atra* (Taiwan), 3) *Naja n. philippinensis* (Luzon), 4) *Naja n. naja* (India), 5) *Naja n. oxiana* (Iran), 6) *Naja n. kaouthia* (Thailand). Antisera: (A) Razi Institute, Iran, (B) Philippine Bureau of Laboratories, Manila, (C) Queen Saovabha Memorial Institute, Thailand, (D) Institute Pasteur, Paris

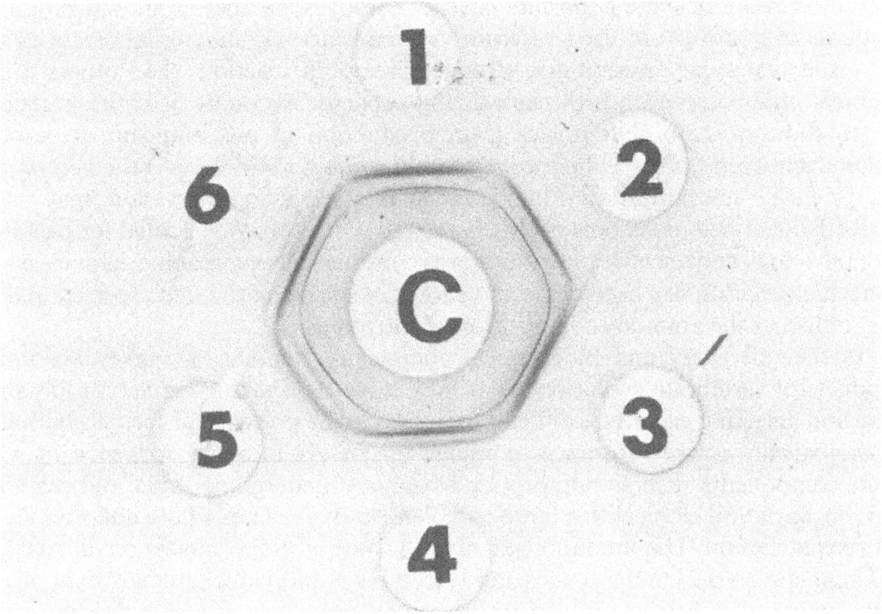
1
2
3
4
5
6
C

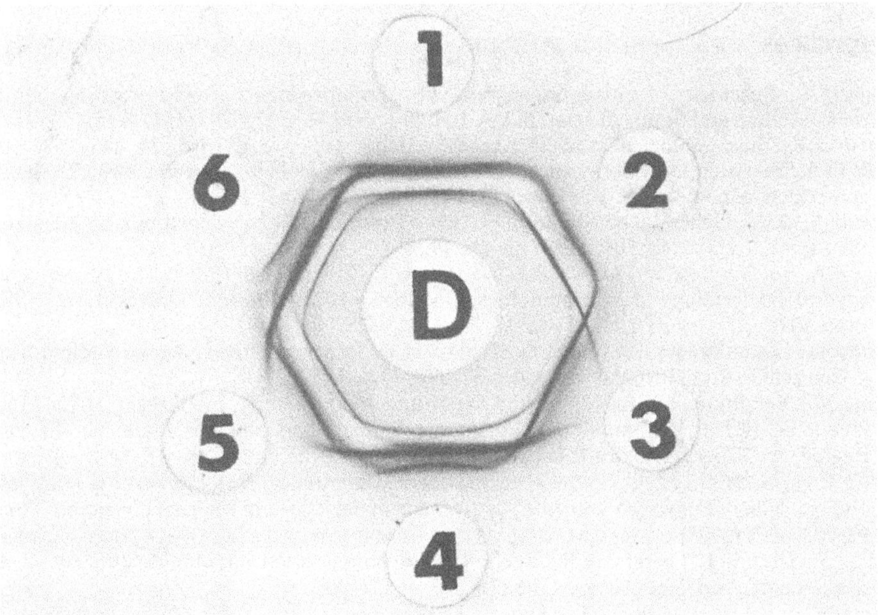
1
2
3
4
5
6
D

should be aware of some important caveats. Firstly, schedules of immunization and methods of treatment of the antiserum vary considerably among laboratories with the result that some antisera give stronger precipitin reactions than others (Fig. 5). There is little correlation with neutralizing capacity. Secondly, it is the practice of some laboratories to shift horses from production of one antivenin to another. Serum from such horses will almost certainly contain antibodies to the venom used for the earlier immunization. Finally, the snakes supplying the venom may not be correctly identified or venoms of closely related species may be pooled for reasons of economy and convenience. Furthermore, considerable geographic and individual antigenic variation has been noted in venoms of snakes of the same species, and this may influence the antibody composition of antivenins.

In their diversity and biochemical complexity, venoms of snakes are unique products of vertebrate evolution. That they serve the snake effectively in obtaining food and deterring enemies is difficult to deny, yet the presence of such a multiplicity of biologically active substances conjures up an evolutionary sequence in which some components such as polypeptide toxins are undergoing rapid and seemingly random variation along with a large complement of enzymes whose adaptive significance is uncertain. The immunologic identification of these substances in snakes of different species and in the tissues and secretions of individual animals may provide some unexpected insights into the evolution of venom in snakes, its synthesis, and its functional significance.

References

Ahuja, M. L.: Specificity of antivenomous sera with special reference to sera prepared with venoms of Indian and South African snakes. Indian J. med. Res. **22**, 479—484 (1935)

Akatsuka, K.: Immunological studies of snake venoms. Jap. J. exp. Med. **14**, 147—183 (1936)

Alper, C. A., Balavitch, D.: Cobra venom factor: evidence for its being altered cobra C3 (the third component of complement). Science **191**, 1275—1276 (1976)

Amaral, A., do: A General Consideration of Snake Poisoning and Observations on Neotropical Pit-Vipers. Cambridge: Harvard Univ. Pr. 1925

Amaral, A., do: Venoms and antivenins. In: Jordan, E. O., Falk, I. S. (Eds.): The Newer Knowledge of Bacteriology and Immunology, pp. 1066—1077. Chicago: University of Chicago Press 1928

Balozet, L.: Les antigénes des venins de *cerastes* et de lébetines étudiés par la precipitation en milieu gélifié. Arch. Inst. Pasteur Algér. **37**, 292—301 (1959)

Barme, M.: Venomous sea snakes of Viet Nam and their venoms. In: Keegan, H. L., Macfarlane, W. V. (Eds.): Venomous and Poisonous Animals and Noxious Plants of the Pacific Region, pp. 373—378. Oxford: Pergamon Press 1963

Baxter, E. H., Gallichio, H. A.: Cross-neutralization by tiger snake *(Notechis scutatus)* antivenene and sea snake *(Enhydrina schistosa)* antivenene against several sea snake venoms. Toxicon **12**, 273—278 (1974)

Boquet, P., Detrait, J., Farzanpay, R.: Recherches biochimiques et immunologiques sur le venin des serpents. Ann. Inst. Pasteur Lille **116**, 522—542 (1969)

Boquet, P., Izard, Y., Jouannet, M., Meaume, J.: Enzymes et toxines des venins de serpents. Recherches biochemiques et immunologiques sur le venin de *Naja nigricollis.* Mem. Inst. Butantan Simp. Intern. **33**, 371—377 (1966)

Calmette, A., Massol, L.: Les précipitines du serum antivenimeux vis-à-vis du venin de cobra. Ann. Inst. Pasteur Lille **23**, 155 (1909)

Carey, J. E., Wright, E. A.: The toxicity and immunological properties of some sea snake venoms with particular reference to that of *Enhydrina schistosa.* Trans. roy. Soc. trop. Med. Hyg. **54**, 50—67 (1960)

Cohen, P., Berkley, W. H., Seligmann, E. B.: Coral snake venoms in vitro relation of neutralizing and precipitating antibodies. Amer. J. trop. Med. Hyg. **20**, 646—649 (1971)

Cohen, P., Dawson, J. H., Seligmann, Jr., E. B.: Cross-neutralization of *Micrurus fulvius fulvius* coral snake venom by anti-*Micrurus carinicauda dumerilii* serum. Amer. J. trop. Med. Hyg. **17**, 308—310 (1968)

Cohen, P., Seligmann, Jr., E. B.: Immunologic studies of coral snake venom. Mem. Inst. Butantan Simp. Intern. **33**, 339—347 (1966)

Coulter, A. R., Sutherland, S. K., Broad, A. J.: Assay of snake venoms in tissue fluids. J. Immunol. Methods **4**, 297—300 (1974)

Detrait, J., Izard, Y., Boquet, P.: Relations antigeniques entre un facteur lethal du venin d'*Echis carinata* et les neutrotoxines des venins de *Naja naja* et *Naja nigricollis*. C. R. Soc. Biol. (Paris) **154**, 1163 (1960)

Fayrer, J.: The Thantophidia of India. London: T. and A. Churchill 1872

Flexner, S., Noguchi, H.: Upon the production and properties of anticrotalus venin. J. med. Res. **11**, 363—376 (1904)

Githens, T. S., Butz, L. W.: Venoms of North American snakes and their relationships. J. Immunol. **16**, 71—80 (1929)

Githens, T. S., Wolff, N. O. C.: The polyvalency of crotalidic antivenins. J. Immunol. **37**, 33—49 (1939)

Grasset, E., Pongratz, E., Brechbuhler, T.: Analyse immunochimique des constituants des venins de serpents par la methode de precipitation en milieu gelifie. Ann. Inst. Pasteur Lille **91**, 162—186 (1956)

Grasset, E., Schaaffma, A. W.: Antigenic characteristics of boomslang *(Dispholidus typus)* venom and preparation of a specific antivenene by means of formalized venom. S. Afr. med. J. **14**, 484—489 (1940)

Hassan, F., El-Hawary, M. F. S.: Immunological properties of antivenins. I. Bivalent *Cerastes cerastes* and *Cerastes vipera* antivenin. Amer. J. trop. Med. Hyg. **24**, 1031—1034 (1975)

Hunter, A.: On the precipitins of snake antivenoms and snake antisera. J. Physiol. (Lond.) **33**, 239—250 (1905)

Kaiser, E., Michl, H.: Chemistry and pharmacology of the venoms of *Bothrops* and *Lachesis*. In: Bücherl, W., Buckley, E. E. (Eds.): Venomous Animals and Their Venoms, Vol. II, pp. 307—318. New York: Academic Press 1971

Kawamura, Y.: Study of the immunological relationships between venom of six Asiatic *Agkistrodons*. Snake **6**, 19—26 (1974)

Keegan, H. L., Weaver, R. E., Matusi, T.: Southeast Asian snakebite anti-venin studies. 406th Med. Lab. Res. Rpt. U.S. Army Med. Command Jap. 1964

Keegan, H. L., Whittemore, F. W., Maxwell, G. R.: Neutralization of ten snake venoms by homologous and heterologous antivenins. Copeia **2**, 313 (1962)

Kellaway, C. H.: The specificity of active immunity against snake venoms. J. Path. Bact. **33**, 157—172 (1930)

Koivastik, T.: Neutralisationsfähigkeit der Schlangengift-Antitoxine gegen homologe und heterologe Gifte. Z. Hyg. Infekt.-Kr. **129**, 373—378 (1949)

Kulkarni, M. E., Rao, S. S.: Antigenic composition of the venoms of poisonous snakes of India. In: Buckley, E. E., Porges, N. (Eds.): Venoms, pp. 175—177. Washington: AAAS Pub. 44, 1956

Lamb, G.: On the precipitin of cobra venom: a means of distinguishing between the proteins of different snake poisons. Lancet **1902 II**, 431—435

Lamb, G.: On the precipitin of cobra venom. Lancet **1904 I**, 916—921

McDowell, S. B.: Notes on the Australian sea-snake *Ephalophis greyi* M. Smith (Serpentes, Elapidae, Hydrophiinae) and the origin and classification of sea snakes. Zool. J. Linn. Soc. **48**, 333—349 (1969)

Mebs, D.: Bißverletzungen durch „ungiftige“ Schlangen. Deutsch. Med. Woch. **102**, 1429—1431 (1977)

Minton, S. A.: An immunological investigation of rattlesnake venoms by the agar diffusion method. Amer. J. trop. Med. Hyg. **6**, 1097—1107 (1957)

Minton, S. A.: Observations on toxicity and antigenic makeup of venoms from juvenile snakes. In: Russell, F. E., Saunders, P. R. (Eds.): Animal Toxins, pp. 211—222. Oxford: Pergamon Press 1967a

Minton, S. A.: Paraspecific protection by elapid and sea snake antivenins. Toxicon **5**, 47—55 (1967b)
Minton, S. A.: Antigenic relationships of the venom of *Atractaspis microlepidota* to that of other snakes. Toxicon **6**, 59—65 (1968a)
Minton, S. A.: Preliminary observations on the venom of Wagler's pit viper (*Trimeresurus wagleri*). Toxicon **6**, 93—97 (1968b)
Minton, S. A.: Common antigens in snake sera and venoms. In: DeVries, A., Kochva, E. (Eds.): Toxins of Animal and Plant Origin, Vol. III, pp. 905—917. New York: Gordon and Breach 1973
Minton, S. A.: Neutralization of Old World viper venoms by American pit viper antivenin. Toxicon **14**, 146—148 (1976)
Minton, S. A., Da Costa, M.: Serological relationships of sea snakes and their evolutionary implication. In: Dunson, W. A. (Ed.): The Biology of Sea Snakes, pp. 33—55. Baltimore: Univ. Park Press 1975
Mitchell, S. W., Reichert, E. T.: Researches upon the venoms of poisonous serpents. Smithson. Contrib. Knowl. **26**, 186 (1886)
Mohamed, A. H., Darwish, M. A., Hani-Ayobe, M.: Immunological studies on Egyptian cobra antivenin. Toxicon **11**, 31—34 (1973a)
Mohamed, A. H., Darwish, M. A., Hani-Ayobe, M.: Immunological studies on *Naja nigricollis* antivenin. Toxicon **11**, 35—38 (1973b)
Munjal, D., Elliott, W. B.: Immunological and histochemical identity of esterases and other antigens in elapid venoms. Toxicon **10**, 47—54 (1972)
Nair, B. C., Nair, C., Elliott, W. B.: Action of antisera against homologous and heterlogous snake venom phospholipases A_2. Toxicon **13**, 453—456 (1975)
Narita, K., Mebs, D., Iwanaga, S., Samejima, Y., Lee, C. Y.: Primary structure of α-bungarotoxin from *Bungarus multicinctus* venom. J. Formosan med. Ass. **71**, 335—343 (1972)
Ouchterlony, O.: Antigen-antibody reactions in gels. Acta path. microbiol. scand. **26**, 516—524 (1949)
Oudin, J.: Methode d'analyse immunochemique par precipitation specifique en milieu gelifie. C. R. Acad. Sci. (Paris) **222**, 115—116 (1946)
Picado, C.: Venom of Costa Rican arboreal vipers. Bull. Antivenin Inst. Am. **4**, 1—3 (1930)
Purananda, C., Lauhatirananda, P., Ganthavorn, S.: Cross immunological reactions in snake venoms. Mem. Inst. Butantan Simp. Intern. **33**, 327—330 (1966)
Schöttler, W. H. A.: Para-specific action of bothropic and crotalic antivenins. Am. J. Trop. Med. **31**, 836—841 (1951)
Schwick, G., Dickgiesser, F.: Probleme der Antigen- und Fermentanalyse im Zusammenhang mit der Herstellung polyvalenter Schlangengiftseren. In: Elwert, N. G. (Ed.): Die Giftschlangen der Erde, pp. 35—66. Marburg (Lahn): Behringwerke-Mitt. 1963
Sewall, H.: Experiments on the preventative inoculation of rattlesnake venom. J. Physiol. (Lond.) **8**, 203—210 (1887)
Stocker, K., Christ, W., Leloup, P.: Characterization of the venoms of various *Bothrops* species by immunoelectrophoresis and reaction with fibrinogen agarose. Toxicon **12**, 415—417 (1974)
Taylor, J., Mallick, S. M. K.: Observations on the neutralization of the hemorrhagin of certain viper venoms by antivenene. Indian J. med. Res. **23**, 121—130 (1935)
Tu, A. T., Adams, B. L.: Phylogenetic relationships among venomous snakes of the genus *Agkistrodon* from Asia and the North American continent. Nature (Lond.) **217**, 760—762 (1968)
Tu, A. T., Ganthavorn, S.: Comparison of *Naja naja siamensis* and *Naja naja atra* venoms. Toxicon **5**, 207—211 (1968)
Tu, A. T., Ganthavorn, S.: Immunological properties and neutralization of sea snake venoms from southeast Asia. Amer. J. trop. Med. Hyg. **18**, 151—154 (1969)
Tu, A. T., Salafranca, E. S.: Immunological properties and neutralization of sea snake venoms. Amer. J. trop. Med. Hyg. **23**, 135—138 (1974)
Wolfenden, R. N.: On the nature and action of the venom of poisonous snakes. J. Physiol. (Lond.) **7**, 326—364 (1886)
Yang, C. C.: Review: Chemistry and evolution of toxins in snake venoms. Toxicon **12**, 1—44 (1974)

CHAPTER 22

Snakes and the Complement System

C. A. ALPER

A. Introduction

Because the study of the interaction between snake venoms and complement began at the very beginnings of complement research, it seems prudent to begin this chapter with a brief history of the development of our knowledge of the complement system. It will be seen that with the very few tools then available, men of great genius and insight were able to gain an impressive understanding of immune cytolysis and of the roles played by antibody and complement. Cobra venom was an important tool in this endeavor and was highly instrumental in the dissection of the complexities of the complement system, a task made far easier in recent years by the availability of methods of protein separation and yet still incomplete. The early work described here spans less than 30 years, from the late 1880's to the eve of World War I. Although occasional studies of the complement system were published between the wars, including a few important contributions, work in this area was not resumed in earnest until after World War II. The past 20 years have seen a remarkable explosion of knowledge in the field, yet some of the newer insights are based (usually unknowingly and very rarely with proper citation) on experiments first performed 70 or 80 years ago.

B. Early Complement Research

It is difficult to date with precision the beginnings of our knowledge of the serum complement system because the earliest evidence for the existence of this system derived from the ability of serum to kill bacteria. That blood has "healing influences" has been known or suspected since antiquity: the oldest written allusion is contained in an Assyrian cuneiform tablet of the first century B.C. (ROTHER et al., 1974). JOHN HUNTER (1817) observed about 1790 that "... (the blood) from the young woman kept quite sweet till the fifth day (at room temperature in England during late June), when it began to smell disagreeably; in this state it continued two days more and then emitted the common odour of putrid blood."

With the discovery of microorganisms and methods for culturing them in the second half of the eighteenth century, closer study of bactericidal activity of blood became possible (LANDAU, 1874). Apparently, the first investigator to show that cell-free blood plasma was capable of killing bacteria and other microorganisms was GROHMANN (1884). This was of particular importance because of the near-contemporaneous recognition of phagocytosis by Metchnikoff. Later workers who injected living organisms into the blood streams of animals and observed rapid clearance of these bacteria from the blood recognized that phagocytosis in the spleen and other organs was primarily responsible (WYSSOKOWITSCH, 1886; VON FODOR, 1886).

NUTTALL (1888) demonstrated the heat lability of the bactericidal activity of serum, showing that this capacity was destroyed by heating at 55° C for 1 h; lower temperatures required longer times for inactivation. It was then shown that keeping serum at 6–8° C preserved bactericidal activity better than 37° C (BUCHNER, 1889a, b). PFEIFFER and ISSAEFF (1894) observed that *Vibrio cholerae* injected intraperitoneally in rabbits granulated and died extracellularly. METCHNIKOFF (1895) confirmed these observations and produced the same phenomenon in vitro with organisms, fresh peritoneal exudate fluid, and antiserum to the vibrio. Whereas Buchner had coined the term "alexin" for the heat-labile bactericidal activity, Metchnikoff called it "cytase."

The important distinction between antibody and complement in immune cytolysis was made by BORDET (1895) who saw that immune serum to the cholera vibrio immobilized and agglutinated the bacteria and (if fresh) killed them. Heating the serum to 55° C destroyed only its bactericidal activity; the other properties remained wholly intact. If fresh serum from a nonimmune animal was added to heated immune serum, bactericidal activity was restored. If a small amount of heated (or fresh) immune serum was added to fresh nonimmune serum, striking bactericidal activity resulted.

A second highly important contribution by BORDET (1898) was his demonstration that fresh immune serum incubated with red cells induced hemolysis and that this system was entirely analogous to the bacteriolysis system. These observations were confirmed and enlarged upon by EHRLICH and MORGENROTH (1899) who noted that erythrocytes exposed to "immune body" at 3° C and then washed would undergo lysis when incubated in fresh nonimmune serum (a source of "addiment") at 37° C. In the following year, they introduced the term "complement" and postulated that antibody must have two combining sites ("haptophore complexes"), one for the red cell and one for complement (EHRLICH and MORGENROTH, 1900). BORDET and GENGOU (1901) published experiments indicating that specificity was a property of antibody and that therefore there were a great multiplicity of antibodies, but only one complement. Ehrlich challenged this view claiming that each immune system had its own complement (EHRLICH and SACHS, 1902), but subsequent work has confirmed Bordet's conclusion.

Proceeding from BUCHNER'S (1893) observation that diluting serum with water or dialyzing it against water destroyed bactericidal (complement) activity, FERRATA (1907) separated the precipitate (euglobulin) formed from serum at low ionic strength from the supernatant (pseudoglobulin) and showed that although neither fraction had hemolytic activity, activity was restored when they were recombined. BRAND (1907) quickly confirmed these findings and further showed that if red cells were first exposed to euglobulin, washed, and then exposed to pseudoglobulin, lysis ensued, but not if the order of exposure was reversed. He therefore called the euglobulin fraction midpiece and the pseudoglobulin fraction end-piece.

C. Early Work on Snake Body Fluids and Complement

MITCHELL (1860) observed that animals given lethal doses of rattlesnake venom died of respiratory paralysis, putrefied rapidly, and had incoagulable blood. These fundamental and thorough observations became the basis for all the work that followed in the ensuing decades on the nature of snake venoms and the interactions of these venoms with blood and other tissues of a wide variety of animals. In later investigations, MITCHELL (1868) showed that rattlesnake venom ingested orally by susceptible animals was without ill effect and that the venom was not toxic for the snake itself. MITCHELL and REICHERT (1883, 1886) clearly established that the toxic materials in snake venoms were proteins and that each was distinct and had different physicochemical properties.

Silas Weir Mitchell, physician, scientist, and poet, also had a personal influence on venom research around the turn of the century. He indirectly instigated the studies of EWING (1894), wherein it was shown that serum from rabbits injected with lethal doses of venom from a rattlesnake *(Crotalus adamanteus)* lost its bactericidal activity for *E. coli* and *B. anthracis*. His part in the highly significant and incisive study of FLEXNER and NOGUCHI (1903) is clear from the introduction by Mitchell: "I have long desired that the action of venoms upon blood should be further examined. I finally indicated in this series of propositions the direction I wished the inquiry to take. Starting from these the following very satisfactory study has been made by Professor Flexner and Dr. Noguchi. My own share in it, although so limited, I mention with satisfaction."

However, before considering the study of FLEXNER and NOGUCHI (1903), we must review the important prior contributions of STEPHENS and MYERS (1898) and STEPHENS (1900). These authors showed that cobra venom incubated with whole human or animal blood produced hemolysis; this effect was specifically prevented by antiserum to the venom. They further observed that at higher doses of venom no hemolysis occurred, but at lower (effective) doses the hemolytic effect was enhanced by serum. STEPHENS and MYERS also studied the extent of hemolysis induced by cobra venom in blood from a variety of warm- and cold-blooded animals and found great variation. They similarly found wide variation in the ability of serum from these animals to mediate cobra venom-induced hemolysis of human erythrocytes. The ability of serum to mediate the hemolytic action of cobra venom was found to be abolished by heating to 58° C for 10 min. It is of interest that among the sera tested were those of the toad, the frog, the eel, the tortoise, and the snake (cobra?), and that direct lysis (without cobra venom) by these sera was observed on incubation with human red cells: sera from warm-blooded animals had little or no direct lysis capacity. Using snake red cells, they found that hemolysis by cobra venom and other animal serum could be inhibited by snake (cobra?) serum. Finally, they showed that the direct hemolytic activity of cobra serum was destroyed by heating at 68° C for 15 min, but this treatment had no effect on the cobra venom hemolytic factor.

In their classic study, FLEXNER and NOGUCHI (1903) pursued some of these questions further and related their findings to complement as it was then understood. They used venom from the rattlesnake *(Crotalus adamanteus)*, water moccasin *(Ancistrodon piscivorus)*, cobra *(Naja tripudians)*, and copperhead *(Ancistrodon contortrix)*. They first observed agglutination but no lysis by the venoms in 0.5% solution of washed red cells from a number of mammals (dog, rabbit, sheep, ox, and pig). When these experiments were carried out with whole blood, both agglutination and later lysis occurred, but only agglutination was observed if the reaction mixture was kept at 0° C. At lower concentrations of venom and at higher temperatures, lysis but no agglutination developed. They found the cobra venom to be most active in producing lysis in the presence of serum, followed by venom from the water moccasin, copperhead, and rattlesnake, in that order. The agglutinating activity was destroyed by heating the venoms to 75–80° C for 30 min but the hemolysis-inducing factor was stable to 96–100° C for 15 min.

They also investigated the relationship between the neurotoxin and hemolysis-inducing activity. They showed that incubation with brain removed the neurotoxin and left the hemolysis-inducing activity intact in copperhead venom. Their experiments also clearly demonstrated that incubation of mammalian serum with snake venom destroyed the bactericidal and hemolytic activities (the latter tested against antibody-sensitized sheep erythrocytes in the usual way) of complement. They concluded that the venoms inactivated complement, but had no effect on antibody. Since heating the mammalian serum to 58° C rendered it incapable of mediating venom-induced passive hemolysis, they felt that this lysis was dependent on complement. Finally, they injected sublethal doses of venoms intravenously into rabbits and confirmed Ewing's findings of destruction of bactericidal activity in vivo.

Further studies by FLEXNER and NOGUCHI (1902) and NOGUCHI (1902, 1903), since they are concerned primarily with serum rather than venoms from snakes and other cold-blooded animals, are at first sight marginal to the main point of this chapter; in fact they are very much to the point, as has become apparent only very recently. FLEXNER and NOGUCHI (1902) found that serum from the rattlesnake was directly lytic for washed mammalian red cells and this activity was destroyed by heating at 58° C for 30 min. They also demonstrated slow hemolysis of some mammalian red cells by certain venoms and postulated that this was by a different mechanism than complement-mediated lysis, speaking of "endocomplements" in the red cells. Finally, they made the interesting observation that antiserum to *Crotalus* serum destroyed the hemolytic action of all venoms in guinea pig serum for mammalian erythrocytes.

In a number of experiments with the sera and red cells of cold-blooded animals at the Marine Biological Laboratories, Woods Hole, Massachusetts, NOGUCHI (1902) found hemolysins for heterologous red cells in a majority of the sera as well as agglutinins and precipitins. Of a great variety of creatures including eels, skates, frogs, fish, turtles, lobster, and the limulus, only limulus, lobster, and box turtle sera failed to produce hemolysis. In an extension of these studies (NOGUCHI, 1903), he showed that hemolysis by many of these sera was inhibited by heating at 40–50° C for 30 min: These results confirmed those of STEPHENS (1900). FRIEDBERGER and SEELIG (1908) observed hemolytic activity in frog (*Rana esculenta* var. *ridibunda*) serum for unsensitized rabbit and human red cells destroyed by heating at 50° C for 20 min. They performed a hepatectomy on a frog and 9 days later (with the frog in seemingly good health!) obtained serum which had lost hemolytic activity. They concluded that the "hemotoxin" was synthesized in the liver. The hemolytic activity of the serum of snakes and other cold-blooded animals for mammalian erythrocytes has been rediscovered a number of times (LAZAR, 1904; LIEFMANN, 1911; MAZZETTI,

1913; REINER and STRILICH, 1929; BOND and SHERWOOD, 1939; LEGLER and EVANS, 1966; DAY et al., 1970).

NOC (1904) studied venoms from members of all families of snakes except the *Hydrophidae* and found hemolytic activity in all that was mediated by heated (58° C) horse serum. This second (noncomplement mediated) manner in which snake venom could induce hemolysis was further investigated (KYES and SACHS, 1903; VON DUNGERN and COCA, 1907, 1908; MORGENROTH and KAYA, 1908) and the "lysolecithin" pathway was defined. Heating the mammalian serum to 65° C or the venom to 70° C destroyed the complement interaction but not the lecithin-mediated hemolysis. Lecithin-mediated hemolysis is unaffected by digesting serum with papain or treating with acid or base, whereas complement activity is destroyed by these agents.

Virtually all subsequent work with snake venom and complement to the present has been done with cobra venom. This is important because very recent evidence, to be described later, suggests very different mechanisms for crotalid and elapid venoms in their effects on complement, although the end results are similar.

In order to determine which of the two known components of complement were destroyed by cobra venom, SACHS and OMOROKOW (1911) tested whether midpiece or end-piece restored hemolytic activity for antibody-sensitized erythrocytes to cobra venom-treated guinea pig serum. They found that either fraction restored activity quantitatively, leading them to suspect the existence of a third component: „Am nächsten würde vielleicht die Annahme liegen, daß zur Komplemente-Wirkung außer den als Mittelstück und Endstück bekannten Komponenten noch ein dritter Faktor erforderlich ist, der eben durch den Einfluß des Cobragiftes inaktiviert wird." RITZ (1912) explored this point further and found that midpiece and end-piece made from cobra venom-inactivated guinea pig serum had the full activities of these fractions when used to "complement" the appropriate fractions from normal guinea pig serum. He further observed that serum heated at 54° C for 30 min, which lacked midpiece and end-piece activity, or heated midpiece or end-piece, could restore hemolytic activity for antibody-sensitized erythrocytes to cobra venom-treated guinea pig serum. It thus contained the "third component" of complement first suggested by SACHS and OMOROKOW. RITZ's observations were confirmed by HUSLER (1912) and by BROWNING and MACKIE (1913). The latter authors also made an observation that was only to be explained many decades later with the elucidation of the properdin or alternative complement pathway. They noted that serum depleted of hemolytic complement by incubation with antibody-sensitized red cells still supported passive hemolysis induced by cobra venom. They concluded: "It is doubtful ... if the assumption of an additional 'third component' can explain all the phenomena above described."

There was yet another line of experimentation that led toward the conclusion that there must be a third component of complement. This began with the observation (VON DUNGERN, 1900) that bacteria and yeast were anticomplementary (destroyed complement on incubation with fresh serum). EHRLICH and SACHS (1902) showed that serum treated with yeast could be restored to full complement activity with either midpiece or end-piece from normal serum. It was COCA (1914) who drew these threads together and showed that the same complement component was inactivated by cobra venom, yeast, and certain bacteria. Moreover, since yeast but not the supernatant from a yeast-serum mixture inactivated complement, there must be an attachment to the yeast surface of the inactivating principle.

A fourth component was discovered 12 years later (GORDON et al., 1926) when it was found that ammonia (or, as shown later, hydrazine) inactivated complement but did not destroy the three known components. In the late 1950s to mid-1960s, it became apparent that Ritz's "third component" was complex and, in fact, consisted of no less than six separate proteins (RAPP, 1958; AMIRAIAN et al., 1958; RAPP et al., 1959; TAYLOR and LEON, 1959; NISHIOKA and LINSCOTT, 1963; KLEIN and WELLENSIEK, 1965; NELSON, 1965).

In the mid-1950's, Pillemer and his co-workers demonstrated the existence of a novel serum protein, properdin (PILLEMER et al., 1954), involved in the inactivation of complement by zymosan (a substance extracted from yeast cell wall). Two other proteins were identified in this system, Factor A which was hydrazine sensitive (PENSKY et al., 1959) and Factor B which was destroyed by heating to 50° C (BLUM et al., 1959). Magnesium ions (Mg^{2+}) but not calcium were essential for activity of the system, which was also activated by endotoxin, a wide variety of polysaccharides, and perhaps other substances. The existence of this separate pathway was cast into doubt by the finding of natural antibody to zymosan and other polysaccharides in normal serum. It was therefore thought by many investigators that C3 consumption proceeded solely by the classical first three complement components (NELSON, 1958). Several lines of investigation around 1970 led to a reevaluation of the properdin pathway and its reacceptance by all in 1971: (1) On repeating the work of PILLEMER and his group (1954), it was found that with modern quantitative assays for individual complement components, C3 and later-acting components were consumed by endotoxin or zymosan without significant consumption of C1, C4, or C2 (GEWURZ et al., 1968). (2) Studies of a patient with repeated bacterial infections and continuous consumption of C3 revealed normal levels of C1, C4, and C2 (ALPER et al., 1970a, b), thereby suggesting "... that there is an alternative physiological mechanism for the inactivation of C3 that bypasses the first three complement components." (ALPER et al., 1970a) (3) Antibodies of the IgGl subclass in guinea pigs activated C3 with little consumption of C1, C4, or C2 (SANDBERG et al., 1970). (4) Serum from guinea pigs with a hereditary deficiency of C4 supported C3 consumption by endotoxin (FRANK et al., 1971). (5) Cobra venom-induced hemolysis and C3 consumption required a protein which proved to be properdin Factor B (GÖTZE and MÜLLER-EBERHARD, 1971). For a fuller description of the alternative pathway and its history, the chapter by Osler is recommended (OSLER, 1976).

D. Present State of Knowledge of the Complement System

We shall for the moment leave the historical approach and consider in broad outline what we know of the nature of the complement system, its constituents, biologic activities generated during activation, and the mechanisms of interaction within the system. There are glaring gaps in our knowledge, but what is known allows us better to understand the interaction of snake venoms and complement.

The classic complement system consists of nine numbered components and four inhibitors. The first component consists of three subcomponents, C1q, C1r, and C1s,

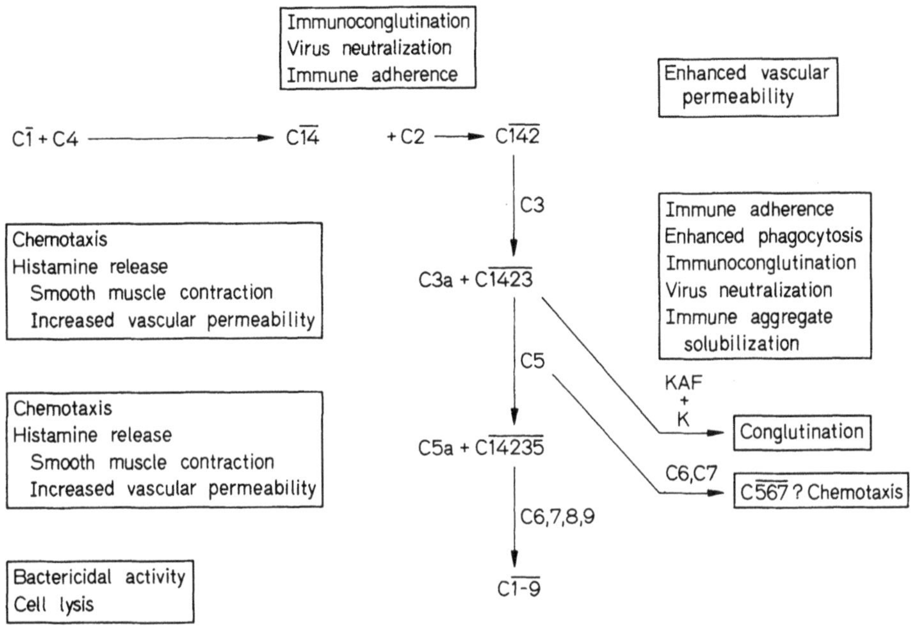

Fig. 1. The classical complement pathway and biologic functions elaborated during activation

and it is the molecular interaction between C1q and aggregated IgG or IgM (as in an antigen-antibody complex) that initiates activation of the classic complement sequence. This interaction of C1q and immunoglobulin leads to conversion, by limited sequential proteolysis, of C1r and C1s to their activated enzymatic forms, C$\overline{1r}$ and C$\overline{1s}$. C$\overline{1s}$ is a protease with C4 and C2 as natural substrates and esterolytic activity for such synthetic amino acid esters as arginyl-L-tyrosinyl ethyl ester (ALTEE) and *p*-toluenesulfonyl arginyl methyl ester (TAME). C4 and C2 are cleaved by C$\overline{1s}$ into two fragments each, the larger of which (C4b and C2a) associate to form a complex called "the classic C3 convertase," C$\overline{42}$. Although C$\overline{1}$ is essential for the formation of this enzyme, its presence or absence is irrelevant for the action of the convertase on C3. Thus, C$\overline{142}$ (Fig. 1) is equivalent to C$\overline{42}$. The classic convertase cleaves C3 to yield a small fragment (C3a) with important biologic properties, and C$\overline{3b}$. C$\overline{423}$ (again, the presence of C$\overline{1}$ is irrelevant) cleaves C5 in a manner analogous to the cleavage of C3, yielding the biologically active small polypeptide C5a and C$\overline{5b}$. C$\overline{5b}$ induces the association of the later-acting components, C6, C7, C8, and C9 with itself, producing a complex (C$\overline{5–9}$) capable of damaging bacterial and animal cell membranes. Although C$\overline{(1)423}$ is necessary for the classic pathway generation of C$\overline{5b}$, it is irrelevant for the generation of C$\overline{5–9}$ either on a surface or in the fluid phase from C$\overline{5b}$ and C$\overline{6–9}$. Thus, activation of the classic complement sequence is characterized by sequential limited proteolysis for the first five components and protein-protein interaction without evident proteolysis in the terminal components.

The known proteins in the alternative or properdin pathway are Factor B, Factor D, and properdin (P) itself (Fig. 2). The activity of Factor $\overline{D}$ is expressed in the

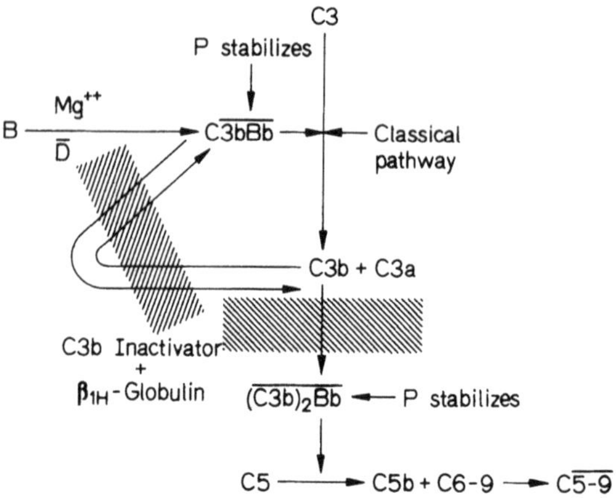

Fig. 2. The alternative complement pathway. Since the parts played by other proteins are uncertain, they are not shown

presence of a cleavage fragment of C3 which is similar to, or identical with, C3b. In the presence of Factor $\overline{\text{D}}$, C$\overline{3\text{b}}$ and the major cleavage fragment of Factor B, $\overline{\text{Bb}}$, form the alternative pathway C3 and C5 convertases, which appear to cleave and activate C3 and C5 in a fashion similar to C$\overline{42}$ and C$\overline{423}$. Properdin stabilizes this alternative pathway convertase.

The presence of a positive-feedback loop in the alternative pathway constitutes an important amplification mechanism for the activation of C3 and later-acting components. It is not absolutely clear whether there are distinct mechanisms for activating the alternative pathway without any activation of the classic pathway, but when added to serum, polysaccharides such as zymosan, inulin, and endotoxin produce large amounts of C3 activation without important consumption of C1, C4, and C2.

The C$\overline{1}$ inhibitor combines stoichiometrically with C$\overline{1\text{s}}$ and C$\overline{1\text{r}}$, inactivating these enzymes and preventing the attack of C$\overline{1}$ on C4 and C2. The C3b inactivator and β_{1H}-globulin form a potent inhibitor of the alternative pathway. Together, these proteins act enzymatically to destroy C3b in antigen-antibody-complement complexes on surfaces and C3b in the fluid phase. In this role, they destroy the B-cleaving activity of Factor D, thereby inhibiting the activity of the alternative pathway (Fig. 2).

A large number of biologic activities important in the inflammatory response and host resistance to infection are elaborated at various points in the complement sequence (Fig. 1). As mentioned, the lytic property for bacterial or animal cells (including bactericidal activity of serum alone) requires the activation of C3 through C9 or C5 through C9. This lytic function of complement probably has some importance in vivo. In contrast, enhancement of phagocytosis is probably of great biologic significance and requires the deposition of C3 on the particle to be ingested. The neutralization of certain viruses occurs after interaction with antibody and only the first two complement components (C1 and C4); other viruses require C2 and C3 in addition for neutralization. Immune adherence, a property whereby certain blood cells, including B lymphocytes, adhere to antigen-antibody complexes, occurs with complement activation through the C4 and C3 steps. Anaphylatoxin activity involving histamine release from mast cells, smooth muscle contraction, and increased vascular permeability are properties of each of the two small fragments, C3a and C5a. C5a is also chemotactic for polymorphonuclear leukocytes. A fragment of C2 increases vascular permeability.

There are a number of excellent reviews of the biochemistry of the complement system (MÜLLER-EBERHARD, 1975; RAPP and BORSOS, 1970; OSLER, 1976) that should be consulted for further details and specific references.

E. Modern Studies of the Interaction Between Snake Venom and Complement

A renewal of interest in the action of cobra venom on human serum resulted from studies of anaphylatoxin carried out by the group in Göttingen, Germany. They (VOGT and SCHMIDT, 1964) carried out the first purification of the *Naja naja* venom protein (CoF) responsible for anaphylatoxin generation in normal mammalian serum, using a salt gradient in DEAE-Sephadex chromatography and gel filtration on Sephadex G-100 to obtain a preparation in 4% yield from whole venom. This material contained at least seven amino acids, was a pseudoglobulin, contained 13% nitrogen, was destroyed by boiling, was stable for months at room temperature at pH 4.0, but was immediately inactivated at pH 2.9. They further showed that anaphylatoxin could be generated by CoF from fractions of rat plasma, that generation occurred in 0.66 M NaCl, and that there was only partial inhibition of generation in EDTA. These characteristics differed from other anaphylatoxin-producing agents such as agar or zymosan.

As part of their studies to define the proteins that made up the "third component" of Ritz and Coca, KLEIN and WELLENSIEK (1965) showed that cobra venom inactivated what we now call C3 and C5 in whole serum. NELSON (1966) purified CoF using salt gradients in DEAE-cellulose and CM-cellulose chromatograpgy of whole cobra venom. He showed that the attack on C3 was indirect, since incubation of purified CoF with functionally pure C3 did not result in destruction of C3, as occurred in whole serum. NELSON (1966) also gave animals purified CoF intravenously and demonstrated a marked decrease in C3 activity within 4 h which persisted for 3–5 days. Animals given a normally lethal dose of Forsmann antigen i.v. during this period of C3 depression showed no ill effects.

MÜLLER-EBERHARD and co-workers (1966; MÜLLER-EBERHARD, 1967) further defined CoF and the normal serum protein involved in the C3 inactivating system. They showed that CoF purified to physicochemical homogeneity by sequential preparative electrophoresis and gel filtration was a 7S β-globulin, that the human serum cofactor was a 5S heat-labile β-mobility pseudoglobulin, and that these two proteins formed a 9S C3-inactivating complex in the presence of divalent cations. JENSEN (1967), again pursuing the nature of anaphylatoxin, obtained evidence that anaphylatoxin could be generated from C5 in rat and guinea-pig serum and from functionally pure C5. Trypsin or antigen-antibody complexes interacted with the first four complement components (SAC$\overline{1423}$) to release anaphylatoxin from the purified C5.

However, CoF required the presence of a non-complement protein for anaphylatoxin generation from C5.

MAILLARD and ZARCO (1968) confirmed that C3 (and C5) were selectively depressed for a prolonged period by the administration in vivo of purified CoF to rats and guinea pigs. They found inhibition of the Arthus reaction but no effect on delayed hypersensitivity, graft rejection, or tolerance-induction in distinction to the findings of others (NELSON, 1966; AZAR et al., 1968). SHIN and co-workers (1969) demonstrated that the interaction of CoF with guinea pig serum resulted in consumption of C3, C5, and later-acting complement components with a complete sparing of C1, C4, and C2. They also found that this interaction generated a chemotactic fragment of 15000 daltons.

In a repetition of the earlier experiments with cobra venom-induced passive hemolysis, which they called a "new mechanism inducing membrane damage by complement," PICKERING et al. (1969) demonstrated that purified CoF produced the phenomenon. They also confirmed that C1, C4, and C2 were neither consumed in, nor required for, the process, and showed that activation of the terminal complement components (C3–C9) was responsible for passive lysis by CoF. By using erythrocytes and serum from the same guinea pig in one set of experiments, these authors effectively ruled out any participation by antibody in CoF-mediated passive hemolysis. They also obtained evidence that CoF destroyed cobra serum complement.

BALLOW and COCHRANE (1969) observed the same passive hemolysis of unsensitized guinea pig erythrocytes and human serum, and confirmed the participation of late-acting complement proteins since C6-deficient rabbit serum gave no hemolysis. They confirmed the formation of a C3-inactivating complex between CoF and a protein in normal guinea pig serum. They also identified an additional protein in cobra venom of 800000 daltons which appeared to inactivate C1 and accounted for 3% of the total anticomplementary activity of the venom.

Studies of the patient with decreased C3 and increased susceptibility to bacterial infections (ALPER et al., 1970a) revealed that C3 circulated primarily as the conversion product, C3b. Hemolytic complement was reduced and complement-mediated functions, such as bactericidal activity, opsonization for smooth gram negative bacilli, and chemotaxis were extraordinarily reduced and could not be restored by the addition of C3 to his serum. Metabolic studies with ^{125}I-labeled C3 revealed a markedly elevated fractional catabolic rate and rapid conversion to C3b in vivo (ALPER et al., 1970b). As mentioned earlier, all complement components except for C3 (and to a lesser extent C5) were in normal concentrations in his serum. On addition of CoF to his serum, no complex-formation and no C3 converting activity occurred. Antibody to a 3.5 S protein termed glycine-rich γ-glycoprotein (GGG) (BOENISCH and ALPER, 1970a), which reacted with a 5S protein in normal serum, glycine-rich β-glycoprotein (GBG) (BOENISCH and ALPER, 1970b), revealed a marked reduction in concentration in the patient's serum (ALPER et al., 1970b). When purified GBG was added to his serum, it was promptly cleaved into the same two fragments that were observed when normal serum was incubated with antigen-antibody aggregates or zymosan (BOENISCH and ALPER, 1970b; ALPER et al., 1971). This led to the identification of GBGase (ALPER and ROSEN, 1971) as a 3S α-euglobulin and the hypothesis that the patient was hereditarily missing an inhibitor of this enzyme. The patient's serum was found to have no detectable C3b-inactivator

Table 1. Amino Acid Composition of Cobra Venom Factor[a]

Residues/1000 residues			
Lysine	65	Alanine	58
Histidine	20	Half cystine (as cysteic acid)	18
Arginine	42	Valine	64
Aspartic	115	Methionine (as methionine sulfone)	15
Threonine	66	Isoleucine	51
Serine	64	Leucine	78
Glutamate	102	Tyrosine	40
Proline	64	Phenylalanine	38
Glycine	60		

[a] From Müller-Eberhard and Fjellström (1971).

(Abramson et al., 1971). This was later shown to be his primary genetic defect, the C3b inactivator functioning as GBGase inhibitor (Alper et al., 1972) by destroying C3b, necessary for the GBG-cleaving activity of GBGase (Müller-Eberhard and Götze, 1972). The patient's defects could be mimicked in vitro by depleting normal serum of the C3b inactivator (Nicol and Lachmann, 1973).

Chemical studies of CoF (Müller-Eberhard and Fjellström, 1971) provided the amino acid analysis given in Table 1. Using sequential preparative electrophoresis and gel filtration for purification, the yield was 0.4%. Based on its gel filtration behavior, CoF was found to have a diffusion constant of 4.17×10^{-7} cm^2/sec. Assuming a partial specific volume of 0.73, the molecular weight was calculated to be 144000 daltons. Carbohydrate analysis revealed 1.3% neuraminic acid, 4.2% hexosamine, and 5.7% hexose (in terms of glucose equivalence). Evidence was presented that the β-globulin was neither C4 nor C2. The CoF-β-globulin complex cleaved C3 in such a fashion that C3a was generated.

Pursuing their studies of the human β-globulin which interacted with CoF to form a C3-cleaving complex, Götze and Müller-Eberhard (1971) isolated this protein, which they termed C3 proactivator or C3PA. They presented evidence that this protein was cleaved in whole serum when the latter was incubated with inulin and that the major (cathodally migrating) fragment of C3PA had C3-cleaving activity. They further found that purified C3PA formed a 9S complex with CoF in the presence of Mg^{2+}. It was established that C3PA was functionally identical to Factor B (Goodkofsky and Lepow, 1971) and immunochemically identical to GBG whose isolation and physicochemical characterization was reported in the previous year (Boenisch and Alper, 1970b). The C3-cleaving activity of Bb has not been found by other workers. At the time, no direct evidence for a complex between CoF and Factor B could be obtained by other investigators (Alper et al., 1973; Hunsicker et al., 1973; Lynen et al., 1973a). Cooper (1973) showed that a CoF·B complex could be formed by the purified proteins providing Factor $\overline{D}$ was present: a conclusion confirmed by others (Fearon et al., 1973; Vogt et al., 1974). The latter workers also showed that Bb was released from the complex and, in the presence of $\overline{D}$ and Mg^{2+}, fresh B could add to the CoF (which was unaltered) to restore the complex and its C3-cleaving activity. Factor D was identified by this group as essential for CoF-induced passive hemolysis (Hunsicker et al., 1973), and it later became apparent that it was the same protein as the previously described GBGase (ALPER and ROSEN, 1971) and C3PAse (MÜLLER-EBERHARD and GÖTZE, 1972).

Continuing their studies of anaphylatoxin generation in guinea pig serum, it became apparent to Vogt's group that their unknown serum factor (UF) was the same as GBG and Factor B (LYNEN et al., 1973a, b). They clearly demonstrated that in whole serum, CoF formed a 9S complex with the major fragment of Factor B, Bb. Similar findings were obtained by BRADE et al. (1972) who found that a heat-labile factor (HLF) in guinea pig serum was necessary for C3 inactivation by CoF. HLF was immunochemically related to human GBG (Factor B) and other serum proteins were necessary for C3 inactivation by CoF.

LACHMANN and NICOL (1973) presented an analysis of the alternative pathway as it was activated by polysaccharides and by CoF and concluded that CoF was C3b-like since it could generate an alternative pathway convertase in the absence of C3. The analogy between CoF and mammalian C3b further extends to the ability of both to generate, with B and D, C5-inactivating complex for which mammalian C3 (or C3b) is not required (JENSEN, 1967; ALPER et al., 1976).

Evidence that CoF was actually a fragment of cobra C3, perhaps C3b, was obtained by ALPER and BALAVITCH (1976) who observed cross-reactivity between rabbit antiserum to CoF and human C3. Anti-CoF also reacted strongly with a β-globulin in cobra serum of slightly different electrophoretic mobility from CoF in the venom of the same snake. The β-globulin in the cobra serum behaved in a manner similar to mammalian C3 in that it converted slowly on storage of serum to a more anodally migrating product. This conversion was hastened by incubation of the cobra serum with endotoxin but not mammalian antigen-antibody complexes. Incubation with hydrazine produced a more cathodally migrating product in agarose gel electrophoresis, as it does in human serum. The striking ability of CoF to convert C3 in mammalian serum could be ascribed to its lack of susceptibility to the mammalian C3b inactivator. On the other hand, a brief incubation with cobra serum inactivated CoF for mammalian serum C3 and caused it to migrate more anodally on electrophoresis. The nature of the inactivation of CoF by cobra serum is not established but a cobra analog of mammalian C3b inactivator could be responsible.

Because of the relationship between CoF and cobra C3, it now becomes germane to consider what is known, in modern terms, of the complement system in snake serum. The existence of a complement system in the serum of cold-blooded animals was well documented, as seen earlier.

DAY and co-workers (1970) studied hemolytic complement and CoF-induced passive hemolysis in a variety of animals, including invertebrates, using sheep and rabbit erythrocytes sensitized with mammalian antibody and a standard complement buffer. They compared direct lysis with passive hemolysis and complement consumption induced by CoF. As an example of snakes, they studied cobra serum. The highest levels of lysis activity for antibody sensitized mammalian erythrocytes were found in the guinea pig and the turtle, whereas the chicken, cobra, frog, carp, paddlefish, and nurseshark had lower levels. No activity was found in the sera of the lamprey, hagfish, limulus, or sipunculid worm. The highest level of CoF-induced passive lysis was obtained in the frog, with lower but definite activity in serum from the guinea pig, chicken, hagfish, and limulus, and possibly some activity in that from the sipunculid worm. No passive lysis by CoF was observed in serum from the cobra, turtle, carp, paddlefish, lamprey, or starfish. In those sera with lytic activity for sensitized erythrocytes, therefore, some produced passive lysis (guinea pig, chicken, and frog) but the remaining sera did not. In three sera without definite activity for sensitized erythrocytes (hagfish, limulus, and possibly the sipunculid worm), passive lysis was detected. Complement consumption by CoF occurred in all sera with complement activity except for the carp and paddlefish. Thus, CoF could produce complement consumption without inducing hemolysis in sera from the cobra and turtle but was without any effect in carp or paddlefish serum.

In studies still being pursued (Calich et al., 1978), the sera and venoms from a variety of Brazilian *Crotalidae* were investigated. The lysis of unsensitized sheep erythrocytes by sera from *Bothrops jararaca*, *B. jararacussu*, *B. moogeni*, and *Crotalus terrificus* was observed to proceed in the presence of Mg EGTA, but not in the presence of EDTA (which chelates both Ca^{2+} and Mg^{2+}). The inclusion of Ca^{2+} in the system or the use of antibody-sensitized sheep red cells did not increase the hemolytic titer of the sera. The hemolytic activity was markedly reduced by prior incubation of the snake serum with *E. coli* 055:B5 endotoxin, zymosan, mammalian antigen-antibody precipitates, or purified CoF *(Naja naja)*. Heating at 52° C for 30 min (which destroys mammalian Factor B and C2) destroyed hemolytic activity. However, incubation with hydrazine, which destroys mammalian C3 and C4, had no effect on hemolytic activity. Antiserum to CoF *(Naja naja)* reacted strongly with a Brazilian snake β-globulin (presumably C3). This protein converted to a more cathodally migrating form when the snake serum was incubated with endotoxin, mammalian antigen-antibody precipitates, zymosan, or CoF *(Naja naja)*, or was stored, but no such conversion was seen when the snake serum was incubated with hydrazine or was heated at 52° C.

The venoms of these snakes contained no material reactive with anti-CoF but did produce C3 conversion in human serum, although to a lesser degree than CoF. These venoms also altered Factor B and C4 in human serum, and on fractionation of the venom preliminary evidence suggested that a single venom protein was responsible. When *Bothrops* serum was examined with antiserum to the corresponding venom, virtually no cross-reacting material was observed, suggesting a primarily local origin for venom proteins.

It thus appears that the mechanisms for anticomplementary activity in cobra venom and the venom of *Crotalidae* are quite different. Moreover, the cobra serum contains a CoF-inactivating protein which is lacking in the serum of *Crotalidae*. The complement activity in the latter sera appears to reside primarily, if not exclusively, in an alternative and common pathway.

F. Epilog

The wheel has now turned full circle with a redirection of scientific interest to the interaction of snake venom and complement after more than half a century of relative dormancy. We can expect further studies to reveal the orderly evolution of the complement system throughout a good part of the animal kingdom. Structural studies of the cobra venom factor may yield clues to the essential functional and structural features of C3. This protein has already been used to depress C3 levels in experimental animals to explore the role of the complement system in allograft rejection (NELSON, 1966; GEWURZ et al., 1967; MAILLARD and ZARCO, 1968), in the antibody response (PEPYS, 1974; DUKOR et al., 1974), and in myocardial damage after infarction (MOROKO and CARPENTER, 1973) as well as in other phenomena (COCHRANE et al., 1970; HENSON and COCHRANE, 1971; DODDS and PICKERING, 1972; GILBERT et al., 1973; MCCALL et al., 1974). The wheel certainly has further to turn.

References

Abramson, N., Alper, C. A., Lachmann, P. J., Rosen, F. S., Jandl, J. H.: Deficiency of C3 inactivator in man. J. Immunol. **107**, 19—27 (1971)

Alper, C. A., Abramson, N., Johnston, R. B., Jr., Jandl, J. H., Rosen, F. S.: Increased susceptibility to infection associated with abnormalities of complement-mediated functions and of the third component of complement (C3). New Engl. J. Med. **282**, 349—354 (1970a)

Alper, C. A., Abramson, N., Johnston, R. B., Jr., Jandl, J. H., Rosen, F. S.: Studies in vivo and in vitro on an abnormality in the metabolism of C3 in a patient with increased susceptibility to infection. J. clin. Invest. **49**, 1975—1985 (1970b)

Alper, C. A., Balavitch, D.: Cobra venom factor: evidence for its being altered cobra C3 (the third component of complement). Science **191**, 1275—1276 (1976)

Alper, C. A., Boenisch, T., Watson, L.: Glycine-rich β-glycoprotein (GBG): evidence for relation to the complement system and for genetic polymorphism in man. J. Immunol. **107** (Abstr.), 323 (1971)

Alper, C. A., Colten, H. R., Gear, J. S. S., Rabson, A. R., Rosen, F. S.: Homozygous human C3 deficiency. The role of C3 in antibody production, $C\overline{1s}$-induced vasopermeability, and cobra venom-induced passive hemolysis. J. clin. Invest. **57**, 222—229 (1976)

Alper, C. A., Goodkofsky, I., Lepow, I. H.: The relationship of glycine-rich β-glycoprotein to factor B in the properdin system and to the cobra factor-binding protein of human serum. J. exp. Med. **137**, 424—437 (1973)

Alper, C. A., Rosen, F. S.: Genetic aspects of the complement system. In: Kunkel, H. G., Dixon, F. J. (Eds.): Advances in Immunology, Vol. XIV, pp. 251—290. New York: Academic Press. 1971

Alper, C. A., Rosen, F. S., Lachmann, P. J.: Inactivator of the third component of complement as an inhibitor in the properdin pathway. Proc. nat. Acad. Sci. (Wash.) **69**, 2910—2913 (1972)

Amiraian, K., Plescia, O., Cavallo, G., Heidelberger, M.: Complex nature of the step in immune hemolysis involving third component of complement. Science **127**, 239—240 (1958)

Azar, M. M., Yunis, E. J., Pickering, R. J., Good, R. A.: On the nature of immunological tolerance. Lancet 1968 **I**, 1279—1281

Ballow, M., Cochrane, C. G.: Two anticomplementary factors in cobra venom: hemolysis of guinea pig erythrocytes by one of them. J. Immunol. **103**, 944—952 (1969)

Blum, L., Pillemer, L., Lepow, I. H.: The properdin system and immunity. XIII. Assay and properties of a heat-labile serum factor (Factor B) in the properdin system. Z. Immun.-Forsch. **118**, 349—357 (1959)

Boenisch, T., Alper, C. A.: Isolation and properties of a glycine-rich γ-glycoprotein of human serum. Biochim. biophys. Acta (Amst.) **214**, 135—140 (1970a)

Boenisch, T., Alper, C. A.: Isolation and properties of a glycine-rich β-glycoprotein of human serum. Biochim. biophys. Acta (Amst.) **221**, 529—535 (1970b)

Bond, G. C., Sherwood, N. P.: Serological studies of Reptilia. II. Hemolytic property of snake serum. J. Immunol. **36**, 11—16 (1939)

Bordet, J.: Les leucocytes et les propriétés actives du sérum chez les vaccinés. Ann. Inst. Pasteur Paris **9**, 462—506 (1895)

Bordet, J.: Sur l'agglutination et la dissolution des globules rouges par le sérum d'animaux injectés de sang défibriné. Ann. Inst. Pasteur Paris **12**, 688—695 (1898)

Bordet, J., Gengou, O.: Sur l'existence de substances sensibilisatrices dans la plupart des sérums antimicrobiens. Ann. Inst. Pasteur Paris **15**, 289—302 (1901)

Brade, V., Schmidt, G., Vogt, W.: Anaphylatoxin formation by contact activation of plasma. III. Fixation of two different anaphylatoxin-forming complexes on zymosan. Europ. J. Immunol. **2**, 180—186 (1972)
Brand, E.: Über das Verhalten der Komplemente bei der Dialyse. Berl. klin. Wschr. **44**, 1075—1079 (1907)
Browning, C. H., Mackie, T. J.: The relationship of the complementing action of fresh serum along with immune body to its haemolytic effect with cobra venom—a contribution on the structure of complement. Z. Immun.-Forsch. **17**, 1—20 (1913)
Buchner, H.: Über die bakterientötende Wirkung des zellenfreien Blutserums. Zentralbl. Bakteriol. (Orig.) **5**, 817—823 (1889a); **6**, 1—11 (1889a)
Buchner, H.: Über die nähere Natur der bakterientötenden Substanz im Blutserum. Zentralbl. Bakteriol. (Orig.) **6**, 561—565 (1889b)
Buchner, H.: Über den Einfluß der Neutralsalze auf Serum-alexine, Enzyme, Toxalbumine, Blutkörperchen und Milzbrandsporen. Arch. Hyg. (Berl.) **17**, 138—178 (1893)
Calich, V. L., Kipnis, T. L., Dias da Silva, W., Alper, C. A., Rosen, F. S.: Brazilian snake serum and venom: studies of the alternative pathway and C3 in man and serpent. J. Immunol. **120** (Abstr.), 1767 (1978)
Coca, A. F.: A study of the anticomplementary action of yeast, of certain bacteria and of cobra-venom. Z. Immun.-Forsch. **21**, 604—622 (1914)
Cochrane, C. G., Müller-Eberhard, H. J., Akin, B. S.: Depletion of plasma complement in vivo by a protein of cobra venom: its effect on various immunologic reactions. J. Immunol. **105**, 55—69 (1970)
Cooper, N. R.: Formation and function of a complex of the C3 proactivator with a protein from cobra venom. J. exp. Med. **137**, 451—460 (1973)
Day, N. K. B., Gewurz, H., Johannsen, R., Finstad, J., Good, R. A.: Complement and complement-like activity in lower vertebrates and in vertebrates. J. exp. Med. **132**, 941—950 (1970)
Dodds, W. J., Pickering, R. J.: The effect of cobra venom factor on hemostasis in guinea pigs. Blood **40**, 400—411 (1972)
Dukor, P., Schumann, G., Gisler, R. H., Dierich, M., König, W., Hadding, U., Bitter-Suermann, D.: Complement-dependent B-cell activation by cobra venom factor and other mitogens. J. exp. Med. **139**, 337—354 (1974)
Dungern, E., von: Beiträge zur Immunitätslehre. Münch. med. Wschr. **47**, 677—680 (1900)
Dungern, E., von, Coca, A. F.: Über Hämolyse durch Schlangengift. Münch. med. Wschr. **54**, 2317—2321 (1907)
Dungern, E., von, Coca, A. F.: Über Hämolyse durch Schlangengift II. Biochem. Z. **12**, 407—421 (1908)
Ehrlich, P., Morgenroth, J.: Zur Theorie der Lysin-Wirkung. Berl. klin. Wschr. **36**, 6—9 (1899)
Ehrlich, P., Morgenroth, J.: Über Haemolysine. Berl. klin. Wschr. **37**, 453—458 (1900)
Ehrlich, P., Sachs, H.: Über die Vielheit der Complemente des Serums. Berl. klin. Wschr. **21**, 297—299 (1902)
Ewing, C. B.: The action of rattlesnake venom upon the bactericidal power of the blood serum. Lancet **1894 I**, 1236—1238
Fearon, D. T., Austen, K. F., Ruddy, S.: Serum proteins involved in decay and regeneration of cobra venom factor-dependent complement activation. J. Immunol. **111**, 1730—1736 (1973)
Ferrata, A.: Die Unwirksamkeit der komplexen Hämolysine in salzfreien Lösungen und ihre Ursache. Berl. klin. Wschr. **44**, 366—368 (1907)
Flexner, S., Noguchi, H.: The constitution of snake venom and snake sera. U. Penn. med. Bull. **15**, 345—362 (1902)
Flexner, S., Noguchi, H.: Snake venom in relation to haemolysis, bacteriolysis, and toxicity. J. exp. Med. **6**, 277—301 (1903)
Fodor, J., von: Bacterien im Blute lebender Thiere. Arch. Hyg. **4**, 129—148 (1886)
Frank, M. M., May, J., Gaither, T., Ellman, L.: In vitro studies of complement function in sera of C4-deficient guinea pigs. J. exp. Med. **134**, 176—187 (1971)
Friedberger, E., Seelig, A.: Zur Hämolyse bei den Kaltblütern. 1. Ein echtes Hämotoxin im Serum des Frosches und der Einfluß der Leberextirpation auf den Giftgehalt des Serums. Zentralbl. Bakteriol. (Orig.) **46**, 421—431 (1908)

Gewurz, H., Clark, D. S., Cooper, M. D., Varco, R., Good, R. A.: Effect of cobra venom-induced inhibition of complement activity on allograft and xenograft rejection reactions. Transplantation **5**, 1296—1303 (1967)
Gewurz, H., Shin, H. S., Mergenhagen, S. E.: Interaction of the complement system with endotoxic lipopolysaccharide: consumption of each of the six terminal complement components. J. exp. Med. **128**, 1049—1057 (1968)
Gilbert, D. N., Barnett, J. A., Sanford, J. P.: *Escherichia coli* bacteremia in the squirrel monkey. I. Effect of cobra venom factor treatment. J. clin. Invest. **52**, 406—413 (1973)
Götze, O., Müller-Eberhard, H. J.: The C3 activator system: an alternate pathway of complement activation. J. exp. Med. **134**, 90s—108s (1971)
Goodkofsky, I., Lepow, I. H.: Functional relationship of Factor B in the properdin system to C3 proactivator of human serum. J. Immunol. **107**, 1200—1204 (1971)
Gordon, J., Whitehead, H. R., Wormall, A.: The action of ammonia on complement. The fourth component. Biochem. J. **20**, 1028—1035 (1926)
Grohmann, W.: Über die Einwirkung des zellenfreien Blutplasma auf einige pflanzliche Microorganismen (schimmel-, spross-, pathogene und nichtpathogene Spaltpilze), p. 34. Dorpat: C. Mattiesen 1884
Henson, P. M., Cochrane, C. G.: Acute immune complex disease in rabbits. The role of complement and of a leukocyte-dependent release of vasoactive amines from platelets. J. exp. Med. **133**, 554—571 (1971)
Hunsicker, L. G., Ruddy, S., Austen, K. F.: Alternate complement pathway: factors involved in cobra venom factor (CoVF) activation of the third component of complement (C3). J. Immunol. **110**, 128—138 (1973)
Hunter, J.: A Treatise on the Blood, Inflammation, and Gun-Shot Wounds, pp. 77—79. Philadelphia: James Webster 1817
Husler, J.: Über die Inaktivierung hämolytischer Komplemente durch Erwärmen. Z. Immun.-Forsch. **15**, 157—171 (1912)
Jensen, J.: Anaphylatoxin in its relation to the complement system. Science **155**, 1122—1123 (1967)
Klein, P. G., Wellensiek, H. J.: Multiple nature of the third component of guinea-pig complement. I. Separation and characterization of three factors a, b, and c, essential for haemolysis. Immunology **8**, 590—603 (1965)
Kyes, P., Sachs, H.: Zur Kenntnis der Cobragift-activierenden Substanzen. Berl. klin. Wschr. **40**, 21—23; 82—85 (1903)
Lachmann, P. J., Nicol, P.: Reaction mechanism of the alternative pathway of complement fixation. Lancet **1973 I**, 465—467
Landau, L.: Über die Beziehung der Fäulnisbacterien zu den Wundfiebern und accidentellen Wundkrankheiten. Jahresbericht der Schlesischen Gesellschaft für Vaterländische Cultur **52**, 190—191 (1874)
Lazar, E.: Über hämolytische Wirkung des Froschserums. Wien. klin. Wschr. **17**, 1057—1059 (1904)
Legler, D. W., Evans, E. E.: Comparative immunology: hemolytic complement in amphibia. Proc. Soc. exp. Biol. (N.Y.) **121**, 1158—1162 (1966)
Liefmann, H.: Über die Hämolysine der Kaltblüterserum. Berl. klin. Wschr. **48**, 1682—1683 (1911)
Lynen, R., Brade, V., Wolf, A., Vogt, W.: Purification and some properties of a heat labile serum factor (UF); Identity with glycine-rich β-glycoprotein and properdin factor B. Hoppe-Seylers Z. physiol. Chem. **354**, 37—47 (1973a)
Lynen, R., Schmidt, G., Vogt, W.: Identification of a heat labile human serum factor (UF) with GBG; participation in anaphylatoxin-forming systems. J. Immunol. **111** (Abstr.), 308 (1973b)
Maillard, J. L., Zarco, R. M.: Décomplémentation par un facteur extrait du venin de cobra. Effet sur plusieurs réactions immune du cobaye et du rat. Ann. Inst. Pasteur Paris **114**, 756—774 (1968)
Mazzetti, L.: Über die hämolytische Wirkung des Serums der Kaltblüter. Z. Immun.-Forsch. **18**, 132—145 (1913)
McCall, C. E., DeChatelet, L. R., Brown, D., Lachmann, P.: New biological activity following intravascular activation of the complement cascade. Nature (Lond.) **249**, 841—843 (1974)

Metchnikoff, E.: Sur la destruction extracellulaire des bactéries dans l'organisme. Ann. Inst. Pasteur Paris **9**, 433—461 (1895)
Mitchell, S. W.: Anatomy, Physiology and Toxicology of the Venomous Organs of the Rattle-Snake. Smithsonian Contribution to Knowledge 1860
Mitchell, S. W.: Experimental contributions to the toxicology of rattlesnake venom. N.Y. State J. Med. **6**, 1—34; 289—322 (1868)
Mitchell, S. W., Reichert, E. T.: Preliminary report on the venoms of serpents. Med. News **42**, 3—14; 461—472 (1883)
Mitchell, S. W., Reichert, E. T.: Researches upon the Venoms of Poisonous Serpents. Smithsonian Contribution to Knowledge 1886, p. 674
Morgenroth, J., Kaya, R.: Über eine komplementzerstörende Wirkung des Kobragiftes. Biochem. Z. **8**, 378—382 (1908)
Moroko, P. R., Carpenter, C. B.: Reduction in infarct size following acute coronary occlusion by the administration of cobra venom factor. Clin. Res. **21** (Abstr.), 950 (1973)
Müller-Eberhard, H. J.: Mechanism of inactivation of the third component of human complement (C3) by cobra venom. Fed. Proc. **26** (Abstr.), 744 (1967)
Müller-Eberhard, H. J.: Complement. In: Annual Review of Biochemistry, Vol. XXXXIV, pp. 697—724. Palo Alto, California: Annual Reviews Inc. 1975
Müller-Eberhard, H. J., Fjellström, K.-E.: Isolation of the anticomplementary protein from cobra venom and its mode of action on C3. J. Immunol. **107**, 1666—1672 (1971)
Müller-Eberhard, H. J., Götze, O.: C3 proactivator convertase and its mode of action. J. exp. Med. **135**, 1003—1008 (1972)
Müller-Eberhard, H. J., Nilsson, U. R., Dalmasso, A. P., Polley, M. J., Calcott, M. A.: A molecular concept of immune cytolysis. Arch. Path. **82**, 205—217 (1966)
Nelson, R. A., Jr.: An alternative mechanism for the properdin system. J. exp. Med. **108**, 515—535 (1958)
Nelson, R. A., Jr.: The role of complement in immune phenomena. In: Zweifach, B. W., Grant, L., McCluskey, R. T. (Eds.): The Inflammatory Process, pp. 819—872. New York: Academic Press. 1965
Nelson, R. A., Jr.: A new concept of immunosuppression in hypersensitivity reactions and in transplantation immunity. Surv. Ophthal. **11**, 498—505 (1966)
Nicol, P. A. E., Lachmann, P. J.: The alternate pathway of complement activation. Immunology **24**, 259—275 (1973)
Nishioka, K., Linscott, W. D.: Components of guinea-pig complement. I. Separation of a serum fraction essential for immune hemolysis and immune adherence. J. exp. Med. **118**, 767—793 (1963)
Noc, F.: Sur quelques propriétés physiologique des différents venins de serpents. Ann. Inst. Pasteur Paris **18**, 387—406 (1904)
Noguchi, H.: The interaction of the blood of cold-blooded animals, with reference to haemolysis, agglutination and precipitation. U. Penn. med. Bull. **15**, 295—307 (1902)
Noguchi, H.: On the heat lability of the complements of cold-blooded animals. Zentralbl. Bakteriol. (Orig.) **34**, 283—285; 286—288 (1903)
Nuttal, G.: Experimente über die bakterienfeindlichen Einflüsse des tierischen Körpers. Z. Hyg. **4**, 353—394 (1888)
Osler, A. G.: Complement Mechanisms and Functions. Englewood Cliffs, New Jersey: Prentice-Hall, Inc. 1976
Pensky, J., Wurz, L., Pillemer, L., Lepow, I. H.: The properdin system and immunity. XII. Assay, properties and partial purification of a hydrazine-sensitive serum factor (Factor A) in the properdin system. Z. Immun.-Forsch. **118**, 329—348 (1959)
Pepys, M. B.: Role of complement in induction of antibody production in vivo. Effect of cobra factor and other C3-reactive agents on thymus-dependent and thymus-independent antibody response. J. exp. Med. **140**, 126—145 (1974)
Pfeiffer, R., Issaeff, R.: Über die spezifische Bedeutung der Choleraimmunität. Z. Hyg. **17**, 355—400 (1894)
Pickering, R. J., Wolfson, M. R., Good, R. A., Gewurz, H.: Passive hemolysis by serum and cobra venom factor: a new mechanism inducing membrane damage by complement. Proc. nat. Acad. Sci. (Wash.) **62**, 521—527 (1969)

Pillemer, L., Blum, L., Lepow, I. H., Ross, O. A., Todd, E. W., Wardlaw, A. C.: The properdin system and immunity. I. Demonstration and isolation of a new serum protein, properdin, and its role in immune phenomena. Science **120**, 279—285 (1954)
Rapp, H. J.: Mechanism of immune hemolysis: recognition of two steps in the conversion of EAC'1,4,2 to E. Science **127**, 234—236 (1958)
Rapp, H. J., Borsos, T.: Molecular Basis of Complement Action. New York: Appleton-Century-Crofts 1970
Rapp, H. J., Sims, M. R., Borsos, T.: Separation of components of guinea pig complement by chromatography. Proc. Soc. exp. Biol. N.Y. **100**, 730—733 (1959)
Reiner, L., Strilich, L.: Beiträge zum Mechanismus der Immunkörperwirkung. Über die Hämolyse mit Warmblüter-Immunserum und Kaltblüter-Komplement und über die Ausführung der Wassermann-Reaktion bei Zimmertemperatur. Z. Immun.-Forsch. **61**, 405—409 (1929)
Ritz, H.: Über die Wirkung des Cobragiftes auf die Komplemente. III. Mitteilung. Zugleich ein Beitrag zur Kenntnis der hämolytischen Komplemente. Z. Immun.-Forsch. **13**, 62—83 (1912)
Rother, K., Hadding, U., Till, G.: Komplement, Biochemie und Pathologie. Darmstadt 1974
Sachs, H., Omorokow, L.: Über die Wirkung des Cobragiftes auf die Komplemente. II. Mitteilung. Z. Immun.-Forsch. **11**, 710—724 (1911)
Sandberg, A. L., Osler, A. G., Shin, H. S., Oliveira, B.: The biological activities of guinea pig antibodies. II. Modes of complement interaction with γ_1 and γ_2 immunoglobulins. J. Immunol. **104**, 329—334 (1970)
Shin, H. S., Gewurz, H., Snyderman, R.: Reaction of a cobra venom factor with guinea pig complement and generation of an activity chemotactic for polymorphonuclear leukocytes. Proc. Soc. exp. Biol. N.Y. **131**, 203—206 (1969)
Stephens, J. W. W.: On the haemolytic action of snake toxins and toxic sera. J. Path. Bact. **6**, 273—302 (1900)
Stephens, J. W. W., Myers, W.: The action of cobra poison on the blood: a contribution to the study of passive immunity. J. Path. Bact. **5**, 279—301 (1898)
Taylor, A. B., Leon, M. A.: Third component of human complement. Resolution into two factors and demonstration of a new reaction intermediate. Proc. Soc. exp. Biol. N.Y. **101**, 587—588 (1959)
Vogt, W., Dieminger, L., Lynen, R., Schmidt, G.: Alternative pathway for the activation of complement in human serum. Formation and composition of the complex with cobra venom factor that cleaves the third component of complement. Hoppe-Seylers Z. physiol. Chem. **355**, 171—183 (1974)
Vogt, W., Schmidt, G.: Abtrennung des anaphylatoxinbildenden Prinzips aus Cobragift von anderen Giftkomponenten. Experientia (Basel) **20**, 207—208 (1964)
Wyssokowitsch, W.: Über die Schicksale der in's Blut injizierten Mikroorganismen in Körper der Warmblüter. Z. Hyg. **1**, 3—46 (1886)

CHAPTER 23

Vaccination Against Snake Bite Poisoning

Y. SAWAI

A. Historic Outlook

Clarification of the principles of immunity and serum therapy were established by studies on the antitoxin against tetanal and diphtherial toxins carried out by BEHRING and KITASATO in 1890. In 1894, CALMETTE incorporated the technique of serum therapy into the field of snake bites, producing antivenin against the venom of Indian cobra. Antivenin proved to be an effective tool for the medical treatment of cobra bites which stimulated many scientists throughout the world and accelerated the production of antivenins against many snake venoms. Thus, the important research at that time was aimed at producing antivenins of high potency.

Prophylaxis against intoxication induced by diphtheria was carried out by GLENNY and HOPKINS (1923) and RAMON (1924, 1925) using formol toxoid. However, it took many years to obtain prophylaxis with venom toxoid, because most scientist believed that antivenin treatment was the best way to overcome snakebites. The detoxification of venoms to increase antigenicity was very difficult even in the immunization of horses to obtain an antivenin of high potency. Moreover, scientists were skeptic about the possibility of prophylaxis against snake venom because there was no evidence of immunity against snake venom, even after repeated bites. In spite of this situation, one of the pioneers in this field (SEWALL, 1887) reported a study on immunity against snake venom entitled "Experiment on the Preventive Inoculation of Rattlesnake Venom." However, this work was not evaluated as a precursor for a vaccination method but only as a guide to serum therapy. Meanwhile, inhabitants of areas infested with venomous snakes and those who became hypersensitive to horse serum antivenin keenly felt the neccessity for a venom toxoid.

Recently, HAAST and WINER (1955) reported that following a series of injections of venom of the Cape copra *Naja flava)*, the subject tolerated an injection of 40 mg of the venom with no ill effects. Later, WIENER (1960) reported the successful immunization of a professional snake handler against the venom of the Australian tiger snake *(Notechis scutatus)* after a series of injections over a 13-month period. FLOWERS (1963, 1965) described his attempt to immunize himself against the venom of the common cobra *(Naja naja)* with an adjuvant of sodium alginate. Following the 17th venom injection, it was found that 1 ml of his globulin neutralized 35 LD_{50} of cobra venom. Near the end of his injection series, he was bitten by a *Naja naja* and suffered no systemic ill effect, although necrosis developed in the bitten finger.

SAWAI et al. (1969b) carried out the first large-scale trial to actively immunize persons in the Amami and Okinawa Islands against habu *(Trimeresurus flavoviridis)* venom. During 3 years (ending in December, 1967), 43,446 volunteers in the

Islands received the toxoid which was prepared with dihydrothioctic acid (DHTA). Statistical analysis of the epidemiologic and clinical data suggested that the toxoid was effective in preventing local lesions caused by the venom. Thereafter, attempts to improve the immunogenicity of the toxoid were made by several workers (SATO, 1965; OKONOGI and HATTORI, 1968; SADAHIRO, 1971a, b; KONDO et al., 1971a; SAWAI et al., 1972). In the meantime, a research committee for habu toxoid was established in 1968 with the aid of the Ministry of Health and Welfare. Minimum requirements for habu toxoid were determined, and a method for titration of the circulating antibodies against HR1 and HR2 (hemorrhagic principles with the main lethal effect) separated from the crude venom was reported. A procedure for calculating the potency of the test specimen relative to that of the reference toxoid was also reported.

The committee examined the potency of several toxoids produced by different methods. On the basis of these results a new toxoid from a mixture of HR1 and HR2 was prepared. A field trial was planned in the Amami Islands to test reactions and immunogenicity of the toxoid; the study is being continued (SOMEYA et al., 1972).

B. Snake Venom Toxoids

I. Habu Toxoids

1. DHTA Toxoid

a) Preparation of the Toxoid

SAWAI et al. (1963, 1967) reported that the hemorrhagic, necrotic, and lethal effects of venoms from snakes of the *Viperidae*, including habu (*Trimeresurus flavoviridis*), could be detoxified by DHTA. Later, SAWAI et al. (1966, 1969a) prepared habu venom toxoid by mixing the crude venom with an equal amount of DHTA and incubated at 37° C for 1 h.

b) Detoxification Tests

Four mice were injected intramuscularly with the toxoid containing 1 mg of the detoxified venom in amounts of 0.2 ml, and all the mice survived without any local reaction such as hemorrhage or necrosis 24 h after the injection of the toxoid. The toxoid was also injected intracutaneously into a rabbit in the amount of 0.1 ml. It was confirmed, 24 h after the injection, that no hemorrhage was observed at the locus of injection. A swelling test of the toxoid was also conducted. The toxoid (0.25 mg) was injected subcutaneously into a plantar side of the leg of mice. The increase of weight of the injected foot was equal to 10% of the weight of the control foot injected 24 h earlier with the same amount of normal saline.

c) Toxicity of the Toxoid

Lethality of the toxoid in mice, calculated by the method of REED and MUENCH (1938), was 221 mg/kg by the intraperitoneal route of injection and 226 mg/kg by subcutaneous injection, whereas the LD_{50} of DHTA was 218 mg by intraperitoneal injection in mice. On the other hand, the LD_{50} of the toxoid separated from DHTA by dialysis was 813 mg. From these results, it is clear that both the lethal and hemorrhagic effects of habu venom were completely detoxified by DHTA.

d) Sterility Test

The sterility test was performed in accordance with the Minimum Requirement of Sterility Test of Biologic Products (Ministry of Health and Welfare, 1965).

e) Safety Test

Four mice were injected intraperitoneally with 0.4 ml of the toxoid, and it was confirmed that no significant changes occurred during the observation period of 7 days.

f) Immunogenicity Test

α) Protection Against the Hemorrhagic Effect of the Venom in Mice

Mice were injected subcutaneously with 0.1 ml of the toxoid containing 0.5 mg of the venom. Three booster shots of increasing strength (1, 1.5, and 2 mg) were given 4 weeks after the injection at intervals of 1 week. One week after the last booster shot, one group of immunized and nonimmunized mice were injected intramuscularly with varying doses of the venom. Mice of both groups were sacrificed 24 h after the injection, and local lesions were investigated. The results indicated that 4.6 mcg (4 minimum hemorrhagic dose, mhds) of the venom were neutralized completely in the immunized mice. The local lesions in immunized mice, challenged with the venom in increasing doses up to 75 mcg, were less severe than those of the control mice.

β) Antivenin Level in Immunized Mice

Pooled sera (0.1 ml) from immunized mice and the same amount of varying doses of the venom were mixed and incubated at 37° C for 1 h and then injected intramuscularly into mice. The local lesions of the mice were observed 24 h later. The results indicated that 0.1 ml of the sera neutralized 16 mcg (16 mhds) of the venom.

γ) Protection Test Against the Hemorrhagic and Necrotic Effects of the Venom in Rabbits

Rabbits were immunized with 2.5 mg of the toxoid, in one dose. After the third booster, varying doses of 0.3, 0.6, 1.2, and 2.4 mg of the venom were injected intramuscularly into the thighs of rabbits. The rabbits were sacrificed 24 h after the injection, and the local lesions were inspected. The results indicated that myolysis at the locus of injection was not found in the immunized rabbits with the exception of one rabbit injected with 2.4 mg of the venom which showed slight myolysis; however, severe myolysis was observed in the nonimmunized rabbits.

δ) Antivenin Level in Immunized Rabbits

Serum (0.1 ml) taken from immunized rabbits 1 week after the last booster neutralized 9.3 mcg (8 mhds) of the venom when injected intramuscularly in mice.

2. Crude Formalin Toxoid (CRF)

A 1% solution of crude habu venom dissolved in M/30 phosphate buffered saline (pH 7.0) was added with formalin initially at a 0.2% concentration and then at concentrations increasing by 0.2% on the 3rd, 5th, and 7th days (SADAHIRO et al.,

1970). The solution was incubated at 37° C for 2 weeks and the pH was adjusted to 7.0 using sodium hydroxide during incubation. After detoxification, the product was dialyzed to remove excess formalin. The hemorrhagic activity of the venom disappeared completely within 10 days and the lethality within 5–7 days (KONDO et al., 1971a). The toxoid was added with the same amount of aluminum phosphate gel as adjuvant. Immunogenicity of the toxoid will be described later.

3. Heat and Alcohol-Treated Formalin Toxoid (HAF)

a) Preparation of the Toxoid

Crude venom (0.5% in distilled water) was incubated at 56° C for 30 min. The precipitate was removed by centrifugation for 10 min at 3000 rpm. The supernatant was mixed with absolute ethanol to 70%, and the ethanol in the solution was removed by centrifugation and the sediment resuspended in normal saline. The suspension was added to 0.5% formalin and allowed to stand at 37° C for 24 h. Later, the formalin was removed by dialysis (OKONOGI et al., 1968).

b) Immunogenicity of the Toxoid

α) Protection Test

Mice were immunized with 300 mcg of the toxoid and 3 weeks later received 100 mcg of the toxoid in a booster shot. They were injected intramuscularly 1 week after the last injection with varying doses of the venom. The results indicated that the local lesions caused by 12.5 mcg of the venom were completely prevented, whereas 1 mcg of the venom induced hemorrhage at the locus of injection in the control mice.

β) Antivenin Level in Blood

1/10ty ml of pooled sera from immunized mice neutralized 12.5 mcg of the venom, and the local lesions due to 50 mcg were less severe than those of the control mice.

4. Alcohol-Precipitated Formalin Toxoid (APF)

a) Purification and Detoxification of the Venom

Habu venom was dissolved in M/60 phosphate buffer solution at pH 7.0 to make a 1% solution. Absolute ethanol was then added (−10° C) into the solution to give a final concentration of 30%. The solution was allowed to stand at −10° C for 5 h and was then centrifuged at 10000 rpm for 20 min at −10° C. The precipitate was redissolved in the same phosphate buffer (double the amount of the original venom solution), mixed with formalin to a concentration of 1%, and allowed to stand at 37° C for 10 days. The solution was ultrafiltrated through a Seitz filter after the formalin was dialyzed. The amount of protein was adjusted to 10 mg per ml of the toxoid.

Detoxification of the toxoid was determined by injecting 0.5 ml of the toxoid intramuscularly into mice and 0.1 ml intracutaneously into rabbits. It was confirmed 24 h after the injections that no hemorrhagic signs appeared at the loci of injection in any of the animals. Finally, the formalin toxoid was added to the same amount of alum (as adjuvant) which consisted of M/5 $AlCl_3 \cdot 6H_2O$ and M/5 $Na_3PO_4 \cdot 12H_2O$. A safety test was undertaken by intraperitoneal injection with 5 ml toxoid into guinea pigs and 0.5 ml into mice. No sign of intoxication due to the venom was observed during 7 days.

b) Immunogenicity of the Toxoid

α) Protection Test

Mice were injected subcutaneously at an interval of 4 weeks with two doses of 0.1 ml of the toxoid containing 0.5 mg protein. They were injected intramuscularly 1 week after the last injection with varying amounts of the venom (100–0.8 mcg). The mice were sacrificed 24 h after the injection and the local lesions inspected. Another group of immunized mice were injected intraperitoneally with varying amounts of the venom and inspected for survival or death. The results indicated that the local lesions in immunized mice were decreased up to a dose of 25 mcg (32 mhds) of the venom, and that the lethality of the venom was also decreased.

β) Antivenin Level in Blood

The circulating antivenin level in immunized mice indicated that 0.1 ml of sera from immunized mice neutralized the hemorrhagic effect from 6 mcg of the venom, whereas in control mice, local hemorrhage was marked when 0.5 mcg of the venom was injected intramuscularly (SAWAI et al., 1972).

5. Mixed Toxoid (MiF)

Two hemorrhagic principles, HR1 and HR2, were separated from habu venom by gel filtration on Sephadex G-100 (OMORI-SATOH et al., 1967). The most lethal activity was found in HR1. The HR2 fraction was further purified by chromatography on Amberlite CG-50 (TAKAHASHI and OHSAKA, 1970). These principles are regarded as the most important factors involved in habu envenomation.

*a) Preparation of MiF Toxoid (*SADAHIRO, 1971a, b; KONDO et al., 1971a)

HR1 and HR2 were treated separately with 0.8% formalin and dialyzed to prepare HR1 and HR2 toxoids. The same amounts of HR1 and HR2 toxoid on a protein basis were mixed to prepare MiF. Alum phosphate was used as adjuvant. The final product contained 2.5 mg of protein (0.8 mg of HR1 and 1.7 mg HR2) and 1.35 mg of aluminum per ml.

b) Safety Test of MiF Toxoid

Mice, rats, and guinea pigs were inoculated intraperitoneally with 0.5, 2, and 5 ml respectively of the toxoid. The inoculated animals showed no pathologic symptoms and the increase in their body weight was comparable to the uninoculated animals. The product passed the Minimum Requirement for Sterility Test for Biologic Products.

c) Immunogenicity of the MiF and CRF Toxoids

α) Antivenin Level in the Blood of Immunized Animals

Guinea pigs received three injections with 0.5 ml of the MiF toxoid at 4-week intervals. Antitoxins in the immunized animals were determined in terms of anti-HR1, anti-HR2, and antilethal (anti-HR1) toxins. Antitoxins against HR1 and HR2 were determined by the rabbit intracutaneous method and the antilethal toxin by the mouse intravenous method (KONDO et al., 1965a, b; 1971a). Guinea pigs were also injected with 0.5 ml of CRF toxoid (5 mg protein/ml) as a reference toxoid by the same method as above. The average titers of anti-HR1 and anti-HR2 sera taken from immunized guinea pigs 10 days after the last injection with MiF toxoid were 28 and 48 u/ml, respectively, whereas 12 and 16 u/ml were obtained with CRF toxoid. On the other hand, antilethal titers of sera from guinea pigs immunized with MiF toxoid were 40 or 80 u/ml, whereas the comparable value for CRF toxoid was 32 u/ml.

β) Protection Test in Guinea-Pigs

Challenges of immunized guinea pig with MiF and CRF toxoids indicated that the hemorrhagic effect of 300–1000 mcg of crude venom was markedly decreased.

γ) Correlation Between Circulating Antivenin Titer and Protective Capacity in Immunized Animals

Challenge experiments with crude venom were carried out with a larger number of guinea pigs immunized with various batches of CRF and MiF toxoids. The results indicated that a certain correlation can be found between the anti-HR1 titer and the amount of venom tolerated.

6. Comparison of Antihemorrhagic, Antinecrotic, and Antilethal Effect of APF, CRF, MiF, and DHTA Toxoids

Guinea pigs were injected subcutaneously with two doses of 1 mg and 0.25 mg of the above toxoids at intervals of 4 weeks. Antihemorrhagic titers of both HR1 and HR2 sera from guinea pigs immunized with APF or DHTA toxoid were lower than those of CRF or MiF toxoid. However, the results of challenges by crude venom to the guinea pigs immunized with each kind of toxoid suggested that both APF and CRF toxoids were more effective in prolonging survival time of guinea pigs which were challenged with 3 mg of the venom. The results also indicated that the necrosis or softening effect of the crude venom on the muscle tissues in guinea pigs immunized with APF or CRF toxoid was prevented, whereas necrosis or softening of the muscle tissues was observed in the guinea pigs immunized by MiF toxoid, although hemorrhagic lesion due to the venom was markedly prevented by MiF toxoid. Those results suggested that the factors which induce hemorrhage, necrosis, and lethal effects are different from each other (SAWAI et al., 1972).

II. Toxoids from Venoms of Other Trimeresurus Species

SAWAI and KAWAMURA (1969) reported that the antigenicity of the venoms of *Trimeresurus mucrosquamatus*, *T. stejnegeri*, and *T. elegans* detoxified by the same amount of DHTA seemed to be similar. The sera of rabbits immunized with one of the three venoms showed cross-protection from the local effects of the other two. Polyvalent DHTA toxoid prepared from venoms of *T. mucrosquamatus*, *T. stejnegeri*, and *Agkistrodon acutus* which are commonly found in Taiwan was a good antigen for protection against the local effects of each venom. The neutralizing antivenin level in the circulating blood increased with repeated immunization. These venoms treated with DHTA produced no toxic signs when injected. HOKAMA (1972) reported

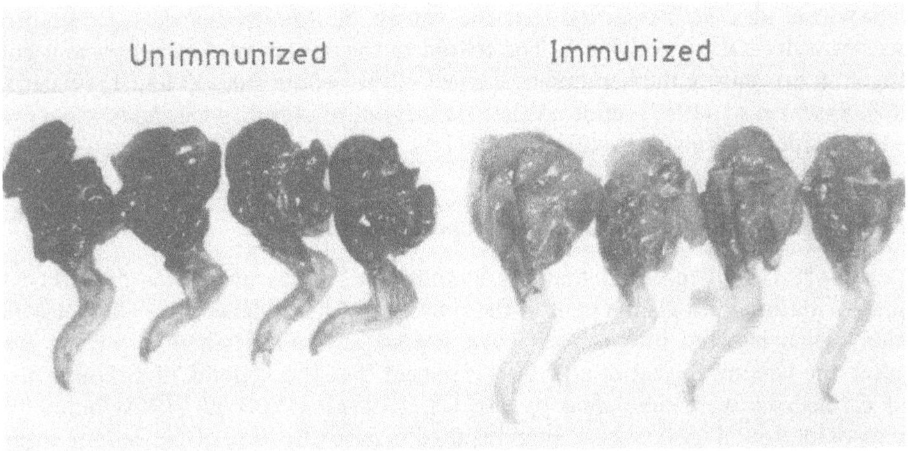

Fig. 1. Protection against local hemorrhage and necrosis. Appearance 24 h after challenge with 1 mg of habu venom injected i.m. into the thighs of four guinea pigs (right) which had been immunized with APF toxoid. Severe hemorrhage and necrosis were seen in the control group (left) which had not received the toxoid

that Sakishima-habu (*Trimeresurus elegans*) venom was detoxified by DHTA. The DHTA, CRF, and APF toxoids were good antigens and some cross-neutralization or cross-protection was observed between the habu venoms. LIN (1972) reported that the antigenicity of APF toxoid from *T. mucrosquamatus* venom was excellent as compared with the CRF or DHTA toxoids. The results of the cross-neutralization test suggested that the venoms of *T. mucrosquamatus*, *T. elegans*, and *T. flavoviridis* are immunologically closely related.

III. Toxoids from Venoms of Agkistrodon Species

SHIMIZU (1967) reported that the venom of mamushi (*Agkistrodon halys blomhoffii*) was detoxified by DHTA. Mice and rabbits were immunized with the toxoid. Four weeks after the first injection, followed by three booster shots. 0.1 ml of the sera of immunized rabbits neutralized 4–16 mhds following intramuscular injection in mice. Local lesions in immunized rabbits which were challenged with the venom were much less as compared with nonimmunized animals. OKUMA et al. (1972) reported that the hemorrhagic activity of mamushi venom was lost by mixing with 0.1 N HCl at pH 2.7; the lethal activity of the venom was lost by treatment with 0.5% formalin. Mice were injected with 0.3 mg toxoid followed by two doses of 0.1 mg at intervals of 1 week. The antisera (0.1 ml) neutralized 25 mcg of the i.m. injected venom in mice. Guinea pigs immunized with the toxoid tolerated 2 mg of the venom when injected intramuscularly.

KOCHOLATY (1966) reported that photo-oxidation of *Agkistrodon piscivorus* venom by visible light in the presence of methylene blue resulted in the detoxification of the venom. FLOWERS (1966) reported that a group of rabbits immunized with venom of *A. piscivorus* pretreated by X-rays suffered no mortality or sloughing of tissues, and local reactions around the site of injection were less severe.

SAWAI et al. (1967) reported that the venom of *Agkistrodon acutus* (Hundred-Pacer) was detoxified by DHTA. The toxoid of the venom of *A. acutus* was a good antigen in preventing the hemorrhagic effect of the venom (SAWAI and KAWAMURA, 1969). SAWAI et al. (1967) reported that the venom of *Agkistrodon rhodostoma* (Malayan pit viper) was also detoxified by DHTA.

IV. Toxoids from Venoms of Other Viperidae Snakes

KOCHOLATY (1966) reported that the venom of *Crotalus atrox* was detoxified by photo-oxidation with visible light in the presence of methylene blue. The detoxified venom when injected into rabbits gave rise to antibodies which protected mice against the venom. SAWAI et al. (1967) reported that the venoms of *Crotalus atrox* and *C. durissus* were detoxified by DHTA. KOCHOLATY et al. (1968) noted that photo-oxidation of *C. durissus* venom resulted in detoxification of the venom. Immunization of rabbits with the toxoid of the venom plus the γ-globulin isolated from the immunized animals gave a very high degree of protection.

KOCHOLATY (1966) reported that immunization of rabbits with venom of *Vipera russellii* detoxified by photo-oxidation resulted in the production of antibodies which protected mice against the venom. SAWAI et al. (1967) reported that the venom of *V. russellii*, *V. xanthina*, *V. ammodytes*, *Bitis arietans*, and *B. nasicornis* were deteoxified by DHTA.

V. Toxoid from Venoms of Elapidae Snakes

1. Toxoid from the Venom of Naja naja atra (Taiwan Cobra)

a) Preparation of the Toxoid

A 1% solution of the crude venom or purified venom fractions (ammonium sulphate fractionation, 0.6–0.9 saturation) was added to 1% formalin (pH 6.5) and 0.05 M L-lysine or L-arginine at 37° C for 3 weeks. The speed of detoxification increased with increasing pH and concentration of formalin. These amino acids were effective in suppressing the heavy precipitate induced during the process of detoxification of the venom by formalin alone, although no precipitations occurred in a solution of cobrotoxin, a purified neurotoxic component from Taiwan cobra venom (YANG, 1965).

After detoxification, excess formalin was removed by dialysis, and the amount of protein was adjusted to 2 mg/ml for the crude or purified toxoid and 4 mg/ml for alum-precipitated toxoid. The latter was adsorbed with the same amount of aluminum phosphate gel and the pH of the mixture was adjusted to 6.5.

A detoxification test was conducted by intraperitoneal injection of 0.2 ml of the toxoid into five mice, and it was confirmed that the mice survived without any paralytic symptoms.

b) Immunogenicity of the Toxoid

α) Antilethal Antivenin

1 ml of the crude or purified toxoid, each containing 2 mg of the venom, was injected subcutaneously into rabbits in four doses at 3-week intervals. The antilethal

effects of sera taken from rabbits immunized with crude venom toxoid indicated that 0.4 ml of the sera neutralized 13–35 mcg (five minimum lethal doses) of the venom. On the other hand, the same amount of sera of rabbits immunized with purified and alum-precipitated toxoid neutralized 25–50 mcg of the venom

β) Protection Against Lethal Effects of the Venom

Most of the rabbits immunized as above which were challenged with the venom in varying amounts ranging from 1.8 to 14 mg survived, whereas all the control rabbits which were injected with 1.3 mg of the venom died within 6 h.

γ) Antinecrotic Effect

Antivenin from immunized rabbits which neutralized the lethal effect of 25–50 mcg of the venom did not inhibit the necrotic effect of 50 mcg (1 minimum necrotic dose, mnd) induced at the site of injection. The immunized rabbits were also not protected from local necrosis due to 50 mcg of the venom injected intracutaneously. Thus, the antilethal antibody could not neutralize the local necrotic effect of the venom (FUKUYAMA and SAWAI, 1974).

c) Relationship Between Antilethal Antibody in the Blood of Immunized Rabbits and Resistance to Challenge with the Venom

From the results of the antigenicity test above, it is suggested that when 1 ml of antivenin of the rabbit immunized with the toxoid neutralizes 5–10 LD_{50} of the venom, the rabbit will resist intramuscular injection of 4–8 mg (2–4 mlds) of the venom. As summarized in Figure 2, a certain correlation can be found between the antilethal antibody and the amount of venom tolerated.

d) Reversion of Toxicity of the Toxoid

It has been reported that diphtheria and tetanus toxoids detoxified by formalin gradually became toxic after storage at room temperature or 37° C (LINGGOOD et al., 1963; AKAMA et al., 1971).

FUKUYAMA and SAWAI (1975) reported that cobra venom toxoid (0.6 mg protein) kept at 37° C for 20 days killed mice by intraperitoneal injection, whereas the toxoid kept at 4° C or freeze-dried toxoid kept at 37° C remained nontoxic. The toxicity of the toxoid became detectable on the 4th day after incubation at 37° C and showed 4 LD_{50} per ml, with 7.1 LD_{50} being observed on the 11th day.

The toxic effect of the reversed toxoid was neutralized by cobra antivenin. The reversal of toxoid into active toxin was not inhibited by the addition of amino acids such as lysine, arginine, sodium glutamate, alanine, cysteine, and glycine during the process of detoxification, whereas addition of 0.16% formalin did inhibit the reversal.

2. Toxoid from the Venom of Bungarus multicinctus

The venom was detoxified by mixing with an equal amount of DHTA at 37° C for 1 h. The toxoid was injected subcutaneously into mice in a quantity of 0.05 mg in 0.1 ml. Three weeks after the injection, 0.05, 0.1, 0.1, and 0.2 mg amounts of the

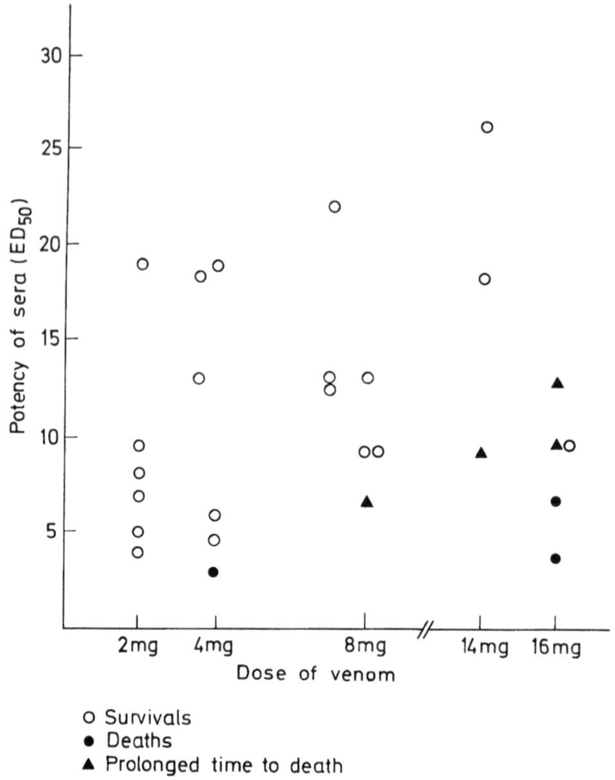

Fig. 2. Relationships between antilethal antibody in serum of rabbits and antilethal effect to challenge with cobra venom

toxoid were given at weekly intervals. One week after the third and last booster, mice were challenged intramuscularly with varying doses of the venom ranging from 2.3 to 75 mcg. The immunized mice were protected from a challenge of 9.3 mcg of venom, whereas untreated mice died at a dose of 4.6 mcg (1 mld). The LD_{50} of the venom against both immunized and nonimmunized mice was 13.5 mcg and 2.7 mcg, respectively (SAWAI et al., 1967, 1969).

3. Toxoid from the Venom of Notechis scutatus

1% of venom solution was added to 6% concentrated hydrochloric acid and the precipitate was removed. The supernatant was dialyzed with distilled water and freeze-dried. Toxoid was prepared by incubating the venom solution, mixed with 0.1% formalin, at 37° C for 13 days. The pH of the solution was increased from 6 to 7.8 by the addition of sodium carbonate in order to hasten the detoxifying process. After a further period of 6 days, the toxicity of the venom was 1/60 of the original value. The toxoid was Seitz-filtered and tested for sterility (WIENER, 1960).

C. Active Immunization

I. Habu Toxoids

1. DHTA Toxoid

a) Dosage and Interval of Injection of the Toxoid

Freeze-dried DHTA toxoid was easily dissolved in distilled water containing 0.25% phenol. For each subcutaneous injection, 0.5 ml of the toxoid containing 2.5 mg of the venom and the same amount of DHTA was used. The same dose was repeated 3 or 4 weeks later (SAWAI et al., 1969b).

b) Reactions

Inquiry cards (2044, 71%) were collected from the participants of the toxoid inoculation. Side reactions after the first shots were as follows: 46 (2%) persons complained of pain which interfered with their work, but 1881 (92%) were able to work without any hindrance, 1594 (78%) persons complained of pain on pressure at the site of injection, and 1413 (69%) persons complained of swelling at the site of injection. The pain persisted for about 7 days and the swelling for 3 days. The degree of side reactions after the second injection was almost the same as that after the first. Generalized symptoms such as itching, lymphadenopathy, fever, headache, arthralgia, and urticaria occurred in a few persons.

c) The Antivenin Level of Circulating Blood

Blood of immunized persons was taken 1 week after the second injection. One-tenth ml of the sera neutralized 1–16 mhds of the venom injected intramuscularly into mice. The booster effect of the toxoid was confirmed in four out of seven persons who received the toxoid 5 months or 1 year before and were reinjected intradermally with 0.1 ml of the toxoid. Antibody level of these four persons rose simultaneously.

d) Clinical Analysis of the Habu Bites After the Immunization

Volunteers (43446) in the Amami and Okinawa Islands received habu toxoid during the period from April, 1965 to December, 1967. Clinical records of 168 patients who had previously received habu toxoid (one or more injections) indicated that of five individuals who suffered from necrosis, three showed deformity or slight motor disturbances. It was found that the lesion which occurred in one of the three was induced by intensive tourniquet pressure which was applied after the bite. On the other hand, of 1542 victims who had not participated in the immunization program, 115 suffered from severe necrosis, out of which 76 had motor disturbances after recovery of the wounds. The rate of occurrence of necrosis was 2.9% in the immunized group, while it was 7.4% in the nonimmunized group. The difference was significant as proved by the chi square test. Two persons who had received the shots previously died, while 19 who did not receive the toxoid died from bites. There was apparently no significant difference in the death rate between the two groups.

e) Hypersensitivity Acquired After Injection of the Toxoid

Seven persons who received DHTA toxoid for one to five times, 5 months to 2 years before were injected with 0.1 ml of the toxoid intradermally in the forearm. An immediate wheal with a pseudopodium and erythema accompanied by oppressive pain occurred at the site of injection in six persons. The reaction in one person who received the toxoid before and two persons who had not received the toxoid was negative. The positive reaction was apparent within 24–48 h and disappeared within a few days (SAWAI, 1969b).

2. APF and MiF Toxoids

a) Dosage and Intervals

Human volunteers were divided into four groups. Each group received three injections of either 0.5 ml or 0.1 ml of APF (1 mg protein per ml) and MiF (0.5 mg) at intervals of 4 weeks and 6 months. Antitoxins in sera from immunized persons, anti-HR1, and anti-HR2 were titrated by the same method described previously (KONDO et al., 1971a). The results indicated that the average antihemorrhagic titers were almost the same with both toxoids (FUKUSHIMA, 1976). It was also reported that most volunteers who received three injections of 0.5 ml of MiF toxoid (0.5 mg/ml protein) at intervals of 5 weeks between the first and the second, and 10 months between the second and the third injections, attained anti-HR1 titers of 1 u or higher after the third injection. Since it is indicated that the administration of 6000 u of habu antivenin is quite effective for the treatment of the bites, it can be stated that any person having a circulating antitoxin titer of about 1.3 u/ml should be protected against the bite (KONDO et al., 1976).

b) Reactions

The main reactions were pain and swelling appearing at the loci of injection. It was also found that the reactions which occurred in the persons who received 0.1 ml of the toxoid were less severe than in those having received 0.5 ml.

II. Tiger Snake Venom and Toxoid

1. Dosage and Intervals

Both purified venom and toxoid were used for inoculation. The course of immunization extended over 13 months during which time 34 injections were given. The initial dose of venom was 0.002 mg and this was gradually increased until 25 mg was administered at the final injection. On four occasions the toxoid was injected in amount of 6, 12, 24, and 36 mg instead of the venom. Usually, injections were given subcutaneously but intracutaneous and intramuscular routes were each used on two occasions. At the begining, injections were given at intervals of approximately 1 week, but thereafter, intervals of up to 4 months elapsed between injections.

2. Level of Circulating Antivenin

The antivenin titer of the sera gradually rose during the first few months of immunizations. By the end of the 4th month, the titer was 5.1 u/ml (1 week after 13th injection of 6 mg of venom). Thus, 1 ml of the serum neutralized 0.05 mg (33 LD_{50}) of the venom following intraperitoneal injection in mice. Further injections of increasing amounts did not result in any appreciable increase in the titer above 5 u.

3. Reactions

After the fifth injection, swelling occurred at the site of injection. Local muscle stiffness, pain, and muscle pain occurred on three occasions and lasted for 24 h. On two occasions (seventh and eighth injections) when the venom was injected intradermally, an immediate wheal with a pseudopodium and erythema resulted, followed by tenderness of the axillar lymph gland (WIENER, 1960).

III. Indian Cobra (Naja naja) Venom

1. Dosage and Intervals

The venom solutions were passed through a millipore filter and then added to an equal volume of 4% sodium alginate adjuvant. A 30-year-old man was given 17 injections over a period of 5 months. The initial dose of the venom was 0.05 mg, and this was gradually increased until 10 mg at the final injection. Injections were given at intervals of 4–14 days and a 30-day rest was taken between the 14th and 15th injections.

2. Antivenin Titer of Serum

Globulin was separated from the serum by ammonium sulphate fractionation, and the antivenin titers were determined by neutralization of the crude venom in mice. The results indicated that 1 ml of the globulin solution (1 g in 8 ml diluent) neutralized 36 LD_{50} (0.244 mg) of the venom. This titer was maintained thereafter by monthly booster injections of 5 mg venom treated in the same manner.

3. Reactions

Examination of the person during and after the injections indicated the absence of pathologic response to the venom except for local swelling and pain, which persisted for 1–3 days in the area of injection.

4. Effectiveness of the Vaccination

Twenty days following the 30th injection, the man was bitten on the left index finger by a 5-foot Indian cobra. The snake remained attached to the finger for a full 3 sec. There were two fang marks over the dorsum of the proximal phalanx with area of hematoma around each. Because of his previous immunization to cobra venom, it was decided not to give antivenin. He developed edema to the elbow within 4 h and to the shoulder within 12 h after the bite, but there were no generalized symptoms. After 48 h, necrosis appeared at the locus of bite. The swelling subsided within 48 h. From the severe local lesions of the patient, it is suggested that a large amount of venom must have been injected into the victim, because one minimum necrotic dose of the Indian cobra venom was 50 mcg in rabbit. Moreover, it is believed that had the patient not been previously immunized, only massive doses of specific antivenin administered immediately after the bite could have saved his life (FLOWERS, 1965).

D. Antigenic Quality of the Prophylactic Toxoid

1. Immunogenicity of the Toxoid

Prophylactic toxoid of snake venom is in principle similar to snake antivenin for medical treatment. Circulating antivenin produced by the active immunization neutralizes the venom introduced into the victims and prevents the development of tissue damage. It is also clear that various toxic factors in snake venom are involved in the pathologic lesions appearing after envenomation. However, very few factors responsible for lesions have been separated from snake venom. For example, cobrotoxin, responsible for the neurotoxic symptoms in cobra bite, has been separated from the venom of *Naja naja atra* (YANG, 1965). The antibody for cobrotoxin could neutralize the neurotoxic effect of the venom. However, cobrotoxin failed to produce local lesions such as swelling or cellulitis induced by the crude venom at the locus of injection (FUKUYAMA, 1973). It has been suggested that cardiotoxin separated from the venom may be responsible for the local lesion (LAI et al., 1972). Since the antibody against crude venom failed to neutralize the local effect of the venom, although it neutralized the neurotoxic effect, studies on toxoids effective in suppressing local lesion due to venom should be carried out.

HR1 and HR2 were separated from habu venom as the main lethal and hemorrhagic principles. However, they could not induce necrotic effects which are observed with the crude venom. It is also reported that the crude habu venom has another lethal effect which cannot be neutralized by anti-HR1 antitoxin. Thus, anti-HR1 and anti-HR2 antitoxins which neutralize the hemorrhagic effect of the venom were not as effective in preventing necrosis or the lethal effect of the venom as the antivenin produced against crude venom, even though the antihemorrhagic titers of the latter are lower than those produced against HR1 and HR2 (SAWAI et al., 1972; YAMAKAWA et al., 1975).

2. Detoxification and Immunogenicity of Toxoid

In habu toxoid, the immunogenicity of DHTA toxoid for hemorrhagic factors was lower than that of CRF toxoid (SAWAI et al., 1972). Detoxification of *Vipera palestinae* venom was pH-dependent. The hemorrhagin separated from the venom was detoxified over a wide pH range (5.5–9.2), but its antigenicity was preserved only at acidic pH (MOROZ-PERLMUTTER et al., 1963).

Although formalin is considered to be a good detoxifying agent for snake venom, heavy precipitation occurred in crude cobra venom solutions when mixed with formalin. It was found that pretreatment of the venom solution with 0.05 M L-lysine or L-arginine before addition formalin was effective in avoiding the occurrence of a precipitate in which some part of the lethal factor may be incorporated (FUKUYAMA and SAWAI, 1974).

3. Differences in Antigenicity of Toxoid for Various Animal Species

KONDO et al. (1971 b, 1976) reported that the immune responses of various animals to a MiF toxoid are different; the anti-HR1 titer was higher than the anti-HR2 in guinea pigs and rabbits, whereas the relation was the reverse in monkeys and humans. On the other hand, the potencies of anti-HR1 and anti-HR2 for APF toxoid were lower than those for MiF toxoid when tested in guinea pigs, whereas the potencies of both APF and MiF were similar in humans (FUKUSHIMA, 1976).

4. Chemical Modification of Antigen

It was found that the lethality of modified cobrotoxin in which a tryptophan residue was converted into N-formyl-kynurenine, oxidized with 2-hydroxy-5-nitrobenzyl bromide (HNB) and 2-nitrophenyl-sulfenyl chloride (NPS), decreased to 6.2 and 3.1% respectively. The neutralizing capacity of anti-tryptophan-modified cobrotoxin was as good as that of unmodified cobrotoxin (CHANG and YANG, 1973). It is noteworthy that cobrotoxin, the main component of neurotoxins in cobra venom, could be detoxified without any changes in its antigenicity.

E. Concluding Remarks

Although active immunization of animals against snake venom originated with the work of SEWALL in 1887, attempts to prepare vaccines for human use are rather recent. Therefore, methods for preparation and testing of various snake venom toxoids are still incomplete.

For improvement of immunogenicity of a toxoid, it is necessary to purify the toxins or separate the venom factors responsible for clinical symptoms due to the bite. More effective toxoid can probably be obtained by mixing the purified and concentrated venom factors after detoxification. However, very few factors have been purified at present and this leaves only crude or partially purified venom as the practical starting material for the preparation of toxoid.

Side effects due to habu toxoids are mild enough to justify vaccination trials among populations that are at high risk. The DHTA toxoid prepared from habu venom was immunogenic in the early trials and reduced the number of necrotic lesions in the rictims. However, reduction in the death rate could not be demonstrated. Vaccination trials with formalin toxoid prepared from a mixture of HR1 and HR2 are in progress in the Amami Islands.

References

Akama, K., Ito, A., Yamamoto, A., Sadahiro, S.: Reversion of toxicity of tetanus toxoid. Jap. J. med. Sci. Biol. **24**, 181—182 (1971)

Behring, E. von, Kitasato, S.: Über das Zustandekommen der Diphtherie-Immunität und der Tetanus-Immunität bei Tieren. Dtsch. med. Wschr. **16**, 1113—1145 (1890)

Calmette, A.: Propriété du sérum des animaux immunités contre le venin de serpents et thérapeutique de l'envenimation. C. R. Acad. Sci. (Paris) **118**, 720—722 (1894)

Chang, C. C., Yang, C. C.: Immunochemical studies on the tryptophan-modified cobrotoxin. Biochim. biophys. Acta (Amst.) **295**, 595—604 (1973)

Flowers, H. H.: Active immunization of human being against cobra *(Naja naja)* venom. Nature (Lond.) **200**, 1017—1018 (1963)

Flowers, H. H.: Cobra bite following immunization against cobra venom. J. Amer. med. Ass. **193**, 625—626 (1965)

Flowers, H. H.: Effect of X-irradiation on the antigenic character of *Agkistrodon piscivorus* (Cottonmouth moccasin) venom. Toxicon **3**, 301—304 (1966)

Fukushima, H., Minakami, K., Koga, S., Higashi, K., Kawabata, H., Yamashita, S., Katsuki, Y., Sakamoto, M., Murata, R., Kondo, S., Sadahiro, S.: Study on prevension of habu snake (*Trimeresurus flavoviridis*) bite by using habu toxoids. Kagoshima Univ. med. J. **28**, 1005—1024 (1976)

Fukuyama, T., Sawai, Y.: Study on the local necrosis induced by the Taiwan cobra (*Naja naja atra*) venom. Snake **5**, 162—167 (1973)

Fukuyama, T., Sawai, Y.: Study on the immunogenicity of alum toxoid of Taiwan cobra (*Naja naja atra*) venom. Snake **6**, 86—88 (1974)

Fukuyama, T., Sawai, Y.: Study on reversion of toxicity of cobra venom toxoid. Snake **7**, 91—94 (1975)

Glenny, A. T., Hopkins, B. E.: Diphtheria toxoid as an immunizing agent. Brit. J. exp. Path. **4**, 283—288 (1923)

Haast, W. E., Winer, M. L.: Complete and spontaneous recovery from the bite of a blue krait (*Bungarus caeruleus*). Amer. J. trop. Med. Hyg. **4**, 1135—1137 (1955)

Hokama, Z.: Experimental study on the toxoid against the venom of Sakishima-habu (*Trimeresurus elegans*). Snake **4**, 23—33 (1972)

Kocholaty, W.: Detoxification of *Crotalus atrox* venom by photooxidation in the presence of methylene blue. Toxicon **3**, 175—186 (1966)

Kocholaty, W., Ashley, B. D.: Detoxification of Russell's viper (*Vipera russellii*) and water moccasin (*Agkistrodon piscivorus*) venom by photooxidation in the presence of methylene blue. Toxicon **3**, 187—194 (1966)

Kocholaty, W., Goetz, J. C., Ashley, B. D., Billings, T. A., Ledford, E. B.: Immunogenic response of the venoms of Fer-de-Lance, *Bothrops atrox asper*, and La cascabella, *Crotalus durissus durissus*, following photooxidative detoxification. Toxicon **5**, 153—158 (1968)

Kondo, H., Kondo, S., Sadahiro, S., Yamauchi, K., Ohsaka, A., Murata, R.: Standardization of antivenine. I. A method for determination of antilethal potency of habu antivenine. Jap. J. med. Sci. Biol. **18**, 101—110 (1965a)

Kondo, H., Kondo, S., Sadahiro, S., Yamauchi, K., Ohsaka, A., Murata, R.: Standardization of antivenine. II. A method for determination of antihemorrhagic potency of habu antivenine in the presence of two hemorrhagic principles and their antibodies. Jap. J. med. Sci. Biol. **18**, 127—141 (1965b)

Kondo, H., Sadahiro, S., Yamauchi, K., Kondo, S., Murata, R.: Preparation and standardization of toxoid from the venom of *Trimeresurus flavoviridis* (habu). Jap. J. med. Sci. Biol. **24**, 281—294 (1971a)

Kondo, H., Sadahiro, S., Kondo, S., Yamauchi, K., Murata, R.: Immunogenicity of a toxoid of habu (*Trimeresurus flavoviridis*) venom in various animal species including man. Jap. J. med. Sci. Biol. **24**, 365—377 (1971b)

Kondo, S., Sadahiro, S., Murata, R.: Relationship between the amount of habu toxoid injected into the monkey and the resulting antitoxin titer in the circulation. In: Animal, Plant and Microbial Toxins. Vol. II, pp. 431—438. New York: Plenum Press 1976

Lai, M. K., Wen, C. Y., Lee, C. Y.: Local lesions caused by cardiotoxin isolated from Formosan cobra venom. J. Formosan med. Ass. **71**, 328—332 (1972)

Lin, Y.-H.: Study on the Taiwan habu (*Trimeresurus mucrosquamatus*) venom toxoid. Snake **4**, 34—43 (1972)

Linggood, F. V., Stevens, M. F., Fulthorpe, A. J., Woiwod, A. J., Pope, C. G.: The toxoiding of purified diphtheria toxin. Brit. J. Exp. Path. **44**, 177—188 (1963)

Ministry of Health and Welfare: Minimum Requirement for Sterility Test for Biologic Products, pp. 256—268. Tokyo: Welfare Ministry 1965

Moroz-Perlmutter, C., Goldblum, N., de Vries, A.: Preparation of *Vipera palestinae* anti-neurotoxin using carboxymethyl-cellulose-bound neurotoxin as antigen. Nature (Lond.) **200**, 697—698 (1963)

Okonogi, T., Hattori, Z.: Attenuation of habu snake (*Trimeresurus flavoviridis*) venom treated with alcohol and its effect as immunizing antigen. Jap. J. Bact. **23**, 137—144 (1968)

Okuma, S., Fukuda, Y., Kabuto, A., Huruta, M.: Study on antigenicity of toxoided mamushi snake (*Agkistrodon halys blomhoffii*) venom. Snake **4**, 108—113 (1972)

Omori-Satoh, T., Ohsaka, A., Kondo, S., Kondo, H.: A simple and rapid method for separation of two hemorrhagic principles in the venom of *Trimeresurus flavoviridis*. Toxicon **5**, 17—24 (1967)

Ramon, G.: Des anatoxines. C. R. Acad. Sc. (Paris) **178**, 1436—1439 (1924)

Ramon, G.: Sur l'anatoxine diphthérique et sur les anatoxines en général. Ann. Inst. Pasteur Lille **39**, 1—21 (1925)

Reed, L. J., Muench, H.: A simple method of estimating fifty per cent end points. Amer. J. Hyg. **27**, 493—497 (1938)

Sadahiro, S.: Studies on toxoids from the venom of habu (*Trimeresurus flavoviridis*), a crotalid. I. Detoxification of habu venom with formalin. Jap. J. Bact. **26**, 214—221 (1971 a)

Sadahiro, S.: Studies on toxoids from the venom of habu (*Trimeresurus flavoviridis*), a crotalid. II. Immunogenicity of toxoids derived from main toxic principles separated from habu venom. Jap. J. Bact. **26**, 319—324 (1971 b)

Sato, M.: Experimental studies on the active immunization of guinea pigs by heated habu snake venom. Kita-Kanto Igaku **15**, 309—316 (1965)

Sawai, Y., Chinzei, H., Kawamura, Y., Fukuyama, T., Okonogi, T.: Studies on the improvement of habu (*Trimeresurus flavoviridis*) bites. 9. Studies on the immunogenicity of the purified habu venom toxoid by alcohol precipitation. Japan. J. Exp. Med. **42**, 155—164 (1972)

Sawai, Y., Kawamura, Y.: Studies on the toxoids against the venoms of certain Asian snakes. Toxicon **7**, 19—24 (1969)

Sawai, Y., Kawamura, Y., Fukuyama, T., Keegan, H. L.: Studies on the inactivation of snake venom by dihydrothioctic acid. Jap. J. exp. Med. **37**, 121—128 (1967)

Sawai, Y., Kawamura, Y., Fukuyama, T., Okonogi, T.: Studies on the improvement of treatment of habu (*Trimeresurus flavoviridis*) bites. 7. Experimental studies on the habu venom toxoid by dihydrothioctic acid. Jap. J. exp. Med. **39**, 109—117 (1969 a)

Sawai, Y., Kawamura, Y., Fukuyama, T., Okonogi, T., Ebisawa, I.: Studies on the improvement of treatment of habu (*Trimeresurus flavoviridis*) bites. 8. A field trial of prophylactic inoculation of the habu venom toxoid. Jap. J. exp. Med. **39**, 197—203 (1969 b)

Sawai, Y., Kawamura, Y., Makino, M., Fukuyama, T., Shimizu, T., Lin, Y-H., Kuribayashi, H., Ishii, T., Okonogi, T.: Experimental studies on habu venom toxoid. I. Antigenicity of the toxoid. Jap. J. Bact. **21**, 32—41 (1966)

Sawai, Y., Makino, M., Kawamura, Y.: Studies on the antitoxic action of dihydrolipoic acid (dihydrothioctic acid) and tetracycline against habu snake (*Trimeresurus flavoviridis* Hallowell) venom. In: Keegan, H. L., MacFarlane, W. V.: Venomous and Poisonous Animals and Noxious Plants of the Pacific Areas, pp. 327—335. New York: Pergamon Press

Sewall, H.: Experiments on the preventive inoculation of rattlesnake venom. J. Physiol. (Lond.) **8**, 203—210 (1887)

Shimizu, T.: Studies on the mamushi (*Agkistrodon halys*) venom toxoid by dihydrothioctic acid. Jap. J. Bact. **22**, 312—320 (1967)

Someya, S., Murata, R., Sawai, Y., Kondo, H., Ishii, A.: Active immunization of man with toxoid of habu (*Trimeresurus flavoviridis*) venom. Jap. J. med. Sci. Biol. **25**, 47—51 (1972)

Takahashi, T., Ohsaka, A.: Purification and some properties of two hemorrhagic principles (HR2a and HR2b) in the venom of *Trimeresurus flavoviridis*; complete separation of the principles from proteolytic activity. Biochim. biophys. Acta (Amst.) **207**, 65—75 (1970)

Wiener, S.: Active immunization of man against venom of Australian tiger-snake (*Notechis scutatus*). Amer. J. trop. Med. Hyg. **9**, 284—292 (1960)

Yamakawa, M., Nozaki, S., Hokama, Z.: Study on habu antivenin. Neutralizing potency of anti-HR1 and anti-HR2 antivenin against crude habu venom. Report on the studies on preparation of anti-Okinawan habu antivenin, No. 2 Okinawa Prefectural Institue of Public Health, Okinawa, Japan, pp. 3—9 (1975)

Yang, C.-C.: Crystallization and properties of cobrotoxin from Formosan cobra venom. J. biol. Chem. **240**, 1616—1618 (1965)

CHAPTER 24

Symptomatology, Pathology and Treatment of the Bites of Elapid Snakes

C. H. CAMPBELL

A venomous snakebite is not always followed by evidence of envenomation and certainly is not always followed by death. Most snakebites are "startled" bites or "defensive" bites as REID (1957) calls them and the snake frequently does not inject venom even though several human lethal doses of venom may be present in the venom glands at the time of the bite (REID, 1957).

A. The Incidence of Envenomation

In a study of 897 cases of venomous snakebites (viper and elapid) in Natal, only 11% were severe and 2.4% were fatal (CHAPMAN, 1968). In Malaya, more than 50% of identified venomous snakebites (viper, elapid, and sea snake) did not give rise to any symptoms of envenomation (REID, 1968). Only three of 11 (27%) patients bitten by American coral snakes developed envenomation and only one (9%) had a serious degree of envenomation and died (PARRISH and KHAN, 1967). At Port Moresby, Papua, in an area where three highly venomous elapid snakes are found, the incidence of envenomation of varying degree after elapid snakebite was 18%. If, however only daytime bites were considered, the incidence of envenomation rose to 32% (CAMPBELL, 1969b). We can quite safely say that 50–60% of patients bitten by elapid snakes will develop no local or systemic effects of envenomation and of the remaining 40–50%, many will develop only local effects or preparalytic symptoms and signs.

B. Snakebite Wound

I. The Wound

It has always been stressed that inspection of the snakebite wound is of great importance in deciding whether a venomous snakebite has occurred; however, the traditional teaching may be misleading (ACTON and KNOWLES, 1915).

Unlike the vipers, the fangs of the elapid snakes are small (SHAW, 1971), e.g., Zaria specimens of the spitting cobra *Naja nigricollis* have fangs of approximately 3 mm in length (WARRELL et al., 1976), while the majority of the important Australian snakes have fangs of 5 mm or less in length (FAIRLEY, 1929b). The fangs of the elapids are of pin thickness. Fang marks from such small structures may not be seen on the skin of the feet and toes of people who go barefooted.

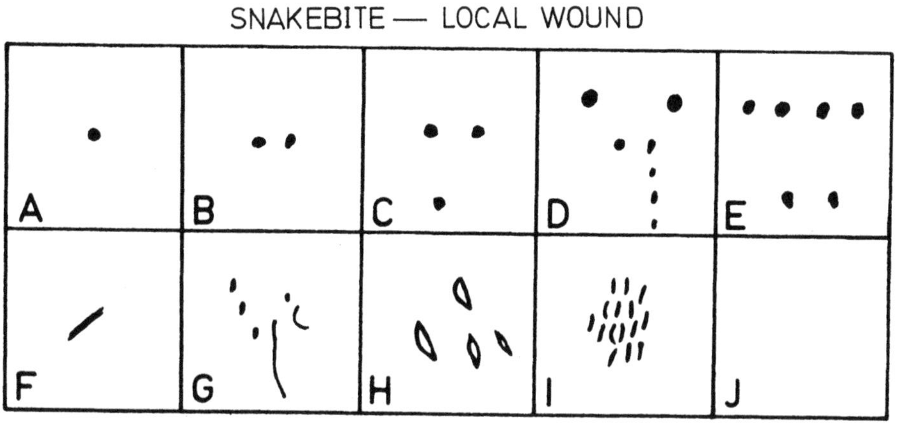

Fig. 1. The variable appearances of the snakebite wound after elapid bite. A—E: puncture wounds; D: palatine teeth marks; E: lower jaw teeth impressions; F: a laceration: G: indefinite marks, scratches; H: four gaping wounds; I: first-aid incisions; J: no wound visible

Fang marks were only found in eight of 14 patients with a proven cobra bite (WARRELL et al., 1976), and FLECKER (1940) found in Northern Queensland that the fang marks were often obliterated by first aid incisions.

Figure 1 is a diagrammatic representation of the different types of local wound found in cases of elapid snakebite observed in the Port Moresby General Hospital (CAMPBELL, 1969b). Over 40% of patients with a proven venomous snakebite had had the wound obliterated by useless first-aid incisions (I). In 10%, despite a careful search of the bitten part, *no snakebite wound could be identified* (J). In only 12% the traditional double puncture mark .. was seen (B). The palatine teeth occasionally marked the skin (D) (see also BENN, 1951), and when the part had been gripped firmly in the snake's jaws, some of the lower jaw teeth impressions (E) were occasionally also seen. These two latter effects produced up to seven puncture wounds. It is not the number of the puncture wounds but their semicircular pattern .·˙·. which indicates that the patient has suffered a nonvenomous snakebite. Repeated bites from a coral snake produced 16–18 puncture wounds (PARRISH and KHAN, 1967). The fangs can also rarely produce a slight scratch (F, G) and even gaping wounds (H). Occasionally, a few millimeter-wide ring of bruising may surround the fang punctures or the teeth marks of nonvenomous snakes.

The study in Port Moresby only confirmed what earlier authorities on Indian snakebite had said; namely, that following a snake bite "any abrasion or scratch however trivial may be dangerous" (FAYRER, 1872). The mark of the teeth are not always a guide because "there may be scarcely a sign on the skin to mark the spot" (WALL, 1883), and "the fine needle-like fangs of the krait may leave no visible mark" (ACTON and KNOWLES, 1915).

Therefore, after inspecting the local wound, one may be able to say quite confidently that an elapid snakebite has occurred, but it is just as likely that one may still be in doubt, because the wounds have been obliterated, because they are "atypical," or because no wound can be seen.

But can one say that envenomation has occurred after an inspection of the bitten area, for we know that after a viper bite the absence of local swelling indicates that envenomation has not occurred?

II. Local Evidence of Envenomation

1. Most Elapids

Pain in the bitten area is an inconstant feature of elapid envenomation probably more often absent than present. Pain may also, of course, be associated with a nonvenomous bite. It is, however, a constant feature of an effective cobra bite, and of the bite of the Australian broad-headed snake *Hoplocephalus bungaroides*.

Local swelling is a constant feature of cobra envenomation but not of Australian elapid, African mamba, Asian krait, or American coral snake envenomation. Usually little or no swelling develops after an Australian elapid bite but occasionally considerable swelling results and would appear to be a constant feature of a mulga snake *Pseudechis australis* bite (CAMPBELL, 1969c; ROWLANDS et al., 1969) and of a broad-headed snakebite where the swelling is sometimes associated with ecchymoses and persists for 6 days (FLECKER, 1952; KREFFT, 1868; ORMSBY, 1947).

Swelling may also occur in a nonenvenomated limb if a tourniquet is used, and thus edema may be present after a nonvenomous snakebite or after a suspected bite. Patients may arrive at the hospital with tourniquets which have been in position for 2–12 h. Considerable swelling may result from this treatment so much so that JUTZY et al. (1953) in Panama were prepared to disregard local swelling as a sign of envenomation.

If a tourniquet has not been used, local swelling indicates that envenomation has probably occurred, but its absence does not indicate that envenomation has not occurred. Particularly is this so, if the patient is seen immediately after, or within an hour or so of, the bite for swelling, if it is going to develop, is not immediately apparent.

An important local sign of envenomation after bites from elapid snakes which have coagulant factors in their venoms (Australian taipan *Oxyuranus scutellatus*, tiger snake *Notechis scutatus*, brown snakes *Pseudonaja* spp., red-bellied black snake *Pseudechis porphyriacus*, rough-scaled snake *Tropidechis carinatus*, spotted black snake *Pseudechis guttatus*) is the fact that the tiny puncture wounds or the incisions continue to bleed or ooze blood for some hours after the bite (CAMPBELL, 1969b; MACDONALD, 1895; SKINNER and MUELLER, 1893).

2. Cobra

While occasionally small areas of necrosis have occurred around the puncture marks after an Australian snakebite (BENN, 1951), REID (1964) drew our attention to the severe local effects of cobra bites, a subject which had been ignored in textbook descriptions of cobra bites but had been recorded in isolated case histories in the Indian literature (GAUDOIN, 1907; HARTY, 1926; HENNESSY, 1918; MACGREGOR, 1906). He, and later WARRELL et al. (1976), further pointed out the infrequency of neurotoxic manifestations after cobra bite, for of 47 identified Malayan cobra bites

(*Naja naja leucodira* or *Naja naja kaouthia*) 20 (43%) developed local necrosis while only 13% developed neurotoxic manifestations and more than half had negligible or no poisoning, while none of 14 envenomated patients bitten by the spitting cobra developed muscle paralyses.

Since REID's paper was published in 1964, papers from Taiwan and Thailand (KUO and WU, 1972; SAWAI et al., 1970, 1972) and from Kenya (DAVIDSON, 1970) Nigeria (WARRELL et al., 1976), and Rhodesia (STROVER, 1973) indicate that local necrosis is not peculiar to cobra bites in India and Malaysia and must now be accepted as the commonest sequela to an effective cobra bite.

Severe local pain, sometimes described as burning in character, is an almost constant feature of an effective cobra bite. The pain commences in the bitten area and frequently radiates up the limb and may last from less than 1 to over 10 days depending on the extent of the local necrosis (REID, 1964).

If venom has been injected, swelling of moderate degree invariably occurs. The swelling commences 2–3 h after the bite and reaches its maximum extent 24–48 h after the bite. A bite on the finger may lead to swelling of the hand and forearm. Limb swelling occasionally spreads to the trunk (WARRELL et al., 1976). The speed of the development and the degree of the swelling is usually less than after viper bites (REID, 1964). Swelling may persist for up to 18 days (WARRELL et al., 1976).

A dusky discoloration around the bite marks, which occasionally ooze serosanguineous fluid (HANNA and LAMB, 1901; AHUJA and SINGH, 1954), extends and darkens until after 3–4 days a greyish black area is present, demarcated by an erythematous margin. Sanguineous blisters may develop. Fluctuation later becomes apparent, and necrosis of skin and subcutaneous tissue is usually evident by the 5th day, the area of skin necrosis may vary from a few cm^2 up to 600 cm^2 (REID, 1964). The extensive skin loss may take several months to heal and may give rise to deformity if inadequately treated (KUO and WU, 1972); chronic relapsing ulceration may also occur and lead to amputation of a limb (WARRELL et al., 1976).

Severe local effects from the bites of unidentified cobras in Africa and Asia have probably been attributed in the past to viper bites (WARRELL et al., 1976).

C. Preparalytic Symptoms and Signs of Envenomation

I. Those Common to Most Elapid Bites

After an inspection of the area bitten by an elapid snake, except in the case of cobra bites, doubt will still exist as to whether venom has been injected or not. The recognition of the preparalytic symptoms and signs of envenomation assumes great importance because, if they are recognized for what they are and antivenene (AV) is given at this stage, it may effectively prevent paralysis developing or may limit its extent. If given after the onset of paralysis, AV will be less effective. They are, however, an inconstant feature of elapid snakebite, frequently absent in cobra and mamba bites and even absent in 10% of patients who subsequently developed paralysis in Papua.

These symptoms may appear within minutes of the bite (FLECKER, 1940, 1944; LE GAC and LEPESME, 1940; TRINCA et al., 1971), even in people who have disregarded the bite as of no consequence (KELLAWAY, 1934; WALLACE, 1954) or may be delayed for some hours. It is important to appreciate just how early after the bite these symptoms can develop for there is a teaching in India that "the universal symptom following snake bite is fright ... The emotional symptoms appear within minutes of the bite whereas symptoms of systemic envenomation rarely appear until half to one hour after the bite" (SETH, 1974). Such a knowledgeable author as REID (1968) lends his support to this Indian error.

1. Vomiting

Vomiting is the commonest of these symptoms, occurring within 5 min of the bite (KNYVETT and MOLPHY, 1959) or not until 12 h or more after the bite. The patient may only vomit once or he may vomit several times. Vomiting was an uncommon symptom after Malayan cobra bite (REID, 1964) but was present in nine of 14 patients bitten by the spitting cobra although its significance was open to question (WARRELL et al., 1976).

2. Headache

Headache may commence within 2 min of the bite (TRINCA et al., 1971). It may only last for $^1/_2$ h or may persist for several hours or even for a day or more (FLECKER, 1952) and may be severe or mild. Although in western communities the importance of this symptom as an indication of envenomation might be questioned, it was rarely reported in patients who thought they had been bitten by snakes or who had been bitten by snakes and developed no signs of envenomation (CAMPBELL, 1969b). The inexperienced in the management of snake envenomation disregards this symptom to the peril of the patient.

3. Loss of Consciousness

This is the least common of these preparalytic symptoms and signs and may also occur within minutes of the bite (ECCLES, 1875; FITZSIMONS, 1962; FLECKER, 1940, 1944; LESTER, 1957; TRINCA et al., 1971) or be delayed for several hours. The period of unconsciousness may last for some minutes (WIENER, 1960) or as long as 12 h (KELLAWAY, 1934). A lack of appreciation of the importance of this symptom as a sign of elapid envenomation probably gave rise to the fear-shock heresy of the Indian snakebite literature which maintained that coma was not a sign of elapid envenomation (RICHARDS, 1885; WALL, 1913) and that syncope was due to fear and could even cause death (WALL, 1913).

A study of Indian literature indicates that syncope is a well-documented symptom of venomous snakebite (BRETON, 1825; ROBSON, 1835; TRESTRAIL, 1855) and of proven elapid (cobra, krait) bite (AHUJA and SINGH, 1954; BEVERIDGE, 1899; BOSE, 1910; BUTTER, 1825; CALMETTE, 1908; GAUDOIN, 1907; SMITH, 1836; WEATHERLY, 1894; WILSON, 1829). The only doubt which exists about this important symptom and sign of envenomation is whether it is always secondary to vasomotor symptoms, i.e., a concomitant of primary venom shock or hypotension or whether it can also occur as a primary effect of the venom in the absence of hypotension (CAMPBELL, 1975).

In this preparalytic comatose state, convulsions may occur (FLECKER, 1940, 1944; PAIN, 1892; SMYTH, 1893; TRESTRAIL, 1855). Respiration may fail and artificial respiration may be required (FORBES, 1891; GARDE, 1890). Yet, despite the severity of these symptoms, the patient although previously "moribund" (REID and FLECKER, 1950) or "dead to all intents and purposes" (EASTON, 1894) recovers and may not even develop a minimal degree of muscle paralysis (EASTON, 1894; FORBES, 1891; GARDE, 1890). During this hypotensive unconscious state, a cerebrovascular accident may occur and result in hemiplegia (CAMPBELL, 1975)

4. Vasomotor Signs (Pallor, Sweating, Weak to Absent Pulse, Hypotension)

A study of the early Australian literature leaves little doubt as to the frequency of the occurrence of these symptoms (Australian Medical Journal, 1875). Patients have been described as being: "ashy pale, cold and sweating profusely" (CONNOR and KELLAWAY, 1934) and comatose, "almost pulseless, and bathed in a cold sweat" (KINGSBURY, 1891). Such symptoms have also been reported after cobra bite (BEVERIDGE, 1899; CALMETTE, 1908; DRAKE-BROCKMAN, 1893; SMITH, 1836), ringhals cobra bite (FITZSIMONS, 1962), and mamba bite (CHAPMAN, 1968; GRAY, 1962).

5. Abdominal Pain

Abdominal pain which may be very severe, variable in its location, persist for hours, and be associated with abdominal tenderness and guarding, occurred in 18/68 (26%) of envenomated patients in Papua. It has also been reported after krait bite (D'ABREU, 1939; HAAST and WINER, 1955; PONNAMBALAM, 1939) and mamba bite (GRAY, 1962).

II. Other Preparalytic Symptoms and Signs

The Australian elapid venoms not only contain potent neurotoxins but some contain potent coagulant factors and potent hemolysins, and one venom at least contains a myotoxin (HARRIS et al., 1973). The presence of these toxic components is associated with symptoms and signs which are perhaps more commonly associated with viper envenomation and which do not usually occur after elapid bites in other countries.

1. Pain in Regional Lymph Nodes — Tenderness and Enlargement

One of the earliest symptoms and the earliest objective sign of envenomation in Papua was the complaint of discomfort or pain in the regional lymph nodes. At times, the pain was quite severe and persisted for over 24 h. The regional lymph nodes should always be palpated because tenderness, even in the absence of pain, was present in 60% of envenomated patients (CAMPBELL, 1969b). This sign does not occur in Asian cobra envenomation (HANNA and LAMB, 1901; REID, 1964) but has been recorded after spitting cobra bites (WARRELL et al., 1976) and krait bite (HAAST and WINER, 1955).

2. Spitting, Vomiting, Coughing of Blood

The spitting of blood or the vomiting of blood occurred in 15% of envenomated patients in Papua. Inspection of the mouth may show that blood is oozing from around the teeth. Rectal bleeding (CHAMPNESS, 1966; FAIRLEY, 1929a) and melena (MUELLER, 1893) have also been described. Some of these symptoms may follow a spitting cobra bite (WARRELL et al., 1976).

3. The Passing of Blood-stained Urine

This very dramatic symptom and sign is usually due to hemoglobinuria, a frequent occurrence after envenomation from *Pseudechis* venoms and may be seen after Australian copperhead *Austrelaps superba* bites (HALL, 1859) and has occurred after rough-scaled snakebites (TRINCA et al., 1971).

Less commonly, bloody urine may be due to frank hematuria; but hematuria, if it occurs after Australian elapid envenomation, is more commonly microscopic. A recent case report indicates that "bloody" urine may also be due to myoglobinuria (HOOD and JOHNSON, 1975).

4. Other Nervous System Symptoms

In addition to these common preparalytic symptoms and signs, there are a variety of symptoms and signs which are described by the more articulate patients. Paraesthesiae affecting the bitten limb, mouth, or other parts of the body have been noted after Australian snakebite (CONNOR and KELLAWAY, 1934; WALLACE, 1954) and krait bite (HAAST and WINER, 1955). Loss of the sense of taste and smell have been noted to occur after Australian taipan bites (FLECKER, 1940; REID and FLECKER, 1950), Australian red-bellied black snake bite, and krait bite (PONNAMBALAM, 1939).

Vertigo suggestive of involvement of the vestibular nerve occurred after a red-bellied black snakebite and persisted for some weeks (CAMPBELL, 1975). Hyperacusis has also been reported (HAAST and WINER, 1955) and convulsions have been the first manifestation of a fatal snakebite (FLECKER, 1944).

Partial or complete loss of vision has been recorded after elapid bite in Australia (EASTON, 1894; TRINCA et al., 1971; WALLACE, 1954; WIENER, 1960; WORRELL, 1963), in India (ALANDIKAR, 1920; WALL, 1914; CROLEY, 1922; GAUDOIN, 1907), and in Africa (CHRISTENSEN, 1955; FITZSIMONS, 1962). Uncertainty exists as to whether this symptom is associated with hypotension or whether it, like unconsciousness, is due to a direct effect of the venom or a venom-induced mediator on nervous tissue. Partial loss of vision has been noted to disappear after the injection of AV (WALLACE, 1954).

5. Drowsiness

Some authorities (REID, 1964) regard drowsiness as one of the cardinal symptoms of elapid envenomation, particularly cobra envenomation. It is a commonly recorded symptom in the early Australian and Indian snakebite literature. Because of its imprecise nature of its own, it would be uncertain evidence of envenomation, and I think it is best not regarded as a cardinal symptom, a view which is shared by WARRELL et al. (1976).

6. Allergic Reaction Following Snakebite

An attack of asthma was the first effect of a tiger snakebite in a snake handler (CONNOR and KELLAWAY, 1934), and urticaria occurred 2 days after a cobra bite in a patient not given antivenene (REID, 1964).

7. Cobra Venom Conjunctivitis

If spitting cobra venom gains access to the eyes, intense pain, congestion, and profuse watering of the eyes may follow. Recovery takes 2–3 days (SINHA, 1972).

D. Clinical Signs of Elapid Envenomation

I. Muscle Paralysis

1. Clinical Picture

Other symptoms are associated with the development of muscle paralysis: difficulty in seeing or double vision, difficulty in opening the mouth, difficulty in swallowing, difficulty in speaking and difficulty in breathing. Occasionally, the first symptom relating to the onset of paralysis has been an inability to get out of bed on the morning after the bite (CAMPBELL, 1969b).

In most elapid bites, there is a latent period from the time of the first indication that absorption of venom has occurred until the time of onset of the paralysis. In the case of mamba and cobra bites, the latent period can be very short, but after krait bite, coral snake bite, and Australian snake bites it can be long. In Port Moresby, paralysis developed 45 min to 9 h after the first symptom of envenomation. On the average, paralysis developed $5^1/_2$ h after the bite, a range of 1–10 h (CAMPBELL, 1969b).

The susceptibility of various muscles to the neurotoxins varies considerably. The extrinsic eye muscles and elevators of the eyelids are the most susceptible; the superficial facial muscles and the diaphragm are the most resistant.

The muscle paralysis is described as if muscle groups were involved one after the other, but several muscle groups are usually involved together; and once swallowing is impaired and respiratory obstruction develops, a "crescendo-like" effect occurs with rapidly progressive paralysis of the muscles of the cranial nerves and cessation of breathing, often before significant limb paralysis is present.

The muscles supplied by the cranial nerves are always affected first and usually the first sign of neurotoxicity is the development of a slight degree of ptosis with or without some impairment of eye movements in a vertical or lateral direction. With small doses of venom, these eye signs may be the only evidence of muscle paralysis (CAMPBELL, 1969b; REID, 1964).

With larger doses of venom, a complete ptosis eventually develops, exposing a small strip of cornea (Fig. 2). A complete external ophthalmoplegia is present, and the eyes become fixed in a central position. The pupils react to light until terminal anoxia develops.

Before the eye signs have progressed very far, there is usually involvement of the muscles—of mastication, of swallowing, and of the tongue. Occasionally, these mus-

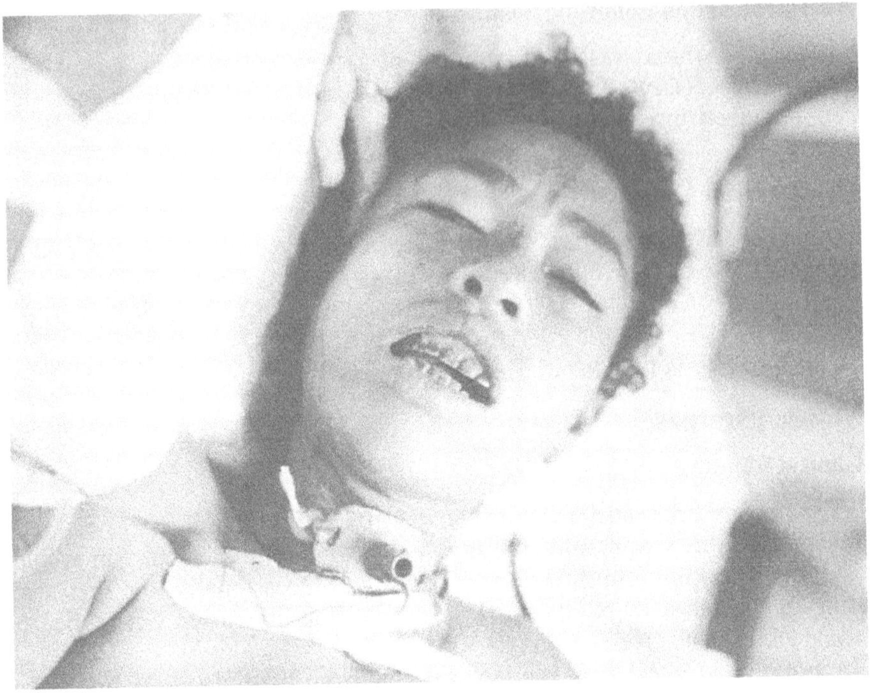

Fig. 2. A Papuan patient 24 h after an elapid bite. Complete ptosis is present. The jaws cannot be separated and there is but slight movement of the facial muscles. A cuffed tracheostomy tube has been inserted

cles develop paralysis before the eye muscles. The patient cannot open his mouth as well as normally, a nasal voice develops, fluids may regurgitate into the nose, and the tongue cannot be protruded much beyond the teeth.

While the bulbar muscles are being involved, some weakness of the intercostal muscles and limb muscles develops. There is at first a generalized limb muscle weakness with preservation of the deep reflexes. Eventually, a complete flaccid quadriplegia develops with loss of the deep reflexes.

There is a progressive reduction in the power to open the mouth with the development of trismus in Australian snakebite, while in cobra and mamba envenomation the lower jaw hangs down. The tongue eventually lies immobile on the floor of the mouth. Secretions, which accumulate in the pharynx and drool from the corner of the mouth, and the paralyzed tongue lead to respiratory obstruction. The patient becomes cyanosed, weakened respiratory muscles fail, consciousnees is lost, convulsions may occur, and eventually the heart stops beating (CAMPBELL, 1964, 1969b; CAMPBELL and YOUNG, 1961; NIGAM et al., 1973).

If, however, respiratory obstruction is relieved by intubation with a cuffed endotracheal tube and, if necessary, respiration is assisted by intermittent positive pressure respiration (IPPR), it may be found that, although the chest muscles are paralyzed completely, the diaphragm is still moving, and it may be able to sustain respiratory exchange unaided or it may become progressively weaker to eventually cease moving some hours after the onset of respiratory obstruction. After Australian elapid bite, the paralysis has continued to extend for up to 61 h after the bite and for 29 h after the administration of antivenene (CAMPBELL, 1969b).

With respiratory support, the most severely paralyzed patients lie immobile but conscious, unable to move except for a slight movement of fingers, toes, corner of mouth, and an ineffectual shrug of the pelvis.

Cutaneous sensation is intact except for some loss in the immediate vicinity of the bite. Bladder and bowel functions are normal. The pregnant uterus is not affected. Cerebrospinal fluid has a normal cell count and no increase in protein content.

If the time at which a tracheostomy was performed gives a rough idea of the death time (time from bite to death), tracheostomy was performed, on the average, 21 h after the bite (range 3–96 h) in 32 Papuan patients (CAMPBELL, 1969b).

2. Duration of Muscle Paralysis

In 29 patients in Port Moresby, all of whom had been given antivenene, the first flicker of eye movement occurred approximately 48 h after the bite (range 35–70 h), and full eye movements were present 69–103 h after the bite. The ability to swallow returned $4^1/_2$ days after the bite, and respiration had to be assisted for an average period of 34 h, range 8–240 h (CAMPBELL, 1969b). The paralysis following cobra bites (antivenene given) lasted 2–3 days (REID, 1964), and following American coral snakebites, respiratory paralysis was said to last "only a few days" (PARRISH and KHAN, 1969).

In general, we may say that following elapid envenomation, the muscle paralysis lasts about 2 days and then recovery occurs over the next 2–5 days.

A longer duration of the paralysis may occur—up to 14 days or more after cobra bite (REID, 1964) and tiger snakebite (FAIRLEY, 1929a). Two patients who were anoxic for a time before intubation was carried out took 1–2 months to recover muscle power (CAMPBELL, 1969b).

Some of the long recovery periods in the Australian literature (FAIRLEY, 1929a; REID, 1894) may be related to the myotoxic action of tiger snake venom.

II. Other Effects of Elapid Envenomation

1. Blood

An elevated white blood cell count due to a neutrophil leukocytosis is an inconstant finding after elapid bite (CAMPBELL, 1969b; REID, 1964; WARRELL et al., 1976). Its presence often relates to the development of necrosis, hemolysis, etc. Absolute neutrophil counts as high as 32000/mm^3 have been recorded after Papuan snakebite (CAMPBELL, 1969b). An elevated erythrocyte sedimentation rate (ESR) is an inconstant phenomenon, and in the presence of a coagulant venom a retarded ESR is to be expected. In 18/21 envenomated patients seen within 12 h of a Papuan snakebite, the ESR was normal (CAMPBELL, 1969b).

Although incoagulable blood due to a defibrination syndrome occurs after the bites of several Australian snakes—tiger snake, eastern brown snake *Pseudonaja textilis*, western brown snake *Pseudonaja nuchalis*, dugite *Pseudonaja affinis*, taipan, rough-scaled snake, red-bellied black snake, and Papuan black snake *Pseudechis papuanus*—clinically it has proved of little importance unless a tracheostomy wound was present. Patients may then ooze blood from wounds and require blood transfusion. But cerebral hemorrhage is a possible complication (FOXTON, 1914), and hematuria and bloody diarrhea seem to be due to this cause (TRINCA, 1969).

The coagulation defect develops early in the course of the envenomation before paralysis is evident (CAMPBELL, 1969b). The bedside coagulation test (REID et al., 1963a) would thus prove useful as a test of envenomation in the case of some Australian elapids. Clinically, the coagulation defect has been analyzed in detail for only one Australian venom (HERRMANN et al., 1972).

Impaired clot retraction after spitting cobra bites was due to a platelet defect and low levels of complement component C3 were also found. The coagulation defect was associated with spontaneous bleeding in 3/14 of patients (WARRELL et al., 1976). No coagulation defect was observed after Malayan cobra bites (REID, 1964). Studies on the blood of coral snake and krait victims have not been reported.

2. Kidney

Proteinuria frequently severe (half to solid on boiling) is a common but inconstant feature of envenomation from some Australian snakes—taipan, tiger snake, rough-scaled snake, Papuan black snake, and probably the red-bellied black snake. Associated with the proteinuria, casts and red blood cells may sometimes be found (CAMPBELL, 1969b). SKINNER (SKINNER and MUELLER, 1893) and later MUELLER (1893) were the first to draw attention to urine findings which had the characteristics of an "acute toxic nephritis" after a tiger snake bite.

Proteinuria was not a feature of death adder envenomation (CAMPBELL, 1966) but was a constant finding in all patients with systemic envenomation due to Malayan cobra bite (REID, 1964), and heavy proteinuria has been recorded after coral snakebite (McCOLLOUGH and GENNARO, 1963). However, in most reported cases of snakebite, no report of urine testing can be found, so the incidence of proteinuria is probably underestimated. Frank hematuria is sometimes present with red cell casts, but microscopic hematuria is more common.

Presumed hemoglobinuria is not uncommonly recorded in the Australian snakebite literature and has followed bites by the red-bellied black snake, mulga snake, Papuan black snake, Papuan taipan, rough-scaled snake, and the copperhead. More recently, myoglobinuria has been reported (FURTADO and LESTER, 1968; HOOD and JOHNSON, 1975), but its delayed onset raises doubts about its relationship to the snakebite. Acute anuria has complicated hemoglobinuria (CAMPBELL, 1967c; KNYVETT and MOLPHY, 1959) and myoglobinuria (HOOD and JOHNSTON, 1975) after Australian snakebite (ROWLANDS et al., 1969).

3. Heart and Blood Pressure

Some venoms contain cardiotoxic factors, and although these may be a factor in causing death, normal electrocardiographs were found in six severely envenomated Papuan patients (CAMPBELL, 1969b). Only one of 17 patients with envenomation due to Malayan cobra bite (REID, 1964) and one of 14 patients bitten by the spitting cobra (WARRELL et al., 1976) had abnormal electrocardiographs.

Blood pressure measurements have not been commonly recorded in the preparalytic phase of envenomation, but if a weak or absent pulse be taken as evidence of hypotension, hypotension (primary hypotension) has been a common occurrence in the preparalytic phase of Australian snakebite. It has also been recorded after Indian cobra (SMITH, 1836; BOSE, 1910), black-necked spitting cobra (STROVER, 1973), ringhals cobra (FITZSIMONS, 1962), and mamba bites (CHAPMAN, 1968; GRAY, 1962).

While untreated, most patients would die from respiratory obstruction and respiratory insufficiency. REID (1964) did not believe that this was always the cause of death after cobra bite as some patients seem to die from pulmonary edema, and one of WARRELL et al., patients (1976) also died from cardiorespiratory failure in the absence of significant paralysis. When life is supported by IPPR, it seems likely that other toxic factors in the venoms like the cardiotoxins of cobra venoms and *Pseudechis* venoms may assume importance. Two badly paralyzed patients in Port Moresby on assisted respiration died of hypotension (secondary hypotension) which was resistant to treatment, and patients with coral snake envenomation may die of cardiovascular failure (RUSSELL et al., 1975).

III. Features of Envenomation from Different Elapid Snakes

1. Cobra

Preparalytic symptoms, apart from the local symptoms of severe pain and swelling, are frequently absent. Headache, vomiting, drowsiness, and loss of consciousness (BOSE, 1910; CALMETTE, 1908; GAUDOIN, 1907; SMITH, 1836) have been reported. Muscle paralysis is not a common sequel to a cobra bite (REID, 1964; WARRELL et al., 1976), but if it occurs, it tends to occur early in the course of envenomation and its progress is frequently rapid. Eye, bulbar, and chest muscles are primarily involved, and limb movement may be present at the time of death. The death time is often quite short (REID, 1964; SAWAI et al., 1972).

2. Krait

There are few reported cases of krait bite (AHUJA and SINGH, 1954; D'ABREU, 1939; GHARPUREY, 1931a, 1932; HAAST and WINER, 1955; KUO and WU, 1972; PEARN, 1971; PONNAMBALAM, 1939; SAWAI et al., 1972; WALL, 1914). Little pain or swelling occurs at the site of the bite. Preparalytic symptoms are common, and there is often a long period before the onset of paralysis. Recovery from severe paralysis must be rare (PEARN, 1971).

3. Mamba

Swelling is slight or absent; local pain is also variable. Mamba bites may be rapidly followed by paralysis and death (CASALE and PATEL, 1974; LEGAC and LEPESME, 1940; GRAY, 1962; KRENGEL and WALTON, 1967; LEFROU, 1951; LOUW, 1967; PHISA-

LIX, 1940; STROVER, 1967). Preparalytic symptoms have been reported in several cases—headache, vomiting, abdominal pain, loss of consciousness, and hypotension.

4. Coral Snake

Coral snakebites resulting in envenomation are uncommon (MCCOLLOUGH and GENNARO, 1963; PARRISH and KHAN, 1967; RAMSEY and KLICKSTEIN, 1962; SHAW, 1971; WILLSON, 1908) local swelling is absent or minimal. Nausea and headache have occurred in the latent phase between bite and onset of paralysis. Symptoms have occurred 1–$7^1/_2$ h after the bite. Paralysis involves eye, bulbar, and limb muscles, and death occurs from respiratory failure but occasionally from cardiovascular collapse (RUSSELL et al., 1975).

E. Pathology

There are few *detailed* published autopsy reports on victims of elapid snake bite (HALL, 1859; ROLLISON, 1928; ROWLANDS et al., 1969).

I. Local Reaction

WALL (1883) stressed the importance of the changes of severe acute inflammation which were to be found in the tissues in the neighbourhood of a cobra bite, changes which KUO and WU (1972) describe as a purulent inflammation and coagulative necrosis. These changes take some time to develop for only edema is found initially (EAKER et al., 1969). At the site of an Australian elapid bite, edema, hemorrhage, or infiltration with polymorphs may sometimes be found (FAIRLEY, 1929a; ROLLISON, 1928; ROWLANDS et al., 1969). Edema with minimal inflammatory reaction has been found after a krait bite (KUO and WU, 1972).

II. Viscera

As a rule, no visceral changes of note are found after elapid bites, but WALL (1883) highlighted the importance of respiratory obstruction by noting that medicines and food were sometimes found in the air passages. The changes found are frequently those associated with asphyxia (HILSON, 1873; FLECKER, 1944); the blood may be fluid (BARKER, 1860; HALL, 1859; ROLLISON, 1928) and generalized congestion of the organs may be present. No visceral abnormality was found after a krait bite (SANT, 1973).

Occasionally, small hemorrhages are sometimes found in the viscera and small subarachnoid hemorrhages have been noted (FOXTON, 1914; SANT, 1973), and a larger subarachnoid hemorrhage has led to death after a spitting cobra bite (WARRELL et al., 1976). Small hemorrhages in the brain stem are thought to have caused death after an Australian eastern brown snake bite (FOXTON, 1914).

Changes of a lower nephron nephrosis were found when renal failure developed in association with hemoglobinuria. Examination of sections of spinal nerves, spinal chord, brain stem, and brain showed no significant changes (KNYVETT and MOLPHY, 1959; ROWLANDS et al., 1969).

III. Lymph Nodes

A lymph node biopsy after a bite from an unidentified Papuan elapid snake showed that the architecture of the lymph node was preserved. There was an accumulation of edema fluid in the peripheral follicles with collections of neutrophils and some histiocytes. The sinuses were dilated and contained an unusual number of neutrophils (CAMPBELL, 1969b). Sinus hyperplasia and degenerative changes in the germinal centers were found at autopsy by ROWLANDS et al. (1969).

IV. Muscles

Massive rhabdomyolysis was found after death from a mulga snake bite (ROWLANDS et al., 1969), and a focal necrotizing myopathy was found on muscle biopsy in a patient admitted in renal failure due to myoglobinuria following tiger snake bite (HOOD and JOHNSON, 1975).

V. Post-Mortem Diagnosis

When the cause of death has been uncertain, radioimmunoassay has detected snake venom in cardiac blood and in the tissues from the bitten area (SUTHERLAND, et al., 1975), and chromatographic analysis of local edema fluid has detected a cobra neurotoxin (EAKER et al., 1969).

F. Treatment of Snakebite

I. First-Aid Treatment

Traditional first-aid measures—ligature, incision, excision, suction—except for ligature, are impractical and of no proven value after elapid bites (RUSSELL, 1967). Even radical measures like amputation (ACTON and KNOWLES, 1914; KNOWLES, 1921) and excision (FAIRLEY, 1929c) may not prevent death after an effective elapid bite.

Ligature may delay the absorption of venom, particularly coagulant venoms, but to be effective it has to obliterate the arterial circulation and should be applied within 30 min of the bite (CHRISTENSEN, 1969; FAIRLEY, 1929c). In practice, most ligatures which have been applied are ineffective.

Complete immobilization of the bitten limb may delay absorption of venoms with large molecular weight toxins but was ineffective in experimental cobra envenomation (BARNES and TRUETA, 1941).

Reassurance (REID, 1970) is the most important first-aid measure, a sound humane measure, based on the firm knowledge of the low incidence of envenomation and of the even lower incidence of death after an elapid bite.

Rest, reassurance, and removal to a hospital are first-aid measures of value. Ligature, if it is used, must be released every 20 min and discarded after 2 h.

If paralysis has commenced, the patient should be watched carefully, and if swallowing is impaired, he should be transported on his side in the "tonsillar position." Assisted respiration with a hand bag and oral airway may be required. Nothing should be given by mouth.

II. Management of a Suspected Venomous Snakebite

In an area where elapid snakes occur, any person who says he has been bitten by a snake should be admitted to hospital *even in the absence of a snakebite wound.* Preventable fatalities will occur if this rule is not followed.

On admission, the history should be taken including specific interrogation about the symptoms of envenomation. Physical examination should include a description of the local wound, examination of the regional lymph nodes for tenderness or enlargement, and examination of the nervous system particularly for ptosis and impaired occular movements. The urine should be examined for protein and blood, and a microscopic examination of the centrifuged deposit should be carried out. Blood should be taken for coagulation studies. Hourly observations should continue for 18 h, and the coagulation studies should be repeated a few hours after admission. Every specimen of urine passed must be examined for protein and blood.

If no symptoms and signs develop, the patient is discharged. If symptoms or signs develop, AV is given—a polyvalent AV or a combination of local monovalent AVs.

III. Definite Elapid Bite—No Evidence of Envenomation

If a person has been bitten by an identified elapid snake but has no symptoms or signs of envenomation when he is admitted to hospital within 6 h of the bite, he should be given specific AV. The risk of dying from the bite is greater than the hazard of anaphylaxis (CAMPBELL, 1963; CHRISTENSEN, 1969). REID (1964, 1968) advocates withholding AV until evidence of systemic envenomation is present. In an institution with a stable staff who are trained to recognize the early symptoms and signs of envenomation and where snakebite is an everyday problem, such a policy might have some theoretical justification, but even in such an institution, this policy can lead to death before AV therapy is started (SAWAI et al., 1972). In a hospital where snakebite is an uncommon problem, it is far safer to give AV immediately if an identified elapid snake has bitten the patient, for the earlier AV is given the more effective it is likely to be (CAMPBELL, 1967b; CHATTERJEE, 1965; CHRISTENSEN, 1955; NIGAM et al., 1973; RUSSELL, 1967; RUSSELL et al., 1975) and the smaller the dose required (CHRISTENSEN, 1969).

After AV is given the patient must still be observed hourly for 24 h.

IV. Antivenene (AV)

The introduction of AV into the therapeutics of snakebite had a sound experimental basis. Because of this, there was initially an uncritical acceptance of the value of AV, in preventing death from snakebite and in counteracting the effects of established envenomation (LAMB, 1904).

The first generally available AV, CALMETTE'S, which had been prepared using a venom mixture containing 80% cobra venom, was claimed to be of value in all forms of snake poisoning but was soon experimentally shown to be ineffective against Australian tiger snake venom (MARTIN, 1897) and the venoms of Indian snakes other than the cobra (LAMB, 1903). In the dosage (10 ml) and by the route (subcutaneous injection) recommended by CALMETTE (1908), CALMETTE'S AV would have been of little value even after a cobra bite, a view which was soon put forward by CARR-WHITE (1902) and LAMB (1904). Notwithstanding this, case histories were published which claimed that CALMETTE'S AV was of value in preventing death from snakebite (BEVERIDGE, 1899; REID, 1901; WORTABET, 1900) including Australian snakebite (BILL, 1902). Indeed, claims for the effectiveness of AV based on the case histories published in CALMETTE'S book (1908) are probably fallacious.

In the individual case, because the dose of venom (if any) is unknown, it is impossible to evaluate whether AV is of value in preventing serious symptoms and signs of envenomation or in preventing death from snakebite. Claims for the effectiveness of AV therapy based on the nonappearance of symptoms and signs of envenomation have to be disregarded (CONNOR and KELLAWAY, 1934; LLOYD, 1932; GHARPUREY, 1931 b; REID, 1901).

The best evaluation of AV therapy would, of course, be obtained by a clinical trial (REID et al., 1963 b), but primarily because of ethical reasons but also because of the small number of identified elapid bites seen in any one institution, a clinical trial of elapid AVs has not been, and probably never will be, carried out.

In the individual patient, AV therapy can only be evaluated by its capacity to shorten the normal duration of the paralysis, the coagulation defect, the hemolytic process, or the normal duration of any other pathological effect of the venom. For most venoms, the normal untreated duration of most of these defects in man is not known.

We can, however, say that the paralysis produced by elapid venoms lasts about 48 h and then slowly reverses over another 2–5 days.

Initially, experience with AV in Port Moresby (CAMPBELL and YOUNG, 1961) induced scepticism as to its value, for after the administration of intravenous AV (a combination of three specific AVs or a polyvalent AV in two to five times the recommended dosages—up to 190 ml of serum), the muscle paralysis did not improve, frequently continued to progress, and even developed after the administration of the AV (even though the paralysis developed after, or progressed after, the injection of AV, AV *may* still have been of considerable value in limiting the extent of the paralysis).

Some years later, two severely paralyzed patients, bitten by death adders *Acanthophis antarcticus*, did recover complete muscle power within 2 h of injecting the AV. The other patients had been bitten by unidentified snakes, probably Papuan black snakes or taipans. The effect of the AV on the muscle paralysis allows the division of the Australian venoms into at least two groups with probably different modes of action of their neurotoxins (CAMPBELL, 1975).

The paralysis induced by the majority of Australian venoms will not respond to AV, and the neurotoxins in these venoms probably have a presynaptic site of action (DATYNER and GAGE, 1973; KAMENSKAYA and THESLEFF, 1974; KARLSSON et al., 1972) while death adder venom was shown to act postsynaptically (MEBS et al., 1976) (but not all postsynaptically acting neurotoxins have a reversible action, e.g., α-bungarotoxin).

AV was considered to be of value in terminating the hemolytic process, the coagulation defect, and the proteinuria (CAMPBELL, 1967 b; 1969 b) but has no effect on the myopathy (HOOD and JOHNSON, 1975).

The predominant site of action of krait venom neurotoxins is on the presynaptic nerve terminal, and experimentally in vitro, AV did not affect the neuromuscular block. Clinically, muscle paralysis due to krait venom appears to be unaffected by

AV therapy (ACTON and KNOWLES, 1915; AHUJA and SINGH, 1954; KUO and WU, 1972; PEARN, 1971; SAWAI et al., 1972), and six krait bites in Taiwan had a 50% case fatality rate (KUO and WU, 1972).

AHUJA and SINGH (1954), FAIRLEY (1933), and STROVER (1955) were enthusiastic about the effects of AV therapy in cobra envenomation. AHUJA and SINGH (1954) claimed that it was never too late to administer AV. Even moribund patients might recover. But were such moribund patients in the preparalytic phase of envenomation from which spontaneous recovery may occur?

For ACTON and KNOWLES (1915) from their considerable experimental work with AV in animals, pointed out that when just a neutralizing dose of AV was given intravenously to cobra-envenomated monkeys and rats, the response was not immediate. Paralysis developed and progressed as in the normal course of envenomation, but breathing remained slow and regular and did not become shallow and rapid as in animals not given AV. However, next morning, the animals would be completely recovered. (When other remedies—corticosteroids, neostigmine—are being evaluated in conjunction with AV, these observations should be kept in mind.)

Cobra venom neurotoxins act postsynaptically, and experimental evidence from nerve-muscle preparations would suggest that AV should be of value if given in adequate doses. Certainly, in some of the published case histories, there is no doubt that cobra AV shortened the duration of paralysis and saved patients whose lives were threatened by paralysis of the muscles of swallowing and respiration (ALANDIKAR, 1920; CROLEY, 1922; HARTY, 1926; KHISTY, 1915).

WARRELL et al. (1976) did not find that two polyvalent AVs were of any value in spitting cobra envenomation, and although improvement followed the administration of AV in patients with neurotoxic manifestations following Malayan cobra bite, REID (1964) did not think that any dramatic effect was evident. AV had no effect in preventing or ameliorating the local necrotic effect of cobra venom (REID, 1964; WARRELL et al., 1976).

Both REID (1964) and WARRELL et al. (1976) have, however, doubts as to whether enough AV was used, and they along with KARUNARATNE and ANANDADAS (1973) wonder what constitutes and adequate dose of AV. WARRELL et al. (1976) caution against accepting evidence that one component of the venom has been neutralized means that all venom components have been neutralized, e.g., blood coagulation tests (KARUNARATNE and ANANDADAS, 1973) and immunologic tests for the presence of venom (WARRELL et al., 1976) have been used to assess the effectiveness of AV therapy.

1. Dosage and Route of Administration

FRASER (1896) and MARTIN (1898) very early pointed out that when venom and AV were injected simultaneously but at different sites, the in vivo neutralizing dose, even if given intravenously, was several times the in vitro neutralizing dose.

There is no argument now about the route of administration. If AV is to be given, it must be given intravenously. Absorption from intramuscular sites is too slow (CHRISTENSEN, 1969) to be of value. The dose of AV required will vary with the amount of venom deposited. As this is unknown, dosage is always empirical.

The dose of specific cobra AV required to neutralize the average venom yield has been estimated to be 330 ml (FRASER, 1896), 350 ml (LAMB, 1904), or 100–200 ml with a more concentrated cobra AV (KNOWLES, 1921). REID (1964) used up to 150 ml of a polyvalent Haffkine AV but felt more should have been used and recommends at least 20 ampules of the Haffkine polyvalant AV-100 ml every 2 h. For South African elapid bites CHRISTENSEN (1969) recommends 3–4 ampules (30–40 ml) of a specific AV but three times this dose if serious envenomation is present.

When dealing with systemic envenomation from an elapid venom whose predominant neurotoxins have a postsynaptic site of action, the AV should be titrated against the patient's signs. Up to 600 ml may be required to treat Thai cobra bite (PURANANANDA, 1967), and after a recent king cobra bite, 1150 ml of serum was required to save the patient (GANTHAVORN, 1971).

The cost of AV must be taken into account. AV can be a dear commodity. (One ampule of Australian polyvalent AV is sold at a cost of $ U.S. 140.) There is no point in using large amounts of VA to treat muscle paralysis due to presynaptic-acting neurotoxins. Twice the recommended dose is a compromise dose.

2. Method of Administration

When the snake has been positively identified, it is preferable to use the homologous monovalent AV. When it is not available and in the case of bites from unidentified snakes, a polyvalent AV should be used. Occasionally, a heterologous monovalent AV may be of value, such as Australian tiger snake AV which has considerable neutralizing powers against cobra and krait venoms and is as effective as, or more effective than, the homologous monovalent AVs (MINTON, 1967).

AV is biological dynamite. It should be given in the expectation that the patient will react to it. Every facility to treat complications must be in the room where the AV is given. The intensive care ward is the best situation for AV administration. In the hospital setting, it must not be given directly into the vein but into the rubber tube of an intravenous infusion. No test for sensitivity is made, for anaphylaxis has followed such tests (SCHAPEL et al., 1971), and the frequency of minor reactions would delay AV administration, but the administration must be commenced very slowly. Other authorities advocate the use of a dilute test dose (CHATTERJEE, 1965; CHRISTENSEN, 1969; REID, 1970; RUSSELL et al., 1975).

If skin reactions occur, adrenaline and an antihistamine drug are injected. If there is no fall in blood pressure, the administration of the AV is continued. If anaphylaxis occurs and envenomation is present, once the blood pressure returns to normal, the remainder of the AV can be given without a reaction occurring. A febrile reaction to the AV frequently follows within 1–2 h of administration.

3. Complications of Antivenene Therapy

As a foreign protein is injected intravenously, a high complication rate could be expected, and the more closely a patient is observed the higher the percentage of side-effects recorded. In 61 administrations of AV, 46% (28/61) were associated with some side-effects. Most of these reactions were mild (itching, urticaria, edema, fever, rigor) and of little clinical significance. In 8% (5/61), the reaction was serious and posed a threat to life; 3% (2/61) developed anaphylaxis (CAMPBELL, 1969a).

The incidence of delayed serum reactions is seldom recorded (PARRISH and KHAN, 1966) because patients are often not seen again, but fever and polyarthralgia have been noted (CAMPBELL and YOUNG, 1961), as well as urticaria (REID and FLECKER, 1950). Recovery from anaphylaxis has been followed by dementia (SYMONS, 1960).

V. Other Modes of Treatment

1. Neostigmine

There is experimental evidence from nerve-muscle preparations that neostigmine can reverse the paralysis produced by pure cobra neurotoxins (LEE et al., 1972) although its ability to reverse the paralysis produced by the crude venom was less clear-cut. It had no effect on the paralysis caused by α-bungarotoxin which also induces a postsynaptic block.

When given in repeated doses after AV, neostigmine was thought to have expedited recovery (KUMAR and USGAONKAR, 1968), and a clinical trial in Indian snakebite suggested that repeated half hourly intravenous 0.5 mg doses of neostigmine with atropine brought about a quicker and better response than AV alone (BANERJEE et al., 1972). Experiments in dogs poisoned with cobra venom indicated that in the completely paralyzed animals neostigmine was without effect, but when administered during the stage of recovery, there was distinct and immediate improvement (GODE et al., 1968).

2. Corticosteroids

Experiments in dogs and clinical evidence suggested that steroids might be of value in cobra envenomation (BENYAJATI et al., 1961), but REID (1964), in a controlled clinical trial, found corticosteroids of no value in Malayan pitviper poisoning, and four patients given prednisone after being bitten by cobras showed no benefit from it nor did one Papuan patient. The routine use of corticosteroids is not recommended. KARUNARATNE and ANANDADAS (1973) used corticosteroids in almost all their cases to reduce and control sensitivity reactions, and GUPTA et al. (1960) thought they had some value in this regard.

3. Intubation, Tracheostomy, IPPR, Intensive Care Nursing

If reliance was placed on AV alone, at least 25% of patients, envenomated by Papuan snakes who might subsequently be saved, would have died (CAMPBELL, 1969a). They were saved with tracheostomy, IPPR, and intensive nursing care.

The indication for intubation and intermittent positive pressure respiration (IPPR) are the same as in any other condition which produces respiratory obstruction and insufficiency. As the paralysis unusally only lasts for less than a week, tracheal intubation with a PVC nasotracheal tube with a low pressure cuff would seem to be preferable to a tracheostomy, but in areas where highly trained staff are not available, a tracheostomy with the insertion of a cuffed endotracheal tube has merit and is easier for such staff to handle.

It cannot be stressed too frequently that the situation in treating envenomated snakebite patients may not be stable until about 48 h after the bite. Up to this time, a careful watch of the patient must be kept for progress in the paralysis and the onset of respiratory obstruction, respiratory failure, secondary shock, or anuria.

VI. Treatment of Local Wound (Cobra Bites)

No local treatment is given initially. Blisters are left alone. When tissue necrosis is apparent, sloughs of skin and subcutaneous tissue are excised. Tendons and muscles are not excised. Local dressings of normal saline are then applied and antibiotics may be necessary. Skin grafting is frequently necessary (REID, 1970). Tetanus antitoxin is not given routinely to snakebite victims.

References

Acton, H. W., Knowles, R.: Studies on the treatment of snake-bite. Indian J. med. Res. **2**, 91—109 (1914)

Acton, H. W., Knowles, R.: Studies on the treatment of snake-bite. Section IV, the present position of antivenene therapy. Indian J. med. Res. **3**, 275—361 (1915)

Ahuja, M. L., Singh, G.: Snake bite in India. Indian J. med. Res. **42**, 661—686 (1954)

Alandikar, K. K.: Cobra poisoning. Indian med. Gaz. **55**, 60 (1920)

Australian Medical Journal: Med. Soc. Victoria **20**. 75—110 (1875)

Banerjee, R. N., Sahni, A. L., Chacko, K. A., Kumar, V.: Neostigmine in the treatment of elapidae bites. J. Ass. Phycns India **20**, 503—509 (1972)

Barker, E.: Aust. med. J. **5**, 146—148 (1860)

Barnes, J. M., Trueta, J.: Absorption of bacteria, toxins and snake venoms from the tissues: importance of the lymphatic circulation. Lancet **1941 I**, 623—626

Benn, K. M.: A further case of snake-bite by a taipan ending fatally. Med. J. Aust. **1**, 147—149 (1951)

Benyajati, C., Keoplung, M., Sribhibhadh, R.: Experimental and clinical studies on glucocorticoids in cobra envenomation. J. trop. Med. Hyg. **64**, 46—49 (1961)

Beveridge, A.: A case of snake bite treated by Dr. Calmette's antivenene. Brit. med. J. **1899 II**, 1732

Bill, G.: Notes on a case of snake-bite, treated with antivenine. Intercolon. med. J. Aust. **7**, 346—348 (1902)

Bose, N.: An interesting case of cobra bite: recovery after treatment. Lancet **1910 I**, 643—644

Breton, P.: Case of the fatal effects of the bite of a venomous snake. Trans. med. Phys. Soc. (Calcutta) **1**, 55 (1825)

Butter, D.: On the treatment of persons bitten by venomous snakes. Trans. med. phys. Soc. (Calcutta) **2**, 220 (1825)

Calmette, A.: Venoms Venomous Animals and Antivenomous Serum—Therapeutics. London: John Bale, Sons and Danielsson 1908

Campbell, C. H.: The treatment of suspected venomous snake bite. Med. J. Aust. **2**, 493—495 (1963)

Campbell, C. H.: Venomous snake bite in Papua and its treatment with tracheotomy, artificial respiration and antivenene. Trans. roy. Soc. trop. Med. Hyg. **58**, 263—273 (1964)

Campbell, C. H.: The death adder *(Acanthophis antarcticus)*. The effect of the bite and its treatment. Med. J. Aust. **2**, 922—925 (1966)

Campbell, C. H.: The taipan *(Oxyuranus scutellatus)* and the effect of its bite. Med. J. Aust. **1**, 735—738 (1967a)

Campbell, C. H.: Antivenene in the treatment of Australian and Papuan snake bite. Med. J. Aust. **2**, 106—110 (1967b)

Campbell, C. H.: The Papuan black snake *(Pseudechis papuanus)* and the effect of its bite. Papua N. Guinea med. J. **10**, 117—121 (1967c)

Campbell, C. H.: Clinical aspects of snake bite in the Pacific Area. Toxicon **7**, 25—28 (1969a)

Campbell, C. H.: A clinical study of venomous snake bite in Papua. M.D. Thesis, University of Sydney, 1969b

Campbell, C. H.: Fatal case of mulga *(Pseudechis australis)* snake bite. Med. J. Aust. **1**, 426 (1969c)

Campbell, C. H.: The effects of snake venoms and their neurotoxins on the nervous system of man and animals. In: Hornabrook, R. W. (Ed.): Topics on Tropical Neurology, Chapt. 10. Philadelphia: Davis 1975
Campbell, C. H., Young, L. N.: The symptomatology, clinical course and successful treatment of Papuan elapine snake envenomation. Med. J. Aust. **1**, 479—486 (1961)
Carr-White, P.: Is antivenine of any value in cobra poising? Indian med. Gaz. **37**, 431—434 (1902)
Casale, F. F., Patel, S. M.: Elapid snake bite: a report of two cases. Brit. J. Anaesth. **46**, 162 (1974)
Champness, L. T.: The defibrination syndrome following elapine snake bites in Papua. Papua N. Guinea Med. J. **9**, 89—94 (1966)
Chapman, D. S.: The symptomatology, pathology, and treatment of the bites of venomous snakes of Central and Southern Africa. In: Bücherl, W., Buckley, E. E., Deulofeu, V. (Eds.): Venomous Animals and Their Venoms, Vol. I, Chapt. 17. New York: Academic Press 1968
Chatterjee, S. C.: Management of snake bite cases. J. Indian med. Ass. **45**, 654—659 (1965)
Christensen, P. A.: South African Snake Venoms and Antivenoms. Johannesburg: S. Afr. Inst. Med. Res. 1955
Christensen, P. A.: The treatment of snakebite. S. Afr. med. J. **43**, 1253—1258 (1969)
Connor, I., Kellaway, C. H.: A case of snake-bite by a tiger snake *(Notechis scutatus)* treated by antivenene. Melbourne Hosp. clin. Rep. **5**, 90—92 (1934)
Croley, V. St. J.: Notes on a case of recovery from the bite of a cobra. Trans. roy. Soc. trop. Med. Hyg. **16**, 57—60 (1922)
D'Abreu, A. R.: Poisoning by bite from *Bungarus caeruleus* with recovery. Indian med. Gaz. **74**, 94—95 (1939)
Datyner, M. E., Gage, P. W.: Presynaptic and postsynaptic effects of the venom of the Australian tiger snake at the neuromuscular junction. Brit. J. Pharmacol. **49**, 340—354 (1973)
Davidson, R. A.: Case of African cobra bite. Brit. med. J. **1970 IV**, 660
Drake-Brockman, H. E.: An interesting case of snakebite-treatment-recovery. Indian med. Gaz. **28**, 373 (1893)
Eaker, D., Karlsson, E., Rammer, L., Saldeen, T.: Isolation of neurotoxin in a case of fatal cobra bite. J. forens. Med. **16**, 96—99 (1969)
Easton, R.: Strychnine in snakebite. Aust. med. Gaz. **13**, 387—388 (1894)
Eccles, T. H.: Professor Halford's intra-venous injection of ammonia. Aust. med. J. **20**, 84—85 (1875)
Fairley, N. H.: The present position of snake bite and the snake bitten in Australia. Med. J. Aust. **1**, 296—313 (1929a)
Fairley, N. H.: The dentition and biting mechanism of Australian snakes. Med. J. Aust. **1**, 313—327 (1929b)
Fairley, N. H.: Criteria for determining the efficacy of ligature in snake bite (the subcutaneous-intravenous index.). Med. J. Aust. **1**, 377—394 (1929c)
Fairley, N. H.: Trans. roy. Soc. trop. Med. Hyg. **27**, 22—24 (1933)
Fayrer, J.: The Thanatophidia of India Being a Description of the Venomous Snakes of the Indian Peninsula, With an Account of the Influence of Their Poison on Life; and a Series of Experiments. London: Churchill 1872
Fitzsimons, V. F. M.: Snakes of Southern Africa. London: MacDonald 1962
Flecker, H.: Snake bite in practice. Med. J. Aust. **2**, 8—13 (1940)
Flecker, H.: More fatal cases of bites of the taipan *(Oxyuranus scutellatus)*. Med. J. Aust. **2**, 383—384 (1944)
Flecker, H.: Bite from broad-headed snake: *Hoplocephalus bungaroides* (Boie) Med. J. Aust. **1**, 368—369 (1952)
Forbes, H. F.: Two cases of snake-bite treated with strychnine. Aust. med. Gaz. **10**, 141 (1891)
Foxton, H. V.: A case of fatal snake-bite (with autopsy). Med. J. Aust. **1**, 108 (1914)
Fraser, T. R.: Immunization against serpents' venom, and the treatment of snake-bite with antivenene. Brit. med. J. **1896 I**, 957—960
Furtado, M. A., Lester, I. A.: Myoglobinuria following snake bite. Med. J. Aust. **1**, 674—676 (1968)
Garde, H. C.: Notes of three cases of snakebite treated by subcutaneous injections of strychnine. Aust. med. Gaz. **9**, 157 (1890)
Ganthavorn, S.: A case of king cobra bite. Toxicon **9**, 293—294 (1971)
Gaudoin, R.: Case of snake-bite. Indian med. Gaz. **42**, 459—460 (1907)
Gharpurey, K. G.: Death from a snake bite (krait poisoning). Indian med. Gaz. **66**, 266 (1931a)
Gharpurey, K. G.: Case of recovery from cobra bite. Indian med. Gaz. **66**, 569—570 (1931b)

Gharpurey, K. G.: Some snake-bite cases. Indian med. Gaz. **67**, 81—82 (1932)
Gode, G. R., Tandan, G. C., Bhide, N. K.: Role of artificial ventilation in experimental cobra envenomation in the dog. Brit. J. Anaesth. **40**, 850—852 (1968)
Gray, H. H.: Green mamba envenomation: case report. Trans. roy. Soc. trop. Med. Hyg. **56**, 390—391 (1962)
Gupta, P. S., Bhargava, S. P., Sharma, M. L.: A review of 200 cases of snake bite with special reference to the corticosteroid therapy. J. Indian med. Ass. **35**, 387—390 (1960)
Haast, W. E., Winer, M. L.: Complete and spontaneous recovery from the bite of a blue krait snake *(Bungarus caeruleus)*. Amer. J. trop. Med. Hyg. **4**, 1135—1137 (1955)
Hall, E. S.: On snake bites. Aust. med. J. **4**, 81—96 (1859)
Hanna, W., Lamb, G.: A case of cobra-poisoning treated with Calmette's antivenine. Lancet **1901 I**, 25—26 (1901)
Harris, J. B., Karlsson, E., Thesleff, S.: Effects of an isolated toxin from Australian tiger snake *(Notechis scutatus scutatus)* venom at the mammalian neuromuscular junction. Brit. J. Pharmacol. **47**, 141—146 (1973)
Harty, A. H.: A case of cobra-bite. Indian med. Gaz. **61**, 178—179 (1926)
Hennessy, P. H.: A snake bite (cobra) case. Indian med. Gaz. **53**, 154 (1918)
Herrmann, R. P., Davey, M. G., Skidmore, P. H.: The coagulation defect after envenomation by the bite of the dugite *(Demansia nuchalis affinis)*, a Western Australian brown snake. Med. J. Aust. **2**, 183—186 (1972)
Hilson, A. H.: Two cases of snake bite treated by injection of liquor ammoniae into the veins, with remarks on the action of snake poison. Indian med. Gaz. **8**, 258—260, 284—286 (1873)
Hood, V. L., Johnson, J. R.: Acute renal failure with myoglobinuria following tiger snake bite. Med. J. Aust. **2**, 638—641 (1975)
Jutzy, D. A., Biber, S. H., Elton, N. W., Lowry, E. C.: A clinical and pathological analysis of snake bites on the Panama Canal Zone. Amer. J. trop. Med. Hyg. **2**, 129—141 (1953)
Kamenskaya, M. A., Thesleff, S.: The neuromuscular blocking action of an isolated toxin from the elapid *(Oxyuranus scutellactus)*. Acta physiol. scand. **90**, 716—724 (1974)
Karlsson, E., Eaker, D., Rydén, L.: Purification of presynaptic neurotoxin from the venom of the Australian tiger snake *Notechis scutatus scutatus*. Toxicon **10**, 405—413 (1972)
Karunaratne, K. E. De S., Anandadas, J. A.: The use of antivenom in snake bite poisoning. Ceylon med. J. **18**, 37—43 (1973)
Kellaway, C. H.: The venom of the ornamented snake *Denisonia maculata*. Aust. J. exp. Biol. med. Sci. **12**, 47—54 (1934)
Khisty, B. R.: Report on a case of bite from *Naia tripudians* treated at the Harda branch dispensary-recovery. Indian. med. Gaz. **50**, 219—220 (1915)
Kingsbury, J.: A case of bite by a tiger snake treated successfully with strychnine. Aust. med. Gaz. **10**, 244 (1891)
Knowles, R.: The mechanism and treatment of snake-bite in India. Trans. roy. Soc. trop. Med. Hyg. **15**, 71—97 (1921)
Knyvett, A. F., Molphy, R.: Respiratory paralysis due to snake-bite: report of two cases. Med. J. Aust. **2**, 481—484 (1959)
Krefft, G.: Remedies for snake-poisoning. The Sydney Morning Herald, May 6, 1868, p. 2
Krengel, B., Walton, J.: A case of mamba bite. S. Afr. med. J. **41**, 1150—1151 (1967)
Kumar, S., Usgaonkar, R. S.: Myasthenia gravis like picture resulting from snake bite. J. Indian med. Ass. **50**, 428—429 (1968)
Kuo, T.-P., Wu, C.-S.: Clinico-pathological studies on snakebites in Taiwan. J. Formosan med. Ass. **71**, 447—466 (1972)
Lamb, G.: Specificity of Antivenomous Sera. Scientific Memoirs by Officers of the Medical and Sanitary Departments of the Government of India, No. 5. Calcutta: Superintendent of Government Printing 1903
Lamb, G.: On the serum therapeutics of cases of snake-bite. Lancet **1904 II**, 1273—1277
Lee, C. Y., Chang, C. C., Chen, Y. M.: Reversibility of neuromuscular blockade by neurotoxins from elapid and sea snake venoms. J. Formosan med. Ass. **71**, 344—349 (1972)
Lefrou, G.: Deux cas de morsure par le serpent *Dendraspis viridis* suivis de guérison. Bull. Soc. Path. exot. **44**, 234—237 (1951)
Le Gac, P., Lepesme, P.: Sur un cas d'envenimation non mortel par morsure de *Dendraspis* (colubridé protéroglyphe) Bull. Soc. Path. exot. **33**, 256—258 (1940)

Lester, I. A.: A case of snake-bite treated by specific taipan antivenene. Med. J. Aust. **2**, 389—391 (1957)
Lloyd, C. H.: Four cases of snake bite. Med. J. Aust. **2**, 360—361 (1932)
Louw, J. X.: Specific mamba antivenom—report of survival of 2 patients with black mamba bites treated with this serum. S. Afr. med. J. **41**, 1175 (1967)
MacDonald, W. C. C.: Some experiences of Queensland snakes. Aust. med. Gaz. **14**, 267—271 (1895)
MacGregor, R. D.: A case of cobra bite-recovery. Indian med. Gaz. **41**, 361—363 (1906)
Martin, C. J.: The curative value of Calmette's antivenomous serum in the treatment of inoculations with the poisons of Australian snakes. Intercolon. med. J. Aust. **2**, 527—536 (1897)
Martin, C. J.: Further observations concerning the relation of the toxin and anti-toxin of snake-venom. Proc. roy. Soc. (Lond.) **64**, 88—94 (1898)
McCollough, N. C., Gennaro, J. F.: Coral snake bites in the United States. J. Fla. med. Ass. **49**, 968—972 (1963)
Mebs, D., Chen, Y. M., Lee, C. Y.: Biochemistry and pharmacology of toxins from Australian snake venoms. Proc. of 5th Int'l. Symp. Animal, Plant and Microbial Toxins, Costa Rica 1976
Minton, S. A.: Paraspecific protection be elapid and sea snake antivenins. Toxicon **5**, 47—55 (1967)
Mueller, A.: On haematuria in snake bite poisoning. Aust. med. Gaz. **12**, 247—249 (1893)
Nigam, P., Tandon, V. K., Kumar, R., Thacore, V. R., Lal, N.: Snake bite—a clinical study. Indian J. med. Sci. **27**, 697—704 (1973)
Ormsby, A. I.: Notes on the broad-headed snake *(Hoplocephalus bungaroides)*. Proc. roy. zool. Soc. N.S.W. **1946—47**, 19—21 (1947)
Pain, F.: Case of snake-bite treated with strychnine. Aust. med. Gaz. **11**, 114—115 (1892)
Parrish, H. M., Khan, M. S.: Bites by foreign venomous snakes in the United States. Amer. J. med. Sci. **251**, 150—155 (1966)
Parrish, H. M., Khan, M. S.: Bites by coral snakes: Report of 11 representative cases. Amer. J. med. Sci. **253**, 561—568 (1967)
Pearn, J. H.: Survival after snake-bite with prolonged neurotoxic envenomation. Med. J. Aust. **2**, 259—261 (1971)
Phisalix, M.: Quelques remarques sur la fréquence des effets rapidement mortels des morsures de colubridés protéroglyphes appartenant au genre Africain *Dendraspis*, Schleg. Bull. Soc. Path. exot. **33**, 258—259 (1940)
Ponnambalam, C.: Notes on a fatal case of krait-poisoning. Ceylon J. Sci. [D] **5**, 37—38 (1939)
Purananda, C.: Personal communication (1967)
Ramsey, G. F., Klickstein, G. D.: Coral snake bite report of a case and suggested therapy. J. Amer. med. Ass. **182**, 949—951 (1962)
Reid, A. S.: The treatment of snake-bite by Calmette's antivenene. Indian med. Gaz. **36**, 372—374 (1901)
Reid, C. C., Flecker, H.: Snake bite by a taipan with recovery. Med. J. Aust. **1**, 82—83 (1950)
Reid, H. A.: Antivenene reaction following accidental sea-snake bite. Brit. med. J. **1957 II**, 26—29
Reid, H. A.: Cobra-bites. Brit. med. J. **1964 II**, 540—545
Reid, H. A.: Symptomatology, pathology, and treatment of land snake bite in India and South-east Asia. In: Bücherl, W., Buckley, E. E., Deulofeu, V. (Eds.): Venomous Animals and Their Venoms, Vol. I, Chapt. 20. New York: Academic Press 1968
Reid, H. A.: The principles of snakebite treatment. Clin. Toxicol. **3**, 473—482 (1970)
Reid, H. A., Chan, K. E., Thean, P. C.: Prolonged coagulation defect (defibrination syndrome) in Malayan viper bite. Lancet **1963 a I**, 621—626
Reid, H. A., Thean, P. C., Martin, W. J.: Specific antivenene and prednisone in viper-bite poisoning: controlled trial. Brit. med. J. 1963b II, 1378—1380
Reid, J. A.: Case of snake-bite. Aust. med. J. **16**, 105—108 (1894)
Richards, V.: The Land-Marks of Snake-Poison Literature, Being a Review of the More Important Researches Into the Nature of Snake-Poisons. Calcutta: Traill 1885
Robson, T.: Case of snake-bite in which bleeding was used as an auxiliary. Trans. med. phys. Soc (Calcutta) **7**, 480 (1835)

Rollison, J. W.: Fatal case of tiger-snake *(Notechis scutatus)* bite. Med. Sci. Arch. Adelaide Hosp. 7, 18—20 (1928)
Rowlands, J. B., Mastaglia, F. L., Kakulas, B. A., Hainsworth, D.: Clinical and pathological aspects of a fatal case of mulga *(Pseudechis australis)* snakebite. Med. J. Aust. **1**, 226—230 (1969)
Russell, F. E.: First-aid for snake venom poisoning. Toxicon **4**, 285—289 (1967)
Russell, F. E., Carlson, R. W., Wainschel, J., Osborne, A. H.: Snake venom poisoning in the United States: experiences with 550 cases. J. Amer. med. Ass. **233**, 341—344 (1975)
Sant, S. M.: Personal communication (1973)
Sawai, Y., Koba, K., Okonogi, T., Mishima, S., Kawamura, Y., Chinzei, H., Bakar, A., Devaraj, T., Phong-Aksara, S., Puranananda, C., Salafranca, E. S., Sumpaico, J. S., Tseng, C.-S., Taylor, J. F., Wu, C.-S., Kuo, T.-P.: An epidemiological study of snakebites in the Southeast Asia. Jap. J. exp. Med. **42**, 283—307 (1972)
Sawai, Y., Tseng, C. S., Kuo, T. P., Wu, C. S.: Snakebites in Kao-Hsiung Prefecture, Taiwan. Snake **2**, 13—17 (1970)
Schapel, G. J., Utley, D., Wilson, G. C.: Envenomation by the Australian common brown snake—*Pseudonaja (Demansia) textilis textilis*. Med. J. Aust. **1**, 142—144 (1971)
Seth, S. D. S.: Snake bite and its treatment. Indian J. med. Sci. **28**, 237—242 (1974)
Shaw, C. E.: The coral snakes, genera *Micrurus* and *Micruroides*, of the United States and Northern Mexico. In: Bücherl, W., Buckley, E. E. (Eds.): Venomous Animals and Their Venoms, Vol. II, pp. 157—172. New York: Academic Press 1971
Sinha, A. K.: Cobra-venom conjunctivitis. Lancet **1972 I**, 1026
Skinner, D., Mueller, A.: A remarkable case of death from snakebite. Aust. med. Gaz. **12**, 74—78 (1893)
Smith, T. J.: Case of snake bite successfully treated by venesection. Trans. med. phys. Soc. (Calcutta) **8**, 95 (1836)
Smyth, T. E.: Strychnine in snakebite. Aust. med. Gaz. **12**, 119—120 (1893)
Strover, H. M.: Snake bite and its treatment. Trop. Dis. Bull. **52**, 421—426 (1955)
Strover, H. M.: Report on a death from black mamba bite (Dendroaspis polylepis). Cent. Afr. J. Med. **13**, 185—186 (1967)
Strover, H. M.: Observations on two cases of snake-bite by *Naja nigricollis ss mossambica*. Cent. Afr. J. Med. **19**, 12—13 (1973)
Sutherland, S. K., Coulter, A. R., Broad, A. J., Hilton, J. M. N., Lane, L. H. D.: Human snake bite victims: the successful detection of circulating snake venom by radioimmunoassay. Med. J. Aust. **1**, 27—29 (1975)
Symons, H. S.: Anaphylactic shock and subsequent dementia following the administration of tiger snake antivenene. Med. J. Aust. **2**, 1010—1011 (1960)
Trestrail, J. C.: Case of snake-bite. Trans. med. phys. Soc. (Bombay) **2**, 303 (1855)
Trinca, J. C.: Report of recovery from taipan bite. Med. J. Aust. **1**, 514—516 (1969)
Trinca, J. C., Graydon, J. J., Covacevich, J., Limpus, C.: The rough-scaled snake *(Tropidechis carinatus)* a dangerously venomous Australian snake. Med. J. Aust. **2**, 801—809 (1971)
Wall, A. J.: Indian Snake Poisons, Their Nature and Effects. London: W.H. Allen 1883
Wall, F.: Treatment of snake poisoning. Indian med. Gaz. **48**, 428—430 (1913)
Wall, F.: Fatal case of ophitoxaemia. Indian med. Gaz. **49**, 253 (1914)
Wallace, I.: Effects of tiger snake bite. Vict. Nat. **70**, 227—228 (1954)
Warrell, D. A., Greenwood, B. M., Davidson, N. McD., Ormerod, L. D., Prentice, C. R. M.: Necrosis, haemorrhage and complement depletion following bites by the spitting cobra *(Naja nigricollis)*. Quart. J. Med. **45**, 1—23 (1976)
Weatherly, A. J.: Snakebite-treatment by strychnine-recovery. Indian med. Gaz. **29**, 220 (1894)
Wiener, S.: Active immunization of man against the venom of the Australian tiger snake *(Notechis scutatus)*. Amer. J. trop. Med. Hyg. **9**, 284—292 (1960)
Willson, P.: Snake poisoning in the United States: a study based on an analysis of 740 cases. Arch. intern. Med. **1**, 516—570 (1908)
Wilson: Account of the effects of a snake bite. Trans. med. phys. Soc. (Calcutta) **5**, 422 (1829)
Worrell, E.: Reptiles of Australia. Sydney: Angus and Robertson 1963
Wortabet, H. G. L.: A case of snake-bite treated by antivenene-recovery. Indian med. Gaz. **35**, 89—91 (1900)

CHAPTER 25

Symptomatology, Pathology and Treatment of the Bites of Sea Snakes

H. A. REID

Sea snakes are the most abundant and widely dispersed of the world's venomous reptiles. Around the coastal seas of the Indian and western Pacific oceans, fishermen encounter sea snakes every day. Sea snake venoms are highly toxic. One "drop" (about 0.03 ml) contains enough venom to kill three adult men; some sea snake species can eject seven to eight such "drops" in a single bite. Fortunately for fishermen, sea snakes are not aggressive, and even when they do bite man, rarely inject much of their highly toxic venom. If this were not the case, deaths from sea snakebite would probably stop all sea fishing in many parts of Asia—and in these vast areas, fish are a most valuable source of high-quality protein.

Apart from their impact on fishing folk, the effects of sea snakes on the tourist trade can be important. In Malaya, as a result of two bathers being fatally bitten in 1954, there was a serious drop in tourist trade which took several years to recover. This aspect is particularly important in view of the greatly increased scale of tourist traffic to tropical countries where sea snakes are known to occur. What is the danger to a bather in such areas? Skin diving as a sport and oil exploration in tropical seas are both increasing; what is the danger of sea snake bite to divers?

In scientific centers throughout the world, venoms are being increasingly recognized as tools for research. In some research fields, venoms are unique because of a highly specific action on vital body processes. Thus, sea snake venom may help to elucidate diseases both of muscles (myopathies) and of nerves (neurologic illnesses). Research on snake venoms has already led to improved treatment of human disease such as thrombosis (REID and CHAN, 1968).

A. Epidemiology

I. Incidence of Sea Snakebite

Despite the known abundance and toxicity of sea snakes, there are few records in medical literature of man being bitten. Reviewing world mortality of snakebite, SWAROOP and GRAB (1952) produced only the observation that fishermen were occasionally bitten by sea snakes. In 1956, my search of the world medical literature revealed mention, or less often records from 1815 until 1942, of only 31 cases (see Sect. C.I). Although the sea snakes are common around northern Australia (SMITH, 1926), I know of only three cases of sea snakebite in Australia, one while skin diving, in 1972–1973 (personal communication, 1974). No poisoning followed these bites. This conforms with SMITH (1926) who quotes a pearl fisher stating that divers in Australian coastal waters were often bitten although symptoms were slight or absent.

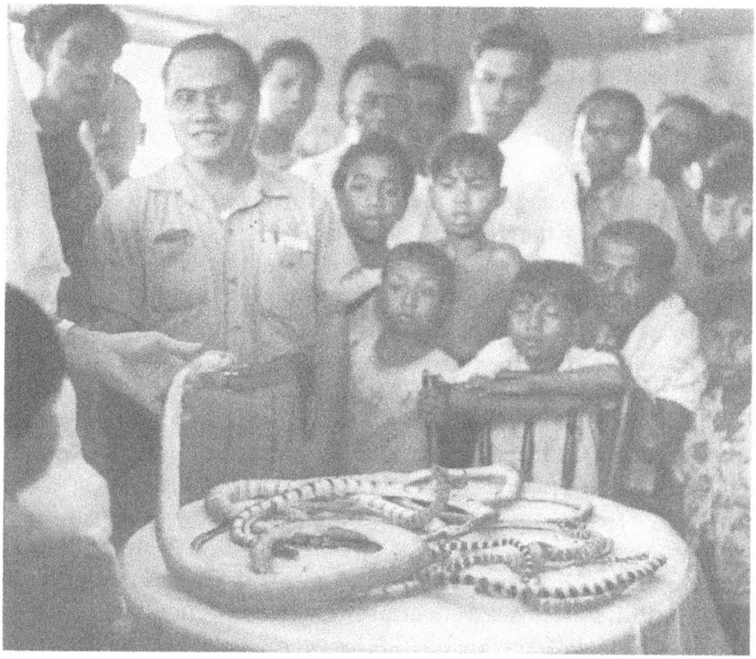

Fig. 1. For superstitious and other reasons, fishing folk are most reluctant to talk about sea snakebite: a casual inquirer would be told that none occurred. But in the survey of Malayan fishing villages, a collection of sea and water snakes in a village coffee shop always attracted an audience, stimulated discussions, and markedly improved communications

In Gato, a small island of the Philippines, enough sea snakes used to breed to maintain a supply of 10000 skins at least 1 m long each year (HERRE and RABOR, 1949). In the 1930s, 30000 were taken every year. Yet during the second world war, no cases of sea snakebite were recorded from the vast American forces operating in that area (personal communications from the Departments of Navy, Army, and Air Force, U.S.A., 1955). BOKMA (1941) in Java found only six fatal cases over 20 years.

However, M'KENZIE (1820) recounted an "epidemic" of sea snakebites, some fatal, in the Coum river mouth at Madras soon after the opening of the bar there in October, 1815. According to ROGERS (1902–1903), deaths were not rare among oyster fishers along the Madras coast. PEAL (1903) was told that three or four fishermen were bitten each year in a fishing village on the Orissa coast and 25% died. During the early 1950s in northern Malaya, Dr. A.A. Wahab succeeded in overcoming the customary reluctance of fishing folk to seek hospital treatment, and by 1953–1954, 30 victims of sea snakebite were being admitted each year from one village alone, a village of about 1200 fishermen. SMITH (1926) wrote of the Gulf of Thailand "... there is hardly a village that cannot tell you of its fatalities." Yet the first medical report of sea snakebite in Thailand was not until 1971 when SITPRIJA et al. recorded two patients treated in Bangkok.

In 1955–1956, a survey of fishing villages was carried out in northwest Malaya, and details of 144 sea snakebites were obtained (REID and LIM, 1957). Because of suspicions and superstitions, the fishing folk were most reluctant to talk about any sea snakebites initially, but after several visits with a display of sea snakes (Fig. 1) in the village coffee shop, communications progressively improved. The number of sea snakes encountered by fishermen varied according to the method of fishing, from nil up to a total of 100 or more each day. The first action on hauling in the catch is to spot sea snakes, pick them up quickly by the tail, and throw them overboard. This responsibility usually rests on one member of the crew, who becomes adept. Malays often used a stick rather than fingers for lifting the snakes. The sea snakes are never killed. Line fishing is not common in the area surveyed, but an average of 20 sea snakes per 300-hook line was quoted by two fishermen using this method in shallow water. Usually, they cut off the line concerned, but one victim was bitten trying to disengage a sea snake and thereby save the hook. He had trivial symptoms following the bite, but thereafter conformed to custom, cutting the lines with sea snakes.

As would be expected, sea snakes were very rare in entangling structures (gill nets). They were not numerous in engulfing structures (drive-in nets), and some entrapping structures (palisade traps, lift nets, falling nets). But a gape net, known by the Chinese as *ch't cheh*, invariably caught 10–20 sea snakes each lift. A conic net with the mouth held open by two poles stuck into the seabed and the tail raised by floats is used in shallow water and lifted two or more times daily according to the tide. However, although this net invariably traps large numbers of sea snakes, only four of the 50 victims bitten whilst handling nets were using this method. The other net in which sea snakes are numerous is a small drag seine called a *kesa* by the Chinese. It is also used in shallow water, being dragged along by two or three fishermen who are in the sea. Of the 50 bitten through handling nets, 27 were handling a *kesa*, 16 (six fatal, five serious, five trivial) being in the sea at the time and 11 (seven serious, four trivial) in the boat pulling in or sorting the net.

All species of sea snake presented during the survey visits were recognized at one or more villages. *Enhydrina schistosa* was considered much the commonest and also the most dangerous. But all fishermen agreed that sea snakes never attacked human beings spontaneously. The only exception was a man who claimed to have been chased by an *E. schistosa* whilst in a fish trap. However, others present laughingly disbelieved him. Several fishermen recounted sea snakes swimming between their vest and body while they stood in fishing nets; all would be well as long as they kept still. As one fisherman put it, if sea snakes *were* aggressive, there would be no more fishing.

It was estimated in the survey report (REID and LIM, 1957) that there was a total of some 150 victims of sea snakebite each year in the villages surveyed. The latter comprised about one-tenth of the Malayan fishing population. Only 18 of the total 144 victims sought orthodox medical help in a hospital. This emphasizes the fact that medical statistics do not accurately reflect the general incidence of sea snakebite.

During 1957–1964, a total of 101 patients with unequivocal sea snakebite were observed under my personal care in Malaya (REID, 1975a). Thirty-one patients with probable or possible sea snakebite (without poisoning) seen during this period were excluded from the series. All victims had been bitten in the northwest Malaya area. In ten bites, the sea snake responsible was brought. In 71 cases, the species biting was reliably identified by the victim or a witness of the bite from the collection of live sea snakes in the Snake and Venom Research Institute, Penang. In 12 bites of fishermen, the sea snake was reliably recognized as such, but the species could not be satisfactorily identified. In eight cases, the cause was not observed, circumstances and bite marks were compatible with those of a sea snake, and typical toxemia ensued. Sea snakebite poisoning was graded:

1. "Nil" when no clinical or laboratory features of poisoning developed.
2. "Trivial" when myalgia was never severe and resolved completely, without antivenom, in 1–3 days. No objective neurologic abnormalities developed. Urine was usually positive for protein, negative for myoglobin; WBC was normal in all cases; serum aspartate aminotransferase was significantly raised.
3. "Serious" when clinical features indicated moderate or severe effects which, without specific antivenom, lasted more than 3 days.
4. "Fatal".

Although this series of 101 unequivocal sea snakebites can give useful information on some epidemiologic aspects, it must be realized that hospital statistics and medical literature can be very misleading on the epidemiology of venomous bites and stings. Doctors, like newspapers, tend to note and report only serious or fatal cases; people bitten without poisoning are ignored. Thus, medical literature exaggerates the severity of snakebite. Also, people bitten by venomous snakes who do not develop poisoning often do not bother to see a doctor—especially if they live in remote rural areas. Hospital patients, therefore, are a selected group, and statistics derived from them underestimate the general incidence of venomous bites and stings and overestimate the general severity of poisoning.

II. Incidence of Poisoning in Sea Snakebites

Although experimental work indicates that sea snake venoms are highly toxic (REID, 1956a), the incidence of serious poisoning in human victims is surprisingly low. In the hospital series, only 22% had serious poisoning (Table 1); in 68% of these unequivocal bites, no poisoning ensued. On the other hand, of the 11 victims with serious poisoning bitten before sea snake antivenom became available, more than one-half died despite nonspecific supportive treatment in a hospital. These facts emphasize how important it is for the clinician to distinguish between sea snakebite without poisoning and sea snakebite with poisoning.

III. Sex, Age, and Race of Victims

Both in the fishing village survey and in the hospital series, 90% of the victims were male, mostly aged 20 years upward, reflecting the groups at risk. But sex, age, and race did not appear to influence the severity of poisoning (Table 2). The youngest patient was an infant aged 16 months, and the oldest, a fisherman aged 70 years.

IV. Occupation of Victims and Circumstances of Bites

In the survey (REID and LIM, 1957), all victims were fishing folk and most were bitten whilst fishing. Five victims were bitten while swimming in a river mouth ("swimming" meaning "feet off the river bed"); one of the five died. Presumably, these five were unlucky enough to hit an oncoming sea snake. Of the 101 hospital patients, 80

Table 1. 1957–1964 hospital series: severity of poisoning before and after sea snake antivenom became available

	Severity of poisoning				Total
	Nil	Trivial	Serious	Fatal	
1957–1961 (no antivenom)	41	6	5	6	58
1962–1964 (specific antivenom available)	27	5	9	2	43

Table 2. 1957–1964 hospital series: sex, age, race, and severity of poisoning

	Severity of poisoning				Total
	Nil	Trivial	Serious	Fatal	
Sex					
Male	63	11	12	8	94
Female	5	—	2	—	7
Age (years)					
0– 9	2	—	2	1	5
10–19	12	2	8	3	25
20–29	18	6	3	1	28
30–39	15	3	—	1	19
40–49	9	—	1	1	11
50 onward	12	—	—	1	13
Race					
Chinese	41	5	6	2	54
Malay	26	5	8	3	42
Other	1	1	—	3	5

Table 3. 1957–1964 hospital series: circumstances of sea snake bites

Activity when bitten	Location when bitten					Total
	In Boat	In sea	In river	On shore	Other	
Handling nets	16	1	—	1	—	18
Sorting fish	13	—	—	5	—	18
Trod on while fishing	6	29	9	—	—	44
Trod on while bathing or washing	—	13	5	—	—	18
Other	—	—	—	2	1	3
Total	35	43	14	8	1	101

were fishermen bitten at their job, and nine were wives or children of fishermen. Of the latter, eight were bitten washing or bathing near their village. The youngest victim, a 16-month infant, was playing with a tin on the shore unseen by her father who was sorting out the catch nearby; he had earlier spotted an *E. schistosa* and put it into the tin. His daughter was bitten on the wrist. Both the daughter and the sea

Table 4. 1957–1964 hospital series: site of bite and severity of poisoning

Site of bite	Severity of poisoning				Total
	Nil	Trivial	Serious	Fatal	
Toe	8	3	—	—	11
Foot	19	6	5	2	32
Leg	9	—	8	2	19
Finger	25	1	1	2	29
Hand	5	1	—	1	7
Arm	1	—	—	1	2
Neck	1	—	—	—	1

snake were brought to me. The *E. schistosa* was a young adult 40 cm long. I "milked" it 2 h after the bite and obtained venom which, after drying, weighed 12 mg. The infant weighed 11 kg and the likely lethal dose of *E. schistosa* venom would be 0.5 mg (Reid, 1956a). The venom obtained was, therefore, equivalent to 24 lethal doses for the patient who had clear fang marks on the wrist. Fortunately, she developed no poisoning.

The circumstances of the bites are summarized in Table 3. Sixty-two of the victims were bitten through treading on the sea snake. This was usually in shallow water either in the sea or in a river mouth. Almost invariably, the victim lifted the bitten limb, bringing the sea snake to the surface, and in many cases, the sea snake continued to cling on until torn or shaken off by the victim. In such cases, poisoning was more likely to be serious than in cases in which the sea snake quickly released its bite. Even so, there were several cases in which the snake clung on obstinately, yet no poisoning followed the bite. Handling nets or sorting fish led to bites on the upper limb, the sea snakes not being seen until the bite. One fisherman was bitten in a boat when his colleague, with the job of finding the sea snakes and throwing them back into the sea, threw a young *E. schistosa* too carelessly so that it hit the victim at the other end of the boat and promptly bit him on the neck.

V. Site of the Bite, Repeated Bites, Other Factors

The site of the bite (Table 4) was determined by the circumstances. Treading on the sea snake caused bites on the toe, foot, or leg and resulted in more cases of serious poisoning (18 of 62 cases, or 29%) than finger, hand, or arm bites (five cases of serious poisoning out of 38 cases, or 13%) which were usually caused by handling nets or sorting fish. One patient had been bitten four times, two patients three times, and five patients had been bitten twice; all these previous bites were in fishermen and had occurred before 1957. In three instances, serious poisoning had followed the previous bites, but in the remainder, trivial effects had ensued. When admitted under my care, serious poisoning was observed in only one patient (his third bite; the first caused serious poisoning and second caused only trivial effects). Trivial poisoning occurred in another patient, and in the remaining six patients no poisoning developed. From these limited observations, it is not possible to judge whether previous bites affect the resistance of the individual to further bites. However, I think this is

Table 5. 1957–1964 hospital series: bite-admission interval and severity of poisoning

Hours between bite and hospital admission	Severity of poisoning				Total
	Nil	Trivial	Serious	Fatal	
$^1/_2$ or less	4	—	—	1	5
Over $^1/_2$ to 1	6	—	2	1	9
Over 1 to 2	11	3	1	—	15
Over 2 to 4	21	2	3	—	26
Over 4 to 6	19	5	3	—	27
Over 6 to 10	6	1	1	3	11
Over 10	1	—	4	3	8
Total	68	11	14	8	101

unlikely because 1) bites so often occur without any envenoming and such bites would have no immunizing effect, 2) even if venom is injected, it is very poorly antigenic as judged by reactions in experimental animals (CAREY and WRIGHT, 1960), and 3) in animals any immunity is short-lived.

The temperature in Malaya varies little, and there is no hibernation among land snakes. Monthly incidence and severity of sea snakebite showed little variation; patients were bitten each month throughout the year. One-seventh (14) of the patients were bitten when it was dark, and the remaining 87 in the daylight. Severity of poisoning showed no significant variation according to the day, the month, or with bites in the dark or light. Observations in the Snake and Venom Research Institute, Penang suggested that sea snakes in Malayan waters mate in January and give birth in May–July, but this appeared to influence neither the frequency nor the severity of bites.

VI. Village Treatment; Bite-Hospital Admission Interval

About half the victims had a tourniquet applied though the description of many ligatures suggested a ritual rather than an effective method of delaying absorption. Amputation was never practiced. The fishermen were unanimous that they would rather risk death than lose a finger or toe. The site of the bite was excised by seven victims. Judging from the victims' descriptions of the procedures (especially the time it took) and the six scars seen (one victim had died of the bite), it seemed unlikely that the excisions affected the issue. Experimentally, in dogs, a lethal dose from a sea snakebite can be absorbed in under 3 min (REID, 1956a). There were no instances of incision or suction being attempted. Thereafter, the treatment depended on the victim's race. If Chinese, a special herbal brandy made from a variety of herbs in rice wine was taken, and for the next 24 h all smoking, talking, and eating were avoided (a sensible measure, because if poisoning develops, there is usually difficulty in swallowing which can lead to fatal choking by inhalation of food, vomit, or secretions). Malays, on the other hand, would consult a *bomor* or medicine man who relied mainly on incantations. Malays and Chinese usually disparaged the other's methods and alleged a resulting high mortality, but the survey figures did not support either advocate.

The severity in relation to time elapsing between the bite and admission to a hospital is summarized in Table 5. Over half the victims were admitted within 4 h of the bite. The most rapid admission was that of the supervisor of the Snake and Venom Research Institute which is in the grounds of the Penang General Hospital. He was accidentally bitten while milking an *E. schistosa*. Fortunately, no poisoning resulted and antivenom did not prove necessary. In the 82 patients coming within 6 h of the bite, serious poisoning developed in only 12 cases (about 15%), whereas of the 19 patients coming more than 6 h after the bite, 11 or 58% developed serious poisoning—a fourfold increase. This emphasizes the potential fallacy of hospital statistics; the longer that time elapses after a bite, the less likely a victim is to seek medical aid unless poisoning is severe. Thus, hospital statistics underestimate the general incidence of sea snakebite but overestimate the number of bites with serious poisoning.

VII. Conclusions on Epidemiology

The findings of the survey of fishing villages (REID and LIM, 1957) and the 1957–1964 Hospital series (REID, 1975a) indicate that sea snakebite is a common occupational hazard to fishing folk in Malayan waters. Both the survey and the Hospital series highlight the difficulty in assessing the incidence, the natural morbidity, and natural mortality of these bites, but they effectively show the surprisingly low incidence of serious poisoning in man relative to the high lethal potential of sea snake venom in experimental animals (see Sect. B.II)—even when no effective antivenom is available. The morbidity and mortality in relation to treatment with sea snake antivenom will be considered later. Do these epidemiologic features in the Malayan area apply also to other areas of the world where sea snakes are found? I do not think they apply to the African or western coasts of America where the sole naturally occurring species is *Pelamis platurus*. This species does not usually live in shallow waters such as *E. schistosa* prefers; fishermen are thus less likely to encounter *P. platurus*. CLARK (1942) recorded that *P. platurus* was ... exceedingly abundant in Panama Bay at some seasons of the year," but he had never heard of anyone being bitten. So far as I am aware, no sea snakebites have been recorded in the western America area; and I know of only three cases recorded in the African area (FITZSIMONS, 1912). But along Asian coasts, wherever *E. schistosa* is common, I think it is highly likely that fishing folk are often bitten, and because of superstitions (REID and LIM, 1957), the casual inquirer at these Asian fishing villages will not be informed of the extent of the problem. In Vietnam, BARME (1963) records that each year fatal cases are numerous but actual numbers remain unknown because of superstitions very similar to those found in the Malayan survey.

What is the risk from sea snakes to bathers? The risk of sea snakebite is certainly much less than the risk of venomous fish stings. During 1957–1959, I observed 13 patients bitten by sea snakes whilst bathing from sea beaches (REID, 1961b) and 140 patients stung by catfish, stingrays, or jelly fish, bathing on the same beaches. Bathers are occasionally bitten by sea snakes when they inadvertently tread on them. Usually, the risk of being bitten is greatly exaggerated. On Penang Island beaches, the risk was statistically assessed at one bite per 270000 man bathing hours. This is in an area where *E. schistosa*, much the most dangerous sea snake to man, is commonly found by fishermen. The risk of sea snakebite to bathers is thus low; the risk of death, even without modern treatment, is very much lower owing to the rarity with which sea snakes inject venom when they bite man. In the Hospital series, 42 of the total 101 patients were admitted during 1957–1961 before specific sea snake antivenom was available, and six died. These 42 patients all had unequivocal sea snakebite; but during 1957–1961, I saw a further 18 patients with probable or possible sea snakebite. The mortality in this selected group, six deaths out of 60 cases, is 10%. And if the victim *is* envenomed, but receives sea snake antivenom within a few hours of the bite, the mortality should be nil (see Sect. G.II.b). The risk of death from sea snakebite is much less than that of accidental drowning. In 1955–1959, only two bathers in Penang Island waters died from sea snakebite, but 21 bathers from the same beaches died from accidental drowning. Along the coastal road adjoining these beaches, there were 724 road accidents during 1955–1959, 14 fatal. The risk of being bitten while swimming is negligible. None of the patients in the 1957–1964 Hospital series who were bitten whilst bathing were swimming at the time; they all trod on the sea snake. The risk to bathers of bites by *P. platurus* appear to be even more remote. On one morning, PICKWELL (1972) counted 22 stranded specimens of *P. platurus* in half a mile on the Playa del Sol, Puerto V Llarta, in Mexico; great numbers of Mexicans thronged to bathe on these beaches, but sea snakebites were unknown.

B. Medically Important Sea Snakes

I. World Distribution

The distribution of sea snake species can differ very markedly within their vast natural habitat in the Indian and Pacific oceans. BARME (1968) and MINTON (1975) give useful tables showing the geographic distribution of the different *Hydrophiidae* species. Further details about species around Australia are given in DUNSON (1975) BARME earlier recorded the capture of several thousand sea snakes along the coasts of Vietnam (BARME, 1963); in south Vietnam, *Lapemis hardwickii* represented 75% of the sea snakes captured, whereas in central Vietnam, *Hydrophis fasciatus* was more frequently taken. *H. cyanocinctus* appears to be the commonest species found around Taiwan (KUNTZ, 1963) and Hong Kong (ROMER, 1972). In the Philippines, large numbers of *H. inornatus* and *L. hardwickii* are caught by fishermen (HERRE and RABOR, 1949). *H. cyanocinctus* is also common (HERRE, 1942). At Surabaia in north-east Java, BERGMAN (1943) collected 984 sea snakes; about one-third were *Thalassophis anomalus* and one-third *L. hardwickii.* TU (1974) captured 14282 sea snakes in the Gulf of Thailand in 1967, 1969, and 1972. Eighty-one per cent were *L. hardwickii*, 3.3% *Praescutata viperina*, 3.3% *Aipysurus eydouxii*, 2.6% *H. cyanocinctus*, 1.8% *H. torquatus diadema*, and 0.9% *E. schistosa*.

E. schistosa has been noted as extremely common in coastal waters of Malaya (CANTOR, 1886), India (DAY, 1869; CANTOR, 1886), Ceylon (WALL, 1921), Pakistan, and the Persian Gulf (BLANFORD, 1876; KNOWLES, 1921). According to SMITH (1926), *E. schistosa* is the commonest sea snake known. It abounds in most localities on Asian coasts from the Persian Gulf to Vietnam and north Australia; but it has not been met with in the Philippines. During the 3 years 1960–1963, a total of 4735 sea snakes were brought alive to the Snake and Venom Research Institute, Penang,

Table 6. Sea snake species and venom yields, Snake and Venom Research Institute, Malaysia, 1960–1963

Species	Number of specimens	Venom yield (mg dry weight)	
		Average	Maximum
Enhydrina schistosa	2403	8.5	79
Hydrophis brookei	262	1.1	2
Hydrophis caerulescens	4	—	—
Hydrophis cyanocinctus	1074	8.2	80
Hydrophis klossi	312	1.0	2
Hydrophis melanosoma	4	—	—
Hydrophis spiralis	349	2.1	8
Kerilia jerdoni	188	2.8	5
Lapemis hardwickii	115	1.9	15
Microcephalophis gracilis	19	—	—
Pelamis platurus	3	—	—
Praescutata viperina	2	—	—
Total	4735		

northwest Malaya. All these snakes were caught in the sea within 10 miles of the coastline of Penang Island. Approximately one-half of these sea snakes were *E. schistosa* and one-quarter *H. cyanocinctus* (Table 6). Although species of *Laticauda* are extremely abundant in the Philippines (HERRE and RABOR, 1949), I am not aware of any record of man being bitten by *Laticaudinae*. In the Philippines, HERRE (1942) recorded fishermen keeping *Laticauda semifasciata* for eating in large jars into which they trust their hands with impunity, pulling out live specimens 1–2 m long. But they never handled *H. cyanocinctus* in this way.

According to WALL (1921), SMITH (1926), and HERRE (1942), sea snakes are gentle, inoffensive creatures which bite only under provocation. CANTOR (1841) referred to *E. schistosa* and wrote "from my own experience" that sea snakes observed in the Bay of Bengal and the Ganges were very ferocious both in and out of the water. Bright light blinded them, otherwise people would be bitten more often. My own observations of sea snakes in captivity in Malaya indicated marked differences of behavior in different species. Thus, *E. schistosa* is much more aggressive than any other species I have observed. When held, it would start snapping long before the spoon used for venom was within its reach. Having bitten the spoon, the jaws contracted repeatedly with very considerable force. *H. cyanocinctus* would also bite readily as a rule, with less pugnacity—but more tenacity, often having to be torn off it or released altogether from my grasp, the spoon still in its mouth. This was in great contrast to specimens of *H. spiralis*, *H. klossi*, *H. melanosoma*, *L. hardwickii*, and *Kerilia jerdoni* which would rarely bite spontaneously. Often the spoon had to be forced between their teeth; even with this, they sometimes refused to bite. Despite these differences amongst species—and, for that matter, amongst individuals of the same species—I agree that, in general, sea snakes are loth to bite man. According to HERRE (1942) and HEATWOLE (1975), sea snakes are more aggressive during the mating season, but neither the incidence of sea snakebite nor the severity of poisoning varied significantly throughout the year in Malaya.

The species of sea snake reliably identified as biting man in the survey (REID and LIM, 1957) and in the Hospital series (REID, 1975a) were: *E. schistosa* 79 cases (14 fatal), *H. cyanocinctus* 24 cases (four fatal), *H. spiralis* 17 cases (two fatal), *H. klossi* 16 cases (one fatal), *K. jerdoni* three cases (nonfatal), *L. hardwickii* four cases (one fatal), and *M. gracilis* three cases (one fatal).

II. Venom Yields and Lethal Toxicity

Venom yields of some common species of sea snakes are summarized in Table 6. It should be realized that venom "milking" by pressure over the venom glands, encouraging the snake to bite through a membrane, electric stimulation, and so on are all very artificial procedures, and the yields obtained may be extremely capricious, varying significantly from species to species, from specimen to specimen, and from time to time in the same individual specimen. It is quite unknown to what extent these figures represent the amount of venom which the sea snake may or may not inject when they bite prey or when they bite man. At most, the venom yields can give an approximate idea of the amount which different species of sea snakes might inject. Probably more valuable is the amount obtained by milking sea snakes soon after they have bitten human victims; I have obtained large amounts of venom in several such cases where the victim developed little or no poisoning (REID, 1957; 1976). It seems that a defensive bite seldom injects much venom. I think this is the main reason for the low mortality and morbidity in sea snakebite.

The lethal toxicity as judged by animal experiments also varies greatly (REID, 1956a). Quite apart from differences according to different species of sea snake, the lethal toxicities can vary according to the method of obtaining the venom, route of injection, types and numbers of animals used, and so on. For example, the LD_{50} of *E. schistosa* venom for mice in μg/kg body weight by various workers are: 107 intraperitoneal injection (CAREY and WRIGHT, 1960), 125 intravenously (BARME, 1963), 150 subcutaneously (MINTON, 1967), and 90 intravenously (TU and GANTHAVORN, 1969). It is notable that the intravenous LD_{50} of sea snake venoms are not very different from the subcutaneous LD_{50}, whereas with viper venoms the intravenous LD_{50} are much lower than subcutaneous LD_{50}. In mice, *E. schistosa* venom was twice as toxic as the venom of the tiger snake, *Notechis scutatus*, in rabbits six times more toxic, but in cats only half as toxic (REID, 1956a). CAREY and WRIGHT (1960) found *E. schistosa* venom four times more toxic than Malayan *Naja naja* venom; venoms of *H. cyanocinctus* and *L. hardwickii* were twice as toxic; venoms of *H. spiralis* and *K. jerdoni* had similar toxicity. BARME (1963) gave minimum intravenous lethal doses for mice of venoms from eight species of sea snake, two species of viper, and one species of cobra, evaluated under the same conditions. The doses in μg/kg were as follows: *E. schistosa* 125, *M. gracilis* 125, *H. fasciatus* 175, *L. hardwickii* 200, *H. cyanocinctus* 350, *P. viperina*, *P. platurus* 500, *Kolpophis annandalei* 550, *Naja haje* 1000, *Trimeresurus gramineus* 1000, and *Agkistrodon piscivorus* 7500. BAXTER and GALLICHIO (1976) record subcutaneous LD_{50} for mice in μg/kg as follows: *Aipysurus laevis* 262, *Astrotia stokesii* 260, *E. schistosa* 111, *H. cyanocinctus* 464, *H. elegans* 262, *H. major* 193, *H. nigrocinctus* 343, *H. stricticollis* 164, *L. hardwickii* 541, *Laticauda semifasciata* 325, *M. gracilis* 480, and *Notechis scutatus* 256.

It is clear from all these findings that sea snake venoms are more toxic than elapid venoms and much more toxic than viper venoms. But this is countered in many instances by vipers having a more efficient injection apparatus and a greater yield of venom; and elapids are midway between vipers and sea snakes in these two aspects. ROGERS (1902–1903) estimated that the minimum lethal dose of *E. schistosa* venom for a 70 kg man would be 3.5 mg. On this basis, the maximum yield of *E. schistosa* venom which I obtained (79 mg) would contain about 22 adult lethal doses. In summary, I regard *E. schistosa* as the most dangerous sea snake to man on the basis of its abundance, the opinion of fishermen, my own observations on aggressiveness (relative only to that of other sea snake species; *E. schistosa* never bites man unless provoked), venom yields, and lethal toxicities. I would rate other species of sea snakes in descending order of potential danger to man as follows: *H. cyanocinctus*, *L. hardwickii*, *M. gracilis*, *H. spiralis*, *K. jerdoni*, *P. platurus*, *H. klossi*.

C. Symptomatology of Sea Snakebite Poisoning

I. Medical Literature

M'KENZIE (1820) reports two victims bitten in the Madras river mouth in 1815; the symptoms suggest hysteric reactions. M'KENZIE mentions 13 other victims with similar symptoms, also three deaths. The species biting were not identified, but in a collection of 300 sea snakes caught, most were *Hydrophis major* or *Microcephalophis gracilis*. DAY (1869) reported a personal bite by *E. schistosa* when wading off the Orissa coast; no poisoning followed. CHEVERS (1870) described a victim dying 4 h after a bite in 1837. BUCKLAND (1879) mentions a fatal bite on board a man-of-war in the Ganges; SMITH (1926) quotes this incident as due to *P. platurus*. FAYRER (1874) records a ship's captain bitten while bathing in a tidal river at Moulmein near Rangoon; he died 71 h after the bite. FORNÉ (1888) reported a French convict dying 15½ h after a bite at Noumea; the sea snake was thought to be a species of *Hydrophis*. PEAL (1903) reported a fisherman bitten by *E. schistosa* at Orissa; mild poisoning developed. FITZSIMONS (1912) mentions three bites in South Africa; one died 2½ h, another 4½ h after the bite, and the third victim recovered. All picked up a *P. platurus* thinking it was an eel. FOSSEN (1940) reported two deaths in Java, one victim dying 6 days and the other 12 h after unidentified bites. BOKMA (1941) reported a fisherman in Java dying 23½ h after a bite by a young *E. schistosa*. BOKMA (1942) reported a second case with moderate poisoning. P. MARTIN (personal communication, 1953) records death 2¾ h after picking up *L. hardwickii* thought to be dead, near Haiphong in 1948. From Malaya, REID (1956 b, c) reported three fatal cases and one recovery. REID (1957) recorded a personal bite by *E. schistosa* with slight poisoning but with a severe neuropathic antivenom reaction. SITPRIJA et al. (1971) reported two recoveries from severe poisoning with renal failure treated by hemodialysis in Thailand. KARUNARATNE and PANNABOKE (1972) from Sri Lanka reported a victim dying 24 days after the bite despite peritoneal dialysis. Clinical accounts of series of cases in Malaya have been published by REID and LIM (1957) and by REID (1961 a, b, 1962, 1975 b, c).

II. Bite Marks: Early Symptoms

Sea snakebites are usually inconspicuous, painless after the initial prick, and without swelling. The fang marks are one, two, or more small dots which are usually circular as though made by a pin or hypodermic needle (Fig. 2), but they can appear as linear scratches. They may be accompanied by teeth marks which are smaller and more

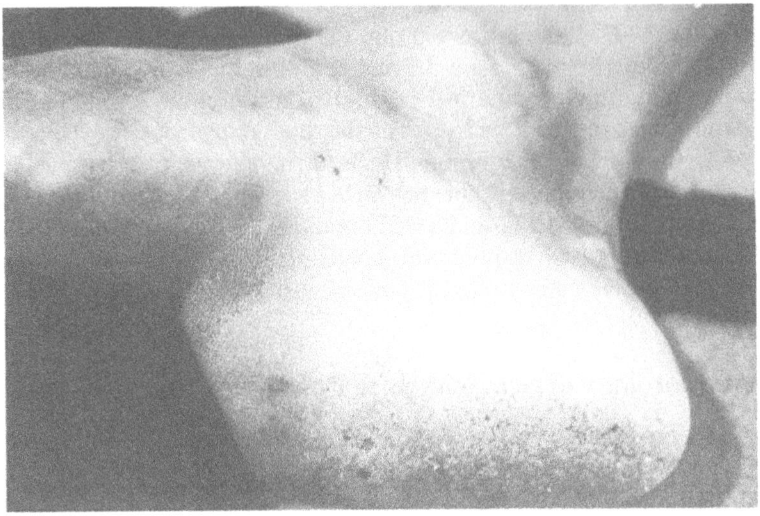

Fig. 2. Sea snakebite on the instep of the foot (two fang marks and one tooth mark). Sea snakebites are inconspicuous, painless, and without swelling. The fang marks are usually circular dots as above but sometimes are mere linear scratches, difficult to make out

likely to be linear. In some cases, there have been no clear fang marks and yet serious, even fatal, poisoning has ensued.

A common symptom in many victims, especially fishermen, regardless of whether venom was injected or not, is a feeling of general coldness coming on soon after the bite. Symptoms due to fright can come on within minutes of the bite and may lead to collapse. The patient may appear semiconscious, with cold clammy skin, feeble pulse, and rapid, shallow breathing. These symptoms resolve dramatically after a placebo injection.

III. Trivial Poisoning

In the most trivial cases of poisoning, there are no symptoms or signs, but the serum aspartate aminotransferase levels are significantly raised for 1–3 days. In other trivial cases, myalgic features start from $^1/_2$–$3^1/_2$ h after the bite with muscle aches, pains, and stiffness on movement in the neck, throat, tongue, shoulders, trunk, or limbs. Occasionally, these myalgic symptoms have been preceded by giddiness, a dry feeling in the throat, vomiting, or general weakness. In about half the trivial cases, the aching stiffness remains confined to one region, such as the neck, shoulders, and so on; in the others, it becomes generalized within $^1/_2$ h of starting. But myalgia in trivial cases is never severe. Examination 1–4 h after the bite reveals moderate pain on passive movement of arm, thigh, neck, or trunk muscles. These myalgic features resolve completely, without antivenom, in 1–3 days. No objective neurologic abnormalities develop, and the electrocardiogram remains normal.

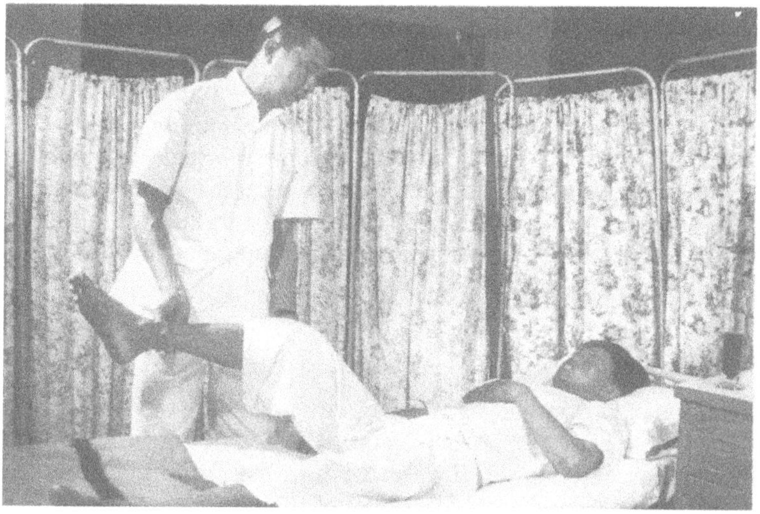

Fig. 3. In sea snakebite poisoning, generalized muscle movement pains start within $\frac{1}{2}$–3 h of the bite. Passive movement of neck, trunk, and limbs—bending as here—becomes very painful. It is a useful clinical diagnostic procedure in determining envenoming

IV. Serious Poisoning

In serious poisoning, the latent period between the bite and the onset of poisoning symptoms never exceeded 2 h, though this would not necessarily have applied if the victim had put on an effective tourniquet immediately after the bite and kept it on. Myalgic symptoms start as in trivial poisoning except that they begin sooner; other early features include headache, a thick feeling of the tongue, constant thirst, episodic sweating, and vomiting. The aching stiffness becomes generalized within $\frac{1}{2}$ h and then the severity increases. Swallowing and speaking become more and more difficult. On examination 1–2 h after the bite, the patient lies in bed with arms flexed and the legs extended. Passive movement of arm, thigh, neck, and trunk muscles is moderately or severely painful (Fig. 3). Muscles may be tender on pressure such as squeezing a limb, but this feature, unlike pain with passive movement, is often absent or unimpressive. At this early stage, neurologic examination, including power and tendon reflexes, is usually normal. The patient is unable (or unwilling owing to the pain entailed) to sit up unaided or to open the mouth fully. In rare cases, the patient has denied muscle pains and stiffness, complaining only of weakness, but on examination passive movement is painful. Myoglobinuria becomes evident on inspection 3–8 h after the bite, first as a dusky yellow color with positive protein tests and then (within the next $\frac{1}{2}$ h) as a red, brown, or black discoloration. In most cases of serious poisoning, the blood pressure on admission is normal. Hypertension on admission is often due to fright but this quickly resolves. When early hypertension is sustained, it may be secondary to nephrotoxic effects. Usually hypertension is a late development of asphyxial origin.

After some hours, true paresis of peripheral type may ensue, and later still, tendon reflexes become depressed, then absent. The paresis becomes flaccid; ptosis, ophthalmoplegia, inability to protrude the tongue or swallow, "broken neck syndrome" (from paresis of neck muscles), and inability to sit up result. But even at a late stage in some patients, active limb movement may be notably preserved. Ptosis may be mistaken for drowsiness; however, the patient is usually mentally alert until respiratory failure is far advanced. There is no clinical evidence of cerebral, cerebellar, or extrapyramidal involvement and sphincter disturbance is unusual. In serious poisoning, the temperature may remain normal throughout the illness but in about half the cases it is slightly raised to 37.5–39° C.

V. Fatal Poisoning

The combination of glossopharyngeal palsy with inhalation of vomit or secretions or both can precipitate early respiratory failure which, if not dealt with promptly, can be rapidly fatal, as early as $2^1/_2$ h after the bite. Respiratory failure from muscle weakness may supervene within a few hours of the bite, or as long as 60 h after the bite. Breathing becomes shallow, the blood pressure rises, and there is increased sweating. The subject becomes drowsy, then comatose. Pupils dilate and their reaction to light fails shortly before death. Other patients succumb from hyperkalemic cardiac arrest or (later) from acute renal failure. Most victims dying do so 12–24 h after the bite. The most rapid death recorded is $2^1/_2$ h after the bite (FITZSIMONS, 1912); the longest period between bite and death is 24 days (KARUNARATNE and PANABOKKE, 1972). In 50 fatal cases (not receiving effective antivenom), 13 died $2^1/_2$–8 h after the bite, 23 died 12–24 h after the bite, and 14 deaths occurred 2 or more days after the bite. Death 48 h or more after the bite is usually due to acute renal failure.

D. Diagnosis

The clinician has to answer two main questions; namely, is it a sea snakebite, and, more important, is there significant poisoning? Fish stings are much more common than sea snakebites, especially among bathers. Severe local pain follows; its presence excludes the possibility of a sea snakebite, which, after the initial prick, is painless. The appearance of the fang and teeth marks at the site of the bite is of little diagnostic help—one or more circular dots as though made by a hypodermic needle. There is no local swelling—unless it is caused by a tight tourniquet. Sometimes there are just a few scratch marks. The inconspicuous local features of a sea snakebite can be deceptive. In one patient, the doctor thought "... it could not be a sea snakebite since there were no fang marks." This led to a fatal delay in admitting the patient. Fangs and teeth may break off and remain embedded in the skin. Fishermen quite often draw a hair over the site to extract teeth, thereby confirming that a bite has been made. But personally, I never found this succeeded by the time the patient reached a hospital. A sea snakebite may be diagnosed when the opportunity for contact with a sea snake has been clearly established, by absence of pain, and by marks compatible with those made by sea snake fangs.

Significant envenoming is shown by the history of myalgic pains and "weakness"; examination 1–2 h after the bite reveals moderate or severe pain on passively moving the patient's arm, thigh, trunk, or neck muscles. Proteinuria, followed by red-brown color indicating myoglobinuria, and a neutrophil leucocytosis confirm the diagnosis of serious poisoning. A high SGOT is a sensitive sign of envenoming, but it is unlikely the result would be received in time to influence treatment (and it is raised even in trivial poisoning).

If a patient should come to a doctor within 1 h of being bitten, before symptoms of poisoning might have started (an uncommon event), judgment must be reserved. But if 2 h have elapsed since the bite and there are no "remote" pains on muscle movement, serious poisoning can be excluded. The only exception to this "2-h clearance" rule would be when a victim has applied an effective tourniquet within a minute or so of the bite and has kept it on until he reaches medical aid.

E. Prognosis

Multiple bite marks suggest a high venom dose, though single marks do not necessarily indicate a small dose. Vomiting, ptosis, weakness of external eye muscles, dilation of pupils with a sluggish light reaction, and a leukocytosis exceeding 20000/mm^3 are all sinister signs. The remaining early clinical features are equally common in patients who subsequently recover (without antivenom), but the tempo is quicker in the potentially fatal cases—a matter of hours rather than days (Fig. 4). Signs of respiratory insufficiency with hypertension and cyanosis indicate the end is near. Serial ECG records are the most practical means of revealing hyperkalemia for prognostic and therapeutic purposes. Tall, peaked T waves in chest leads V 2, V 3, and V 4 are a danger sign. After the first 3 or 4 days following the bite, renal failure is the chief hazard and may cause death with remarkably few warning symptoms. A "fixed" specific gravity of 1.010–1.013 together with a low urine volume output, and progressively rising blood urea, indicate the need for urgent treatment.

In severe poisoning, when the patient has not received effective antivenom, recovery may take up to 6 months (REID, 1961a). Myalgia and myoglobinuria reach a peak during the 1st week and recede early in the 2nd week. Paresis becomes more complete during this week. Improvement in power starts slowly during the 3rd week. Tendon reflexes return during the 3rd or 4th week. The patient is now able to lift his head off the bed and sits up by rolling onto his side and helping himself up with his arms. For the next month, the clinical resemblance to muscular dystrophy is striking—the patient "climbs up himself." During the following few months, hand grip, "press ups," and sitting up spontaneously from the lying position slowly return to normal. The best guide to the rate of recovery is the duration of myoglobinuria—each day myoglobin is visible on inspecting the urine means approximately 1 week of illness. Full recovery occurs in 3–4 weeks in moderate cases; within a few days in trivial poisoning.

Permanent renal damage can result from sea snakebite poisoning and some muscle weakness has still been detectable 1½ years after the bite. But none of those long-term effects should occur if the patient receives effective antivenom treatment. No evidence of long-term liver damage has been found.

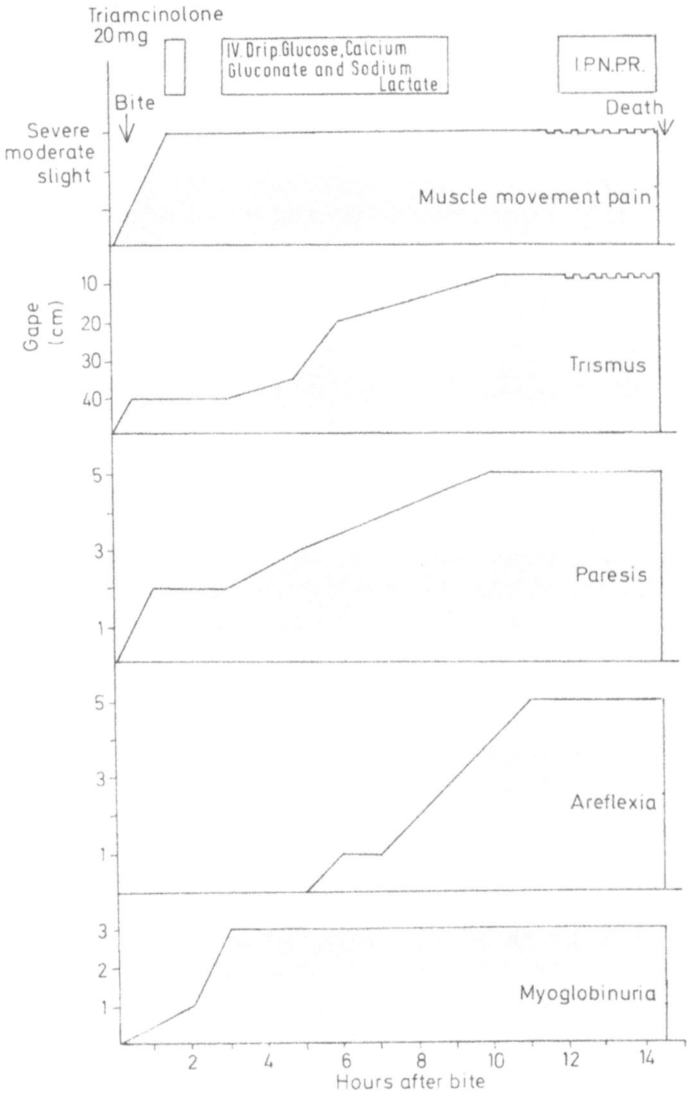

Fig. 4. Clinical course to death before sea snake antivenom was available. Paresis follows muscle-movement pains; death occurred despite adequate artificial respiration. I.P.N.P.R. = Intermittent positive/negative-pressure artificial respiration. Paresis: 5 = respiratory failure, 4 = unable to lift one or more limbs, 3 = unable to lift head, 2 = unable to sit up spontaneously, 1 = objective weakness less than 2. Areflexia: 5 = 7–8 tendon reflexes absent, 4 = 5–6 absent, 3 = 3–4 absent, 2 = 1–2 absent, 1 = present but weak. Myoglobinuria; 3 = dark brown, red, or black, spectroscopically positive, 2 = light brown or dark yellow, spectroscopically positive, 1 = benzidine-positive, spectroscopically negative

F. Pathology

I. Clinical Pathology

In trivial poisoning, the white blood cell count is normal, but in serious poisoning, moderate neutrophil leukocytosis is usual. The degree and duration of the neutrophil leukocytosis correlate approximately with the severity of the toxemia. In fatal cases, the leukocytosis usually exceeds 20000/mm^3. Serial (differential) leukocyte counts are, therefore, important in monitoring patients with sea snakebite poisoning, although the neutrophils do not start rising until several hours after myalgic poisoning symptoms begin. And I have seen fatal poisoning with a white blood cell count of only 12600/mm^3. In severe envenoming not treated by effective antivenom, the neutrophil leukocytosis continues for 1–2 weeks. Eosinophils have not been increased. No evidence of abnormal hemolysis or coagulation defect has been found. Reticulocytes, platelets, saline fragility of red blood cells, serum bilirubin, urinary urobilinogen, bleeding time, coagulation time, one-stage prothrombin time, direct Coombs, Schumm's, Donath-Landsteiner, and Kahn tests were always normal.

In trivial poisoning, the urine is often positive for protein on the 1st day but negative for myoglobin. Heavy proteinuria, numerous granular casts, and some erythrocytes in early urine specimens indicate serious kidney damage. Myoglobinuria is an important sign of serious poisoning. It is easily overlooked or mistaken for hemoglobinuria. The simplest distinction is observation of the plasma color which is normal with myoglobinuria (because the myoglobin molecule is much smaller than hemoglobin and is rapidly excreted); with hemoglobinuria the plasma is pink or red during the phase of acute hemolysis. Other confirmatory tests of myoglobinuria include spectroscopy (preferably after conversion to carboxymyoglobin), electrophoretic mobility (WHISHNANT et al., 1959), and immunoassay (FARMER et al., 1961). The most sensitive test of sea snake envenoming is the serum aspartate aminotransferase (SGOT). The marked elevation of SGOT is due to release of the enzyme from damaged skeletal muscle, and similar changes have been recorded in idiopathic myoglobinuria (PEARSON et al., 1957). SGOT has been grossly raised in patients with no myalgic symptoms and no abnormal clinical signs; it is thus a very sensitive confirmatory test of sea snakebite poisoning, but the level does not necessarily reflect the severity of the lesions. The serum alanine aminotransferase may also be raised if there is liver dysfunction (REID, 1962). Lumbar puncture has revealed normal cerebrospinal fluid.

Plasma urea, creatinine, and potassium are usually raised in severe poisoning, and become progressively raised in the terminal stages of fatal cases. The electrocardiogram (ECG) is particularly useful for detecting and monitoring hyperkalemia. Apart from the changes due to hyperkalemia, ECG abnormalities, especially in the right chest leads, are common in severe sea snakebite poisoning (REID, 1961a), although clinical, radiologic, and pathologic evidence of direct cardiovascular damage is conspicuously absent.

II. Pathophysiology in Experimental Animals

When I investigated the rate of absorption of *E. schistosa* venom in dogs whose tails were bitten by adult specimens of *E. schistosa* (bites involving strong jaw contractions and in all cases resulting in fang marks), I found, by amputating the tail at intervals timed by a stopwatch, that a lethal dose could be absorbed within 3 min or less (REID, 1956a). I also observed that sea snakes may bite without injecting any significant amounts of venom even when immediate subsequent milking confirmed the presence of more than enough venom to kill the dogs.

In animals, ROGERS (1902, 1903), FRASER and ELLIOT (1905), KELLAWAY et al. (1932), CAREY and WRIGHT (1960, 1961), and CHEYMOL et al. (1967) considered that sea snake venom was "neurotoxic" acting mainly at the neuromuscular junction. CHEYMOL et al. (1967) investigated the venoms of *E. schistosa*, *H. cyanocinctus*, and *L. hardwickii*. Paralysis in preparations from rats, cats, and frogs was peripheral. Nerve fibers did not seem to be affected and muscle fibers were not directly blocked. Specific receptors of the postsynaptic membrane were blocked almost irreversibly. A synergistic action with D-tubocurarine was demonstrated, but neostigmine did not antagonize the paralytic action of the venoms. In doses capable of paralyzing skeletal muscle, the venoms did not affect cardiac contractions in isolated heart preparations from rats and frogs. The authors considered that the action of sea snake venom is practically identic to that of cobra venoms. LAMB and HUNTER (1907) injected *E. schistosa* venom subcutaneously into five monkeys and described degenerative changes in the central nervous system and peripheral nerves. ROGERS (1902), NAUCK (1929), and CAREY and WRIGHT (1960) found little at necropsy. In a later publication, CAREY and WRIGHT (1961) reported a direct myotoxic action following injection of *E. schistosa* venom into the femoral artery of rabbits. In 1959, I injected 0.1 mg *E. schistosa* venom per kg body weight subcutaneously into two dogs. Two further dogs received the equivalent of 0.04 mg dried *E. schistosa* venom per kg body weight. All four dogs died 1–4 h later; at necropsy, necrosis was evident in 33–75% of the skeletal muscle fibers from each of eight regions examined (REID, 1975c). Experimental work on biochemistry and pharmacology of sea snake venoms has been recently reviewed by LEE (1972), TU (1973), CAMPBELL (1975), and TAMIYA (1975).

III. Pathophysiology in Man

The clinical paradox of trismus yet flaccid paresis elsewhere originally stimulated my investigations of sea snakebite (REID, 1956a). The medical literature then available indicated that sea snake venom was "neurotoxic" and therefore in two of my fatal cases, tissues of the nervous system were referred to a neuropathologist. No histologic abnormality was found; at this stage, skeletal muscle was not examined. Experimentally, sea snake venom had been reported as only feebly hemolytic; theoretically, a dose of venom sufficient to cause hemoglobinuria should inevitably be fatal. Yet I knew of patients surviving despite apparent "hemoglobinuria." These anomalies were resolved in 1957 when I realized that the urinary pigment was myoglobin from muscle and not hemoglobin (REID, 1961a). This clarified many of the clinical features, and complementary to the clinical studies, we found the chief pathologic lesions of sea snakebite poisoning in man were in skeletal muscle, kidney, and liver (MARSDEN and REID, 1961).

In necropsy studies of seven fatal cases and biopsy studies of a patient with very severe nonfatal poisoning, macroscopic changes were deceptively absent, apart from brown or black urine in the bladder. In particular, the color and consistency of

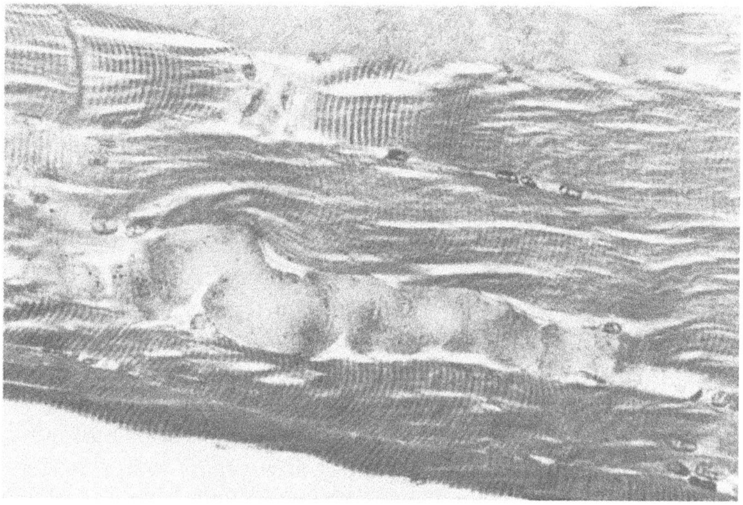

Fig. 5. Sea snake venom is primarily myotoxic in man. Skeletal muscle biopsy from a patient with severe poisoning shows necrotic fibers which are pale and have no striations. Other fibers retain striations and are apparently healthy

skeletal muscles were normal. But histologically, there were widespread hyaline necroses in skeletal muscles. The toxin picks out individual muscle fibers, leaving a healthy fiber next to a necrosed one and affects only one or more segments of varying length in a fiber, usually with an abrupt transition to normal muscle. The number of fibers with focal necroses varies from muscle to muscle; in the same patient there may be necroses in 20% or less of the fibers of one muscle while in another muscle, every fiber shows necroses. The affected segment of a muscle fiber first becomes greatly swollen and the sarcoplasm undergoes coagulation necrosis. At this stage, the nuclei and swollen myofibrils can still be distinguished, but the disks of the myofibrils soon lose their differential staining, and both nuclei and myofibrils disappear as they become fused into an amorphous hyaline mass (Fig. 5). This necrotic material contracts, leaving an empty space beneath the sarcolemma, which remains intact although it may slightly collapse. Necrotic segments stain more intensely with acid dyes, but this is not conspicuous in routine sections and could easily be overlooked by casual or inexperienced observation. The myonecroses become very obvious with special stains.

Soluble products, notably myoglobin, enzymes, and electrolytes, are rapidly absorbed into the blood stream. Insoluble necrotic fragments are phagocytosed by histiocytes and macrophages. Regeneration and repair begin 1–2 weeks after the bite with multiplication of surviving muscle nuclei. The muscle fiber is thus regenerated within its original sarcolemmal sheath and repair is remarkably complete, probably because very few muscle fibers are entirely necrosed. Biopsy 6 months after the bite showed only a little fine scarring.

Renal damage often results from sea snake envenoming as with other types of myonecrosis and other types of envenoming. Distal tubular necrosis was found in all three patients dying more than 48 h after the bite. There is extensive necrosis of the epithelium of the loop of Henle, the second convoluted tubule, and the collecting tubules. Desquamated cells with granular and amorphous debris fill the lumen and form casts in the distal and collecting tubules. Pigment giving a positive benzidine reaction is deposited in most of the cases and even in some of the desquamated cells. The boundary zone is still intensely congested and the interstitial tissue is now edematous, as well as showing both a diffuse and a focal cellular infiltration.

The reactionary or healing stage is not often seen because victims usually die too quickly. Our only example was a patient who died 12 days after the bite. There may be considerable proliferation of the capsular cells of the glomeruli, presumably a reaction to the excreted myoglobin or its breakdown products. The first convoluted tubules appear normal, but, from the loop of Henle downward, degenerating and regenerating epithelial cells crowd into the lumen, while some of the collecting tubules and excretory ducts are filled with a mass of proliferating cells. The interstitial tissue of the boundary zone and medulla is still edematous and infiltrated with plasma cells, lymphocytes, and histiocytes but now begins to appear more fibrous. SITPRIJA et al. (1971) studied two patients with severe poisoning and renal failure. In both patients, biopsies confirmed necrosis in the kidney tubules and in skeletal muscles.

In the liver there are no specific changes, but there is usually a centrilobular degeneration with a round or mixed-cell infiltration of the portal areas. The lungs showed patchy edema, small areas of collapse with compensatory emphysema, and early inflammatory changes in some bronchi were evident, but in no case did it appear likely that the lesions would play an important part in the clinical picture. In cardiac and smooth muscle, no significant lesions have been found.

Apart from the above pathologic studies in man, the following clinical observations strongly suggest in my opinion that sea snake venom in man is primarily myotoxic rather than neurotoxic:

1. Muscle-movement pains may precede objective paresis by 3–24 h.

2. Initially, much of the paresis is apparent rather than real. The patient may say that he is unable to move his limbs when objectively limb power is normal—the patient is unwilling to move the limbs himself because this is painful.

3. Similarly, the difficulty in opening the mouth is really pseudotrismus. It differs strikingly from the true trismus of tetanus which is neurogenic. Sustained pressure on the lower jaw does not increase the gape in tetanus at all, but will do so in sea snake envenoming (though this is very painful for the patient). Secondly, the jaw jerk is very brisk in tetanus, but becomes sluggish or absent in sea snakebite poisoning.

4. No muscle fibrillation or fasciculation is seen.

5. There is no qualitative change in response to faradic and galvanic stimulation—this is typical of a myopathic lesion (WALTON and ADAMS, 1958). Electromyograms in a patient with severe poisoning also indicated a myopathic disturbance (SITPRIJA et al., 1971).

6. Myoglobinuria appears before paresis and occurs in minimal poisoning, with no paresis.

7. Neostigmine is ineffective in "unblocking" myoneural junctions (see Sect. G.II.a).

8. Without antivenom, natural recovery following severe sea snakebite poisoning is slow (months), whereas it is rapid (days) in neurotoxic elapid poisoning.

9. SGOT is greatly raised in minimal poisoning with no myalgia or paresis; SGOT levels are normal in severe neurotoxic poisoning by Malayan cobra bite.

Myonecrosis can explain the generalized muscle movement pains, hyperkalemia, myoglobinuria, and much of the paresis in severe sea snakebite poisoning. Hyperkalemia, uremia, and other factors may also contribute to the paresis since SITPRIJA et al. (1971) found that hemodialysis produced a rapid improvement of the muscular activity. It is probable that sea snake venom attacks the cell membrane of skeletal muscle directly in human victims. But the patchy distribution of visible damage to skeletal muscles and the absence of lesions in cardiac and smooth muscle are not explained—except that it is increasingly apparent that venoms can be very highly specific in their biologic actions; hence their great value as research tools. In victims dying more than 48 h after the bite, acute renal failure appeared to be the immediate cause of death. Experimentally, BYWATERS and STEAD (1944) showed that myoglobin injected into healthy rabbits caused no renal damage unless the urine was acidified. It is, therefore, unlikely that the myoglobin released in sea snake poisoning is solely responsible for the renal lesions. Is the venom nephrotoxic? REID and JENKINS (1948) showed that cobra venom acted directly on the kidney of eviscerated adrenalectomized cats, causing liberation of renin. Early sustained hypertension was observed in two cases; progressive hyperkalemia was the immediate cause of death in another two patients. Renal damage may be mainly responsible for these two features—a renal pressor factor leading to hypertension while progressive hyperkalemia arose because diminished renal excretion failed to cope with the extra load from cellular release of potassium.

There is, thus, a great challenge to pharmacologists to resolve the anomaly of the actions of sea snake venoms—their "neurotoxic" action in experimental animals and their "myotoxic" action in man. It is easy for the clinician to overlook myoglobinuria or to mistake it for hemoglobinuria or even hematuria. In 1960, on the basis of reported clinical features, I suggested that venom of land snakes, such as the tiger snake, *Notechis scutatus*, might be myotoxic in man (REID, 1960). HOOD and JOHNSON (1975) confirmed myoglobinuria and renal failure after *N. scutatus* bite. Experimentally in rats, HARRIS et al. (1975) reported that notexin, a purified basic toxin derived from *N. scutatus* venom, had a direct myotoxic effect which preferentially damaged mitochondria-rich skeletal muscle fibers. It is also notable that *N. scutatus* antivenom is highly effective against sea snake venoms (see Sect. G.II.b). Recently, a phospholipase fraction of *E. schistosa* venom has been reported as myotoxic in guinea pigs (GEH and TOH, 1976) and in mice (FOHLMAN and EAKER, 1976). Could these venoms in man cause mitochondrial calcium overload leading to muscle-cell necrosis as suggested by WROGEMANN and PENA (1976) for a wide variety of muscle diseases?

G. Treatment

I. First-Aid Measures

First-aid comprises the measures taken by the victim or associates before receiving medical treatment. A firm ligature should be applied at the base of the toe or finger, or, if the bite is higher up, around the thigh or arm. The purpose of the ligature is to compress the underlying tissues and thus delay absorption of venom *if* venom has been injected (as will be seen from the above, this is an unlikely event, but there is no reliable way of knowing shortly after the bite whether venom has in fact been injected or not). The tourniquet should not be so tight that the arterial pulses are obliterated, and it should be left on until the patient reaches medical aid. If the victim is able to reach a hospital or a medical center holding effective antivenom within an hour, there is no point in applying a tourniquet. Incision and suction are ineffective and not recommended. The victim should go to a hospital as quickly as possible. Experimentally, muscle movements entailed by walking and so on can accelerate absorption of venom (again, *if* venom is injected). Because of this, some writers have advised that all exertion must be avoided. Such advice, in my opinion, is ill-founded because it is quite impracticable, and if attempted would be highly likely to increase emotional reactions of fear. Experiments have also shown that amputation of a bitten part, if performed within 3 min of a bite, could effectively prevent poisoning. It might be possible to do this in the case of a toe or finger bite, but almost certainly the toe or finger would be sacrificed unnecessarily.

On the rare occasions the sea snake has been killed, it should be taken to a hospital. Otherwise, no attempt should be made to recover the sea snake; I know of three instances when associates of the victim tried to catch the sea snake and another bite resulted.

Antivenom should play no part in first-aid treatment. It is strictly medical treatment and if wrongly used can be more dangerous than the sea snakebite. Antivenom is only needed in a small proportion of sea snakebites and to be effective has to be given by intravenous infusion under expert medical supervision. The only exception to this important matter might be a sophisticated expedition with no hospital available within 5–6 h of the bite. Provided the expedition included a doctor or a medical assistant especially trained in the administration of antivenom, it might be sensible to carry antivenom. But in this event, antivenom administration would constitute a medical and not a first-aid procedure.

II. Medical Treatment

1. Supportive Treatment

It is important not to panic. In virtually every case, there will be abundant time to administer antivenom effectively *if* it is indicated; on the other hand, one should never dismiss a case of possible sea snakebite as trivial without proper observation. When first seen by a doctor, many patients with sea snakebite will pass the "2-h clearance test," having no myalgia etc (see Sect. D), and thus require only reassurance which is best achieved by a prompt injection of a placebo. Any ligature that has been applied should be released. If the doctor has any doubt about poisoning subsequently developing (for example, if the victim has presented very shortly after the bite, or has applied a tourniquet which could delay absorption of venom), the patient should be detained for several hours and carefully observed for signs of poisoning. The following observations should be charted frequently: 1) myalgic pains on active movement by the patient or pains on passive movement by the doctor, 2) ptosis, dysphagia, dysphonia, vomiting, 3) blood pressure, respiration rate, neutrophil leukocyte count, 4) urine color, protein, myoglobin, 5) serum creatinine phosphokinase or aspartate aminotransferase, and 6) electrocardiogram.

If signs of poisoning develop, or are already present when the patient is first seen, then antivenom is indicated. If symptoms do not develop within a few hours, the patient can be discharged.

As soon as significant toxemia is apparent (see Sect. C, D, E), antivenom should be given and general supportive measures adopted. Removal of sea snake venom from the site of the bite by incision, suction, and so on, would not be effective as hospital treatment. It is not known whether appreciable venom is excreted by the kidneys in man. When I injected into animals urine from patients with severe sea snake envenoming, the results were equivocal, although some animals died suggesting renal excretion of venom. It is, therefore, rational to promote a diuresis, both to encourage excretion of venom and secondary toxic products and to minimize renal damage. The patient should drink a liter of water as quickly as possible or be given a rapid intravenous infusion of a liter of a mixture of 25% glucose, 10% calcium gluconate, and molar sodium lactate. Postural treatment is vital to prevent inhalation of vomit or secretions, or both; the patient should be kept off his back so that gravity will assist tracheal drainage of chest secretions; infection and lung collapse are thus prevented. Physical rest is important in severe poisoning to avoid tearing the fragile sarcolemmal sheaths which normally guide the regenerating muscle fibers. I used to give steroid therapy as a nonspecific antitoxemic drug, as a muscle strengthener, and as a means of increasing potassium excretion by the kidneys (REID, 1961 b), but this was before effective antivenom became available. In practice, it was not notably successful, and I would no longer recommend its use except for delayed antivenom reactions. I also tried neostigmine in five patients in the hope that it might "unblock" the myoneural junctions; no discernible improvement resulted. Tracheostomy and artificial respiration may still be needed if patients present themselves late and are already in respiratory failure. But this supportive measure should no longer be needed provided effective antivenom can be given in an adequate dose. Hyperkalemia sometimes improves with insulin, and if this does not succeed in shifting the potassium back into the cells, a potassium-removing ion-exchange resin should be given by gastric tube. In this type of case, where the ECG shows the tall, peaked T waves of hyperkalemia, hemodialysis can be dramatically successful (SITPRIJA et al., 1971). Peritoneal dialysis has also been tried (KARUNARATNE and PANABOKKE, 1972); the patient improved temporarily but eventually died 24 days after the bite. However, the dialysis was not started until 10 days after the bite and was done under adverse conditions. Effective antivenom was not available for these patients.

2. Antivenom

Specific antivenom is the most important therapeutic agent available for the effective treatment of systemic snakebite poisoning. If it is used correctly, it can be effective even though it is not given until hours, or sometimes days after the bite.

The two main disadvantages of antivenom are cost and adverse reactions. Adequate antivenom treatment is expensive, and this is particularly important in those parts of the world where snakebite is a major medical problem, in the developing areas of the tropics. Five ampules of sea snake antivenom, which may be needed for adequate treatment of a patient with severe sea snake envenoming, may cost the equivalent of 700 US dollars. With unrefined antivenom, the overall incidence of adverse serum reactions is about 30%. Severe immediate reactions are, of course, less common, perhaps about 3%. Three therapeutic antivenoms have been shown to be effective for sea snakebite poisoning—*Enhydrina schistosa* antivenom (REID, 1962; 1975b) and *Notechis scutatus* (tiger snake) antivenom from the Commonwealth Serum Laboratories, Melbourne, Australia, and *Lapemis hardwickii* antivenom made in Vietnam (BARME et al., 1962). The latter antivenom is no longer available. The two Australian antivenoms are available commercially and both are refined so that adverse serum reactions are much less likely to occur than with unrefined antivenoms. Nevertheless, anaphylactic reactions can occur and may be fatal (REID, 1957; LANCET, 1957). In other words, antivenom can be lethal.

We have already seen that only a small minority of human beings bitten by sea snake do in fact develop poisoning (less than one-third of the patients coming to Penang Hospital in 1962–1964). It should, therefore, be obvious that at least two-thirds do *not* require antivenom. And yet the idea unfortunately still persists for many people, including doctors, that antivenom should automatically be injected in every single case of sea snakebite, or even in cases where sea snakebite is merely suspected. Indiscriminate use of sea snake (or other) antivenom can easily bring it into disrepute, firstly by unnecessarily increasing the number of serum reactions, secondly, by encouraging inadequate dosage in the few patients who really could benefit from antivenom, and thirdly, by the unnecessary, even harmful, waste of money.

A controlled trial of specific antivenom in patients with Malayan pit viper envenoming showed highly significant benefit in systemic poisoning (REID et al., 1963). Disappointingly, the antivenom did not appear to benefit the local effects of envenoming, especially local necrosis. In land snakebite, the adequate treatment of local necrosis remains a major problem. In the trial, the antivenom was given by intramuscular injection; recent work suggests that intravenously infused antivenom can prevent or lessen local necrosis, if given soon after the bite. Fortunately, this problem does not arise in sea snakebites because local effects are negligible. Thus, the only indication for giving effective antivenom in sea snakebites is *clinically evident systemic poisoning.*

The first refined therapeutic sea snake antivenom to be made has been produced at the Commonwealth Serum Laboratories (CSL) by hyperimmunizing horses with *E. schistosa* venom supplied from the Snake and Venom Research Institute, Penang. Hyperimmunization is carried out by a series of injections of increasing doses of *E. schistosa* venom over a period of 2–6 months, followed by maintenance "booster" doses. The horse develops immunity and its serum is removed and purified—a process for separating the antitoxic immunoglobulins from unwanted proteins. The incidence of allergic reactions in human beings is thus reduced from 30% (with unpurified antivenom) to about 10%. The CSL sea snake antivenom is in liquid form, each ampule containing 1000 units (sufficient to neutralize 10 mg *E. schistosa* by in vitro tests). The volume may vary but is usually 36 ml per ampule. If it is kept in an ordinary refrigerator at 4° C, loss of potency is negligible, even though the ampule is marked with a 2-year "expiry date" (stored at 4–15° C, loss of potency is under 3% p.a., at 20° C under 5% p.a., at 37° C, 10–20% p.a.). It should, therefore, be realized

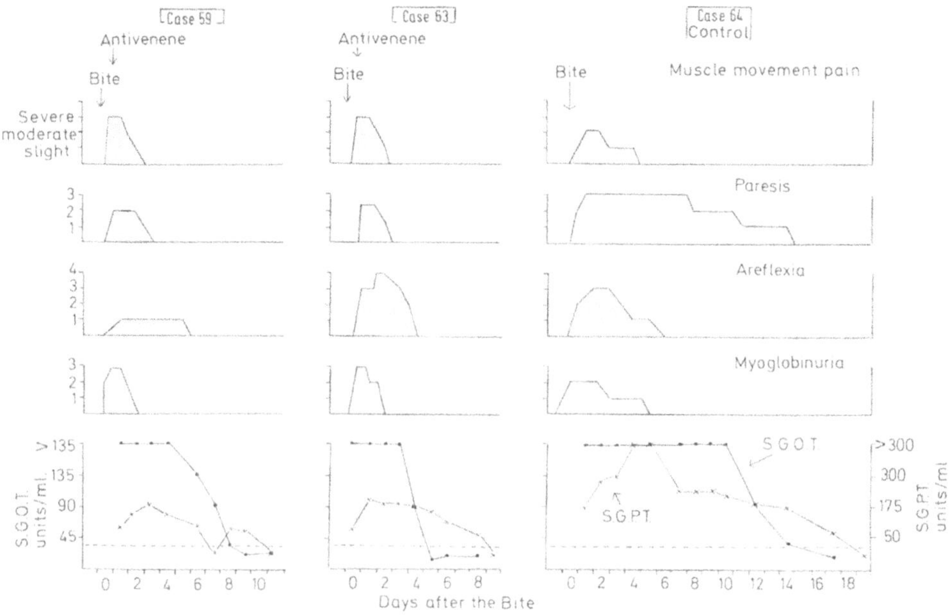

Fig. 6. Rapid recovery after administration of sea snake antivenom in two severely poisoned patients (Cases 59 and 63 in Table 7). Recovery in Case 64 with only moderate poisoning and no antivenom (because supply was very restricted) was by comparison much delayed. Notation as in Figure 4

that antivenom does not become useless immediately after the expiration date (CHRISTENSEN, 1975). Provided the solution is clear on inspection, it is safe to use, but if it has become cloudy or opaque, the antivenom should be discarded since the neutralizing potency will be reduced and there will be a much greater danger of unwanted reactions.

Shortly after I first received this CSL sea snake antivenom in Penang, I was able to use it to treat two victims with severe poisoning (REID, 1962). In at least one of them (Fig. 6), the poisoning was likely—by comparison with previous cases—to have been fatal. Without antivenom, severely poisoned victims have invariably taken weeks or months to recover (REID, 1961 a). The improvement following antivenom in these two subjects was by comparison dramatic; clinical recovery took only 6 days and 3 days, respectively. A third patient seen at this time with moderate poisoning was not given antivenom because the supply was then so severely restricted. He took 2 weeks to recover. During 1962 to early 1964, I treated ten patients with serious sea snake envenoming by the CSL sea snake antivenom (REID, 1975 b). Seven received either 1000 or 2000 units and responded dramatically, recovering completely in a few days (Table 7). One patient was admitted moribund 45 h after the bite. The delay in admission was mainly due to a doctor dismissing the possibility of sea snakebite because he could not make out definite fang marks. The patient received 2000 units of antivenom (the total stock at that time), and temporarily improved, but he died 59 h after the bite. Another patient, admitted 8 h after the bite in advanced poisoning,

Table 7. Clinical course in serious poisoning before and after antivenom became available

Patient				Snake	Course			Recovery time (days)		*Antivenom Dose (units)*
Case No.	Age (years)	Bather (B) or Fisherman (F)	Where bitten	Species of snake	Bite/myalgia interval (min)	Bite/hospital admission interval (h)	Bite/death interval (h)	Clinical	SGOT	
1957–1961 (Antivenom not available)										
6	17	B	Leg	—	60	$1^1/_4$	—	180	—	
7	11	B	Foot	—	60	99	—	90	—	
8	21	B	Foot	—	60	24	—	30	—	
9	44	F	Leg	*E. sch.*	60	1	—	30	—	
52	20	F	Foot	*H. cy.*	90	96	—	12	14	
1	32	B	Leg	*E. sch.*	35	$^1/_2$	13	—	—	
2	10	B	Foot	—	40	$^3/_4$	$14^1/_2$	—	—	
3	50	F	Foot	*E. sch.*	60	36	52	—	—	
4	41	F	Hand	*E. sch.*	35	12	$18^1/_2$	—	—	
5	17	F	Finger	*E. sch.*	60	$6^1/_4$	$14^1/_2$	—	—	
56	7	B	Leg	*E. sch.*	90	$7^1/_4$	$7^1/_2$	—	—	
1962–1964 (Antivenom available)										
64	16	F	Thumb	*E. sch.*	90	4	—	15	14	Nil
59	16	F	Foot	—	30	$3^1/_2$	—	6	8	1000
63	8	B	Leg	—	60	7	—	4	5	1000
70	10	B	Arm	*E. sch.*	60	45	59	—	—	2000
81	28	F	Leg	—	60	$4^1/_2$	—	1	3	1000
83	13	B	Leg	—	90	3	—	1	6	1000
87	17	F	Foot	*E. sch.*	120	7	—	4	4	1000
94	11	B	Leg	*E. sch.*	120	6	—	2	5	2000
95	16	F	Leg	*E. sch.*	60	3	—	4	3	2000
96	29	F	Finger	*E. sch.*	60	8	19	—	—	5000
99	9	B	Leg	—	30	47	—	25	13	5000

E. sch. = *Enhydrina schistosa*.
H. cy. = *Hydrophis cyanocinctus*.

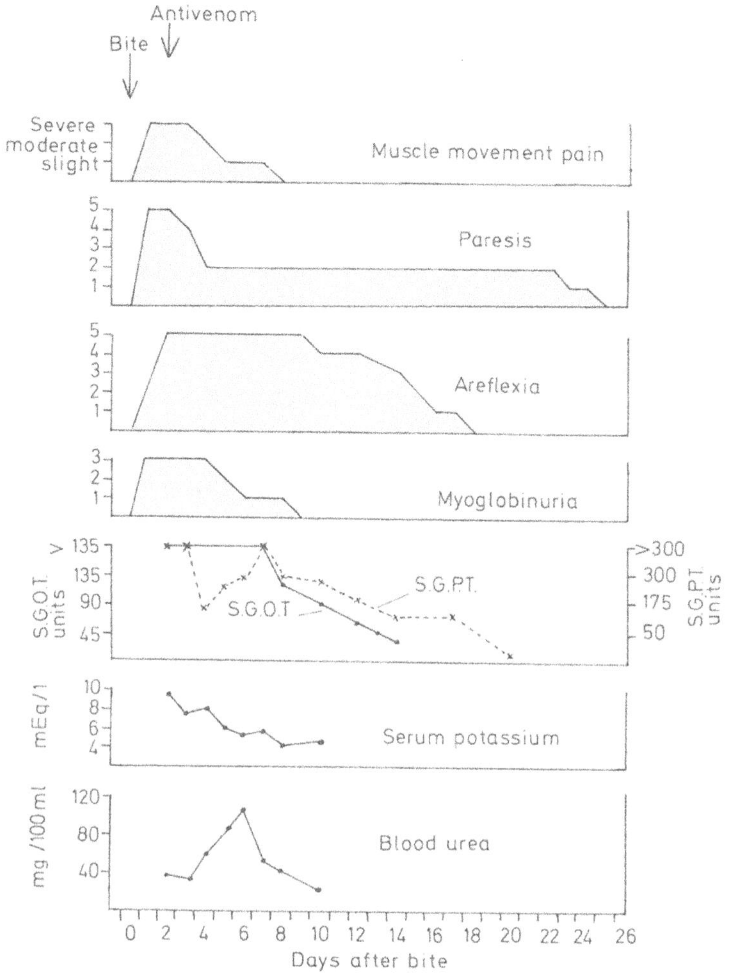

Fig. 7. Recovery in Case 99 even though the patient delayed admission so that antivenom was not started until 47 h after the bite when poisoning seemed very likely to be fatal. Notation as in Figure 4

received 5000 units of antivenom and greatly improved so far as the myotoxic signs were concerned. But he developed increasing hyperkalemia which did not respond to insulin and he died 19 h after the bite. The tenth patient was admitted with severe poisoning 46 h after the bite. He was given 5000 units of antivenom. He steadily improved and had fully recovered 25 days after the bite (Fig. 7). In all 10 cases, the antivenom was given solely by intravenous infusion. A mild urticarial skin eruption occurred in four patients but quickly responded to antihistamine treatment. No hypotensive serum reactions occurred. If more antivenom had been available, it is likely that these two deaths would have been prevented and the recovery of the tenth patient would have been expedited.

One of the most important aspects of these cases is the fact that antivenom was successful although not given until up to 2 days after the bite (the earliest it was given was 3 h after the bite). It is, therefore, not only safe but very desirable to wait until there is clear evidence of poisoning before giving sea snake antivenom. In the minority needing antivenom, the intravenous route is mandatory. It is much more effective than other parenteral routes; it is also safer because, if serum reactions occur, administration can be slowed or stopped, whereas the whole dose is already in the patient with an intramuscular or subcutaneous injection. Serum sensitivity tests are not advised because they can mislead; reactions may occur in patients with negative sensitivity tests and in some patients with a positive test, antivenom was subsequently infused without any reaction.

The intravenous infusion is started slowly (15 drops per minute). If a reaction occurs the drip should be temporarily stopped and 0.5 ml adrenaline 1:1000 solution should be injected subcutaneously. If adrenaline is injected at the first sign of anaphylaxis, it is quickly effective and usually the drip can be cautiously restarted. In the ten cases recorded above, no patient developed hypotensive anaphylactic reactions, whereas treating patients with land snake envenoming by unrefined antivenom, anaphylactic reactions were fairly common. I found adrenaline (if given promptly) much more effective than steroids or antihistamine drugs for this type of reaction. In some cases, several injections of adrenaline are needed. In trivial or mild cases of sea snakebite poisoning, 1000–2000 units of antivenom should suffice; in later or more severe cases 3000–10000 units would be more suitable. The speed of administration is progressively increased so that the infusion is completed within about an hour. If by then there has been little significant improvement, further antivenom should be given. The myotoxic symptoms will quickly resolve in successful treatment but for the next few days, the possibility of hyperkalemia and renal failure should be constantly monitored by ECG, renal output, and blood urea estimations. Late serum reactions may also occur up to 2 weeks after the bite and are best treated by steroids (REID, 1957).

The CSL sea snake antivenom is made by using *E. schistosa* venom as antigen. By in vitro tests, CAREY and WRIGHT (1960) found that *E. schistosa* antivenom significantly neutralized venoms of *H. cyanocinctus* and *H. spiralis*; similarly, TU and GANTHAVORN (1969) found it neutralized venoms of *H. cyanocinctus*, *L. hardwickii*, and *P. platurus*. MINTON (1967) found that *N. scutatus* (tiger snake) antivenom, also from CSL, neutralized *E. schistosa* venom as effectively as the specific antivenom. BAXTER and GALLICHIO (1974) studied in vitro neutralization of venoms of *Aipysurus laevis*, *Astrotia stokesii*, *E. schistosa*, *H. cyanocinctus*, *H. elegans*, *H. major*, *H. spiralis*, *L. hardwickii*, *L. semifasciata*, and *N. scutatus* by *E. schistosa* antivenom and *N. scutatus* antivenom. Both antivenoms neutralized all these venoms. More recently, BAXTER and GALLICHIO (1976) compared the neutralizing potency of four antivenoms, monovalent tiger snake *(N. scutatus)*, monovalent sea snake *(E. schistosa)*, polyvalent sea snake (*L. hardwickii*, *L. semifasciata*, and *H. cyanocinctus*), and *N. scutatus* combined with *E. schistosa* antivenom. Potency against sea snake venoms and tiger snake venom was determined by injecting the venom subcutaneously into mice and then injecting the antivenom intravenously. Tiger snake (monovalent *N. scutatus*) antivenom proved to be the antivenom of choice. The following amounts of venom were neutralized by tiger snake and *E. schistosa* antivenoms, respectively:

Venom	Mg neutralized by 1 ampule (8.4 ml) *tiger snake antivenom*	Mg neutralized by 1 ampule (36 ml) *E. schistosa antivenom*
Aipysurus laevis	2.59	3.97
Astrotia stokesii	12.77	13.60
Enhydrina schistosa	3.43	7.30
Hydrophis cyanocinctus	17.46	26.31
Hydrophis elegans	12.78	13.60
Hydrophis major	4.90	10.42
Hydrophis nigrocinctus	21.69	11.56
Hydrophis stricticollis	2.80	2.97
Lapemis hardwickii	19.90	35.66
Laticauda semifasciata	4.45	3.37
Notechis scutatus	58.36	22.66

At the time of writing (March, 1976). 1 ampule of tiger snake antivenom costs about U.S. $ 30.00 compared with U.S. $ 140.00 for 1 ampule of sea snake antivenom. These important studies require clinical confirmation but they suggest that tiger snake antivenom is now the antivenom of choice for all sea snakebite poisoning. Judging by the clinical results with *E. schistosa* antivenom (Reid, 1975b), a suitable dosage of tiger snake antivenom would be 2–4 ampules for trivial or mild poisoning, 6–20 ampules in later and more severe cases.

H. Summary

The world medical literature, a survey of Malayan fishing villages, and a hospital series of 101 unequivocal sea snakebites are considered in relation to the epidemiology of sea snakebite. There is a high incidence among Asian fishing folk. Bathers are sometimes bitten when they tread on a sea snake. The risk to divers throughout the world and to bathers or fishing folk in east African or western American coastal waters is remote. The hospital series confirmed a low mortality considering the high lethal toxicity of sea snake venom—a mortality of only 10% before effective antivenom became available. Trivial or no poisoning followed in 80% of these unequivocal bites. On the other hand, of 11 patients with serious poisoning, over half (six patients) died. These facts emphasize the importance of distinguishing sea snakebite without poisoning from sea snakebite with poisoning.

On the basis of its abundance, the opinion of fishermen, my own observations on aggressiveness relative to that of other sea snakes, venom yields and lethal toxicities, and my observations on human victims, I regard *Enhydrina schistosa* as the most dangerous sea snake to man. I would rate other species of sea snakes in descending order of potential danger to man as follows: *Hydrophis cyanocinctus, Lapemis hardwickii, Microcephalophis gracilis, Hydrophis spiralis, Kerilia jerdoni, Pelamis platurus*, and *Hydrophis klossi.*

The symptomatology of sea snakebite is reviewed. The majority of victims suffer only from the effects of fright. In mild poisoning, myalgia begins within 3 h of the bite but is never severe and resolves without antivenom in 1–3 days. No objective neurologic abnormalities develop. The urine is usually positive for protein but negative for myoglobin. In serious poisoning, myalgia starts within 2 h of the bite and within $1/2$ h becomes generalized and of increasing severity. Myoglobinuria becomes visible a few hours after the bite. Flaccid paresis follows later and especially involves the eyes, lids, tongue, swallowing, neck, and breathing muscles. Respiratory failure can occur early from a combination of glossopharyngeal palsy with inhalation of vomit or secretion. Respiratory failure from muscle weakness may supervene within a few hours of the bite, or as long as 60 h after the bite. In fatal cases, most victims die 12–24 h after the bite, either from respiratory failure or from hyperkalemic cardiac arrest, or a combination of these features. If the victim survives 48 h, he may still die from acute renal failure.

Diagnosis is considered; especially the most important question, is there significant poisoning? In prognosis, vomiting, ptosis, weakness of external eye muscles, dilated pupils with poor light reactions, abnormal electrocardiogram findings, and a leukocytosis exceeding $20000/mm^3$ are all sinister signs. Myalgia merges into true paresis in a matter of hours.

The laboratory features of envenoming are reviewed. Experimentally in animals, a lethal dose of *E. schistosa* venom can be absorbed within 3 min or less of the bite. The effects in animals have been observed to be "neurotoxic," acting mainly at the neuromuscular junction. But, in man, both clinical and pathologic observations clearly show that sea snake venom is primarily myotoxic. In fatal cases, there is widespread necrosis of skeletal muscle and the changes are described in detail. Renal damage is common. The liver shows nonspecific changes. In cardiac and smooth muscles, there is a notable absence of lesions.

In medical treatment, most patients do not develop significant poisoning and require only reassurance. But if there is *any* doubt about envenoming, the patient should be detained for several hours and frequently observed for signs of poisoning. As soon as significant toxemia is apparent (in most cases, it will already be apparent when the patient presents himself if he is one of the unfortunate few with envenoming), effective antivenom should be given. Sea snake antivenom has proved highly successful even when given 2 days after the bite. Recent work suggests that *Notechis scutatus* (tiger snake) antivenom is the antivenom of choice. Details of dosage, administration, and so on are discussed.

In conclusion, it is fortunate for fishermen that sea snakes are not usually aggressive and when they do bite man it is unusual that they inject their highly toxic venom. But even in the comparatively rare cases of serious sea snakebite poisoning, death should not now occur if the victim receives proper medical treatment within a few hours of the bite.

Acknowledgements. I thank numerous colleagues for help with clinical and research work in Malaya, and Mrs. Heather HUXLEY for her secretarial help.

References

Barme, M.: Venomous sea snakes of Viet Nam and their venoms. In: Keegan, H. L., Macfarlane, W. V. (Eds.): Venomous and Poisonous Animals and Noxious Plants of the Pacific Ocean, pp. 373—378. New York: Macmillan 1963

Barme, M.: Venomous sea snakes *(Hydrophiidae)*. In: Bücherl, W., Buckley, E., Deulofeu, V. (Eds.): Venomous Animals and Their Venoms, Vol. I, pp. 285—308. New York: Academic Press 1968

Barme, M., Huard, M., Nguyen, X. M.: Preparation d'un serum anti-venin d'Hydrophiides. Premiers essais therapeutiques. Ann. Inst. Pasteur Lille **102**, 497—500 (1962)

Baxter, E. H., Gallichio, H. A.: Cross neutralisation by tiger snake *(Notechis scutatus)* antivenene and sea snake *(Enhydrina schistosa)* antivenene against several sea snake venoms. Toxicon **12**, 273—278 (1974)

Baxter, E. H., Gallichio, H. A.: Protection against sea snake envenomation: comparative potency of four antivenenes. Toxicon **14**, 347—355 (1976)

Bergman, A. M.: The breeding habits of sea snakes. Copeia **3**, 156—160 (1943)

Blanford, W. T.: Eastern Persia: An Account of the Journeys of the Persian Boundary Commission, 1870—1872. Vol. II, Zoology and Geology, p. 427. London: Macmillan and Comp. 1876

Bokma, H.: Doodelijke vergiftiging door den beet van een zeeslang, *Enhydrina schistosa* (Daudin). Geneesk. Tijdschr. Ned. Ind. **81**, 1926—1931 (1941)

Bokma, H.: Nog eens een beet van een zeeslang, door. Geneesk. Tijdschr. Ned. Ind. **82**, 87 (1942)

Buckland, F.: Land Water **27**, 414 (1879)

Bywaters, E. G. L., Stead, J. K.: The production of renal failure following injection of solutions containing myohemoglobin. Quart. J. exp. Physiol. **33**, 53—70 (1944)

Campbell, C. H.: The effects of snake venoms and their neurotoxins on the nervous system of man and animals. In: Hornabrook, R. W. (Ed.): Topics on Tropical Neurology. Philadelphia: F. A. Davis 1975

Cantor, T.: On pelagic serpents. Trans. Zool. Soc. **2**, 303—311 (1841)

Cantor, T.: Miscellaneous Papers Relating to Indo-China, Vol. II, pp. 112—257. London, 1886

Carey, J. E., Wright, E. A.: The toxicity and immunological properties of some sea snake venoms with particular reference to that of *Enhydrina schistosa*. Trans. roy. Soc. trop. Med. Hyg. **54**, 50—67 (1960)

Carey, J. E., Wright, E. A.: The site of action of the venom of the sea snake *Enhydrina schistosa*. Trans. roy. Soc. trop. Med. Hyg. **55**, 153—160 (1961)

Chevers, N.: A Manual of Jurisprudence for India Including the Outline of a History of Crime Against the Person in India, p. 372—373. India: Thacker Spink 1870

Cheymol, J., Barme, M., Bourillet, F., Roch-Arveiller, M.: Action neuromusculaire de trois venins d'Hydrophiides. Toxicon **5**, 111—119 (1967)

Christensen, P.: The stability of refined antivenin. Toxicon **13**, 75—77 (1975)

Clark, H. C.: Venomous snakes. Some Central American records: incidence of snake-bite accidents. Amer. J. trop. Med. **22**, 37—39 (1942)

Day, F.: On the bite of the sea-snake. Ind. med. Gaz. **4**, 92 (1869)

Dunson, W. A.: The Biology of Sea Snakes. Baltimore-London-Tokyo: Univ. Park Press 1975

Farmer, T. A., Hammack, W. J., Frommeyer, Jr., W. B.: Idiopathic recurrent rhabdomyolysis associated with myoglobinuria. Report of a case. New Engl. J. Med. **264**, 60—66 (1961)

Fayrer, J.: The Thanatophidia of India, 2nd Ed., pp. 45—46. London: J. and A. Churchill 1874

Fitzsimons, F. W.: The Snakes of South Africa, pp. 159—160. Cape Town: T. Maskew Miller 1912

Fohlman, J., Eaker, D.: Isolation and characterization of a lethal myotoxic phospholipase A from the venom of the common sea-snake *Enhydrina schistosa* causing myoglobonuria in mice. Toxicon **15**, 385—393 (1977)

Forné, F.: Note Sur un Cas de Mort par Morsure de Serpent de Mer. Noumea, 1888

Fossen, A.: Vergiftiging door den beet van zeeslangen. Geneesk. Tijdschr. Ned. Ind. **80**, 1164—1166 (1940)

Fraser, T. R., Elliot, R. H.: Contributions to the study of the action of sea snake venoms. Part I: Venoms of *Enhydrina valakadien* and *Enhydrina curtus*. Phil. Trans. roy. Soc. [B] **197**, 249—279 (1905)

Geh, S. L., Toh, H. T.: The effect of sea-snake neurotoxins and a phospholipase fraction on the ultrastructure of mammalian skeletal muscle. Abstract 33, SEA/WP Regional Meeting of Pharmacologists, Singapore, May, 1976

Harris, J. B., Johnson, M. A., Karlsson, E.: Pathological responses of rat skeletal muscle to a single subcutaneous injection of a toxin isolated from the venom of the Australian tiger snake, *Notechis scutatus scutatus*. Clin. exp. Pharm. Phys. **2**, 383—404 (1975)

Heatwole, H.: Attacks by Sea Snakes on Divers. In: Dunson, W. A. (Ed.): The Biology of Sea Snakes, pp. 503—516. Baltimore-London-Tokyo: Univ. Park Press 1975
Herre, A. W. C. T.: Notes on Philippine sea snakes. Copeia **1**, 7—9 (1942)
Herre, A. W. C. T., Rabor, D. S.: Notes on Philippine sea snakes of the genus *Laticauda*. Copeia **4**, 282—284 (1949)
Hood, V. L., Johnson, J. R.: Acute renal failure with myoglobinuria after tiger snake bite. Med. J. Aust. **2**, 638—641 (1975)
Karunaratne, K. E. S., Panabokke, R. G.: Sea snake poisoning. Case report. J. trop. Med. Hyg. **75**, 91—94 (1972)
Kellaway, C. H., Cherry, R. O., Williams, F. E.: The peripheral action of the Australian snake venoms. II. The curare-like action in mammals. Aust. J. exp. Biol. med. Sci. **10**, 181—194 (1932)
Knowles, R.: The mechanism and treatment of snake bite in India. Trans. R. Soc. trop. Med. Hyg. **15**, 72—92 (1921)
Kuntz, R. E.: Snakes of Taiwan. U.S. Naval Med. Res. Unit. No. 2, Taipei, Taiwan, 1963
Lamb, G., Hunter, W. K.: On the action of venoms of different species of poisonous snakes on the nervous system. VI. Venom of *Enhydrina valakadien*. Lancet **1907 II**, 1017—1019
Lancet: Death after adder bite. Lancet **1957/I**, 1095
Lee, C. Y.: Chemistry and pharmacology of polypeptide toxins in snake venoms. Ann. Rev. Pharmacol. **12**, 265—286 (1972)
Marsden, A. T. H., Reid, H. A.: Pathology of sea snake poisoning. Brit. med. J. **1961 I**, 1290—1293
M'Kenzie: An account of venomous sea snakes on the coast of Madras. Asiatic Res. **13**, 329—336 (1820)
Minton, S. A.: Paraspecific protection by elapid and sea snake antivenins. Toxicon **5**, 47—55 (1967)
Minton, S. A.: Geographic Distribution of Sea Snakes. In: Dunson, W. A. (Ed.): The Biology of Sea Snakes, pp. 21—31. Baltimore: Univ. Park Press 1975
Nauck, E. G.: Untersuchungen über das Gift einer Seeschlange *(Hydrus platurus)* des Pazifischen Ozeans. Arch. Schiffts. Trop. Hyg. **33**, 167—170 (1929)
Peal, H. W.: Antivenine as an antidote for sea snake bite. Ind. med. Gaz. **37**, 276—277 (1903)
Pearson, C. M., Beck, W. S., Bland, W. H.: Idiopathic paroxysmal myoglobinuria; detailed study of a case including radioisotope and serum enzyme evaluations. Arch. intern. Med. **99**, 376—389 (1957)
Pickwell, G. V.: The venomous sea snakes. Fauna **4**, 17—32 (1972)
Reid, G., Jenkins, G.: The liberation of renin from the kidney by tissue injury with cobra venom. Aust. J. exp. Biol. med. Sci. **26**, 215—222 (1948)
Reid, H. A.: Sea snake bite research. Trans. roy. Soc. trop. Med. Hyg. **50**, 517—542 (1956a)
Reid, H. A.: Sea snake bites. Brit. med. J. **1956 b II**, 73—78
Reid, H. A.: Three fatal cases of sea snake bite. In: Buckley, E. E., Porges, N. (Eds.): Venoms, pp. 367—371. Washington, D.C.: Am. Assoc. Adv. Sci. 1956c
Reid, H. A.: Antivenene reaction following accidental sea snake bite. Br. Med. J. **2**, 26—29 (1957)
Reid, H. A.: The natural history of sea-snake bite and poisoning: a clinical study. M.D. thesis, University of Edinburgh, 1960
Reid, H. A.: Myoglobinuria and sea snake bite poisoning. Br. med. J. **1961 a I**, 1284—1289
Reid, H. A.: Diagnosis, prognosis and treatment of sea snake bite. Lancet **1961 b II**, 399—402
Reid, H. A.: Sea snake antivenene: successful trial. Brit. med. J. **1962 II**, 576—579
Reid, H. A.: Epidemiology of sea snake bites. J. trop. Med. Hyg. **78**, 106—113 (1975a)
Reid, H. A.: Antivenom in sea snake bite poisoning. Lancet **1975 b II**, 622—623
Reid, H. A.: Epidemiology and Clinical Aspects of Sea Snake Bites. In: Dunson, W. A. (Ed.): The Biology of Sea Snakes, pp. 417—462. Baltimore: Univ. Park Press 1975c
Reid, H. A.: Venom yields from snakes biting man. (Unpublished data) (1976)
Reid, H. A., Chan, K. E.: The paradox in therapeutic defibrination. Lancet **1968 I**, 485—486
Reid, H. A., Lim, K. J.: Sea-snake bite: a survey of fishing villages in north-west Malaya. Brit. med. J. **1957 II**, 1266—1272
Reid, H. A., Thean, P. C., Martin, W. J.: Specific antivenene and prednisone in viper-bite poisoning: controlled trial. Brit. med. J. **1963 II**, 1378—1380

Rogers, L.: On the physiological action of the poison of the *Hydrophiidae*. Proc. roy. Soc. **71**, 481—496 (1902—1903)

Rogers, L.: On the physiological action of the poison of the *Hydrophiidae*. Part II. Action on the circulatory, respiratory, and nervous systems. Proc. roy. Soc. **72**, 305—310 (1903—1904)

Romer, J. D.: Illustrated Guide to the Venomous Snakes of Hong Kong. Hong Kong: Government Pr. 1972

Sitprija, V., Sribhibhadh, R., Benyajati, C.: Haemodialysis in poisoning by sea snake venom. Brit. med. J. **1971 III**, 218—219

Smith, M. A.: Monograph of the Sea Snakes *(Hydrophiidae)*. London: British Museum (Natural History) 1926

Swaroop, S., Grab, B.: Snake bite mortality in the world. Bull. Wld. Hlth. Org. **10**, 35—76 (1954)

Tamiya, N.: Sea Snake Venoms and Toxins. In: Dunson, W. A. (Ed.): The Biology of Sea Snakes, pp. 385—415. Baltimore: Univ. Park Press 1975

Tu, A. T.: Neurotoxins of animal venoms: snakes. Ann. Rev. Biochem. **42**, 235—258 (1973)

Tu, A. T.: Sea snake investigation in the Gulf of Thailand. J. Herpetol. **8**, 201—210 (1974)

Tu, A. T., Ganthavorn, S.: Immunological properties and neutralization of sea snake venoms from southeast Asia. Amer. J. trop. Med. Hyg. **18**, 151—154 (1969)

Wall, F.: The Snakes of Ceylon. Colombo: H. R. Cottle 1921

Walton, J. N., Adams, R. D.: Polymyositis. Edinburgh: Livingstone 1958

Whishnant, C. L., Owings, R. H., Cantrell, C. G., Cooper, G. R.: Primary idiopathic myoglobinuria in a negro female: its implications and a new method of laboratory diagnosis. Ann. intern. Med. **51**, 140—150 (1959)

Wrogemann, K., Pena, S. D.: Mitochondrial calcium overload: a general mechanism for cell-necrosis in muscle disease. Lancet **1976 I**, 672—674

CHAPTER 26

Symptomatology, Pathology and Treatment of the Bites of Viperid Snakes

P. EFRATI

A. Introduction

The present chapter deals with clinical problems concerning bites of certain viperid snakes, often included in the subfamily of *Viperinae*, such as *Atractaspis*, *Bitis*, *Cerastes*, *Echis*, and *Vipera*. Bites by crotalid snakes are discussed in Chapter 27.

B. Incidence

The real incidence of bites by venomous snakes in general can be only roughly estimated, as in most of the countries where snake bites occur usually no official registration of snakebites is required. It is even more difficult to obtain reliable information about bites of single families of snakes in countries where a mixed population of venomous snakes exists, as the snakes inflicting bites are only rarely available for identification.

Our discussion is based, therefore, on some random series of cases published by different authors.

The incidence of snakebites depends mainly on the density of population of the venomous snakes, as well as on the frequency of contact between them and human beings. This is why the incidence of snakebites in developing countries decreases accordingly, as the snake population usually diminishes. This was clearly to be observed in Israel in the years following the establishment of the State.

CORKILL (1956) reported 337 snakebites in Sudan in the period 1933–1946. Only 41 of them were caused by viperid snakes.

AHUJA and SINGH (1956) reviewed 1231 cases of snakebite in India which occurred in the years 1940–1953. The bites were inflicted by venomous and nonvenomous snakes, and 261 of them by viperid snakes.

CHAPMAN (1968) reviewed 1007 bites of venomous snakes observed in Southern Africa during the years 1957–1963. Of them, 210 were caused by *Bitis lachesis*.

REID (1976) recently reviewed 95 cases of adder (*Vipera berus*) bite that have occurred in Britain over the past 100 years.

The present author published two series on bites inflicted by *Vipera xanthina palestinae* (EFRATI and REIF, 1953; EFRATI, 1962) which, together with unpublished cases mentioned in the present Chapter, amount to some 300 cases.

In Israel, until the late 1960s, cases of bites inflicted by *Vipera xanthina palestinae* Werner were mainly known. In recent years, however, cases were published presenting bites by viperid snakes other than *V. xanthina palestinae*, such as *Atractaspis engaddensis* Haas (CHAJEK et al., 1974), *Echis colorata* Gunther (RAVINA et al., 1965; FAINARU et al., 1970), and *Vipera aspis* (PATH and RAVID, 1971; SHARGIL et al., 1973).

According to reports reaching the Ministry of Health in the period 1969–1975, 615 cases of snakebite occurred in Israel. In 165 cases, the snake was identified as *V. xanthina palestinae*, in nine cases as *E. colorata*, and in five cases as nonvenomous snake. The mortality totaled eight cases. The incidence of bites decreased from 165 in 1969 to 37 in 1975.

C. Symptomatology

It is customary to describe manifestations of snakebite as local versus general ones. This classification is certainly justified, mainly for didactic reasons, but it does not mean that the chronologic order of appearance of the manifestations is necessarily such that general manifestations follow local ones. Often, general manifestations precede local changes by as much as $^1/_2$ h or more.

The following description of symptomatology is based on observations in nearly 300 hospitalized cases of bite by *V. xanthina palestinae*. When the symptomatology differs in bites inflicted by viperid snakes other than *V. xanthina palestinae*, this will be pointed out in the discussion.

I. Natural History

We had the sad opportunity to observe the natural course of envenomation in many cases of bite by *V. xanthina palestinae* as no specific antiserum was available in Israel until the late 1950s. Only supportive treatment was given—usually nonspecific antishock treatment which, unfortunately, had no influence whatsoever on the subsequent course of the envenomation.

The clinical evolution of the envenomation could be best observed in severe cases. In a previous publication (EFRATI, 1966), we gave a short outline of this evolution. A more elaborate discussion follows.

The victim experiences pain at the site of the bite 15–20 min after the bite and soon becomes overwhelmed by weakness and restlessness. He vomits repeatedly, perspires profusely, and complains of abdominal pains. Often diarrhea sets in, the feces turn sanguinolent or, more often, watery and profuse like in cholera. At this stage, the victim is usually in severe peripheral circulatory failure. Hypotension is present and often the blood pressure cannot be measured. No pulse is palpable and the heart rate is rapid. On examination one may find—besides the features already mentioned—angioneurotic edema of the upper lip and face. Often the tongue is swollen. Simultaneously with the symptoms described, local changes at the site of the bite and adjacent areas make their appearance. Typical fang marks are rarely encountered. Usually, a single skin puncture or scratch is present. Soon swelling of the bitten extremity sets in. The swollen part is tender and painful to palpation. The swelling subsequently increases and spreads centripetally, reaching tremendous dimensions during the following days (Fig. 1). It may extend up to the trunk and even pass over to the opposite side of the body. Several hours after local swelling appears one can observe ascending lymphangitis and lymphadenitis on the affected extrem-

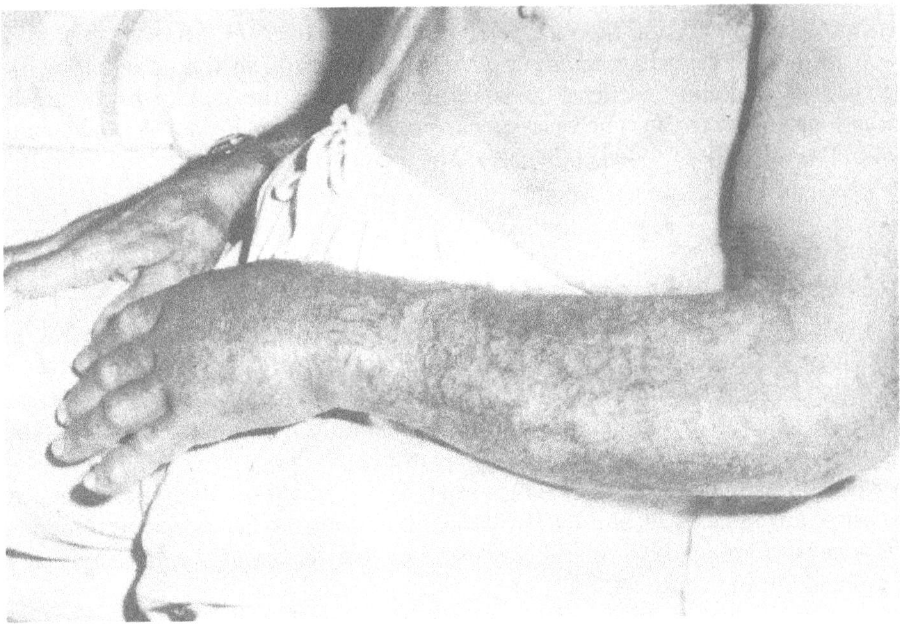

Fig. 1. Typical swelling of bitten extremity

ity. A few days later, the reddening of the skin increases in width, and blisters may appear similar to those in burns (Fig. 2). The skin changes color, it becomes dark violet and later yellow, like the discoloration seen in disintegrating blood in a bruise. The swelling usually clears after 1–2 weeks. As to the general condition of the victim: if he recovers, the primary circulatory failure ("anaphylactoid shock" as will be explained later) disappears, the swelling clears, and the patient can leave the hospital after 2–3 weeks. This anaphylactoid shock may, however, pass over to hypovolemic shock caused by extravasation of blood into the soft tissues. Another consequence of the exsanguination is a severe anemia developing a few days after the envenomation and/or bleeding into some internal organs and intestines. Circulatory failure or bleeding is the frequent cause of death.

The typical course of a severe envenomation will be demonstrated in a case reported in extenso, representing the natural course of the envenomation.

Case Report 1

A 44-years-old farmer was admitted to the Kaplan Hospital at Rehovot on the 30th of July, 1953 at midnight. At 8.00 p.m., while walking on the field, he was bitten by a snake in his left foot, in the vicinity of the ankle. He had to walk another 100 meters to reach his home. He felt no pain. However, 10 min after the accident, he felt weak and vomited. He also had diarrhea and his left leg became swollen. He was transferred to a military camp nearby. A doctor saw him about half an hour after the accident and found him in a severe circulatory failure, with a blood pressure of 65/20 mm-Hg. He was given an infusion of plasma and a glucose-saline solution i.v. Superficial incisions were carried out and a tourniquet was applied. The blood pressure rose to 85/55 mm-Hg and the patient was transferred to the hospital. On arrival, the blood pressure was 70/50 mm-

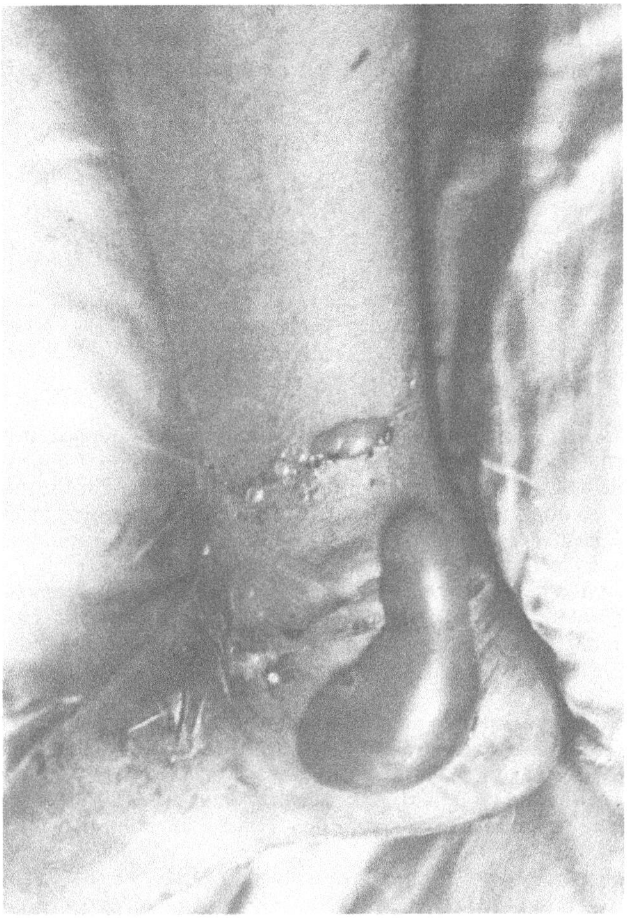

Fig. 2. Blisters in the skin near the site of the bite

Hg and the pulse rate 130/min. The patient was apathetic, covered by cold perspiration, complained of general weakness and of pain in his left leg.

In the region of his left ankle, a soft swelling was found extending to the distal part of the leg. In the skin, some superficial incisions could be seen and dark discoloration around them. The tongue of the patient was swollen. Laboratory examination revealed severe hemoconcentration and normal blood urea concentration. In the urinary bladder, only a small quantity of urine was found (15 ml). Test for albumin was positive. In the sediment, some blood cells were seen as well as a few hyaline casts. An unexpected finding was thrombocytopenia—16000 platelets in 1 mm^3 of blood. ECG revealed sinus tachycardia. About half an hour after admission, the patient again had diarrhea, he passed watery stools with some blood admixture. Blood transfusion was given and drop infusion of glucose saline started.

July 31, 1953. In the morning, the swelling increased considerably and covered the left leg and a part of the thigh. It later progressed and at noon time reached the left inguinal region. In the evening, the whole left lower extremity was swollen. The difference in circumference between the bitten extremity and the normal one was 9 cm in the leg and 8 cm in the thigh. In the skin of the bitten extremity blisters and ecchymotic patches were observed. The patient was conscious and complained of weakness and pain in the bitten leg. Blood pressure was 105/70 mm Hg. The treatment by fluid infusion was continued. During the day, the patient passed 280 ml of urine.

Table 1. Blood count

Date	Hb. gm%	RBC $10^6/mm^3$	WBC $10^3/mm^3$	Neutro $10^3/mm^3$	Eos. $10^3/mm^3$	Thr. $10^3/mm^3$	Ret. %
30.7.53	19	6.1	21.2	17.3	0	16	—
2.8.53	6.5	2.4	18.4		0.184	20	nor-
5.8.53	5.5	1.5	21.7		0.508		mal
10.8.53	7.0	2.0	13			368	
13.8.53	7.5	3.1	9.1			450	
25.8.53	10		7				

Hb. = hemoglobin, RBC = red blood cells, WBC = white blood cells, Neutro. = neutrophils, Eos. = eosinophils, Thr. = platelets, Ret. = reticulocytes.

August 1, 1953. In the early morning hours, drop infusion was stopped for technical reasons. The patient lapsed immediately into a state of shock. Blood pressure dropped to 85/50 mm Hg, the pulse was rapid and weak, and the sensorium became clouded. After the infusion of fluid was reinstalled and blood transfusion started, the patient's condition improved quickly. At noon time the patient complained of weakness and pain in his left leg. The swelling progressed up to his left shoulder. The blisters increased in size and from one of them 50 ml of serous fluid was aspirated. In the afternoon, while receiving infusion of plasma, the patient again complained of weakness and his blood pressure dropped to 85/50 mm Hg. Blood was given and blood pressure rose, reaching 130/70 mm Hg in the evening. During the day, the patient passed 500 ml of urine.

August 2, 1953. The patient felt well but appeared pale. The blood count revealed severe anemia (Table 1).

August 3, 1953. The patient had satisfactory diuresis. His blood pressure remained stable—130/70 mm Hg. Hemoglobin concentration was still low, in spite of repeated blood transfusions. The temperature—which had remained within normal limits—rose to 38.5° C. Blood urea concentration was 60 mg-% and total bilirubin concentration in blood 0.83 mg-%. The difference in circumference of the thighs reached 12 cm. For the last 3 days the patient was given 100 mg cortisone daily.

August 4, 1953. The patient still had severe pains in his bitten leg. The swelling increased again and passed to the opposite side of the thorax. The circumference of the thorax was found to be 107 cm. Hemoglobin concentration dropped to 5 gm-%. Treatment including blood transfusions was continued.

August 5, 1953. The patient was still pale. Hemoglobin concentration remained low. In blood smears, anisocytosis of the red blood corpuscles and some normoblasts were found. There was also thrombocytopenia: 20000 platelets in 1 mm^3. The blisters in the skin pealed off. This resulted in a large skin surface void of epidermis. The dark blue patches in the skin turned yellowish. Swelling then also embraced the genitalia.

August 6, 1953. The patient was still pale and weak. The fever continued. Large ecchymotic patches appeared in the skin of the right upper extremity. The blood pressure was stable. Drop infusion was stopped.

August 8, 1953. The general condition of the patient improved considerably. The blood pressure rose to 160/80 mm Hg. Rapid clearing of the swelling started. The difference in circumference of the thighs decreased to 9 cm, and the circumference of the thorax was now 102 cm. The patient was still pale and the fever continued.

August 10, 1953. The patient complained of severe pains in the bitten leg and from time to time required injection of pethedine. The temperature dropped to within normal limits. Subicterus of the sclerae appeared and blood bilirubin concentration was found to be 10 mg-%–1.2 mg-% direct. Platelet count returned to normal and reached 368000/1 mm^3. Diuresis increased and the patient passed huge amounts of urine—4–5 l per day.

August 13, 1953. The general condition of the patient remained good. Blood pressure was stable. Blood urea concentration was 95 mg-% despite the copious diuresis. The circumference of the thorax dropped to 100 cm.

August 19, 1953. The general condition of the patient was good. The swelling decreased considerably. The difference in circumference of the thighs was found to be 3 cm. Bilirubin concentration in the blood dropped to 0.75 mg-% total.

August 25, 1953. The patient left his bed for the first time. He felt weak and was unable to walk. While being in a vertical position, the skin of the whole left lower extremity reddened considerably. Blood count improved (Table 1).

September 7, 1953. The patient felt well all the time. Blood pressure was stable—130/70 mm Hg. Swelling of the extremity cleared almost completely. The patient was now able to walk. On the skin, dark blue and yellow discoloration could be observed. The sore skin became covered by regenerated epidermis. The patient left the hospital.

On follow-up examination—a year after dismissal—the patient was found to be in good health. He complained of intermittent claudication in his left leg. No peripheral pulse could be felt in this extemity.

The salient features in the case presented were: primary anaphylactoid shock, swelling of the tongue, lymphangitis, lymphadenitis, pain and swelling in the bitten extemity extending to remote parts of the body, secondary hypovolemic shock, extravasation of plasma and blood, anemia, thrombocytopenia, and—as late sequela—occlusion of artery in the bitten extremity. In the 2nd week following envenomation, subicterus of the sclera was observed with increased blood bilirubin concentration.

An interesting feature concerning the course of envenomation in children was reported recently by SADAN et al. (1970).

Contrary to the generally prevalent opinion that the effect of snake venom is more severe in children than in adults, they were impressed by the relatively small number of severe cases in children they saw. They compared the course of envenomation in 65 children aged 1–12 years to a group of adults—comprising 165 cases—treated in the Department of Medicine. All the patients were admitted from the same geographic region—Valley of Yezreel—under comparable circumstances. Whereas 41 adults (25.4%) showed severe envenomation, only nine (13.8%) children were in a similar condition. There were three deaths among the adults but none among the children. These results may reflect the diminished disposition of children to anaphylactoid reactions.

The described severe condition representing the natural course of envenomation disappeared almost completely when treatment with specific antivenom was started in 1956.

A case of comparable severity on admission will be presented to demonstrate the changed pattern of the course of envenomation in patients treated with specific antivenom.

Case Report 2

A Bedouin, approximately 40 years old, was admitted to the hospital about 3 h after having been bitten by a big snake in his left hand while working in the field. A kind of tourniquet was applied above the wrist. After a few minutes, the patient became very restless. No vehicle was available and he had to walk about a kilometer until he reached the road. After a delay of almost 3 h, he was brought to the hospital. Upon arrival—at 11:45 a.m.—he was unconscious, restless, pale, in deep shock, and covered by cold perspiration. Blood pressure could not be measured and a weak filiform pulse was palpated. Tachycardia was present and the ECG revealed idioventricular rhythm. In the dorsal part of his left hand, some scratches could be observed in the vicinity of the fourth finger. The whole dorsum of the hand up to the middle of the forearm was swollen. Blood count revealed normal hemoglobin concentration, leukocytosis, and a normal platelet count.

Blood taken from the vein clotted normally but after an hour became fluid again. While waiting for results of a skin sensitivity test for horse serum, adrenaline was given i.m. and i.v. drop infusion was started. The patient then received noradrenaline and hydrocortison (100 mg) i.v. An hour after his arrival, 80 cm^3 of specific antivenom was given i.v. The tourniquet was gradually loosened. At 13:10 the blood pressure reached 55 mm Hg (systolic) and after half an hour 105 mm Hg under continuous drop infusion of noradrenaline. In the course of the 1st day, the patient vomited several times.

A few hours later consciousness returned. While in shock, blood transfusion was additionally given.

The following day the patient felt well, and the swelling progressed somewhat. Two days after the bite, the i.v. drop infusion could be stopped. On the 5th day, the swelling diminished. After a week, the patient was discharged.

II. Review of Recent Literature

The symptomatology of viper bites in other countries is, in general, similar to that described in bites of *V. xanthina palestinae*, the difference being mainly in the severity of symptoms.

CHAPMAN (1968) described the clinical features encountered in bites of *Bitis lachesis* in Southern Africa. They were mainly local. In 210 cases, only nine showed general effects separate from any influence of the local lesion. He divided cases of local swelling into two groups: 1) those without evidence of surface extravasation, and 2) those in which hemorrhages are evident as ecchymoses and bleeding from fang marks. In the second group, the swelling is usually more solid and often massive. Necrosis may be found in either group but is usually found in the second one. He also described instances of sudden and often fatal circulatory collapse which occurred when the subject had been doing well. Such cases were always encountered in patients with extensive extravasation, and CHAPMAN ascribes them to concealed fluid loss. According to him, venous thrombosis is a more important entity in the development of the local lesion than hitherto has been realized. General effects included vomiting, abdominal colic, dizziness, sweating, urticaria, hyperpyrexia, and drowsiness. These were considered to be sensitivity reactions to venom before any antivenin had been given. In three cases, hemorrhages distant from the site of the bite (conjunctiva, urinary tract) were found.

REID (1968) reported on snakebites in India and in southeast Asia. He regards the Malayan pit viper, Russell's viper, and *Echis carinatus* as of serious medical importance. Dealing with local effects, he stressed swelling which starts within a few minutes of the bite and may continue to increase for 24–72 h according to the venom dose. Extravasation of blood into subcutaneous tissues results in discoloration going through the same color changes as a bruise. Blisters around the bite site were also common. When extending up the limb, it is usually an indication of a large dose of venom injected. Hemorrhage is, according to REID, the outstanding symptom of systemic viper poisoning. Clotting defect usually accompanies hemorrhage and may be an aggravating factor. The commonest and earliest hemorrhagic manifestation in his experience is hemoptysis which may be seen as early as 20 min after the bite. There is continual oozing from the fang marks. Hematemesis, melena, and hematuria may occur but are less common. Bleeding into the brain or other vital organs may be fatal. In severe cases, loss of blood may lead to hypovolemic shock. Tourniquet test for hemorrhagic tendency is usually positive.

In a recent paper—after returning to England—REID (1976) summarized the clinical problems in bites of *Vipera berus* in Britain. He reviewed 95 cases of bite that have occurred in Britain over the past 100 years. Fifty-five cases reported from 1876 to 1971 were collected from the literature, and in 40 cases, the author was involved through consultation or correspondence from 1957 to 1975. It seems that from all viper bites reported, the bites of *Vipera berus*—as described by REID—show the closest similarity to the symptomatology of bites by *V. xanthina palestinae*. Interestingly enough, REID found in 12 out of 29 cases of severe poisoning, besides local changes, swelling of the face and lips or tongue which sometimes appeared immediately after the bite and lasted for up to 2 days. To the best of my knowledge, this is the only instance of appearance of angioneurotic edema in viper bite in a snake other than *V. xanthina palestinae*. REID also mentioned vomiting and diarrhea as initial manifestations in adder bite. Shock started in severe cases within 10 min after the bite or not until 10 h after the bite. Edema and hemorrhage were also prominent.

Ten cases of bite by puff adder—*Bitis arietans*—were reported recently by WARREL et al. (1975) from Nigeria. All of the ten patients presented were observed in a hospital. Six of them showed severe local signs and four had in addition evidence of systemic envenomation. Local pain and swelling were noticed by all the patients within 20 min after being bitten. Local swelling was maximal 1–2 days after the bite and it took 5 days to 3 weeks to resolve. Local blistering was seen in five cases and necrosis in three. Popliteal artery thrombosis was a complication in one case. Systemic envenomation included evidence of spontaneous bleeding with thrombocytopenia, hypotension, and bradycardia. Two patients died after developing circulatory collapse and renal failure; one of them showed—as already mentioned—occlusion of popliteal artery and a delayed amputation was carried out. Five patients had fever on admission. The time from the bite to admission was 2–5$^1/_2$ h in eight cases, 3–4 h in one case, and 5 weeks in another. Laboratory investigations of interest revealed leukocytosis in five out of six cases examined, anemia in three, and thrombocytopenia in three. No disturbances in the clotting mechanism were detected in the few cases examined.

In addition to the occlusion of peripheral artery mentioned in our case and that in the preceding one, AMERATUNGA (1972) published a case in which neurologic deficit was found in the form of hemiplegia within 24 h following a bite by Russell's viper. The arteriogram showed a partial middle cerebral artery occlusion.

Recently, several cases of renal insufficiency were published following viper bite. SITPRIJA (1974) described two patients bitten by Russell's viper who developed renal insufficiency. No antivenom had been given. SEEAT et al. (1974) reported two cases of acute renal failure following a bite by *Bitis arietans*. Both were maintained on hemodialysis and recovered. In neither case was antivenom given.

CHUGH et al. (1975) described eight patients with acute renal failure following snakebite. In three of them, intravascular hemolysis and disseminated intravascular clotting (DIC) contributed to the development of acute renal failure. Three patients had histopathologic lesions of acute symmetric cortical necrosis. None of them survived. Five patients had acute tubular necrosis, all of them recovered, three with the help of dialysis and two with conservative management.

III. Envenomation Caused by Other Genera of Viperid Snakes

1. Echis colorata

The first case of envenomation by *E. colorata* in Israel was published by RAVINA et al. in 1965. In this case, no severe local or general symptoms were observed in the beginning. At this stage, laboratory examination showed normal hemoglobin concentration (15 gm-%); the number of platelets was 150000/mm^3. Prothrombin activity was diminished: 25% of normal and fibrinogen concentration was found to be 50 mg-%. After an hour, slight gingival hemorrhage started.

Laboratory examination—2 h after the bite—revealed a further drop in fibrinogen concentration (30 mg-%) and no prothrombin activity at all could be detected. The blood did not clot. The number of platelets remained within normal limits (250000/mm^3). In the 2 subsequent days, the hemorrhagic tendency increased. Hematuria appeared and continuous bleeding followed each vein puncture when blood was taken for examination. The blood values did not change essentially in spite of blood transfusions and administration of ε-amino caproic acid. Interestingly enough, the general condition remained good. The bitten extremity swelled and a bloody blister appeared at the site of the bite. The patient complained of pain in his bitten hand. The patient was bitten in the morning and only in the evening of the following day was specific antivenom available (produced in the Rogoff Institute at Petah Tiqua, Israel), and 50 ml was injected i.v. The effect was dramatic. Two hours after the administration of antivenom, the hemorrhagic tendency stopped. The following day, prothrombin activity was already 50% of normal and fibrinogen concentration rose to 112 mg-%. Subsequently all the blood values returned to normal.

Recently, several additional cases were reported (FAINARU et al., 1970, 1974; DVILANSKY and BIRAN, 1973; YATZIV et al., 1974). In most of the cases, no severe general manifestations were present. In some of them, mild hypotension, vomiting, renal failure, etc. were observed. The patients usually revealed swelling of the bitten extremity, slight local hemorrhage around the site of the bite, and they complained of pains. The most remarkable feature in the majority of cases was the discrepancy between the severe alterations in the clotting mechanism and the absence of significant clinical manifestations. As to the nature of those alterations, a heated argument is still going on between the hematologists who claim that the cause of the disturbances in coagulation is primary fibrinolysis and those who try to explain it by assuming that DIC is the cause. The main difficulty is that patients are examined at different stages of envenomation and their findings may not be comparable.

A single case of death following a bite by *E. colorata* was recently mentioned in a doctoral thesis at the University of Jerusalem (MAN, 1976). The 44-year-old man was asymptomatic for 24 h after a bite by *E. colorata* when hemorrhages set in and he died in acute renal failure. On postmortem examination, skin necrosis was found at the site of the bite on the finger as well as serosanguinolent swelling in different regions of the body: skin, subendocardial tissues, retroperitoneum, etc. The cause of the renal failure was found to be acute interstitial nephritis. In some countries, bites by snakes of the genus *Echis* are more frequent. In a recent report by WARRELL et al. (1974) it was stated that in an enormous area comprising Africa north of the equator, the Middle East, Pakistan, India, and Sri Lanka, *Echis carinatus* is the most important cause of morbidity and mortality from snakebite in man. In parts of Nigeria, more than 150 victims are treated each year with an overall mortality of 7–15%. Local swelling, spontaneous bleeding, and alterations in coagulation seemed to be the most frequent manifestations. The authors compared the effect of the treatment by two specific antivenoms. Forty-six patients were given *Echis* antivenom and a simple test of blood coagulability was used to assess whether an adequate neutralizing dose had been given. Comparison of the results showed that S.A.I.M.R. antivenom (South Africa Institute for Medical Research antivenom) was the more effective one. Recently, a case was reported from the United States (WEISS et al., 1973) in which DIC developed in a 28-year-old man who was bitten by a saw-scaled viper (*Echis carinatus*). The patient became severely anemic, probably due to hemorrhage and microangiopathic hemolysis. He also developed swelling of the arm. Treatment with fibrinogen and 100 ml i.v. of antivenom (monovalent *Echis* antivenin, Pasteur Institute, Paris) on the 1st day and 10 ml and 20 ml on the 2nd and 3rd days failed to control the coagulation defects and heparin was given. The patient recovered rapidly. In vitro studies showed that the venom of this snake activates prothrombin directly and may lead to DIC.

2. Atractaspis

Information on bites of snakes belonging to the genus *Atractaspis* is scanty. CORKILL et al. (1959) summarized the information which was available at that time. The clinical data were presented. They were in part characteristic of viper bite and in part differed greatly. The most common features were: local pain, swelling, local hemorrhage, discoloration, lymphadenitis, abdominal pain, fever, tachycardia, sweating, vomiting, vertigo, salivation, coma, etc. He also described the ability of the snake to inflict bites with one fang independently with its mouth practically closed.

Recently, a small series of three cases was published by CHAJEK et al. (1974) from Israel in which the culprit was *Atractaspis engaddensis* Haas. The patients were admitted to a hospital and thoroughly investigated. Pain and numbness at the site of the bite were present in all the patients. Two presented swelling and necrosis progressing in one of them to gangrene necessitating amputation of a thumb. Vomiting and diarrhea appeared in two patients. One patient was admitted in a state of severe respiratory failure. He was unconscious and cyanotic. Examination of arterial blood revealed hypoxia (PO_2—45 mm Hg), hypercapnia (pCO_2—140 mm Hg), and a pH of 6.9. He also had hypertension (160/110 mm Hg). In the ECG alterations of S–T segment and T wave were found. On energetic treatment, including intubation, administration of oxygen through the intratracheal tube, hydrocortison, and aminophyllin i.v., the patient improved and eventually recovered.

In two patients, laboratory examination revealed mild disturbances in the function of the liver. Liver biopsy was carried out in one of them. On histologic examination, necrosis of some cells was found. Interestingly enough, in all the cases only one fang mark was found, in accordance with the view expressed by CORKILL et al. (1959).

No recent information could be found on bites inflicted by snakes belonging to the genus *Cerastes*.

Recently, several cases of bite by *Aspis cerastes* were reported from Israel (PATH and RAVID, 1971; SHARGIL et al., 1973). Seven cases were described presenting mani-

Table 2. Clinical manifestations of bites by viperid snakes

Local	Systematic			
Pain Fang marks Swelling Blisters Ecchymoses Lymphangitis Lymphadenitis Discoloration	*Anaphylactoid manifestations:* Primary shock Hypotension Tachycardia Perspiration Angioneurotic edema Urticaria	*Gastrointestinal disturbances:* Abdominal pain Nausea Vomiting Diarrhea	*Disturbances in clotting of blood:* Primary fibrinolysis? DIC? Thrombocytopenia	*Extravasation of blood* Anemia

festations resembling those in mild cases of bites by *Vipera xanthina palestinae.* In one case, a necrotic lesion progressing to gangrene necessitated amputation of the bitten finger. Usually only swelling was present. General manifestations were also mild. In most of the cases, nausea, and vomiting were observed. Besides hemorrhages in the skin, hematuria was observed in four patients.

As in the bite by *E. colorata,* disturbances in blood clotting were observed, although less severe ones. There were some drop in fibrinogen concentration, diminished prothrombin activity, and in one case a mild DIC appeared.

Clinical manifestations of bites caused by viperid snakes are summarized in Table 2.

D. Prognosis and Sequela

There is no reliable information on the true mortality rate in patients with viper bite. The percentage of mortality found in the literature is around 7–8%, but the composition of the series is not comparable. If one separates the cases who were admitted in a severe state, the mortality in them will obviously be very high. Mild cases included in statistical evaluation tend to lower the mortality rate.

The progress in treatment of the envenomation changed the outcome—in Israel—quite radically.

As the quantity of venom injected by the snake is unknown, the course of the envenomation can hardly be predicted. Fortunately, most of the victims of viper bite recover eventually. On the other hand, the high doses of serum used in the modern treatment of snakebite increased considerably the incidence of serum sickness. In two patients observed by us, severe neuritis of the brachial plexus occurred, accompanying a reaction to the serum. In general, patients who recover from the envenomation show no sequela. In bites located in the hand, however, late complications may sometimes occur.

In the past 10 years, KESSLER (1976) treated nine patients with problems in the hand after viper bite. The snakes were identified in four cases: in three of them the bite was inflicted by *V. xanthina palestinae* and in one by *E. colorata.* In five cases, the snake has not been identified. Stiffness of the metacarpophalangeal joints, sensory disturbances and adduction contracture of the thumb were the main problems. According to him, the adduction contracture of the thumb could be minimized by using a proper splint in the acute stage.

E. Pathology

I. Gross Anatomy

EFRATI and REIF (1953) found swelling and hemorrhages in the subcutaneous soft tissues and deep muscles. Hemorrhages were also found in most of the internal organs, in the serous and mucous membranes, and in the brain. REIF (1962) reported edema, hemorrhages, and blisters containing serous or serosanguinous fluid. The changes were usually located proximal and distal to the site of the bite, sometimes covering a very large area. The hemorrhages involve—besides the skin—muscles and fascia. The regional lymph nodes are always swollen, usually with hemorrhages. Hemorrhages are also found in various organs, particularly in the heart (epicard, subendocardial tissue, and myocard), in the gastrointestinal tract, and in the brain. In a case of ours, severe headache and restlessness found explanation in a massive edema of the brain. There are also hemorrhages in the serous cavities and in the lungs. In a patient in whom clinically pulmonary edema was suspected, intra-alveolar hemorrhages were found (Fig. 3).

II. Histology

On microscopic examination, the hemorrhagic diathesis stands out. There is blurring and swelling of endothelial cells in capillaries and precapillaries. Also, tears in the walls of capillaries could be observed with hemorrhages around them. A small hemorrhage from a damaged vessel in the pons resulted in the death of a patient 7 days after the bite. LEFFKOWITZ et al. (1960) described aneurysmal dilatation of glomerular loops in the kidney. We observed hemorrhages in the lumen of the tubuli (Fig. 4), in the myocard (Fig. 5), in the adrenal gland (Fig. 6), and in the brain (Fig. 7).

In skeletal muscles in the vicinity of the site of the bite, sanguineous edema was often seen (Fig. 8). The described changes were usually found in victims of a bite by *V. xanthina palestinae*. Recently, a case of a bite by *E. colorata* was reported in whom post-mortem examination was carried out (MAN, 1976). The 44-year-old patient remained asymptomatic for 24 h after the bite, when hemorrhages set in, and he died with symptoms of renal failure. The gross pathologic changes were similar to those described in the bite of *V. xanthina palestinae*, and tiny hemorrhages were also seen in several internal organs, including the renal pelvis and calyces. On microscopic examination of the kidneys, changes compatible with acute interstitial nephritis were found. Proliferative nephritis (epithelial crescents) was found in biopsy specimens of kidneys in two patients following the bite of *Bitis arietans* in southern Africa (SEEAT et al., 1974).

In two other patients, who lapsed into acute renal failure after a bite by Russell's viper, tubular necrosis and arteritis was found on renal biopsy (SITPRIJA et al., 1974). In neither of the cases was antivenom given.

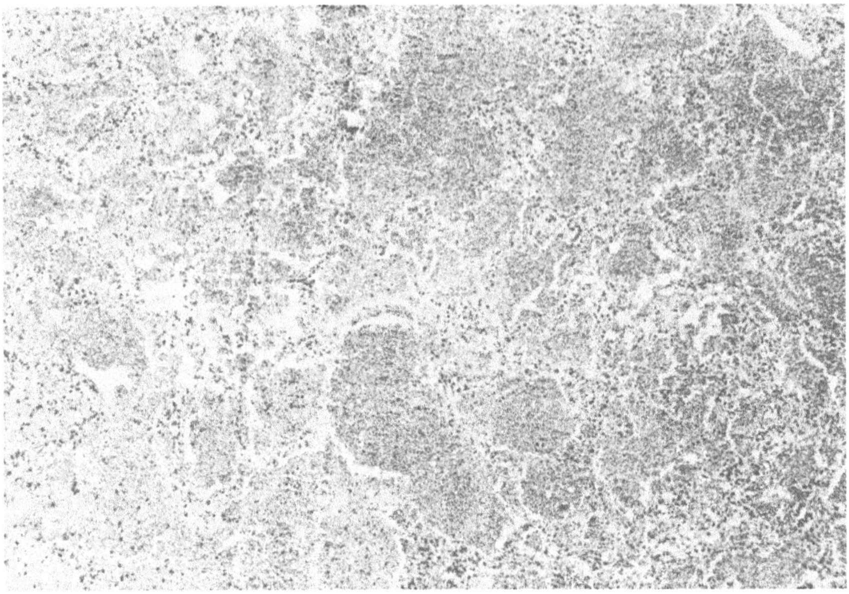

Fig. 3. Intraalveolar hemorrhage in the lung (magnification 100 ×)

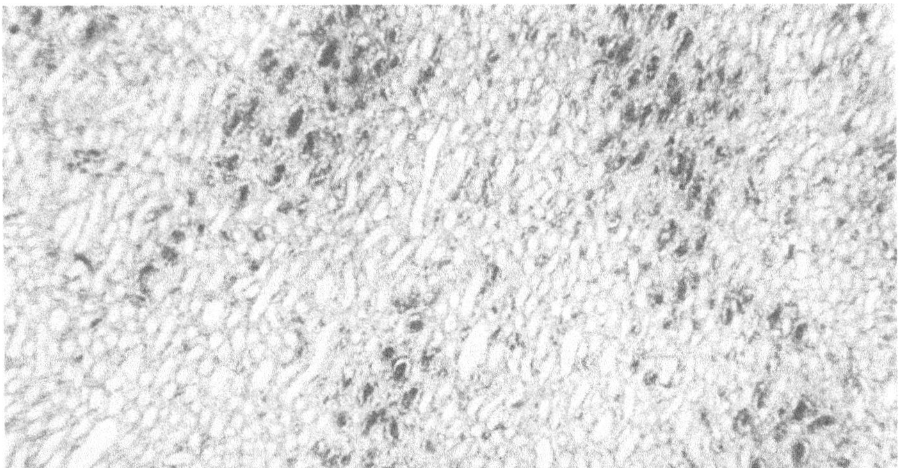

Fig. 4. Hemorrhage in the renal tubuli (magnification 250 ×)

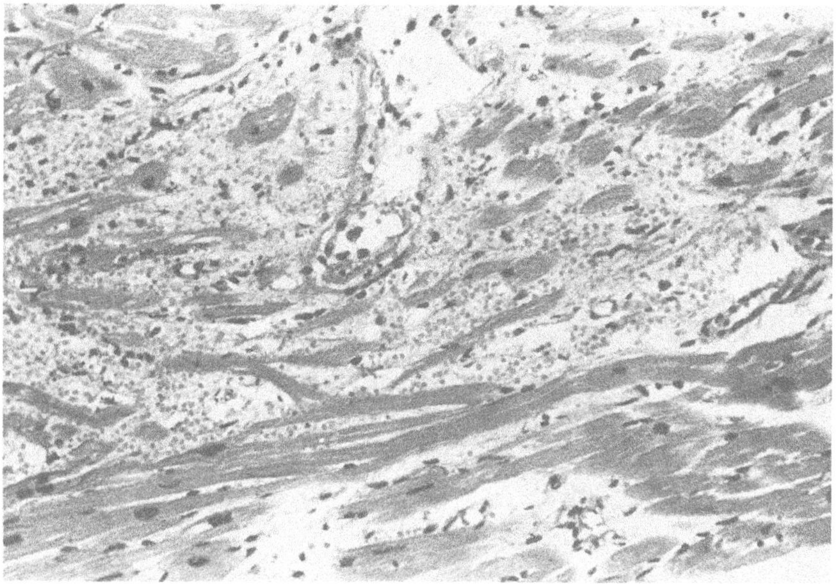

Fig. 5. Hemorrhage in the myocard (magnification 250 ×)

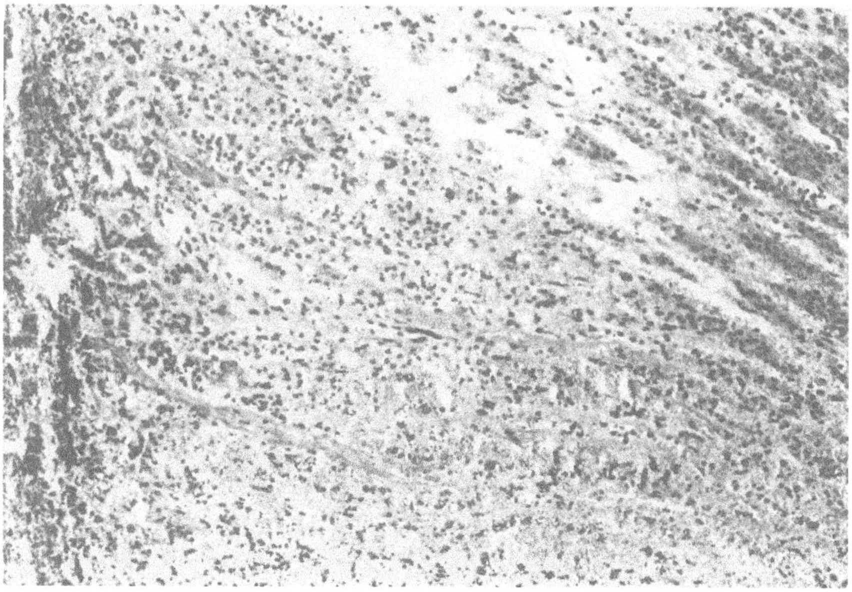

Fig. 6. Hemorrhage in the adrenal gland (magnification 100 ×)

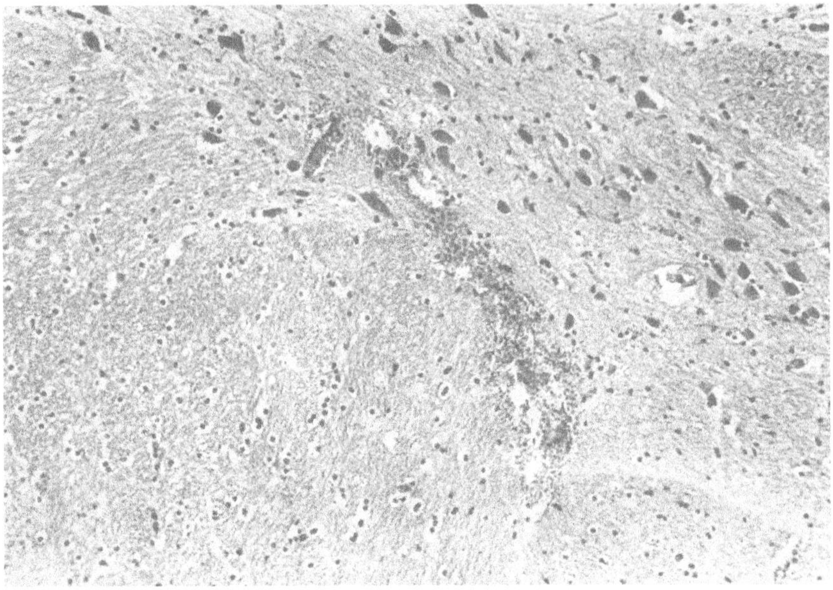

Fig. 7. Hemorrhage in the brain (magnification 100 ×)

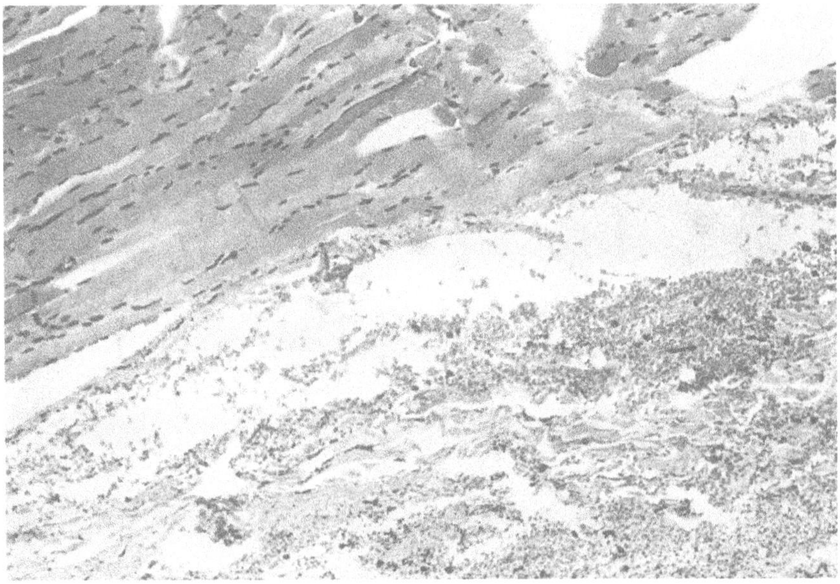

Fig. 8. Hemorrhage in skeletal muscle (magnification 100 ×)

III. Laboratory Examinations

Information on results of laboratory investigations are scanty. Patients with snakebite are usually admitted as emergency cases, often at night and in peripheral hospitals where laboratory facilities are only rarely available. In most of our cases, the laboratory examinations were carried out in the ward.

In cases of shock, blood count showed hemoconcentration, hemoglobin sometimes reaching values as high as 20 gm-% and hematocrit up to 58%. Usually, leukocytosis was also observed. Thrombocytopenia was found only in patients who were in shock. In some cases, eosinophilia could be observed with or without angioneurotic edema or urticaria. In several cases, the clotting time of blood was within normal limits, but within 45–60 min fibrinolysis occurred and the blood again became fluid. The sedimentation rate of the red blood corpuscles was greatly delayed in the phase of hemoconcentration.

In the severe cases, hemoglobin concentration usually decreased in the subsequent days, as a result of bleeding into the tissues, reaching at the end of the 1st week values as low as 5 gm-%. Only at this time could mild jaundice be observed, and in the serum, an increase of indirect bilirubin concentration was found. Discoloration appearing simultaneously in the ecchymotic patches could explain the appearance of jaundice as caused by disintegration of red blood cells. Coagulation disturbances in vitro were investigated by DE VRIES et al. (1957, 1962). Recently, the influence of the venom of *E. colorata* on the coagulation in vitro and in vivo was extensively investigated (DVILANSKY and BIRAN, 1973; BIRAN et al., 1972; FAINARU et al., 1970, 1974; YATZIV et al., 1974). No close correlation could be found between the changes in vitro and the clinical manifestations.

Immunologic methods were used for diagnosis of the species of snake inflicting the bite. GREENWOOD et al. (1974) applied immunodiffusion to detect traces of snake venom in wound aspirates, blister fluids, sera, and urine samples from patients with snakebite. A positive species diagnosis was made in 40 out of 101 patients. SUTHERLAND et al. (1975) reported on a new solid-phase radioimmunoassay which allows positive identification of the type of snake venom in human tissue and fluids and its accurate quantitation. The method is not proposed as an emergency procedure since an incubation period of 24 h at 0–4° C has been found to be optimal. However, it has been modified to give a positive or negative result when used on serum or tissue fluids within 1 h of commencement of the assay.

For the time being, no further information is available. One cannot know whether the immunologic methods will be useful for routine diagnosis of snakebite in order to exclude bites by other animals or nonvenomous snakes, or whether the main use will be the recognition of the species in countries with a mixed population of venomous snakes.

F. Pathogenesis of the Envenomation

In our earlier publications (EFRATI and REIF, 1953; EFRATI, 1966), we proposed anaphylactoid reaction as a possible explanation for the primary shock observed in viper bite because of the similarity to the anaphylactic reaction, without any preceding sensitization. We based our assumption on the literature cited which was available at that time. Interestingly enough, cases of true anaphylaxis are also known to occur due to previous sensitization by snake venom (ELLIS and SMITH, 1965).

It was known for many years that snake venoms release histamine from animal tissues. Accordingly, we tried to treat patients in early stages of envenomation by i.v. injection of antihistaminic drugs but without success.

Research carried out subsequently by different investigators (KAISER and RAAB, 1966) showed that, in addition to histamine, some slow-reacting substances were also released from the plasma, the most potent being bradykinin. Its effect closely imitates the systemic manifestations of the early stage of viper bite, such as vasodilatation, hypotension, increased permeability of the vessels in the microcirculation causing edema, contraction of smooth muscles and pain (see Chap. 16).

Enzymic inactivation of the plasma kinins is very rapid and their half-life is approximately 15 seconds. Bradykinin is probably released as long as circulating snake venom is available. Early treatment with specific antivenom will bind free venom and will stop—in this way—further release of bradykinin.

The severe anemia appearing in the 1st week has been explained by extravasation of blood. We found correlation between the increase of volume of the bitten extremity and the drop in hemoglobin concentration (EFRATI and REIF, 1953). No hemolysis was present at this time and mild jaundice with an increase of the indirect bilirubin concentration in the serum appeared later, when the extravasated blood in the tissues started to disintegrate.

Bleeding was caused by the hemorrhagin present in the venom, and it could also occur in sites remote from the vicinity of the bite.

We found no explanation for the fibrinolysis. It was observed only in severe cases and was often associated with thrombocytopenia. No clear evidence of DIC was found.

The lymphangitis and lymphadenitis starting at the site of the bite seem to be a direct effect of the venom.

G. Treatment of Viper Bite

The principles of the local treatment of snakebite, as practiced at present, were already known in the Middle Ages. An admirable summary of them can be found in a treatise by MOSHE BEN MAIMON (MAIMONIDES, 1135–1206), "Poisons and Their Antidotes," written originally in Arabic and translated into Hebrew by IBN TIBBON (edited by MUNTER, S.: "Maimonides' Medical Works," Rubin Mass Edition, Jerusalem, 1947).

I shall quote from this work some relevant passages:

> Immediately after having been bitten one has to tie up above the bite to prevent the poison from spreading. Another person should—at the same time—make cuts with a knife in the site of the bite and to suck, as forcibly as he can, and to spit out what he sucked. The one who sucks must not have any sores or bad teeth in his mouth. When no sucker is available put cupping glasses with or without fire; those with fire are stronger.

Unfortunately, no information was given about the results. The long list of drugs advocated, including the "great theriac," as well as local application of different plasters, and in severe cases of young, newly slaughtered pigeons with slit bellies, blood still warm, may indicate that those preventive measures were not always effective. In recent times, doubts arose as to the soundness of the measures mentioned, although one can still find some enthusiasts. In general, the less personal experience the physician has, the more obstinately he tends to stick to the old principles. Especially authors of popular guides to first-aid used to copy firm rules from each other. Results of animal experiments are not always transferable to human beings. On the other hand, there are very few controlled clinical studies available. The main difficulty lies in the fact that one can never know how much venom has been injected. Interesting studies were carried out by ALLON and KOCHVA (1974). They offered seven specimens of *V. xanthina palestinae* injected with ^{14}C amino acids—in order to label the venom—three pairs of one mouse and one rat each. The amounts of venom injected to either prey were variable, ranging from zero to more than 220 mg. In most cases, 50 mg were injected, approximately 8% of the total venom available in the glands. The size of the prey did not influence markedly the amount of the venom injected by the snake.

In a previous publication, KOCHVA (1962) showed that in successive bites by the same snakes the amount of venom injected varied considerably. Although, in general, the amount decreased after multiple bites, it occurred frequently that in the first few bites no venom was injected at all, followed by quantities as high as 64 mg, 48 mg, etc. in subsequent bites.

The application of a tourniquet is still a matter of intense argument. Theoretically one can classify tourniquets as arterial, venous, and lymphatic. Nobody would contest that arterial occlusion has no place in the prevention of venom resorption. In a swollen extremity, where the arterial flow is already compromised, the application of an arterial tourniquet could lead to disaster. A venous tourniquet, if properly applied, will inevitably raise the back pressure in the veins, thus increasing extravasation of fluid and promoting lymph flow. A lymphatic tourniquet—to the best of my knowledge—does not exist and one can hardly imagine anatomically how it could work. It is astonishing to read instructions, given to uninformed persons, on how to apply a tourniquet, when even physicians have difficulty distinguishing between the different kinds of vascular occlusion.

As to "incision and suction," most of the authors emphasize that it can be useful only in the very early time after the bite. In addition, one has to take into consideration the opening of lymph channels by the incision, encouraging in this way the resorption of venom. At least one experimental study points in the same direction (LEOPOLD and MERRIAM, 1960). SHULOV et al. (1969) studied the efficacy of incision and suction in removal of venom of *V. xanthina palestinae* from adult rabbits injected subcutaneously and intramuscularly. In the case of s.c. injection, they could recover 30–35% of venom injected if suction was carried out early enough and continued 15–30 min. Even a delay of 15 min reduced the amount of venom that could be removed. In the case of i.m. injection, the immediate application of suction removed only very small amounts of venom. After a delay of a few minutes, the amount of venom removed was negligible. No significant difference was noted in the amount of venom obtained whether a tourniquet was employed or not.

The use of cold in the treatment of snakebite is nowadays rarely advocated. A vigorous debate on this subject went on in the USA in the mid-1960s (RUSSELL and QUILLIGAN, 1966).

In recent years, surgical methods of treatment of snakebite have been proposed in face of the danger of severe anaphylactic reactions which sometimes follow serotherapy. GLASS (1973), dealing with pit viper bite, reported on immediate debridment and fasciotomy (when indicated) combined with large doses of hydrocortisone (1 gm, i.v.). Patients were selected for this treatment if there were toxic symptoms, severe pain at the bite site, rapid spread of swelling, and ecchymoses during the 1st hour after the bite. After debridment, fasciotomy, or both, no blistering or skin necrosis developed in any of the 84 patients treated. Hospitalization was shortened considerably.

HUANG et al. (1974) used excisional therapy in 54 patients bitten by snakes. The advocated method is based upon the finding that the bulk of the injected venom will remain in the area of the bite, and mechanical removal of the tissue containing the venom injected can conceivably aid in eliminating the local toxic effects and reducing the magnitude of systemic intoxication. The authors, treating 54 patients over a 3-year period, support this concept of treatment.

Criticizing the current methods of local treatment of snakebite, ARNOLD (1975) summarizes his view on emergency treatment by proposing to limit it to reassurance and rapid transport to a medical facility. Definite treatment consists of fluid administration, control of pain, and specific serotherapy if the patient is not allergic to horse serum. Fourteen patients with *Crotalus* bite were treated, ten being severe enough to require antivenom. No deaths occurred and there were no tissue sloughs or amputations. In our opinion the most important first-aid measure is transfer of the patient—as soon as possible—to the nearest medical facility, where proper management of the case is feasible. It is necessary to immobilize the bitten extremity before transport in order to slow down the absorption of the venom by the lymphatic channels.

It was shown by BARNES and TRUETA (1941) that snake venom with high molecular weight is absorbed by lymphatic vessels and complete elimination of muscle contractions considerably reduces the lymph flow.

The most important single measure in the definite treatment of viper bite is undoubtedly the serotherapy. The antivenom must be highly specific, purified as far as possible, and given in slow intravenous injection in adequate quantities. We use a locally produced antivenom against the venom of *V. xanthina palestinae* and inject 50–80 ml i.v. according to the size of the patient and the severity of the envenomation. Usually a single application suffices. No serum is given i.m. nor injected around the site of the bite. We carry out an intracutaneous sensitivity test, but it cannot predict the subsequent appearance of serum sickness. Fortunately, no primary hypersensitivity was encountered up to now.

Patients treated by serum improved rapidly and their hospitalization was shortened considerably. The use of serum is only indicated in cases in whom symptoms of systemic envenomation appear, such as hypotension, vomiting and/or diarrhea, soon after the bite. Specific antivenom is also available against the venom of *E. colorata*, and it proved to be useful in combating hemorrhagic features.

As supportive treatment, we propose i.v. infusion of a glucose-saline solution or similar solutions (Ringer, etc.) in iso-osmotic concentration in cases of prolonged hypotension. In addition, vasopressor substances are sometimes employed.

Most of the patients also need analgetics for the severe pains often complained of.

Use of corticosteroid hormones has no place in the treatment of snakebite. Its administration is usually a sign of "alarm reaction" of the physician. No convincing evidence of influence on shock in general has been shown (GOODMAN and GILMAN, 1975). In anaphylactic reactions their effect is doubtful. In our experience corticosteroid hormones started in the early stages of envenomation and continued until the 2nd week did not even prevent serum sickness on the 7–9th day after administration of antivenom. In severe—usually untreated—patients, anemia often develops and blood transfusion is indicated.

H. Summary of Management of Snakebites

I. *Early treatment* (including "first-aid")
   1. Reassurance of the victim
   2. Immunobilization of the bitten extremity
   3. Transport to a medical facility
   4. Identification of the snake, if available

II. *Definite treatment* (in the admission room)
   1. Installation of an intravenous drop infusion set
   2. Intracutaneous sensitivity test to horse serum
   3. Alleviation of pain
   4. Intravenous administration of specific antivenom in adequate quantities (in cases of bite inflicted by *Vipera xanthina palestinae* 50–80 ml)
   5. Intravenous drop infusion of physiologic solution with or without vasopressor drugs until hypotension is overcome
   6. Transfer to the ward
   7. Monitoring blood pressure, blood count, coagulation studies, and observation for edema
   8. Blood transfusion if anemia develops

References

Ahuja, M. L., Singh, G.: Snakebite in India. In: Venoms, pp. 341—351. Washington, D.C.: Amer. Ass. Advanc. Sci. 1956

Allon, N., Kochva, E.: The quantities of venom injected into prey of different size by *Vipera palestinae* in a single bite. J. exp. Zool. **138**, 71—75 (1974)

Ameratunga, B.: Middle cerebral occlusion following Russell's viper bite. J. trop. Med. Hyg. **75**, 95—97 (1972)

Arnold, R. E.: Results of treatment of *Crotalus* envenomation. Amer. Surg. **41**, 643—647 (1975)

Barnes, J. M., Trueta, J.: Absorption of bacterial toxin and snake venoms from the tissues. Lancet **1941**, 623—626

Biran, H., Stern, J., Dvilansky, A.: Impaired platelet aggregation after *Echis colorata* bite in man. (Letter to the editor). Israel J. med. Sci. **8**, 1257 (1972)

Chajek, T., Rubinger, D., Alkan, M., Melmed, R. M., Gunders, A. E.: Anaphylactoid reaction and tissue damage following bite by *Atractaspis engaddensis*. Trans. roy. Soc. trop. Med. Hyg. **68**, 333—337 (1974)

Chapman, D. S.: The Symptomatology, pathology, and treatment of the bites of venomous snakes of Central ans Southern Africa. In: Bücherl, W., Buckley, E., Denlofen, V. (Eds.): Venomons Animals and Their Venoms, Vol. I, pp. 463—527. New York: Academic Press 1968

Chugh, K. S., Aikat, B. K., Sharma, B. K., Dash, S. C., Matthew, M. Th., Dash, K. C.: Acute renal failure following snakebite. Amer. J. trop. Med. Hyg. **24**, 692—697 (1975)
Corkill, N. L.: Snake poisoning in the Sudan. In: Buckley, E., Porges, N. (Eds.): Venoms, pp. 331—339, Washington, D.C.: Amer. Ass. Adv. Sci. 1956
Corkill, N. S., Jonides, Jr., C., Pitma, C. R. S.: Biting and poisoning by the mole vipers of the genus *Atractaspis*. Trans. roy. Soc. trop. Med. Hyg. **53**, 95—101 (1959)
Dvilansky, A., Biran, H.: Hypofibrinogenemia after *Echis colorata* bite in man. Acta Haemat. **49**, 123—127 (1973)
Efrati, P.: Observations on 125 cases of viper bite. (In Hebrew). Harefuah **63**, 1—10 (1962)
Efrati, P.: Clinical manifestations of snake bite by *Vipera xanthina palestinae* (Werner) and their pathophysiological basis. Mem. Inst. Butantan **32**, 189—191 (1966)
Efrati, P., Reif, L.: Clinical and pathological observations on sixty five cases of viper bite in Israel. Amer. J. trop. Med. Hyg. **2**, 1085—1108 (1953)
Ellis, E. F., Smith, R. T.: Systemic anaphylaxis after rattle snake bite. J. Amer. med. Ass. **193**, 401—402 (1965)
Fainaru, M., Eisenberg, S., Manny, N., Hershko, C.: The natural course of defibrination syndrome caused by *Echis colorata* venom in man. Thromb. Diathes. hemorrh. (Stuttg.) **31**, 420—428 (1974)
Fainaru, M., Manny, N., Hershko, C., Eisenberg, S.: Defibrination following *Echis colorata* bite in man. Israel J. med. Sci. **6**, 720—725 (1970)
Glass, Jr., T. G.: Early debridment in pit viper bite. Surg. Gynec. Obstet. **136**, 774—776 (1973)
Goodman, S. S., Gilman, A.: The Pharmacological Basis of Therapeutics, 5th Ed. New York: Mac Millan 1975
Greenwood, B. M., Warrell, D. A., Davidson, N. Mc.D., Ormerod, S. D., Reid, H. A.: Immunodiagnosis of snake bite. Brit. med. J. **1974 VI**, 743—745
Huang, T. T., Lynch, J. B., Larson, D. S., Lewis, S. R.: Management of snakebite. Ann. Surg. **179**, 598—607 (1974)
Kaiser, E., Raab, W.: Liberation of pharmacologically active substances from mast cells by animal venoms. Mem. Inst. Butantan **33**, 461—466 (1966)
Kessler, I.: Personal communication (1976)
Kochva, E.: On the anatomy of the venom apparatus in snakes and venom secretion by *Vipera palestinae*. Dapin Refuiim (Folia Medica) **21**, 593—607 (In Hebrew) (1962)
Leffkowitz, M., Casper, J., Gitter, S., Kochwa, S., de Vries, A.: The bite of the *Vipera palestinae* in Israel. Abstracts of the Sixth Internat. Congress of Int. Med., Basle, 1960, p. 246
Leopold, R. S., Merriam, T. W.: The effectiveness of tourniquet, incision and suction in snake venom removal. Naval Med. Field Res. Lab. **10**, 211—240 (1960)
Man, G.: Snake bites in Israel, M.D.Thesis University of Jerusalem (In Hebrew) 1976
Munter, S. (Ed.): Maimonides' Medical Works. Jerusalem: Rubin Mass 1947
Path, J., Ravid, M.: *Aspis cerastes* bite—Case report (In Hebrew) Harefuah **81**, 85—86 (1971)
Ravina, A., Lehman, E., Gottfried, J., Stern, J.: *Echis colorata* bite and treatment with specific antiserum (In Hebrew) Harefuah **69**, 309—310 (1965)
Reid, H. A.: Symptomatology and treatment of land snake bites in India and southeast Asia. In: Bücherl, W., Buckley, E., Deulofeu, V. (Eds.): Venomous Animals and Their Venoms, Vol. I, pp. 611—642. New York: Academic Press 1968
Reid, H. A.: Adder bites in Britain. Brit. med. J. **1976 II**, 153—156
Reif, L.: Snake bite, a pathologic—anatomical study (In Hebrew with English summary). Dapim Refuiim (Folia Medica) **21**, 651—654 (1962)
Russell, F. E., Quilligan, Jr., J. J.: Snakebite. J. Amer. med. Ass. **195**, 596—597 (1966)
Sadan, N., Soroker, B.: Observations on the effects of the bite of a venomous snake on children and adults. J. Pediat. **76**, 711—715 (1970)
Seeat, J. K., Reddy, J., Edington, D. R.: Acute renal failure due to proliferative nephritis from snake bite poisoning. Nephron **13**, 455—463 (1974)
Shargil, A., Shabaton, D., Rosenthal, T.: Clinical and laboratory findings in *Aspis cerastes* snake bite (In Hebrew with English summary) Harefuah **85**, 504—508 (1973)
Shulov, A., Ben Shaul, D., Rosin, R., Nitzan, M.: The efficacy of suction as a method of treatment in snake venom poisoning. Toxicon **7**, 15—18 (1969)

Sitprija, V., Benyajati, C., Boonpucknavig: Further observations of renal insufficiency in snake bite. Nephron **13**, 396—403 (1974)

Sutherland, S. K., Coulter, A. R., Broad, A. J., Hilton, J. M. N., Lane, L. H. D.: Human snake bite victims: the successful detection of circulating snake venom by radioimmunoassay. Med. J. Aust. **1**, 27—29 (1975)

Vries, A., de, Condrea, E., Klibanski, C., Rechnic, J., Moroz, C., Kirschman, C.: Hematological effects of the venoms of two Near Eastern snakes: *Vipera palestinae* and *Echis colorata* (In Hebrew with English summary). Dapim Refuiim (Folia Medica) **21**, 614—625 (1962)

Vries, A., de, Gitter, S.: The action of *Vipera xanthina palestinae* venom on blood coagulation in vitro. Brit. J. Haemat. **3**, 379—386 (1957)

Warrell, D. A., Davidson, N. McD., Ormerod, L. D., Pope, H. M., Watkins, B. J., Greenwood, B. M., Reid, H. A.: Bites by the saw-scaled or carpet viper *(Echis carinatus)*: Trial of two specific antivenoms. Brit. med. J. **1974 IV**, 437—440

Warrell, D. A., Ormerod, L. D., Davidson, N. McD.: Bites by Puff adder *(Bitis arietans)* in Nigeria and value of antivenom. Brit. med. J. **1975 IV**, 697—700

Weiss, H. J., Phillips, L. L., Hopewell, W. S., Phillips, G., Christy, N. P., Nitti, J. F.: Heparin therapy in a patient bitten by a saw-scaled viper *(Echis carinatus)*, a snake whose venom activates prothrombin. Amer. J. Med. **54**, 653—662 (1973)

Yatziv, S., Manny, N., Ritchie, J., Russell, A.: The indication of afibrinogenemia by *Echis colorata* snake bite. J. trop. Med. Hyg. **77**, 136—138 (1974)

CHAPTER 27

The Clinical Problem of Crotalid Snake Venom Poisoning

F. E. RUSSELL

A. Introduction

Bites by snakes of the family Crotalidae are usually medical emergencies requiring immediate attention and the exercise of considerable judgment. Delayed or inadequate treatment may result in undue harm to the patient and may result in tragic consequences. On the other hand, the failure to differentiate between the bite of a nonvenomous snake and a venomous one can lead to the use of measures that may not only cause discomfort to the patient but may provoke serious complications. Before any treatment is instituted, it is essential that a working diagnosis be established. In making this diagnosis, it must always be kept in mind that a venomous snake may bite a person without injecting venom.

While the word *snakebite* is commonly used to denote bites by venomous snakes, it is more properly applied to bites by all snakes, whether venomous or not. The two terms, snakebite and snake venom poisoning, are commonly confused in both the medical and lay literature, and the confusion has sometimes led to errors in clinical judgment. Bites by any snake, whether venomous or not, and in which there is no evidence of poisoning, might be called *snakebite*, whereas bites by venomous snakes in which poisoning does not occur might more appropriately be called *venomous snake bite without envenomation*. Finally, those bites in which poisoning does occur are best termed *snake venom poisoning*.

In snake venom poisoning, the diagnosis is established on the basis of the presence of fang marks and symptoms and signs. Professional identification of the offending reptile, if available, should be noted on the patient's chart. Diagnoses based on fang marks alone are precarious, as teeth marks vary widely in venomous and nonvenomous snakes. It must also be remembered that one may be bitten by a nonvenomous snake and in the excitement develop symptoms and signs which to the untrained eye may appear to resemble snake venom poisoning. Hyperventilation, weakness, anxiety, nausea, and swelling of a part behind a tourniquet have all been mistaken for poisoning, following bites by nonvenomous snakes.

It is also well-known that rattlesnakes and other crotalids can bite, even bite twice, and not eject venom. In a series of 600 cases of bites by venomous snakes seen by the author, 20% showed no evidence of poisoning (RUSSELL et al., 1975). Colleagues in the southeastern part of the United States, and in Central and South America, have indicated by correspondence that approximately 30% of all cases of bites by venomous snakes seen by them do not result in envenomation. In the author's experiences in South America, at least 35% of the bites by crotalids showed no effects of poisoning. The Old World pit vipers, such as *Agkistrodon* species and the various *Trimeresurus* species, also appear to bite without ejecting venom in 30–50% of their strikes.

It is easy to understand that the physician faced with his first case of a bite by a venomous snake, or even his first several cases, may not appreciate the possibility of nonenvenomation, and may make a diagnosis and institute treatment that is not indicated. There appears to be little doubt that many of the "cures" noted in the literature (RUSSELL and SCHARFFENBERG, 1964) can be attributed to the fact that the treatment was successful because there was no poisoning involved, and the puncture wound healed of its own accord. This often overlooked observation is perhaps best expressed by FONTANA (1781).

> The physician regards as a remedy for a disorder, that medication which has been followed by recovery, when in sound logic no other deduction can be drawn than that the vaunted remedy has not killed the patient; and we see the physician quietly reasons and believes that the sick person would have certainly died had he not been treated by him, and with this, supposes that which he does not know, and which is most likely altogether untrue.

This Chapter will concern itself with the medical problem of envenomation by Crotalidae and, in particular, envenomation by the New World species. However, in the cases of bites by Old World species treated or seen by the author, there appears to be a sufficient degree of similarity in the overall clinical syndrome to warrant some generalizations, but some important differences must also be considered.

B. Identification

In Table 1 are shown the New World Crotalidae. The common names may vary with different areas. The Table is modified from a previous paper (RUSSELL, 1969). The data are taken from a number of sources, including KLAUBER (1956a), KLEMMER (1963), HOGE (1965), DOWLING et al. (1968), and from collections noted elsewhere (RUSSELL, 1969). It should be noted that this Table is based on more than the morphologic characteristics of the crotalids. It is based on some considerations of the differences in the chemical composition of the venoms. The reader is referred to the Chapter by UNDERWOOD in this volume for a more thorough review of the Old World Crotalidae.

In North America, the clinically important crotalids include: *Agkistrodon bilineatus, contortrix*, and *piscivorus; Crotalus adamanteus, atrox, basiliscus, cerastes, horridus, mitchelli, molossus, ruber, scutulatus*, and *viridis;* and *Sistrurus catenatus* and *miliarius*. The taxonomy, distribution, and general biology of these snakes have been reviewed by CONANT (1958), GLOYD (1940), KLAUBER (1956a), SHAW and CAMPBELL (1974), STEBBINS (1954), and WRIGHT and WRIGHT (1957).

In Central and South America, the clinically important crotalids include: *Bothrops alternatus, atrox, bilineatus, jararaca, jararacussu, neuwiedi, nummifer*, and *schlegeli; Crotalus durissus* and *viridis;* and *Lachesis mutus*. Texts on these snakes include those by HOGE (1965), LAZELL (1964), MERTENS (1952), PETERS (1960), and SANTOS (1955).

The Old World Crotalidae do not appear to be as well worked out as the New World species, although the works of BELLAIRS (1970), GLOYD (1972), HAILE (1958), KUNTZ (1963), LEVITON (1961), LIM (1971), POPE (1935), REID et al. (1963c), SAWAI (1973), UNDERWOOD (1967), and WERLER and KEEGAN (1963) are references of value

Table 1. New World *Crotalidae*

Name	Common Name	Canada	U.S.A.	Mexico	C. America	S. America
Agkistrodon bilineatus Günther	Cantil or Mexican moccasin			×	×	
Agkistrodon bilineatus taylori Burger and Robertson	Taylor's moccasin			×		
Agkistrodon contortrix contortrix (Linnaeus)[a]	Southern copperhead		×			
Agkistrodon contortrix laticinctus Gloyd and Conant	Broad-banded copperhead		×			
Agkistrodon contortrix mokeson (Daudin)	Northern copperhead		×			
Agkistrodon contortrix pictigaster Gloyd and Conant	Trans-Pecos copperhead		×			
Agkistrodon piscivorus piscivorus (Lacépède)	Eastern cottonmouth		×			
Agkistrodon piscivorus leucostoma (Troost)	Western cottonmouth		×			
Bothrops albocarinatus Shreve						×
Bothrops alternatus Duméril, Bibron and Duméril	Urutu or Yarara					×
Bothrops alticola Parker	Parker's pit viper					×
Bothrops ammodytoides Leybold	Patagonian pit viper or Snouted Lance-Head					×
Bothrops andianus Amaral	Andian pit viper					×
Bothrops atrox atrox Linnaeus	"Fer-de-lance"				×	×
Bothrops atrox asper Garman				×	×	×
Bothrops karbouri (Dunn)	Barbour's pit viper			×		
Bothrops barnetti Parker	Barnett's pit viper					×
Bothrops bicolor Bocourt	Bocourt's pit viper			×	×	
Bothrops bilineatus bilineatus (Wied)						×
Bothrops bilineatus smaragdinus						×
Bothrops brazili Hoge[b]	Brazil's pit viper					×
Bothrops caribbeaus (Garman)	Caribbean pit viper	St. Lucia Island				
Bothrops castelnaudi (Duméril, Bibron and Duméril)	Castelnau's pit viper					×
Bothrops cotiara (Gomes)	Cotiara					×
Bothrops dunni (Hartweg and Oliver)	Dunn's pit viper			×		
Bothrops erythromelas Amaral[c]						×
Bothrops fonsecai Hoge and Belluomini	Fonseca's pit viper					×
Bothrops godmanni (Günther)	Godmann's pit viper			×	×	
Bothrops hypoprorus Amaral						×

Bothrops iglesiasi Amaral[c]	Iglesiasi pit viper				×
Bothrops insularis Amaral[d]	Island jararaca	Queimada Grande Island			
Bothrops itapetiningae (Boulenger)	Cotiarinha				×
Bothrops jararaca (Wied)[d]	Jararaca				×
Bothrops jararacussu Lacerda	Jararacussu				×
Bothrops lanceolatus (Lacépède)	Fer-de-lance	Martinique Island			
Bothrops lansbergii lansbergii Schlegel	Lansberg's pit viper		×	×	
Bothrops lansbergii annectens (Schmidt)				×	
Bothrops lansbergii venezuelensis Roze					
Bothrops lateralis (Peters)				×	×
Bothrops lichenosus Roze					
Bothrops lojanus Parker	Lojan pit viper				×
Bothrops marajoensis (see Hoge)					×
Bothrops medusa (Sternfeld)					×
Bothrops melanurus (Müller)	Black-tailed viper		×		×
Bothrops microphthalmus microphthalmus Cope					
Bothrops microphthalmus colombianus					×
Rendahl and Vestergren					×
Bothrops moojeni (see Hoge)					
Bothrops nasutus Bocourt	Hog-nosed pit viper		×	×	×
Bothrops neuwiedi neuwiedi Wagler[e]	Jararaca pintada or Wied's lance-head				×
Bothrops neuwiedi bolivianus Amaral[e]					×
Bothrops neuwiedi meridionalis Müller					×
Bothrops neuwiedi diporus Cope					×
Bothrops neuwiedi lutzi (Miranda-Ribeiro)	Lutz pit viper				×
Bothrops neuwiedi piauhyensis Amaral					×
Bothrops neuwiedi pubescens (Cope)					×
Bothrops neuwiedi urutu Lacerda					×
Bothrops nigroviridis nigroviridis (Peters)				×	×
Bothrops nigroviridis aurifer (Salvin)			×	×	
Bothrops nummifer mexicanus (Duméril, Bibron and Duméril)			×	×	
Bothrops nummifer occiduus Hodge			×	×	
Bothrops oligolepis (Werner)					×
Bothrops orphryomegas Bocourt				×	
Bothrops peruvianus (Boulenger)					×
Bothrops picadoi (Dunn)				×	
Bothrops pictus (Tschudi)					×

Table 1 (continued)

Name	Common Name	Canada	U.S.A.	Mexico	C. America	S. America
Bothrops pifanoi Sandner Montilla and Römer						×
Bothrops pirajai Amaral	Pirajá's pit viper, Jararacuçu					×
Bothrops pradoi (Hoge)						×
Bothrops pulcher (Peters)						×
Bothrops punctatus (Garcia)					×	×
Bothrops roedingeri Mertens						×
Bothrops sanctaecrucis Hoge						×
Bothrops schlegelii (Berthold)	Schlegel's pit viper			×	×	×
Bothrops sphenophrys Smith				×		
Bothrops supraciliaris Taylor					×	
Bothrops undulatus (Jan)				×		
Bothrops xanthogrammus (Cope)						×
Bothrops yucatanicus (Smith)	Yucatan pit viper			×		
Crotalus adamanteus Beauvois	Eastern diamond rattlesnake		×			
Crotalus atrox Baird and Girard	Western diamond rattlesnake		×	×		
Crotalus basiliscus basiliscus (Cope)	Mexican west-coast rattlesnake			×		
Crotalus basiliscus oaxacus Gloyd	Oaxacan rattlesnake			×		
Crotalus catalinensis Cliff	Santa Catalina Island rattlesnake			×		
Crotalus cerastes cerastes Hallowell	Mojave Desert sidewinder		×	×		
Crotalus cerastes cercobombus Savage and Cliff	Sonoran Desert sidewinder		×	×		
Crotalus cerastes laterorepens Klauber	Colorado Desert sidewinder		×	×		
Crotalus durissus durissus Linné	Central American rattlesnake			×	×	×
Crotalus durissus culminatus Klauber	Northwestern neotropical rattlesnake			×		
Crotalus durissus terrificus (Laurenti)	South American rattlesnake					×
Crotalus durissus totonacus Gloyd and Kauffeld	Totonacan rattlesnake			×		
Crotalus durissus tzabcan Klauber	Yucatan neotropical rattlesnake			×	×	
Crotalus durissus vegrandis Klauber	Uracoan rattlesnake					×
Crotalus enyo enyo (Cope)	Lower California rattlesnake			×		
Crotalus enyo cerralvensis Cliff	Cerralvo Island rattlesnake			×		
Crotalus enyo furvus Lowe and Norris	Rosario rattlesnake			×		
Crotalus exsul Garman	Cedros Island diamond rattlesnake			×		
Crotalus horridus horridus Linné[f]	Timber rattlesnake		×			
Crotalus horridus atricaudatus Latreille	Canebrake rattlesnake		×			
Crotalus intermedius intermedius Troschel	Totalcan small-headed rattlesnake			×		

Crotalus intermedius omiltemanus Günther	Omilteman small-headed rattlesnake			×	
Crotalus lepidus lepidus (Kennicott)	Mottled rock rattlesnake		×	×	
Crotalus lepidus klauberi Gloyd	Banded rock rattlesnake		×	×	
Crotalus lepidus morulus Klauber	Tamaulipan rock rattlesnake			×	
Crotalus mitchellii mitchellii (Cope)	San Lucan speckled rattlesnake			×	
Crotalus mitchellii muertensis Klauber	El Muerto Island speckled rattlesnake			×	
Crotalus mitchellii pyrrhus (Cope)	Southwestern speckled rattlesnake		×	×	
Crotalus mitchellii stephensi Klauber	Panamint rattlesnake		×		
Crotalus molossus molossus Baird and Girard	Northern black-tailed rattlesnake		×	×	
Crotalus molossus nigrescens Gloyd	Mexican black-tailed rattlesnake			×	
Crotalus molossus estebanensis Klauber	San Esteban Island rattlesnake			×	
Crotalus polystictus (Cope)	Mexican lance-headed rattlesnake			×	
Crotalus pricei pricei Van Denburgh	Arizona twin-spotted rattlesnake		×	×	
Crotalus pricei miquihuanus Gloyd	Miquihuanan twin-spotted rattlesnake			×	
Crotalus pusillus Klauber	Tancitaran dusky rattlesnake			×	
Crotalus ruber ruber Cope	Red diamond rattlesnake		×	×	
Crotalus ruber lucasensis Van Denburgh	San Lucan diamond rattlesnake			×	
Crotalus scutulatus scutulatus (Kennicott)	Mojave rattlesnake		×	×	
Crotalus scutulatus salvini Günther	Huamantlan rattlesnake			×	
Crotalus stejnegeri Dunn	Long-tailed rattlesnake			×	
Crotalus tigris Kennicott	Tiger rattlesnake		×	×	
Crotalus tortugensis Van Denburgh and Slevin	Tortuga Island diamond rattlesnake			×	
Crotalus transversus Taylor	Cross-banded mountain rattlesnake			×	
Crotalus triseriatus triseriatus (Wagler)	Central-plateau dusky rattlesnake			×	
Crotalus triseriatus aquilus Klauber	Queretaran dusky rattlesnake			×	
Crotalus unicolor van Lidth de Jeude	Aruba Island rattlesnake				×
Crotalus viridis viridis (Rafinesque)	Prairie rattlesnake	×	×	×	
Crotalus viridis abyssus Klauber	Grand Canyon rattlesnake		×		
Crotalus viridis caliginis Klauber	Coronado Island rattlesnake			×	
Crotalus viridis cerberus (Coues)	Arizona black rattlesnake		×		
Crotalus viridis decolor Klauber	Midget faded rattlesnake		×		
Crotalus viridis helleri Meek	Southern Pacific rattlesnake		×	×	
Crotalus viridis lutosus Klauber	Great Basin rattlesnake		×		
Crotalus viridis nuntius Klauber	Arizona prairie rattlesnake		×		
Crotalus viridis oreganus Holbrook	Northern Pacific rattlesnake		×		
Crotalus willardi willardi Meek	Arizona ridge-nosed rattlesnake		×	×	
Crotalus willardi meridionalis Klauber	Southern ridge-nosed rattlesnake			×	
Crotalus willardi silus Klauber	Chihuahuan ridge-nosed rattlesnake			×	

Table 1 (continued)

Name	Common Name	Canada	U.S.A.	Mexico	C. America	S. America
Sistrurus catenatus catenatus (Rafinesque)	Eastern massasauga	×	×			
Sistrurus catenatus tergeminus (Say)	Western massasauga		×	×		
Sistrurus miliarius miliarius (Linné)	Carolina pigmy rattlesnake		×			
Sistrurus miliarius barbouri Gloyd	Southeastern pigmy rattlesnake		×			
Sistrurus miliarius streckeri Gloyd	Western pigmy rattlesnake		×			
Sistrurus ravus (Cope)	Mexican pigmy rattlesnake			×		
Lachesis mutus mutus (Linnaeus)	Bushmaster				×	×
Lachesis mutus stenophrys Cope					×	
Lachesis mutus noctiuaga Hoag						×

[a] Could be expected to occur south of the U.S. border.
[b] Venom of single specimen indicated its pattern very different from other species of the general area.
[c] Venom patterns very similar.
[d] Venom patterns almost identic.
[e] Venom patterns almost identic.
[f] Possibly extinct in Canada.

to the clinician. Of particular medical importance are *Agkistrodon acutus, blomhoffii, elegans, halys*, and *rhodostoma;* and *Trimeresurus albolabris, flavoviridis, gramineus, monticola, mucrosquamatus, popeorum purpureromaculatus, stejnegeri*, and *wagleri.*

Recent general reference works on crotalid snakes and snakebites of importance to the clinician include those by DOWLING et al. (1968), KLEMMER (1963), MINTON and MINTON (1969), MINTON (1974), RUSSELL et al. (1975), and SAWAI (1973).

Whenever possible, positive identification of the snake should be made by a trained person. The proper identification of a venomous crotalid is not always easy, and when the offending snake is not captured, or even seen, the physician will need to give most careful attention to the development of the symptoms and signs. There are some distinguishing features of note for identifying poisonous snakes. The crotalids are distinguished from the nonvenomous snakes in their areas by their two elongated, canaliculated, upper maxillary teeth, which can be rotated from their resting position, in which they are folded against the roof of the mouth to their biting position, where they are almost perpendicular to the upper jaw. Each fang is shed periodically and replaced by the first reserve fang. In the crotalids and vipers, the pupils are vertically elliptic, but a few nonvenomous snakes also have such pupils. Most dangerous elapids have round pupils. In the pit vipers, there is a deep, easily identifiable pit between the eye and the nostril. This is a heat-receptor organ. The somewhat triangular shape of the head of most of the crotalids may also help to distinguish them from nonvenomous snakes, and, of course, the rattlesnake is distinguished by its rattles. Color and pattern are the most deceptive criteria for identification. Unfortunately, these are the characteristics most uninformed persons will present. Correct identification of a crotalid at the species level is highly desirable, for among other things, species identification may be an important factor in determining the amount of antivenin to be used.

The venom apparatus of Crotalidae consists of the two venom glands, the two venom ducts, and two or more upper maxillary teeth or fangs. The venom glands are homologous with the mammalian salivary parotids. Their size, shape, and location vary with the genus of the snake. In the pit vipers, the venom glands lie posterior to the eyes and near the outer edge of the upper jaw. The innervation of these muscles is different from that controlling the biting mechanisms; thus, the snake can control the amount of venom to be ejected. It can discharge venom from one fang, from both, or from neither. Snakes rarely, if ever, eject the full contents of their glands. The amount of venom injected in the process of obtaining food appears to be related to the size of the prey. In the case of bites on humans, or in situations where the snake strikes in quick defense, the amount of venom may vary from 0–90% of the gland content.

C. Epidemiology

More than 45000 people in the United States are bitten by snakes each year (RUSSELL, 1968). However, only about 8000 of these bites are inflicted by venomous snakes, and just under 7000 cases of snake venom poisoning are reported (PARRISH, 1966). Fewer than 12 persons a year now die from snakebite in the United States. The majority of these deaths are in children, untreated or undertreated cases, or in members of religious sects who handle venomous serpents as part of their worship exercises. Almost all of the deaths are attributed to rattlesnakes, which account for about 60% of all bites by venomous snakes in the United States. Most other bites are attributed to the other crotalids, the copperhead and cottonmouth. Coral snakes inflict less than 1% of all bites. In a series of 600 cases seen at the Los Angeles County-University of Southern California Medical Center over a 20-year period, the ages of the patients were as follows:

Age	Number of cases	Age	Number of cases
1–9	46	21–25	122
10–15	140	26–30	80
16–20	153	31+	59

Snakebites are generally divided into "legitimate" and "illegitimate" categories. The former is applied to those cases in which the patient had no "intention of indulging in so unnecessary a risk," while the latter includes cases in which the patient, by his own decision, chose to handle the snake. Further study of the above figures indicates the following:

Age	% Legitimate	Age	% Legitimate
1–9	81	21–25	62
10–15	51	26–30	69
16–20	48	31+	83

These statistics obviously vary from one country to another. The relatively high incidence of illegitimate bites in this series reflects children's interest in snakes and the desire to capture them for pets or sale. With respect to bite location, more than 95% were on the hands or feet and 90% of the legitimate bites occurred between March 15 and October 15.

Recent comprehensive statistics on crotalid bites outside the United States are not available. MINTON and MINTON (1969) note an earlier figure of approximately 200 snakebite fatalities annually in Mexico, of which most were certainly caused by Crotalidae. This figure is far in excess of the present number of deaths from snakebite in that country. However, personal correspondence from knowledgeable persons in Mexico would indicate that the number of cases of snake venom poisoning by crotalids exceeds 5000. In Central America, no recent statistics on snakebite are available, but a review of the literature from the countries of this area, along with personal observations in Nicaragua, data by MINTON and MINTON (1969), and letters from the United Fruit Company would appear to place the annual number of snake venom poisoning cases between 2000–3000, most of which are inflicted by crotalids. ROSENFELD (1971) notes that during the 12-year period 1954–1965, 1718 cases of snakebite were seen at the Hospital Vital Brazil at the Instituto Butantan. There were 30 deaths. A total figure of 3000 cases of crotalid bites for South America seems reasonable, although this number may certainly be low if a count of unreported cases was available.

With respect to crotalid bites in the Old World, no comprehensive statistics are available, but reliable figures on some areas can be obtained from the many fine papers by REID and SAWAI. SAWAI (1973) notes 3510 habu bites on Amami Oshima during the 13-year period 1959–1971. During the 12-year period, 1959–1970, there were approximately 3852 habu bites on Okinawa. These statistics are indeed startling. One wonders what the incidence of snake venom poisoning might be in the whole of Asia if the statistics were as carefully recorded as these by SAWAI.

On Taiwan, 108 patients died of snake venom poisoning during the 3-year period 1966–1968. Approximately 65% of these deaths were caused by crotalids. In the Philippines, 300 patients died from snakebite in 1968, but most of these deaths were caused by the Philippine cobra. In Thailand during 1968, there were 4107 snakebite cases reported, with 273 deaths (SAWAI, 1973). Most of these deaths were caused by the cobra, but the Malayan pit viper and Pope's tree viper accounted for many. REID et al. (1963c) note 2114 cases of snakebite during a 3-year period. Of 1159 of these, 733 were caused by *Agkistrodon rhodostoma*, and at least 40 additional bites were inflicted by other Crotalidae. They note that in more than half of the 824 cases in which the snake was identified, there was either no or only very slight poisoning.

D. Clinical Manifestations

The symptoms, signs, and gravity of snake venom poisoning are dependent upon a number of factors: 1) the age and size of the victim, 2) the nature, location, depth, and number of bites, 3) the length of time the snake holds on, 4) the extent of anger or fear that motivates the snake to strike, 5) the amount of venom injected, 6) the species and size of the snake involved, 7) the condition of his fangs and the venom glands, 8) the victim's sensitivity to the venom, 9) the pathogens present in the snake's mouth, and 10) the degree and kind of first-aid treatment and subsequent medical care. It can be seen that snakebites may vary in severity from trivial to extremely grave. Whenever possible, positive identification of the snake should be made by a trained person. The proper identification of a venomous crotalid is not always easy, and when the offending snake is not captured, or even seen, the physician will need to give most careful attention to the development of the symptoms and signs. Much has been written about "typical" fang mark patterns, based on the anatomy of the snake's jaw and laboratory experiments, but these patterns are infrequently seen under field conditions. Crotalidae may leave one or two fang marks, as well as some other teeth marks. Single fang punctures are very common, and they are not uncommon in bites by some nonvenomous snakes. Some insight to the identity of the offending snakes can be obtained from the puncture wounds. However, they should never be relied upon for positive identification. Positive diagnosis of snake venom poisoning is dependent upon identification of the snake and evidence of envenomation.

Grading of rattlesnake bites by numbers, as sometimes described in the literature, may serve some useful purpose, but it is of limited value in grading envenomation by many species of snakes. It seems far more practical to describe cases as *minor*, *moderate*, or *severe*, based on all symptoms, all signs, and all laboratory findings, including changes in the blood cells, blood chemistry, deficiencies in neuromuscular transmission, changes in motor and sensory functions, and the like, rather than grading the bite on one or several parameters, such as the amount of swelling and pain. Bites by the Mojave rattlesnake, for instance, may give rise to minimal edema, few local tissue changes, and pain (and be graded as 1); the result, as has happened, is that the physician gives an insufficient amount of antivenin. In California and Ari-

Table 2. Rattlesnake venom poisoning

Fang marks	100/100[a]
Swelling and edema	80/100
Pain	72/100
Ecchymosis	60/100
Vesiculations	51/100
Changes in pulse rate	60/100
Weakness	72/100
Sweating and/or chill	54/100
Numbness or tingling of tongue and mouth, or scalp or feet	63/100
Faintness or dizziness	52/100
Nausea, vomiting, or both	48/100
Blood pressure changes	46/100
Increased body temperature	22/100
Swelling regional lymph nodes	40/100
Fasciculations	33/100
Increased blood clotting time	32/100
Sphering of red blood cells	29/100
Tingling or numbness of affected part	41/100
Necrosis	38/100
Respiratory rate changes	30/100
Decreased hemoglobin	37/100
Abnormal electrocardiogram	26/100
Cyanosis	20/100
Hematemesis, hematuria, or melena	22/100
Glycosuria	32/100
Proteinuria	21/100
Unconsciousness	20/100
Thirst	24/100
Increased salivation	19/100
Swollen eyelids	7/100
Retinal hemorrhage	5/100
Blurring of vision	12/100
Convulsions	1/100
Increased blood platelets	4/100
Decreased blood platelets	47/100

[a] Times: Symptoms or signs observed/total number of cases.

zona prior to 1955, there were more deaths attributed to this species than any other, probably because of an insufficient dose of antivenin, which had been based on the relatively minor local tissue reactions on which the case had been graded.

Table 2 shows the symptoms and signs following bites by rattlesnakes. The table is based on the author's experience with 85 treated and 15 untreated patients in a series of 600 cases. These symptoms and signs are representative for approximately 15 subspecies of rattlesnakes. Bites by the eastern diamondback rattlesnake tend to produce more swelling and edema, more necrosis, and more tissue and blood loss. Paralysis also appears to be more commonly reported following bites by the eastern diamondback than most other species. This may be due, in part, to the more severe edema and hemorrhage produced by the venom of this snake, which in turn causes localized ischemia of nerve tissues. In most cases of rattlesnake venom poisoning, some degree of swelling is a constant finding and usually seen in the injured area within 5 min after the bite. In the absence of treatment, the swelling progresses rapidly and may involve the entire injured extremity within an hour. Generally, however, the edema spreads more slowly, and usually over a period of 8–36 h. As noted, the swelling is most marked following bites by the eastern diamondback rattlesnake. It is less marked following western diamondback bites, and even less severe following bites by the prairie, timber, red, Pacific, Mojave, and black-tailed rattlesnakes, and the sidewinders. It is least marked following bites by copperheads, massasaugas, and pygmy rattlesnakes. Ecchymosis and discoloration of the skin can appear in the area of the bite within several hours. The skin may appear tense and shiny. In the untreated case, vesiculations may be found within 3 h; they are generally present by the end of 24 h. Petechiae and hemorrhagic vesiculations are not uncommon, and thrombosis in the superficial vessels and sloughing of the injured tissues is also not uncommon in untreated cases. Necrosis develops in a large percentage of cases in which an insufficient amount of antivenin, or no antivenin, has been given. Amputation of an extremity or part of an extremity is much less common today than it was even a decade ago. However, the use of a measure known as cryotherapy has been associated with a high incidence of amputation. Pain immediately following the bites is a complaint in most cases of poisoning by the North American rattlesnake. It is most severe following eastern and western diamondback bites, less severe following bites by the prairie and other *viridis* rattlesnakes, and least severe following copperhead and massasauga bites. Weakness, sweating, faintness and nausea are commonly reported. Skin temperature usually is elevated immediately following the bite. Regional lymph nodes may be enlarged, painful, and tender. A very common complaint following bites by the southern Pacific rattlesnake, and one sometimes reported following other pit viper bites, is tingling or numbness over the tongue and mouth or scalp and paresthesia about the wound. Hematemesis, melena, increased or decreased salivation, and muscle fasciculations may be seen. Hematologic findings may show hemoconcentration early, then a decrease in red cells and platelets. Urinalysis may reveal hematuria, glycosuria, and proteinuria. Bleeding and clotting times are usually prolonged.

In bites by Central and South American crotalids seen at our Medical Center, the clinical manifestations have varied considerably. In general, bites by South American *Crotalus* species have given rise to far less edema and local tissue changes than those inflicted by North American species, but there have been far greater neurologic deficits, and in the case of *C. durissus terrificus*, greater intravascular hemolysis.

Pain is usually an immediate complaint, and within 20 min there is often parasthesia of the involved part and some muscular weakness. Subsequently, there may be pain in the large muscle masses, particularly those of the back and neck. Edema is minimal and it is far more difficult to identify the wound site than in North American crotalid bites. Visual disturbances may occur within 90 min of the envenomation and with the usual lid lag the patient presents, the facies is diagnostic. It has been described in detail by ROSENFELD (1966). Increasing respiratory distress, headache, dizziness, and weakness are often reported. Deep reflexes usually are hypoactive and superficial reflexes are abnormal. Methemoglobinuria with progressive anuria may develop. The hemolysis gives rise to some degree of anemia.

Bites by the large lancehead vipers, particularly *Bothrops alternatus* and *B. jararacussu*, produce edema and local tissue changes similar to those caused by the venoms of North American *Crotalus* species, as well as scattered petecchiae. They are more scattered than those observed following North American crotalid bites. Nausea and vomiting, and sometimes hematemesis, hematuria, and melena are not uncommon, and hemorrhage from the nose and gums is often observed. Bleeding time is usually prolonged. The hematologic changes are often more marked than those observed following North American crotalid envenomation, but they respond to supportive treatment. These observations appear to confirm the clinical observations of ROSENFELD (1971).

In most bites by Asiatic Crotalidae, particularly the habus, severe pain and edema are common and necrosis is frequently seen in the untreated or undertreated cases, or those in which the use of antivenin has been delayed. Nausea, vomiting, abdominal pain, and diarrhea and oozing from the wound appear to be more common in Old World than New World crotalid bites, but the incidence of shock and cyanosis does not appear to be remarkably greater. Swelling of the regional lymph nodes and lymphadenitis are reported more frequently following North American than Asian crotalid bites, but this may be more related to reporting than fact.

Hemorrhagic manifestations are very common following Old World crotalid bites, particularly after Malayan pit viper bites, where hemoptysis may occur within 20 min of the bite. It is a valuable diagnostic sign of systemic involvement (REID, 1968). Bleeding from the gums, spontaneous ecchymoses over any part of the body, particularly where there has been trauma or infection, hematemesis, hematuria, and melena may occur following many Old World crotalid bites (REID et al., 1963a). Defects in blood coagulation are not uncommon in crotalid bites. In 1958, the author treated a *Crotalus viridis helleri* bite in which there was a coagulation defect for over 12 days (until the patient was discharged from the hospital). When he returned, 1 month later, the hematologic findings were normal. REID et al. (1963b) observed a coagulation abnormality for 26 days in a patient bitten by a Malayan pit viper. Excellent reviews on the clinical problem of Old World crotalid envenomation can be found in the papers by KUO and WU (1972), REID et al. (1963a, c), SAWAI (1973), and TATENO et al. (1963).

E. Laboratory Tests

The type of laboratory test of value to the physician in both establishing the diagnosis and guiding the therapeutic regime will depend upon the species of snake involved and the facilities available. It has been our practice in Crotalidae envenomations to carry out the following immediate procedures: typing and cross-matching, bleeding, blood clotting and clot retraction times, complete blood count, hematocrit, platelet count, and urinalysis. RBC indices, sedimentation rate, prothrombin time, arterial blood gases, sodium, potassium, and chloride determinations may be necessary. An electrocardiogram is indicated in severe cases. Serum proteins, fibrinogen titer, partial thromboplastin time, and renal function tests are often useful. In severe envenomation, the hematocrit, blood count, hemoglobin concentration, and platelet count should be carried out several times during the first several days, and all urine and stool samples should be examined, particularly for blood.

F. Treatment

Snake venom poisoning is an emergency requiring immediate medical attention and the exercise of considerable judgment. Remember, also, that if one has been bitten by a venomous snake it does not necessarily follow that he or she has been envenomated by it. Finally, do not forget that one is treating a complex poisoning in a complex biologic system. Do not depart on vague new uncontrolled trials with steroids, heparin, or homogenized barnacle juice, based on some observation in a primitive Porifera without a thorough consideration of the physiopharmacology of the venom in mammals, good experimental and clinical evidence for your trial, and a conviction that what you are doing is superior to the standard of procedure. Standards of procedures are not always the best, but they are far superior to most of the material one is likely to scrounge from the throwaway medical journals, and from that rather impressive number of nonmedical people who write so voluminously on the therapeutics of snake venom poisoning. There are two kinds of patients in snake venom poisoning, those in beds and those in the literature, and the clinician will do best who gives his full attention to the patient before him.

For a treatment to be effective, it must be instituted immediately following the bite and must include measures 1) to remove as much venom as possible from the wound, 2) to retard absorption of the venom, 3) to neutralize the venom, 4) to mitigate the effects produced by the venom, and 5) to prevent complications, including secondary infection (RUSSELL, 1962).

I. First Aid

In bites by the North American rattlesnake and the cottonmouth, if the patient arrives at the hospital within 20 min of the injury and there is evidence of envenomation (swelling, ecchymosis, weakness, paresthesias, and/or pain), a constriction band should be placed immediately above the first joint proximal to the bite. The band should be tight enough to occlude the superficial venous and lymphatic return but not tight enough to impede deep venous or arterial flow. It can be moved in advance of progressive swelling. It should be used in conjunction with incision and suction in *Crotalus* bites, and removed as soon as antivenin has been started or suction discontinued. In elapid envenomations, the tourniquet is of questionable value. However, in cases of severe envenomation by cobras, kraits, mambas, tiger snakes, death adders, and taipans, a tight tourniquet should be applied immediately proximal to the bite and left in place until antivenin is given. It should be released for 90 s every 10 min. When the tourniquet is released, the physician should be prepared to treat immediate circulatory collapse. Incision through the fang marks and suction are of definite value when applied immediately following bites by the pit vipers of North America. They are of lesser value following bites by the South American vipers and Asiatic vipers, and probably of little value subsequent to envenomation by the elapids and sea snakes. In rattlesnake bites, incisions of 3–6 mm in length should be made through the fang marks. The incisions should be about 4 mm deep, or as deep as the fang penetration, which in most rattlesnake bites is just through the skin. Suction should then be applied and continued for the 1st hour following the bite. Multiple incisions over the involved extremity or in advance of progressive edema are not advised. To be effective, suction must be started within the first few minutes following the bite. The injured part should be immobilized in a physiologic position at the level or slightly below the heart but not in a completely dependent position. It should not be elevated at this time. If the wound is on the body, keep the patient in a sitting or lying position, depending on the location of the bite. The patient should be kept warm and given reassurance. Activity should be kept at a minimum.

II. Medical Treatment

On admission to the hospital, and in the presence of envenomation, and if the use of antivenin seems warranted, skin or conjunctiva tests for sensitivity to horse serum should be done, following the instructions on the antivenin brochure. The amount of antivenin to be given will depend on a number of factors, most important of which is the severity of the symptoms and signs and their progression. The importance of early antivenin administration, preferably intravenously for many types of venom poisoning, cannot be overemphasized. The choice of antivenin, the route of injection, and the amount to be given will depend upon the species and size of snake involved, the site of envenomation, the size of the patient, and a number of other factors (RUSSELL, 1960).

In the United States, the dose of antivenin appears to be rather standardized for the three grades of Crotalidae envenomation—minimal, moderate or severe. In minimal rattlesnake venom poisoning, 1–4 U (vials or packages) of antivenin will usually suffice. In moderate cases, 4–7 U may be required, whereas in severe cases, up to 15 U or even more may be needed. Poisoning by water moccasins usually requires lesser doses, whereas in copperhead bites antivenin is usually required only for children and the elderly. Antivenin should be given intravenously in saline in most cases. The longer the delay, the more urgent the need for intravenous antivenin. In all cases of shock the antivenin should be given intravenously. If necessary to inject intramuscularly, give in the buttocks. Under *no* circumstances should antivenin be injected into a finger or toe.

Unfortunately, there does not appear to be any standard of procedure with respect to antivenin dosages for Central and South American, nor for Old World crotalid bites. This is due, in part, to the differences in antivenins in the different areas, some of which are more specific than others and, in part, to a considerable difference in opinions. The amounts generally employed in both South America and the Orient are much smaller than those employed in the United States, and based on neutralization titers from the manufacturers (RUSSELL and LAURITZEN, 1966), the doses reported in the medical literature for these areas would seem to be insufficient. This opinion appears to be shared by ROSENFELD (1971). It seems best, therefore, in the absences of controlled clinical trials, that the instructions on the brochure for the specific antivenin be followed.

It is not known how long after envenomation antivenin can still be used effectively. Recent studies indicate efficacy when given within 4 h of a bite; it is of less value if delayed for 8 h, and of questionable value after 24 h, except perhaps in poisoning by certain elapids. However, it seems advisable to recommend its use up to 24 h in all severe cases of crotalid venom poisoning. As a guide to antivenin administration, measure the circumference of the involved extremity proximal to the bite and at a second and third area proximal to this, and record measurements every 15–30 min. Tourniquet, oxygen, epinephrine, and other drugs and equipment for treating anaphylaxis should be available during antivenin administration. If further antivenin is needed, add this to the i.v. drip over 3–4 h. The amount of i.v. fluids, however, should be kept to a minimum, except where shock or hypovolemia is present.

There are more than 30 producers of antivenins throughout the world and in most countries there is a central laboratory or agency which advises on the appropriate serum and its availability. In the United States, when the offending snake is an imported species, the physician should consult the nearest Poison Control Center for guidance on the availability and choice of antivenin. The larger zoos of the country usually stock supplies of antivenins, have emergency programs for dispensing them, and provide addresses of consulting physicians. A national Antivenin Index is maintained by the Oklahoma City Zoo (405-424-3344).

A decrease in circulating blood volume and perfusion failure is a common finding in all severe and most moderate cases of crotalid venom poisoning. There may also be a concomitant lysis of red blood cells and loss of platelets, necessitating transfusions and parenteral fluids. In cases with hypovolemia, plasma or albumin may be used to restore circulatory blood volume. If there is evidence of a decrease in red cell mass, either from lysis of red cells or bleeding, packed cells or whole blood should be given. Where these complications are accompanied by defects in hemostasis, i.e., abnormal clotting or lysis of cells or clots or a disturbance of platelet activity, then replacement with specific clotting factors, fresh frozen plasma, or platelet transfusions may be indicated.

The appropriate antitetanus agent should always be administered and a broad-spectrum antimicrobial given in all severe and moderate cases. Aspirin or codeine may be used to alleviate pain or meperidine hydrochloride if the pain is severe. At the first signs of respiratory distress, oxygen should be given and preparations made to apply intermittent positive-pressure artificial respiration. Tracheal intubation or tracheostomy may be indicated, particularly if trismus, laryngeal spasm, or excessive salivation is present. The routine measures for the treatment of acute renal failure should be followed if this develops. Renal dialysis may be necessary. Peritoneal dialysis has been of little value in the author's experience; however, it is said to have been used successfully in severe cobra venom poisoning. Mild sedation is indicated in all severe bites and when respiratory depression is not a problem. Sedation will usually reduce the amount of analgesic necessary to control the pain. Atropine can be used as a parasympatholytic drug, if needed. Recent clinical experiences with hyperbaric oxygen indicate its value in some cases. The daily application of oxygen to the wound area is advised. Isolation perfusion of an extremity and intra-arterial infusion with antivenin have been tried with indifferent results.

Antihistamines are of no proven value during the acute stages of poisoning, except when it might be decided to give one intravenously before administering antivenin in a sensitive person. In such cases, diphenhydramine hydrochloride (benadryl) should be given intravenously 10 min prior to administration of the antivenin, if it is decided that use of the antivenin is necessary. In all cases when the patient is found to be sensitive to antivenin, cardiovascular parameters must be carefully monitored during the serum administration. In most cases, the antivenin can be given safely if administered slowly and with periodic doses of benadryl. If the patient reacts to the infusion, the antivenin should be halted for a 10-min period and then started again, usually more slowly, following further benadryl. Oxygen, epinephrine, and other drugs for treating anaphylaxis should be available. The author has been surprised at the few serum reactions to intravenous antivenin he has seen in horse serum-sensitive patients. However, do not use horse serum antivenin in a sensitive patient, unless it is determined that without the antivenin the patient's life or a limb might be lost.

Corticosteroids are of unproven value during the acute states of the poisoning, and may be contraindicated. They should not be used as substitutes for catecholamines and fluids in a venom shock state. Continued use of corticosteroids with antivenin, or even without antivenin, is not advised. It is the clinical impression of most toxinologists that steroids have no effect on the local tissue reaction caused by crotalid venoms. Local infiltration of small amounts of 0.05 M ethylenediaminetetraacetic acid (EDTA) in saline around the bite area may reduce some of the local tissue effects of the venom, if done within 30 min of the bite, but EDTA should not be used intravenously.

The wound should be cleansed and covered with a sterile dressing. The injured part should be immobilized in a physiologic position. Ice bags, isolated from the skin by towels, afford some local pain relief, but they should never be applied while antivenin is being given or for the first few hours thereafter. Under no circumstances should an extremity be placed or packed in ice or left in ice. Surgical debridement of blebs, bloody vesicles, and superficial necrosis may have to be performed between the 3rd and 10th days. Most of these changes appear between the 2nd and 5th days, and usually have reached maximal development by the 5th to 9th days. Debridement may need to be done in stages. If it is tried too early, the underlying tissues will continue to lose fluid and blood and be more susceptible to infection. If the debridement is done too late, the clots and superficial necrotic tissues become difficult to remove.

Often neglected but of the utmost importance is the follow-up care. Contractures can be reduced by initiating early corrective measures and exercises. The use of fasciotomy should be discouraged. In most cases, it is unnecessary and reflects the use of an insufficient amount of antivenin during the first 12 h of the poisoning. It may be necessary when there is substantial proof of severe vascular impairment. Within 4 days of the injury, a complete physical therapy evaluation should be made: joint motion, muscle strength, sensation, and girth measurements. Immobilization is then interrupted by frequent periods of gentle exercise, progressing from passive exercises to active exercises. Follow-up care should include sterile whirlpool treatment, debridement as indicated, daily cleansing of the wound with hydrogen peroxide followed by 15-min soaks in 1:20 Burow's solution, and daily painting of the wound with an aqueous dye consisting of brilliant green 1:400, gentian violet 1:400, and n-acriflavine 1:1000. A 5% scarlet red ointment or antimicrobial ointment can be applied at bedtime. Daily exposure of open lesions to continuous oxygen flow while the part is immobilized in a plastic bag is of value. Hyperbaric oxygen is of value in some cases. The lesion should be covered with a loose sterile bandage when the patient is supine. This should be reasonably firm when the patient is ambulatory.

References

Bellairs, A.: The Life of Reptiles, Vol. II. New York: Universe Books 1970

Conant, R.: A Field Guide to Reptiles and Amphibians of the United States and Canada East of the 100th Meridian, 1st Ed. Boston: Houghton Mifflin 1958

Dowling, H., Minton, S. A., Jr., Russell, F. E.: Poisonous Snakes of the World. Washington: U.S. Govt. Printing Office 1968

Fontana, F.: Traite Sur le Venin de la Vipere, Vol. II, Paris, 1781

Gloyd, H. K.: The Rattlesnake, Genera *Sistrurus* and *Crotalus*. Chicago: Chicago Academy of Sciences 1940

Gloyd, H. K.: The Korean snakes of the genus *Agkistrodon* (Crotalidae). Proc. biol. Soc. (Wash.) **85**, 557—578 (1972)

Haile, N. S.: The snakes of Borneo with a key to the species. Sarawak. Mus. J. **8**, 743—771 (1958)

Hoge, A. R.: Preliminary account on neotropical Crotalinae (Serpentes, *Viperidae*). Mem. Inst. Butantan **32**, 109—184 (1965)

Klauber, L. M.: Rattlesnakes. Their Habits, Life Histories and Influence on Mankind, Vol. II. Berkeley: Univ. Calif. Pr. 1956a

Klauber, L. M.: Some factors affecting the gravity of rattlesnake bite. In: Venoms. Washington: A.A.A.S. 1956b

Klemmer, K.: Liste der rezenten Giftschlangen: *Elapidae, Hydrophidae, Viperidae* und *Crotalidae*. In: Die Giftschlangen der Erde. Marburg (Lahn): N. G. Elwert 1963

Kuntz, R. E.: Snakes of Taiwan. Taipei: U.S. Naval Medical Research Unit No. 2, 1963

Kuo, T.-P., Wu, C.-S.: Clinico-pathological studies on snakebites in Taiwan. Snake **4**, 1—22 (1972)

Lazell, J. D., Jr.: The lesser Antillean representatives of *Bothrops* and *Constrictor*. Bull. Mus. Comp. Zool. **132**, 245—273 (1964)

Leviton, A. E.: Keys to the dangerously venomous terrestrial snakes of the Philippine Islands. Silliman J. **8**, 98—106 (1961)

Lim, B. L.: Venomous snakes of Southeast Asia. Stheast. Asian J. Trop. Med. Publ. Health **2**, 56—64 (1971)

Mertens, R.: Die Amphibien und Reptilien von El Salvador, auf Grund der Reisen von R. Mertens und A. Zilch. Abh. Senckenbergischen Ges. **487**, 1—120 (1952)

Minton, S. A., Jr.: Venom Diseases. Springfield (Illinois): Charles C. Thomas 1974

Minton, S. A., Minton, M. R.: Venomous Reptiles. New York: Scribners 1969

Parrish, H. M.: Incidence of treated snakebite in the United States. Publ. Health Rep. **81**, 269—276 (1966)

Peters, J. A.: The snakes of Ecuador: A check list and key. Bull. Mus. Comp. Zool. **122**, 491—541 (1960)

Pope, C.: The reptiles of China. Amer. Mus. Nat. Hist. 1935

Reid, H. A.: Symptomatology, pathology, and treatment of land snake bite in India and Southeast Asia. In: Venomous Animals and Their Venoms, Vol. I. New York: Academic Press 1968

Reid, H. A., Chan, K. E., Thean, P. C.: Prolonged coagulation defect (defibrination syndrome) in Malayan viper bite. Lancet **1963a I**, 621—626

Reid, H. A., Thean, P. C., Chan, K. E., Baharam, A. R.: Clinical effects of bites by Malayan viper (*Ancistrodon rhodostoma*). Lancet **1963b I**, 617—621

Reid, H. A., Thean, P. C., Martin, W. J.: Epidemiology of snake in North Malaya. Brit. med. J. **1963c I**, 992—997

Rosenfeld, G.: In: Trattato Italiano di Medicina Interna, Part XI. Roma: Sadea & Sansoni 1966

Rosenfeld, G.: Symptomatology, pathology, and treatment of snake bites in South America. In: Venomous Animals and Their Venoms, Vol. II. New York: Academic Press 1971

Russell, F. E.: Rattlesnake bites in Southern California. Amer. J. med. Sci. **239**, 1—10 (1960)

Russell, F. E.: Snake venom poisoning. In: Cyclopedia of Medicine, Surgery and the Specialties, Vol. II. Philadelphia: F. A. Davis 1962

Russell, F. E.: Snakebite. In: Current Therapy. Philadelphia: W. B. Saunders 1968

Russell, F. E.: Crotalidae of the western hemisphere. Herpeton **4**, 1—8 (1969)

Russell, F. E., Carlson, R. W., Wainschel, J., Osborne, A. H.: Snake venom poisoning in the United States. Experiences with 550 cases. JAMA **233**, 341—344 (1975)

Russell, F. E., Lauritzen, L.: Antivenins. Trans. roy. Soc. trop. med. Hyg. **60**, 191—810 (1966)

Russell, F. E., Scharffenberg, R. S.: Bibliography of Snake Venoms and Venomous Snakes. California: Bibliographic Associates 1964

Santos, E.: Anfibios e Repteis do Brasil (Vide e Costumes), 2nd Ed. Rio de Janeiro: F. Briguiet 1955

Sawai, Y.: A historical outlook of the study on the treatment of snakebites. Snake **5**, 15—27 (1973)

Shaw, C. E., Campbell, S.: Snakes of the American West. New York: Alfred Knopf 1974

Stebbins, R. C.: Amphibians and Reptiles of Western North America. New York: McGraw-Hill 1954

Tateno, I., Sawai, Y., Makino, M.: Current status of mamushi snake *(Agkistrodon halys)* bite in Japan with special reference to severe and fatal cases. Jap. J. exp. Med. **33**, 331—346 (1963)

Underwood, G.: A Contribution to the Classification of Snakes. England: Staples Printers 1967

Werler, J. E., Keegan, H. L.: Venomous snakes of the Pacific area. In: Venomous and Poisonous Animals and Noxious Plants of the Pacific Region. Oxford: Pergamon 1963

Wright, A. H., Wright, A. A.: Handbook of Snakes, Vol. II. New York: Comstock/Cornell 1957

CHAPTER 28

Snake Venoms and Nephrotoxicity

V. SITPRIJA and V. BOONPUCKNAVIG

A. Introduction

The clinical syndromes which are associated with snakebite are variable. While minor reactions consist only of local pain and swelling, severe reactions may include muscular weakness or paralysis, respiratory failure, hemorrhage, hypotension, shock, and death. Hematologic changes predominate in crotalid and viperid envenomation. Elapid venom produces neuromuscular symptoms with or without local tissue necrosis. There is usually little cardiodepressor effect. Sea snake venom, on the other hand, is not only neurotoxic but also myotoxic, causing myonecrosis which is responsible for muscular pains and paresis.

The kidney is one of the organs frequently involved in snakebite. However, there are rather few data on this subject. Scattered reports concerning the renal lesions include glomerulitis (SANT and PURANDARE, 1972), glomerulonephritis (SEEDAT et al., 1974), arteritis (SITPRIJA et al., 1974), interstitial nephritis (SANT and PURANDARE, 1972), tubular necrosis (SITPRIJA et al., 1973, 1974), cortical necrosis (ORAM et al., 1963; VARAGUNAM and PANABOKKE, 1970), and renal infarct (RAAB and KAISER, 1966). Among the renal manifestations, renal failure is most common. The others consist of hematuria, myoglobinuria, hemoglobinuria, and proteinuria. Nephrotic syndrome has also been described (STEINBECK, 1960).

In reviewing the literature tubular necrosis was noted at autopsy by AMORIM and MELLO (1954) in three patients bitten by crotalid snakes. DANZIG and ABELS (1961) described a patient bitten by a rattlesnake who had convulsions, collapsed, and developed acute renal failure. The patient was successfully treated by hemodialysis. There was no pathologic diagnosis, but the clinical course resembled that of tubular necrosis. Similar findings and results were experienced by FRAZIER and CARTER (1962). In a series of 15 patients bitten by unidentified poisonous snakes reported by VISUVARATNAM et al. (1970), renal failure was observed in four cases. The clinical findings included drowsiness, restlessness, and hemoglobinuria. SILVA et al. (1966) noted acute tubular necrosis in three patients bitten by *Crotalus terrificus*. Cortical necrosis has been observed in patients bitten by *Bothrops jararaca* (DE AZEVEDO and DE CASTRO TEIXEIRA, 1938; SILVA et al., 1966), *Agkistrodon kypnale* (VARAGUNAM and PANABOKKE, 1970), *Echis carinatus* (ORAM et al., 1963), and Russell's viper (CHUGH et al., 1975). Acute renal failure with tubular necrosis was recently described by SITPRIJA et al. (1973, 1974, 1976) in patients bitten by Russel's vipers. This was later confirmed by CHUGH et al. (1975). Of nine cases of sea snakebite studied by MARSDEN and REID (1961), tubular necrosis was noted in three patients. Recently, renal failure is sea snake poisoning attributed to myoglobinuria has been described by SITPRIJA et al. (1971). FURTADO and LESTER (1968) noted tubular necrosis at autopsy in a patient bitten by a small-eyed blacksnake *(Cryptophis nigrescens)*. Besides tubular necrosis, proliferative glomerulonephritis has been reported by SEEDAT et al. (1974) as being responsible for renal failure in their patients bitten by *Bitis arietans*.

In our series of 400 patients bitten by poisonous tropical snakes, renal failure was observed in 5% of cases, mild proteinuria was noted in 4%, and hematuria in 35%. Renal involvement in snakebite is thus not uncommon. Therefore, it seems necessary to scrutinize in detail the pathologic changes, pathogenesis, and manifestations of renal involvement caused by snake venoms.

B. Renal Pathologic Changes

I. Glomerular Lesions

Glomerulitis, glomerulonephritis, and even nephrotic syndrome have been described in patients with snakebite. Glomerular changes described consist essentially of proliferation of the endothelial and mesangial cells, fibrin deposition, and occasional epithelial crescents. The basement membrane usually shows no remarkable changes. Our experience to be described here emphasizes mainly the lesions seen in tropical snakebite. Glomerular changes are rather inconspicous. This is not surprising since several mechanisms are involved in its pathogenesis. The predominant lesions consist of mild proliferation of mesangial cells with an increase in the amount of basement membrane-like matrix (Fig. 1). Segmental thickening of the basement membrane is more prominent in cobra bite than green pit viper bite or Russell's viper bite. Occasionally, there are polymorphonuclear cells in the glomerular capillaries. By Masson's trichome stain, there is deposition of fuchsinophilic granular material in some mesangial areas. In puff adder *(Bitis arietans)* bite proliferative glomerulonephritis with epithelial crescents has been reported (SEEDAT et al., 1974).

In rabbits injected with the venom of *Crotalus adamanteus*, glomerular changes of both hemorrhagic and exudative natures have been found (PEARCE, 1909). The hemorrhagic lesion is confined mostly to the glomerular tuft, while the exudative lesion involves the capsular space. In dog experiments with crotoxin, glomerular congestion and deposition of PAS-positive material between capillary loops have been observed (HADLER and BRAZIL, 1966).

The common immunopathologic findings are tabulated in Table 1. Diffuse fine granular deposition of IgM and the third component of complement (C3) in the mesangial areas with extension along the capillary wall is detected (Figs. 2 and 3). The intensity of the deposition varies from one group to another. The deposition of IgM is more dense in Russell's viper cases than green pit viper or cobra cases. Interestingly, cases with cobra bite are found to have more C3 deposition than the others. Late in the course of the disease, IgM disappears, and only C3 is seen (SITPRIJA et al., 1976). Focal deposition of fibrin in the glomerular tufts and within the Bowman's space is detectable in a few cases of green pit viper bite (Fig. 4).

By electron microscopy, occasional narrowing of the glomerular capillary lumen is observed. This is due to mesangial hyperplasia with an increase in the amount of

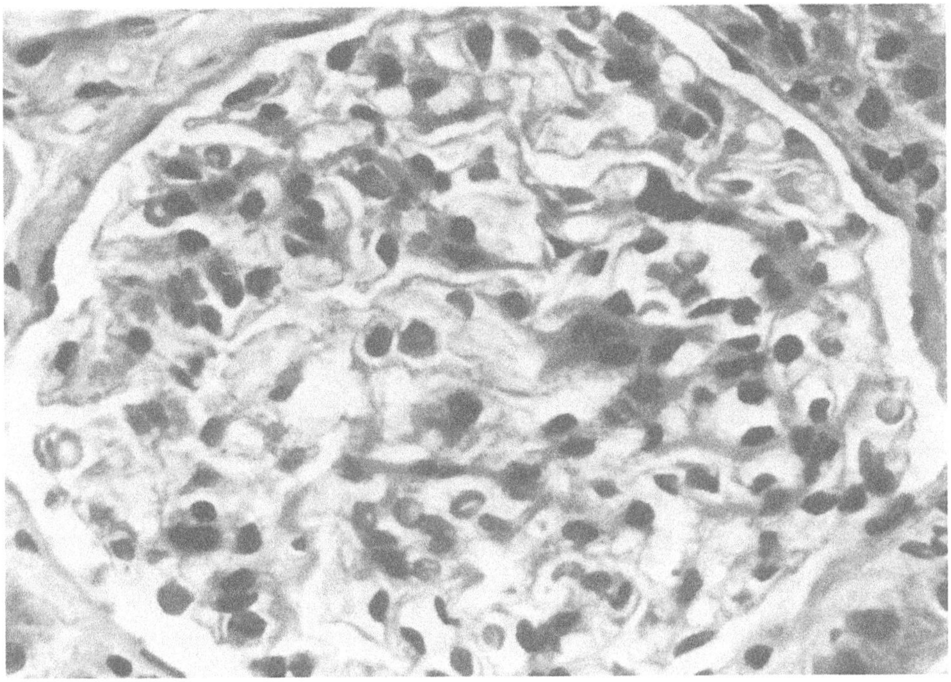

Fig. 1. A glomerulus in a cobra bite case showing mild mesangial cell proliferation. Some capillary walls are thickened. (H & E original magnification × 400, reduced to 75%)

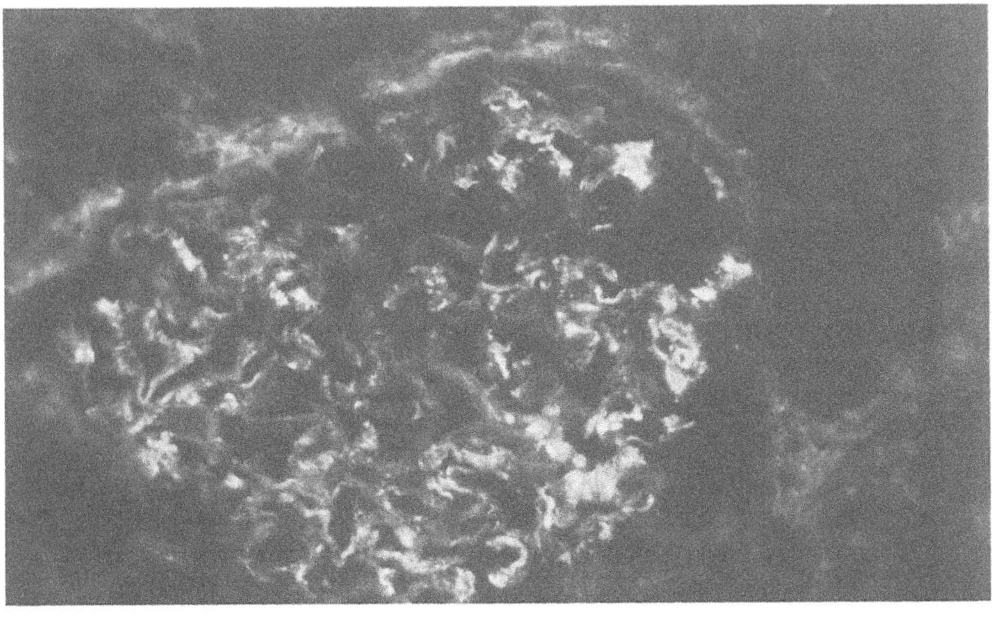

Fig. 2. A glomerulus in a Russell's viper case showing granular deposition of IgM in some mesangial area and along capillary walls. (Fluorescent anti-IgM, original magnification × 252)

Table 1. Summary of immunopathology, histopathology, and electron-microscopic findings of the kidney in snakebite

Type of snake	Immunopathologic findings Location of deposits			Histopathologic findings				Electron-microscopic findings		
	Glomerular capillary	Arteriolar wall	Arterial wall	Proliferation of glomerular mesangial cells	Tubular necrosis and regeneration	Necrotizing arteritis	Thrombo-phlebitis	Glomerular electron-dense deposits	Glomerular basement membrane alteration	Tubular degeneration, necrosis and regeneration
Russell's viper	IgM (+ to + +) C3 (+)	C3 (+)	C3 (+)	+	+ +	+	+	+	—	+
Green pit viper	IgM (trace to +) C3 (+) Fibrin[a]	C3 (+)	No deposit	+ to + +	+	—	+	+[b]	—	+
Cobra	IgM (+) C3 (+ to + +)	C3 (+)	No deposit	+	—	—	—	+	+	—

— = Negative.
+ = Mild.
+ + = Moderate.
[a] Focal deposition.
[b] With deposition of fibrin.

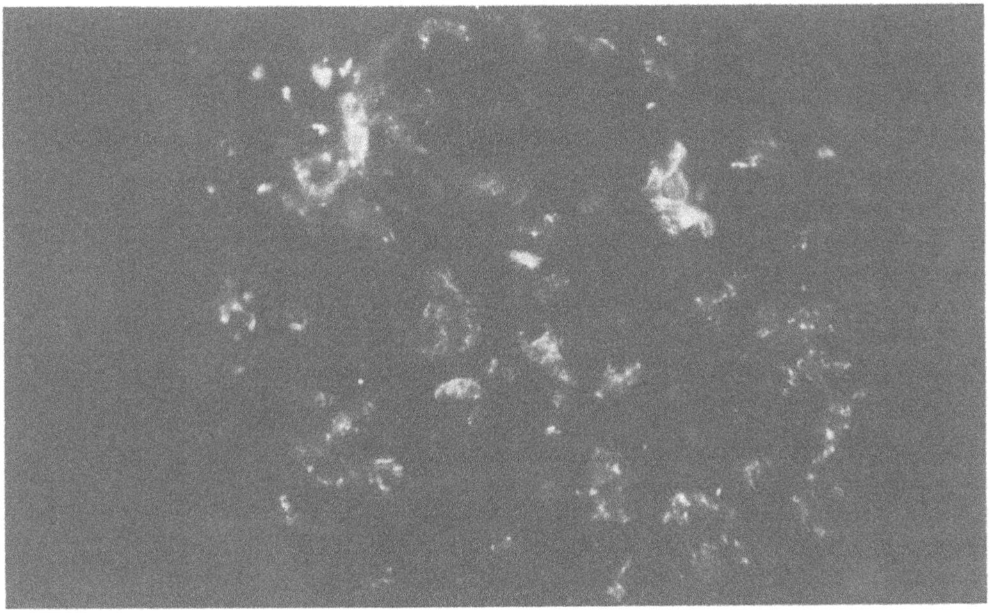

Fig. 3. A glomerulus in a cobra bite case showing granular deposition of C3. (Fluorescent anti-C3, original magnification × 252)

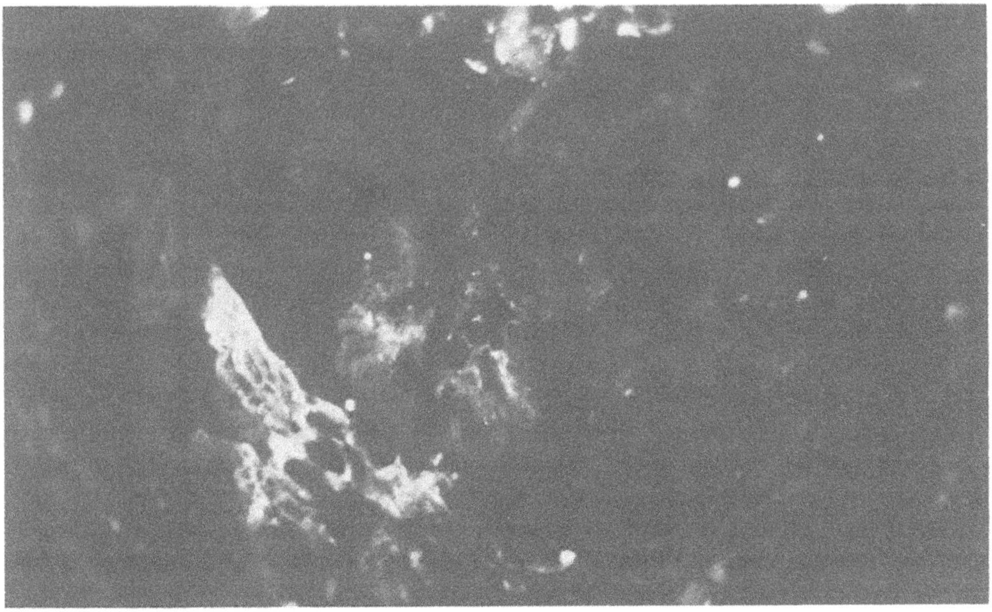

Fig. 4. Focal deposition of fibrin in glomerular tufts and Bowman's capsule in green pit viper bite. (Fluorescent antifibrin, original magnification × 252)

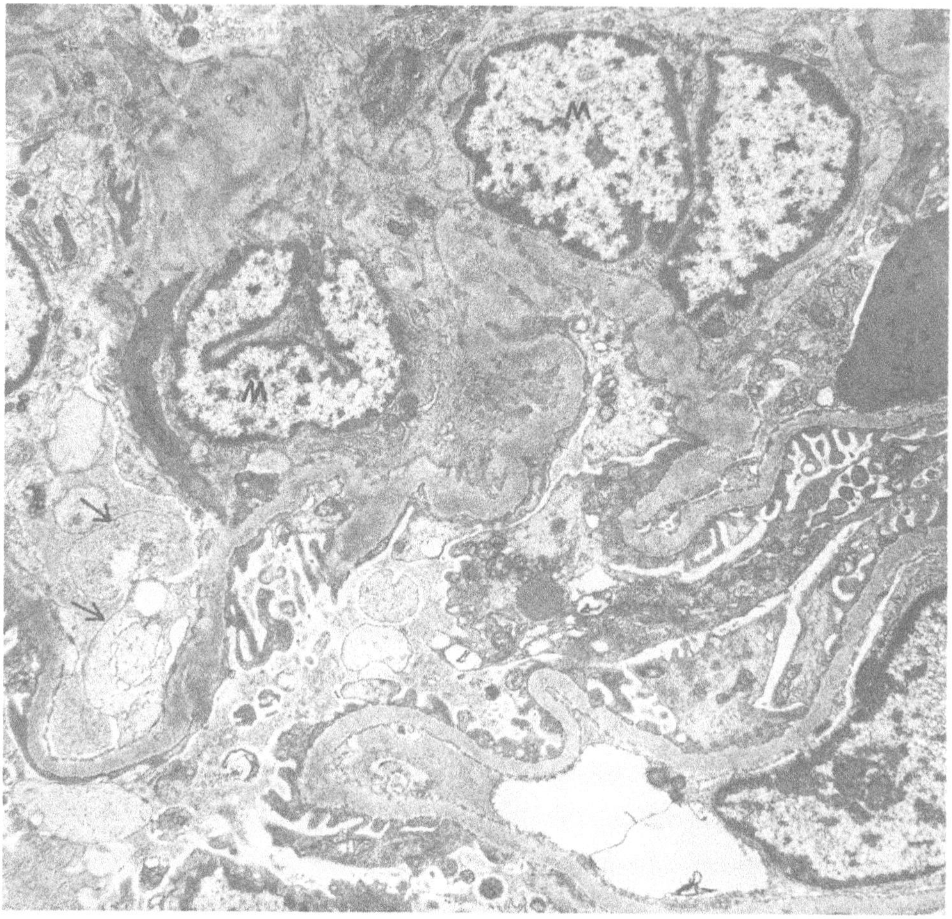

Fig. 5. Electron micrograph of the glomerular structure in green pit viper bite showing proliferation of mesangial cell (*M*) and endothelial cytoplasmic blebs (arrows) (×9750, reduced to 70%)

basement membrane-like matrix and the swelling of the attenuate portion of the endothelial cytoplasm (Fig. 5). In a few cases of green pit viper bite, some capillary lumens are filled with fibrin and degenerating platelets (Fig. 6).

Electron-dense deposits are usually seen in the basement membrane-like matrix. The thickness of the peripheral capillary wall is usually normal except in cobra bite cases in which some capillary walls show irregular thickening. Some of these thickened walls present the spikes projecting from the epithelial side of the basement membrane. Occasionally, the striated membranous structure is seen at the bottom of the basement membrane crater (Fig. 7). The origin of this structure is unknown. The other common finding is the wrinkling of the *lamina interna* of the basement membrane (Fig. 8).

Focal absence of the epithelial foot processes is seen in the area where the basement membrane changes are obvious. The cytoplasm of the visceral epithelial cells shows two compartments (Fig. 9). In one compartment, there is increased den-

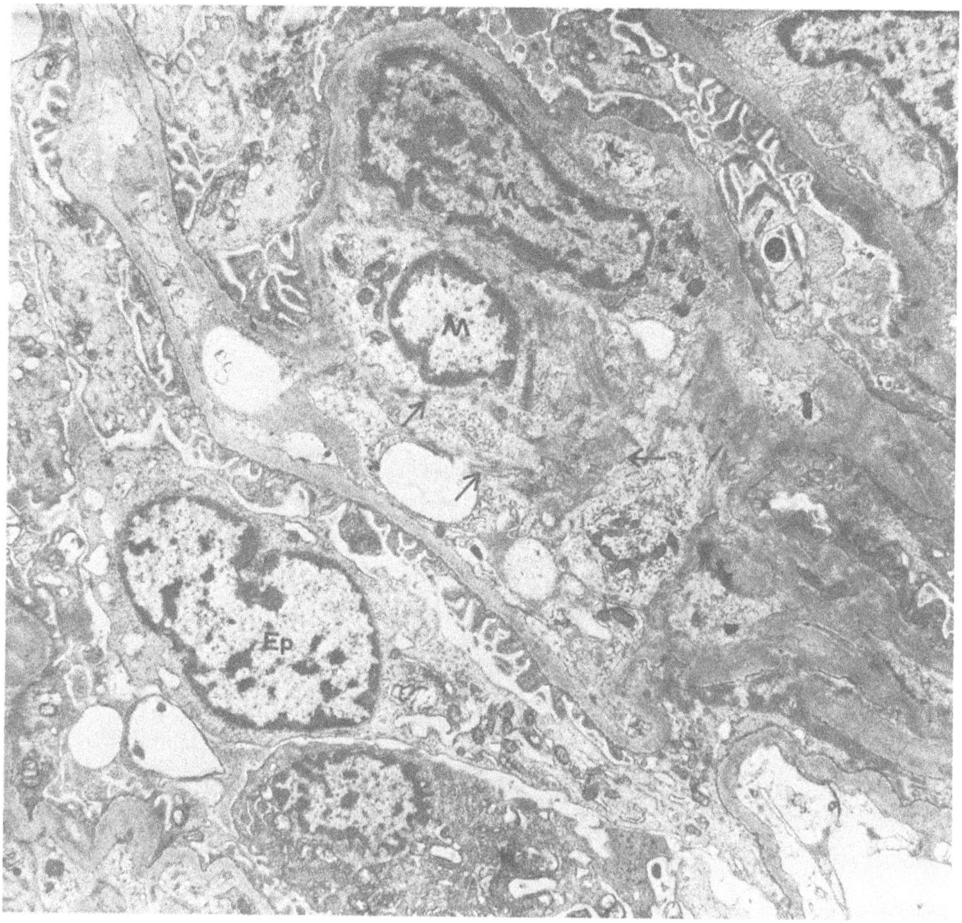

Fig. 6. Electron micrograph of the glomerular structure in green pit viper bite showing deposition of fibrin (arrows) in paramesangial area. (*Ep*) epithelial cell, (*M*) mesangial cell (×9750, reduced to 70%)

sity of the cell sap that is devoid of cytoplasmic organelles. The plasma membrane of this compartment shows lack of microvilli. The other compartment has the cell sap of less density and contains abundant mitochondria with considerable amount of fibrillary structure with or without increased endoplasmic reticulum. The Bowman's space contains microvillous structure and debris of cells.

II. Vascular Lesions

The arterial lesions are seen strikingly in Russell's viper bite. The most obvious alteration is necrotizing arteritis of the interlobular arteries (Fig. 10). The lesion is found segmentally. Thrombophlebitis of the arcuate vein and its tributaries is present in both Russell's viper cases and green pit viper cases (Fig. 11). The lesion is also segmental. There is no vascular change in cobra cases.

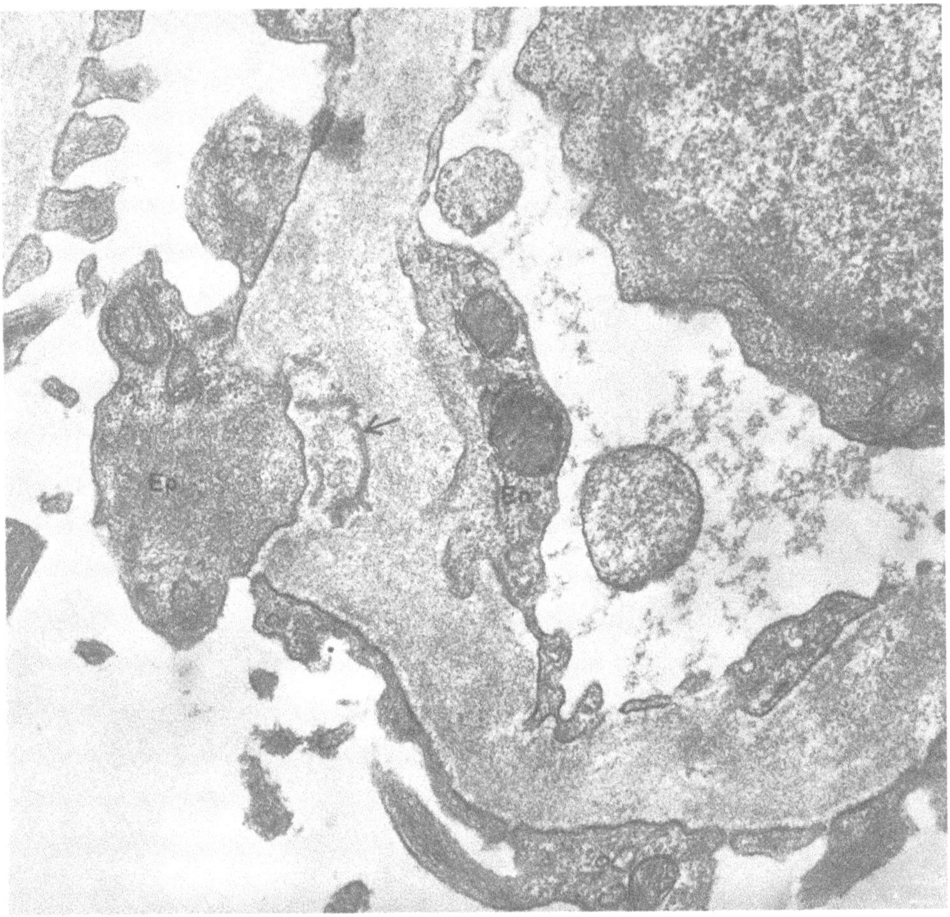

Fig. 7. Electron micrograph of the glomerular capillary wall in cobra bite showing irregular thickening of the basement membrane. Striated membranous structures (arrow) are present. (*Ep*) epithelial cell, (*En*) endothelial cytoplasm (×47500, reduced to 70%)

Dense deposit of C3 in the walls of afferent and efferent arterioles is observed (Fig. 12). In addition, in Russell's viper cases, the arterial wall of the necrotized artery shows deposition of C3 without immunoglobulins.

Electron microscopy shows no remarkable changes.

III. Tubulointerstitial Lesions

Tubulointerstitial changes vary among each group of snakebites. In cobra bite, the tubules and interstitium show no obvious changes. Severe tubulointerstitial lesions are noted in cases of green pit viper bite with renal failure. In viper bite, as demonstrated by the Puchtler-Sweat method (LUNA, 1960), there are hemoglobin casts in the lumen of distal convoluted tubules and collecting tubules (Fig. 13). In sea snakebite, the tubular lumens contain myoglobin. This has also been observed in a

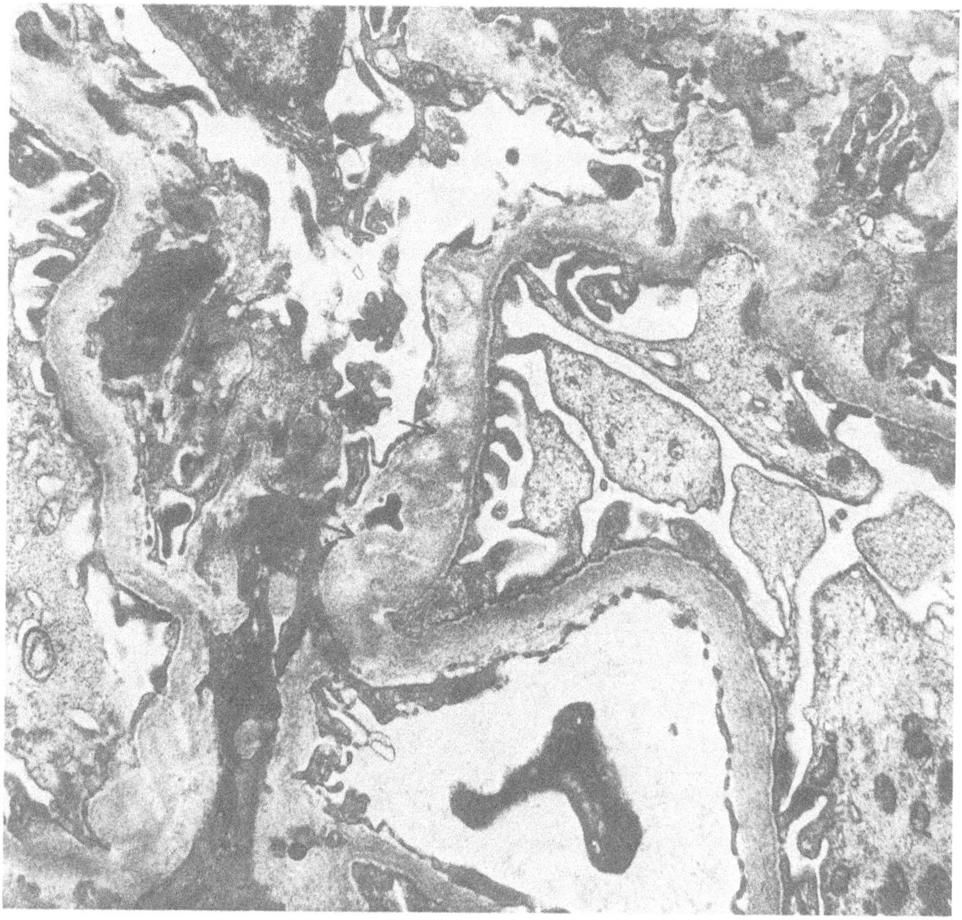

Fig. 8. Electron micrograph of the glomerular structure in cobra bite showing irregularity in thickness and wrinkling of *lamina interna* of the basement membrance (arrows) (×20250, reduced to 70%)

patient bitten by a small-eyed blacksnake *(Cryptophis nigrescens)*. Degeneration, necrosis, and regeneration of epithelial cells are more prominent in distal tubules and collecting tubules than the proximal ones. The tubular basement membrane in the severely involved area may be ruptured. The presence of necrotic epithelial cells may or may not be associated with the presence of hemoglobin casts in the lumen.

Interstitial changes are observed only in cases with renal failure. Interstitial edema is a constant finding and is more pronounced in the cortical portion. Inflammatory cells including lymphocytes, plasma cells, and mononuclear cells are more dense in the interstitial tissue of corticomedullary junction (Fig. 14) and always located around the necrotic collecting tubules. Some of these cells even penetrate into the wall of such tubules (Fig. 15). Interstitial lesions are in fact secondary to tubular necrosis. Pure interstitial nephritis has not been observed in our experience.

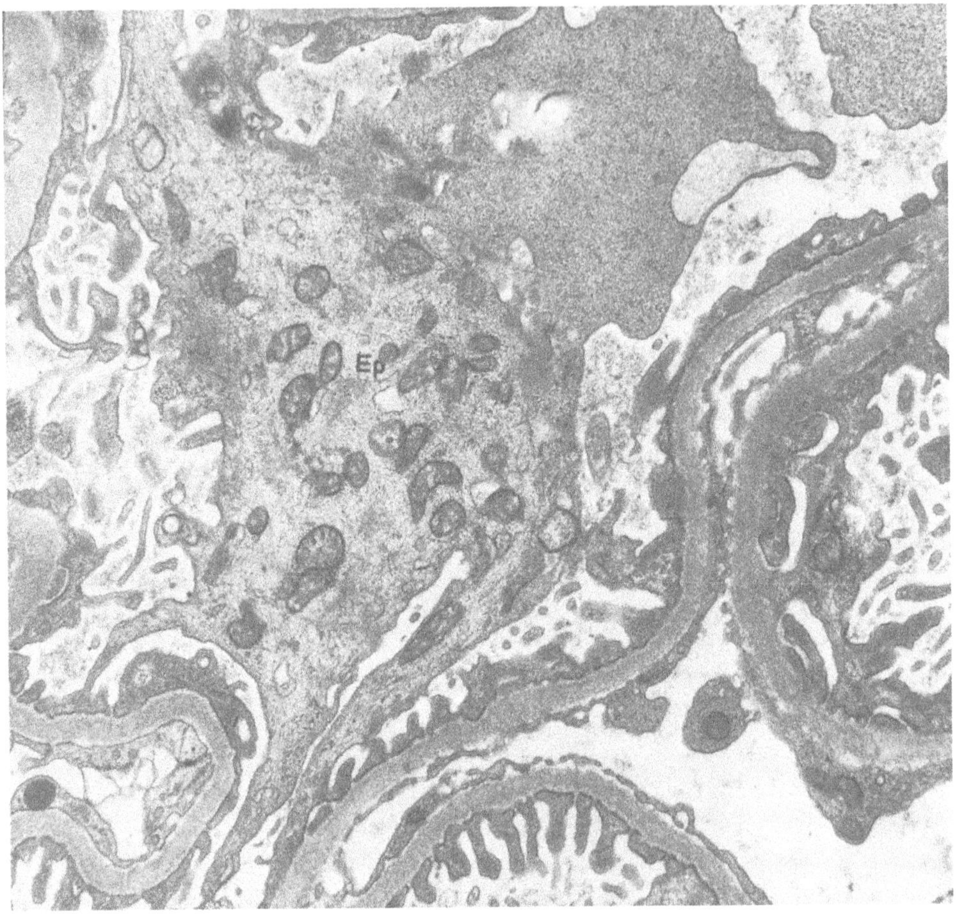

Fig. 9. Electron micrograph of the glomerular structure in Russell's viper bite showing two compartments of a visceral epithelial cell (*Ep*) (× 20250, reduced to 70%)

Electron microscopy of the tubules confirms the light microscopic findings. The epithelial cells of the distal and collecting tubules are in varying stages of degeneration, necrosis, and regeneration. Edema of interstitial tissue with dilatation of the peritubular capillaries is seen (Fig. 16). By immunofluorescent study, the tubules and interstitium show no immune deposit.

IV. Cortical Necrosis

Necrosis of the renal cortex has been observed following the bite of *Bothrops jararaca* (DE AZEVEDO and DE CASTRO TEIXEIRA, 1938; SILVA et al., 1966), *Echis carinatus* (ORAM et al., 1963), *Agkistrodon hypnale* (VARAGUNAM and PANABOKKE, 1970), and Russell's viper (CHUGH et al., 1975). This is summarized in Table 2. The lesion is usually associated with severe disseminated intravascular coagulation with fibrin deposition in the renal vascular bed. In some of the cases in which recovery has

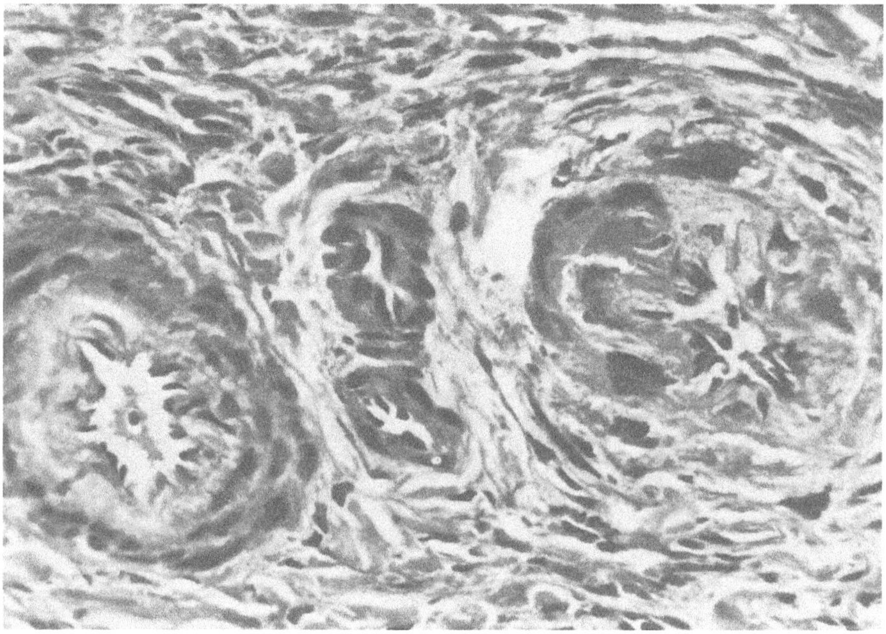

Fig. 10. Necrotizing arteritis of an interlobular artery in Russell's viper bite. Note that the other segment of the same sized artery shows no change. (H & E, original magnification × 252, reduced to 70%, from Nephron, **13**, 396—403 (1974) with the permission of S. Karger)

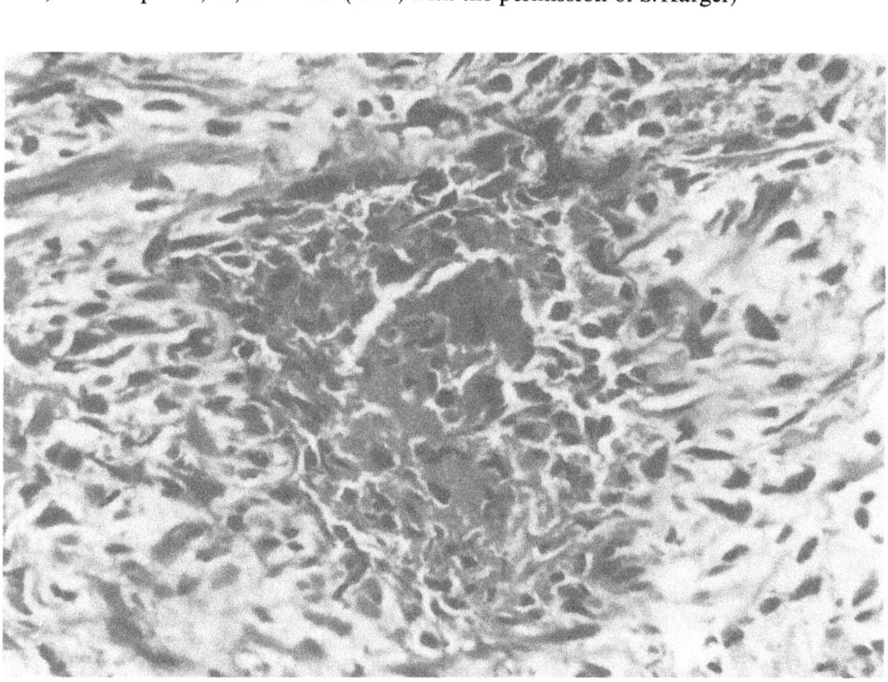

Fig. 11. Thrombophlebitis in Russell's viper bite case. (H&E, original magnification × 252, reduced to 70%)

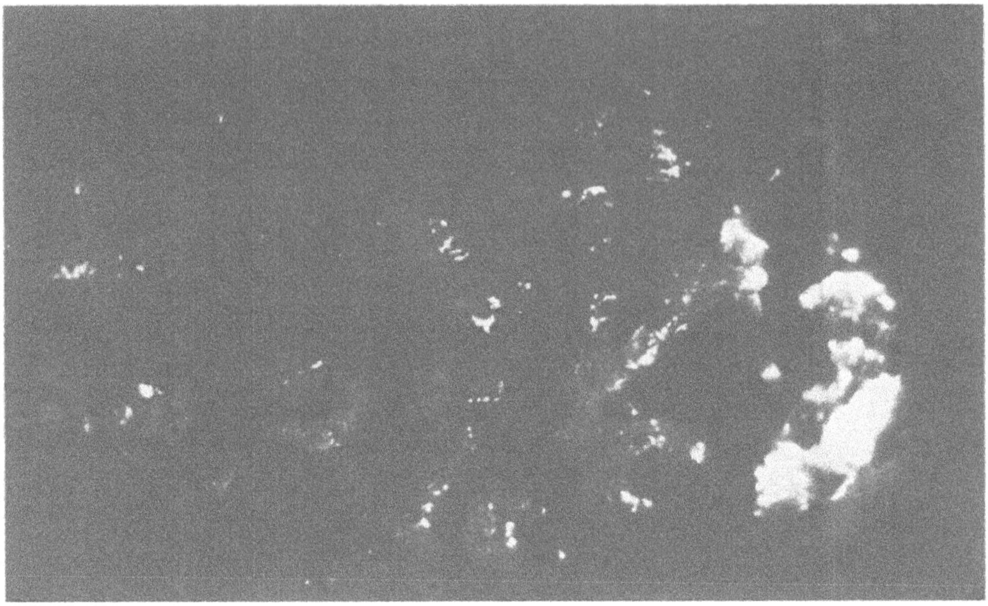

Fig. 12. Dense deposition of C3 in the arteriolar wall and in mesangial areas in cobra bite. (Fluorescent anti-C3, original magnification ×252)

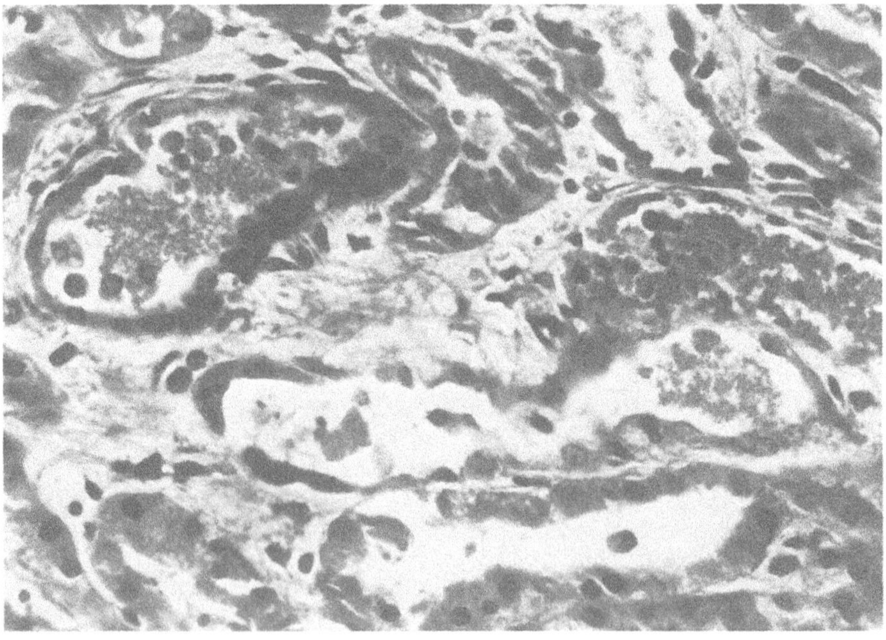

Fig. 13. Necrotic tubules containing hemoglobin casts in Russell's viper case. (H&E, original magnification ×252, reduced to 70%)

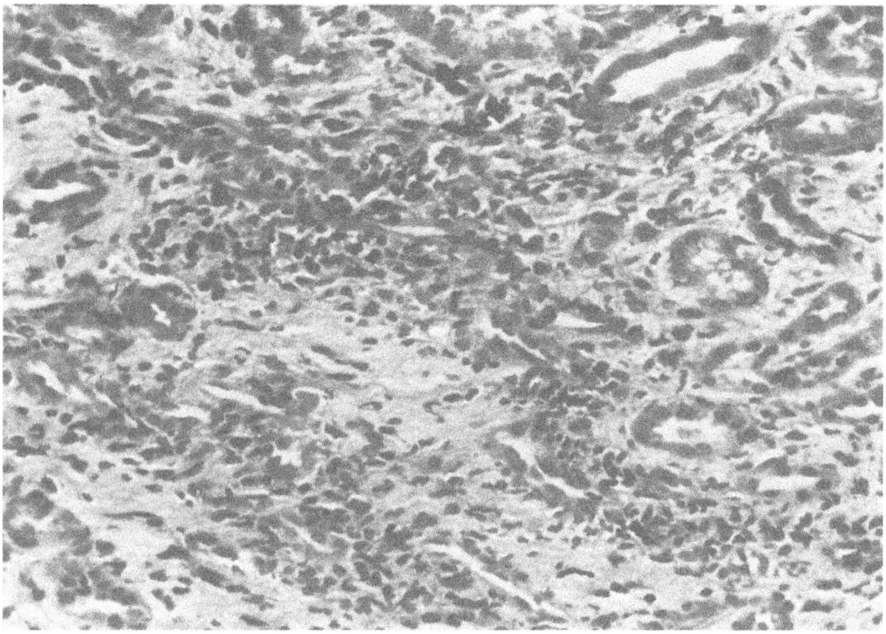

Fig. 14. Tubular necrosis with dense inflammatory cell infiltration in the corticomedullary area in green pit viper case. (H&E, original magnification × 200, reduced to 70%)

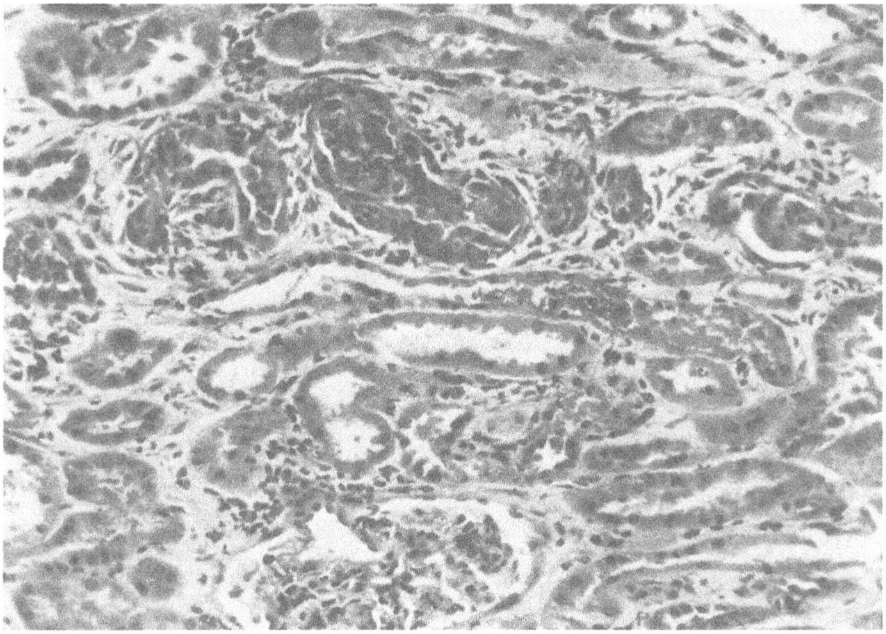

Fig. 15. Necrotic distal tubules are infiltrated by acute and chronic inflammatory cells in a case with Russell's viper bite. (H & E, original magnification × 126, reduced to 70%)

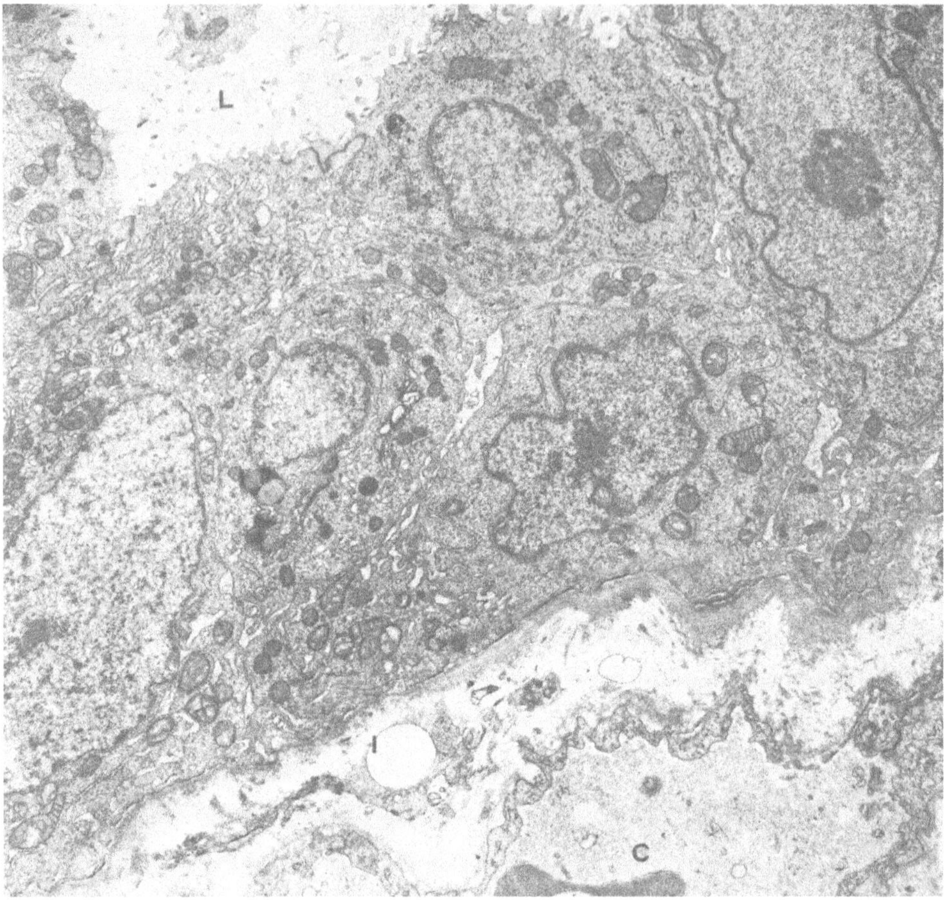

Fig. 16. Electron micrograph of a collecting duct in green pit viper bite showing interstitial edema and regeneration of epithelial cells. (*L*) lumen, (*I*) interstitium, (*C*) capillary (×9750, reduced to 70%)

occurred, calcification of the necrotic cortex may be evident by radiography. This has been observed in a case of *Echis carinatus* bite by ORAM et al. (1963).

C. Pathogenesis

The pathogenesis of the renal lesions is shown in Figure 17.

I. Glomerular Lesions

At least three theories have been proposed to explain the glomerular lesions in snakebite.

1. Direct Irritation by Snake Venom

The venom may cause direct injurious effect to the glomeruli similar to the effect of cantharidin which is an irritant. The vasculotoxic effect of viper venom is well-

Table 2. Renal failure with known renal lesions in various snakebites[a]

Snake	Renal lesion	Reference
Crotalus terrificus	Tubular necrosis	AMORIM and MELLO (1954) SILVA et al. (1966)
Cryptophis nigrescens	Tubular necrosis	FURTADO and LESTER (1968)
Sea snake	Tubular necrosis	MARSDEN and REID (1961) SITPRIJA et al. (1971)
Russell's viper	Tubular necrosis	SITPRIJA et al. (1973, 1974) CHUGH et al. (1975)
	Cortical necrosis	CHUGH et al. (1975)
Echis carinatus	Cortical necrosis	ORAM et al. (1963)
Bothrops jararaca	Cortical necrosis	SILVA et al. (1966) DE AZEVEDO and DE CASTRO TEIXEIRA (1938)
Agkistrodon hypnale	Cortical necrosis	VARAGUNAM and PANABOKKE (1970)
Bitis arietans	Proliferative glomerulonephritis	SEEDAT et al. (1974)

[a] Cases with renal failure without known snake or known renal lesion are not included.

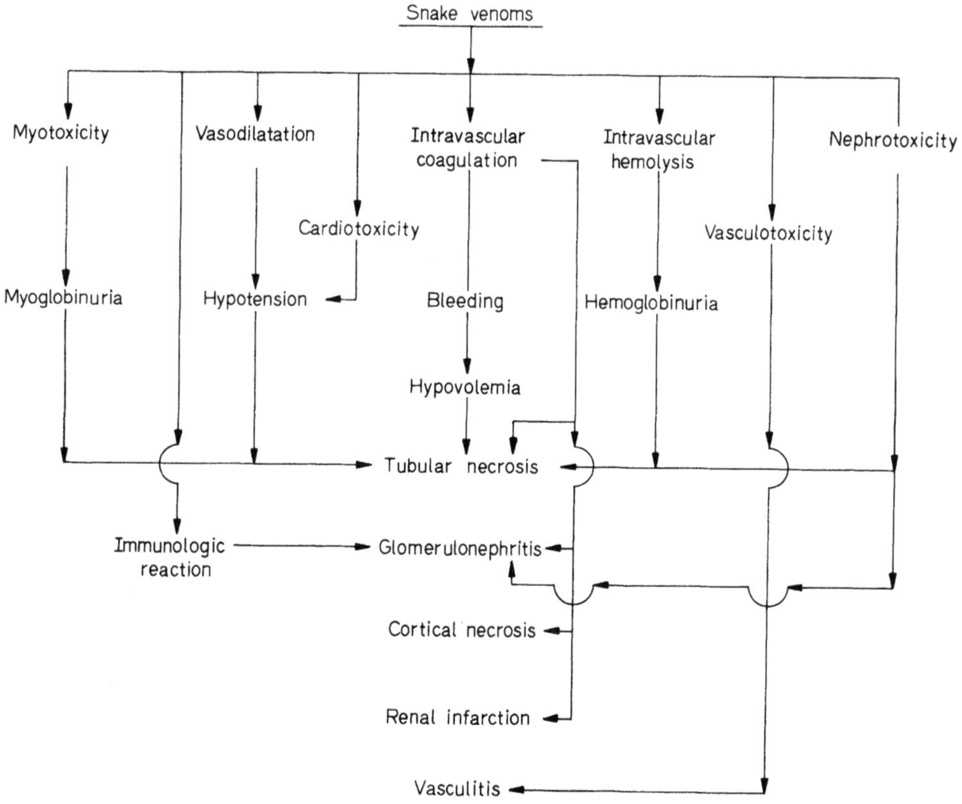

Fig. 17. A diagram showing the pathogenesis of renal lesions caused by snake venoms

known (JIMÉNEZ-PORRAS, 1970), and this effect might extend to the glomerular capillaries. The toxic effect of hemorrhagic principles to the glomerular basement membrane has been shown (OHSAKA et al., 1973).

2. Fibrin Deposition

The induction of intravascular coagulation may lead to glomerular damage. The principal changes are swelling and proliferation of endothelial and mesangial cells (VASSALLI and MCCLUSKEY, 1965). This, in fact, appears to be the basis for the glomerular changes found in toxemia of pregnancy in which slow intravascular coagulation is present. Since intravascular coagulation is a frequent finding in viper and crotalid bites, it is conceivable that the glomerular lesion could be explained by fibrin deposition.

3. Immunologic Reaction

It is well-established that glomerulonephritis can be produced by immunologic mechanisms. In snakebite, the antigen-antibody complex may trigger the immunologic reactions leading to the development of glomerular lesions similar to those observed in infectious diseases. The presence of immunoglobulin and C3 in the glomeruli supports the immunologic mechanism. The serum complement is also decreased. The venom could serve as an antigen, and its combination with antivenom given in the treatment could give rise to an immune complex. Since there is no difference in glomerular changes between cases that receive antivenom therapy and cases in which antivenom is not given, it would seem that the antibody to venom can be naturally acquired although this is a transient phenomenon.

It is, in general, felt that all three mechanisms operate in concert in the pathogenesis of glomerular changes. However, the present evidence from our study, based on glomerular deposition of the immune complex, indicates the importance of the immunologic mechanism. Since humoral immunity to snake venom is of short duration, glomerular lesions are, therefore, mild and transient in most cases. Severe glomerulonephritis could be predominantly due to direct glomerular irritation by specific components of snake venom. Intravascular coagulation may play a contributory role in severe cases.

II. Vascular Lesions

Necrotizing arteritis in Russell's viper bite differs from Arthus phenomenon in that there is deposition of C3 in the arterial wall without immunoglobulins. The finding suggests the injurious effect of the venom which could be mediated through complement activation (SITPRIJA et al., 1974). At the arteriolar level, although no morphologic change is visible both by light microscopy and electron microscopy, there is deposition of C3 in the arteriolar wall. No immunoglobulins are detectable. The significance of the finding is not understood. Nevertheless, complement activation without the participation of immunoglobulins is well-recognized (BRUNINGA, 1971; RUDDY et al., 1972). Complement deposition could also be the result of complement trapping in the kidney which is the organ rich in venom concentration. The finding bears close resemblance to that observed in the loin pain and hematuria syndrome recently described (NAISH et al., 1975).

III. Renal Failure

Renal hemodynamic study in the patient during the period of renal failure has shown a decrease in renal cortical blood flow similar to the changes seen in renal failure due to other causes.

Several factors are considered as being responsible for the development of renal failure.

1. Role of Hypotension

Hypotension may occur as a reaction to viper and crotalid venoms, since the venoms are known to cause the release of histamine and kinins which have profound effects on the peripheral circulation (BRAZIL et al., 1966). Continuous intravenous infusion of rattlesnake venom can produce a fall in cardiac output, hypotension, hemoconcentration, and hypoventilation known as "crotalin shock" (HALMAGYI et al., 1965). Hypotension may also result from volume depletion secondary to hemorrhage which frequently occurs. However, in some cases, especially in our experience with Russell's viper bite, renal failure has been noted even without hypotention.

2. Role of Intravascular Coagulation

The close association between tubular necrosis and intravascular coagulation has been shown (CLARKSON et al., 1970; MCKAY and MARGARETTEN, 1967). In severe disseminated intravascular coagulation, renal blood flow may be greatly diminished to produce cortical necrosis. Since some viper and crotalid venoms can cause intravascular coagulation, it is not surprising that renal failure can occur either in the form of tubular necrosis or cortical necrosis.

3. Role of Intravascular Hemolysis

Intravascular hemolysis of varying degrees with hemoglobinuria may occur in snakebite Severe intravascular hemolysis, by virtue of tubular obstruction by hemoglobin casts, may cause renal failure. Alarming hemolysis has been observed in Russell's viper bite (PEIRIS et al., 1969). Intravascular hemolysis can also cause intravascular clotting (DEYKIN, 1970) which in turn would enhance intravascular hemolysis (BRAIN et al., 1957), thus creating a vicious cycle.

4. Role of Myoglobinuria

Myoglobinuria secondary to myonecrosis is common in sea snakebite. Renal failure in sea snakebite is attributed to tubular obstruction by myoglobin (MARSDEN and REID, 1961; SITPRIJA et al., 1971). The same explanation is true for renal failure caused by the bite of the small-eyed blacksnake *(Cryptophis nigrescens)* described by FURTADO and LESTER (1968).

5. Role of Arteritis

Renal blood flow may be compromised by narrowing of the arterial lumen due to arteritis. In addition, arterial lesions could further accelerate intravascular coagulation and further decrease the renal blood flow. This has been observed in Russell's viper bite (SITPRIJA et al., 1974).

6. Role of Glomerular Lesions

Renal failure may also be a result of severe proliferative glomerulonephritis. This has not been our experience, but has been documented by other authors (SEEDAT et al., 1974).

7. Nephrotoxic Effect of the Venom

In a study of the effect of *Agkistrodon piscivorus* venom in rats, RAAB and KAISER (1966) found increased activity of alkaline phosphatase and leucine aminopeptidase in the urine. They believed that the venom had a direct cytotoxic effect on renal tubular cells. HADLER and BRAZIL (1966) in a study on crotoxin attributed the renal tubular lesions partly to the effect of lysolecithin formed by the activity of phospholipase A. In contrast, FIDLER et al. (1940) found no renal lesion in monkeys injected with rattlesnake venom. Clinical experience by our group in renal failure due to Russell's viper bite suggests direct nephrotoxicity of Russell's viper venom (SITPRIJA et al., 1976).

Although acute tubular necrosis by itself may be enough to explain renal failure and oliguria, ureteric obstruction either by edema or a blood clot should be considered as a contributing factor (SITPRIJA et al., 1973).

D. Clinical Manifestations

I. General Manifestations

Besides local symptoms at the site of bite, bleeding attributed to hemotoxicity and capillary injury is most common in viper and crotalid bites. In Russell's viper bite, there is a decrease in platelets and coagulation factors. Clotting factors commonly decreased are fibrinogen and factors II, V, and VIII. Serum fibrin degradation products are elevated. There may be intravascular hemolysis of varying degrees. In some cases, hemolysis may be severe enough to cause jaundice.

The blood pressure in most cases is normal. Hypotension has been observed on occasions in the patient bitten by a rattlesnake (AMORIM and MELLO, 1954; DANZIG and ABELS, 1961). Muscular symptoms are noted in sea snakebite (MARSDEN and REID, 1961; SITPRIJA et al., 1971). They have also been reported in some cases of Russell's viper bite (PEIRIS et al., 1969) and small-eyed blacksnake bite (FURTADO and LESTER, 1968). The symptoms include muscular pains and paresis affecting the proximal muscular groups more than the distal. Hyperkalemia may aggravate the muscular symptoms. Ptosis has been observed in both sea snakebite and Russell's viper bite. The size of pupils varies. While dilated pupils have been described in some cases of sea snake poisoning (MARSDEN and REID, 1961), pinpoint pupils have been noted in a single case of rattlesnake bite (FRAZIER and CARTER, 1962). Convulsions have been experienced in the patient bitten by crotalid snakes (DANZIG and ABEL, 1961; FRAZIER and CARTER, 1962). Drowsiness and restlessness have been described. Neuromuscular symptoms are common in cobra bite.

Of interest is the decrease in serum complement (C3) in victims of green pit viper, Russell's viper, and cobra. It takes about 1 week for C3 to return to the normal value. The decrease could be due to the decreased production as well as the increased metabolism or consumption. Recent investigations have shown the interrelation between blood coagulation, snake venom, and complement system. Serum complement can be depleted by injection of cobra venom (MIESCHER and MÜLLER-EBERHARD, 1968). A protein fraction in cobra venom does not act directly on C3 but combines in serum with β-globulin to form a stable protein-protein complex known as C3 inactivator which cleaves C3 to F(a)C3 and F(b)C3. Significant hemolytic complement depletion has been observed in animals after the injection of cobra venom along with significant prolongation of one-stage prothrombin time and partial thromboplastin time (DODDS and PICKERING, 1972). In viper bite, the decrease in C3 might be related to disseminated intravascular coagulation since both plasmin and thrombin are capable of activating complement (BOKISCH et al., 1969; DONALSON, 1968), although it is possible that viper venom activates the complement system through the alternate pathway. The deposition of C3 and IgM in the glomeruli in our study rather suggests immunologic consumption of complement. This is also true for cobra bite. However, the increased metabolic breakdown of complement and the decreased production from the effect of venom cannot be excluded.

II. Renal Manifestations

Renal symptoms in snakebite varyl widely. The renal manifestations include mild to heavy proteinuria, nephrotic syndrome, microscopic and gross hematuria, and renal failure. Hemoglobinuria is not uncommon. Myoglobinuria is observed in sea snakebite and small-eyed blacksnake bite *(Cryptophis nigrescens)*. In our series of 400 cases of poisonous snakebite, mild and transient proteinuria with urinary protein ranging from 150 to 500 mg/24 h was noted in 4%, all of which were cobra cases. Although nephrotic syndrome may occur, this has not been our experience. Gross hematuria was observed in 35%, all being viper cases. Renal failure occurred in 5%. They were patients with Russell's viper bite and sea snakebite. Oliguria in all cases were noticeable on the 1st day of the bite. The clinical course of renal failure does not differ from renal failure due to other causes. In renal failure due to sea snakebite, hyperkalemia secondary to myonecrosis may be alarming and requires special attention. Renal failure and renal lesions in relation to the types of snakes are summarized in Table 2.

In cobra bite, the renal function, based on creatinine clearance, paraaminohippurate (PAH) clearance, concentration and dilution tests, is normal. There is a decrease in urine concentration power and PAH clearance in green pit viper bite, but the creatinine clearance and the dilution ability are normal. Renal function changes are thus in agreement with histopathologic alterations.

E. Treatment

The management of renal failure in snakebite does not differ from the standard treatment of acute renal failure in other conditions. Dialysis is indicated when uremia ensues. Hyperkalemia must be watched for and treated in sea snakebite. Recovery is usually complete unless there is cortical necrosis. Because of the high molecular weight of most of the venom components and the rapid tissue fixation (EFRATI and REIF, 1953), dialysis may not be able to remove them and would not improve the clinical symptoms except uremia. However, many postsynaptic neurotoxins and cardiotoxins with smaller molecular weight could be dialyzed somewhat. In sea snake poisoning, dramatic improvement of the muscular symptoms by hemodialysis has been observed (SITPRIJA et al., 1971). The improvement is believed to be due to the correction of hyperkalemia which worsens the muscular symptoms. Exchange transfusion of blood performed earlier after the bite may be of help in relieving the symptoms. In fact, clinical improvement by exchange blood transfusion in Russell's viper bite has been reported by PEIRIS et al. (1969).

Heparin should be given when there is evidence of active disseminated intravascular coagulation. In our experience, the patient is usually admitted in the hospital a few days after the bite when bleeding has already ceased. Heparin is thus never required. Antivenom therapy does not seem to prevent renal failure although it improves the general condition of the patient. This might reflect a delay in its institution. Most important is the conventional treatment to prevent renal failure by proper fluid load, blood transfusion when there is hemorrhage, and diuretic administration. These measures should be started promptly in any patient bitten by a snake known to cause renal failure. Alkalinization of urine should be attempted when there is hemoglobinuria or myoglobinuria.

References

Amorim, M.F., Mello, R.F.: Intermediate nephron nephrosis from snake poisoning in man. Amer. J. Path. **30**, 479—499 (1954)

Azevedo, A., de, Castro Teixeira, J., de: Intoxicacao pro veneno de cobra. Necrose symetrica da cortex renal uremia. Mem. Inst. Cruz. **33**, 23—38 (1938)

Bokisch, V., Müller-Eberhard, H.J., Cochrane, C.G.: Isolation of a fragment (C 3a) of the third component of human complement containing anaphylatoxin and chemotactic activity and description of an anaphylatoxin inactivator of human serum. J. exp. Med. **129**, 1109—1130 (1969)

Brain, M.C., Esterly, J.R., Beck, E.A.: Intravascular hemolysis with experimentally produced vascular thrombi. Br. J. Haematol. **13**, 868—891 (1957)

Brazil, O.V., Farina, R., Yoshida, L., Oliveira, V.A. de: Pharmacology of crystalline crotoxin. III. Cardiovascular and respiratory effects of crotoxin and *Crotalus durissus terrificus* venom. Mem. Inst. Butantan **33**, 993—1000 (1966)

Bruninga, G.L.: Complement: A review of the chemistry and reaction mechanism. Amer. J. clin. Path. **55**, 273—282 (1971)

Chugh, K.S., Aikat, B.K., Sharma, B.K., Dash, K.C., Mathew, M.T., Das, K.C.: Acute renal failure following snakebite. Amer. J. trop. Med. Hyg. **24**, 692—697 (1975)

Clarkson, A.R., MacDonald, M.K., Fuster, V., Cash, J.D., Robson, J.S.: Glomerular coagulation in acute ischaemic renal failure. Quart. J. Med. **39**, 585—599 (1970)

Danzig, L.E., Abels, G.H.: Hemodialysis of acute renal failure following rattlesnake bite, with recovery. J. Amer. med. Ass. **175**, 136—137 (1961)

Deykin, D.: The clinical challenge of disseminated intravascular coagulation. New Engl. J. Med. **283**, 636—644 (1970)
Dodds, W. J., Pickering, R. J.: The effect of cobra venom factor on hemostasis in guinea pigs. Blood **40**, 400—411 (1972)
Donaldson, V. H.: Mechanism of activation of C1 esterase in hereditary angioneurotic edema plasma in vitro. The role of Hagemen factor, a clot-promoting agent. J. exp. Med. **227**, 411—429 (1968)
Efrati, P., Reif, L.: Clinical and pathological observation on sixty-five cases of viper bite in Israel. Amer. J. trop. Med. Hyg. **2**, 1085—1108 (1953)
Fidler, H. K., Glasgow, R. D., Carmicheal, E. B.: Pathological changes produced by subcutaneous injection of rattlesnake *(Crotalus)* venom into *Macaca mullata* monkeys. Amer. J. Path. **16**, 355—364 (1940)
Frazier, D. B., Carter, F. H.: Use of the artificial kidney in snakebite. Calif. Med. **97**, 177—178 (1962)
Furtado, M. A., Lester, I. A.: Myoglobinuria following snakebite. Med. J. Aust. **1**, 674—676 (1968)
Hadler, W. A., Brazil, O. V.: Pharmacology of crystalline crotoxin. IV. Nephrotoxicity. Mem. Inst. Butantan **33**, 1001—1008 (1966)
Halmagyi, D. F., Starzecki, B., Horner, G. J.: Mechanism and pharmacology of shock due to rattlesnake venom in sheep. J. appl. Physiol. **20**, 709—718 (1965)
Jiménez-Porras, J. M.: Biochemistry of snake venoms (a review). Clin. Toxicol. **3**, 389—431 (1970)
Luna, G.: Manual of Histologic Staining Methods of the Armed Forces Institute of Pathology, 3rd Ed. New York: McGraw-Hill 1960
Marsden, A. T. H., Reid, H. A.: Pathology of sea-snake poisoning. Brit. med. J. **1961 I**, 1290—1293
McKay, D. G., Margaretten, W.: Disseminated intravascular coagulation in virus diseases. Arch. intern. Med. **120**, 129—152 (1967)
Miescher, P. A., Müller-Eberhard, H. J.: Textbook of Immunopathology, Vol. I, 1st Ed. New York-London: Grune & Stratton 1968
Naish, P. F., Aber, G. M., Boyd, W. N.: C3 deposition in renal arterioles in the loin pain and haematuria syndrome. Brit. med. J. **1975 III**, 746
Ohsaka, A., Just, M., Habermann, E.: Action of snake venom hemorrhagic principles on isolated glomerular basement membrane. Biochim. biophys. Acta (Amst.) **323**, 415—428 (1973)
Oram, S., Ross, S., Pell, L., Winteler, J.: Renal cortical calcification after snakebite. Brit. med. J. **1963 I**, 1647—1648
Pearce, R. M.: An experimental glomerular lesion caused by venom *(Crotalus adamanteus)*. J. exp. Med. **11**, 532—540 (1909)
Peiris, O. A., Wimalaratne, K. D. P., Nimalasuriya, A.: Exchange transfusion in the treatment of Russell's viper bite. Postgrad. med. J. **45**, 627—629 (1969)
Raab, W., Kaiser, E.: Nephrotoxic action of snake venom. Mem. Inst. Butantan **33**, 1017—1020 (1966)
Ruddy, S., Giglo, I., Austen, K. F.: The complement system in man. Part IV. New Engl. J. Med. **287**, 642—646 (1972)
Sant, S. M., Purandare, N. M.: Autopsy study of cases of snake bite with special reference to renal lesions. J. postgrad. Med. **18**, 181—188 (1972)
Seedat, Y. K., Reddy, J., Edington, D. A.: Acute renal failure due to proliferative nephritis from snake bite poisoning. Nephron **13**, 455—463 (1974)
Silva, H. B., Brito, T., Lima, P. R., Penna, D. O., Almeida, S. S., Mattar, E.: Acute anuric renal insufficiency due to snake, waxbee and spider bites. Clinical and pathological observations in 8 cases. Abstract II. Free communications. 3rd International Congress of Nephrology, 1966
Sitprija, V., Benyajati, C., Boonpucknavig, V.: Further observations of renal insufficiency in snakebite. Nephron **13**, 396—403 (1974)
Sitprija, V., Benyajati, C., Boonpucknavig, V.: Renal involvement in snakebite. In: Ohsaka, A., Hayashi, K., Sawai, Y. (Eds.): Animal, Plant, and Microbial Toxins. Vol. 2, p.p. 483—495, New York: Plenum 1976
Sitprija, V., Sribhibhadh, R., Benyajati, C.: Haemodialysis in poisoning by sea-snake venom. Brit. med. J. **1971 III**, 218—219
Sitprija, V., Sribhibhadh, R., Benyajati, C., Tangchai, P.: Acute renal failure in snakebite. In: de Vries, A., Kochva, E. (Eds.): Toxins of Animal and Plant Origins, Vol. 3. London: Gordon and Breach 1973

Steinbeck, A. W.: Nephrotic syndrome developing after snakebite. Med. J. Aust. **1**, 543—545 (1960)
Varagunam, T., Panabokke, R. G.: Bilateral cortical necrosis of the kidneys following snakebite. Postgrad. med. J. **46**, 449—451 (1970)
Vassalli, P., McCluskey, R. T.: The coagulation process and glomerular disease. Amer. J. Med. **39**, 179—182 (1965)
Visuvaratnam, M., Vinayagamoorthy, C., Balakrishnam, S.: Venomous snakebite in North Ceylon: a study of 15 cases. J. trop. Med. Hyg. **73**, 9—14 (1970)

Author Index

Page numbers in *italics* indiate References

* Chang, Chuan-Chiung
** Chang, Chun-Chang

Subject Index

Handbuch der experimentellen Pharmakologie
Handbook of Experimental Pharmacology

Heffter-Heubner/ New Series

Herausgeber:
G.V.R. Born, O. Eichler, A. Farah, H. Herken, A.D. Welch

Band 48

Springer-Verlag
Berlin
Heidelberg
New York

Arthropod Venoms

Editor: S. Bettini
1978. 293 figures. XXXIII, 977 pages
Cloth DM 450,–; US $ 225.00
ISBN 3-540-08228-X

Contents: Introduction to Venomous Arthropods Systematics. – Venoms of Crustacea and Merostomata. – Defensive Secretions of Millipeds. – Secretions of Centipedes. – Secretions of Opilionids, Whip Scorpions and Pseudoscorpionids. – Review of the Spider Families with Notes on the Lesser Known Poisonous Forms. – Venoms of Dipluridae. – Venoms of Theridiidae, Genus Latrodectus. – Venoms of Theridiidae Genus Steatoda. – Venoms of Ctenidae. – Venoms of Scytodidae, Genus Loxosceles. – Venoms of Isometrinae & Rhopalurinae. – Venoms of Buthinae. – Venoms of Tityinae. – Chactoid Venoms. – Tick Paralysis. – Toxins of Blattaria. – Venoms of Rhyncota (= Hemiptera) Venoms of Coleoptera. – Venoms of Lepidoptera. – Venoms of Apidae. – Venoms of Sphecidae, Pompilidae, Multilidae, Bethylidae. – Venoms of Vespidae. – Venoms of Braconidae. – Venom and Venom Apparatuses of the Formicidae.

The 25 chapters of this volume are written by 43 authors and coauthors, chosen from among the best specialists from all over the world, and covers all arthropod groups which include toxic species. It offers all available information and pertaining literature on arthropod venoms, i.e. venomous apparatus secretions toxic substances originating from other glands or tissues, and substances capable of modifying other species behavior. Each chapter deals mainly with the chemistry, toxicology, pharmacology and venom mode of action. The systematics, distribution and biology species involved and is treated. Information given on the epidemiology, symptomatology and therapy of envenomizations.

Preisänderungen vorbehalten.

Handbook of Experimental Pharmacology

Continuation of "Handbuch der experimentellen Pharmakologie"

Heffter-Heubner, New Series

Volume 25
Bradykinin, Kallidin and Kallikrein

Volume 26
H. Fischer: **Vergleichende Pharmakologie von Überträgersubstanzen in tiersystematischer Darstellung**

Volume 27
Anticoagulantien

Volume 28: Part 1
Concepts in Biochemical Pharmacology I

Part 3
Concepts in Biochemical Pharmacology III

Volume 29
Oral wirksame Antidiabetika

Volume 30
Modern Inhalation Anesthetics

Volume 32: Part 1
Insulin I

Part 2
Insulin II

Volume 34
Secretin, Cholecystokinin, Pancreozymin and Gastrin

Volume 35: Part 1
H. E. Voss, G. Oertel:
Androgene I

Part 2
Androgens II and Antiandrogens/ Androgene II und Antiandrogene

Volume 36
Uranium – Plutonium – Transplutonic Elements

Volume 37
Angiotensin

Volume 38: Part 1
Antineoplastic and Immunosuppressive Agents I

Part 2
Antineoplastic and Immunosuppressive Agents II

Volume 39
Antihypertensive Agents

Volume 40
Organic Nitrates

Volume 41
Hypolipidemic Agents

Volume 42
Neuromuscular Junction

Volume 43
Anabolic-Androgenic Steroids

Volume 44
Heme and Hemoproteins

Volume 45: Part 1
Drug Addiction I

Part 2
Drug Addiction II

Volume 46
Fibrinolytics and Antifibrinolytics

Volume 47
Kinetics of Drug Action

Volume 48
Arthropod Venoms

Volume 49
Ergot Alkaloids and Related Compounds

Volume 50: Part 1
Inflammation

Part 2
Anti-Inflammatory Drugs

Volume 51
Uric Acid

Volume 52
Snake Venoms
(In preparation)

Volume 53
Gangliomic Transmission
(In preparation)

Springer-Verlag
Berlin
Heidelberg
New York

www.ingramcontent.com/pod-product-compliance
Ingram Content Group UK Ltd.
Pitfield, Milton Keynes, MK11 3LW, UK
UKHW052255220926
475870UK00007B/269
* 9 7 8 3 6 4 2 6 6 9 1 5 6 *